D1298974

Pediatric Medications
A Handbook for Nurses

Suanne Miller, MS, RN, CS, PNP

Assistant Professor of Clinical Nursing
University of Rochester School of Nursing
Pediatric Nurse Practitioner—Primary Care
Children's Hospital at the University of Rochester Medical Center
Rochester, New York

Joanne Fioravanti, MS, RN, PNP

Assistant Professor of Clinical Nursing
University of Rochester School of Nursing
Pediatric Nurse Practitioner—Pediatric Cardiology
Children's Hospital at the University of Rochester Medical Center
Rochester, New York

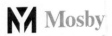 Mosby

St. Louis Baltimore Boston
Carlsbad Chicago Naples New York Philadelphia Portland
London Madrid Mexico City Singapore Sydney Tokyo Toronto Wiesbaden

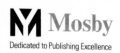
Mosby
Dedicated to Publishing Excellence

A Times Mirror
Company

Vice President and Publisher: Nancy L. Coon
Editor: Robin Carter
Developmental Editor: Jeanne Allison
Project Manager: John Rogers
Senior Production Editor: Lavon Wirch Peters
Design Coordinator: Yael Kats
Manufacturing Manager: Theresa Fuchs
Cover art: © David Hanover/Tony Stone Images

A NOTE TO THE READER
The authors and publisher have made every attempt to check dosages
and nursing content for accuracy. Because the science of pharmacology
is continually advancing, our knowledge base continues to expand.
Therefore we recommend that the reader always check product information for changes in dosage or administration before administering
any medication. This is particularly important with new or rarely used
drugs. The authors and publisher disclaim responsibility for any adverse effects resulting directly or indirectly from suggested procedures,
undetected errors, or reader's misunderstanding of the text.

Copyright © 1997 by Mosby–Year Book, Inc.

All rights reserved. No part of this publication may be reproduced,
stored in a retrieval system, or transmitted, in any form or by any
means, electronic, mechanical, photocopying, recording, or otherwise,
without prior written permission from the publisher.

Permission to photocopy or reproduce solely for internal or personal use
is permitted for libraries or other users registered with the Copyright
Clearance Center, provided that the base fee of $4.00 per chapter plus
$.10 per page is paid directly to the Copyright Clearance Center, 27
Congress Street, Salem, MA 01970. This consent does not extend to
other kinds of copying, such as copying for general distribution, for ad-
vertising or promotional purposes, for creating new collected works, or
for resale.

Printed in the United States of America
Editing and project management by Graphic World Publishing Services
Composition by Graphic World, Inc.
Printing/binding by Western Graphic Communications

Mosby–Year Book, Inc.
11830 Westline Industrial Drive
St. Louis, Missouri 63146

International Standard Book Number 1-55664-482-5

97 98 99 00 01 / 9 8 7 6 5 4 3 2 1

CONTRIBUTORS

Leslie R. Babbitt, MS, RD, CD
Clinical Nutrition Specialist
Swedish Medical Center
Fred Hutchinson Bone
    Marrow Unit
Seattle, Washington

Patricia Corbett-Dick, MS, RN,
    CS, PNP
Instructor of Clinical Nursing
University of Rochester
    School of Nursing
Pediatric Nurse
    Practitioner—Primary Care
Children's Hospital at the
    University of Rochester
    Medical Center
Rochester, New York

Carolyn V. Diagneau, MS, RN,
    CS, PNP
Pediatric Nurse
    Practitioner—Neurology
Department of Pediatrics
University of Houston
Health Science Center
Houston, Texas

Irene Dutko Fioravanti, MS,
    RN, CS, PNP, M.Ed
Assistant Professor of
    Clinical Nursing
University of Rochester
    School of Nursing
Clinical Nurse
    Specialist—Pediatrics
Children's Hospital at the
    University of Rochester
    Medical Center
Rochester, New York

Michelle Gullace, MS, RN
Clinical Associate
Instructor of Clinical Nursing
University of Rochester
    School of Nursing
Clinical Nurse
    Specialist—Pediatric
    Oncology
Children's Hospital at the
    University of Rochester
    Medical Center
Rochester, New York

Fran London, MS, RN
Health Education Specialist
Phoenix Children's Hospital
Phoenix, Arizona

Jean Mack-Fogg, MS, RN, CS,
    PNP
Instructor of Clinical Nursing
University of Rochester
    School of Nursing
Pediatric Nurse
    Practitioner—Endocrinology
Children's Hospital at the
    University of Rochester
    Medical Center
Rochester, New York

Kathleen McGrath, MS, RN, CS,
    PNP
Instructor of Clinical Nursing
University of Rochester
    School of Nursing
Pediatric Nurse
    Practitioner—Cardiology
Children's Hospital at the
    University of Rochester
    Medical Center
Rochester, New York

Pamela Myers, MS, RN, CS, PNP

Instructor of Clinical Nursing
University of Rochester
  School of Nursing
Pediatric Nurse
  Practitioner—Primary Care
Children's Hospital at the
  University of Rochester
  Medical Center
Rochester, New York

Veronica Perrone Pollack,
  MS, RN

Assistant Professor
Yale University School of
  Nursing
Clinical Nurse
  Specialist—Pediatric
  Gastroenterology
Yale-New Haven Hospital
New Haven, Connecticut

Cindy B. Proukou, MS, RN, CS,
  PNP

Clinical Associate
University of Rochester
  School of Nursing
Pediatric Nurse
  Practitioner—Pediatric
  Oncology
Children's Hospital at the
  University of Rochester
  Medical Center
Rochester, New York

Kathy Rideout, EdD, RN

Assistant Professor of
  Clinical Nursing
University of Rochester
  School of Nursing
Clinical Nurse
  Specialist—Adolescent
  Nursing
Children's Hospital at the
  University of Rochester
  Medical Center
Rochester, New York

Consultants

Donna Babao, MA-Ed, MSN, RN
Nursing Instructor
Yuba College
Maryville, California

Donna L. Betcher, MSN, RN, PNP
Pediatric Oncology
Mayo Clinic
Rochester, Minnesota

Janice Bush, BSN, RN
Nursing Instructor
South Arkansas Community
  College
El Dorado, Arkansas

Ellen M. Chiocca, MSN, RNC
Instructor, Maternal-Child
  Health
Loyola University
Chicago, Illinois

Laura H. Clayton, MSN, RN, FNP
Instructor of Nursing
  Education
Shepherd College
Shepherdstown, West
  Virginia
Staff Nurse
Intensive Care Unit
City Hospital, Inc.
Martinsburg, West Virginia

Teresa A. Free, PhD, RN
Pediatric Nurse Practitioner
Associate Professor
College of Nursing
University of Kentucky
Lexington, Kentucky

Kathleen Jarvis, MSN, RN, PhD
Professor of Nursing
Division of Nursing
California State University
  at Sacramento
Sacramento, California

Tom LeMaster, RN, NREMT-P
MS Coordinator
Children's Hospital
Cincinnati, Ohio

Lori A. Martell, PhD
Pharmacologist
Durham, North Carolina

J. Maria Mikuta, PharmD
Pediatric Clinical Pharmacist
Methodist Hospital
Indianapolis, Indiana

Kathy Modene, MSN, RN
Associate Professor
Deaconess College of Nursing
St. Louis, Missouri

Joyce Mulholland, MA, MS, RNC, ANP
Alliance Medical Professional
  Services
Faculty Member
Gateway Community College
Phoenix, Arizona

Marilyn M. Rowe, MA, RN
Instructor, Nursing of
  Children
South Suburban College
South Holland, Illinois

vii

Margaret A. Tufts, MS, RNC
Assistant Professor
Department of Nursing
Luinnipiac College
Hamden, Connecticut

Carla Wallace, PharmD
Assistant Professor of
Pharmacy Practice
St. Louis College of
Pharmacy
St. Louis, Missouri

Kirsten West, MA, RNC
Clinical Specialist
Neonatal Intensive Care Unit
Saint Francis Hospital
Tulsa, Oklahoma

Sarah E. Whitaker, DNS(c), RN
Lecturer and Nursery Staff
Nurse
College of Nursing and
Health Sciences
University of Texas at El
Paso
R.E. Thomason General
Hospital
El Paso, Texas

Patricia D. Wilcox, MSN, RN
Professor of Nursing
Owens Community College
Toledo, Ohio

We dedicate this book to our children

David and Jared Lippman
Meghan Makielski

and to all children
cared for and loved
by pediatric nurses

PREFACE

Pediatric Medications: A Handbook for Nurses is written specifically for nurses who care for infants, children, and adolescents. Pediatric patients differ from adults in several ways, both physiologically and psychologically, and this book was created with such differences in mind. The book is an invaluable resource for nurses who work in a variety of settings—in acute and chronic care inpatient units, in neonatal and pediatric intensive care units, with ambulatory and specialty-based outpatient care, with community health care and homecare, and in schools, colleges, and camps—basically everywhere you find children. Student nurses will find this book to be instrumental during pediatric, obstetric-gynecologic, and ambulatory care clinical rotations. Nurses who occasionally care for children will also want to have this book available to ensure safe medication administration. This portable resource provides nurses with quick facts about doses, routes of administration, and side effects in a user-friendly format. In-depth information about prescribing, administering, and evaluating drug therapy is included, as well as a comprehensive section on patient and family education.

Because the book was written by advanced practice nurses who prescribe and administer these drugs in their everyday practice, readers can be assured that each monograph contains current, accurate information and useful facts that will benefit the nurse as well as the patient. It contains many drugs for special diagnoses, such as chemotherapeutic agents, antiviral medications, and cardiac and respiratory drugs. This book uses a family-centered approach, acknowledging that drug therapy without the full understanding and cooperation of family members will not be successful.

Three introductory chapters precede the drug monographs. Chapter 1, "Basic Pharmacokinetics in Children," introduces the reader to the basic principles of pharmacology and drug therapy in the pediatric population. Chapter 2, "Pediatric Medication Administration: Guidelines and Techniques," supplies the reader with useful information about drug administration (including an important section on how a child's developmental and cognitive levels affect medication therapy). The experience of pain in children is discussed, as well as useful strategies to ameliorate it. Chapter 3, "Medication Administration in Special Settings," will prove invaluable to nurses who practice in such settings. Drug therapy in special settings reflects the current trends in health care as children previously hospitalized with complex health needs are sent home and even to school. Nurses in these settings must also be knowledgeable about a wide variety of drugs and devices used to deliver them.

The drug monographs are organized to make key information readily available to the user. The following sections are provided:

- **Generic name** of drug is shown in lower case letters.
- **Brand names** of drugs manufactured in the United States and Canada (signified with a maple leaf, ✤) are listed.
- **Classification** of each drug is included as the functional class.
- **Controlled substance schedules** are included (if appropriate)—see Appendix C.
- **Pregnancy categories** are stated for all drugs—see Appendix B.
- **Available preparations** are listed, including oral, injectable, topical, otic, and ophthalmologic preparations (as appropriate).
- **Routes and dosages** are listed, and are based on weight, body surface area, or age (where appropriate). If multiple indications exist for a particular drug, each is listed separately.
- **IV administration** describes what fluids each drug can be administered with, at what concentration each should be administered, and the rate of drug administration.
- **Mechanism and indications** are described and listed.
- **Pharmacokinetic** processes are discussed when that information is known.
- **Contraindications and precautions** to specific drug therapy are described.
- **Interactions** between specific drugs, as well as alterations in lab values and nutrition that occur because of drug therapy, are listed.
- **Incompatibilities** between drugs and solutions are described.
- **Side effects** are listed by system, with most commonly occurring side effects listed first.
- **Toxicity and overdose** information is included (when known), as are the clinical signs and treatment of toxicity.
- **Patient care management** information is discussed, including how to assess patients for appropriateness of drug therapy, how to provide that therapy, how to evaluate patients receiving medication(s), and how to provide the patient or family with critical information about specific drug therapy.

The following appendixes are included to enhance the usefulness of this text for pediatric nurses: Appendix A, a table for determining body surface area; Appendix B, FDA pregnancy risk categories; Appendix C, DEA controlled substances classification; Appendix D, childhood immunization schedules and dosages; Appendix E, oral contraceptives for adolescents; Appendix F, table of recommended daily dietary allowances; Appendix G, a table of nonprescription medications; Appendix H, American Heart Association guidelines for bacterial endocarditis prophylaxis; Appendix I, bibliographic information; and Appendix J, patient and family education.

We sincerely hope this new pediatric reference enables nursing professionals to practice more effectively and efficiently in today's health care environment. We welcome comments from users on how we can make improvements in future editions of this book.

Suanne Miller
Joanne Fioravanti

ACKNOWLEDGMENTS

The authors would like to acknowledge and thank the following individuals whose combined efforts brought this handbook from its early conception to its completion:

- Robin Carter, editor, for her vision and expertise throughout the writing process
- Jeanne Allison, developmental editor, who was always knowledgeable, available, and supportive during manuscript preparation
- Tim Gillison, production editor, for his excellent editing skills and patient, friendly manner
- The many nursing and pharmacology professionals who reviewed and edited this work (especially Maria Mikuta, PharmD, for her thorough assessment)
- Nancy Kita, Dale Smialek, and Mabel Meloche for their help in preparing the manuscript
- Our family, friends, and colleagues who supported our work over the past 3 years
- Special thanks are extended to our husbands, Wade Lippman and Tom Makielski, who were always available to help in any way we asked

CONTENTS

CHAPTER 1

Basic Pharmacokinetics in Children

Providing drug therapy to infants and children presents a unique set of challenges. Physiological differences exist between infants, children, and adults, including differences in vital organ maturity and body composition. The pharmacokinetic processes of absorption, distribution, metabolism, and excretion are therefore altered in infants and children as compared to those of adults. Altered pharmacokinetic processes impact the action, safety, and effectiveness of drug therapy in children.

Further complicating drug therapy safety is the fact that, for a variety of reasons, detailed pharmacokinetic studies are not frequently performed on the pediatric population. Historically, ethical constraints have limited the performance of clinical research, including pharmacokinetic studies, in the pediatric population. (The wisdom of this argument is lost on those who are advocates for children. Indeed, many feel it is unethical to perpetuate the current lack of understanding of drug effects in children and to deny them potentially beneficial drugs.) Another limiting factor is that parents may be reluctant to allow their children to participate in a research study testing drugs that have not been approved for children. Frequent blood draws to measure drug levels in the blood cause discomfort to children, also making parents reluctant to consent to research. And finally, the pharmaceutical industry has been less motivated to do clinical pharmacokinetic studies in children due not only to the ethical and parental issues noted above, but also to the perceived lack of market share the pediatric population would contribute to drug sales. Lower profits from drug sales to the pediatric population as compared to the adult population are not perceived by drug companies to outweigh the costs of research and development. For these reasons, many drugs currently lack FDA approval for safe and effective use in children.

The following discussion will help the reader understand how and why pharmacokinetic processes differ in the pediatric population. In providing drug therapy to children, careful attention must be paid when choosing an administration route, calculating a drug dose, administering the drug, and monitoring drug effects and response.

PHARMACOKINETICS

Pharmacokinetics is the study of the concentration of a drug within the body during the processes of *absorption, distribution, metabolism,* and *excretion.* After oral administration of a drug, it is *absorbed,* primarily through the gastrointestinal system into the circulatory system. After parenteral administration, drugs are absorbed at the site of administration (IM or SC) or directly by the blood (IV). Once absorbed, molecules of the drug are *distributed* throughout the body to various sites of action. The distribution process also enables delivery of drug molecules to sites where they can be chemically changed or metabolized. *Metabolism,* which most often takes place in the liver, is the process whereby drugs are changed or biotransformed into other active or inactive compounds or metabolites. Metabolites are then *excreted,* most commonly by the kidneys.

DEFINITION OF PHARMACOKINETIC PROCESSES

Absorption

Absorption is the process that involves drug movement from the site of entry in the body to the bloodstream. The rate of drug absorption is important because it determines how quickly a drug will become available to exert its pharmacological effect(s). The rate of drug absorption is affected by the route of administration (Table 1-1), the dosage of the drug, and the form of the dose (Table 1-2). Absorption of drugs given by mouth is affected by gastric transit time, gastric acidity, levels of intestinal flora, enzyme function, and gastric emptying time. When drugs are given orally, they are most commonly absorbed through the stomach and small intestine. Parenteral drugs are absorbed at the site of injection.

Distribution

Distribution is defined as the transport of a drug in body fluids from the bloodstream to various tissues of the body and, ultimately, to its site of action (McKenry, 1995). Distribution is affected by body water content, body fat content, the degree of drug binding to plasma proteins, and the efficacy of barriers to drug distribution (i.e., skin, blood–brain barrier). The increased total body water percentage of infants and young children (as compared to adults) leads to a decreased concentration of drug in

TABLE 1.1
Rate of Drug Absorption by Route of Administration

ROUTE OF ADMINISTRATION	ABSORPTION CHARACTERISTICS
Enteral (oral)	Absorption of drug is variable and will depend on gastric pH and transit time, empty or full stomach, and simultaneous use of other drugs that may interact to decrease or increase absorption.
	Generally considered to be the most unreliable and slowest route of drug administration with respect to absorption.
Parenteral Subcutaneous	Rate of absorption is rapid with aqueous solutions.
	Rate of absorption is slow with oily or depot preparations.
Intramuscular	Absorption is rapid due to increased blood flow.
Intravenous	Absorption is immediate due to direct injection into bloodstream, bypassing absorption process.
Intrathecal	Absorption is rapid in the CNS due to bypass of blood brain barrier.
Inhalation	Absorption is rapid due to large surface area of lungs.
	Vascularity of lungs promotes ready entry into bloodstream.
Transdermal	Absorption is erratic unless drug is specifically formulated for this use; in this case, absorption is slow but prolonged and consistent over time.
Rectal	Absorption is generally erratic.
Sublingual, buccal	Absorption is rapid and complete as long as tablet is retained at administration site.
	Food or drink will interfere with absorption.
Topical	Absorption is somewhat erratic but more complete in children due to smaller body surface area.

the body. This means that relatively larger doses of water-soluble drugs may be necessary to achieve the desired therapeutic effect. In contrast, the lower level of body fat in this population as compared to adults results in less fat-soluble drug being stored in adipose tissue. This results in higher circulating levels of fat-soluble drugs which may necessitate giving lower doses of fat-soluble medications. Before 1 year of age, the number of plasma proteins is low. This results in a decrease in the amount of

TABLE 1.2
Rate of Enteral Absorption

Solution	Fastest
Suspension	
Capsules	↑
Tablets	↕
Enteric coated tablets	↓
Sustained release capsules or tablets	Slowest

Adapted from McKenry and Salerno: *Pharmacology in nursing,* St. Louis, 1995, Mosby.

protein-bound drug and a corresponding increase in the concentration of free drug in the circulation. In infants, glial cells are immature and do not protect the central nervous system like the blood–brain barrier does in children and adults. This means that drugs have ready access to the brain in infants, increasing the potential for toxicity. Likewise, the skin of infants is not an effective barrier, resulting in enhanced absorption of topically applied agents.

Metabolism

Metabolism is the process by which drugs are chemically inactivated (biotransformed) and converted into a water-soluble compound, or metabolite, that can then be excreted readily from the body. The liver is the primary site of drug metabolism. The kidneys, lungs, and intestinal mucosa can also play a role in metabolism.

Excretion

Excretion is the process whereby metabolized drugs are removed from their sites of action and eliminated from the body. Excretion most commonly takes place in the kidneys. Drugs may also be excreted by the intestine, lungs, and sweat, salivary, and mammary glands.

PHARMACOKINETICS IN INFANTS

Drug actions in infants are variable because of the infant's physiological attributes (Table 1-3). These include small body mass, high relative body water content, low body fat, greater membrane permeability of the skin and blood–brain barrier, and reduced plasma protein-binding abilities.

Absorption

Rates of drug absorption in the infant are lower than absorption rates in children and adults. Prolonged gastric transit time and variable gastric pH lead to diminished absorption. Frequent feedings impede drug absorption because the stomach is often full

TABLE 1.3

Physiologic Attributes of Infants and Implications for Drug Therapy

ATTRIBUTE	IMPLICATION
Increased total body water	Increased distribution of drug, decreased blood levels of water-soluble drugs
Increased membrane permeability, skin and blood-brain barrier	Increased CNS distribution and likelihood of neurotoxicity, enhanced topical absorption
Decreased body fat	Increased absorption of fat-soluble drugs
Immature kidney, liver function	Prolonged excretion or metabolism of certain drugs
Immature temperature regulation	May dehydrate readily, increasing concentration of drugs

Adapted from Shlafer: *The nurse, pharmacology, and drug therapy,* Menlo Park, Calif, 1993, The Benjamin/Cummings Publishing Company.

and thus drugs must compete with nutrients for absorption. Low levels of intestinal flora and reduced enzyme function, both of which are necessary for active transport of some drugs, can result in decreased absorption. Low peripheral perfusion rates and immature heat regulatory mechanisms can also decrease absorption when drugs are given IV, IM, or SC (Shlafer, 1993).

Distribution

Infants have a low concentration of plasma proteins and a diminished protein-binding capacity (Shlafer, 1993). This means that drugs are less bound to protein in infants and therefore are more available in the circulation to exert their pharmacological effects. This can result in serious adverse drug effects and toxicities. Additionally, immature glial cell development results in greater permeability of the blood–brain barrier, allowing rapid access of drugs to the central nervous system.

In newborns, total body water is 80% of body weight for full-term infants and 70% of body weight for preterm infants, as compared to adult values of approximately 50% of body weight. Increased body water content in infants (as compared to adults) results in increased volume of distribution for water-soluble drugs. A higher dosage of water-soluble drugs relative to that of adults may be necessary to achieve therapeutic effects.

Metabolism

Drug-metabolizing enzymes in the liver of infants are immature. Certain enzyme functions responsible for drug metabolism do not mature until 1 to 2 months of age. Drugs are thus not biotransformed into inactive compounds as readily as they are in children and adults, resulting in higher levels of circulating active drug and greater potential for toxicity. Full pediatric dosages of some drugs (e.g., chloramphenicol) can produce severe adverse or toxic reactions in infants. Drug dosages for infants must therefore be calculated very carefully and drug levels and clinical response monitored closely.

Excretion

The kidneys of infants function immaturely. Infant kidneys have a higher resistance to blood flow, imcomplete Henle's loops, incomplete glomerular and tubular development, low glomerular filtration rate, and a decreased ability to concentrate urine. Consequently infants excrete drugs more slowly. Because renal excretion is inadequate, drug accumulation can occur, leading to toxicity. Response to drug therapy must be closely monitored in the infant. This is accomplished by monitoring clinical response and drug serum levels. Drug dosages must be altered appropriately to avoid toxicity.

Summary

In summary, absorption of water-soluble drugs in the infant is slightly diminished as compared to that of children. This may necessitate giving a higher dosage of oral and, in some cases, parenteral medication to infants. Once absorbed, however, drugs are metabolized and excreted less effectively, placing the infant at high risk for developing drug toxicities. Drug dosages for infants must be adjusted based on clinical response and serum drug levels.

PHARMACOKINETICS IN CHILDREN

Several physiological factors affect drug administration in children. Biological maturity and growth gradually enable the drug response of children to approximate that of adults. As growth occurs, body mass increases, fat content increases, the percentage of body water volume decreases, and the number of plasma proteins for drug binding increases. The blood-brain barrier and the skin become more effective drug barriers as children mature. Growth spurts during childhood and adolescence also affect drug response. All of these factors affect the absorption, distribution, metabolism, and excretion of drugs.

Absorption

Gastric pH in children does not approximate adult pH values by 2 to 3 years of age. Until then, this relative lack of acidity results in increased absorption of medications that are normally inactivated by gastric acid. Gastric emptying rates are faster than in infants, enabling drugs to move more rapidly to the small intestine where absorption is enhanced. The skin and blood-brain barrier become more effective, making the child less vulnerable to drug toxicities.

Distribution

The concentration of plasma proteins reaches adult levels by approximately age 1. This means that more of the drug can bind to the increased number of protein-binding sites in 1-year-olds as compared to infants, resulting in a decreased distribution of active drug. Young children (up to about age 2) continue to have a higher relative body water content compared to older children and adults, and thus may require higher dosages of water-soluble drugs than those over age 2.

Metabolism

As children mature, liver enzymes are able to effectively metabolize most drugs. Because the basal metabolic rate in children is higher than in adults, drugs are metabolized more rapidly. Thus drug dosages relative to body weight may need to be higher for children than for adults. Drug dosages for certain drugs that are metabolized very quickly in some children, (e.g., theophylline) should be tailored to the individual based on drug levels and clinical response.

Excretion

Kidney and liver function do not reach mature levels until about 6 to 12 months of age. Until then, dosages of drugs that are excreted by the kidney should be carefully calculated to minimize the chance of drug toxicity. Children over 12 months of age are able to excrete drugs effectively from their more mature kidneys, preventing drug effects from lasting too long.

Summary

In summary, absorption rates of drugs in children are higher than absorption rates in infants. This can result in lower drug dosages relative to weight in children than in infants. Drugs are distributed in the body, in a manner similar to that of adults. However, drugs are metabolized more readily in children, requiring careful dosage per weight and necessitating attention to serum drug levels and clinical response.

PHARMACOKINETICS AND DRUG RESPONSE RELATIONSHIPS

Serum Drug Levels

As described above, each drug administered to children will have its own rate of absorption, distribution, metabolism, and excretion. These processes can be measured by obtaining plasma or serum levels of the drug in blood. Monitoring serum levels of a drug enables the care provider to determine the most appropriate dosage, scheduling, and route of administration in individual patients. One can also determine if drug levels are approaching toxicity or are too low to provide a therapeutic response. Because pharmacokinetic processes are so variable in infants and children, drug serum levels are especially important tools in providing drug therapy for this population.

Using serum level analysis, peak and trough levels also can be determined. *Peak level* is the highest concentration a drug reaches after a number of doses have been administered. *Trough level* refers to the lowest concentration a drug reaches between doses. Peak and trough levels help to determine if the drug is in the desired range for therapeusis and safety. If peak and trough levels are too high or too low, drug dosages are modified.

Half-Life

The rate of metabolism and excretion of a drug determines its *half-life*. The half-life of a drug is the length of time it takes for 50% of the drug dose to be excreted. The half-life of each drug is different and will vary somewhat depending on the age and size of the patient. Knowing a drug's half-life will help the provider determine how often a drug should be administered. For example, a drug with a half-life of 3 to 4 hours will have to be given more frequently than one with a half-life of 12 hours.

Therapeutic Index, Lethal Dose, Effective Dose

The *therapeutic index* (TI) is the concentration of a drug necessary to produce the desired therapeutic effect without causing toxicity. The TI represents a ratio between the dosage of the drug that is lethal in 50% of lab animals (LD_{50}) and the dosage required to provide a therapeutic effect in 50% of a similar study population (ED_{50}). As the LD_{50} and ED_{50} approach one another and their ratio is closer to 1, the drug will have a greater chance of producing toxic effects. For example, if the LD_{50} of a drug is 95 and the ED_{50} is 100, the TI is 0.95. Because the TI is close to 1, a different dosage or drug will be necessary to avoid toxicity.

Steady State

The *steady state concentration* of a drug refers to the state in which the drug's distribution is in equilibrium with the body (i.e., the amount of drug taken is equal to the amount excreted). The steady state occurs only after repetitive drug dosing and is affected by the half-life of the drug. The longer a drug's half-life, the longer it will take that drug to reach a steady state concentration.

Loading Dose

The *loading dose* is a relatively high dose used with some drugs to start therapy to shorten the length of time it takes for that drug to reach a steady state concentration. For example, a loading dose is commonly used when starting digoxin and is called, in this case, a digitalizing dose. Once the loading dose has been given, the drug dosage is decreased to the *maintenance dose* and given on a regular schedule.

DRUG DOSING IN INFANTS AND CHILDREN

The determination of accurate drug dosages for infants and children is critical since they do not have the mature physiological responses to compensate for drug errors that could lead to overdosage, toxicity, and even death. Recommended doses for FDA-approved drugs are contained within this text and must be computed based on the individual child's weight.

When there is not a specifically recommended pediatric dosage available, the dosage must be extrapolated based on the adult dosage. The most accurate method of extrapolating pediatric drug dosages is determined by a formula using the body surface area (BSA) and basal metabolic rate (Shlafer, 1993). The BSA is determined from a nomogram (Appendix A). The formula is as follows:

$$\text{Child's dose} = \frac{\text{Body surface area (m}^2)}{1.7} \times \text{Adult dose}$$

The calculation of a drug dosage using this formula is based on the correlation of BSA and basal metabolic rate rather than on size alone. It should be used only when standard pediatric dosages based on weight are not available. The reliability of this method is based on the accuracy with which the BSA is calculated.

SUMMARY

This chapter is designed to reintroduce the reader to the principles of basic pharmacokinetics. The four processes of absorption, distribution, metabolism, and excretion are described. Physiological differences between infants, children, and adults are reviewed, as is the impact that these differences have on pharmacokinetic processes. Key terminology used in pharmacokinetics and drug response relationships is defined. This chapter is meant to help readers understand the unique challenges they will encounter in prescribing, administering, and monitoring safe and effective drug therapy in children.

BIBLIOGRAPHY

Beer CL, Williams BR: *Clinical pharmacology and nursing,* Philadelphia, 1992, Springhouse.

Clark JB, Queener JB, Karb VB: *Pharmacological basis of nursing practice,* St Louis, 1993, Mosby.

McKenry L, Salerno E: *Pharmacology in nursing,* St Louis, 1995, Mosby.

Peck C, Conner DP, Murphy MG: *Bedside clinical pharmacokinetics,* Vancouver, 1990, Applied Therapeutics, Inc.

Radde IC: *Pediatric pharmacology and therapeutics,* St Louis, 1993, Mosby.

Shlafer M: *The nurse, pharmacology, and drug therapy: a prototype approach,* Redwood City, Calif, 1993, Addison-Wesley.

CHAPTER 2

Pediatric Medication Administration: Guidelines and Techniques

Administration of medications to infants, children, and adolescents can be a challenging experience, requiring not only knowledge of a child's physiological development but also knowledge of cognitive and psychosocial development. In addition, all care providers responsible for administering medications must possess a certain degree of patience, creativity, and, at times, a compassionate sense of humor.

This chapter focuses on cognitive and psychosocial developmental considerations of pediatric medication administration. Routes of administration are also discussed with specific emphasis on strategies for success. Finally, special attention is briefly given to another challenge facing all pediatric nurses, the assessment and treatment of pain in children. (The term *parent* is used frequently in this chapter; however, it represents not only the child's biological or adoptive parent but also the child's significant care provider, recognizing that they are not always the same. This term was chosen to simplify the discussion.)

COGNITIVE AND PSYCHOSOCIAL DEVELOPMENTAL CONSIDERATIONS

Before discussing each age group individually, we must briefly address two issues that relate to all age groups: biological age vs. developmental age and temperament of the child.

It is important to note that, although a child might have reached a certain biological age, his or her level of development may be quite different. Therefore it is imperative to determine, to the greatest possible extent, the developmental age and functioning of the child. Nurses must use strategies consistent with the child's

11

developmental age to ensure safe and effective medication administration.

Discussions with the parent about the child's temperament can also provide significant information that may help to achieve successful administration of the medication. The "easy" child generally will present minimal difficulty, whereas the "slow-to-warm-up" and "difficult" child may require more careful planning and ingenuity (Chess and Thomas, 1985; Johnson, 1992; McClowry, 1992). The slow-to-warm-up child may need more preparation before medication administration and may need to be an active participant in the process (e.g., holding the cup of water, adhesive bandage) in order to "warm up" to what is going to happen. In contrast, the difficult child may become much more intense and upset if too much preparation time is allowed. The nurse's expectations for cooperation and compliance from a temperamentally difficult child need to be realistic. Enlistment of parent and staff support and identification of appropriate limit-setting strategies with rewards must be done before administering the medication.

Premature Infants

This group of children obviously does not have the cognitive ability to understand what is happening to them, what is expected of them (e.g., swallowing, holding still), or the importance of cooperating with the process. The focus of administering to premature infants should be on providing comfort and security before, during, and after the medication has been administered. The infant's sucking and gag reflex may be very weak, if present at all; therefore precautions against aspiration must be taken when administering oral medications (Bindler and Howry, 1991).

Infants (Birth to 12 Months)

The cognitive limitations previously described are still present in this age group; however, as the infant reaches some developmental milestones, the process of administration will vary. All infants should be physically supported to ensure safe administration. For example, an infant with poor head control needs his or her head supported during oral medication administration, whereas an infant who has developed new strengths in gross motor movements may need gentle restraint.

For young infants unfamiliar with taking oral medications, the initial reaction may be to spit or drool the medication from his or her mouth. The person administering the medication may want to gently hold the child's chin up, talking calmly and encouraging the child to swallow. The older infant may be more familiar with taking medications and therefore may have a more intense reaction to the administration. One person can administer the

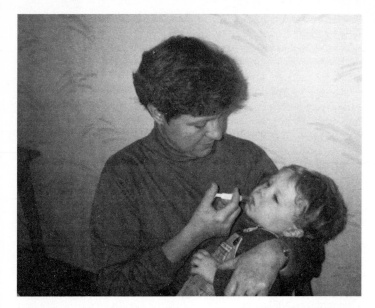

Technique for oral administration of medication to an infant.

medication by using a technique similar to that shown in the illustration above.

Separation anxiety can begin as early as 8 months; therefore familiarity with the person administering the medication may be a factor. When present, parents can provide invaluable support to allay the child's fears; however, the parents should be used only to provide emotional support and comfort to the child, not to restrain him or her. Some parents may choose not to be a part of the medication administration process, particularly if it is perceived as painful (e.g., intramuscular or intrathecal injection). They can then be used to provide comfort immediately after the medication has been administered.

Toddler: 12 to 36 Months

The achievement of increased expressive and receptive language skills and ambulation at this age creates more challenges for medication administration. The approach used will directly affect the outcome of the present experience and can affect future experiences as well. Positively portraying an air of confidence and expectation for success will help the toddler feel more secure and comfortable.

Separation anxiety continues to be a concern with toddlers. The same strategies discussed previously should be enlisted for this age group as well. Communication with this group of children should be succinct, using words that are familiar and understandable to them. Lengthy discussion as to what the medication is and why it is important for them to take is irrelevant. It can even be detrimental to a successful outcome, as this discussion can prolong the experience and increase anxiety for the child. Simple and brief explanations are helpful, always ensuring they are developmentally appropriate. Using a technique called *forced choice* can be successful with this age group (e.g., "Do you want to sit on mommy's or daddy's lap?", "Do you want to drink it from this cup or with a straw?"). The use of dolls and stuffed animals to simulate taking medication allows the child to use new skills in imaginative play and can increase cooperation, even making the experience enjoyable.

Preschool-Age: 3 to 6 Years

Prior experience with taking medications, the temperamental profile of the child, and the child's cognitive ability become more important in this developmental age group. In general, preschool-age children are fairly cooperative as their level of understanding begins to increase and they begin to realize the importance of taking medications. However, if a preschooler has had significant negative experiences with taking medications in the past or possesses a very difficult temperament, the child's resistance is far more physically challenging for the nurse and parent. At times, the nurse may have more success than the parent because the nurse is viewed as an authority figure whom the child wants to please.

Explanations about the purpose of the medication and the importance of cooperation may be a little more detailed than those given to the toddler, but still need to be short and simple. Preschoolers still respond well to forced choices, and they can now choose, when applicable, among oral preparations (e.g., elixir, chewable, or tablet). Continued use of therapeutic play with dolls and stuffed animals is also essential for this age group.

School-Age: 6 to 12 Years

The school-age child is usually cooperative with taking medications, particularly if careful attention is given to ensuring that the child has at least a minimal understanding of the purpose and importance of the medication. It is important for this age group to have a sense of control over the situation; therefore, allow the child to have as much control as possible. Fears of bodily injury are also prominent for school-age children; therefore the nurse should assess the fears of the child and intervene accordingly. Side effects of medications should be reviewed with the child to help allay any future fears the child may have if side effects do occur.

Adolescents: 12 to 19 Years

As adolescents' cognitive abilities expand, so does their need to have more explicit information about medications. Adolescents continue to have fears of bodily injury, have increased concerns about body image, and begin to have fears about death. The extent to which these issues must be discussed with the adolescent will obviously depend on the medication being administered. Ensuring privacy is also important because adolescents are experiencing many physiological changes in addition to the formation of their personal identity. Decisions regarding medications may be discussed with adolescents since they now are becoming more responsible and autonomous.

All Age Groups

The following few principles need to be adhered to for all age groups:

- Honesty is always a priority; children must always be told the truth (e.g., how much discomfort is involved with administration of the medication, taste of oral medications).
- Careful attention to vocabulary used is essential when giving explanations so as not to frighten the child.
- Forceful restraint should never be used. Physical injury could occur in addition to psychological trauma from loss of control over the process. If a child is demonstrating such an intense response as to warrant forceful restraint, then the care provider must stop and reevaluate the situation (except in an emergency).
- Praising the child after successful administration of medication, regardless of behavior during the process, helps to build a child's self-esteem while allaying any guilty feelings. Any resistive behavior should be ignored and forgotten once the experience is over.
- Never threaten or shame a child into taking a medication; thoughtful limit-setting only is acceptable. Communicate to the child using developmentally appropriate language what behavior will and will not be tolerated.

ROUTES OF ADMINISTRATION

Many routes for medication administration are available for pediatric patients; the choice of route is dependent upon the drug's dosage form, available preparations, frequency of administration, and the child's developmental age and physical condition. The amount of education and training required by nursing personnel prior to administering medications by a particular route is generally dependent on institutional and state-defined practice

TABLE 2.1

General Guidelines for Nursing Personnel Who Can Administer Medications by Various Routes*

ROUTE	LVN/LPN	RN	ADVANCED RN†
Oral (PO)	Yes	Yes	Yes
Intravenous (IV)	No	Yes	Yes
Intramuscular (IM)	Yes‡	Yes	Yes
Subcutaneous (SC)	Yes‡	Yes	Yes
Intraosseous	No	No	Yes
Intrathecal	No	No	Yes
Epidural	No	No	Yes
Rectal	Yes	Yes	Yes
Ophthalmic/Otic/Nasal	Yes	Yes	Yes
Inhalants	Yes	Yes	Yes
Transdermal	Yes	Yes	Yes
Topical	Yes	Yes	Yes
Vaginal	Yes	Yes	Yes

*These are general guidelines. Nursing personnel are responsible for following their specific institutional and state practice policies.

†RNs administering by these routes need additional education (graduate level) or advanced training.

‡Ability to administer medication by this route may be medication-dependent.

policies. Table 2-1 identifies generally accepted practice guidelines for the routes described below.

Oral

Oral medications have a variety of preparations: liquid (elixirs, syrups, and suspensions), tablets (some may be chewable), and capsules. Careful attention must be given to accurate dose administration when using liquid preparations. The use of a calibrated oral syringe or spoon device or scored droppers ensures the accuracy of the dose; the use of medicine cups for small doses may result in an inaccurate dose. Parents should be told not to use regular silverware for medication administration since the amount that can be held in household teaspoons or tablespoons is quite variable. Some tablets may be crushed and mixed with a palatable liquid to ease administration; however, this may decrease the effectiveness of the drug (e.g., sustained-release medications). A pharmacist should always be consulted before changing the preparation form of the medication.

Infants and young children must be positioned upright to prevent aspiration during oral medication administration. Swallowing of medication can be facilitated in infants up to 11 months of age by blowing a small puff of air into their face once the

TABLE 2.2
Calculation of Fluid Volume Maintenance

Total fluid volume require- ments for 24 hours	100 ml/kg for first 10 kg of weight 50 ml/kg for second 10 kg of weight 20 ml/kg for each additional kg
Example	Child's weight = 25 kg 100 ml × 10 kg = 1000 ml 50 ml × 10 kg = 500 ml 20 ml × 5 kg = 100 ml TOTAL: 25 kg = 1600 ml/day

medication has been placed in their cheeks (Orenstein, 1988). *Never* pinch the nose of an infant or child shut to facilitate swallowing; this can easily cause choking or aspiration.

Intravenous

Intravenous administration is now frequently used in pediatrics as it is often the most effective route. The following key issues should be addressed for safe and effective IV administration:
• Type of diluent needed
• Dilution amount required
• Compatibility for admixtures
• Rate of infusion
• Stability of the solution once diluted
• Degree of irritability to venous walls
• Extravasation precautions
• Fluid volume needs of the child
    For infants and young children (as well as children of all ages with cardiopulmonary difficulties), the amount and rate of diluent must be carefully calculated to prevent fluid volume excess (Table 2-2). The IV site and rate of infusion must be frequently monitored for signs of infiltration or phlebitis and for potential fluid overload, respectively. For children less than 40 kg, a calibrated volume control chamber should be used to decrease the possibility of fluid volume overload. The amount of fluid in the tubing must be considered when calculating the rate of infusion when a specific time for medication infusion is indicated. Warm compresses may be applied to the IV site during the administration of irritating medications to decrease discomfort.

Intramuscular

The use of IM injection has significantly decreased over recent years, particularly as a result of the increased safety and acceptance of the IV route. It should only be used when no other route of administration is applicable or available. The correct site for IM administration, the amount of medication or solution permitted for each site, the type of needle to be used, and the irritability of the medication to the tissues must be determined before administration.

In determining the appropriate IM site, the following factors should considered (Whaley and Wong, 1994):

• Characteristics of medication to be injected
• Condition of child's muscle mass
• Expected frequency and duration of IM-administered medications
• Accessibility of site
• Safety of administration

Controversy continues as to the preferred IM injection site; there is general agreement, however, that the vastis lateralis site should be used at least until the child has been walking for 1 year (Table 2-3). The volume of solution that can be safely given per injection site and the size of needle recommended is also quite variable depending on the child's age and the medication to be administered (Table 2-3 and Table 2-4).

Administration of IM medications is almost always a traumatic experience for infants and young children, nor is it a favorite of older children either. The placement of an anesthetic cream such as EMLA cream (Eutetic Mixture of Local Anesthetics) on the injection site before administration can decrease the discomfort. However, for toddlers and preschoolers the sight of EMLA may increase their anxiety as they anticipate the injection from the time the EMLA cream was placed. (EMLA cream requires application at least one hour before injection for maximum anesthetic effects.) Therapeutic play, in addition to other adjunctive pain management strategies, can be used before and after the injection to enhance coping in toddlers and preschoolers (Table 2-5) (Kane and Sugarman, 1995).

Subcutaneous

As with IM injections, SC administration is reserved for use only when absolutely necessary (administration of insulin, heparin). The same issues discussed with IM injections apply to this route as well.

Intraosseous

Intraosseous administration is only indicated in an emergency situation when IV access is not available or accessible. Fluids and medications can be administered by this route. Insertion into the bone marrow through the anteromedial surface of the proximal tibia is made with a large bore needle (Baer and Williams, 1992). If the child is awake, a local anesthetic should be used prior to

TABLE 2.3
IM Injection Sites for Children

SITE	DISCUSSION
Vastus Lateralis GREATER TROCHANTER* Sciatic nerve Femoral artery **Site of injection** (Vastus lateralis) Rectus femoris KNEE JOINT* G.J.Wassilchenko	**Location*** Palpate to find greater trochanter and knee joints; divide vertical distance between these two landmarks into quadrants; inject into middle of upper quadrant. **Needle insertion and size** Insert needle at 45-degree angle toward knee in infants and in young children or needle perpendicular to thigh or slightly angled toward anterior thigh. 22-25 gauge, ⅝-1 in.† **Advantages** Large, well-developed muscle that can tolerate larger quantities of fluid (0.5 ml [infant] to 2.0 ml [child]) No important nerves or blood vessels in this location Easily accessible if child is supine, side lying, or sitting A tourniquet can be applied above injection site to delay drug hypersensitivity reaction if necessary **Disadvantages** Thrombosis of femoral artery from injecton in midthigh area Sciatic nerve damage from long needle injected posteriorly and medially into small extremity

From Wong, DL: *Whaley and Wong's nursing care of infants and children,* ed 5, St Louis, 1995, Mosby. *Continued.*

TABLE 2.3
IM Injection Sites for Children—cont'd

SITE	DISCUSSION
Ventrogluteal	**Location***

Location*
Palpate to locate greater trochanter, anterior superior iliac tubercle (found by flexing thigh at hip and measuring up to 1-2 cm above crease formed in groin), and posterior iliac crest; place palm of hand over greater trochanter, index finger over anterior superior iliac tubercle, and middle finger along crest of ilium posteriorly as far as possible; inject into center of V formed by fingers.

Needle insertion and size
Insert needle perpendicular to site but angled slightly toward iliac crest.
22-25 gauge, ½-1 in.

Advantages
Free of important nerves and vascular structures
Easily identified by prominent bony landmarks
Thinner layer of subcutaneous tissue than in dorsgluteal site, thus less chance of depositing drug subcutaneously rather than intramuscularly
Can accommodate larger quantities of fluid (0.5 ml [infant] to 2.0 ml [child])
Easily accessible if child is supine, prone, or side lying
Less painful than vastus lateralis

Disadvantages
Health professionals' unfamiliarity with site
Not suitable for use of a tourniquet

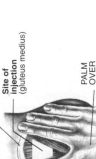

ANTERIOR SUPERIOR ILIAC SPINE POSTERIOR ILIAC CREST

Site of injection (gluteus medius)

PALM OVER GREATER TROCHANTER*

G.J.Wassilchenko

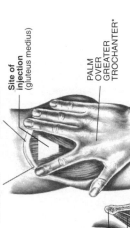

Iliac crest
Gluteus medius
Gluteus minimus
Greater trochanter

Ventrogluteal site of injection

Dorsogluteal

Location*

Locate greater trochanter and posterior superior iliac spine; draw imaginary line between these two points and inject lateral and superior to line into gluteus maximus or medius muscle.

Needle insertion and size

Insert needle perpendicular to surface on which child is lying when prone.

20-25 gauge, ½-1½ in.

Advantages

In older child, large muscle mass; well-developed muscle can tolerate greater volume of fluid (up to 2.0 ml)

Child does not see needle and syringe

Easily accessible if child is prone or side lying

Disadvantages

Contraindicated in children who have not been walking for at least 1 year

Danger of injury to sciatic nerve

Thick subcutaneous fat, predisposing to deposition of drug subcutaneously rather than intramuscularly

Not suitable for use of a tourniquet

Inaccessible if child is supine

Exposure of site may cause embarrassment in older child

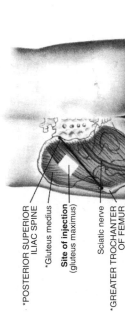

*POSTERIOR SUPERIOR ILIAC SPINE

*Gluteus medius

Site of injection (gluteus maximus)

Sciatic nerve

*GREATER TROCHANTER OF FEMUR

G. J. Wassilchenko

Continued.

TABLE 2.3
IM Injection Sites for Children—cont'd

SITE	DISCUSSION
Deltoid 	**Location*** Locate acromion process; inject only into upper third of muscle that begins about 2 fingerbreadths below acromion. **Needle insertion and size** Insert needle perpendicular to site but angled slightly toward shoulder. 22-25 gauge, ½-1 in. **Advantages** Faster absorption rates than gluteal sites Tourniquet can be applied above injection site Easily accessible with minimum removal of clothing Less pain and fewer local side effects from vaccines as compared with vastus lateralis **Disadvantages** Small muscle mass; only limited amounts of drug can be injected (0.5-1.0 ml) Small margins of safety with possible damage to radial nerve and axillary nerve (not shown, lies under deltoid at head of humerus)

*Locations are indicated by asterisks on illustrations.

†Research has shown that a 1-in. needle is needed for adequate muscle penetration in infants 4 mo. old and possibly in infants as young as 2 mo. (Hicks, and others, 1989). Other recommendations for needle size and volume of fluid are based on traditional practice and have not been verified by research.

TABLE 2.4
Maximum IM Solution Volumes for Children by Age and Muscle Site

| | | | MUSCLE SITE | |
AGE	VASTUS LATERALIS	VENTROGLUTEAL	DORSOGLUTEAL	DELTOID
0-1½ yr	0.5-1.0 ml	Not recommended	Not recommended	Not recommended
1½-3 yr	1.0 ml	1.0 ml (Use only when other sites unavailable)	1.0 ml (Use only when other sites unavailable)	0.5 ml (Use only when other sites unavailable)
3-6 yr	1.5 ml	1.5 ml	1.5 ml	0.5 ml
6-15 yr	1.5-2.0 ml	1.5-2.0 ml	1.5-2.0 ml	0.5 ml
>15 yr	2.0-2.5 ml	2.0-2.5 ml	2.0-2.5 ml	0.5 ml

TABLE 2.5
Adjunctive Pain Management Strategies (Summary Table—See Specific Recommendations in Text)

AGE LEVEL	PREPARATION	RELAXATION	FOCUSED ATTENTION	IMAGERY*
Birth–2 years	Prepare parents Review history of strategies that have worked in past Explain role of parental anxiety to reduce its transmission to child	Oral stimulation Sucking Rhymes Rocking Massage Holding personal comfort items Singing Talking	Cause-and-effect toys Singing Rattles Music Pop-up toys, books	Not beneficial in this age group
Preschool 2–5 years old	Review history of strategies that have worked in past Prepare just before procedure History of temperament, coping abilities Discuss sensory aspects Use teaching dolls, transitional objects	This age rarely uses physical relaxation to cope, may be counter-productive Holding Massaging Singing Nursery rhymes Holding personal comfort items Breathing rhythm, focus on exhalation	Pop-up toys, books Stories Video tapes, games Counting ABC's Manipulatives Blowing Massage Eye fixation	Use external, concrete stimuli Pop-up books Stuffed animals Puppets Video/audio tapes

| School-Age 6-11 years old | Prepare as early as 1 day in advance of procedure Use teaching dolls, transitional objects Discuss sensory aspects Offer choices of strategies Use medical play Rehearse strategies Discuss parents' roles with child | See preschool methods Eye fixation Progressive relaxation Relatively indirect methods more effective than suggestions to "relax" | Preschool methods Audio/video tapes Humor | "Favorite place" Enjoyable memories "Dimmer switch" Revivify anesthetic experiences (cold, gloves) Dissociation Use pain scale Peer demonstration |
| Adolescent 11-18 years old | Prepare in advance Use body outlines Use correct terminology Give written material Offer choices of strategies Rehearse strategies Discuss parents' roles | Talking Music Video Audio tapes Massage Eye fixation Progressive relaxation | School age methods of appropriate sophistication | Elaborate upon school age techniques Music tapes Books on tape Peer demonstration |

Developed by Kane T, Sugarman L: unpublished document, 1995. Used with permission.

*Clinicians require training in clinical hypnosis to employ advanced forms of imagery.

insertion. This route can only be used for children 5 years of age or younger.

Intrathecal

Antineoplastic agents are the most common medications administered intrathecally. The child needs to be placed in the same position used for lumbar punctures: side-lying position with knees flexed to chest and head flexed downward. EMLA cream or other local anesthetics should be used before insertion to minimize discomfort.

Epidural

Epidural administration is used for anesthesia and analgesia, and most recently has been used for patient-controlled epidural analgesia (PCEA) (Caudle and others, 1993). Specialized training is required to initiate access into the caudal or epidural space. Medications can be given either by bolus or continuous infusion. Careful monitoring of the access site is necessary to ensure patency and placement.

Rectal

Significant consideration should be given to the developmental age of the child for rectal administration. This route is considered invasive and threatening by most age groups and must be carefully explained and demonstrated before administration. Doll play should be used with toddlers and preschoolers to facilitate their cooperation, and drawings or diagrams can be used with older children. Late school-age children and adolescents may want to insert the suppository themselves. Infants and young children may lie on their backs with knees held up in a flexed position for insertion, whereas older children can lie on their side with top leg flexed. Suppositories need not be lubricated before insertion; however, moistening with water can ease insertion.

Ophthalmic, Otic, and Nasal

Depending on the child's age, two persons may be needed to administer ophthalmic ointments or drops because it is difficult to stabilize the child's head and administer the medication at the same time. An older child may be able to assist in the administration by helping to pull down the lower lid or by looking up when the medication is being administered. Hyperextension of the child's head is usually necessary to ensure proper dispersal of the medication. Sterile technique should always be used.

Ear drops may be warmed before administration to minimize discomfort for the child. Otic administration techniques will vary depending on the age of the child; however, it is not a sterile procedure. For children under age 3, pull the earlobe down and back; for children over age 3, pull up and back. After administration, gently rub the anterior ear to facilitate the drops entering the ear canal. Cotton may be used to help hold drops in the ear.

Administration of nasal medications is not a sterile technique; again some restraint or assistance may be needed. The most significant concern is to ensure that the drops have as much contact with the nasal passages as possible before entering the throat. Only slight hyperextension of the head should be used; if the child is very small, the head may be held in a "football" position against the care provider. The child should remain in this position for at least 1 minute after administration.

Inhalants

There are several administration devices that can be used for inhalants (e.g., tents, oxyhoods, nebulizers, metered dose inhalers, and spacers). The length of time for administration and technique is determined by the device used. Education of the parent or older child in proper use of the device is very important. If more than one inhalant is being administered at the same time, mixing of the medications or sequence of the medications (which one to give first) is determined by the type of medication.

Transdermal

Placement of the transdermal patch is dependent on three issues: the age of the child, the number of patches to be used, and the indication for medication. The developmentally young child may try to take the patch off or accidentally ingest it, whereas the older child may want to conceal the patches on areas of the body less exposed (for self-esteem reasons). If several patches are needed to obtain full medication potential, it may be necessary to use several areas of the body at the same time. The type of medication may require a specific patch placement; therefore, consult specific medication instructions before administration.

Topical

Meticulous skin assessment is needed before topical application of any medications. The area to be treated should be observed for skin integrity and appearance. The technique used (sterile vs. clean) is determined based on the integrity of the skin and the type of agent to be used. For the very young child, careful attention must be given to the amount of agent used; toxic systemic reactions can occur because of their relatively large body surface area.

Vaginal

Consideration of the child's developmental level is crucial before use of vaginal medications, as this route can cause significant psychological trauma. Therapeutic play should be used for toddlers and preschoolers and specific explanations given for older children and adolescents. The older child may be able to administer the medication by herself with only guidance from the care provider.

PAIN ASSESSMENT AND MANAGEMENT

The following facts about pediatric pain should be stated before discussion of assessment and management:

- Infants as young as 24 weeks gestation have sufficient development of the central nervous system to transmit a painful stimulus (Fitzgerald and McIntosh, 1989; Lawrence and others, 1993).
- Infants do have memory of painful experiences (Schechter and others, 1993).
- Children do not always tell the truth about pain (for a variety of reasons).
- Activity level is not an indicator for the degree of pain a child is experiencing (McCready and others, 1991).
- Children do not become addicted faster to narcotics than adults (Schechter and others, 1993).
- Narcotics are not too dangerous to use with any age group; however, careful dosage calculation and monitoring are necessary.

Pain is difficult to assess as it is truly a subjective experience. There are, however, three types of assessments to be made: assessment of physiologic parameters, behavioral indices, and subjective reports. Each age group will exhibit slight differences in each of these categories. Physiological and behavioral changes are far more crucial in the very young, preverbal, or developmentally delayed child. Subjective reports should include the use of rating scales in addition to parent or care provider assessment. Multiple assessment scales exist to rate pediatric pain (AHCPR, 1992). The important concern is that an assessment scale be adopted and used consistently. Obtaining a pain history can also assist in management of the current pain experience.

Management of pain should always include the use of non–pharmacological strategies, with pharmacological therapies when necessary. Non–pharmacological strategies include the following:

- Maximizing comfortable positions
- Holding, rocking, cuddling
- Application of heat or cold

- Relaxation techniques, guided imagery, focused attention, and hypnotherapy.

The use of hypnotherapy does require specialized training, and credentialing as a clinical hypnotherapist may be required.

When pharmacological therapies are employed, several guidelines should be addressed. IV is the route of choice, when available. IM injections should be avoided unless absolutely necessary. For acute postoperative pain, morphine sulfate is the drug of choice and Dilaudid is the second choice. Postoperative pain, and some acute medical pain (e.g., otitis media), should be managed with routine scheduling of medications and should no longer be managed on a prn (as needed) basis (AHCPR, 1992; Schechter, 1995). Knowledge of medication side effects is critical to ensure proper monitoring. Children (particularly adolescents) and their parents need to be reassured that addiction is not a concern when managing acute pain. And finally, allowing children and adolescents as much control over their pain management as possible is integral to successful alleviation of their pain. Encourage the use of patient-controlled analgesia (for children as young as 7, maybe younger depending on developmental age) for postoperative pain, episodes of acute pain with underlying chronic pain (e.g., sickle cell crisis), and for terminal pain (AHCPR, 1992).

In summary, there are many challenges that face pediatric nurses; medication administration and pain assessment and management are only two of them. Understanding the child's development and adhering to the general principles and guidelines outlined in this chapter will result in a successful endeavor.

BIBLIOGRAPHY

Agency for Health Care Policy and Research (AHCPR): *Acute pain management in infants, children and adolescents: operative and medical procedures,* AHCPR Pub. #92-0020, Rockville, Md., 1992, Agency for Health Care Policy and Research, Public Health Service, U.S. Department of Health and Human Services.

Baer CL, Williams BR: The pediatric patient. In *Clinical pharmacology and nursing,* ed 2, Springhouse, Penn., 1992, Springhouse Corp.

Bindler RM, Howry LB: *Pediatric drugs and nursing implications,* Norwalk, Conn., 1991, Appleton & Lange.

Caudle CL, Freid EB, Bailey AG, and others: Epidural fentanyl infusion with patient-controlled epidural analgesia for postoperative analgesia in children, *J Pediatr Surg* 28 (4):554, 1993.

Chess S, Thomas A: Temperamental differences: a critical concept in child health care, *Pediatr Nurs* 3:167, 1985.

Fitzgerald M, McIntosh N: Pain and analgesia in the newborn, *Arch Dis Childhood* 64(4):441, 1989.

Johnson JM: The tendency for temperament to be "temperamental": conceptual and methodological considerations, *J Pediatr Nurs* 7(5):347, 1992.

Kane T, Sugarman L: *Adjunctive pain management strategies,* University of Rochester Pediatric Pain Subcommittee, unpublished document, 1995.

Lawrence J, Alcock D, McGrath P, and others: The development of a tool to assess neonatal pain, *Neonatal Network* 12(16):59, 1993.

McClowry SG: Temperament theory and research, *IMAGE: J Nurs Scholarship* 24(4):319, 1992.

McCready M, MacDavitt K, O'Sullivan KK: Children and pain: easing the hurt, *Orthop Nurs* 10(6):33, 1991.

Orenstein S: The Santmyer swallow: a new and useful infant reflex, *Lancet* 8581(1):345, 1988.

Schechter NL: Common pain problems in the general pediatric setting, *Pediatr Ann* 24(3):139, 1995.

Schechter NL, Berde CB, Yaster M: Pain in infants, children and adolescents: an overview. In Schechter NL, Berde CB, Yaster M, editors, *Pain in infants, children, and adolescents,* Baltimore, 1993, Williams & Wilkins, pp 3-9.

Wong DL: Whaley and Wong's *nursing care of infants and children,* ed 5, St Louis, 1995, Mosby.

CHAPTER 3

Medication Administration in Special Settings

Administration of medications to children in non–hospital settings has become commonplace as health care for children with special needs has rapidly moved into outpatient settings (e.g., home, early intervention programs, day care, and schools). Nurses who administer medication to children or are responsible for coordinating the administration of medication to children in special settings must consider the unique needs of the child as well as the setting. This chapter focuses on a discussion of the characteristics of special settings, common medication regimes, special devices used to administer medications, and useful tips to facilitate safe and effective medication administration. As discussed in Chapter 2, attention to the developmental age and temperament of the child and collaboration with primary caretakers is essential, regardless of the setting. References to child also refer to the child's primary caretaker and family as indicated.

The transition of care from hospital to home requires careful predischarge planning and collaboration between hospital staff and all health care discipline, agency, and school personnel who will provide care to the child. Similar planning is essential for children with special health care needs managed by their families at home as they make the transition into day care or school settings. Involvement of the family as active participants in this process is essential to developing a plan for a successful transition. Identification of a care coordinator, particularly for children with complex care needs, can facilitate the development of a holistic plan to address all health care needs. Planning takes into account specific goals of the child and family, primary care provider, specialists, home care agencies, and other involved community resources (e.g., schools or day care). The discipline acting in the care coordinator role (medicine, nursing, or social work) may vary based on the identification of the child's health and home care needs and the region in which he lives. It is imperative that the roles and responsibilities of all involved be clearly delineated before the child's transition either from hospital to home or from home into a day care or school setting. This is especially important when several specialists or disciplines are involved in the child's care.

Regardless of the setting a concerted attempt should be made to consider the developmental needs of the child, including eating, sleeping, play, and school routines, when planning medication schedules. A medication plan should be made based on the needs of the child and family with a minimum of disruption of the usual activities and routines.

CHARACTERISTICS OF SPECIAL SETTINGS

Early Intervention Programs

Early intervention programs provide educational and therapeutic services to children from birth to age 3 who are at risk for developmental delay due to biological or environmental factors. (Savage and Culbert, 1989). Services are provided by an interdisciplinary team of specialists who collaborate to provide input into the development of an individualized family service plan (IFSP). The family is an integral part of the planning process. Early intervention programs can be center-based, home-based, or a combination of both. Center-based programs provide services to the child and family within a center-based facility. In home-based programs, services are provided within the child's home.

At least 50% of mothers of children under age 6 are employed outside of the home. Thus it is reasonable to assume that increasingly young children with special health care needs will be cared for by non–family members in a variety of settings.

Day Care Homes

Day care in a home setting may be of three general types: several children within a caretaker's home (with or without the caretaker's own children), a non–family caretaker providing care in the child's home, and children cared for in a home setting by multiple caretakers. Home care allows the child to spend time in a home-like setting while his or her parents are working. Licensing requirements (including specific skills of caregivers) vary from state to state (Betz, 1994).

Day Care Center

This type of care is usually provided in its own facility and provides care for many children, typically those from age 6 to 8 weeks through preschool age. Although the quality of care can vary greatly among day care centers, individual states have established minimum standards for day care centers. Many are run as business enterprises on a for-profit basis. Many day care centers have trained staff and established programs designed to meet the physical, social, cognitive, and emotional needs of children (Betz, 1994).

Home Care

Technology-dependent children who are deemed stable enough for discharge from the hospital yet continue to require ongoing medical services may be cared for in a home setting. This group may include ventilator-dependent children as well as children with other complex health care needs. Based on individual needs of the child and family, care may be required for a limited time only or long term.

Schools

The passage of Education for All Handicapped Children (Public Law 94-142) in 1975 brought sweeping reforms into school systems, particularly special education programs. Mandated reforms included establishment of the rights of children with disabilities to receive educational services in the least-restrictive environment. This translates into a process of including students with disabilities in settings with non–disabled students.

COMMON MEDICATION REGIMES IN SPECIAL SETTINGS

Regardless of the setting, medication regimes should be scheduled around the needs of the child. Day care and school activities should be interrupted as little as possible. Children should not routinely be scheduled to receive medications during recess or special activity times. They can easily perceive this as a type of punishment and thus develop resentment toward taking medications. Children may be very sensitive about taking medications since it may cause them to see themselves as different from their peers. Privacy may be important, and public reminders for the child to take medication or go to the nurse may be embarrassing. These issues should be discussed openly with the child. Involving the child in planning can facilitate cooperation and a sense of control. Timing of many medications is essential; medication effectiveness may depend on when it is given (such as with or without meals, before exercise or activity, or prn) based on specific needs of the child. Special attention is required when children participate in field trips. Medication may need to be taken or dosages readjusted based on a change in the day's scheduled activities. It is important to identify who will be responsible in a given setting for giving medications or making assessments that medication is indicated. Nurses may not be present in all settings, yet they may be responsible for coordinating medication scheduling and teaching non–medical personnel to safely administer medications.

CHILDREN RECEIVING MEDICATIONS TO TREAT CARDIAC DISORDERS

The majority of children receiving medications to improve cardiac function have some type of congenital cardiac defect. The most common medications used to treat children with congenital cardiac disease are digoxin and diuretics; these are most often used before palliative or corrective surgical treatment. Medications are typically used to treat congestive heart failure that may be present before surgical intervention. Digoxin is a potentially lethal medication; careful monitoring for side effects and meticulous care in administration are essential. Digoxin is given at regular intervals to maintain serum levels. Specific instructions from the child's physician regarding missed or vomited doses are an important part of the plan of care. The child should be monitored for signs of digoxin toxicity, including nausea and vomiting, anorexia, listlessness, dysrhythmias, and bradycardia. It is critical to report these symptoms to the child's physician promptly. Digoxin levels may be altered by vomiting, diarrhea, or elevated temperature; thus careful communication with the child's physician is indicated with these symptoms.

Diuretics such as Lasix, Diuril, or Edecrin are frequently used to decrease total body fluids and increase urine output. Children receiving diuretics must be monitored for decreased potassium levels, and they may require potassium supplements. Staff working with children receiving diuretics must be sensitive to the child's potential need for extra trips to the bathroom and must develop extra reminders for the child who may have an increased potential for medication-induced enuresis.

CHILDREN WITH DIABETES RECEIVING INSULIN

Children with Type I diabetes produce little or no insulin and are classified as having insulin-dependent diabetes. Treatment centers around a regime of planned meals and meal times, exercise (including organized sports and gym schedule), or anticipated periods of high activity level and insulin dosing. The insulin regime typically consists of a daily combination of regular (short acting) and NPH (long acting) insulin. Maintaining blood glucose levels within an acceptable range is dependent on careful planning of meals, exercise, and insulin doses. Any change in insulin, food intake, or exercise will affect the child's blood glucose level. Nurses working with children must be knowledgeable about the interaction of food, exercise, and insulin, and they must anticipate the impact that a change in any one these will have on blood glucose levels. Nurses must be aware of peak times and duration of insulin action, able to monitor blood glucose levels, and able to recognize and treat hypoglycemia and hyperglycemia. Nurses may be in a position of responsibility to ensure that day care or school staff who come into contact with the child are knowledgeable about the child's needs related to his or her diabetes; at a minimum, all staff, including teachers, teacher aides, gym teachers, bus drivers, and others, must be able to recognize and treat hypoglycemia, including severe episodes in which the child may be unconscious. They should also be aware that skipped or late meals or snacks and skipped or unplanned exercise may change the child's blood glucose to potentially dangerous levels.

Older school-age children and adolescents may receive insulin using an insulin pump. Insulin dosage remains dependent on planned meals or snacks and exercise to maintain an acceptable blood glucose level. Typically, these children do *not* have activity restrictions associated with the use of the pump. During some activities (such as swimming), the pump may be disconnected while the tubing connected to the child is covered and secured. Insulin pumps are generally not used with younger children because dosage rates could be altered by a young child playing with the pump.

CHILDREN RECEIVING MEDICATIONS TO CONTROL A NEUROLOGIC DISORDER

Seizures

Seizures are a symptom of a central nervous system condition associated with a variety of etiologies. The terms *epilepsy* and *seizure disorder* are used synonymously to describe a tendency toward recurrent seizures in which the seizure discharge develops spontaneously. It is estimated that as many as one in ten children may have epilepsy. Staff providing care to children with seizures must have baseline information on management regarding the type and characteristics of the seizure disorder, medication side effects and response, maintenance of a safe environment (including any activity restrictions), and interventions to manage a seizure. The child with partial seizures may become dizzy, confused, or even angry, which may be mistaken for emotional disturbance or mental illness. Generalized seizures may cause the child to lose consciousness and convulse. The child with absence seizures may stare as if daydreaming.

Staff should be familiar with the medication regime prescribed, including any side effects, as well as the child's response to the medication. Medication management is based on choosing the drug with the fewest adverse effects that will effectively control the seizures. Familiarity with specific medications and their adverse effects is essential. Balancing these two objectives may be difficult; thus it is imperative that the child be monitored closely for changes in seizure frequency as well as for any adverse effects. Children may become drowsy at certain times of the day, requiring attention to scheduled activities and expectations, particularly within a school setting. In general, children whose seizures are well controlled may be able to participate in most extracurricular activities. Although some children may be restricted from activities that pose a risk for falling (e.g., climbing), the emotional and physical benefits of the child participating in sports and exercise should not be ignored. Identifying precipitating events that may trigger a seizure in a particular child can assist staff members to provide a safe environment. Suitable types of activity for the individual child should be built into his or her routine.

ADHD

Attention deficit hyperactivity disorder (ADHD) is thought to be a result of decreased activity of the neurotransmitters that stimulate the parts of the brain responsible for concentration and attention. Attention deficit hyperactivity disorder is subdivided into two categories. The first is primarily characterized by impulsivity and hyperactivity with subsequent inattention. The second type is characterized primarily by inattentiveness. A multimodal approach to the treatment of children with both types of ADHD has been shown to have the most success in increasing positive behavioral changes, improving self-esteem, and facilitating academic progress. This often includes the use of specific behavioral strategies, environmental changes to facilitate child's attention, and the use of stimulant medication (including most commonly methylphenidate (Ritalin), dextroamphetamine (Dexedrine), and pemoline (Cylert). They are referred to as stimulants because they stimulate the parts of the brain that control concentration and attention. In addition they can decrease the impulsive behavior characteristic of children with hyperactive impulsive ADHD. Ritalin and Dexedrine are the most commonly used stimulants; they are available in both regular and sustained-release preparations. Regular preparations are typically given bid in the morning and at lunch time, with each dose lasting approximately 4 hours. Sustained-release preparations are typically given qd in the morning and last throughout the school day. Metabolism varies in individual children, and alternative timing or additional doses may be indicated. The child on bid regular Ritalin who routinely has increased difficulty focusing or staying seated in the classroom an hour before the next scheduled dose may need his or her midday dose of medication earlier. Alternatively, the child who does well on a sustained-release preparation until the last period of the day or the bus trip home may benefit from an additional dose of regular Ritalin in the early afternoon. Some children experience rebound irritability with increased inattentiveness and impulsive behavior as the medication wears off. This frequently is seen after school, when the child returns home or to an after-school program, but it also may be seen in school or on the bus trip home. Again, a small dose of additional medication may be indicated.

School nurses may frequently be asked to assist in monitoring side effects as well as the effectiveness of medication. Common side effects of stimulant medications seen during the school day include headache, stomachache, tics, and appetite suppression. Appetite should be monitored at lunch time in children receiving bid doses of Ritalin or Dexedrine who have lunch after receiving their midday medication. In addition, complaints of headache and stomachache should be evaluated to determine if they are indeed medication-induced side effects or are infact the result of appetite suppression and the lack of eating. Complaints of headache and stomachache that occur in early afternoon may frequently be caused by the child's skipping or eating little at lunch time. Arranging to increase planned snacks during the day may be necessary to facilitate ongoing growth and diminish poor appetite-induced headache or stomachache. Monitoring for medication response also includes assessing the impact of integration of non-medication strategies into the child's school activities, including classroom, gym, and other planned activities. Acute or chronic stress in either the home or school setting may increase inattentiveness and negative behavior in the child. Evaluating non-medication strategies and identifying the non-ADHD causes of increased inattentiveness and problem behavior is essential in making decisions related to the child's medication dosage and the timing of administration.

CHILDREN RECEIVING MEDICATIONS TO IMPROVE RESPIRATORY FUNCTION

Children with respiratory difficulties (e.g., upper and lower respiratory tract infections, otitis, bronchopulmonary dysplasia, and asthma) are the most common group receiving medications. Nurses must have good assessment skills and be able to recognize the signs and symptoms of increasing respiratory difficulty and impending respiratory failure. They should always keep in mind that oxygen, when available, may be the most important respiratory "medication" for a child in acute respiratory difficulty.

The group of children most commonly receiving medication to

improve respiratory function are those with asthma. Approximately 5% of children in the United States suffer from chronic asthma. Asthma (or reactive airway disease) is characterized by smooth muscle contraction in the airway, tracheobronchial mucosa edema, and excessive secretion of submucosal glands; combined, these result in a narrowing of the airway and varying degree of respiratory difficulty. Asthma management is based on avoidance of known triggers, such as exercise, allergy, or infection, that might precipitate an asthma attack combined with the use of medications to prevent attacks and reduce airway hypersensitivity. Medication therapy is aimed at decreasing both airway inflammation and bronchoconstriction. Thus children with asthma are often treated with a combination of bronchodilators, smooth muscle relaxants, and antiinflammatory agents.

Bronchopulmonary dysplasia (BPD) is an iatrogenic chronic lung disease that may develop in premature infants following respiratory therapy. Contributing factors can include mechanical ventilation, oxygen therapy, meconium aspiration, and pulmonary edema from a persistent ductus arteriosus. Reported incidence varies based on the criteria used and the severity of the disease. Overall, the incidence is rising as technological advances increase the survival rate of premature infants. As these children enter the toddler and preschool-age years, it is not unusual for them to develop reactive airway disease requiring management with medication.

Treatment of reactive airway disease includes the use of β-adrenergic agents such as albuterol or terbutaline, which are often prescribed in an aerosolized preparation that is effective in relaxing smooth muscle with fewer significant systemic side effects than oral preparations. Oral preparations such as theophylline work as bronchodilators, and they are available in sustained-release and liquid preparations. Children receiving oral preparations must be monitored closely for systemic side effects and toxicity; periodic blood samples are obtained to determine serum concentrations. Medications used to decrease inflammation, enhance bronchodilation, and decrease edema include glucocorticosteroids in both oral and aerosolized preparations. Steroids are used to prevent inflammation and during acute exacerbation to reduce inflammation. The use of aerosolized preparations can decrease systemic effects and is particularly effective for preventive maintenance. However, during an acute exacerbation, systemic oral steroid preparations may be indicated to maximize effects. Non-steroidal antiinflammatory agents such as cromolyn sodium are used exclusively as a preventive measure and are *not* effective in opening the airway during an asthma attack. The use of medications to treat children with asthma is individualized based on the severity of disease, known triggers, and the frequency of exacerbation. Some children require daily steroid and β-adrenergic preparations, whereas others require use of medications episodically with seasonal triggers, respiratory infections, or exercise.

Nurses caring for children with reactive airway disease should be aware of the child's history, including specific triggers (if known), typical treatment, and expected response to medications. Giving aerosolized medications with either a nebulizer or a metered dose inhaler (MDI) may cause coughing; thus routine medications should be given before lunch. Children using aerosolized steroid preparations should be taught to rinse their mouth and throat after use to decrease irritation to the pharynx and airways. Children on bronchodilators requiring postural drainage and cupping (PD&C) should receive medication first to facilitate drainage. Inhaled steroids are typically given after PD&C. Deaths have occurred from asthma related to the improper use of medication. The overuse of medication, including the use of over-the-counter preparations, can be fatal. Staff members must understand the correct use of medications, be familiar with the pathophysiology of the course of an acute exacerbation, recognize impending respiratory distress and failure, and comprehend the institution of emergency measures should they become necessary. It is not infrequent for a child who has initially improved with treatment to develop significant respiratory difficulty hours later.

DEVICES AND INSTRUCTIONS FOR USE

Respiratory Devices

There are a number of devices used to facilitate delivery or monitoring of inhaled medications. The correct use of these devices is essential to ensuring effective medication delivery.

Inhalers. Metered dose inhalers consist of a metal canister containing medication that fits into a plastic holding device with a mouthpiece. MDIs provide a premeasured amount of aerosolized medication with each depression or "puff" of the canister. It is important that the canister be shaken thoroughly to mix the medication with the propellant. It is also important to check periodically that the canister contains medication and not just propellant. Simply shaking the canister does not give accurate information regarding the amount of medication left in the canister. To check to see that medication remains in the canister, remove the metal canister from the plastic holding device. Place the canister in a bowl of water. If the canister remains vertical, it still contains medication; if the canister floats horizontally or is nearly horizontal (like a dead fish), it is empty or nearly empty. Any time that a child does not respond to medication as anticipated, a caregiver must check to ensure that medication is present in the canister. This may be important, particularly in a school setting with medication used on a prn basis.

Spacers. MDIs used improperly leave medication in the oral–pharyngeal area or in the air outside the child's mouth. A spacer or a holding device can be used to increase the delivery of medication into the lower airway. A spacer is a cylinder chamber that attaches to the MDI. The spacer holds medication long enough for the child to draw it out by taking long, slow breaths. There are a variety of spacer devices that can be used. General instructions include placing the MDI on the spacer, shaking the MDI, pressing the MDI to release medication into the holding chamber (one puff), placing the mouthpiece of the spacer in the child's mouth with the lips tightly sealed (masks are available for younger child), having the child inhale slowly, holding the breath for a few seconds, and exhaling. Repeat breathing cycles and administer additional puffs of medication per prescriber's instructions. General instructions include waiting between additional puffs of medication. The amount of time may vary depending on the type of medication and the level of respiratory distress the child may be experiencing.

Nebulizers. A nebulizer is an electrically powered device that vibrates using a transducer, producing small particles that the child inhales through a tent or face mask. Medication is inhaled along with an aerosolized mist that can loosen secretions and facilitate medication delivery. Children with very thick secretions (such as those seen with cystic fibrosis or the acute exacerbations of reactive airway disease) may benefit from the use of this form of medication delivery system.

Pulmonary Flow Meters. Pulmonary flow meters measure peak expiratory flow rates. They can provide an objective way to measure the severity of an individual child's respiratory difficulty, to detect airway obstruction before wheezing and other symptoms occur, and to evaluate the effectiveness of the treatment. The effectiveness of pulmonary flow meters relies on correct technique when using the meter and appropriate interpretation of readings. A log should be kept to record an individual child's peak expiratory flow rates over time so that the child's personal-best values can be determined. Once individual values have been determined, the meter can then be used to monitor for early changes in respiratory status and changes in response to medication administration.

Central Venous Access Devices—Central Venous Catheters

A central venous catheter (CVC) is a long-term IV catheter that is surgically inserted into a deep large vein in the chest or neck, usually close to the heart. The access site or port of the CVC may be visible through an exit site, usually on the chest, or may be implanted and covered by skin. A CVC is placed to provide long-term access to the bloodstream for medications, total parenteral nutrition, fluids, chemotherapy, or blood transfusions. Nurses must be aware of the child's underlying or potential problems and associated complications. Potential problems related to the catheter include blood in the tubing, tubing that breaks or cracks, chest pain or difficulty breathing related to air that has entered the catheter, a catheter that becomes dislodged or falls out, and signs and symptoms of infection (e.g., fever, redness at the CVC site, fatigue, or irritability). Dressing changes needed for a CVC with an exit port require meticulous technique. Several different types of catheters are available, and nurses must be aware of the nature of care required based on the type of catheter present. Although many routine activities may not be restricted, the nurse must be aware of activities or physical education restrictions that are present and ensure that the child and those working with the child adhere to them.

Gastrointestinal Tubes

A gastrostomy tube is a flexible rubber catheter inserted through a surgical opening into the stomach through the abdominal surface. A balloon or a widened "mushroom" at the tip of the tube holds the tube in place in the stomach. Liquid or pureed food, medication, and fluids can be given through the tube directly into the stomach. The tube remains in place at all times and can be clamped between uses to prevent stomach contents from leaking out. Some children requiring access for gastrostomy feedings or medications have had a gastrostomy button inserted. This allows the actual catheter, which provides access for food or medications, to be removed between use (Huddleston, 1990).

Nurses caring for children with a gastrostomy tube used for feeding should be aware of the type of feeding the child receives (continuous or bolus), the method of feeding (gravity or continuous pump), the activity restrictions or positioning needs during or after feedings, the need for venting of the tube, the need to check for residuals, and typical problems that may be encountered by the child. Vomiting, abdominal distention, or cramping may occur related to the rate and temperature of feeding. A tube may be blocked due to inadequate flushing or the infusion of thick fluid. If the tube becomes dislodged or falls out, arrangements to have the tube replaced may need to be made quickly since the gastrostomy tract in some children can close within 1 to 2 hours.

Liquid medications may be given directly through the tube. It is important to flush the tube after giving medication to ensure that all of the medication reaches the stomach and to prevent medication from sticking to the tube, leading to clogging. Some medications may be crushed and mixed with liquid and given through the tube. It is important to be aware of medications in which crushing or mixing with certain types of liquids may alter the effectiveness of or increase the toxicity of the medication; for example, sustained-release preparations should not be crushed or removed from their gelatin capsules for administration through the tube. Recommendations in giving medications related to the timing of meals should be followed with all medication given through the GI tract. The nurse should be alert to medication orders that require contact with the mouth and upper GI tract for effectiveness (e.g., oral antifungal medications).

Infusion Pumps

A variety of medications (including insulin, chemotherapy, total parenteral nutrition [TPN] and liquid feedings) may be infused through an infusion pump. Although infusion pumps can vary, they basically allow for a controlled infusion at a preset rate and volume. It is important that infusion pumps are accurately set to deliver the correct fluid or medication at the correct volume or dosage within the predetermined time frame. Nurses must be aware of and use built-in safety mechanisms that are part of many infusion pumps. These are designed to decrease or prevent accidental or intentional tinkering with the device by an inquisitive child.

SUMMARY

Nurses working with children in a variety of settings are responsible for the coordination of medication regimes. Knowledge of the child's underlying medical condition, the rationale for medication administration, familiarity with the prescribed medication (including the impact of medication on the child's daily routine), and restrictions related to the underlying medical condition or medication itself are essential. The nurse must be aware of the need for normalizing the child's day with medication planning and must communicate and educate all personnel in contact with the child to ensure a safe, effective, and child-centered approach to medication management.

REFERENCES

Baer CL, Williams BR (editors): The pediatric patient. In *Clinical pharmacology and nursing,* ed 2, Springhouse, Penn., 1992, Springhouse Corp.

Barry K, Teixeira S: The role of the nurse in the diagnostic classification and management of epileptic seizures, *Neurosurg Nurs* 15(4):243, 1983.

Basel Pharmaceuticals: *Starting school: a guide for parents of children with epilepsy,* Summit, N.J., 1992, CIBA-Geigy Corporation.

Betz CL, Hunsberger MM, Wright S: *Family-centered nursing care of children,* ed 2, Philadelphia, 1994, WB Saunders.

Crowley A: Health services in child day care center: a survey, *Pediatr Hlth Care* 4(5):252, 1990.

Faro B: Students with diabetes: implications of the diabetes control and complications trial for the school setting, *School Nurs* 11(1):16, 1995.

Ferry PC, Banner W, Wolf RA: *Seizure disorders in children,* Philadelphia, 1986, J.B. Lippincott.

Finston P: Parent and teacher equal healthy child: bring your child's teacher aboard the diabetes team, *Diabetes Forecast* 47(9):27, 1994.

Gates JR, Spiegel R: Epilepsy, sports and exercise, *Sports Med,* 15(1):1, 1993.

Haynie M, Porter S, Palfrey J: *Children assisted by medical technology in educational settings: guidelines for care,* Boston, 1989, The Children's Hospital, Project School Care.

Huddleston KC, Palmer KL: A button for gastrostomy feedings, *Am J Maternal Child Nurs* 15(5):315, 1990.

Jornsay D, Carney T: Diabetes care in school: guidelines for health-care providers who care for school-aged children, *Diabetes Spectrum* 5(5):260, 1992.

Marshall RM, Cupoli JM: Epilepsy and education: the pediatrician's expanding role, *Adv Pediatr* 3:159, 1986.

McCarren M: Diabetes Control and Complications Trial (DCCT): intensive therapy: it works, *Diabetes Forecast* (Special report), 49(9):1, 1993.

Miller D, Miller H: Giving meds through tube, *RN* 8(1):44, 1995.

Rostain AL: Attention deficit disorder in children and adolescents, *Pediatr Clin North Am* 38(3):607, 1991.

Savage T, Culbert C: Early intervention: the unique role of nursing, *J Pediatr Nurs* 4(5):339, 1989.

Schmitt BD: The child with a short attention span (ADD), *Contemporary Pediatr* January, 10(1):57, 1993.

Schwab N, Haas M: Delegation and supervision in school settings: standards, issues, and guidelines for practice (Part 1), *J School Nurs* 11(1):26, 1995.

Sheffer AL, Chairman Expert Panel on the Management of Asthma: Executive summary: guidelines for the management of asthma, Bethesda, Md., U.S. Department of Health and Human Services, 1991, Publication No 91-3042A.

Smitherman CH: A drug to ease attention deficit disorder, *Am J Matern Child Nurs* 15(6):362, 1990.

Snyder A, Clarke W: The diabetes control and complications trial: new challenges for the school nurse, *J School Nurs* 11(1):22, 1995.

Travis LB: *An instructional aid on insulin dependent diabetes mellitus,* ed 10, Austin, Tex., 1995, Designer's Ink.

Voeller K: Clinical management of attention deficit hyperactivity disorder, *Child Neurol* 6(Supplement):S51-S67, 1991.

Walker O and others: Mainstreaming children with handicaps: implications for pediatricians, *J Dev Behav Pediatr,* 10:151, 1989.

acetaminophen

Brand Name(s): Abenol🍁, Acephen, Aceta, Anacin-3, Apacet, Banesin, Dapa, Datril, Genapap, Halenol, Myapap Drops, Neopap, Panadol🍁, Tempra🍁, Tylenol🍁

Classification: Analgesic (non-narcotic), antipyretic

Pregnancy Category: B

AVAILABLE PREPARATIONS
Drops: 48 mg/ml, 100 mg/ml
Elixir: 120 mg/ml, 160 mg/ml, 167 mg/ml, 325 mg/ml
Liquid: 160 mg/5 ml
Oral susp: 100 mg/ml, 160 mg/ml
Tabs (chewable): 80 mg, 160 mg
Tabs: 325 mg, 500 mg, 650 mg
Caplet: 160 mg, 325 mg, 500 mg
Rectal suppos: 120 mg, 125 mg, 325 mg, 650 mg

ROUTES AND DOSAGES
Children: PO/rectal 10-15 mg/kg/dose q4-6h prn (max. 5 doses/24 hr)
or
0-3 mo, 40 mg; 4-11 mo, 80 mg; 1-2 yr, 120 mg; 2-3 yr, 160 mg; 4-5 yr, 240 mg; 6-8 yr, 320 mg; 9-10 yr, 400 mg; 11 yr, 480 mg
Adults: 325-650 mg q4-6h prn or 1000 mg tid-qid (max. 4 g/24 hr)

MECHANISM AND INDICATIONS
Mechanism: Inhibits synthesis of prostaglandins (believed to serve as mediators of pain, fever); acts on hypothalamus to cause antipyresis and on CNS to provide analgesia
Indications: Used in treatment of mild-to-moderate pain, fever

PHARMACOKINETICS
Onset of action: PO: 30-45 min
Peak: PO: 60-120 min
Duration: 4-6 hr
Metabolism: Liver
Excretion: Urine

CONTRAINDICATIONS AND PRECAUTIONS
• Contraindicated with known hypersensitivity to acetaminophen, sulfites; preparations containing aspartame contraindicated in pts with phenylketonuria
• Use cautiously with hepatic or renal dysfunction, history of GI disease or bleeding, anemia, pregnancy, lactation

INTERACTIONS
Drug
• Severe hypothermia possible when used with phenothiazine antipsychotics
• Additive risk of hepatotoxicity when administered with other hepatotoxic substances (including alcohol)
• Increased risk of hepatotoxicity possible in overdose with concurrent use of phenobarbital
• Decreased absorption with cholestyramine and colestipol
• Increased anticoagulant effect with coumarins occurs with chronic acetaminophen use
Lab
• False positive for 5-hydroxyindoleacetic acid
• False decrease in BG
• False increase in urine glucose, serum uric acid
• Interferes with bentiromide test for pancreatic function
Nutrition
• Decreased absorption with high carbohydrate meal

SIDE EFFECTS
CNS: Mental changes, stupor, confusion, agitation with toxic doses, weakness
DERM: Rash, urticaria, pruritus, bruising, erythema
EENT: Sore throat
GI: Nausea, vomiting, diarrhea, abdominal pain, anorexia, severe liver damage with toxic doses
GU: Hematuria, renal dysfunction with chronic use
HEME: Bleeding, bruising, hemolytic anemia, neutropenia, leukopenia, pancytopenia, thrombocytopenia, methemoglobinemia

Other: Anaphylaxis, hypoglyce-mia, jaundice, unexplained fever

TOXICITY AND OVERDOSE

Clinical signs: Cyanosis, anemia, jaundice, rash, fever, vomiting, CNS stimulation, delirium, met-hemoglobinemia, coma, vascular collapse, seizures, death; stage 1 (12-24 hr post-ingestion), nausea, vomiting, diaphoresis, anorexia; stage 2 (24-48 hr post-ingestion), clinically improved, elevated liver function tests; stage 3 (72-96 hr post-ingestion), peak hepatotoxic-ity; stage 4 (7-8 days post-inges-tion), recovery

Treatment: Empty stomach by in-duced vomiting or gastric lavage; administer activated charcoal via NG tube; acetylcysteine most ef-fective within 10-12 hr after in-gestion; can be administered within 24 hr after ingestion; re-move charcoal before administer-ing acetylcysteine; hemodialysis; supportive care

PATIENT CARE MANAGEMENT

Assessment

• Assess history of hypersensitiv-ity to acetaminophen, sulfites
• Assess pain (type, location, se-verity), fever, VS
• Assess renal function (BUN, cre-atinine), hepatic function (ALT, AST, bilirubin), especially with long-term use

Interventions

• Tablets may be crushed, mixed with food or fluid
• Administer with food or milk to decrease GI irritation; do not ad-minister with high carbohydrate meal, which can decrease absorp-tion
• Determine dosing interval based on patient response; administer when pain is not too severe to en-hance effectiveness

NURSING ALERT

Accidental ingestion or over-dose occur frequently

Overdose can result in hepato-toxicity

Evaluation

• Evaluate therapeutic response (decrease pain, fever)
• Evaluate VS, renal function (BUN, CrCl, I&O), hepatic func-tion (ALT, AST, bilirubin) for long-term use

PATIENT AND FAMILY EDUCATION

Teach/instruct

• To take as directed at prescribed intervals for prescribed length of time
• Best time to take medication if ordered prn

Advise/warn

• To notify care provider of hyper-sensitivity, side effects
• To limit infants and children to 5 doses/24 hr
• To notify care provider if fever is over >39.5° C (103.1° F), if fever or illness persists >3 days, if fever is recurrent, or if no relief is obtained
• To avoid OTC medications un-less prescribed by health care pro-vider
• To keep out of reach of children; acetaminophen is frequently in-gested accidentally
• To avoid alcohol if on chronic or high-dosage therapy

STORAGE

• Store rectal suppository form in refrigerator
• Store all other forms at room temp

---

acetaminophen (with codeine)

Brand Name(s): Acet Co-deine♣, Empracet-30♣, Empracet-60♣, PMS-Acetaminophen with Codeine♣, Tylenol #1, Tylenol #2, Tylenol #3, Tylenol #4

Classification: Narcotic analgesic, opiate agonist, antipyretic

Controlled Substance Schedule III

Pregnancy Category: C

♣ Available in Canada.

AVAILABLE PREPARATIONS

Elixir: Acetaminophen 120 mg, codeine 12 mg/5 ml
Caps: Acetaminophen 325 mg, codeine 15 mg; acetaminophen 325 mg, codeine 30 mg; acetaminophen 325 mg, codeine 60 mg
Tabs: Tylenol #1, acetaminophen 300 mg, codeine 7.5 mg; Tylenol #2, acetaminophen 300 mg, codeine 15 mg; Tylenol #3, acetaminophen 300 mg, codeine 30 mg; Tylenol #4, acetaminophen 300 mg, codeine 60 mg

ROUTES AND DOSAGES

Analgesia: Dose is based on the codeine component
Children and adults: PO: acetaminophen 10-15 mg/kg/dose; codeine 0.5-1 mg/kg/dose q4-6h prn

MECHANISM AND INDICATIONS

Acetaminophen: Inhibits synthesis of prostaglandins (believed to serve as mediators of pain and fever); acts on hypothalamus to cause antipyresis and on CNS to provide analgesia
Codeine: Acts on CNS using neurotransmitters to create analgesia; binds to opiate receptors in CNS; alters perception of, response to painful stimuli
Indications: Used to treat mild to moderate pain with accompanying treatment of fever

PHARMACOKINETICS

Onset of action: PO: 30-45 min
Peak: PO: 60-120 min
Duration: 4-6 hr
Half-life: 1-4 hr
Metabolism: Liver
Excretion: Urine

CONTRAINDICATIONS AND PRECAUTIONS

• Contraindicated with known hypersensitivities, pregnancy, and lactation; do not give preparations with sulfite to those with sulfite allergy
• Use cautiously with the following: head trauma; increased ICP; severe renal, hepatic, pulmonary disease; hypothyroidism; adrenal insufficiency; alcoholism; undiagnosed abdominal pain; respiratory depression, altered mental status, anemia

INTERACTIONS

Drug

Acetaminophen
• Severe hypothermia possible when used with phenothiazine antipsychotics
• Additive risk of hepatotoxicity when administered with other hepatotoxic substances (including alcohol)
• Increased liver toxicity in overdose possible with concurrent use of phenobarbital
• Increased anticoagulant effect with coumarins occurs with chronic acetaminophen use
• Decreased absorption, effectiveness with cholestyramine and colestipol
Codeine
• Additive CNS effects with alcohol, antihistamines, sedative/hypnotics
• Increased metabolism (may decrease analgesic effectiveness when smoking)
• Precipitates narcotic withdrawal when administered with partial antagonist (e.g., buprenorphine, butorphanol, nalbuphine, pentazocine)
• Antagonized action possible with phenothiazines
• Increased effects with dextroamphetamine
• Increased effects of neuromuscular blocking agents possible
• Decreased effects of diuretics in CHF possible

Lab

Acetaminophen
• False positive for 5-hydroxyindoleacetic acid
• False decrease in BG
• False increase in urine glucose, serum uric acid
• Interferes with bentiromide test for pancreatic function
Codeine
• Increased serum amylase, lipase; decrease blood drawing time for these tests until 24 hours after administration of drug

---

✤ Available in Canada.

• Decreased serum and urine 17-KS, 17-OHCS

Nutrition

Acetaminophen

• Decreased absorption with high carbohydrate meal

SIDE EFFECTS

CNS: Sedation, confusion, behavior changes, dizziness, depression, coma, euphoria, restlessness, insomnia, floating feeling, unusual dreams, hallucinations, dysphoria, agitation, lethargy

CV: Circulatory depression, orthostatic hypotension, palpitation, bradycardia, tachycardia

DERM: Rash, erythema, urticaria, pruritus, facial flushing (indicating hypersensitivity reaction), sweating

EENT: Miosis, diplopia, blurred vision

GI: Nausea, vomiting, diarrhea, constipation, anorexia, biliary spasm, increased serum amylase/lipase, hepatic necrosis (with acetaminophen overdose)

GU: Urinary retention, oliguria, impotence, hematuria, renal damage and dysfunction in those with renal disease

HEME: Bleeding, ecchymosis, anemia, thrombocytopenia, leukopenia, pancytopenia (all are more common with long term use of acetaminophen)

RESP: Respiratory depression, respiratory paralysis

Other: Tolerance, physical or psychological dependence

TOXICITY AND OVERDOSE

Clinical signs: Acetaminophen: symptoms of hepatotoxicity; *codeine:* respiratory/circulatory depression

Treatment: Acetaminophen: acetylcysteine; *codeine:* naloxone

PATIENT CARE MANAGEMENT

Assessment

• Assess history of hypersensitivity to acetaminophen, codeine, related drugs

• Assess pain (type, location, severity)

• Assess baseline VS, I&O

Interventions

• Administer with food or milk to decrease GI irritation

• Determine dosing interval based on pt response

• Administer when pain is not too severe to enhance its effectiveness

• Institute safety measures (e.g., supervise ambulation, raise side rails, ensure call light is within reach)

> **NURSING ALERT**
> Physical dependency may result if used for extended periods of time

Evaluation

• Evaluate therapeutic response (decrease pain without significant alteration in LOC, respiratory status)

• Evaluate VS, hepatic and renal functioning with long-term use

• Evaluate side effects, hypersensitivity

PATIENT AND FAMILY EDUCATION

Teach/instruct

• To take as directed at prescribed intervals for prescribed length of time

• To take with food or milk to decrease GI irritation as needed

• Best time to take medication if ordered prn

Warn/advise

• To notify care provider of hypersensitivity, side effects

• To make position changes slowly and seek assistance with ambulation until effects of medication are known; may cause drowsiness, dizziness, orthostatic hypertension

• To avoid hazardous activities

• To avoid alcohol, other CNS depressants (unless prescribed), smoking

STORAGE

• Store at room temp, protect from light

✚ Available in Canada.

acetazolamide

Brand Name(s): Diamox✸, Acetazolamide, Apo-Acetazolamide✸, Cetazol, Dazamide

Classification: Diuretic, antiglaucoma agent, anticonvulsant

Pregnancy Category: C

AVAILABLE PREPARATIONS
Tabs: 125, 250 mg
Caps: Sus rel 500 mg
Inj: 500 mg/vial

ROUTES AND DOSAGES
Edema
Children: PO, IM, or IV 5 mg/kg qd in AM
Adults: PO, IM, or IV 250-375 mg qd in AM
Seizures
Children: PO, IM, or IV 8-30 mg/kg tid-qid; maximum daily dose 1.5 g
Adults: PO, IM, or IV 375 mg qd; up to 250 mg qid
Glaucoma
Children: PO 8-30 mg/kg/24 hr divided q6-8h; IM/IV 20-40 mg/kg/24 hr divided q6h
Adults: PO 1000 mg/24 hr divided q6h
IV administration
• Maximum concentration: Dilute 500 mg in at least 5 ml SW
• IV push rate: 100-500 mg/min
• Intermittent infusion rate: over 4-8 hr

MECHANISM AND INDICATIONS
Diuretic: Inhibits carbonic anhydrase production, promoting excretion of bicarbonate, Na, K, H_2O from kidneys
Anticonvulsant: Decreases carbonic anhydrase levels in CNS, increasing seizure threshold
Antiglaucoma: Decreases formation of aqueous humor, decreasing intraocular pressure
Indications: For use in treatment of glaucoma, seizures, edema

PHARMACOKINETICS
Onset of action: PO: 1-1½ hr; IV: 2 min
Peak: PO: 2-4 hr; IV: 15 min
Half-life: 4-10 hr
Metabolism: Liver
Excretion: Urine

CONTRAINDICATIONS AND PRECAUTIONS
• Contraindicated with hypersensitivity to sulfonamides, hepatic insufficiency, severe renal disease, electrolyte imbalances (e.g., hyponatremia, hypokalemia, hyperchloremia)
• Use cautiously with respiratory acidosis, diabetes, cardiac glycosides, other diuretics, pregnancy, lactation

INTERACTIONS
Drug
• Increased action of amphetamines, procainamide, quinidine, flecainide
• Decreased action of salicylates, phenobarbital, lithium
Lab
• False positive for proteinuria, 17-OHCS

SIDE EFFECTS
CNS: Drowsiness, confusion, decreased alertness in children, dizziness
DERM: Rash, photosensitivity, Stevens-Johnson syndrome
EENT: Myopia (transient), tinnitus
ENDO: Hyperglycemia
GI: Nausea, vomiting, anorexia, transient diarrhea, poor oral feeding
GU: Crystalluria, hematuria, renal calculi, glucosuria
HEME: Aplastic anemia, hemolytic anemia, leukopenia, agranulocytosis
Local: Pain at injection site

TOXICITY AND OVERDOSE
Clinical signs: Paresthesias, hypokalemia, hyperchloremia, acidosis
Treatment: Induce emesis, gastric lavage, correct fluid/electrolyte imbalances

✸ Available in Canada.

PATIENT CARE MANAGEMENT

Assessment
- Assess history of hypersensitivity
- Assess wt daily
- Assess I&O daily
- Assess baseline electrolytes, liver and renal studies, CBC and differential
- Assess B/P lying and standing

Interventions
- Administer IV or PO when possible (IM painful)
- Administer K+ replacement if K+ <3.0
- Administer with food to minimize GI distress

Evaluation
- Evaluate therapeutic response (decrease seizure activity, edema; decrease intraocular pressure)
- Monitor electrolytes (Na, K+), CBC and differential, liver function (AST, ALT, bilirubin), renal function (BUN, creatinine, I&O)
- Monitor for edema
- Monitor for signs of hypokalemia, especially if taking digoxin
- Monitor for signs of toxicity

PATIENT AND FAMILY EDUCATION

Teach/instruct
- To take as directed at prescribed intervals, for prescribed length of time
- About rationale for diuretic therapy
- About side effects—call care provider

Warn/advise
- To supervise activities of children closely to prevent falls or injuries secondary to drowsiness, dizziness
- To eat foods rich in K+
- To report increased edema, wt gain
- About importance of regular follow-up care while taking drug

STORAGE
- Store in dark, cool area; use reconstituted sol within 24 hr

---

acetylcysteine

Brand Name(s): Mucomyst✿, Mucosol, Parvolex✿

Classification: Mucolytic agent, antidote for acetaminophen overdose

Pregnancy category: B

AVAILABLE PREPARATIONS

Sol: 10% (100 mg/ml); 20% (200 mg/ml)

ROUTES AND DOSAGES

Acetaminophen Poisoning

Children and adults: PO 140 mg/kg loading dose, then 70 mg/kg q4h for 17 doses (best to mix at 1:4 ratio with carbonated beverage)

Mucolytic

Infants: INH 1-2 ml 20% sol or 2-4 ml 10% sol via nebulizer tid-qid

Children: INH 3-5 ml 20% sol or 6-10 ml 10% sol via nebulizer tid-qid

Adolescents: INH 5-10 ml 10%-20% sol via nebulizer tid-qid

Meconium Ileus

Infants: PO, PR 5-30 ml 10% sol 3-6 times/24 hr; usual dose 10 ml qid

MECHANISM AND INDICATIONS

Mechanism: Decreases viscosity of secretions by breaking disulfide links of mucoproteins; may act by increasing hepatic glutathione, which inactivates toxic metabolites in acetaminophen overdose

Indications: For use as an adjunctive therapy in patients with abnormal or thick mucous secretions accompanying acute or chronic pulmonary disease, (e.g., cystic fibrosis, pneumonia, emphysema, tuberculosis); decreases viscosity of stool in meconium ileus; used as an antidote for acute acetaminophen toxicity

PHARMACOKINETICS

Onset of action: 5-10 min

Duration: Approximately 1 hr

Half-life: Reduced acetylcysteine 2 hr; total acetylcysteine 5.5 hr

---

✿ Available in Canada.

Metabolism: Liver
Excretion: Urine

CONTRAINDICATIONS AND PRECAUTIONS
• Contraindicated with known hypersensitivity, increased ICP, status asthmaticus
• Use cautiously with reactive airway disease (bronchospasm), hypothyroidism, Addison's disease, CNS depression, brain tumor, hepatic or renal disease, psychosis, alcoholism, seizure disorder

INTERACTIONS
• Decreased absorption with activated charcoal (prevents absorption of acetylcysteine)

INCOMPATIBILITIES
• Tetracyclines, erythromycin, amphotericin-B, sodium ampicillin, iodized oil, chymotrypsin, trypsin, hydrogen peroxide

SIDE EFFECTS
CNS: Dizziness, drowsiness, HA, fever, chills
DERM: Urticaria, rash, fever
EENT: Rhinorrhea
GI: Nausea, vomiting, stomatitis, anorexia, constipation
RESP: Bronchospasm

TOXICITY AND OVERDOSE
• No information available

PATIENT CARE MANAGEMENT
Assessment
• Assess history of hypersensitivity to drug
• Assess VS, cardiac rhythm, ABGs
• Assess breath sounds before and after treatment
• Assess acetaminophen levels as soon as possible after ingestion
• Assess liver function tests
• Assess for nausea, vomiting, rash
Interventions
• Have patient cough or use aerosolized bronchodilator before treatment

• Administer 1-1½ hr before meals for better absorption, to decrease vomiting/nausea
• Have suction equipment standing by
• As acetaminophen antidote, administer within 24 hr of acetaminophen ingestion with carbonated beverage or juice; dilute 1:4 to mask taste
• Provide assistance with nebulization as necessary
• May be administered in croup tent; use up to 300 ml of 10% or 20% sol to maintain heavy mist; can be constant or intermittent treatment
Evaluation
• Evaluate therapeutic response (decreased viscosity of secretions)
• Evaluate cough for frequency, type, characteristics of secretions
• Evaluate breath sounds, respiratory rate; discontinue drug if bronchospasm occurs
• For antidotal use, evaluate liver function tests, decreases in hepatic encephalopathy
• Evaluate ABGs for CO_2 retention

PATIENT AND FAMILY EDUCATION
Teach/instruct
• To take as directed at prescribed intervals for prescribed length of time
• To avoid alcohol, other CNS depressants; will increase sedating properties of drug
• That drug has foul odor (sulfurous egg odor)
• About side effects
• To rinse mouth after nebulizer treatment
• That discoloration of sol after bottle is opened does not affect drug effectiveness

STORAGE
• Store at room temp
• Refrigerate after opening

acyclovir

Brand Name(s): Avirax✤, Zovirax, Zorivax Cream✤, Zorivax Ointment✤, Zorivax Oral✤

Classification: Antiviral (synthetic purine nucleoside)

Pregnancy Category: C

AVAILABLE PREPARATIONS
Oral susp: 200 mg/5 ml
Tabs: 800 mg
Caps: 200 mg
Inj: 50 mg/ml
Top oint: 5%

ROUTES AND DOSAGES
Herpes Zoster in Immuno-compromised Patients
Children: PO 250-600 mg/m^2/dose 4-5 times/24 hr; IV 7.5 mg/kg/dose q8h for 7-14 days
Adults: PO 800 mg q4h (5 times/24 hr) for 7-10 days; prophylaxis 400 mg (5 times/24 hr); IV 7.5 mg/kg/dose q8h for 7-14 days
Varicella Zoster in Immuno-compromised Patient
Adults and children: PO 20 mg/kg/dose qid; maximum 800 mg/dose for 5 days; begin treatment at earliest sign or symptom; IV 1500 mg/m^2/24 hr divided q8h or 30 mg/kg/24 hr divided q8h for 7 days
Genital Herpes Infection
Adults: PO 200 mg q4h while awake (5 times/24 hr); treat for 7-10 days for first infection, 5 days for recurrence; prophylaxis 200 mg tid-qid or 400 mg bid (maximum duration 12 mo)
HSV Infection
Neonates: IV 1500 mg/m^2/24 hr divided q8h or 30 mg/kg/24 hr divided q8h for 10-14 days
Mucocutaneous HSV Infection
Children and adults: IV 750 mg/m^2/24 hr divided q8h or 15 mg/kg/24 hr divided q8h for 5-7 days
HSV Encephalitis
Children and adults: IV 1500 mg/m^2/24 hr divided q8h or 30 mg/kg/24 hr divided q8h for 14-21 days

Prophylaxis of Bone Marrow Transplant Patients, HSV-sero-positive
Children and adults: IV 150 mg/m^2/dose q12hr; with clinical symptoms of herpes simplex, 150 mg/m^2/dose q8h
Prophylaxis of Bone Marrow Transplant Patients, CMV-sero-positive
Children and adults: IV 500 mg/m^2/dose q8h; for clinically symptomatic CMV infection, consider ganciclovir instead of acyclovir
Herpes Genitalis: Non–life-threatening Herpes Simplex in Immunocompromised Patient:
Children and adults: TOP Apply ½" strip of ointment for a 4" square surface area q3h (6 times/24 hr) for 7 days
IV Administration
• Recommended concentration: ≤7 mg/ml in D$_5$NS, D$_5$W, LR, NS
• Maximum concentration: 7-10 mg/ml; infusion of sol >10 mg/ml increases risk of phlebitis
• IV push rate: Not recommended
• Intermittent infusion rate: over 1 hr

MECHANISM AND INDICATIONS
Antiviral mechanism: Interferes with DNA synthesis, inhibits viral replication
Indications: Used in treatment of initial and prophylaxis of recurrent mucosal and cutaneous herpes simplex infections (HSV-1 and HSV-2); herpes simplex encephalitis; herpes zoster and varicella-zoster infections in healthy non-pregnant patients over age 13 years; children over age 12 months who have chronic dermatologic or respiratory disorders or who are receiving long-term aspirin therapy; and immunocompromised patients

PHARMACOKINETICS
Peak: PO 1.5-2.0 hr
Distribution: Widely throughout body
Half-life: Terminal phase, neo-

✤ Available in Canada.

nates 4 hr; children 2-3 hr; adults 2-3.5 hr
Metabolism: Liver
Excretion: Urine

CONTRAINDICATIONS AND PRECAUTIONS
• Contraindicated with known hypersensitivity to acyclovir
• Use cautiously with renal or hepatic impairment, dehydration, underlying neurologic disease, hypoxia, electrolyte abnormalities, pregnancy, and lactation

INTERACTIONS
Drug
• Increased risk of neurotoxicity with use of interferon, methotrexate
• Decreased renal clearance with use of probenecid
Lab
• Increased serum creatinine, BUN levels
Incompatabilities
• Dobutamine, dopamine, protein-containing solutions, all blood products

SIDE EFFECTS
CNS: Headache, lethargy, tremors, coma, dizziness, seizures, insomnia
CV: Hypotension
DERM: Rash, pruritus
GI: Nausea, vomiting, diarrhea, elevated liver enzymes
GU: Hematuria, crystalluria, reversible renal dysfunction
HEME: Bone marrow depression
Local: Phlebitis at IV injection site

TOXICITY AND OVERDOSE
Clinical signs: Nephrotoxicity, renal failure
Treatment: Supportive care; hemodialysis

PATIENT CARE MANAGEMENT
Assessment
• Assess history of hypersensitivity to acyclovir
• Obtain cultures to confirm diagnosis; may begin therapy before obtaining results
• Assess renal function (BUN, creatinine, I&O), hepatic function (AST, ALT, bilirubin), hematologic function (CBC, differential, platelet count)
• Assess skin lesions by characteristics, number
• Assess possibility of sexual assault or abuse if otherwise healthy young child is infected
Interventions
• May administer PO without regard to meals; shake susp well before administering each dose; tabs may be crushed, caps taken apart, mixed with food or fluid
• Ensure adequate hydration before, during IV infusion
• Do not administer IV push, SC, IM, ID
• Do not mix with other medications in syringe or solution
• Use large vein with small-bore needle to reduce local reaction; rotate site q48-72h
• Top, wash hands before/after application; before application, cleanse area with soap, water, then dry well; apply ointment (using gloves) to cover lesions completely
• Begin treatment at first sign of lesions
• Maintain age-appropriate fluid intake
• Notify social services if otherwise healthy young child is infected

> **NURSING ALERT**
> Discontinue if hypersensitivity or encephalopathic reactions occur
>
> Do not administer by IV push, IM, SC, ID

Evaluation
• Evaluate therapeutic response (absence of lesions, symptoms)
• Monitor renal status (BUN, creatinine, I&O), hepatic status (AST, ALT, bilirubin), hematologic status (CBC, differential, platelet count)
• Monitor for CNS side effects (tremor, confusion, seizures)
• Evaluate IV site for vein irritation

PATIENT AND FAMILY EDUCATION
Teach/instruct
• To take as directed at prescribed intervals for prescribed length of time
• To initiate therapy as soon as itching, tingling, pain develop at site
• About comfort measures (e.g., keeping infected areas clean, wearing loose clothing)
• About sexual transmission of herpes; patient should avoid sexual activity if either partner has symptoms of herpes; condom use may help prevent herpes spread; acyclovir will not prevent transmission; female patients should have annual or semiannual PAP test because of increased risk of cervical cancer from herpes
Warn/advise
• To notify care provider of hypersensitivity, side effects
• To avoid use of OTC creams, ointments, lotions unless directed to do so by care provider
• Not to share towels, wash cloths, linens with family member being treated
• To maintain good dental hygiene to avoid gingival hyperplasia

STORAGE
• Store caps, tabs, oint at room temp, protected from light, moisture
• Reconstituted parenteral solution stable at room temp for 24 hr; refrigeration may result in formation of a precipitate, which will redissolve at room temp

---

adenosine
Brand Name(s): Adenocard
Classification: Antiarrhythmic
Pregnancy Category: C

AVAILABLE PREPARATIONS
Inj: 6 mg/2 ml (3 mg/ml)
ROUTES AND DOSAGES
Children: IV 0.1 mg/kg; may increase dose by 0.05 mg/kg q2min to total of 3 doses; maximum dose 12 mg
Adults: IV 6 mg; may follow after 2 min with 12 mg; maximum single dose 12 mg; may repeat 12 mg dose 1 time
IV administration
• Recommended concentration: ≤3 mg/ml in NS
• Maximum concentration: 3 mg/ml
• IV push rate: rapid IV bolus
• Continuous infusion rate: 0.05 mcg/kg/min to 0.3 mcg/kg/min

MECHANISM AND INDICATIONS
Antiarrhythmic mechanism: Slows conduction time through AV node; interrupts reentry pathways associated with supraventricular tachycardia
Indications: Supraventricular tachycardia, including that associated with Wolff-Parkinson-White syndrome

PHARMACOKINETICS
Onset of action: 1-2 sec
Peak: <10 sec
Half-life: <10 sec
Metabolism: Erythrocytes
Excretion: Vascular endothelial cells

CONTRAINDICATIONS AND PRECAUTIONS
• Contraindicated with known hypersensitivity, 2nd- or 3rd-degree AV block, or sick sinus syndrome unless artificial pacemaker is in place
• Use cautiously with asthma

INTERACTIONS
Drugs
• Decreased effectiveness with aminophylline, caffeine
• Increased effects with dipyridamole
• Increased heart block possible with carbamazepine

INCOMPATIBILITIES
• Incompatible with any drug in solution or syringe

SIDE EFFECTS
CNS: Lightheadedness, dizziness,

✤ Available in Canada.

paresthesias, apprehension, neck and back pain, headache
CV: PACs, PVCs, sinus bradycardia, sinus tachycardia, asystole, chest pain, hypotension, flushing, diaphoresis
DERM: Burning sensation
EENT: Blurred vision, metallic taste, tightness in throat
GI: Nausea
RESP: Dyspnea, hyperventilation, shortness of breath

TOXICITY AND OVERDOSE
Clinical signs: Life-threatening arrhythmias, asystole
Treatment: Treat symptoms as appropriate; resuscitate as necessary

PATIENT CARE MANAGEMENT
Assessment
• Assess history of hypersensitivity to drug
• Assess baseline VS, B/P
• Identify supraventricular tachycardia in conjunction with physician
Interventions
• Have emergency equipment readily available
• Inject rapidly directly into vein or proximal IV injection site

NURSING ALERT
Crystal formation occurs when adenosine is refrigerated; do not store in refrigerator.

Evaluation
• Evaluate therapeutic response (supraventricular tachycardia converted to normal sinus rhythm)
• Evaluate for side effects, hypersensitivity
• Monitor VS, ECG continuously

PATIENT AND FAMILY EDUCATION
Teach/instruct
• To perform vagal maneuvers prior to medication administration to attempt to convert rhythm
• That close monitoring is necessary during administration
Warn/advise
• To notify care provider of hypersensitivity, side effects

Encourage
• To provide emotional support as indicated

STORAGE
• Store at room temp

---

albumin, human serum
Brand Name(s): Albuminar 5%, Albuminar 25%, Albutein 5%, Albutein 25%, Buminate 5%, Buminate 25%, Plasbumin 5%, Plasbumin 25%, Plasbumine-5✤, Plasbumine-10✤

Classification: Blood derivative/plasma volume expander

Pregnancy Category: C

AVAILABLE PREPARATIONS
Inj: 5% (50 mg/ml) in 50 ml, 250 ml, 500 ml, 1000 ml vials: 25% (250 mg/ml) in 20, 50, 100 ml vials

ROUTES AND DOSAGES
Hypoproteinemia
Children: 0.5-1 g/kg/dose IV over 30-120 min
Adults: 25 g/dose IV over 30-120 min
Shock
Children: 1 g/kg/dose IV rapid infusion; maximum dose 6 g/kg/24 hr
Adults: 25 g/dose IV rapid infusion
IV administration
• Concentration for administration: Dilute in D_5W, $D_{10}W$, LR, NS, ½NS, R
• Maximum concentration: May give undiluted
• IV push rate: Rapid
• Intermittent infusion rate: Hypoproteinemia: 2-3 ml/min (25%) adults; shock: 1 ml/min (25%) adults

MECHANISM AND INDICATIONS
Mechanism: Causes fluid shift from interstitial space to circulation; increases plasma volume
Indications: For use in shock, hy-

---

poproteinemia, burns, hyperbili-rubinemia

PHARMACOKINETICS

Distribution: Intravascular space, extravascular sites (e.g., skin, muscle, bone)
Metabolism: As protein/energy source

CONTRAINDICATIONS AND PRECAUTIONS

• Contraindicated with severe anemia, heart failure
• Use cautiously with severe salt restriction; dehydration; decreased cardiac reserve; liver, pulmonary, or kidney disease; pregnancy

INTERACTIONS

Lab
• False increase: Alk phos
• Increased plasma albumin

SIDE EFFECTS

CNS: Headache
CV: Vascular overload, hypotension, tachycardia, dilution anemia
DERM: Urticaria
GI: Nausea, vomiting, excess salivation
RESP: Pulmonary edema, altered respiration
Other: Chills, fever

TOXICITY AND OVERDOSE

Clinical signs: Circulatory overload, pulmonary edema
Treatment: Decrease rate of IV infusion, reevaluate therapy, may need to discontinue

PATIENT CARE MANAGEMENT

Assessment
• Assess history of hypersensitivity
• Assess VS, B/P, Hct, Hgb, serum protein, electrolytes
• Assess I&O
• Assess central venous pressure
Interventions
• Use 5 micron or larger filter for IV
• May be administered without blood typing, cross matching

NURSING ALERT
Monitor for signs of allergic reaction while giving

Evaluation
• Evaluate therapeutic response (increase B/P, increase serum protein)
• Evaluate pt for dyspnea, hypoxemia
• Evaluate pt for adverse allergic reaction

PATIENT AND FAMILY EDUCATION

Teach/instruct
• That drug is blood derivative, risk of blood-borne infection is low
Provide
• Support during acute phase

STORAGE

• Store at room temp, do not use if cloudy or containing sediment
• Discard unused portion after 4 hr

---

albuterol sulfate

Brand Name(s): Asmavent✤, Gen-Salbutamol✤, Novo-Salbutamol✤, PMS-Salbautamol✤, Proventil, RHO-Salbutamol✤, Ventolin

Classification: Bronchodilator (adrenergic)

Pregnancy Category: C

AVAILABLE PREPARATIONS

Syr: 2 mg/5 ml
Tabs: 2, 4 mg
Tabs (EXT): 4 mg
Aerosol (oral): 90 mcg/metered spray
Inh (sol): 0.083%, 0.5%

ROUTES AND DOSAGES

Children 2-6 yr: PO 0.1-0.2 mg/kg/dose tid; maximum dose 4 mg tid
Children 6-12 yr: PO 2 mg/dose tid-qid; maximum dose 24 mg/24 hr

---

✤ Available in Canada.

Children under 12 yr: 1-2 inhalations qid using aerosol inhal and tube spacer; nebulizer inhal 1.25-2.5 mg q4-6h (Safety and effectiveness not established. Dosage represents accepted standard practice recommendations.)

Children over 12 yr and adults: PO 2-4 mg/dose tid-qid (maximum 32 mg/24 hr); ext rel tabs 4-8 mg q12h; aerosol inhal 1-2 inhalations q4-6h; nebulizer inhal 2.5 mg tid-qid

MECHANISMS AND INDICATIONS

Bronchodilator mechanism: Selectively stimulates β_2-adrenergic receptors of lungs, uterus, and vascular smooth muscle, resulting in bronchodilation, mild vasodilation, slight decreases in B/P; relaxation of bronchial muscles relieves bronchospasm, reduces airway resistance

Indications: Used to prevent/treat reversible obstructive bronchospasm of asthma, bronchitis, cystic fibrosis; also used to prevent exercise-induced bronchospasm

PHARMACOKINETICS

Onset of action: PO 30 min; aerosol inhal 5-15 min; nebulization 5 min

Peak: PO 2-3 hr; aerosol inhal 0.5-2 hr; nebulization 1-2 hr

Distribution: Does not cross blood-brain barrier

Half-life: PO 2.7-5 hr; inhal 3.8 hr

Metabolism: Liver

Excretion: Urine, feces

CONTRAINDICATIONS AND PRECAUTIONS

• Contraindicated with known hypersensitivity to albuterol sulfate or any adrenergic amine

• Use cautiously with hyperthyroidism, DM, CV disorders (including coronary insufficiency or hypertension), pregnancy, and lactation

INTERACTIONS

Drug

• Increased action, risk of toxicity with use of epinephrine, other orally inhaled sympathomimetic amines

• Increased risk of serious CV effects with use of MAOIs, tricyclic antidepressants

• Decreased effectiveness possible with use of propranolol, other β-adrenergic blocking agents

SIDE EFFECTS:

CNS: Tremors, nervousness, insomnia, hyperactivity, headache, dizziness, restlessness, hallucinations, irritability

CV: Palpitations, tachycardia, hypotension, hypertension, arrhythmias

EENT: Dry or irritated nose, throat; dilated pupils

ENDO / METAB: Hypokalemia

GI: Nausea, vomiting

RESP: Paradoxical bronchospasm

Other: Muscle cramps

TOXICITY AND OVERDOSE

Clinical signs: Exaggeration of common reactions, particularly angina, hypertension, tachycardia, hypokalemia

Treatment: Cautiously administer selective β_1-adrenergic blocker (metaprolol tartrate); severe bronchospasm may occur; supportive care; monitor electrolyte levels; hemodialysis not recommended

PATIENT CARE MANAGEMENT

Assessment

• Assess history of hypersensitivity to albuterol sulfate, adrenergic amines

• Assess respiratory status, baseline VS

Interventions

• Administer PO with meals to reduce gastric irritation; tabs may be crushed, mixed with food or fluid; do not crush or chew ext rel tabs

• Aerosol inhal (see Chapter 3 for discussion of inhaler) instructions; shake canister well before using

• Manufacturers recommend allowing 2 min between first and second inhalations

• Nebulization (see Chapter 3 for discussion of nebulizer use)

• Maintain age-appropriate fluid intake

• Offer sips of fluids, gum for dry mouth

NURSING ALERT

Discontinue if hypersensitivity or paradoxical bronchospasm occur

Do not use with other sympathomimetic agents

Evaluation
• Evaluate therapeutic response (decreased dyspnea, wheezing)
• Monitor respiratory status, VS
• Monitor for dyspnea that persists 1 hr after treatment, for return of symptoms within 4 hr, or for worsening respiratory status

PATIENT AND FAMILY EDUCATION:
Teach/instruct
• To take as directed at prescribed intervals for prescribed length of time
• To start treatment at first sign of bronchospasm
• About proper use, care of inhaler or nebulizer
Warn/advise
• To notify care provider of hypersensitivity, side effects
• To discontinue albuterol, notify care provider if paradoxical bronchospasm occurs
• To notify care provider if symptoms persist >1 hr or worsen
• Not to use more than prescribed
• Not to use other adrenergic medications unless directed by care provider
• To wait 1-2 min before assessing need for second dose of inhalation
• To wait 20-30 min after inhalation before using inhal steroids
• To avoid getting aerosol in eyes
• To rinse with or drink water to avoid dry mouth
• That sputum, saliva may appear pink after inhalation
• To avoid smoking, contact with second-hand smoke, or persons with respiratory infections

STORAGE
• Store syr and tabs at room temp in tight, light-resistant container

• Store aerosol canisters at room temp away from heat, direct sunlight
• Do not puncture canisters

---

allopurinol

Brand Name(s): Apo-Allopurinol♣, Lopurin, Purinol♣, Zyloprim, Zyloprin Oral♣

Classification: Antilithic (agent that prevents formation of urinary or biliary calculi)

Pregnancy Category: C

AVAILABLE PREPARATIONS
Tabs: 100 mg, 300 mg

ROUTES AND DOSAGES
Prevention of Uric Acid Nephropathy during Chemotherapy:
Children: 10 mg/kg/24 hr or 200-300 mg/m^2/24 hr divided tid to maximum 800 mg/24 hr
OR
Children <6 yr: PO 150 mg/24 hr divided tid
Children 6-10 yr: PO 300 mg/24 hr divided bid-tid
Adult: PO 600-800 mg qd for 2-3 days with high fluid intake
• Dosages >300 mg/24 hr should be administered in divided doses

MECHANISM AND INDICATIONS
Mechanism: Blocks xanthine oxidase enzyme (catalyzes conversion of hypoxanthine to xanthine and xanthine to uric acid), prevents excessively high blood and urine levels of uric acid
Indications: Prevent complications of acute hyperuricemia occurring in tumor lysis syndrome, a side effect of cytoreductive chemotherapy in diseases (e.g., lymphoma, leukemia) with large tumor burden

PHARMACOKINETICS
Onset of action: 2-3 days
Peak: Peak concentrations (allopu-

♣ Available in Canada.

rinol, acute metabolites) 2-6 hr
Distribution: 80%-90% of oral dose absorbed from GI tract
Half-life: Allopurinol, 1-3 hr; oxypurinol metabolite, 18-30 hr (less enzymatic inhibitory activity, but responsible for most antihyperuricemic effects because of longer half-life)
Metabolism: Liver
Excretion: Urine, feces

CONTRAINDICTIONS AND PRECAUTIONS
• Contraindicated with pregnancy or lactation; hypersensitivity (as evidenced by fever, chills, leukopenia, leukocytosis, eosinophilia, arthralgias, nausea, vomiting, renal failure, uremia); idiopathic hemochromatosis
• Use cautiously with impaired renal or hepatic function

INTERACTIONS
Drug
• Potentiated myelosuppressive action of 6-mercaptopurine, azathioprine
• Increased incidence of skin rashes with amoxicillin or ampicillin
• Prolonged half-life of dicumarol, warfarin, theophylline, oral hyperglycemic drugs
• Increased neurotoxicity when combined with vidarabine
Lab
• Increased serum alk phos, AST, ALT

SIDE EFFECTS
CNS: Headache, peripheral neuropathy, neuritis, paresthesia, somnolence, vertigo, depression, confusion
CV: Necrotizing angiitis, vasculitis
DERM: Rash, Stevens-Johnson syndrome, toxic epidermal necrolysis, alopecia, erythema multiforme, ichthyosis, purpuric lesions, vesicular bullous dermatitis, eczematous dermatitis, pruritus, urticaria
EENT: Cataracts, retinopathy, furunculosis (nose), retinitis, iritis, conjunctivitis, amblyopia, tinnitus, epistaxis, optic neuritis
GI: Nausea, vomiting, diarrhea, intermittent abdominal pain, gastritis, dyspepsia, metallic taste, loss of taste, aggravation of peptic ulcer, hepatomegaly, hyperbilirubinemia, cholestatic jaundice
HEME: Agranulocytosis, anemia, aplastic anemia, leukopenia, pancytopenia, thrombocytopenia
MS: Myopathy
Other: Fever

TOXICITY AND OVERDOSE
• Overdose has not been reported

PATIENT CARE MANAGEMENT
Assessment
• Assess history of hypersensitivity to allopurinol
• Assess I&O, keeping urinary output >1-2 ml/kg/hr
• Assess CBC, serum uric acid, renal function (BUN, creatinine, urine CrCl) and liver function (alk phos, AST, ALT)
• Assess wt daily
• Assess for evidence of tumor lysis syndrome
Interventions
• Maintain alkaline urine
• Minimize GI effects by administering medicine with or immediately after meals; tab may be crushed, mixed with food or fluids
• Encourage oral fluid intake, supplement with IV fluid
Evaluation
• Evaluate therapeutic response through maintenance of normal serum chemistry, electrolytes, urinary output
• Evaluate CBC, serum uric acid, renal function (BUN, creatinine, urine CrCl, I&O) and liver function (alk phos, AST, ALT)

PATIENT/FAMILY EDUCATION
Teach/instruct
• To take as directed at prescribed intervals for prescribed length of time
• About importance of hydration, alkalinization of urine, medicine to prevent renal complications of chemotherapy
• To avoid alcohol intake

✤ Available in Canada.

Warn/advise
• To report fever, chills, nausea, vomiting, arthralgias to care provider

Encourage
• To increase oral fluid intake

STORAGE
• Tabs should be stored in tightly closed container at room temp

---

alprostadil

Brand Name(s): PGE_1, Prostaglandin E_1, Prostin-VR✤

Classification: Prostaglandin

Pregnancy Category: X

AVAILABLE PREPARATIONS
Inj: 500 mcg/ml

ROUTES AND DOSAGES
Neonates: IV 0.05-0.1 mcg/kg/min as initial dose, then reduce infusion to lowest dose that will maintain therapeutic response; maintenance dose 0.01-0.4 mcg/kg/min

IV administration
• Recommended concentration: Add 500 mcg ampule to 50 ml dextrose or NS, concentration will be 10 mcg/ml
• Maximum concentration: Not established

MECHANISM AND INDICATIONS
Mechanism: Relaxes or dilates rings of smooth muscle of the patent ductus arteriosus to maintain patency in neonates before natural closure
Indications: For maintenance of patency of ductus arteriosus in pts with ductal dependent congenital heart disease until surgery can be performed

PHARMACOKINETICS
Metabolism: Oxidation through lungs
Half-life: 5-10 min
Excretion: Lungs, urine

CONTRAINDICATIONS AND PRECAUTIONS
• Contraindicated in respiratory distress syndrome or persistent fetal circulation, pregnancy and lactation
• Use cautiously with tendency to bleed

INTERACTIONS
Drug
• None known
Lab
• Inhibits platelet aggregation

INCOMPATIBILITIES
• Do not mix in sol or syringe with other drugs

SIDE EFFECTS
CNS: Fever, seizure-like activities, hyperirritability, hypothermia
CV: Bradycardia, rhythm disturbances, flushing, edema, hypotension, shock
GI: Diarrhea, nausea, vomiting, regurgitation
GU: Oliguria, hematuria, anuria
HEME: Disseminated intravascular clotting, thrombocytopenia, bleeding, anemia, decreased platelet aggregation
RESP: Apnea, wheezing, respiratory distress, bronchospasm
Other: Sepsis, hypokalemia, hyperkalemia, hypoglycemia

TOXICITY AND OVERDOSE
Clinical signs: Similar to side effects (e.g., apnea, bradycardia, hypotension, pyrexia)
Treatment: Discontinue drug, provide supportive care (including ventilation) if indicated; reposition intraarterial catheter if flushing occurs

PATIENT CARE MANAGEMENT
Assessment
• Assess VS closely when taking medication
• Monitor arterial pressure
• Monitor ABGs, continuous ECG
Interventions
• Administer CONT INF through pump in an ICU
• 0.01 ml/kg/min = 0.1 mcg/kg/min; sol may be further diluted
• Administer only in an ICU with trained personnel and life support available

---

✤ Available in Canada.

- Flushing may respond to repositioning of catheter

Evaluation
- Evaluate therapeutic response (increased PaO$_2$)
- Monitor for side effects; apnea, bradycardia may signal overdose; stop infusion, call care provider; have ventilatory assistance available
- Evaluate pH, B/P, urinary output, respiratory rate, heart rate

PATIENT AND FAMILY EDUCATION
Teach/instruct
- About diagnosis, treatment
Provide
- Support, reassurance

STORAGE
- Refrigerate alprostadil ampules
- Discard unused prepared sol after 24 hr

---

amantadine hydrochloride

Brand Name(s): Gen-Amantadine✤, PMS-Amantadine✤, Symmetrel✤

Classification: Antiviral (tricyclic amine)

Pregnancy Category: C

AVAILABLE PREPARATIONS
Syr: 50 mg/5 ml
Caps: 100 mg

ROUTES AND DOSAGES
Children 1-8 yr: PO 5-9 mg/kg/24 hr divided bid; maximum 200 mg/24 hr
Children 9-12 yr: PO 100-200 mg/24 hr divided bid; maximum 200 mg/24 hr
Adults: 200 mg/24 hr qd or divided bid
- After first influenza A virus vaccine dose, prophylaxis may be administered for up to 6 wk or until 2 wk after second vaccine dose
- Prophylaxis should start as soon as possible after initial exposure, continue for 10 days
- For symptomatic treatment, administer within 1-2 days of onset of symptoms, continue therapy for 2-7 days

MECHANISM AND INDICATIONS
Antiviral mechanism: Interferes with penetration of influenza A virus into susceptible cells, blocks viral uncoating by RNA
Indications: Active only against influenza type A virus; reduces duration of fever/other systemic symptoms when administered within 24-48 hr of onset of illness

PHARMACOKINETICS
Peak: 1-4 hr
Half-life: 10-28 hr
Excretion: Urine

CONTRAINDICATIONS AND PRECAUTIONS
- Contraindicated in infants <1 yr, with known hypersensitivity to amantadine, pregnancy, lactation
- Use cautiously with history of hepatic or renal disease, seizures, psychosis, recurrent eczematoid dermatitis, cardiovascular disease, peripheral edema, orthostatic hypotension, or pts receiving CNS stimulant medications
- Consider contraceptive options for women of childbearing age

INTERACTIONS
Drug
- Increased confusion, hallucinations from anticholinergic drugs (e.g., trihexyphenidyl, benztropine)
- Increased stimulation from CNS stimulants
- Increased CNS effects with use of alcohol

SIDE EFFECTS
CNS: Dizziness, confusion, headache, insomnia, difficulty concentrating, anxiety, depression, restlessness, irritability, hallucinations
CV: Edema, orthostatic hypotension, CHF
DERM: Livedo reticularis with prolonged care

✤ Available in Canada.

GI: Nausea, vomiting, dry mouth, constipation
GU: Urinary retention

OVERDOSE AND TOXICITY
Clinical signs: Nausea, vomiting, anorexia, hyperexcitability, tremors, slurred speech, blurred vision, lethargy, anticholinergic symptoms, seizures, ventricular arrhythmias, dyspnea
Treatment: Gastric lavage or induced emesis, supportive care, increased fluids, urine acidification, physostigmine to counteract CNS toxicity

PATIENT CARE MANAGEMENT
Assessment
• Assess history of hypersensitivity to amantadine
• Assess for influenza A virus exposure
• Assess renal function (BUN, creatinine, I&O), bowel pattern
Interventions
• Administer PO after meals for optimal absorption, reduced GI irritation; divided doses may reduce CNS effects; administer at least 4 hr before hs to prevent insomnia
• Caps may be taken apart, mixed with food or fluid

NURSING ALERT
Discontinue drug if signs of hypersensitivity develop

Evaluation
• Evaluate therapeutic response (decrease in or absence of fever, malaise, cough, dyspnea during viral infection)
• Monitor renal function (BUN, creatinine, I&O), bowel pattern
• Monitor respiratory function (wheezing, dyspnea), skin eruptions, CNS symptoms
• Monitor activities requiring mental alertness, changes in position

PATIENT AND FAMILY EDUCATION
Teach/instruct
• To take as directed at prescribed

intervals for prescribed length of time
Warn/advise
• To notify care provider of hypersensitivity, side effects
• To avoid hazardous activities (e.g., biking, skating, skateboarding) because mental alertness may be impaired; change positions slowly to reduce orthostatic hypotension
• To avoid alcohol, medications containing alcohol during therapy

STORAGE
• Store at room temp in light-resistant containers

---

amikacin sulfate
Brand Name(s): Amikin ♣
Classification: Antibiotic (aminoglycoside)
Pregnancy Category: D

AVAILABLE PREPARATIONS
Inj: 50 mg/ml, 250 mg/ml

ROUTES AND DOSAGES
Neonates: Wt <1200 g, age 0-4 wk 7.5 mg/kg/dose q18-24h; wt 1200-2000 g, age 0-7 days 7.5 mg/kg/dose q12-18h; wt 1200-2000 g, age >7 days 7.5 mg/kg/dose q8-12h; wt >2000 g, age 0-7 days 10 mg/kg/dose q12h; wt >2000 g, age >7 days 10 mg/kg/dose q8h
Infants and children: 15-22.5 mg/kg/24 hr divided q8-12h; maximum 1.5 g/24 hr
Adults: 15 mg/kg/24 hr divided q8-12h
Meningitis and ventriculitis
Infants and children: Systemic therapy as above; may also give 1-2 mg/24 hr IT
Adults: Systemic therapy as above; may also give up to 20 mg/24 hr IT or intraventricularly
IV administration
• Recommended concentration: Dilute in sufficient volume of D_5 ¼ NS, D_5 ½ NS, D_5W, LR, or NS to infuse over 30 min

---

- Maximum concentration: 5 mg/ml
- IV push rate: Not recommended
- Intermittent infusion rate: Over 30 min
- Continuous infusion: Not recommended

MECHANISM AND INDICATIONS

Antibiotic mechanism: Bactericidal; inhibits bacterial protein-synthesis by binding directly to 30S ribosomal subunit

Indications: Active against gram-positive and gram-negative bacteria including *Escherichia coli* and *Staphylococcus, Enterococcus, Klebsiella,* and *Enterobacter* species; amikacin may act against some organisms resistant to other aminoglycosides such as *Proteus, Serratia,* and *Pseudomonas* species, although some strains may be resistant to amikacin; used to treat otitis media, UTIs, septicemia, meningitis, and infections of burns and bone

PHARMACOKINETICS

Peak: IM 0.5-2.0 hr; IV, end of infusion or 30 min
Distribution: Primarily into extracellular fluid; poor penetration into blood–brain barrier (even with inflamed meninges)
Half-life: Neonates 4.0-8.0 hr; children and adults 2.0-2.5 hr
Metabolism: Not metabolized
Excretion: Urine
Therapeutic levels: Peak 15-30 mcg/ml; trough: 5-10 mcg/ml

CONTRAINDICATIONS AND PRECAUTIONS

- Contraindicated with known hypersensitivity to amikacin or other aminoglycosides and with renal failure
- Use cautiously in neonates and infants because of renal immaturity, with impaired renal function, dehydration, eighth cranial nerve impairment, myasthenia gravis, parkinsonism, hypocalcemia, pregnancy, and lactation

INTERACTIONS

Drug

- Increased risk of nephrotoxicity, ototoxicity, neurotoxicity with use of amphotericin B, loop diuretics, methoxyflurane, polymyxin B, capreomycin, cisplatin, cephalosporins, other aminoglycosides
- Increased risk of ototoxicity with use of ethacrynic acid, furosemide, bumetanide, urea, mannitol
- Masked symptoms of ototoxicity with use of dimenhydrinate and other antiemetic or antivertigo drugs
- Increased risk of neuromuscular blockade with use of general anesthetics or neuromuscular blocking agents such as succinylcholine, tubocurarine
- Increased respiratory depression with use of opioids, analgesics
- Inactivated when administered with penicillin, carbenicillin, ticarcillin

Lab

- Increased LDH, BUN, non-protein N, serum creatinine levels
- Increased urinary excretion of casts
- Decreased serum Na

INCOMPATIBILITIES

- Do not mix in sol or syringe: carbenicillin, ticarcillin, amphotericin B, cephalothin, erythromycin, heparin, ampicillin, cefazolin, chlorothiazide, phenytoin, thiopental, vitamin B complex with vitamin C, warfarin, methicillin

SIDE EFFECTS

CNS: Headache, lethargy, neuromuscular blockade with respiratory depression
EENT: Ototoxicity (tinnitus, vertigo, hearing loss)
GI: Diarrhea; transient hepatomegaly, elevated hepatic enzymes
GU: Nephrotoxicity (cells or casts in urine, oliguria, proteinuria, decreased CrCl, elevated BUN, serum creatinine, non-protein N levels)
HEME: Blood dyscrasias, purpura in infants

♣ Available in Canada.

Other: Hypersensitivity reactions (eosinophilia, fever, rash, urticaria, pruritus), bacterial or fungal superinfections

PATIENT CARE MANAGEMENT
Assessment
• Assess history of hypersensitivity to amikacin or other aminoglycosides
• Obtain C&S; may begin therapy before obtaining results
• Assess renal function (BUN, creatinine, I&O), baseline weight, hearing tests before beginning therapy

Interventions
• Sol should be clear and colorless to very pale yellow; do not use if dark yellow, cloudy, or precipitates
• Administer amikacin at least 1 hr before or after other antibiotics
• Administer IM; inject deeply into large muscle mass, rotate injection sites; do not administer more than 2 g of drug per injection site
• Do not premix IV sol with other medications; infuse separately and flush line with D_5W or NS
• Use large vein with small-bore needle to reduce local reaction; rotate site q48-72h
• Maintain age appropriate fluid intake; keep patient well hydrated to reduce risk of renal toxicity
• Supervise ambulation, other safety measures with vestibular dysfunction
• Obtain drug levels after 3rd dose, sooner in neonates or pts with rapidly changing renal function; peak levels drawn after end of 30-min IV infusion; 1 hr after IM injection; trough levels drawn within 30 min before next dose

---

NURSING ALERT
Discontinue drug if signs of ototoxicity, nephrotoxicity, or hypersensitivity develop

Do not give IV push

Evaluation
• Evaluate therapeutic response (decreased symptoms of infection)

• Evaluate renal function (BUN, creatinine, I&O), daily wt, hearing evaluations
• Monitor for signs of respiratory depression with IV infusion
• Observe for signs of superinfection (perineal itching, diaper rash, fever, malaise, redness, pain, swelling, drainage, rash, diarrhea, sore throat, change in cough or sputum)
• Evaluate IM site for tissue damage, IV site for vein irritation

PATIENT AND FAMILY EDUCATION
Teach/instruct
• To take as directed at prescribed intervals for prescribed length of time
Warn/advise
• To notify care provider of hypersensitivity, side effects, superinfection

STORAGE
• Store at room temp; reconstituted IV sol potent at room temp for 24 hr

---

aminocaproic acid
Brand Name(s): Amicar✽
Classification: Fibrinolysis inhibitor
Pregnancy Category: C

AVAILABLE PREPARATIONS
Tabs: 500 mg
Syrup: 250 mg/ml
Inj: 5 g/20 ml for dilution; 24 g/96 ml for infusion

ROUTES AND DOSAGES
Adults: PO 5-30 g/24 hr q3-6h
Children: IV 100 mg/kg or 3 g/m² first hr, followed by constant infusion of 33.3 mg/kg/hr or 1 g/m²/hr; maximum dose 18 g/m²/24 hr
IV administration
• Recommended concentration: Dilute doses up to 5 g with at least 250 ml of NS, D_5W, LR; dilute doses >5 g with at least 500 ml of NS, D_5W, LR
• IV push rate: Not recommended

✽ Available in Canada.

MECHANISM AND INDICATIONS
Mechanism: Inhibits plasminogen activators, inhibits fibrinolysis
Indications: For use in hemorrhage from hyperfibrinolysis and for chronic bleeding tendency

PHARMACOKINETICS
Peak: 2 hr
Duration: < 3 hr
Metabolism: Insignificant
Excretion: Urine

CONTRAINDICATIONS AND PRECAUTIONS
• Contraindicated with intravascular clotting, disseminated intravascular clotting, abnormal bleeding, burns
• Use cautiously in neonates, with kidney disease, liver disease, thrombosis, pregnancy, and lactation

INTERACTIONS
Drug
• Increased coagulation with estrogens and OCPs
Lab
• Increased serum K^+ in pts with impaired renal function
• Increased CPK, AST, ALT

INCOMPATIBILITIES
• Na lactate sol

SIDE EFFECTS
CNS: Headache, dizziness, delirium, seizures, hallucinations
CV: Hypotension, bradycardia, arrhythmias
DERM: Rash
EENT: Nasal congestion, tinnitus, conjunctival suffusion
GI: Nausea, vomiting, diarrhea, abdominal cramps
GU: Dysuria, menstrual irregularities, ejaculatory failure
HEME: Thrombosis
Other: Skeletal myopathy

TOXICITY AND OVERDOSE
Clinical signs: Nausea, delirium, thrombotic episodes
Treatment: Discontinue drug immediately

PATIENT CARE MANAGEMENT
Assessment
• Assess hypersensitivity history
• Assess VS, B/P
• Assess I & O
• Assess blood studies (platelets, serum K^+, PT or activated clotting time), baseline and ongoing
Interventions
• Use infusion pump for IV
• Discontinue drug if signs of allergy or thrombosis occur
Evaluation
• Evaluate therapeutic response (decreased bleeding)
• Evaluate bleeding, especially mucus membrane, epistaxis, GI bleeding, ecchymosis, petechiae, hematuria

PATIENT AND FAMILY EDUCATION
Teach/instruct
• To take as directed at prescribed intervals for prescribed length of time
• To report signs of bleeding, myopathy
• To change position slowly to avoid dizziness

STORAGE
• Store in tight container in cool environment

---

aminophylline (theophylline ethelenediamine)
Brand Name(s): Aminophyllin, Somophyllin, Phyllocontin✤, Phyllocontin-350✤, Truphylline
Classification: Bronchodilator (xanthine derivative)
Pregnancy Category: C

AVAILABLE PREPARATIONS
Sol: 105 mg/5 ml (86% theophylline)
Tabs: 100 mg, 200 mg (79% theophylline)
Sus Rel Tabs: 225 mg (79% theophylline)
Inj: 25 mg/ml (79% theophylline)

✤ Available in Canada.

ROUTES AND DOSAGES
Bronchial Asthma, COPDs
Loading dose: PO 0.8 mg/kg/dose for each 2 mg/L desired increase in serum theophylline level

Maintenance dose: *Children:* 0-2 mo, 3-6 mg/kg/24 hr divided q8h; 2-6 mo, 6-15 mg/kg/24 hr divided q6h; 6-12 mo, 15-22 mg/kg/24 hr divided q4-6h; 1-9 yr, 22 mg/kg/24 hr divided q4-6h; 9-16 yr, 18 mg/kg/24 hr divided q6h

Adults: 12 mg/kg/24 hr divided q6h; maximum 900 mg/24 hr

Acute Bronchospasm
• Loading dose (in all patients not receiving aminophylline or theophylline): IV 5-7.5 mg/kg over 20-30 min

• Maintenance (before serum concentration monitoring): <14 days, 2.5 mg/kg q12h; ≥14 days, 4 mg/kg q12h; 6-52 wk:

$$\frac{[0.3 \text{ (age in wk)} + 8]/24}{0.8} = \text{mg/kg/hr}$$

or

$$\frac{[0.008 \text{(age in wk)} + 0.21]}{0.8} = \text{mg/kg/hr}$$

1-9 yr, 1 mg/kg/hr; 9-12 yr, 0.9 mg/kg/hr; 12-16 yr (non-smoker), 0.6 mg/kg/hr; 12-16 yr (smoker), 0.9 mg/kg/hr

• Dosages should be individualized based on serum concentration monitoring; total daily doses may also be administered IV q4-6h; infants and children may require q4h dosing due to enhanced metabolism; each 1 mg/kg dose raises serum theophylline concentration 2 mg/L

Neonatal Apnea
Loading dose: IV or PO 5-6 mg/kg; maintenance dose: preterm (<36 wk) IV or PO 1-2 mg/kg/dose q8-12; term (1 mo) PO 2-4 mg/kg/24 hr divided q8-12h

IV administration:
• Recommended concentration: 1-25 mg/ml in D-LR, D-R, D-S, D_5LR, D_5NS, D_5 ¼ NS, D_5W, $D_{10}W$, $D_{20}W$, LR, NS, ½NS, or R

• Maximum concentration: 25 mg/ml

• IV push rate: ≤25 mg/min faster administration may result in excessive peak serum concentrations and circulatory failure

• Intermittent infusion rate: Over 15-30 min q4-6h (intermittent infusion preferred for neonates)

• Continuous infusion: See following maintenance doses

MECHANISM AND INDICATIONS
Bronchodilator mechanism: Relaxes smooth muscle particularly bronchial airways and pulmonary blood vessels, producing a reversal of bronchospasm, increasing respiratory flow rates and vital capacity; increases sensitivity of the medullary respiratory center to CO_2, decreasing apneic episodes in neonates; prevents diaphragmatic fatigue thereby improving contractility in pts with COPD

Indications: Used to treat bronchospasm associated with bronchial asthma; to treat bronchitis, pulmonary emphysema, other COPDs; and to treat neonatal apnea

PHARMACOKINETICS
Peak: PO, sol 1 hr; tabs 2 hr; chewable tabs 1-1.5 hr; enteric coated 5 hr; EXT or caps 4-7 hr; IV, within 30 min

Half-life: Premature 30 hr; newborn-6 mo >25-30 hr; infant over 1 yr 6.9 hr; children 3.4-3.7 hr; adult non-smoker, uncomplicated asthma 6.5-10.9 hr; smoker 1-2 packs/day 4-5 hr; COPD, cardiac failure, liver disease >24 hr

Metabolism: Liver

Excretion: Urine

Therapeutic serum level: Bronchodilation 10-20 mcg/ml; respiratory stimulation 6-13 mcg/ml; toxic concentration >20 mcg/ml. Therapeutic response may be seen at 5-10 mcg serum level and some toxicity noted at 15-20 mcg/ml; therefore close monitoring and individualized dose adjustment is indicated

Guidelines for assessing therapeutic serum level:
• IV bolus, 30 min after end of 30

✤ Available in Canada.

min infusion; IV continuous infusion, 12-24 hr after initiation of infusion; PO (liquid, fast-release tab), peak 1 hr after a dose after at least 1 day of therapy, trough just ā dose after at least 1 day of therapy; PO (slow release product) peak 4 hr after a dose after at least 1 day of therapy, trough just ā dose after at least 1 day of therapy. In patients with a prolonged half-life, assess after 48-72 hr of therapy

CONTRAINDICATIONS AND PRECAUTIONS
• Contraindicated with ethelene-diamine hypersensitivity, uncontrolled arrhythmia, xanthine (caffeine) hypersensitivity, active peptic ulcer disease, seizure disorder (unless on appropriate anticonvulsants)
• Use cautiously with compromised circulatory or cardiac function, diabetes, glaucoma, hyperthyroidism, peptic ulcer, gastroesophageal reflux; renal or hepatic disease, cor pulmonale, hypoxemia; smokers and those who have quit within previous 2 yr; sulfite sensitivity; sustained high fever; infants <1 yr, children, adolescents; lactation (since drug is excreted in breast milk and may cause insomnia, fretfulness, irritability, known potential for toxicity in the breastfed infant exists)

INTERACTIONS
Drug
• Increased serum concentration of theophylline with allopurinol, cimetidine, ciprofloxacin, ephedrine, other sympathomimetics, β-agonists, erythromycin, oral contraceptives, propranolol, ranitidine, thiabendazole, troleandomycin (because of decreased hepatic clearance of theophylline)
• Decreased serum concentration of theophylline with corticosteroids, lithium, barbiturates, phenytoin, carbamazepine, primidone, rifampin, IV isoproterenol; tobacco, marijuana
• Antagonistic effect with β adrenergic blockers (e.g., proprano-

lol) and bronchospasm may result if combination used
• Antagonistic effect when used with propofol; decreases sedative effect of propofol
• Increased potential for toxicity with cardiac glycosides
• Decreased effect of lithium and furosemide
• Increased potential for seizures with ketamine
Nutrition
• Increased serum concentration of theophylline with high carbohydrate diet
• Decreased serum concentration of theophylline with high protein/low carbohydrate diets and charcoal broiled foods
Lab
• Increased serum uric acid possible
• Falsely elevated theophylline levels if furosemide, phenbutazone, probenecid, theobromine, caffeine, tea, chocolate, cola drinks, or acetaminophen present (depending on analytical methods used)

INCOMPATIBILITIES
• Acid solutions
• Alkali sensitive drugs (penicillin G, isoproterenol, thiamine)
• Codeine, chlorpromazine, dobutamine, epinephrine, erythromycin, insulin, meperidine, methadone, methylprednisolone, morphine, phenytoin, tetracycline, vancomycin
• Vitamin B complex; vitamin B with vitamin C
• Others; check with pharmacy before mixing with any other medications

SIDE EFFECTS
CNS: Anxiety, restlessness, headache, dizziness, nervousness, depression, irritability, insomnia, muscle twitching, seizure
CV: Palpitations, arrhythmias, sinus tachycardia, extrasystoles, chest pain, flushing, decreased B/P, circulatory failure, cardiac arrest
DERM: Urticaria, exfoliative dermatitis, rash, alopecia
GI: Nausea, GI upset, vomiting,

---

anorexia, bitter aftertaste, epigastric pain, diarrhea, gastroesophageal reflux
GU: Urinary retention
Local: Redness, pain at IV site
RESP: Tachypnea, respiratory arrest
Other: Hyperglycemia, inappropriate ADH levels, fever

TOXICITY AND OVERDOSE
Clinical signs: Behavior changes, insomnia, headaches, flushing, dizziness, increasing irritability, anorexia, severe nausea or vomiting, seizure, abdominal pain, increased respiratory or heart rate, irregular heart beat, weakness, black or bloody stools, vomiting of dark (dry blood) emesis or blood, urinary urgency, falling B/P; onset of toxicity may be sudden and severe, with seizure, arrhythmia, even death as first sign.
Treatment: Charcoal hemoperfusion may be indicated in severe overdose (level >40 mcg/ml); otherwise induce emesis, (except in patients with impaired consciousness), then give activated charcoal every 4 hr (taking precautions to prevent aspiration) and cathartics; treat seizure with IV diazepam; treat arrhythmias with lidocaine; support cardiac and respiratory systems, provide adequate hydration

PATIENT CARE MANAGEMENT
Assessment
• Assess hypersensitivity to theophylline (and related drugs)
• Assess respiratory status
• Assess baseline VS
• Assess for risks of toxicity: age, lifestyle (smoking, drug use, medical history, medication history—especially any theophylline, time of last dose)
• Obtain height/wt
Interventions
• Administer PO at equally spaced intervals
• Do not crush or allow patient to chew timed release preparations
• Plain tablets may be crushed, administered with food or fluids; can administer with food if GI distress occurs
• Chewable form should be chewed, not swallowed whole
• Maintain age-appropriate fluid intake.
• PO dose can be administered via NG tube
• Avoid rectal forms, if possible, because of erratic and unreliable absorption patterns
• Calculate drug dosage on lean body weight (drug does not distribute to fatty tissue)
• Notify provider for levels ≥20 mcg/ml
• Monitor closely if changing from one route of administration to another; wait 4-6 hr after discontinuing IV therapy to start oral therapy

---

NURSING ALERT

Rapid IV dosing can lead to severe or fatal acute circulatory failure

Serious toxicity is not reliably preceded by less severe side effects

Do not attempt to maintain any dosage that is not well tolerated

Dosage individualization necessary

Some commercial products contain sulfites which may produce hypersensitivity reactions in sensitive individuals

---

Evaluation
• Evaluate therapeutic response (improved respiratory effort)
• Evaluate peak serum levels frequently in infants, young children at least q 6 mo for maintenance therapy, more frequently for acute indications
• Evaluate respiratory status, VS, I&O, ABGs or capillary blood gases (if appropriate)
• Evaluate for signs or symptoms of toxicity
• Evaluate number, severity of apnea spells (if used to treat neonatal apnea)

✤ Available in Canada.

- Evaluate children closely for CNS effects (nervousness, restlessness, insomnia, hyperreflexia, twitching, convulsions)
- Evaluate IV site for pain, inflammation

PATIENT AND FAMILY EDUCATION
Teach/instruct

- To use only prescribed amount of drug; carefully review dosage schedule and preparation with patient and family
- To avoid other medications (especially those for pulmonary disorders) unless prescribed
- To take any missed dose as soon as possible, but *not* to double the dose
- To take drug at regular intervals to maintain blood levels
- To take oral preparations with a full glass of water
- Not to crush or chew sustained- or extended-release tablets; plain tablets may be crushed and given with food or fluid
- That some timed-release capsules can be opened and sprinkled on a spoonful of applesauce or pudding, then swallowed without chewing, followed with juice or water
- To take medication with food if GI upset occurs with liquid or non–sustained-release forms
- About follow-up appointments, lab appointments for monitoring blood levels; emphasize importance of compliance
- That some elixir preparations contain alcohol

Warn/advise

- About adverse effects, signs of toxicity (nausea or vomiting, restlessness, tachycardia, irregular heartbeat, seizure); advise to contact provider immediately if any of these occur
- To avoid drinking large amounts of coffee, tea, cola, cocoa, or eating large amounts of chocolate while on this medication to avoid increased potential for adverse effects

- That smoking decreases drug's effectiveness
- That dizziness may occur; to take precautions to avoid falls
- To not change brands because not all forms are equivalent
- To notify provider if flu symptoms occur; a dose change may be indicated

STORAGE

- Store at room temp
- Protect parenteral form from light, freezing
- Keep out of reach of children

---

amitriptyline hydrochloride

Brand Name(s): Amitril, Apo-Amitriptyline✤, Elavil✤, Endep, Enovil, Amitril

Classification: Tricyclic antidepressant

Pregnancy Category: D

AVAILABLE PREPARATIONS
Tabs: 10 mg, 25 mg, 50 mg, 75 mg, 100 mg, 150 mg

DOSAGES AND ROUTES
Enuresis
Children <6 yr: PO 10 mg at hs
Children >6 yr: PO 10-25 mg at hs

Chronic Pain Management
Children: PO initial 0.1 mg/kg at hs; may advance as tolerated over 2-3 wk to 0.5-2 mg/kg at hs

Depression
Children 6-12 yr: Investigational use PO 10-30 mg/day or 1-1.5 mg/kg/24 hr divided tid
Adolescents: Initial PO 25-50 mg/24 hr qd or divided tid; increase gradually up to 100 mg/24 hr in divided doses; maximum dose 200 mg/24 hr
Adult: 30-100 mg/24 hr as single dose hs or divided tid; may increase gradually to maximum of 300 mg/24 hr

- Safety, effectiveness for use with children <12 have not been established

---

MECHANISM AND INDICATIONS

Mechanism: Amitriptyline inhibits reuptake of serotonin and norepinephrine at presynaptic neuronal membrane, increasing the action of norepinephrine, serotonin in nerve cells

Indications: Used in treating depression, especially depression with insomnia, and in treatment of enuresis

Unlabeled uses: To treat chronic and neuropathic pain; to treat anorexia, bulimia, attention deficit disorder, enuresis and pruritus in cold urticaria; to prevent the onset of cluster/migraine headaches; and to treat pathologic weeping and laughing in people with bilateral forebrain disease due to stroke, MS, trauma, or other causes

PHARMACOKINETICS

Onset of action: Therapeutic antidepressant effects begin in 7-21 days; maximum effects may not occur for 2 wk; however, adequate response may require continual use for 4-6 wk or longer

Therapeutic reference range: Therapeutic level 110-250 ng/ml; analgesia levels >120 ng/ml

Peak: 2-12 hr; PO, 45 mins

Half-life: Adults 9-50 hr, 15 hr average

Metabolism: Liver

Excretion: Mainly in urine, small amounts in feces

CONTRAINDICATIONS AND PRECAUTIONS

• Contraindicated with hypersensitivity to amitriptyline or any component of this medication, any other tricyclic antidepressant or maprotiline; pts receiving MAOI antidepressants within past 14 days; angina; recent heart attack; asthma; electroshock therapy; lactation; untreated narrow-angle glaucoma

• Use cautiously with children and adolescents; treated narrow-angle glaucoma; increased intraocular pressure; bipolar disorder; diabetes; cardiac conduction disturbances; cerebrovascular disease; heart failure; hyperthyroidism (or those receiving thyroid hormone replacement); kidney disease; liver disease; GI problems; severe depression; paranoia; pregnancy; prostate gland enlargement; schizophrenia; suicidal tendencies; surgery under general anesthesia; spasms of ureter or urethra; history of urinary retention; pregnancy; lactation

INTERACTIONS

Drug

• Increased sedation with alcohol, antihistamines, antipsychotics, barbiturates, glutethimide, chloral hydrate, sedatives, benzodiazepines, CNS depressant drugs

• Increased hypotension with methyldopa, β-adrenergic blockers, clonidine, diuretics

• May lead to a hypertensive crisis with clonidine and may decrease effects of clonidine

• Additive cardiotoxicity with quinidine, thioridazine, mesoridazine

• Additive anticholinergic toxicity with antihistamines, antiparkinsonians, thioridazine, OTC sleeping medications, GI antispasmodics and antidiarrheals

• Increased effects of warfarin, dicumarol, barbiturates, benzodiazepines, CNS depressants, phenothiazines, adrenergic agents (e.g., epinephrine, isoproterenol), anticholinergic agents, atropine-like drugs

• Possible decreased effects of antihypertensives and guanethidine possible; indirect acting sympathomimetics, such as ephedrine

• Impaired heart rhythm and function possible with thyroid preparations; thyroid dosage may have to be adjusted

• Increased risk of hyperpyretic crisis, convulsions, hypertensive episode with MAOIs; hyperpyrexia, tachycardia, hypertension, confusion, seizures, and death have been reported

• Decreased metabolism of ami-

triptyline with cimetidine, methylphenidate
• Increased gastric emptying time, therefore absorption may be slowed, causing inactivation of some drugs in stomach

Nutrition
• Do not drink alcohol

Lab
• Increased alk phos, ALT/GPT, AST/GOT, eosinophils, serum bilirubin, BG, transaminase
• Decreased white cells and platelets, VMA, 5-HIAA, blood glucose
• Falsely elevated urinary catecholamines
• Results of the metyrapone test may be affected by this medicine
• Liver toxicity may be confused with viral hepatitis

SIDE EFFECTS
• Anticholinergic effects may be more pronounced with amitriptyline than other tricyclic antidepressants; moderate to marked sedation can occur; tolerance to these effects usually develops
CNS: Dizziness, drowsiness, agitation, anxiety, ataxia, impaired cognitive function, confusion, disorientation, EPS, fainting, fatigue, unsteady gait, incoordination, hallucinations, headache, insomnia, lethargy, mood changes, nightmares, increased psychiatric symptoms, restlessness, sedation, seizures, stimulation, tremor, weakness
CV: Orthostatic hypotension, arrhythmias, ECG changes, particularly in children with AV dissociation, prolonged PR intervals, widened QRS; CHF, heart block; heart palpitations, hypertension, sudden death, tachycardia, thrombosis, ventricular flutter and fibrillation
DERM: Erythema, hives, itching, petechiae, photosensitivity, rash, sweating, swelling of face or tongue
EENT: Blurred vision, dysphagia, increased intraocular pressure, irritation of tongue or mouth, stomatitis, mydriasis, ophthalmoplegia, peculiar taste, ringing in ears

GI: Dry mouth, diarrhea, anorexia, increased appetite, constipation, cramps, decreased lower esophageal sphincter tone with GE reflux, GI distress, hepatitis, indigestion, jaundice, altered liver function tests, nausea, paralytic ileus, stomatitis, vomiting, weight gain
GU: Urinary retention, impotence, decreased libido, inhibited female orgasm, inhibited ejaculation, galactorrhea, gynecomastia, swelling of testicles (usually disappears 2-10 days after discontinuation of this medication), kidney damage
HEME: Agranulocytosis, bone marrow depression, eosinophilia, leukopenia, thrombocytopenia
Other: Allergic reactions, dysarthria, peripheral neuritis, syndrome of inappropriate antidiuretic hormone, fluctuation of BS levels, neuroleptic malignant syndrome, conversion of depression to mania in bipolar disorders

TOXICITY AND OVERDOSE
• Toxic >0.5 mcg/ml (500 ng/ml)
Clinical signs: Agitation, arrhythmias, coma, confusion, disturbed concentration, severe drowsiness, fever, hallucinations, heart palpitations, hypotension, hypothermia, dilated pupils, restlessness, seizures, shortness of breath, deep sleep, stupor, tachycardia, tremor, urinary retention, vomiting, weakness
Treatment: Maintain normal temperature, monitor ECG, induce emesis, lavage, administer activated charcoal, administer anticonvulsant; correct acidosis with $NaHCO_3$ to increase protein binding, decrease free fraction; correction of acidosis may decrease CV toxicities; avoid disopyramide, procainamide, quinidine; lidocaine, phenytoin, or propranolol may be necessary; reserve physostigmine for refractory life-threatening anticholinergic toxicities
• For life-threatening arrhythmias or seizures in *children,* slow IV, physostigmine 0.01-0.03 mg/

kg/dose up to 0.5 mg/dose over 2-3 min, repeat in 5 min; maximum total dose 2 mg; *adolescents and adults,* 2 mg/dose physostigmine, may repeat 1-2 mg in 20 min and give 1-4 mg slow IV over 5-10 min if signs and symptoms recur

PATIENT CARE MANAGEMENT
Assessment
• Assess history of hypersensitivity to drug
• Obtain careful history to identify CV, blood, and other diseases
• Obtain baseline wt, VS, CBC counts with differential, AST, ALT, bilirubin
• Obtain baseline ECG for flattening of T wave, bundle branch block, AV block, arrhythmias
• Assess mental status (mood, sensorium, affect, impulsiveness, suicidal tendencies, psychiatric symptoms, panic)

Interventions
• Tab may be crushed for administration; if GI symptoms occur, administer with food or milk
• May be administered without regard to meals
• May administer entire dose hs if oversedation occurs during the day
• Increase fluids, fiber in diet if constipation or urinary retention occurs
• Rinse with water, take sips of fluid, sugarless gum, hard candy for dry mouth
• Withhold this drug if electroconvulsive therapy (ECT) is to be used to treat depression
• Help with ambulation when therapy is begun; dizziness or drowsiness may occur
• Taper medication before surgery
• Record nightly wettings if using for enuresis

NURSING ALERT

IM not to be used in children

Do not use at the same time as or within 14 days of administration of MAO type A inhibitor drugs

---

Evaluation
• Evaluate therapeutic response (ability to function in daily activities, ability to sleep throughout the night, symptoms of depression, enuresis)
• Evaluate mental status (mood, sensorium, affect, impulsiveness, suicidal tendencies, psychiatric symptoms, panic)
• Monitor VS, including orthostatic B/P; if systolic B/P drops 20 mm Hg, hold amitriptyline and notify care provider
• Monitor wt
• Evaluate cardiac enzymes with long-term therapy
• Evaluate for urinary retention, constipation
• Evaluate for other side effects, especially if pt has history of seizures, allergies, or cardiac disease
• Evaluate need for continuing medication at least q 6 mo
• Withdrawal symptoms may occur if amitriptyline is discontinued abruptly (headache, nausea, vomiting, muscle pain, weakness)

PATIENT AND FAMILY EDUCATION
Teach/instruct
• To take as directed at prescribed intervals for prescribed length of time
• That medicine sometimes must be taken for 3-4 wk before improvement is noticed
• That medication is most helpful when used as part of comprehensive multimodal treatment program
• To make sure medication is swallowed
• Not to discontinue medication without prescriber approval
• About rationale for follow-up visits
• To avoid ingesting alcohol, other CNS depressants
• Not to use OTC drugs without consulting prescriber
• That smoking may speed elimination of amitriptyline; if pt smokes, dosage may need to be increased

---

✤ Available in Canada.

Warn/advise
• That medication may cause drowsiness; be careful on bicycles, skates, skateboards, while driving, with other activities requiring alertness
• To stay out of direct sunlight (especially between 10 AM and 3 PM) if possible; if pt must be outside, wear protective clothing, hat, sunglasses; put on sun block that has skin protection factor (SPF) of at least 15
• That amitriptyline can inhibit sweating, impair the body's ability to cope with hot environments, increasing the risk of heat stroke; avoid saunas, hot tubs, steam baths
• To not stop medication suddenly after long-term use; may cause nausea, headache, vomiting, muscle pain, weakness
• That the effects of medicine may last for 3-7 days after discontinuation

STORAGE
• Store at room temp in tightly closed container
• Do not freeze inj sol
• Protect inj sol from light

---

amobarbital sodium

Brand Name(s): Amobarbital Sodium, Amytal✚, Amytal Sodium, Amytal Sodium Pulvules

Classification: Sedative, intermediate-acting hypnotic-barbiturate

Controlled Substance Schedule II (USA)

Pregnancy Category: B

AVAILABLE PREPARATIONS
Tabs: 30 mg, 50 mg, 100 mg
Caps: 65 mg, 200 mg
Inj: As powder in 250 mg/vial, 500 mg/vial

DOSAGES AND ROUTES
Sedation
PO 2-5 mg/kg/24 hr divided qid

Insomnia
IM 3-5 mg/kg at hs
Anticonvulsant/psychiatry
Child <6 yr: IM, IV 3-5 mg/kg
Children >6 yr and adults: IV 65-500 mg
IV administration
• Recommended concentration: Dilute 125 mg in 1.25 ml SW, results in 10% sol
• IV push rate: Child, give by direct IV at 60 mg/m^2/1 min; adult, 100 mg or less/min
• Do not exceed 1 ml of 10% sol/min

MECHANISM AND INDICATIONS
Mechanism: Depresses activity in the posterior hypothalamus, limbic structures, reticular activating system of the brain stem; decreases seizure activity by inhibiting nerve impulses
Indications: Used as preanesthetic sedation, as an adjunct in psychiatry, to treat insomnia, after trying conservative measures, in treating seizures

PHARMACOKINETICS
Onset of action: When used to treat insomnia, clinical effects may take 2 nights; PO 45-60 min; IV 5 min
Duration: PO 6-8 hr; IV 3-6 hr
Half-life: 16-40 hr
Metabolism: Liver
Excretion: Urine (as inactive metabolites)

CONTRAINDICATIONS AND PRECAUTIONS
• Contraindicated with hypersensitivity to amobarbital, any component of this medication, or barbiturates; history of addiction to barbiturates; severe liver impairment; porphyria; respiratory depression
• Use cautiously with severe anemia; history of asthma; history of alcohol abuse, drug abuse, or dependence; acute or chronic pain; anemia; mental depression; DM; emphysema; children with hyperactivity; hypertension; hyperthyroidism; kidney disease; liver disease; underactive adrenal gland; pregnancy; lactation

---

INTERACTIONS
Drug
• Increased half-life of doxycycline
• Increased CNS depression with alcohol, MAOIs, sedatives, narcotics
• Decreased effects of oral anticoagulants, oral contraceptives, corticosteroids, estrogens, griseofulvin, quinidine
Nutrition
• Do not drink alcohol
Lab
• Falsely elevated sulfobromophthalein
• Inaccurate metyrapone test

INCOMPATIBILITIES
• Incompatible in sol or syringe with cefazolin, cephalothin, chlorpromazine, cimetidine, clindamycin, codeine, dimenhydrinate, droperidol, hydrocortisone, hydroxyzine, insulin, levarterenol, levorphanol, meperidine, pentazocine, penicillin G, phytonadione, procaine, prochlorperazine, streptomycin, tetracycline, thiamine, trifluoperazine, vancomycin

SIDE EFFECTS
CNS: CNS depression, physical dependence, mental depression, dizziness, drowsiness, hangover, lethargy, light-headedness, slurred speech, stimulation in children
CV: Bradycardia, hypotension
DERM: Abscess at injection site, angioedema, hives, pain, rash, Stevens-Johnson syndrome, thrombophlebitis
GI: Constipation, diarrhea, nausea, vomiting
HEME: Agranulocytosis, thrombocytopenia, megaloblastic anemia with long-term treatment
RESP: Apnea, bronchospasm, laryngospasm, respiratory depression

TOXICITY AND OVERDOSE
Clinical signs: Cold, clammy skin; coma; severe confusion; CNS depression; severe drowsiness; cyanosis of lips; delirium; hallucinations; hypotension; nausea; pulmonary constriction; pupillary constriction; shortness of breath, or slow or troubled breathing; slow heartbeat; slurred speech; staggering; vomiting; weakness; possibly death
Treatment: Supportive care, administer activated charcoal, lavage, alkalinize urine, give IV volume expanders/IV fluids, dialysis

PATIENT CARE MANAGEMENT
Assessment
• Assess history of hypersensitivity to drug
• Obtain baseline VS
Interventions
• Administer PO on empty stomach for best absorption
• Make sure PO dose was swallowed
• Mix with SW for IM injection; inject within 30 min of mixing preparation
• Administer IM inj deep in large muscle mass to prevent tissue sloughing, abscesses
• Administer IV only with resuscitative equipment available
• Administer ½-2 hr before hs for insomnia
• Provide assistance with ambulation after administration
Evaluation
• Evaluate therapeutic response (ability to sleep at night, decreased amount of early morning awakening or decrease in seizures)
• Evaluate mental status (mood, sensorium, affect, short and long-term memory)
• Evaluate for signs, symptoms of toxicity
• Monitor Hct, Hgb, RBCs, blood dyscrasias, serum folate, vitamin D, AST, ALT, bilirubin if on long-term therapy
• Amobarbital is usually discontinued if liver function tests are increased
• Monitor PT in patients receiving anticoagulants
• Monitor character, rate, rhythm of respirations; hold amobarbital if respirations <10/min, if pupils dilated
• Monitor for physical dependency; signs include more frequent

requests for medication, shakes, anxiety

PATIENT AND FAMILY EDUCATION
Teach/instruct
• To take as directed at prescribed intervals for prescribed length of time
• To make sure PO medication is swallowed
• To tell all care providers that amobarbital is being taken
• Not to discontinue medication without prescriber approval
• That hangover is common, dreaming may increase
• About complementary methods to improve sleep (exercise several hr before hs, warm bath, quiet time, reading, TV, warm milk, self-hypnosis, deep breathing)
• That amobarbital is only for short-term treatment of insomnia, is generally ineffective after 2 wk
• That withdrawal insomnia may occur after short-term use
Warn/advise
• To avoid ingesting alcohol, other CNS depressants, e.g., antihistamines or medicine for allergies or colds, sedatives, tranquilizers, sleeping medicine, prescription pain medicine or narcotics, medicine for seizures, muscle relaxants, anesthetics (including some dental anesthetics)
• That medication may cause drowsiness
• To be careful on bicycles, skates, skateboards, while driving, during other activities requiring alertness
• That medication may become habit-forming if too much is used or if used for 45-90 days

STORAGE
• Store away from heat, direct light
• Do not store amobarbital in damp places; heat or moisture may cause medicine to break down
• Do not keep medicine which is no longer needed

---

amoxicillin and clavulanate potassium
Brand Name(s): Augmentin, Clavulin✤
Classification: Antibiotic (aminopenicillin)
Pregnancy Category: B

AVAILABLE PREPARATIONS
Oral susp: 125 mg amoxicillin, 31.25 mg clavulanic acid/5 ml; 250 mg amoxicillin, 62.5 mg clavulanic acid/5 ml
Chewable tabs: 125 mg amoxicillin, 31.25 mg clavulanic acid; 250 mg amoxicillin, 62.5 mg clavulanic acid
Tabs: 250 mg, 500 mg amoxicillin each with 125 mg clavulanic acid

ROUTES AND DOSAGES
Children: 40 mg/kg/24 hr of amoxicillin component divided q8h
Adults: 250-500 mg q8h; maximum dose 2 g/24 hr

MECHANISM AND INDICATIONS
Antibiotic mechanism: Amoxicillin is bactericidal; inhibits bacterial cell wall synthesis by adhering to bacterial penicillin-binding proteins. Clavulanate has a weak antibacterial effect; binds irreversibly with certain β-lactamase, prevents them from inactivating amoxicillin, thus enhancing its bactericidal activity
Indications: Effective against some gram-positive and gram-negative bacteria, including *Neisseria meningitidis, Haemophilus influenzae, Escherichia coli, Proteus mirabilis, Citrobacter diversus, Klebsiella pneumoniae, Proteus vulgaris, Salmonella,* and *Shigella;* used to treat infections of lower and upper respiratory tracts, ear, GU tract, soft tissue, skin

PHARMACOKINETICS
Peak: 1.0-2.5 hr
Distribution: Diffuses into most body fluids and tissues, except

---

CSF (unless meninges are inflamed) and synovial fluid
Half-life: Amoxicillin 1.0-1.5 hr; clavulanate 1.0-1.5 hr
Metabolism: Liver
Excretion: Urine

CONTRAINDICATIONS AND PRECAUTIONS
• Contraindicated with known hypersensitivity to amoxicillin, penicillins, or cephalosporins, and with infectious mononucleosis (rash may develop during therapy)
• Use cautiously with renal impairment and pregnancy

INTERACTIONS
Drug
• Decreased effectiveness with use of erythromycin, tetracycline, chloramphenicol
• Increased serum concentrations of drug with use of probenecid
• Increased serum concentrations of methotrexate
• Increased incidence of skin rash from both drugs with use of allopurinol
Lab
• False positive for urine protein
• False positive Coombs' test
• False decrease of serum aminoglycoside concentrations possible

SIDE EFFECTS
GI: Nausea, vomiting, diarrhea, pseudomembranous colitis
GU: Acute interstitial nephritis
HEME: Anemia, thrombocytopenia, thrombocytopenic purpura, eosinophilia, leukopenia
Other: Hypersensitivity (erythematous maculopapular rash, urticaria, anaphylaxis), bacterial or fungal superinfection

TOXICITY AND OVERDOSE
Clinical signs: Neuromuscular sensitivity, seizures
Treatment: If treated within 4 hr of ingestion, empty stomach by induced vomiting or gastric lavage, follow with activated charcoal to reduce absorption; supportive care; hemodialysis

PATIENT CARE MANAGEMENT
Assessment
• Assess history of hypersensitivity to amoxicillin, penicillins, cephalosporins
• Obtain C&S; may begin therapy before obtaining results
• Assess renal function (BUN, creatinine, I&O), bowel pattern
Interventions
• Administer penicillins at least 1 hr before bacteriostatic antibiotics (tetracyclines, erythromycins, chloramphenicol)
• May administer PO without regard to meals; administer with food if GI distress occurs; shake susp well before administering
• Tabs may be crushed, cap taken apart and mixed with food or fluid
• To avoid doubling dose of clavulanic acid, do not administer two 250 mg tabs in place of one 500 mg tab; there is 125 mg clavulanic acid in each 250 mg tab and each 500 mg tab
• Maintain age-appropriate fluid intake
• For group A β-hemolytic streptococcal infection, provide 10-day course of treatment to prevent risk of acute rheumatic fever, glomerulonephritis

> **NURSING ALERT**
> Discontinue drug if hypersensitivity, bone marrow toxicity, pseudomembranous colitis, acute interstitial nephritis develops

Evaluation
• Evaluate therapeutic response (decreased signs of infection)
• Monitor signs of superinfection (perineal itching, diaper rash, fever, malaise, redness, pain, swelling, drainage, rash, diarrhea, sore throat, change in cough or sputum)
• Observe for hypersensitivity reactions (wheezing, tightness in chest, urticaria), especially within 15-20 min of first dose

---

♣ Available in Canada.

• Monitor bowel pattern; diarrhea may be symptomatic of pseudo-membranous colitis

• Monitor renal functions (BUN, creatinine, I&O), hepatic functions (ALT, AST, bilirubin), and hematologic functions (CBC, differential, platelet count) with prolonged (and/or high dose) therapy or with premature infants or neonates

PATIENT AND FAMILY EDUCATION
Teach/intruct
• To take as directed at prescribed intervals, for prescribed length of time
Warn/advise
• To notify care provider of hypersensitivity, side effects, superinfection

STORAGE
• Store tabs or powder at room temp
• Reconstituted susp stable when refrigerated for 14 days or when kept at room temp for 7 days; label date, time of reconstitution

---

amoxicillin trihydrate
Brand Name(s): A-cillin, Amoxil♣, Apo-Amoxi♣, Larotid, Novamoxin♣, Nu-Amoxi♣, Polymox, Trimox, Ultimox, Wymox

Classification: Antibiotic (aminopenicillin)

Pregnancy Category: B

AVAILABLE PREPARATIONS
Drops: 50 mg/ml
Oral susp: 125 mg/5 ml, 250 mg/5 ml
Caps: 250 mg, 500 mg
Chewable tabs: 125 mg, 250 mg

ROUTES AND DOSAGES
Children: 40 mg/kg/24 hr divided q8h
Adults: 250-500 mg q8h; maximum 2-3 g/24 hr

Acute, Uncomplicated Gonorrhea Caused by *N. gonorrhoeae*:
Children >2 yr, <45 kg: PO 50 mg/kg as single dose with probenecid 25 mg/kg; maximum probenecid dose 1 g
Children >45 kg: PO 3 g as single dose with probenecid 1 g
Prophylaxis of Bacterial Endocarditis
Children <30 kg: PO 50 mg/kg 1 hr before procedure and 25 mg/kg 6 hr later (maximum 3 g initial dose; 1.5 g follow-up dose)
Children >30 kg: PO 3 g 1 hr before procedure and 1.5 g 6 hr later

MECHANISM AND INDICATIONS
Antibiotic mechanism: Bactericidal; adheres to bacterial penicillin-binding proteins, thus inhibiting bacterial cell wall synthesis
Indications: Active against gram-positive cocci (including *Streptococcus pneumoniae*, *Str. pyogenes*, *Staphylococcus aureus*, *Neisseria gonorrhoeae*, *N. meningitidis*, *Escherichia coli*), gram-negative bacilli (including *Corynebacterium diphtheriae*, *Listeria monocytogenes*), and gram-negative bacilli (including *Haemophilus influenzae*, *Proteus mirabilis*, and *Salmonella*). Used to treat upper respiratory and GU tract; ear, skin, and soft tissue infections; and bacterial endocarditis prophylaxis

PHARMACOKINETICS
Peak: 1.0-2.5 hr
Distribution: Diffuses into most body fluids and tissues, except CSF (unless meninges are inflamed) and synovial fluid
Half-life: 1.0 hr
Metabolism: Liver
Excretion: Urine

CONTRAINDICATIONS AND PRECAUTIONS
• Contraindicated with a history of hypersensitivity to amoxicillin, penicillins, or cephalosporins, with infectious mononucleosis (many develop a rash during therapy)

♣ Available in Canada.

• Use cautiously with impaired renal function; history of colitis (or other GI disease); pregnancy

INTERACTIONS
Drug
• Synergistic antimicrobial activity against some strains of enterococci and group B streptococci with aminoglycosides
• Increased serum concentrations of drug with use of probenecid
• Increased serum concentrations of methotrexate
• Decreased effectiveness with use of tetracyclines, erythromycins, chloramphenicol
• Enhanced effect with use of clavulanate potassium
• Increased incidence of skin rash from both drugs with use of allopurinol

Lab
• False decrease of serum aminoglycoside concentrations
• False positive for urine protein
• False positive for Coombs' test

Incompatibilities
• Aminoglycosides

SIDE EFFECTS
GI: Nausea, vomiting, diarrhea, pseudomembranous colitis
GU: Acute interstitial nephritis
HEME: Anemia, thrombocytopenia, thrombocytopenic purpura, eosinophilia, leukopenia
Other: Hypersensitivity (erythematous maculopapular rash, urticaria, anaphylaxis), bacterial or fungal superinfection

TOXICITY AND OVERDOSE
Clinical signs: Neuromuscular hypersensitivity, seizures
Treatment: If treated within 4 hr of ingestion, empty stomach by induced vomiting or gastric lavage, follow with activated charcoal; supportive care; hemodialysis

PATIENT CARE MANAGEMENT
Assessment
• Assess history of hypersensitivity to amoxicillin, penicillins, cephalosporins
• Obtain C&S; may begin therapy before obtaining results

• Assess renal function (BUN, creatinine, I&O), bowel pattern
Interventions
• Administer penicillins at least 1 hr before bacteriostatic antibiotics (tetracyclines, erythromycins, chloramphenicol)
• May administer PO without regard to meals; administer with food if GI distress occurs; shake susp well before administering; tabs may be crushed, caps taken apart and mixed with food or fluid
• Maintain age-appropriate fluid intake
• For group A β-hemolytic streptococcal infection, provide 10-day course of treatment to prevent risk of acute rheumatic fever or glomerulonephritis

> **NURSING ALERT**
> Discontinue drug if hypersensitivity, bone marrow toxicity, pseudomembranous colitis, acute interstitial nephritis develop

Evaluation
• Evaluate therapeutic response (decreased symptoms of infection)
• Monitor signs of superinfection (perineal itching, diaper rash, fever, malaise, redness, pain, swelling, drainage, rash, diarrhea, sore throat, change in cough or sputum)
• Observe for signs of hypersensitivity (respiratory change, urticaria) especially within 30 min of first dose
• Monitor bowel pattern; diarrhea may be symptomatic of pseudomembranous colitis
• Monitor renal functions (BUN, creatinine, I&O), hematologic functions (CBC, differential, platelet count), and hepatic functions (ALT, AST, bilirubin) with prolonged (and/or high dose) therapy or with premature infants or neonates

PATIENT AND FAMILY EDUCATION
Teach/instruct
• To take as directed at prescribed

intervals, for prescribed length of time

Warn/advise
• To notify care provider of hypersensitivity, side effects, superinfection

STORAGE
• Store tabs, caps, or powder at room temp
• Reconstituted susp is stable when refrigerated for 14 days or when kept at room temp for 7 days; label date, time of reconstitution

---

amphotericin

Brand Name(s): Fungizone, Fungizone Intravenous♣

Classification: Antifungal agent

Pregnancy Category: B

AVAILABLE PREPARATIONS
Inj: Powder for reconstitution 50 mg
Top: 3% cream, lotion, oint

ROUTES AND DOSAGES
IV
Infants and children: Test dose: 0.1 mg/kg/dose up to max 1 mg; infuse over 30-60 min; follow with initial dose of 0.25 mg/kg/24 hr; increment: increase as tolerated by 0.125-0.25 mg/kg/24 hr qd or qod; maintenance dose 0.25-1 mg/kg/24 hr qd or 1-1.5 mg/kg/dose qod; infuse over 2-6 hr; maximum 1.5 mg/kg/24 hr
Adults: Test dose 1 mg infused over 20-30 min; initial dose 0.25 mg/kg, increase as tolerated by 0.25 mg/kg/24 hr; maintenance dose 0.25-1 mg/kg/dose qod or 1-1.5 mg/kg/dose qod; infuse over 2-6 hrs
Infants and children: IT 25-100 mcg q48-72h; increase to 500 mcg as tolerated
Adult: IT 100 mcg q48-72 hrs, increase to 500 mcg as tolerated
Bladder Irrigation
Children and adults: 5-15 mg amphotericin/100 ml SW irrigation solution at 100-300 ml/24 hr;

instill fluid into bladder, clamp catheter for 60-120 min, drain bladder; irrigate tid-qid for 2-5 days (Note: smaller volume may be used for smaller children because of smaller bladder size)

TOP
Apply to affected areas bid-qid for 7-21 days or longer if needed

IV administration
• Recommended concentration: 0.1 mg/ml in D_5W, $D_{10}W$, $D_{15}W$, $D_{20}W$
• Maximum concentration: 0.1 mg/ml
• Intermittent infusion rate: over 2-6 hr

MECHANISM AND INDICATIONS
Mechanism: Binds to ergosterol, altering cell membrane permeability in fungi and causing leaking of cell components with cell death resulting
Indications: Used to treat severe systemic infections caused by susceptible fungi

PHARMACOKINETICS
Peak: 1-2 hr after infusion
Distribution: Minimal amounts enter CNS, eye, bile, pleural, pericardial, synovial, or amniotic fluids
Half-life: 24 hr; increased in small neonates
Metabolism: Liver
Excretion: Urine, breast milk
Absorption: Absorbed poorly from GI tract

CONTRAINDICATIONS AND PRECAUTIONS
• Contraindicated with hypersensitivity to amphotericin or any component, severe bone marrow depression
• Use cautiously with other nephrotoxic drugs, in infants (because of lower elimination), and with pregnancy

INTERACTIONS
Drug
• Additive toxic effects with use of nephrotoxic drugs
• Increased K^+ depletion because of amphotericin with use of corticosteroids

---

♣ Available in Canada.

• Increased risk of toxicity with use of cardiac glycosides, skeletal muscle relaxants because of hypokalemia
• Antagonism: miconazole

Lab
• Increased BUN, serum creatinine, alk phos, bilirubin levels possible
• Hypokalemia, hypomagnesemia possible
• Decreased WBC, RBC, platelet counts possible

SIDE EFFECTS
CNS: Fever, delirium, headache, chills, vertigo, paresthesia, peripheral neuropathy
CV: Hypotension, hypertension, arrhythmias, flushing
DERM: With top: dryness, irritation, pruritus, dermatitis
EENT: Vision changes, tinnitus, deafness
GI: Anorexia, nausea, vomiting, diarrhea, cramps, hemorrhagic gastroenteritis, acute liver failure
GU: Renal tubular acidosis, renal failure, azotemia, anuria, oliguria
HEME: Leukopenia, thrombocytopenia, anemia, agranulocytosis, eosinophilia
METAB: Hypokalemia, hyponatremia, hypomagnesemia
Local: Phlebitis, necrosis, irritation at injection site
Other: Arthralgia, myalgia, weakness

TOXICITY AND OVERDOSE
Clinical signs: CV, respiratory function affected
Treatment: Supportive care

PATIENT CARE MANAGEMENT
Assessment
• Assess history of hypersensitivity to amphotericin B, drug components
• Obtain C&S before starting medication
• Assess baseline renal status (BUN, creatinine, I&O), hepatic status (ALT, AST, bilirubin), hematologic status (CBC, differential, platelet count)

Interventions
• Prepare IV infusion exactly as manufacturer directs
• Administer test dose as ordered to avoid anaphylactic reaction
• Use an inline filter with a pore size ≥1 micron
• Do not mix with other medications; infuse separately; do not mix with Na sol, or diluent with preservatives
• Reduce pain at injection site by adding 1 U heparin/ml of sol
• Hydration, Na repletion before administration may reduce risk of nephrotoxicity
• Use distal veins; rotate site frequently
• Premedicate with acetaminophen, diphenhydramine as ordered to reduce risk of adverse reactions; administer meperidine as ordered to reduce rigors; administer corticosteroids as ordered to reduce febrile response
• Top: cleanse area as ordered; use cream or ointment for groin, neck, axillae; apply sparingly; do not use occlusive dressings

---

NURSING ALERT
Cardiovascular collapse has been reported after rapid IV infusion

Premedicate as ordered with acetaminophen, diphenhydramine, meperidine, corticosteroids to reduce adverse reactions with IV infusion

---

Evaluation
• Evaluate therapeutic response (decreased fever, malaise, rash, negative C&S for infecting organism
• Monitor VS q 30 min for first 4 hr after start of IV infusion; q1h if afebrile; febrile reaction may start 1-2 hr into infusion; usuually subsides within 4 hr of discontinuing drug
• Monitor renal status (BUN, creatinine, I&O), hepatic status (ALT, AST, bilirubin), hematologic status (CBC, differential, platelet count), electrolyte status (K⁺, Mg)

A

- Monitor for allergic reaction (rash)
- Monitor for hypokalemia (anorexia, drowsiness, weakness, decreased reflexes, dizziness, increased urinary output, increased thirst, paresthesias)
- Monitor for ototoxicity (tinnitus, vertigo, loss of hearing)
- Evaluate IV site for extravasation, vein irritation

PATIENT AND FAMILY EDUCATION
Teach/instruct
- To take as directed at prescribed intervals for prescribed length of time
Warn/advise
- To notify care provider of hypersensitivity, side effects
- To notify care provider if no improvement is noted in 2 wk
- That top forms may discolor skin, clothing; remove by using soap and water or standard cleaning fluid
- To use careful personal hygiene to prevent spread of lesions
- To avoid use of OTC creams, lotions unless prescribed by care provider
- To comply with follow-up care; therapy may require several mos

STORAGE
- Store powder in refrigerator, protected from light, moisture
- Reconstituted sol stable for 1 wk in refrigerator
- Store top forms at room temp

---

ampicillin, ampicillin sodium

Brand Name(s): Amcill, Ampicin✤, Amplin, Omnipen, Penamp, Polycillin, Polycillin-N, Principen, Totacillin, Totacillin-N

Classification: Antibiotic (aminopenicillin)

Pregnancy Category: B

AVAILABLE PREPARATIONS
Pediatric drops: 100 mg/ml
Oral susp: 125 mg/5 ml, 250 mg/5 ml
Tabs, caps: 250 mg, 500 mg
Inj: 125 mg, 250 mg, 500 mg; 1 g, 2 g, 10 g

ROUTES AND DOSAGES
PO
Infants and children: 50-100 mg/kg/24 hr divided q6h (maximum: 2-3 g/24 hr)
Adults: 250-500 mg q6h
Acute uncomplicated gonorrhea caused by N. gonorrhoeae: Wt ≥45 kg, 3.5 g as single dose with probenecid 1.0 g
IM/IV
Neonates: Wt <1200 g, age 0-4 wk, for meningitis or severe infections 50 mg/kg/dose q12h, for mild infections 25 mg/kg/dose q12h; wt 1200-2000 g, age 0-7 days, for meningitis or severe infections 50 mg/kg/dose q12h, for mild infections 25 mg/kg/dose q12h; wt 1200-2000 g, age >7 days, for meningitis or severe infections 50 mg/kg/dose q8h, for mild infections 25 mg/kg/dose q8h; wt >2000 g, age 0-7 days, for meningitis or severe infections 50 mg/kg/dose q8h, for mild infections 25 mg/kg/dose q8h; wt >2000 g, age >7 days, for meningitis or severe infections 50 mg/kg/dose q6h, for mild infections 25 mg/kg/dose q6h
Infants and children: For meningitis and severe infections 200-400 mg/kg/24 hr divided q4-6 (maximum 12 g/24 hr); for mild infections 100-200 mg/kg/24 hr divided q4-6h
Adults: 500 mg-3 gm q4-6h
Bacterial Endocarditis Prophylaxis (see Appendix H)
Children <27 kg: For dental surgery, IM/IV 50 mg/kg (maximum 2 g) 30-60 min before procedure and 8 hours later; administer with gentamycin 2 mg/kg IM/IV (maximum 80 mg); for GI, GU, biliary tract surgery, IM/IV 50 mg/kg (maximum 2 g) 30-60 min before procedure and 8 hr later; administer with gentamycin IM/IV 2 mg/kg (maximum 80 mg)

Children >27 kg: for dental surgery, IM/IV 2 g 30-60 min before procedure and 1 g 8 h later; administer with gentamycin IM/IV 1.5 mg/kg (maximum 80 mg); for GI, GU, biliary tract surgery, IM/IV 2 g 30-60 min before procedure and 1 g 8 h later; administer with gentamycin IM/IV 1.5 mg/kg (maximum 80 mg)

IV administration
• Recommended concentration: ≤30 mg/ml in LR, NS, or SW for IV infusion
• Maximum concentration: 100 mg/ml in NS or SW for IV push
• IV push rate: Over 3-5 min; not to exceed 100 mg/min in adults
• Intermittent infusion: Over 10-15 min for larger doses

MECHANISM AND INDICATIONS

Antibiotic mechanism: Bactericidal; inhibits bacterial cell wall synthesis by adhering to bacterial penicillin-binding proteins
Indications: Effective against many gram-positive and gram-negative organisms, including *Haemophilus influenzae, Escherichia coli, Proteus mirabilis, Salmonella, Shigella, Neisseria gonorrhoeae, N. meningitidis, Staphylococcus aureus, Streptococcus pneumoniae,* and *Str. pyogenes;* used to treat ear, meningeal, upper respiratory, GU, skin, and soft tissue infections

PHARMACOKINETICS

Peak: PO 1-2 hr; IM 1 hr
Distribution: To most body tissues; high CNS penetration only with inflamed meninges
Half-life: 1.0-1.5 hr
Metabolism: Liver
Excretion: Urine

CONTRAINDICATIONS AND PRECAUTIONS

• Contraindicated with known hypersensitivity to ampicillin, penicillins, or cephalosporins; with infectious mononucleosis (many develop a rash during therapy)
• Use cautiously with impaired renal function, history of colitis or other GI disorders, and pregnancy

INTERACTIONS

Drug
• Synergistic antimicrobial activity against some strains of enterococci and group B streptococci with use of aminoglycosides
• Increased serum concentrations of drug with use of probenecid
• Increased serum concentrations of methotrexate
• Decreased effectiveness with use of tetracyclines, erythromycins, chloramphenicol
• Enhanced effect with use of clavulanate potassium
• Increased incidence of skin rash from both drugs with use of allopurinol
• Increased bleeding with use of oral anticoagulants
• Decreased effectiveness of oral contraceptives

Lab
• False decrease of serum aminoglycosides concentrations
• False positive for urine protein
• False positive Coombs' test

Nutrition
• Slightly reduced absorption if given with meals, acidic fruit juices, citrus fruits, acidic beverages such as cola drinks

INCOMPATABILITIES

• Aminoglycosides; do not add or premix with other drugs

SIDE EFFECTS

GI: Nausea, vomiting, diarrhea, glossitis, stomatitis, pseudomembranous colitis
GU: Acute interstitial nephritis
HEME: Anemia, thrombocytopenia, thrombocytopenic purpura, eosinophilia, leukopenia
Local: Pain at injection site; vein irritation, thrombophlebitis with IV injection
Other: Metabolic alkalosis, hypersensitivity (erythematous maculopapular rash, urticaria, anaphylaxis), bacterial or fungal superinfection

TOXICITY AND OVERDOSE

Clinical signs: Neuromuscular sensitivity, seizures
Treatment: If within 4 hr of ingestion, empty stomach by induced

---

✦ Available in Canada.

vomiting or gastric lavage, follow with activated charcoal to reduce absorption; supportive care; hemodialysis

PATIENT CARE MANAGEMENT
Assessment
• Assess history of hypersensitivity to ampicillin, penicillins, cephalosporins
• Obtain C&S; may begin therapy before obtaining results
• Assess renal function (BUN, creatinine, I&O), bowel pattern

Interventions
• Administer penicillins at least 1 hr before bacteriostatic antibiotics (tetracycline, erythromycins, chloramphenicol)
• Administer PO 1 hr ac or 2 hr after meals; administer with water; avoid acidic beverages; shake susp well before administering; tabs may be crushed, caps taken apart and mixed with food or fluid
• Do not use bacteriostatic IM preparations containing benzyl alcohol for reconstitution in neonates; use reconstituted sol within 1 hr
• Do not premix IV with other medications
• Use large vein with small-bore needle to reduce local reaction; rotate site q48-72hr
• Maintain age-appropriate fluid intake
• For group A β-hemolytic streptococcal infection, provide 10-day course to prevent risk of acute rheumatic fever, glomerulonephritis

---

NURSING ALERT

Discontinue drug if signs of hypersensitivity, bone marrow toxicity, acute interstitial nephritis, pseudomembranous colitis develop

---

Evaluation
• Evaluate therapeutic response (decreased symptoms of infection)
• Monitor signs of superinfection (perineal itching, diaper rash, fever, malaise, redness, pain, swelling, drainage, rash, diarrhea, sore throat, change in cough or sputum)
• Monitor bowel pattern; diarrhea may be symptomatic of pseudomembranous colitis
• Observe for signs of allergic reaction (respiratory changes, urticaria), especially within 15-30 min of first dose
• Monitor renal function (BUN, creatinine, I&O), hepatic function (ALT, AST, bilirubin), hematologic function (CBC, differential, platelet count) during high-dose (or prolonged) therapy and with neonates
• Evaluate IM site for tissue damage, IV site for vein irritation.

PATIENT AND FAMILY EDUCATION
Teach/instruct
• To take as directed at prescribed intervals for prescribed length of time
Warn/Advise
• To notify care provider of hypersensitivity, side effects, superinfection

STORAGE
• Store powder, caps, tabs at room temp
• Reconstituted susp stable refrigerated for 14 days; room temp for 7 days; label date, time of reconstitution
• Reconstituted parenteral form stable for 1 hr at room temp

---

ampicillin sodium and sulbactam sodium

Brand Name(s): Unasyn

Classification: Antibiotic (aminopenicillin)

Pregnancy Category: B

AVAILABLE PREPARATIONS
Inj: 1.5 g (1 g ampicillin, 0.5 g sulbactam); 3.0 g (2 g ampicillin, 1 g sulbactam)

ROUTES AND DOSAGES

Children: IM/IV 100-200 mg ampicillin/kg/24 hr divided q6h; maximum dose 8 g ampicillin/24 hr)

Adults: IM/IV 1-2 g ampicillin q6-8hr; maximum dose 8 g ampicillin/24 hr)

IV administration:
• Recommended concentration:
• 3-45 mg/ml in D_5W, NS, LR, D_5 ½ NS
• Maximum concentration: 45 mg Unasyn (30 mg ampicillin, 15 mg sulbactam)/ml
• Intermittent infusion rate: Over 15-30 min

MECHANISM AND INDICATIONS

Antibiotic mechanism: Bactericidal; ampicillin inhibits bacterial cell wall synthesis by adhering to bacterial penicillinase-binding proteins; sulbactam improves bactericidal activity of ampicillin against β lactamase-producing strains resistant to penicillins, cephalosporins

Indications:
Effective against *Staphylococcus aureus, Escherichia coli, Klebsiella, Proteus mirabilis, Bacillus fragilis, Enterobacter, Acinetobacter calcoaceticus;* used to treat lower respiratory tract, skin, soft tissue, intraabdominal, GU, bone, and joint infections

PHARMACOKINETICS

Peak: At end of infusion
Distribution: To most body tissues; high CNS penetration only with inflamed meninges
Half-life: 50-110 min
Metabolism: Liver
Excretion: Urine

CONTRAINDICATIONS AND PRECAUTIONS

• Contraindicated with known hypersensitivity to ampicillin, penicillins, or cephalosporins and with infectious mononucleosis (many develop a rash during therapy)
• Use cautiously in neonates, with impaired renal function, and pregnancy

INTERACTIONS
Drug
• Synergistic antimicrobial activity against enterococci with use of aminoglycosides
• Increased serum concentrations of drug with use of probenecid
• Increased serum concentrations of methotrexate
• Decreased effectiveness with use of tetracyclines, erythromycins, chloramphenicol
• Increased incidence of skin rash from both drugs with use of allopurinol
• Increased bleeding with use of oral anticoagulants
• Decreased effectiveness of oral contraceptives

Lab
• False decrease of serum aminoglycoside concentrations
• False positive for urine protein
• False positive for Coomb's test

INCOMPATABILITIES
• Aminoglycosides; do not add or premix with other drugs

SIDE EFFECTS

GI: Nausea, vomiting, diarrhea, abdominal pain, glossitis, pseudomembranous colitis, elevated liver function tests
GU: Acute interstitial nephritis
HEME: Anemia, thrombocytopenia, thrombocytopenic purpura, eosinophilia, leukopenia
Local: Vein irritation, thrombophlebitis with IV injection
Other: Metabolic alkalosis, hypersensitivity (erythematous maculopapular rash, urticaria, anaphylaxis), bacterial or fungal superinfection

TOXICITY AND OVERDOSE

Clinical signs: Neuromuscular hypersensitivity, seizures
Treatment: Supportive care, hemodialysis

PATIENT CARE MANAGEMENT
Assessment
• Assess hypersensitivity history to ampicillin, penicillins, or cephalosporins

---

✤ Available in Canada.

• Obtain C&S; may begin therapy before obtaining results
• Assess renal function (BUN, creatinine, I&O), bowel pattern

Interventions
• Administer penicillins at least 1 hr before bacteriostatic antibiotics (tetracyclines, erythromycins, chloramphenicol)
• Do not premix IV with other medications
• Use large vein with small-bore needle to reduce local reaction; rotate site q48-72h
• Maintain age-appropriate fluid intake

> **NURSING ALERT**
> Discontinue drug if signs of hypersensitivity, bone marrow toxicity, acute interstitial nephritis, pseudomembranous colitis develop

Evaluation
• Evaluate therapeutic response (decreased symptoms of infection)
• Monitor signs of superinfection (perineal itching, diaper rash, fever, malaise, redness, pain, swelling, drainage, rash, diarrhea, sore throat, change in cough or sputum)
• Monitor bowel pattern; diarrhea may be symptomatic of pseudomembranous colitis
• Observe for signs of allergic reaction (wheezing, tightness in chest, urticaria), especially within 15-30 min of first dose
• Monitor renal functions (BUN, creatinine, I&O), hepatic functions (ALT, AST, bilirubin), hematologic functions (CBC, differential, platelet count)
• Evaluate IV site for vein irritation

PATIENT AND FAMILY EDUCATION
Teach/instruct
• To take as directed at prescribed intervals for prescribed length of time
Warn/advise
• To notify care provider of hypersensitivity, side effects, superinfection

STORAGE
• Store at room temp; stability of reconstituted sol depends on sol used for dilution; check package insert

---

amrinone lactate
Brand Name(s): Inocor✤
Classification: Inotropic
Pregnancy Category: C

AVAILABLE PREPARATIONS
Inj: 5 mg/ml
ROUTES AND DOSAGES
Neonates, infants, children, adults: IV loading dose 0.75 mg/kg; maintenance 5 mcg/kg/min to 10 mcg/kg/min; may repeat loading dose 30 min after initial loading dose; maximum dose 10 mg/kg/24 hr
IV administration
• Recommended concentration: ≤1-3 mg/ml in NS or ½ NS
• Maximum concentration: May administer undiluted
• IV push rate: 2-3 min
• Continuous infusion rate: Neonates 3-5 mcg/kg/min; infants/children/adults 5-10 mcg/kg/min

MECHANISMS AND INDICATIONS
Inotropic mechanism: Reduces preload, afterload by directly relaxing vascular smooth muscle; increases cardiac output without measurable increase in myocardial oxygen consumption; vasodilator characteristics
Indications: Short-term management of pts with CHF who have not responded to digoxin, diuretics, or vasodilators; may be used in conjunction with digoxin

PHARMACOKINETICS
Onset of action: 2-5 min
Peak: 10 min
Half-life: 4-6 hr
Metabolism: Liver
Excretion: Urine (drug and metabolites)

✤ Available in Canada.

CONTRAINDICATIONS AND PRECAUTIONS
• Contraindicated with known sensitivity to medication or bisulfites, severe aortic disease, severe pulmonary valve disease, acute MI
• Use with caution with renal disease, hepatic disease, atrial flutter and fibrillation

INTERACTIONS
Drug
• Excessive hypotension possible when used with antihypertensives
• Additive effect possible when used with digoxin

INCOMPATABILITIES
• Furosemide or dextrose sols (other than for direct dilution)

SIDE EFFECTS
CNS: Headache
CV: Arrhythmias, hypotension, chest pain
DERM: Allergic reactions, thrombocytopenia
GI: Abdominal pain, anorexia, nausea, vomiting, hepatotoxicity, ascites, jaundice, hiccups
Local: Burning at injection site
RESP: Pleuritis, pulmonary densities, hypoxemia

TOXICITY AND OVERDOSE
Clinical signs: Severe hypotension
Treatment: Discontinue drug, support circulation

PATIENT CARE MANAGEMENT
Assessment
• Assess history of hypersensitivity to drug, bisulfites
• Assess baseline VS, B/P, weight, hydration status
• Assess baseline labs: electrolytes, Ca, BUN, creatinine, CBC, platelet count, bilirubin, AST, ALT
Interventions
• Do not mix IV sol directly with glucose solutions; may administer through Y-connector
• Always use infusion pump (except when administering boluses)

> **NURSING ALERT**
> Do not mix with furosemide

Evaluation
• Evaluate for therapeutic response (improved cardiac function)
• Monitor IV site carefully
• Evaluate labs frequently (electrolytes, Ca, BUN, creatinine, CBC, platelet count), daily bilirubin, AST, ALT;
• Evaluate side effects, hypersensitivity

PATIENT AND FAMILY EDUCATION
Teach/instruct
• About illness, need for IV infusion
Warn/advise
• To notify care provider of side effects, hypersensitivity
Provide
• Emotional support as indicated

STORAGE
• Store at room temp
• Protect from light

---

antihemophilic factor (AHF)

Brand Name(s): Hemofil T, Factorate, Humafac, Koate-HT, Koate-HS, Kogenate (recombinant), Profilate

Classification: Antihemophilic agent (blood derivative)

Pregnancy Category: C

AVAILABLE PREPARATIONS
Inj: Single dose vials with varied units; 10 ml, 20 ml, 30 ml

ROUTES AND DOSAGES
IV; dose individualized based on coagulation studies; usually 20-50 U/kg/dose q12-24h; dilute with NS, D₅W, LR, roll bottle gently to mix

IV administration
• Continuous infusion rate: <2 ml/min if infusion >34 U AHF/ml; 3 ml/min if infusion <34 U AHF/ml

---

✤ Available in Canada.

MECHANISM AND INDICATIONS

Mechanism: Replaces deficient clotting factor responsible for converting prothrombin to thrombin
Indications: Used for treatment of hemophilia A

PHARMACOKINETICS

Half-life: 4-24 hr (average 12 hr)
Metabolism: Drug cleared rapidly from plasma, consumed during blood clotting

CONTRAINDICATIONS AND PRECAUTIONS

• Contraindicated with hypersensitivity to mouse protein
• Use cautiously with neonates, older infants, pts not immunized against hepatitis B, hepatic disease

INTERACTIONS

Drug
• No significant interactions
Lab
• No interactions reported

INCOMPATIBILITIES

• Do not mix with other drugs in syringe

SIDE EFFECTS

CNS: Headaches, paraesthesia
CV: Hypotension, tachycardia, possible intravascular hemolysis with blood type A, B, or AB
DERM: Erythema, urticaria
EENT: Blurred vision
Local: Stinging at infusion site
Other: Chills, fever, flushing, chest pain

TOXICITY AND OVERDOSE

Clinical signs: None reported

PATIENT CARE MANAGEMENT

Assessment
• Assess history of hypersensitivity
• Assess coagulation studies before, during therapy
• Assess for signs of allergic reaction
• Assess baseline HR, B/P; monitor during therapy
• Assess Hct, Coomb's test with blood types A, B, AB

Interventions
• Discontinue IV therapy if signs of allergic reaction occur
• Dilute with NS, D₅W, LR; roll bottle gently to mix
Evaluation
• Evaluate therapeutic response (decreased bleeding)
• Evaluate for signs of bleeding, joint pain

PATIENT AND FAMILY EDUCATION

Teach/instruct
• To take as directed at prescribed intervals for prescribed length of time
• To report any signs of bleeding
• About correct way to administer drug at home
• To avoid salicylates
Encourage
• To be immunized against hepatitis B
• To have regular HIV screening

STORAGE

• Refrigerate AHF concentrate
• Use reconstituted sol within 3 hr; do not refrigerate after reconstitution

---

ascorbic acid (vitamin C)

Brand Name(s): Ascorbicap, C-Crystals, Cecon, Ce-Vi-Sol, Dull-C, Flavorcee, Vita-C

Classification: Water soluble vitamin

Pregnancy Category: A (C if dosage exceeds RDA)

AVAILABLE PREPARATIONS

Liquid: 35 mg/0.6 ml, 100 mg/ml
Syr: 500 mg/5 ml
Powder: 4 g/tsp
Crystals: 4 g/tsp, 5 g/tsp
Tabs: 25 mg, 50 mg, 100 mg, 250 mg, 500 mg, 1000 mg
Tabs (chewable): 100 mg, 250 mg, 500 mg
Tabs (time release): 500 mg, 1000 mg, 1500 mg
Caps (time release): 500 mg

ROUTES AND DOSAGES
Dietary Supplementation
See Appendix F, Table of Recommended Daily Dietary Allowances
Urinary Acidification
Children: PO 500 mg tid-qid
Adults: PO 4-12 g/24 hr divided tid-qid
Delayed Wound Healing
Children: PO 100-200 mg/24 hr
Adults: PO 300-500 mg/24 hr
Treatment of Deficiency
Infants: IV/IM 50-100 mg qd
Children: IV/IM 100-300 mg qd
Adults: IV/IM 100-250 mg qd-bid
Burns
Individualize dose; severe burns may require 1-2 g/24 hr
IV administration
• Direct IV: 100 mg undiluted over at least 1 min
• IV infusion: Over 15 min diluted in D_5W, D_5NS, NS, LR, R

MECHANISM AND INDICATIONS
Mechanism: Vitamin C is involved in many physiologic functions, such as carbohydrate metabolism; formation of fats and proteins, maintenance of blood vessels; promotion of growth; tissue repair; wound healing; tooth and bone formation; increases iron absorption; collagen formation; and oxidation-reduction reactions
Indications: Treatment, prevention of vitamin C deficiency (scurvy) and to acidify the urine

PHARMACOKINETICS
Metabolism: Liver
Excretion: Urine

CONTRAINDICATIONS AND PRECAUTIONS
• No contraindications reported
• Use cautiously with anticoagulant therapy, diabetes, kidney stones, or Na-restricted diets, pregnancy
• Some products may contain tartrazine, use with caution for pts with allergies to yellow dye #5
• Prolonged use of large doses followed by intake of normal levels may potentiate rebound scurvy

INTERACTIONS
Drug
• Greater than 2 g/24 hr may affect urine pH; changes in urine acidification may alter effectiveness of other medications
• Use with iron (30 mg) recommended to increase iron absorption
• Crystallization may occur with use of sulfonamides
• Increased intensity, duration of dicumarol effects
• Increased vitamin C requirements with use of oral contraceptives
• Increased vitamin C requirements with smoking
Lab
• Doses >500 mg may cause false negative in urine glucose test results
• May alter tests because of oxidation-reduction reactions

INCOMPATIBILITIES
• Aminophylline, bleomycin, chloramphenicol, chlordiazepoxide, chlorthiazide, estrogens, dextran, erythromycin, hydrocortisone, nafcillin, phytonadione, sulfisoxazole, trifluopromazine, vitamin $B_{12,}$ warfarin, $NaHCO_3$

SIDE EFFECTS
CNS: Faintness, dizziness, headache
CV: Flushing
DERM: Discomfort at IV site
GI: Nausea, vomiting, gastroesophageal reflux, diarrhea, mouth sores, stomach upset
GU: Hyperoxaluria, increased urination, kidney stones
Other: Dental erosion with prolonged use of chewable tabs

TOXICITY AND OVERDOSE
Excessively high doses of vitamin C are excreted in the urine and toxicity is very uncommon. However, excessively high doses should be decreased gradually or deficiency symptoms may occur as listed above.

PATIENT CARE MANAGEMENT
Assessment
- Assess history of hypersensitivity to vitamin C
- Obtain baseline serum vitamin C levels
- Assess dietary history for inadequate nutrient intake, inappropriate formulas, fad diets, alcoholism, or other intolerance
- Assess for conditions which may increase vitamin C requirements, such as fever, infection, burns, wound healing, severe trauma
- Assess use in pts with renal disease, as excess is excreted in urine

Interventions
- Administer large PO doses (>1 g/24 hr) in divided doses to maximize absorption and use
- Dissolve effervescent tabs in water immediately before administering
- Administer IV slowly
- Maintain age-appropriate fluid intake

NURSING ALERT
Use cautiously in pts with renal disease since excess is excreted in the urine

Evaluation
- Evaluate therapeutic response (absence of anorexia, irritability, pallor, joint pain, hyperkeratosis, petechiae, poor wound healing)
- Evaluate serum vitamin C levels
- Evaluate side effects, hypersensitivity, including (but not limited to) nausea, vomiting, diarrhea, GI discomfort, flushing, dizziness, injection sites for infection

PATIENT AND FAMILY EDUCATION
Teach/instruct
- To take as directed at prescribed intervals for prescribed length of time
Warn/advise
- To use supplements with caution; pts with diabetes, kidney stones, on Na-restricted diets, or on oral anticoagulant therapy should consult care provider and follow recommendations closely

Encourage
- A balanced diet should include a variety of fruits, vegetables, should provide adequate amounts of vitamin C; most people do not require supplements unless there is an increased requirement; see Appendix F for daily requirement
- Common sources of vitamin C include citrus fruits, tomatoes, potatoes, leafy vegetables

STORAGE
- Store oral forms at room temp in airtight container, protect from light
- Store IV form in refrigerator

---

asparaginase
Brand Name(s): Elspar, Oncaspar (conjugated form)
Classification: Antineoplastic enzyme, cell cycle phase specific (G_1 phase)
Pregnancy Category: C

AVAILABLE PREPARATIONS
Inj: Drug isolated from *Escherichia coli* (Elspar), 10,000 U/vial
Inj: Drug isolated from *Erwinia carotovorum,* 10,000 U/vial (investigational use only)
Inj: Modified drug isolated from *E. coli* and conjugated to monomethoxypolyethylene glycol (Oncaspar), 750 U/ml in 5 ml vial

ROUTES AND DOSAGES
- Dosage may vary in response to diagnosis, extent of disease, concurrent or previous therapy, protocol guidelines, physiological parameters; consult current literature, protocol recommendations
Multiple Dosing Regimens for Elspar Preparation
IM 1000 U/kg/24 hr for 10 days starting on day 22 of induction, or 6000 U/m²/dose × 9 injections administered every third day, or 25,000 U/m²/dose weekly × 30 wk

during consolidation phase of therapy

Dosing for Oncaspar
IM 2000 U/m²/dose every 2 wk

Dosing for Erwinia Preparation (Used If Hypersensitive to Elspar)
Dosages generally set according to Elspar recommendations (although there is no clinical evidence to support practice)

• Skin testing recommended by manufacturer before administration; this is difficult in clinical practice because of additional injections, the proposed timing of skin testing relative to asparaginase dosing schedules, and the disclaimer that allergic reactions may occur despite negative skin testing

• May be administered IV or IM (usually IM to decrease the number of allergic reactions)

• Maximum amount of drug injected IM should be 2 ml

MECHANISM AND INDICATIONS

Mechanism: Derived from defect in metabolic pathway of certain malignant cells dependent on exogenous source of asparagine for protein synthesis; drug is an enzyme that hydrolyzes asparagine in bloodstream depriving tumor cells of an essential amino acid; this deprivation acts to inhibit asparagine-dependent protein synthesis, tumor cell proliferation, and it causes delayed inhibition of DNA and RNA synthesis

Indications: Induction and consolidation treatment for acute lymphocytic leukemia, in combination with other chemotherapy; may be of some use in non-Hodgkin's lymphoma, acute myelogenous leukemia, and chronic myelogenous leukemia

PHARMACOKINETICS

Onset of action: Asparagine levels in plasma become immeasurable immediately after drug administration

Peak action: Peak following IM administration is approximately ½ that for IV, although clinical significance is uncertain; peak follows IM administration by about 14-24 hr

Distribution: Primarily within intravascular space, with detectable levels in cervical and thoracic lymph fluid; crosses blood–brain barrier minimally

Duration: 23-33 days

Half-life: 1.4-1.8 days

Excretion: Small amounts found in urine

CONTRAINDICATIONS AND PRECAUTIONS

• Contraindicated with severe hypersensitivity reaction (pts may be able to tolerate a different asparaginase preparation); active infections (especially chicken pox and herpes zoster); pancreatitis; pregnancy, lactation

• Use cautiously with IV administration (drug is derived from gram-negative bacteria, can contain potentially antigenic proteins that precipitate severe allergic reactions; anaphylaxis occurs in approximately 20% of pts; IM administration significantly reduces incidence of anaphylactic reactions), liver dysfunction, DM

INTERACTIONS

Drug

• Increased possibility of hyperglycemia with corticosteroid use

• Increased incidence of neurotoxicities possible with concomitant administration of vincristine; might be avoided by administration of asparaginase after vincristine, and may be lessened with delay in peak action with IM administration

• Decreased production of coagulation factors caused by asparaginase may result in bleeding tendencies when administered concurrently with chemotherapy drugs that cause thrombocytopenia

• Synergistic cytotoxic activity when used with cytarabine

• Effect of concomitant methotrexate therapy may theoretically be blocked (asparaginase markedly decreases number of rapidly

---

dividing cells on which methotrexate exerts action); no clinical evidence

Lab
• Decreases total protein and albumin, with subsequent effect on serum Ca and PO$_4$; this reverses following cessation of asparaginase therapy
• Transient increase in AST, ALT, alk phos, bilirubin, ammonia
• Transient decrease in serum fibrinogen
• Increase in serum cholesterol, triglycerides
• Interference with thyroid function tests (decreased thyroxine, increased thyroxine-binding globulin index)

SIDE EFFECTS
CNS: Lethargy, somnolence that may progress to coma; disorientation, confusion, confabulation, recent memory loss, focal neurological signs, depression, headache, irritability, dizziness, hallucinations; thrombotic hemorrhagic events involving cortical infarction, capsular infarction, intracerebral hemorrhage, cerebral venous and dural sinus thrombosis; most pediatric patients recover from neurological events
ENDO: Hypoalbuminemia, hyperglycemia, glycosuria, polyuria
GI: Increased AST, bilirubin, alk phos, serum cholesterol; decreased serum albumin; abdominal pain secondary to acute pancreatitis; malaise, anorexia, mildly emetogenic (effects may be more pronounced in Oncaspar preparation)
GU: Azotemia, renal insufficiency, transient proteinuria, hyperuricemia, glycosuria, polyuria
HEME: Decreased PT fibrinogen, Factors V, VII, VIII, IX; Oncaspar causes increased PTT, decrease in fibrinogen not associated with increased bleeding

TOXICITY AND OVERDOSE
Clinical signs: Acute pancreatitis (nausea, vomiting, abdominal pain, increased serum amylase and lipase), CNS events
Treatment: Blood transfusions, hydration, nutritional supplementation, broad spectrum antibiotic therapy if febrile, electrolyte replacement; CNS events, acute pancreatitis indicated discontinuing therapy

PATIENT CARE MANAGEMENT
Assessment
• Assess hypersensitivity reaction to asparaginase preparation
• Assess baseline BG, albumin, amylase, Ca, P, alk phos, AST, ALT, bilirubin, ammonia, cholesterol, triglycerides
• Assess baseline PT, PTT, fibrinogen
• Assess baseline neurologic exam
• Assess history of previous chemotherapy, radiation therapy
• Assess previous success with antiemetic therapy
• Assess baseline CBC, differential, platelet count

Intervention
• Administer dose IM to decrease risk of anaphylaxis
• Observe for signs or symptoms of allergic reaction at least 30 min after injection
• Provide supportive therapy to maintain hematologic status

Evaluate
• Evaluate therapeutic response (remission of ALL, AML, decreased tumor size, spread of malignancy)
• Evaluate CBC, differential, platelet count weekly
• Evaluate BUN, creatinine, alk phos, AST, ALT, bilirubin regularly
• Evaluate amylase before each dose
• Evaluate BG, urine glucose before each dose
• Evaluate for signs or symptoms of bleeding
• Evaluate serum albumin, Ca, PO$_4$ regularly
• Evaluate neurologic status (including inquiry into short-term memory status)

PATIENT AND FAMILY EDUCATION
Teach/instruct
• To have pt well hydrated before and after chemotherapy
• About the importance of follow-up visits to monitor blood counts and serum chemistry values, for urinalysis
• To take an accurate temp; taking temp rectally contraindicated
• To notify care provider of signs of bleeding (bruising, epistaxis, bleeding gums), signs of infection (fever, sore throat, fatigue)
Warn/advise
• About impact of body changes that may occur (hair loss, hyperpigmentation, nail ridging), how to minimize changes (wigs, caps, scarves, long sleeves)
• To avoid OTC preparations containing aspirin
• To report any alterations in behavior, sensation, perception; help to develop a plan of care to manage side effects, stress of illness, and treatment
• That dental work should be delayed until blood counts return to baseline
• To notify care provider of any delayed hypersensitivity reaction
• To avoid people with known bacterial or viral illnesses
• To report exposure to chicken pox in susceptible child immediately
• To report activation of herpes zoster (shingles) immediately
• That household contacts of child not be immunized with live polio virus; use inactivated form
• That pts should not receive immunizations while on therapy or until immune system can mount appropriate antibody response
• To report any nausea, vomiting, abdominal pain immediately
• To report any mental status changes immediately
• To report polyuria, polydipsia immediately
Encourage
• Provision of nutritious food intake; consider nutrition consultation

• To use topical anesthetics to control discomfort of mucositis; avoid spicy foods, commercial mouthwashes

STORAGE
• May be stored in refrigerated conditions for lot life
• After reconstitution, sol should be used within 8 hr

---

astemizole
Brand Name(s): Hismanal✤
Classification: Antihistamine
Pregnancy Category: C

AVAILABLE PREPARATIONS
Tabs: 10 mg

ROUTES AND DOSAGES
Children <6 yr: PO 0.2 mg/kg/24 hr qd
Children 6-12 yr: PO 5 mg qd
Children >12 yr and adults: PO 10-30 mg qd; give 30 mg on first day, 20 mg on second day, followed by 10 mg qd

MECHANISM AND INDICATIONS
Antihistamine mechanism: Competitively antagonizes histamine at H_1-receptor site; reduced sedative potential results from preferential binding to peripheral H_1, not central H_1-receptor sites
Indications: Used to treat seasonal and perennial allergic rhinitis, other allergic symptoms

PHARMACOKINETICS
Peak: After 1 hr
Half-Life: Biphasic: distribution 20 hr; elimination 7-11 days
Metabolism: Liver
Elimination: Eliminated after drug is metabolized in liver

CONTRAINDICATIONS AND PRECAUTIONS
• Contraindicated with hypersensitivity to astemizole or any component; with severe hepatic dysfunction; with concomitant use of erythromycin, ketoconazole, and itraconazole

---

✤ Available in Canada.

• Use cautiously with lower airway diseases, renal or hepatic impairment, narrow-angle glaucoma, prostatic hypertrophy, pregnancy

INTERACTIONS
Drug
• Reduced hepatic metabolism resulting in life-threatening cardiac arrhythmias with use of erythromycin, ciprofloxacin, cimetidine, ketoconazole, disulfiram
• Increased CNS depression with use of alcohol, other CNS depressants, procarbazine
• Increased anticholinergic effects with use of MAOIs
• Decreased action of oral anticoagulants
Lab
• False negative for skin allergy tests
Nutrition
• Reduced absorption when taken with food

SIDE EFFECTS
CNS: Headache, drowsiness, dizziness, nervousness
CV: Life-threatening arrhythmias
GI: Increased appetite, dry mouth
Other: Weight increase

TOXICITY AND OVERDOSE
Clinical signs: Syncope, cardiac arrhythmias
Treatment: Induce vomiting or perform gastric lavage; supportive care

PATIENT CARE MANAGEMENT
Assessment
• Assess history of hypersensitivity to astemizole, any component
• Assess renal status (BUN, creatinine, I&O), hepatic status (ALT, AST, bilirubin), hematologic status (CBC, differential, platelet count) for long-term therapy
Interventions
• Administer PO 1 hr ac or 2 hr after meals; tab may be crushed, mixed with food or fluid
• Provide sugarless hard candy, gum, frequent oral care for dry mouth

---

NURSING ALERT
Do not exceed recommended dose; life-threatening arrhythmias may develop

---

Evaluation
• Evaluate therapeutic response (decreased allergy symptoms)
• Monitor respiratory status (change in secretions, wheezing, chest tightness)

PATIENT AND FAMILY EDUCATION
Teach/instruct
• To take as directed at prescribed intervals for prescribed length of time
Warn/advise
• To notify care provider of hypersensitivity, side effects
• Not to exceed recommended dosage
• To avoid hazardous activities if drowsiness occurs (bicycles, skateboards, skates)
• To avoid use of alcohol, medications containing alcohol, or CNS depressants

STORAGE
• Store at room temp in tight, light-resistant container

---

atenolol
Brand Name(s): Apo-Atenolol♣, Atenolol, Novo-Atenol♣, Nu-Atenol♣, Tenormin♣

Classification: β-blocker, antihypertensive, antiarrhythmic

Pregnancy Category: C

AVAILABLE PREPARATIONS
PO: Tabs 25 mg, 50 mg, 100 mg
Inj: 5 mg/10 ml ampule

ROUTES AND DOSAGES
Antihypertensive/Antiarrhythmic
Children: PO 0.8-1.5 mg/kg/24 hr qd, maximum dose 2 mg/kg/24 hr
Adults: PO 25-50 mg qd, increase q

♣ Available in Canada.

1-2 wk to 100 mg qd for hypertension

Angina
Adults: PO 200 mg qd

Early Treatment of MI
- IV 5 mg slowly; may repeat in 10 min if initial dose tolerated

IV administration
- Recommended concentration: 0.5 mg/ml or dilute in NS, D_5W
- Maximum concentration: 0.5 mg/ml
- IV push rate: Over 5 min, not to exceed 1 mg/min

MECHANISM AND INDICATIONS
β-*blocker mechanism:* Blocks β-adrenergic receptors in vascular smooth muscle; decreases rate of SA node discharge; increases recovery time; slows conduction of AV node; decreases heart rate; decreases O_2 consumption in myocardial cells; decreases renin–aldosterone–angiotensin system; inhibits bronchial $β_2$ receptors
Indications: Hypertension, arrhythmias, angina, suspected or known MI

PHARMACOKINETICS
Onset of action: Immediate
Peak: PO 2-4 hr; IV 5 min
Half-life: 6-7 hr
Metabolism: None, remains unchanged
Excretion: Urine

CONTRAINDICATIONS AND PRECAUTIONS
- Contraindicated with hypersensitivity to β-blockers, cardiogenic shock, second- or third-degree heart block, bradycardia, CHF, cardiac failure
- Use cautiously with diabetes, renal disease, thyroid disease, asthma, COPD, well-compensated heart failure, after major surgery

INTERACTIONS
Drug
- Increased hypotension and bradycardia with reserpine, hydralazine, methyldopa, prazosin, anticholinergics, digoxin
- Increased hypoglycemia with insulin
- Decreased antihypertensive effects with indomethacin
- Decreased bronchodilatation effects of theophyllines
- Paradoxical hypertension with clonidine
- Mutual inhibition with sympathomimetics

Lab
- Interference with glucose/insulin tolerance test

INCOMPATIBILITIES
- May not be mixed with any other medication in sol or syringe

SIDE EFFECTS
CNS: Drowsiness, fatigue, lethargy, insomnia, dizziness, mental changes, mental loss, depression, hallucinations, dreams, catatonia, visual disturbances, emotional lability
CV: Hypotension, bradycardia, CHF, cold extremities, second- or third-degree heart block
DERM: Rash, fever, alopecia
EENT: Dry, burning eyes, sore throat
GI: Nausea, diarrhea, vomiting, mesenteric arterial thrombosis, colitis
GU: Impotence
RESP: Wheezing, bronchospasm, dyspnea
Other: Agranulocytosis, purpura, thrombocytopenia

TOXICITY AND OVERDOSE
Clinical signs: Lethargy, bradycardia, second- or third-degree heart block, hypotension, bronchospasm, wheezing, cardiac failure, hypoglycemia
Treatment: Gastric lavage, IV atropine, IV theophylline, proventil aerosol, digoxin, O_2 therapy, diuretics, isoproteronol, hemodialysis

PATIENT CARE MANAGEMENT
Assessment
- Assess hypersensitivity to drug, β blockers
- Assess baseline VS, weight, hydration status
- Assess baseline labs BUN, creatinine, AST, ALT, bilirubin

✤ Available in Canada.

Interventions
- Administer ac, hs
- Tablets may be crushed
- Decrease dosage in renal dysfunction
- Begin PO dose 10 min after IV dose

Evaluation
- Evaluate therapeutic response (decreased B/P, arrhythmias)
- Evaluate labs (BUN, creatinine, AST, ALT, bilirubin) regularly
- Evaluate VS, hydration status regularly
- Evaluate side effects, hypersensitivity

PATIENT AND FAMILY EDUCATION
Teach/instruct
- To take as directed at prescribed intervals for prescribed length of time
- Not to discontinue drug abruptly; taper over 2 wk period
- To teach family about weight control, diet, Na intake, exercise

Warn/advise
- Not to use OTC medications unless directed by care provider
- To notify care provider of hypersensitivity, side effects
- To inform care provider of any dizziness, bradycardia, confusion, depression, fever
- To avoid alcohol, smoking
- To avoid hazardous activities if dizziness is present

Provide
- Emotional support as indicated

STORAGE
- Store at room temp
- Protect from light, moisture

---

atracurium besylate

Brand Name(s): Tracrium

Classification: Neuromuscular blocking agent (nondepolarizing)

Pregnancy category: C

AVAILABLE PREPARATIONS
Inj: 10 mg/ml

ROUTES AND DOSAGES
Neonates ≤1 mo: IV initial dose 0.2-0.5 mg/kg; maintenance dose 0.08-0.1 mg/kg prn to maintain neuromuscular blockade
Infants and children 1 mo-2 yr: IV initial dose 0.3-0.4 mg/kg; maintenance dose 0.08-0.1 mg/kg prn to maintain neuromuscular blockade
Children >2 yr and adults: IV initial dose 0.4-0.5 mg/kg; maintenance dose 0.08-0.1 mg/kg prn to maintain neuromuscular blockade

IV administration
- Recommended concentration: 0.2 or 0.5 mg/ml in D_5NS, D_5W, or NS for IV inf; 10 mg/ml (commercially available) for IV push or infusion
- Maximum concentration: 10 mg/ml for IV push or infusion
- IV push rate: 1 min
- Continuous infusion rate: Following loading dose, 0.3-0.6 mg/kg/hr (5-10 mcg/kg/min) continuous inf has been administered to infants, children, adults for prolonged surgical procedures
- Possible need for increased dosages with prolonged administration

MECHANISM AND INDICATIONS
Mechanism: Interrupts transmission of nerve impulse at skeletal neuromuscular junction; antagonizes acetylcholine by competitively binding to cholinergic sites on motor endplates, resulting in muscle paralysis; reversible with edrophonium, neostigmine, physostigmine
Indications: Used as an adjunct in surgical anesthesia; used to facilitate endotracheal intubation and skeletal muscle relaxation during mechanical ventilation or surgery

PHARMACOKINETICS
Onset: Within 2 min
Peak: 3-5 min (range 1.7-10 min)
Recovery: 20-35 min when anesthesia is balanced
Half-life: 20 min (terminal)
Metabolism: In plasma by nonspecific esterases, nonenzymatic reactions
Excretion: Urine, bile

CONTRAINDICATIONS AND PRECAUTIONS
• Contraindicated with known hypersensitivity to atracurium; injectable solution may contain benzyl alcohol as a preservative (administration of benzyl alcohol in doses ranging from 99-234 mg/kg has been associated with fatal gasping syndrome in neonates; clinical signs include metabolic acidosis, hypotension, CNS depression, cardiovascular collapse)
• Use cautiously with pregnancy, lactation, renal and hepatic disease, children <2 yr, fluid and electrolyte imbalances, neuromuscular disease, dehydration, respiratory disease

INTERACTIONS
Drug
• Increased neuromuscular blockade when used with aminoglycosides, bacitracin, clindamycin, lincomycin, quinidine, local anesthetics, polymyxin antibiotics, lithium, narcotic analgesics, thiazides, enflurane, isoflurane, verapamil, magnesium sulfate, furosemide
• Use with theophylline may result in arrhythmias

INCOMPATIBILITIES
• Do not mix with barbiturates in syringe or solution; do not dilute in LR; unstable in alkaline sol

SIDE EFFECTS
CV: Brachycardia, tachycardia, increased or decreased BP
DERM: Rash, flushing, pruritus, urticaria
EENT: Increased secretions, salivation
MS: Weakness
RESP: Prolonged apnea, bronchospasm, cyanosis, respiratory depression
Other: Endogenous histamine release may occur; noted clinically as erythema, hypotension, and either brachycardia or tachycardia

TOXICITY AND OVERDOSE
Clinical signs: Prolonged apnea, bronchospasm, cyanosis, respiratory depression
Treatment: Supportive care; mechanical ventilation may be required; use Anticholinesterases to reverse neuromuscular blockade; edrophonium or neostigmine, atropine

PATIENT CARE MANAGEMENT
Assessment
• Assess history of hypersensitivity to atracurium
• Assess for preexisting conditions requiring caution (pregnancy, lactation, renal or hepatic disease, fluid or electrolyte imbalance, neuromuscular disease, dehydration, respiratory disease)
• Assess electrolytes (Na, K^+) before procedure; electrolyte imbalances may increase the action of drug
Interventions
• Monitor vital signs (pulse, respirations, airway, B/P) until fully recovered; characteristics of respirations (rate, depth, pattern); strength of hand grip
• Monitor therapeutic response (paralysis of jaw, eyelid, head, neck, rest of the body)
• Monitor I&O for urinary frequency, hesitancy, retention
• Monitor for allergic reactions (rash, fever, respiratory distress, pruritus); *drug should be discontinued if these reactions occur*
• Instill artificial tears (q2h), covering to eyes to protect the cornea

NURSING ALERT
Injectible solution may contain
benzyl alcohol as a preservative; administration of benzyl
alcohol in doses ranging from
99-234 mg/kg has been associated with a fatal gasping syndrome in neonates; clinical
signs include metabolic acidosis,
hypotension, CNS depression,
cardiovascular collapse

Should be administered only
by experienced clinicians
familiar with drug's actions,
complications

Administer only in facilities
where intubation, artificial respiration, O$_2$ therapy, antagonists are immediately available

Evaluation
• Monitor effectiveness of neuromuscular blockade (degree of paralysis, using nerve stimulator)
• Monitor for recovery (decreased
paralysis of face, diaphragm, arm,
rest of the body)
General
• Should be administered only by
experienced clinicians familiar
with drug's actions, complications
• Administer only in facilities
where intubation, artificial respiration, O$_2$ therapy, antagonists are
immediately available

**PATIENT AND FAMILY
EDUCATION**
Warn/advise
• Provide reassurance to pt if communication is difficult during the
recovery; inform pt that postoperative stiffness often occurs, is normal, and will subside

STORAGE
Refrigerate drug

atropine sulfate

Brand Name(s): Atropine✤,
Atropine-care, Atropine
Injection✤, Atropine Oint-
ment✤, Atropine Sulfate
Injection✤, Atripisol✤,
Atropisol, Dioptic's Atro-
pine✤, Isopto Atropine✤,
I-Tropine

Classification: Antiarrhythmic, anticholinergic, vago-
lytic

Pregnancy Category: C

AVAILABLE PREPARATIONS
Tabs: (PO) 0.4 mg, 0.6 mg
Inj: 0.05 mg/ml, 0.1 mg/ml, 0.3
mg/ml, 0.4 mg/ml, 0.5 mg/ml, 0.6
mg/ml, 0.8 mg/ml, 1 mg/ml, 1.2
mg/ml
Nebulizer: 0.2%, 0.5%

ROUTES AND DOSAGES
CPR
Children: IV/intratracheal 0.02
mg/kg/dose q 5 min × 2-3 prn;
minimum dose 0.1 mg, maximum
dose 1 mg in children or 2 mg in
adolescents
Adult: IV/intratracheal 0.5-1 mg/
dose q 5 min; maximum dose 2 mg
Insecticide Poisoning
Children: IM/IV 0.05 mg/kg; may
repeat q 10-30 min as needed;
maintenance dose 0.01 mg/kg,
maximum dose 0.25 mg
Adult: IM/IV 2 mg q 20-30 min
until muscarinic symptoms disappear; maximum dose 6 mg/hr
Preanesthesia
Children: SC/IM/IV 0.01 mg/kg/
dose; minimum dose 0.1 mg, maximum dose 0.4 mg
Adult: IV 0.4-0.6 mg 30-60 min
before anesthesia
Bronchospasm
Children and adults: Inh 0.05 mg/
kg/dose in 2.5 ml NS q4-6h prn;
minimum dose 0.25 mg, maximum
dose 1 mg q6-8h
IV administration
• Recommended concentration:
0.05 mg/ml, 0.1 mg/ml, 0.3 mg/ml,
0.4 mg/ml, 0.5 mg/ml, 0.8 mg/ml, 1
mg/ml

✤ Available in Canada.

- Maximum concentration: 1 mg/ml
- IV push rate: Over 1 min

MECHANISM AND INDICATIONS

Antiarrhythmic mechanism: Blocks acetylcholine effects on SA and AV node; shortens PR interval; increases cardiac output, HR by blocking vagal stimulation of heart

Anticholinergic mechanism: Decreases action of parasympathetic nervous system on bronchial, salivary, and sweat glands, causing decrease in secretions; decreases cholinergic effects on iris, ciliary body, intestinal and bronchial smooth muscle; blocks cholinomimetic effects of pesticides

Indications: Symptomatic bradycardia, bradyarrhythmias, anticholinesterase insecticide poisoning; to block cardiac vagal responses, decrease secretions before surgery, and decrease smooth muscle contractions of GI and GU tract; occasionally used as bronchodilator

PHARMACOKINETICS

Onset of action: Immediate
Peak: IV 2-4 min; IM 30 min; PO 60 min
Half-life: 2-3 hr
Metabolism: Liver
Excretion: Urine

CONTRAINDICATIONS AND PRECAUTIONS

- Contraindicated with known hypersensitivity to belladonna alkaloids, glaucoma, GI obstruction, myasthenia gravis, thyrotoxicosis, tachycardia/tachyarrhythmias, asthma
- Use cautiously with acute MI, CHF, Down syndrome, spastic paralysis, fever, hyperthyroidism, hypertension, hepatic disease, renal disease

INTERACTIONS
Drug
- Increases effects of anticholinergics, MAOIs, antidepressants, amantadine
- Decreases effects of phenothiazines

Lab
- Interferes with gastric acid secretion test, PSP excretion test

INCOMPATIBILITIES
- Amobarbital, ampicillin, chloramphenicol, chlortetracycline, cimetidine, epinephrine, heparin, isoproterenol, levarterenol, metaraminol, methicillin, methohexital, nitrofurantoin, pentobarbital, promazine, thiopental, warfarin, $NaHCO_3$ in sol or syringe

SIDE EFFECTS
CNS: Headache, dizziness, confusion, psychosis, anxiety, coma, drowsiness, insomnia, combativeness, weakness, hallucination, excitement, agitation
CV: Tachycardia, palpitations, angina, bradycardia, hypotension, hypertension
DERM: Flushing, urticaria, rash, dermatitis, dry skin
EENT: Dry mouth, thirst, blurred vision, photophobia, mydriasis, glaucoma, eye pain, nasal congestion
GI: Constipation, nausea, vomiting, abdominal pain, anorexia, abdominal distention, paralytic ileus
GU: Urinary retention, hesitancy, impotence, dysuria
Other: Decreased sweating, lactation suppression, fever, leukocytosis

TOXICITY AND OVERDOSE
Clinical signs: Excessive CV, CNS stimulation
Treatment: Administer physostigmine to reverse anticholinergic activity; supportive measures including O_2, ventilation, dopamine for circulatory depression, anticonvulsants, antiarrhythmics

PATIENT CARE MANAGEMENT
Assessment
- Assess history of hypersensitivity to drug, other belladonna alkaloids
- Assess baseline VS

Interventions
- Have pt void before administration
- Provide sugarless hard candy, mouth wash, frequent rinsing for complaints of dry mouth.
- Increase fluid intake, increase bulk, or administer laxatives for constipation

---

NURSING ALERT

Atropine may be given via endotracheal tube or intraosseous during an emergency when IV access has not yet been obtained

---

Evaluation
- Evaluate therapeutic response (decreased arrhythmias, decreased secretions, relief of muscarinic symptoms, decreased GI and GU symptoms)
- Evaluate side effects, hypersensitivity
- Evaluate I&O, check for urinary retention
- Monitor bowel sounds

PATIENT AND FAMILY EDUCATION
Teach/instruct
- To increase fluids, dietary fiber
- About monitoring for irregular heartbeat, to report immediately to health care provider
Warn/advise
- To notify care provider of hypersensitivity, side effects
- To avoid alcoholic beverages because of possibility of additive CNS effects
- That drug may cause sensitivity or intolerance to high temp, causing dizziness
- To watch for signs of confusion
Encourage
- By providing emotional support as indicated

STORAGE
- Store at room temp in tightly sealed, light-resistant container

---

azithromycin
Brand Name: Zithromax✤
Classification: Antibiotic (macrolide)
Pregnancy Category: C

A

AVAILABLE PREPARATIONS
Oral susp: 100 mg/5 ml, 200 mg/5 ml
Caps: 250 mg

ROUTES AND DOSAGES
Infants >6 mo and children: PO day 1, 10 mg/kg qd; maximum dose 500 mg/24 hr; day 2-5, 5 mg/kg qd; maximum dose 250 mg/24 hr
Adults: PO 500 mg day 1, then 250 mg qd for 2-5 days; total dose 1.5 g
Non-Gonococcal Urethritis or Chlamydia
1.0 g one time only

MECHANISM AND INDICATIONS
Antibiotic mechanism: Binds to 50S subunit of ribosome, inhibiting bacterial protein synthesis
Indications: Active against *Moraxella catarrhalis, Streptococcus pneumoniae, Str. pyogenes, Str. agalactiae, Staphylococcus aureus, Haemophilus influenzae, Clostridium, Legionella pneumophila,* non-gonococcal urethritis or cervicitis because of *Chlamydia trachomatis;* used to treat mild-to-moderate infections of the upper/lower respiratory tact, otitis media, uncomplicated skin and tissue infections

PHARMACOKINETICS
Peak: 12 hr
Distribution: Extensive, into most tissues
Half-life: 11-57 hr
Metabolism: Liver
Excretion: Bile, feces

CONTRAINDICATIONS AND PRECAUTIONS
- Contraindicated with known hypersensitivity to azithromycin, erythromycins
- Use cautiously in children <16, elderly, and with hepatic, renal, or

---

cardiac disease, pregnancy, lactation

INTERACTIONS
Drug
• Increased action, potential toxicity of oral anticoagulants, digoxin, theophylline, methylprednisolone, cyclosporine, bromocriptine, disopyramide, carbamazepine
• Decreased action of clindamycins
Lab
• False elevations in urinary catecholamines and steroids, AST, ALT
• False decrease in folate assay
Nutrition
• Reduced absorption if taken with meals, Al- or Mg-containing antacids, acidic fruit juices, citrus fruit, acidic beverages (such as cola drinks)

SIDE EFFECTS
CNS: Dizziness, headache, vertigo, somnolence
CV: Palpitations, chest pain
DERM: Rash, urticaria, pruritus, photosensitivity
GI: Nausea, vomiting, diarrhea, hepatotoxicity, abdominal pain, stomatitis, heartburn, dyspepsia, flatulence, melena
GU: Vaginitis, moniliasis, nephritis
Other: Overgrowth of nonsusceptible bacteria or fungi, anaphylaxis, fever

PATIENT CARE MANAGEMENT
Assessment
• Assess history of hypersensitivity to azithromycin, erythromycins
• Obtain C&S; may begin therapy before obtaining results
• Assess renal function (BUN, creatinine, I&O), hepatic function (ALT, AST, bilirubin)
Interventions
• Administer PO 1 hr ac or 2 hr after meals with full glass of water; shake susp well before administering
• Maintain age-appropriate fluid intake

NURSING ALERT
Discontinue drug if hypersensitivity reaction develops

Evaluation
• Evaluate therapeutic response (decreased symptoms of infection).
• Observe for signs of allergic reaction (rash, pruritus, wheezing, tightness in chest)
• Monitor bowel pattern
• Monitor renal function (BUN, creatinine, I&O), hepatic function (ALT, AST, bilirubin)
• Observe for signs of superinfection (perineal itching, diaper rash, fever, malaise, redness, pain, swelling, drainage, rash, diarrhea, sore throat, change in cough or sputum)

PATIENT AND FAMILY EDUCATION
Teach/instruct
• To take as directed at prescribed intervals for prescribed length of time
Warn/advise
• To notify care provider of hypersensitivity, side effects, superinfection

STORAGE
• Store oral susp and caps at room temp

---

azlocillin sodium
Brand Name(s): Azlin
Classification: Antibiotic (extended-spectrum penicillin)
Pregnancy Category: B

AVAILABLE PREPARATIONS
Inj: 2 g, 3 g, 4 g

ROUTES AND DOSAGES
Premature neonates <7 days: IM/IV 50 mg/kg q12h (Safety and effectiveness not established. Dosage represents accepted standard practice recommendations.)
Full-term neonates <7 days: IM/IV 100 mg/kg q12h (Safety and effec-

---

tiveness not established. Dosage represents accepted standard practice recommendations.)
Infants and children: IV 240-350 mg/kg/24 hr divided q4-6h
Children with acute exacerbation of cystic fibrosis: IV 75 mg/kg q4h; maximum dose 24 g/24 hr
Adults: IV 200-350 mg/kg q4-6h; maximum dose 24 g/24 hr

IV administration
• Recommended concentration: 10-50 mg/ml in D_5 ¼ NS, D_5 ½ NS, D_5W, LR, NS, or SW for IV infusion
• Maximum concentration: 100 mg/ml in D_5W, NS, or SW for IV push
• IV push rate: Over ≥5 min
• Intermittent infusion rate: Over 20-50 min

MECHANISM AND INDICATIONS
Antibiotic mechanism: Bactericidal; inhibits bacterial cell wall synthesis by adhering to bacterial penicillin-binding proteins
Indications: Effective against gram-positive and gram-negative organisms including *Staphylococcus aureus, Streptococcus pyogenes, Str. faecalis, Bacteroides, Pseudomonas aeruginosa, Escherichia coli, Haemophilus influenzae, Proteus mirabilis, Clostridium perfringens, C. tetani;* used to treat septicemia, lower respiratory (cystic fibrosis), urinary tract, skin, and bone infections

PHARMACOKINETICS
Half-life: Prematures 2.6-4.4 hr; full-term neonates 2.5-3.4 hr; infants 1-3 mo 1.9 hr; children 0.93-0.97 hr
Distribution: Throughout body tissues, fluids including CSF (especially with inflamed meninges)
Metabolism: Liver
Excretion: Urine, bile

CONTRAINDICATIONS AND PRECAUTIONS
• Contraindicated with known hypersensitivity to azlocillin, penicillins, cephalosporins
• Use cautiously in neonates, with impaired renal function, pregnancy

INTERACTIONS
Drug
• Synergistic antimicrobial activity against certain organisms with use of aminoglycosides, clavulanic acid
• Increased serum concentrations of azlocillin with use of probenecid
• Increased serum concentrations of methotrexate
• Decreased effectiveness with use of tetracyclines, erythromycins, chloramphenicol
• Increased risk of bleeding with use of anticoagulants
Lab
• False positive for urine protein with all tests (except those using bromophenol blue—Albustix Abutest, Multistix)
• Decreased serum uric acid levels

INCOMPATABILITIES
• Aminoglycosides, amphotericin B, chloramphenicol, lincomycin, oxytetracycline, polymyxin B, promethazine, tetracycline, vitamins B and C

SIDE EFFECTS
CNS: Neuromuscular irritability, headache, dizziness
ENDO/METAB: Hypokalemia
GI: Nausea, diarrhea, vomiting, pseudomembranous colitis
HEME: Bleeding with high doses, neutropenia, eosinophilia, leukopenia, thrombocytopenia
Local: Phlebitis, vein irritation with IV injection
Other: Hypersensitivity (edema, fever, chills, rash, pruritus, urticaria, anaphylaxis), overgrowth of nonsusceptible organisms

TOXICITY AND OVERDOSE
Clinical signs: Neuromuscular hypersensitivity; seizures may result from high CNS concentrations
Treatment: Supportive care; hemodialysis

PATIENT CARE MANAGEMENT
Assessment
• Assess hypersensitivity history to azlocillin, penicillins, or cephalosporins

- Obtain C&S; may begin therapy before obtaining results
- Assess renal function (BUN, creatinine, I&O), hepatic function (ALT, AST, bilirubin), hematologic function (CBC, differential, platelet count); bowel pattern, K⁺ levels if on long-term therapy

Interventions

- Administer penicillins at least 1 hr before bacteriostatic antibiotics (tetracyclines, erythromycins, chloramphenicol)
- Darkening of powder, solutions with storage does not affect potency; if refrigerated, reconstituted sol forms precipitate, redissolve by raising solution temp to 37° C in warm water bath for 20 min; agitate vigorously
- Do not premix IV sol with other medications, particularly aminoglycosides; infuse separately
- Use large vein with small-bore needle to reduce local reaction; rotate site every 48-72 hr
- Maintain age-appropriate fluid intake

> **NURSING ALERT**
> Discontinue drug if signs of hypersensitivity, bleeding complications, pseudomembranous colitis develop

Evaluation

- Evaluate therapeutic response (decreased symptoms of infection)
- Monitor for signs of superinfection (perineal itching, diaper rash, fever, malaise, redness, pain swelling, drainage, rash, diarrhea, sore throat, change in cough or sputum)
- Observe for signs of allergic reaction (wheezing, tightness in chest, urticaria) especially within 20-30 min of first dose
- Monitor bowel pattern; diarrhea may be symptomatic of pseudomembranous colitis
- Monitor renal function (BUN, creatinine, I&O), hepatic function (ALT, AST, bilirubin), electrolytes, particularly K⁺ and Na
- Monitor for signs of bleeding (ecchymosis, bleeding gums, hematuria, daily stool guaiac); monitor prothrombin times, platelet counts
- Evaluate IV site for vein irritation

PATIENT AND FAMILY EDUCATION

Teach/instruct

- To take as directed at prescribed intervals for prescribed length of time

Warn/advise

- To notify care provider of hypersensitivity, side effects, superinfection

STORAGE

- Store powder at room temp
- Consult package insert for storage
- Stability varies with strength and dilution

---

bacampicillin hydrochloride

Brand Name(s): Spectrobid

Classification: Antibiotic (aminopenicillin)

Pregnancy Category: B

AVAILABLE PREPARATIONS

Oral susp: 125 mg/5 ml
Tabs: 400 mg

ROUTES AND DOSAGES

Children <25 kg: PO 25 mg/kg/dose q12h
Children >25 kg/adults: PO 400-800 mg q12h

Neiserria gonorrhoeae

Children >25 kg/adults: PO 1.6 g with 1 g probenecid as single dose

MECHANISM AND INDICATIONS

Antibiotic mechanism: Precursor of ampicillin which is bactericidal; inhibits bacterial cell wall synthesis by adhering to bacterial penicillin-binding proteins
Indications: Effective against *Streptococcus faecalis, Str. pneumoniae, N. gonorrhoeae, N. meningitidis, Haemophilus influenzae,*

✤ Available in Canada.

B

Esherichia coli, Proteus mirabilis, Salmonella, Shigella; used to treat upper and lower respiratory tract, urinary tract, and skin infections

PHARMACOKINETICS
Peak: 0.5-1.5 hr
Distribution: To most body tissues
Half-life: 0.5-1.5 hr
Metabolism: Liver
Excretion: Urine

CONTRAINDICATIONS AND PRECAUTIONS
• Contraindicated with known hypersensitivity to bacampicillin, other penicillins, or cephalosporins; in neonates; with infectious mononucleosis (many develop rash during therapy)
• Use cautiously with impaired renal function, history of colitis or other GI disorders, pregnancy

INTERACTIONS
Drug
• Synergistic antimicrobial activity against certain organisms with use of aminoglycosides
• Increased serum concentrations with use of probenecid
• Increased serum concentrations of methotrexate
• Increased incidence of skin rash from both drugs with use of allopurinol
• Decreased effectiveness with use of tetracyclines, erythromycins, chloramphenicol
• Increased bleeding with use of oral anticoagulants
• Decreased effectiveness of oral contraceptives
Lab
• False positive for urine protein
• Falsely decreased serum aminoglycoside concentrations
• False positive Coombs' test
Nutrition
• Reduced absorption of oral susp when taken with food

INCOMPATIBILITIES
• Do not administer with disulfiram

SIDE EFFECTS
GI: Nausea, vomiting, diarrhea, glossitis, stomatitis, pseudomembranous colitis

GU: Acute interstitial nephritis
HEME: Anemia, thrombocytopenia, thrombocytopenic purpura, eosinophilia, leukopenia
Other: Hypersensitivity (erythematous maculopapular rash, urticaria, anaphylaxis), bacterial or fungal superinfection

TOXICITY AND OVERDOSE
Clinical signs: Neuromuscular hypersensitivity, seizures
Treatment: If ingestion within 4 h, empty the stomach by induced emesis or gastric lavage, followed with activated charcoal; supportive care, hemodialysis

PATIENT CARE MANAGEMENT
Assessment
• Assess history of hypersensitivity to bacampicillin, penicillins, cephalosporins
• Obtain C&S; may begin therapy before obtaining results
• Assess renal function (BUN, creatinine, I&O) bowel pattern
Interventions
• Administer penicillins at least 1 hr before bacteriostatic antibiotics (tetracycline, erythromycin, chloramphenicol)
• Administer oral susp 1 hr ac or 2 hr after meals; tabs may be administered without regard to meals; shake susp well before administering; tabs may be crushed, mixed with food or fluid
• Maintain age-appropriate fluid intake

> **NURSING ALERT**
> Discontinue drug if signs of hypersensitivity, bone marrow toxicity, acute interstitial nephritis, pseudomembranous colitis develop

Evaluation
• Evaluate therapeutic response (decreased symptoms of infection)
• Monitor signs of superinfection (perineal itching, diaper rash, fever, malaise, redness, pain, swelling, drainage, rash, diarrhea, sore

throat, change in cough or sputum)

• Monitor bowel pattern; diarrhea may be symptomatic of pseudomembranous colitis

• Observe for hypersensitivity (wheezing, tightness in chest, urticaria), especially within 15-30 min of first dose

• Monitor renal function (BUN, creatinine, I&O), hepatic function (ALT, AST, bilirubin), hematologic function (CBC, differential, platelet count)

PATIENT AND FAMILY EDUCATION
Teach/instruct
• To take as directed as prescribed intervals for prescribed length of time
Warn/advise
• To notify care provider of hypersensitivity, side effects, superinfection
Storage
• Store powder or tabs at room temp
• Reconstituted susp stable refrigerated for 14 days, at room temp for 7 days
• Label date, time of reconstitution

---

bacitracin

Brand Name(s): Ak-tracin, Baci-IM, Bactin✤, Baciguent (Bacitracin Compound)✤

Classification: Antibiotic (polypeptide)

Pregnancy Category: C

AVAILABLE PREPARATIONS
Inj: 10,000 U, 50,000 U
Ophth oint: 500 U/g
Top oint: 500 U/g

ROUTES AND DOSAGES
Infants <2.5 kg: IM 900 U/kg/24 hr divided q8-12h; do not administer for more than 12 days
Infants > 2.5 kg: IM 1000 U/kg/24 hr divided q8-12h; do not administer for more than 12 days

Children: IM 800-1200 U/kg/24 hr divided q8h
Adults: IM 10,000-25,000 U q6h for 7-10 days (maximum 100,000 U/24 hr)
• IM route not recommended
Infants, children, and adults: Ophth, instill small strip into conjunctival sac qd-bid; top, apply sparingly to affected area bid-tid

MECHANISM AND INDICATIONS
Antibiotic mechanism: Bactericidal or bacteriostatic; impairs bacterial cell wall synthesis, thus damaging bacterial plasma membrane and making the cell more vulnerable to osmotic pressure
Indications: Effective against many gram-positive organisms (including streptococci, staphylococci, *Corynebacterium,* and *Clostridium);* used to treat staphylococcal pneumonia, empyema, pseudomembranous colitis; topical, ophth forms used to treat short-term, superficial infections

PHARMACOKINETICS
Peak: 1-2 hr
Distribution: Widely distributed
Metabolism: Not significantly metabolized
Excretion: Urine

CONTRAINDICATIONS AND PRECAUTIONS
• Contraindicated with known hypersensitivity to bacitracin, with severe renal impairment; pts with allergy to neomycin may be allergic to bacitracin; top oint contraindicated for application in external ear canal if tympanic membrane is perforated
• Use cautiously with preexisting renal dysfunction, neuromuscular disease, and pregnancy

INTERACTIONS
Drug
• Increased nephrotoxicity, neurotoxicity with use of aminoglycosides, amphotericin B, capreomycin, methoxyflurane, polymyxin B sulfate, vancomycin
• Increased neuromuscular block-

✤ Available in Canada.

ade with use of neuromuscular blocking agents, anesthetics

Lab

• Increased urinary protein/cast excretion
• Increased serum creatinine/BUN levels

SIDE EFFECTS

DERM: Urticaria, rash, stinging, itching, burning, swelling of lips or face with top forms
EENT: Ototoxicity
GI: Nausea, vomiting, anorexia, diarrhea, rectal itching or burning
GU: Nephrotoxicity (albuminuria, cylinduria, oliguria, anuria, increased BUN, tubular and glomerular necrosis)
HEME: Blood dyscrasias, eosinophilia
Local: Pain at injection site
Other: Fever, anaphylaxis, neuromuscular blockage, allergic reactions, chest tightness, hypotension, bacterial or fungal superinfection

TOXICITY AND OVERDOSE

Clinical signs: Nephrotoxicity with parenteral administration; nausea, vomiting, minor GI upset with oral overdose
Treatment: Supportive care

PATIENT CARE MANAGEMENT

Assessment

• Assess history of hypersensitivity to bacitracin, neomycin
• Obtain C&S; may begin therapy before obtaining results
• Assess renal function (BUN, creatinine, I&O)

Interventions

• IM injection may be painful; administer deeply, rotate injection sites
• Wash hands before/after ophth instillation; cleanse crusts or discharge from eye before instillation; wipe excess medication from eye; do not flush medication from eye
• Wash hands before/after top application; cleanse wound; apply sparingly
• Maintain age-appropriate fluid intake

NURSING ALERT

Discontinue drug if signs of hypersensitivity, nephrotoxicity, neuromuscular blockage develop

Do not administer IV

Evaluation

• Evaluate therapeutic response (decreased symptoms of infection)
• Evaluate renal function (BUN, creatinine, I&O); urine pH (maintain pH >6)
• Monitor for signs of nephrotoxicity, neuromuscular blockade with parenteral form; monitor for rash, itching, swelling with ophthal or top forms
• Observe for signs of superinfection (perineal itching, diaper rash, fever, malaise, redness, pain, swelling, drainage, rash, diarrhea, sore throat, change in cough or sputum)
• Evaluate IM site for tissue damage

PATIENT AND FAMILY EDUCATION

Teach/instruct

• To take as directed at prescribed intervals for prescribed length of time

Warn/advise

• To notify care provider of hypersensitivity, side effects, superinfection
• Not to share towels, wash cloths, linens, eye makeup with family member being treated with ophth form

STORAGE

• Store sterile powder in refrigerator protected from direct sunlight
• Aqueous sol stable in refrigerator for 2 wk
• Store ophth, top oint at room temp

beclomethasone dipropionate

Brand Name(s): Beclodisk, Beclodisk Inhaler, Becloforte, Beclovent, Beclovent Inhaler, Beclovent Rotocaps, Beclovent Rotohaler, Beconase, Beconase AZ, Propaderm, Vancenase, Vanceril

Classification: Antiinflammatory (glucocorticoid); antiasthma

Pregnancy Category: C

AVAILABLE PREPARATIONS

Aerosol inh: 42 mcg/inhalation
Nasal inh: 42 mcg/inhalation
Nasal spray: 42 mcg/dose (aqueous)

ROUTES AND DOSAGES

Asthma

Children 6-12 yr: Aerosol inhaler, 1-2 inhalations q6-8h, or 4 inhalations bid; maximum dose 10 inhalations/24 hr
Children >12 yr and adults: 2 inhalations q6-8h, for severe asthma, 12-16 inhalations/24 hr initially, then decrease dose based on pt's response; maximum dose 20 inhalations/24 hr

Allergic Rhinitis

Children 6-12 yr: Nasal inhaler, 1 spray each nostril tid
Children >12 yr and adults: Nasal inhaler, 1 spray each nostril bid-qid; nasal spray, 1-2 sprays each nostril bid

MECHANISM AND INDICATIONS

Antiinflammatory mechanism: Precise mechanisms unclear, but it likely inhibits activation of and mediator release from inflammatory cells associated with asthma; increases responsiveness of β-receptors in airway smooth muscle; decreases bronchial activity with chronic use
Indications: Used to treat steroid-dependent asthma, asthma not well controlled with non-steroid treatment; used increasingly as a first-line drug for treatment of mild-to-moderate asthma; used to treat seasonal or perennial rhinitis unresponsive to conventional therapy; also used to prevent recurrence of nasal polyps after surgical removal

PHARMACOKINETICS

Onset of action: 1-4 wk (aerosol inh); few days-2 wk (nasal spray/inh)
Peak: Rapidly absorbed
Half-life: 15 hr
Metabolism: Liver
Excretion: Feces, urine (<10%)

CONTRAINDICATIONS AND PRECAUTIONS

• Contraindicated for primary treatment of acute bronchospasm, status asthmaticus when intensive measures are required; with hypersensitivity to any component of preparation
• Use cautiously with pts transferred from systemically active corticosteroids to beclomethasone (deaths because of adrenal insufficiency and rebound bronchospasm have occurred in asthmatic pts during/after transfer) in severe stress, asthma, emergency situations, infection or trauma; systemic steroids may be indicated; with long term treatment; with pulmonary tuberculosis, other untreated pulmonary infections; with ocular herpes simplex; with recent nasal septal ulcers, oral/nasal surgery or trauma (wait until healing occurs); with untreated infections of nasal mucosa; with lactation (since safety has not been established)

SIDE EFFECTS

CNS: Headache
CV: Flushing
DERM: Urticaria, angioedema, rash
EENT: Irritation, burning of nose, sneezing, stuffiness, rhinorrhea, epistaxis, bloody nasal discharge, ulceration and nasal septal perforation (rare), local infection of

---

nose; increased intraocular pressure, tearing eyes

GI: Nausea, candidal infection of mouth, throat, larynx, dry mouth, sore mouth, altered taste, tongue irritation

RESP: Bronchospasm, cough, tracheal irritation, wheezing

Other: Hypersensitivity reactions; suppression of hypothalamic–pituitary–adrenal function

TOXICITY AND OVERDOSE

• Acute overdose is unlikely

Clinical signs: Hypercorticism (bruising, weight gain, mental disturbances, cushingoid features, acneiform lesions, menstrual irregularities), hypothalamic–pituitary–adrenal suppression (decreased height, wt) may occur when used at excessive dosages

Treatment: Discontinue drug slowly (consistent with accepted procedures for discontinuing oral steroid therapy)

PATIENT CARE MANAGEMENT

Assessment

• Assess history of hypersensitivity to beclomethasone, related drugs

• Assess respiratory status, HEENT

• Assess baseline VS

• Review other medications used

• Measure baseline height, wt

Interventions

• Follow manufacturer instructions for aerosol inh use; see Chapter 3 for information regarding inh use

• Shake inh before use

• Administer bronchodilator (if prescribed) 5-15 min before beclomethasone

• Administer second inhalation of beclomethasone (if prescribed) 1 min after first inhalation

• Have pt rinse mouth, offer oral care (do not allow pt to swallow water used for rinsing)

• Follow manufacturer instructions for use of nasal spray

• Have pt clear nose before intranasal use

NURSING ALERT

Deaths because of adrenal insufficiency have occurred in asthma pts during, after transfer to beclomethasone dipropionate from systemic corticosteriods

Not recommended for children under 6 yr

Evaluation

• Evaluate therapeutic response (lessened respiratory, nasal symptoms, decreased need for systemic steroids, bronchodilators, decongestants)

• Evaluate side effects, hypersensitivity

• Evaluate respiratory status during treatment

• Evaluate compliance with regime

• Evaluate height, wt, development for any signs of growth retardation

• Evaluate oropharynx daily for symptoms of fungal infection

• Evaluate response, reduce dose to smallest amount necessary to control symptoms after consulting prescriber

• Evaluate need for oral steroids; reduce oral steroid gradually (if transferring from oral to aerosol/inh, and only under care of prescriber)

• Evaluate for symptoms of systemic steroid withdrawal (if transferred from oral to inhaled steroid)

• Evaluate pts receiving treatment for several months (or more) for possible changes in nasal mucosa

• Evaluate for diminished response to medication; report to provider for possible dosage change

• Evaluate for systemic effects of beclomethasone (steroid effects) such as mental disturbance, wt gain, bruising, cushingoid features, decreased growth velocity; report to prescriber for possible dosage change or slow discontinuation

---

✽ Available in Canada.

PATIENT AND FAMILY EDUCATION
Teach/instruct
• To shake aerosol inh, nasal spray before use
• About proper use of aerosol inh, nasal sprays
• To rinse/dry inh between uses
• That mild transient nasal stinging, burning common with intranasal use
• To check nose, mouth, throat daily; local fungal infections of oropharynx, larynx, esophagus possible; report symptoms to provider
• To rinse mouth, use good oral hygiene to prevent infections; to not swallow water used for rinsing mouth
• That therapeutic effect of medication may be diminished if canister is cold

Warn/advise
• To contact provider if no clinical improvement is seen within 3 wk (for nasal spray) or 4 wk (for aerosol inh); drug will gradually be discontinued
• That compliance with regime is necessary, regular use required to achieve full benefit
• About need to work closely with provider to titrate drug to the lowest maintenance dose needed to control symptoms
• That drug is *not* a bronchodilator, not indicated for rapid relief of bronchospasm
• To not exceed recommended dosage to prevent systemic effects, hypothalamic–pituitary–adrenal axis suppression
• That symptoms of steroid withdrawal may occur (lassitude, muscle or joint pain, depression, nausea or vomiting, low blood pressure) if pt had been taking oral steroids; hypothalamic–pituitary–adrenal axis suppression may last up to 1 yr; pt should carry a card indicating potential need for supplemental systemic steroids (because of hypothalamic–pituitary–adrenal axis suppression) in stress, acute asthma, trauma, surgery, infection (especially gastroenteritis); provider should be no-

tified immediately; transfer to inhaled steroids from oral steroids may unmask symptoms suppressed by oral dose (e.g., eczema)
• To administer bronchodilator (if prescribed) *before* use of drug for maximum penetration into bronchial tree and allow several min to elapse between inhalation of the two drugs
• That administration of an oral decongestant or nasal vasoconstrictor may be indicated, to contact provider if pt's nasal passages are blocked
• To avoid exposure to chicken pox or measles, report any exposure to provider
• To report immediately any wheezing that does not respond to treatment with bronchodilators and beclomethasone since systemic steroids may be indicated
• To observe for symptoms of hypercorticism and hypothalamic–pituitary–adrenal axis suppression; notify provider if these occur
• That long-term effects of drug are unknown

STORAGE
• Store aerosol at room temp; do not puncture, use/store near heat, open flame; temperatures >120° F may cause bursting
• Store nasal spray at room temp
• Keep out of reach of children

---

benztropine mesylate
Brand Name(s): Apo-Benztropine✤, Cogentin✤, PMS-Benztropine✤

Classification: Anticholinergic

Pregnancy Category: C

AVAILABLE PREPARATIONS
Tabs: 0.5 mg, 1 mg, 2 mg
Inj: 1 mg/ml

ROUTES AND DOSAGES
Drug-induced Extrapyramidal Reactions
Children >3 yr: PO/IM/IV 0.02-0.05 mg/kg/dose qd-bid

✤ Available in Canada.

Adults: PO/IM/IV 1-4 mg/kg/dose qd-bid

IV administration
• Recommended concentration: Administer undiluted
• Intermittent infusion rate: Over 1-2 min

MECHANISM AND INDICATIONS
Mechanism: Blockade of acetylcholine receptors
Indications: For use in treatment of drug-induced extrapyramidal effects, acute dystonic reactions

PHARMACOKINETICS
Onset: IM/IV 15 min; PO 1 hr
Duration: 6-10 hr

CONTRAINDICATIONS AND PRECAUTIONS
• Contraindicated with hypersensitivity, narrow-angle glaucoma, myasthenia gravis, children less than 3 yr, peptic ulcer, megacolon
• Use cautiously in hot weather, tachycardia, renal or hepatic disease, hypertension, hypotension, arrhythmias, pregnancy, lactation

INTERACTIONS
Drug
• Increased anticholinergic effect with antihistamines, phenothiazines, amantadine
• Decreased effect of levodopa
• Increased schizophrenic symptoms with haloperidol

INCOMPATIBILITIES
• Unknown

SIDE EFFECTS
CNS: Confusion, restlessness, irritability, hallucinations, headache, sedation, dizziness
CV: Tachycardia, bradycardia, hypotension, palpitations
DERM: Rash, urticaria, decreased sweating, flushing, increased temp
EENT: Blurred vision, dry eyes, dilated pupils, photophobia, increased intraocular tension
GI: Dry mouth, constipation, nausea, vomiting, abdominal distress, paralytic ileus
GU: Urinary retention, hesitancy, dysuria

TOXICITY AND OVERDOSE
Clinical signs: Delirium, coma, shock, seizures, respiratory distress; hyperthermia, glaucoma
Treatment: Antidote is physostigmine

PATIENT CARE MANAGEMENT
Assessment
• Assess history of hypersensitivity drug
• Assess VS, B/P, I&O
• Assess mental status
Interventions
• Administer IV/IM undiluted
• Keep pt lying flat for 1 hr after IV dose
• Administer PO with or after meals
Evaluation
• Evaluate therapeutic response (decreased involuntary movements)
• Evaluate for side effects (especially GI and GU); treat prn

PATIENT AND FAMILY EDUCATION
Teach/instruct
• To take as directed at prescribed intervals for prescribed length of time
Warn/advise
• To use caution in hot weather, limit time outdoors, drink fluids
• To avoid OTC medications (especially those with antihistamines and alcohol)
• Not to discontinue drug abruptly; taper over one week

STORAGE
• Store at room temp

---

beractant
Brand Name(s): Survanta
Classification: Lung surfactant
Pregnancy Category: X

AVAILABLE PREPARATIONS
Susp: 200 mg phospholipids/8 ml (25 mg/ml)

ROUTES AND DOSAGES
Prophylactic Treatment
Intratracheal 4 ml/kg as soon as possible; up to 4 doses can be administered during first 48 hr of life; maximum frequency q6h; repeat doses with evidence of continued respiratory distress (mechanical ventilation, PaO_2 <80, FIO_2 >30%), no sooner than 6 hr after previous dose

Rescue Treatment
Intratreacheal 4 ml/kg as soon as diagnosis of RDS is made

MECHANISM AND INDICATIONS
Mechanism: Replaces deficient endogenous lung surfactant; prevents alveoli from collapsing during expiration by lowering surface tension between air and alveolar surfaces

Indications: For use in prevention, treatment of respiratory distress syndrome in neonates

PHARMACOKINETICS
Absorption: Following intratracheal administration, drug is absorbed from alveoli, catabolized, and reused for further synthesis and secretion in lung tissue

CONTRAINDICATIONS AND PRECAUTIONS
• Contraindications: none known
• Use cautiously with bradycardia, rales, infections; administer only in highly supervised areas with trained clinicians experienced in intubation and mechanical ventilation of premature infants, neonates; arterial measurement of PO_2 and PCO_2 should be performed before, during, after treatment

INTERACTIONS
Lab
• None

INCOMPATIBILITIES
• No information available

SIDE EFFECTS
CV: Transient bradycardia, vasoconstriction, hypotension, hypertension, pallor
RESP: Decreased O_2 saturation, rales during treatment; apnea, air leaks, PIE
Other: ET tube reflex, blockage, increased chance of nosocomial (post-treatment) infections

TOXICITY AND OVERDOSE
• Not reported in humans

PATIENT CARE MANAGEMENT
Assessment
• Assess respiratory rate, rhythm, ABGs, color
• Assess ET tube placement before dosing
• Assess for apnea after dosing
• Assess for reflux of drug into ET tube; if reflux occurs, stop drug administration, increase peak inspiratory ventilation pressure until ET tube is clear

Interventions
• Suction infant before administration
• Inspect beractant visually for discoloration before administration; should be off-white to light brown; if settling occurs during storage, swirl vial *gently* (do not shake) to redisperse
• Administer using 5F ng tube cut to length of ET tube; 4 equal aliquots are given with the infant in 4 different positions (order does not matter): head, body down, head turned to right; head, body down, head turned to left; head, body up, head turned to right; head, body up, head turned to left; bed can be adjusted to place infant in "up" or "down" position
• Ventilate the infant mechanically during dosing after each aliquot (do not use hand-bagged ventilation); duration of ventilation between aliquots should be at least 30 sec (or longer) until infant stable
• Do not suction infants for at least 1 hr unless ET tube occlusion is suspected

Evaluation
• Evaluate therapeutic response (improvement in respiratory status)
• Monitor VS, ECG, and O_2 saturation continuously

- Evaluate for repeat dosing using chest x-ray results, clinical status, monitoring parameters

PATIENT AND FAMILY EDUCATION

Teach/instruct
- About rationale for treatment
- About treatment protocol

Provide
- Support to family

STORAGE

- Must be refrigerated
- Beractant should be stored in refrigerator; before administration, it should be warmed by allowing it to stand at room temp for at least 20 min or by warming in hand for at least 8 min
- Unopened, unused vials of beractant that have been warmed to room temp may be returned to refrigerator within 8 hr and stored for future use (this may be done only once)

---

betamethasone dipropionate, betamethasone valerate, betamethasone benzoate

Brand Name(s): Betamethasone dipropionate: Diprolene, Diprosone, Alphatrex
Betamethasone valerate: Betatrex, Betacort, Betaderm, Valisone
Betamethasone benzoate: Uticort

Classification: Topical anti-inflammatory

Pregnancy Category: C

AVAILABLE PREPARATIONS

Top betamethasone dipropionate: Lotion, ointment, cream 0.05%
Top betamethasone valerate: Lotion, ointment 0.1%; cream 0.01%, 0.1%
Top betamethasone benzoate: Lotion, ointment, gel, cream 0.025%

ROUTES AND DOSAGES

Children and adults: Top, apply lotion, ointment, cream, gel qd-tid

MECHANISMS AND INDICATIONS

Mechanism: Stimulates production of enzymes needed to reduce inflammatory response; decreases cell proliferation
Indications: For use in topical dermatoses (e.g., eczema, psoriasis, seborrheic, contact, or atopic dermatitis)

PHARMACOKINETICS

Absorption: Amount absorbed depends on amount applied; effectiveness of action depends on vehicle used (highest to lowest effectiveness: ointment, gel, cream, sol); amount absorbed depends on nature of skin at site of application; on thick skin (palms, soles, elbows, knees), absorption minimal; on thin skin (face, eyelids, genitals), absorption high; any absorbed drug removed rapidly from circulation, distributed into muscle, skin, liver, intestines, kidney
Distribution: Distributed, metabolized primarily in skin
Metabolism: Liver
Excretion: Urine, feces

CONTRAINDICATIONS AND PRECAUTIONS

- Contraindicated with known hypersensitivity to drug or its components; with viral, fungal, tubercular lesions
- Use cautiously with impaired circulation (because of risk of skin ulceration), pregnancy, lactation; in children (because of increased systemic absorption, which could lead to Cushing syndrome, intracranial hypertension, hypothalamic–pituitary–adrenal axis suppression)

INTERACTIONS

Drug
- Decreased antiinflammatory effects with barbiturates, phenytoin, rifampin

Lab
- Suppressed reaction to skin tests

INCOMPATIBILITIES
• None significant

SIDE EFFECTS
CNS: Significant systemic absorption may cause euphoria, insomnia, headache, pseudotumor cerebri, mental changes, restlessness
CV: Significant systemic absorption may cause edema, hypertension
Local: Burning, pruritis, hypopigmentation, atrophy, striae, allergic contact dermatitis

TOXICITY AND OVERDOSE
Clinical signs: No information available

PATIENT CARE MANAGEMENT
Assessment
• Assess skin to ensure application is appropriate; do not apply to skin with ulcerations or viral, fungal, or tubercular lesions
• Assess skin after application for side effects (especially striae, increased inflammation, atrophy, infection)

Interventions
• Apply small amount sparingly to clean, dry skin lesion(s) for as short a period of time as possible; stop drug if signs of systemic absorption appear; do not apply occlusive dressings, since this will increase absorption

> **NURSING ALERT**
> In children, limit topical application to least effective amount

Evaluation
• Evaluate therapeutic response (decreased skin inflammation)
• Inspect skin for infection, striae, atrophy

PATIENT AND FAMILY EDUCATION
Teach/instruct
• To take as directed at prescribed intervals for prescribed length of time; do not over-apply
• To apply drug sparingly, using a light film; rub into affected area(s) gently

• Not to use occlusive dressing over area of application; a diaper may be used if changed regularly and not in place longer than 16 hr
• To call provider if side effects occur or if skin not improved within 1 wk
• About side effects of drug, especially if over-applied
• To wash/dry hands before, after application
• To avoid prolonged application on face, skin folds, genital area; to notify care provider of hypersensitivity reactions

STORAGE
• Store at room temp

---

bleomycin
Brand Name: Blenoxane❧
Classification: Antineoplastic, antibiotic; cell cycle phase specific (G_2 and M)
Pregnancy Category: D

AVAILABLE PREPARATIONS
Inj: 15 U powder

ROUTES AND DOSAGES
• Dosages may vary in response to diagnosis, extent of disease, concurrent or previous therapy, protocol guidelines, and physiological parameters; consult current literature and protocol recommendations

Single Agent
IM/SC/IV 10-20 U/m^2 or 0.25-0.5 U/kg 1-2 times/wk; after a 50% reduction in tumor size, dosage may be decreased to 1 U/24 hr or 5 U/wk

Combination Regimens
IM/SC/IV 10-15 U/m^2 q 2-3 wk or several lower dose regimens of 3-4 U/m^2

Malignant Effusions
Intracavitary, drainage catheter placed, fluid removed, 60 U bleomycin in 30-60 ml preservative-free diluent placed, catheter withdrawn; response rates, defined as freedom from reaccumulation for 3-6 mo, 50%-70%

❧ Available in Canada.

• A test dose of bleomycin (0.5-1 U) has been recommended to assess for hypersensitivity; this practice is controversial because hypersensitivity may occur at any time during treatment with bleomycin; the decision to give test dose must be made by individual clinicians

• Cumulative dose should not exceed 400 U total dose in a lifetime; use caution when administering doses >300 U, since higher doses significantly increase risk of life-threatening pulmonary toxicity

• Generally administered in combination chemotherapy regimens

• May be administered IM, IV, SC, intraarterial, intratumor, by intracavitary routes

IV administration

• Maximum concentration: 3 U/ml

• IV push rate: 1 U/min

• Continuous infusion rate: 15 $U/m^2/24$ hr for 4 days

MECHANISM AND INDICATIONS

Mechanism: Appears to interact with iron, O_2 to form superoxide anions that cause scission of DNA; inhibits DNA synthesis and (to a lesser degree) RNA and protein synthesis; exerts action during G_2 and M phases of cell cycle; perhaps most effective during G phase when it causes arrest in prophase chromosomal maturation, thus inhibiting cell progression out of G_2 phase; may be used to synchronize cells kinetically in multi-agent therapy

Indications: Hodgkin's and non-Hodgkin's lymphoma; squamous cell cancer, testicular cancer, mycosis fungoides, and osteosarcoma; sclerotherapy for malignant effusions

PHARMACOKINETICS

Distribution: Widely in total body water (skin, lungs, kidneys, peritoneum, lymphatic tissue)

Half-life: Terminal plasma elimination half-life 2-4 hr

Metabolism: Inactivation appears to occur as result of bleomycin hydrolase, an enzyme system that prevents bleomycin from binding to a metal ion, which causes loss of cytotoxic potential for drug; this occurs in all tissues, but enzyme activity is lowest in lungs and skin, which demonstrates increased potential for toxicity

Excretion: Drug, metabolites excreted primarily in urine

CONTRAINDICATIONS AND PRECAUTIONS

• Contraindicated with pregnancy, lactation, history of hypersensitivity, idiosyncratic reactions to drug; with evidence of pulmonary fibrosis, mucocutaneous toxicity; with active infections (especially chicken pox, herpes zoster)

• Use cautiously with impaired renal or pulmonary function; pts who have previously received pulmonary radiation

INTERACTIONS

Drug

• Synergistic with other antineoplastic drugs because bleomycin causes synchrony of cells in G_2 phase

• Increased antitumor activity possible with drugs that deplete cellular glutathione

• Exacerbated pulmonary toxicity possible with concomitant use of pulmonary radiation or in presence of a hyperoxic condition

• Decreased excretion of bleomycin, increased toxicities possible with use of other nephrotoxic drugs

• Increased oral bioavailability of digoxin possible

• Altered phenytoin levels possible

• Suppressed ability of body to respond to immunizations

Lab

• Increased concentration of uric acid in blood and urine possible

INCOMPATIBILITIES

• Aminophylline, ascorbic acid, carbenicillin, cefazolin, cephalothin, diazepam, hydrocortisone sodium succinate, methotrexate, mitomycin C, nafcillin, penicillin, terbutaline

✤ Available in Canada.

SIDE EFFECTS

CNS: Headache

CV: Hypotension with rapid infusion

DERM: Most frequently encountered toxicity because of decreased activity of bleomycin hydrolase in skin; rash; erythema; vesiculation; hardening and discoloration of palmar and plantar skin; desquamation of hands, feet, and pressure areas; acne; hyperpigmentation; urticaria; facial flushing; pruritus; thickening of nail beds

EENT: Mild stomatitis

GI: Nausea, vomiting, diarrhea, prolonged anorexia

HEME: Minimal myelosuppression

MS: Swelling of interphalangeal joints, Raynaud's phenomena

RESP: Pulmonary fibrosis, potentially lethal progressive compromise with clinical picture of fine crackles, rales, fever, dyspnea, nonproductive cough

Other: Fever in about 50% of pts approximately 4-10 hr after drug administration; anaphylactoid reaction (lymphoma pts may be at greater risk)

TOXICITY AND OVERDOSE

Clinical signs: Evidence of pulmonary disease consistent with pulmonary fibrosis; cutaneous lesions

Treatment: Stop bleomycin at first sign of end inspiratory rales or pulmonary compromise; pulmonary fibrosis must be treated aggressively with local and systemic corticosteroids; antioxidants (such as vitamin E) may also be helpful; topical steroids may help cutaneous lesions

PATIENT CARE MANAGEMENT

Assess

• Assess history of hypersensitivity to bleomycin

• Assess history of previous treatment with radiation therapy or antineoplastics, especially those that may predispose pt to increased risk of pulmonary toxicity

• Assess baseline VS, oximetry, pulmonary function tests, breath sounds, chest radiograph

• Assess skin, oral mucosa

• Assess baseline CBC, differential, platelet count

• Assess baseline liver function (AST, ALT, bilirubin) and renal function (BUN, creatinine)

Interventions

• Have epinephrine, diphenhydramine, corticosteroids, O$_2$ available in event of anaphylactoid reaction; reaction can occur immediately or several hr later; symptoms are decreased BP, fever, chills, confusion, wheezing

• Premedicate with acetaminophen, steroid, diphenhydramine if necessary

• Provide supportive measures to maintain homeostasis, fluid and electrolyte balance, nutritional status

> **NURSING ALERT**
> Bleomycin can cause progressive, potentially fatal pulmonary fibrosis; frequent assessment of respiratory status by chest auscultation, oximetry readings is necessary; follow-up of any untoward respiratory symptom or physical examination finding is imperative

Evaluate

• Evaluate therapeutic response through radiologic or clinical demonstration of tumor regression

• Evaluate respiratory status; auscultation of fine end-inspiratory rales may be first clinical finding of pulmonary fibrosis

• Evaluate pulmonary function tests, chest radiographs; in presence of pulmonary fibrosis, pulmonary function tests reveal arterial hypoxemia, decreased diffusing capacity, restrictive ventilatory changes; radiograph changes may run continuum from interstitial changes to fibrosis

• Assess VS, oximetry for evidence of increased HR, respiratory rate, decreased O$_2$ saturation

• CBC, platelet count, differen-

B

tial, renal function (BUN, creatinine) and liver function (AST, ALT, bilirubin)

PATIENT AND FAMILY EDUCATION
Teach/instruct
• To have pt well hydrated before and after chemotherapy
• About the importance of follow-up to monitor blood counts, serum chemistry values, urinalysis
• To take an accurate temp; rectal temp contraindicated
• To notify care provider of signs of bleeding (bruising, epistaxis, bleeding gums); signs of infection (fever, sore throat, fatigue)
Warn/advise
• About impact of body changes that may occur (hair loss, hyperpigmentation, nail ridging) and how to minimize changes (wigs, caps, scarves, long sleeves)
• To avoid OTC preparations containing aspirin
• To report any alterations in behavior, sensation, perception; help to develop a plan of care to manage side effects, stress of illness or treatment
• To report any respiratory symptoms such as coughing, dyspnea, fever, chills that occur within 3-6 hr after dose
• To report immediately any shortness of breath, persistent cough
• To avoid contact with bacterial or viral illnesses
• That good oral hygiene with very soft toothbrush is imperative
• That dental work be delayed until CBC returns to normal, with permission of care provider
• That close household contacts of child not be immunized with live polio virus; use inactivated form
• That children on chemotherapy not receive immunization until immune system recovers sufficiently to mount necessary antibody response
• To report exposure to chicken pox in susceptible child immediately

• To report reactivation of herpes zoster virus (shingles) immediately
• About ways to preserve reproductive patterns and sexuality, if appropriate (sperm banking, contraceptives)
Encourage
• Provision of nutritious food intake; consider nutritional consultation
• To use top anesthetics to control discomfort of mucositis; to avoid spicy foods, commercial mouthwashes

STORAGE
• Sterile powder stable for 2 yr when refrigerated
• Reconstituted sol stable for 14 hr at room temp and 96 hr refrigerated; long-term storage not recommended because of possibility of bacterial contamination

---

bretylium tosylate
Brand Name(s): Bretylate✤, Bretylol

Classification: Ventricular antiarrhythmic

Pregnancy Category: C

AVAILABLE PREPARATIONS
Inj: 50 mg/ml

ROUTES AND DOSAGES
Ventricular Fibrillation
Children and adults: IV 5 mg/kg/dose undiluted, rapid IV; may increase to 10 mg/kg/dose q 15-30 min until total dose of 30 mg/kg is administered
Ventricular Arryhthmias and Maintenance Dose for Ventricular Fibrillation
Children and adults: IV dilute 500 mg in 50 ml (minimum) D_5W or NS, 5-10 mg/kg/dose q6h
IV administration
• Recommended concentration: 10 mg/ml in D_5LR, D_5NS, D_5 ½ NS, D_5W, LR, NS
• Maximum concentration: 50 mg/ml

• IV push rate for ventricular fibrillation: Undiluted over 1 min
• Intermittent infusion rate: Over >8 min
• Continuous infusion rate: 1-2 mg/min for 6 hr

MECHANISM AND INDICATIONS

Mechanism: Transient release of norepinephrine accounts for increase in successful defibrillation threshold, increase B/P and HR; prolongs action potential duration, effective refractory period
Indications: For use in ventricular tachycardia, ventricular fibrillation, cardioversion; short-term use only

PHARMACOKINETICS

Onset of action: Within mins
Half life: 5-10 hr
Peak action: 6-9 hr
Excretion: Urine

CONTRAINDICATIONS AND PRECAUTIONS

• Contraindicated in digitalis toxicity
• Use cautiously in aortic stenosis, pulmonary hypertension, renal disease, pregnancy

INTERACTIONS

Drug
• Toxicity with digitalis
• Hypotension with antihypertensives
• Increased or decreased effects of bretylium with antiarrhythmics
Lab
• Decreased urine epinephrine, norepinephrine, VMA epinephrine

INCOMPATIBILITIES

• Phenytoin

SIDE EFFECTS

CNS: Syncope, vertigo, dizziness, confusion, lightheadedness
CV: Hypotension, bradycardia, PVCs, angina, chest pain
GI: Nausea, vomiting
RESP: Respiratory depression
Local: IV extravasation may cause tissue necrosis

TOXICITY AND OVERDOSE

Clinical signs: Severe hypotension
Treatment: Administer vasopressors, volume expanders, position changes, supportive care

PATIENT CARE MANAGEMENT

Assessment
• Assess VS, B/P, and ECG throughout infusion
• Assess I&O
Interventions
• Infuse IV with pump
• Place patient on monitor, watch for hypotension

> **NURSING ALERT**
> Bretylium is not a first line treatment for ventricular arrhythmias

Evaluation
• Evaluate therapeutic response: absence of ventricular arrhythmias
• Evaluate cardiac status, HR, and rhythm
• Evaluate BP, ECG throughout infusion

PATIENT AND FAMILY EDUCATION

Provide
• Support to pt, family during acute stage of pt's condition

STORAGE

• Store at room temp

---

bumetanide

Brand Name(s): Bumex, Burinex✤

Classification: Loop diuretic

Pregnancy Category: C

AVAILABLE PREPARATIONS

Tabs: 0.5 mg, 1 mg, 2 mg
Inj: 0.25 mg/ml

ROUTES AND DOSAGES

Children: PO, IM, IV 0.02-0.1 mg / kg/24 hr divided q12hr; maximum dose 2 mg qd
Adults: PO 0.5-2 mg qd-bid; maximum dose 10 mg qd; IV/IM 0.5-1 mg, may repeat at 2-3 hr intervals; maximum dose 10 mg qd

---

✤ Available in Canada.

IV administration
- Recommended concentration: Dilute in D_5W, LR, or NS
- Maximum concentration: 0.25 mg/ml
- IV push rate: Over 1-2 min
- Intermittent infusion rate: Over 5 min
- Continuous infusion rate: Adults, after 1 mg loading dose, 0.912 mg/hr for 12 hr

MECHANISM AND INDICATIONS
Diuretic mechanism: Acts on the ascending loop of Henle to excrete Na, Cl, K^+

Indications: Used for treatment of edema associated with CHF, liver disease with ascites, kidney disease (nephrotic syndrome), acute pulmonary edema, hypertension

PHARMACOKINETICS
Onset of action: PO ½ to 1 hr; IM 40 min; IV 5 min
Peak: PO/IM 1-2 hr; IV 15-30 min
Half-life: 1-1½ hr
Metabolism: Liver
Excretion: Urine

CONTRAINDICATIONS AND PRECAUTIONS
- Contraindicated with known hypersensitivity, anuria, hepatic coma, oliguria, with increasing BUN and creatinine
- Use cautiously with allergy to sulfa drugs, dehydration, ascites, cardiac glycosides (may produce hypokalemia leading to digoxin toxicity); in neonates (use pediatric dose, extend intervals); in pregnancy, lactation

INTERACTIONS
Drug
- Increased hypotensive effects with other diuretics, antihypertensives
- Increased K^+ loss with other K^+-depleting drugs (e.g., amphotericin B, steroids)
- Increased ototoxicity with other ototoxic drugs (e.g., cisplatin, aminoglycosides, amphotericin B)
- Increased serum levels of β blockers, lithium

- Decreased diuretic effect with indomethacin, probenecid

INCOMPATIBILITIES
- Dobutamine, milrinone

SIDE EFFECTS
CNS: Headache, dizziness, weakness
CV: Chest pain, hypotension, ECG changes
EENT: Hearing loss, tinnitus, blurred vision
GI: Nausea, vomiting, anorexia, dry mouth
GU: Polyuria, glycosuria
HEME: Transient thrombocytopenia, leukopenia
METAB: Hypokalemia, hyperchloremic alkalosis, hypocalcemia, hyperglycemia, hyponatremia, hypomagnesemia

TOXICITY AND OVERDOSE
Clinical signs: Profound volume and electrolyte depletion, circulatory collapse
Treatment: Lavage if taken PO; supportive care; replace fluids, electrolytes

PATIENT CARE MANAGEMENT
Assessment
- Assess history of hypersensitivity to drug
- Assess baseline VS, wt, B/P (lying, standing), electrolytes, CBC, creatinine

Interventions
- Administer IVP undiluted over at least 1-2 min
- Monitor I&O
- Administer PO dose in AM to avoid nighttime diuresis
- Monitor electrolytes, provide K^+ replacement prn
- Ensure safe environment in case hypotension, dizziness occur

Evaluation
- Evaluate therapeutic response (decreased edema)
- Evaluate for edema (sacral, dependent extremities) and ascites
- Evaluate ongoing electrolytes, if $K^+ < 3.5$, notify provider
- Evaluate for signs of hypokalemia, leg cramps, fatigue, muscle weakness

✦ Available in Canada.

PATIENT AND FAMILY EDUCATION
Teach/instruct
- To take as directed at prescribed intervals for prescribed length of time
- About rationale for drug therapy, diuretic effect
- To provide K^+ rich foods (e.g., citrus fruits, bananas, raisins, potatoes)

Warn/advise
- About adverse effects; to call care provider if they occur
- To rise slowly from lying or sitting position
- To return for regular follow-up care

STORAGE
- Use diluted drug within 24 hr
- Store inj and tabs in light resistant containers, avoid freezing

---

bupropion

Brand Name(s): Wellbutrin

Classification: Nontricyclic antidepressant

Pregnancy Category: B

AVAILABLE PREPARATIONS
Tabs: 75 mg, 100 mg

DOSAGES AND ROUTES
Adolescents: 150 to 375 mg/24 hr divided bid maximum < 450 mg/24 hr (Safety and effectiveness not established. Dosage represents accepted standard practice recommendations.)
Adult: PO 100 mg bid initially; increase after 3 days to 100 mg tid (if needed); may increase after 1 mo to 150 mg tid

MECHANISM AND INDICATIONS
Mechanism: Bupropion inhibits reuptake of dopamine; also inhibits reuptake of serotonin, norepinephrine, but blocks these more weakly than tricyclic antidepressants do
Indications: For use in treating major depressive disorder in adolescents and adults, ADD and ADHD in children, adolescents

PHARMACOKINETICS
Onset of action: 2-4 wk
Half-life: 12-14 hr
Metabolism: Liver

CONTRAINDICATIONS AND PRECAUTIONS
- Contraindicated in pts with hypersensitivity to this or any component of this medication, eating disorders, history of seizure disorder
- Use cautiously with cranial trauma, liver disease, recent MI, kidney disease, pregnancy, lactation

INTERACTIONS
Drug
- Increased adverse reactions with use of alcohol, benzodiazepines, levodopa, MAOIs, phenothiazines, tricyclic antidepressants

Nutrition
- If GI upset occurs, take with or following food, milk

SIDE EFFECTS
CNS: Agitation or restlessness, confusion, headache, akathisia, delusions, insomnia, precipitation of mania, sedation, seizures (bupropion's potential for precipitating seizures is as much as four times that of other antidepressants), sweating, tremors
CV: Arrhythmias, hypertension, hypotension, palpitations, tachycardia
DERM: Pruritus, rash, sweating
EENT: Auditory disturbance, blurred vision
GI: Appetite increase or decrease, constipation, dry mouth, GI distress, nausea, weight loss, vomiting
GU: Impotence, urinary frequency, urinary retention

TOXICITY AND OVERDOSE
Clinical signs: Induction of seizures with doses >450 mg/24 hr
Treatment: Monitor VS, ECG; induce emesis; lavage; administer activated charcoal, anticonvulsant

---

✢ Available in Canada.

PATIENT CARE MANAGEMENT
Assessment
• Assess history of hypersensitivity to drug
• Assess general physical condition
• Assess for history of seizures
• Assess baseline CBC and diff, AST, bilirubin, ALT, ECG
Interventions
• Administer medication in AM; may cause insomnia if administered hs
• Administer with food or milk if GI symptoms occur
• Rinse mouth with water, or provide sugarless gum or hard candy for dry mouth; suggest sips of fluid
• Increase fluids, fiber in diet if constipation occurs
Evaluation
• Evaluate therapeutic response (ability to function in daily activities, ability to sleep throughout the night, activity level, impulsivity, distractibility, attending; if taken for attention deficit, obtain parent, teacher reports about attention, behavioral performance of the child; if taken for depression, evaluate for symptoms of depression)
• Evaluate mental status (mood, sensorium, affect, impulsiveness, suicidal ideation, psychiatric symptoms)
• Monitor wt, obtain general physical examination results, liver function (bilirubin, AST, ALT) test results at regular intervals during therapy
• Monitor cardiac enzymes with long-term therapy
• If medication is discontinued abruptly, withdrawal symptoms may occur (headache, nausea, vomiting, muscle pain, weakness)

PATIENT AND FAMILY EDUCATION
Teach/instruct
• To take as directed at prescribed intervals for prescribed length of time
• That medication is most helpful when used as part of a comprehensive multimodal treatment program
• Not to stop taking this medication without prescriber approval
• That therapeutic effects may take 2-4 wk
• To increase fluids, fiber in diet if constipation occurs
Warn/advise
• To avoid alcohol, other CNS depressants
• Not to stop taking medication quickly after long-term use; this might cause headache, nausea, vomiting, muscle pain or weakness

STORAGE
• Store at room temp in light resistant containers

---

busulfan
Brand Name(s): Myleran✤
Classification: Alkylating Agent
Pregnancy Category: D

AVAILABLE PREPARATION
Tabs: (PO) 2 mg

ROUTES AND DOSAGES
• Drug may vary in response to diagnosis, extent of disease, concurrent or previous therapy, protocol guidelines, physiologic parameters; consult current literature, protocol recommendations
Chronic Myelogenous Leukemia
Children and adults: PO 0.06-0.12 mg/kg/24 hr or 1.8-4.6 mg/m^2/24 hr; dosage is adjusted to maintain WBC count at 20,000/mm^3, but never < 10,000/mm^3; therapy stopped at WBC count of ≤10,000/mm^3 because count will continue to decrease for 2-3 wk without further busulfan therapy
• Dosage based on clinical, hematologic response and tolerance of pt to obtain optimum therapeutic results with minimal adverse effects

---

MECHANISM AND INDICATIONS

Mechanism: Cell cycle nonspecific and cytotoxic selective for granulocytic WBCs; forms carbonium ions by releasing a methane sulfonate group; cross-links strands of cellular DNA and interferes with RNA transcription, causing an imbalance of growth that leads to cell death

Indications: Used to treat chronic myelogenous leukemia (CML); used in very high doses as marrow ablative conditioning regimen before bone marrow transplant (BMT) in antileukemia regimen in combination with VP-16 or Cytoxan

PHARMACOKINETICS

Onset of action: About 1-2 wk

Half-life: Duration half-life about 2½ hr

Absorption: Well-absorbed orally from GI tract; blood concentration obtained within ½-2 hr after oral administration

Metabolism: Liver

Excretion: Urine (10%-50% of dose excreted as metabolites within 24-48 hr)

CONTRAINDICATIONS AND PRECAUTIONS

• Contraindicated with history of hypersensitivity to busulfan, pregnancy, lactation

• Use cautiously with other myelosuppressive agents or radiation therapy; with already-depressed neutrophil or platelet counts because of the risk of busulfan-induced aplastic bone marrow reactions; with history of seizure disorder or head trauma (because seizure threshold may be lowered)

INTERACTIONS

Drug

• Increased risk of bleeding with use of aspirin, anticoagulants

• Possible hepatotoxicity, esophageal varices, portal hypertension with use of thioguanine

INCOMPATIBILITIES

• Should not be mixed with other drugs during administration

SIDE EFFECTS

CNS: Seizures, unusual tiredness or weakness

DERM: Hyperpigmentation of skin creases may occur because of increased melanin production; rash, urticaria, anhidrosis, dryness of skin and mucus membranes

GI: Nausea, vomiting, diarrhea, glossitis, anorexia

GU: Amenorrhea, testicular atrophy, sterility, azoospermia, uric acid nephropathy, renal stones, acute renal failure, hyperuricemia

HEME: Thrombocytopenia, anemia, leukopenia; WBC may continue to fall for a month or more after stopping busulfan

RESP: Persistent cough, dyspnea, rales, fever, and anorexia, which may lead to irreversible pulmonary fibrosis or bronchopulmonary dysplasia commonly called "busulfan lung"

Other: Alopecia, Addison-like wasting syndrome (hypotension, wt loss, fatigue, apathy, confusion), gynecomastia, glossitis, hepatic dysfunction, infertility, amenorrhea, melanoderma, asthenia

TOXICITY AND OVERDOSE

Clinical signs: Pancytopenia with hypoplastic marrow will develop if treatment is maintained with falling counts; in some cases, WBC may continue to fall for a month or more after drug is stopped

Treatment: Busulfan should be stopped as soon as WBC reaches 15,000-20,000; this is generally a reversible situation and pts can be given sustained support (blood products and antibiotics) through this period

PATIENT CARE MANAGEMENT

Assess

• Assess history of hypersensitivity to busulfan, related drugs

• Assess baseline CBC, differential, platelet count, renal function (BUN, creatinine, I&O), hepatic function (ALT, AST, LDH, bilirubin, alk phos), pulmonary function

---

• Assess hydration status, urinary frequency, dysuria
• Assess success of previous antiemetic therapy
• Assess history of previous treatment with special attention to other therapies that may predispose pt to renal or pulmonary dysfunction

Interventions
• Premedicate with antiemetics; continue periodically through chemotherapy
• Administer 1 hr ac or 2 hr after meals
• Encourage small, frequent feedings of foods that pt likes
• Administer IV fluids until pt is able to resume normal PO intake
• Provide supportive measures to maintain hemostasis, fluid and electrolyte balance, nutritional support

---

NURSING ALERT

Hyperpigmentation, especially at skin creases may occur because of increased melanin production

Do not administer any aspirin, products containing aspirin

Evaluate
• Evaluate therapeutic response (decreased exacerbations of CML)
• CBC, differential, platelet count, renal function (BUN, creatinine), hepatic function (ALT, AST, LDH, bilirubin, alk phos) at given intervals after chemotherapy; dosage adjustment or discontinuation of drug based on WBC
• Evaluate for signs or symptoms of infection (fever, fatigue, sore throat), signs of bleeding (easy bruising, nose bleeds, bleeding gums)
• Evaluate I&O carefully; check wt regularly
• Evaluate for side effects, response to antiemetic regimen
• Evaluate for persistent cough, progressive dyspnea with alveolar exudate (suggestive of pneumonia, may be the result of drug toxicity);

report any respiratory symptoms to provider so dosage adjustments can be made

PATIENT AND FAMILY EDUCATION
Teach/instruct
• To have pt well-hydrated before and after chemotherapy
• About importance of follow-up to monitor blood counts, serum chemistry values, drug blood values, pulmonary function
• To take accurate temp; rectal temp contraindicated
• To notify care provider of signs of bleeding (bruising, epistaxis, bleeding gums), signs of infection (fever, sore throat, fatigue)
• To notify care provider of signs, symptoms of respiratory problems (cough, dyspnea)

Warn/advise
• About impact of body changes that may occur (hair loss, hyperpigmentation, nail ridging), how to minimize changes (wigs, caps, scarves, long sleeves)
• To avoid OTC products containing aspirin
• To report any alterations in behavior, sensation, perception; help to develop plan of care to manage side effects, stress of illness and treatment
• To manage bowel function; to call care provider if abdominal pain, constipation noted
• That good oral hygiene with very soft toothbrush is imperative
• That dental work be delayed until blood counts return to baseline, with permission of care provider
• To avoid contact with known viral, bacterial illnesses
• That household contacts of pt not be immunized with live polio virus; inactivated form should be used
• That pt not receive immunizations until immune system recovers sufficiently to mount needed antibody response
• To report exposure to chicken pox in susceptible pt immediately
• To report reactivation of herpes

---

zoster virus (shingles) immediately
• Ways to preserve reproductive patterns, and sexuality, if appropriate (sperm banking, contraceptives)

Encourage
• Provision of nutritional food intake; consider nutritional consultation
• To comply with bowel management program
• To use top anesthetics to control discomfort of mucositis; to avoid spicy foods, commercial mouthwashes

STORAGE
• Store in tight-fitting containers at room temp

---

caffeine

Brand Name(s): caffeine, citrated caffeine

Classification: Respiratory stimulant

Pregnancy Category: B

AVAILABLE PREPARATIONS
Tabs: (PO) 65 mg
Extemporaneous preparation: Oral sol 10 mg/ml, 20 mg/ml
Inj: 125 mg/ml with sodium benzoate

ROUTES AND DOSAGES
Neonatal Apnea
PO/IV/IM loading dose 5-10 mg/kg maintenance dose 2.5-5 mg/kg qd
• Dosages for caffeine citrate are twice the listed dosages
IV administration
• Recommended concentration: May be administered undiluted
• IV push rate: Over 1-2 min

MECHANISM AND INDICATIONS
Mechanism: Increases muscle contractile force, decreases fatigue of skeletal muscle
Indications: For use in neonatal apnea (unlabeled use)

PHARMACOKINETICS
Peak: 60-90 min

Absorption: Rapid with PO, IV
Half-life: Neonates, 100 hr
Excretion: Neonates < 1 mo, urine; infant and adult, liver

CONTRAINDICATIONS AND PRECAUTIONS
• Contraindicated with hypersensitivity to caffeine or citrate
• Use with caution with peptic ulcer, cardiac arrhythmias, pregnancy, lactation

INTERACTIONS
Drug
• Increased effects of caffeine with cimetidine, OCPs, disulfiram
• Increased stimulant effects with theophylline
• Increased cardiac effects with β agonists (albuterol/terbutaline)
Lab
• Increased glucose levels
• False positive for pheochromocytoma or neuroblastoma based on urine catecholamines
Nutrition
• Caffeine may inhibit Ca absorption

SIDE EFFECTS
CNS: Restlessness, agitation, insomnia, twitches, irritability, tremor, seizures with toxic doses
CV: Tachycardia, bradycardia, palpitations, decreased B/P, flushing
GI: Nausea, vomiting, diarrhea, gastric irritation
GU: Diuresis
RESP: Tachypnea, respiratory depression

TOXICITY AND OVERDOSE
Clinical signs: Hypertonicity, hypotonicity, tremors, bradycardia, hypotension, acidosis, opisthotonoid posture, seizures
Treatment: Gastric lavage, activated charcoal with oral use, monitor ECG, fluid and electrolyte balance, treat seizures with anticonvulsants

PATIENT CARE MANAGEMENT
Assessment
• Assess ECG, B/P, respiratory rate, HR
• Assess baseline respiratory, cardiac, and neurologic status

---

Interventions
• Administer drug IM, IV, or PO
• Monitor serum drug levels: therapeutic levels = 5-25 mcg/ml; toxic levels = 40-50 mcg/ml
Evaluation
• Evaluate therapeutic response (decreased frequency apnea spells)
• Evaluate pt for side effects

PATIENT AND FAMILY EDUCATION
Teach/instruct
• About rationale for treatment
Provide
• Support, reassurance

STORAGE
• Store at room temp

---

calcitriol

Brand Name(s): Calciject, Calcijex♣, Rocaltrol♣

Classification: Antihypocalcemic or vitamin D analog

Pregnancy Category: A (D if dosage exceeds RDA)

AVAILABLE PREPARATIONS
Caps: 0.25 mcg, 0.5 mcg
Inj: 1 mcg/ml, 2 mcg/ml

ROUTES AND DOSAGES
Renal Failure
Children: PO 0.25-2 mcg/24 hr with hemodialysis; PO 0.014-0.041 mcg/kg/24 hr without hemodialysis; increase at 4-8 wk intervals; IV 0.01-0.05 mcg/kg/24 hr three times/wk with hemodialysis
Adults: PO 0.25-1 mcg/24 hr as qd or qod dose; increased at 4-8 wk intervals; IV 0.5-3 mcg/24 hr three times/wk with hemodialysis
Cystic Fibrosis
Children and adults: PO 0.25 mcg/24 hr
Hypoparathyroidism
Children <1 yr: PO 0.04-0.08 mcg/kg/24 hr
Children 1-5 yr: PO 0.25-0.75 mcg/24 hr
Children >6 yr and adults: PO 0.5-2 mcg/24 hr

Vitamin D-dependent Rickets
Children and adults: PO 1 mcg/24 hr
Vitamin D-resistant Rickets
Children and adults: PO initial 0.015-0.02 mcg/kg/24 hr; maintenance 0.03-0.06 mcg/kg/24 hr; maximum 2 mcg/day
Hypocalcemia
Premature infants: PO 1 mcg/24 hr for 5 days

MECHANISM AND INDICATIONS
Mechanism: As activated cholecalciferol, promotes intestinal absorption and renal retention of Ca, thereby increasing serum Ca levels; decreases excessive serum phosphatase levels and parathyroid hormone levels
Indications: Used in the management of hypocalcemia in pts on chronic renal dialysis; used to reduce elevated parathyroid hormone level

PHARMACOKINETICS
Peak: 3-6 hr
Half-life: 3-6 hr
Metabolism: Liver, kidney
Excretion: Bile, feces

CONTRAINDICATIONS AND PRECAUTIONS
• Contraindicated with hypersensitivity to calcitriol, hypercalcemia, hypercalcuria, vitamin D toxicity
• Use cautiously with pts who are dehydrated, pregnancy, lactation

INTERACTIONS
Drug
• Decreased absorption with use of cholestyramine
• Altered absorption with use of thiazide diuretic, colestipol, corticosteroids
• Increased risk of cardiac arrhythmias with use of cardiac glycosides
• Possible altered absorption with use of Mg-containing antacids
Lab
• Falsely elevated cholesterol levels
• Altered electrolyte levels

• Altered serum phosphatase levels

SIDE EFFECTS
CNS: Weakness, headache, somnolence
CV: Hyperthermia, increased B/P, cardiac arrhythmias
DERM: Pruritus
EENT: Rhinorrhea, conjunctivitis
GI: Nausea, vomiting, constipation, anorexia, wt loss, dry mouth, pancreatitis
Local: Photophobia
Other: Bone pain, metallic taste, myalgia, hyperthermia

TOXICITY AND OVERDOSE
Clinical signs: Signs of hypercalcemia (weakness, increased B/P, cardiac arrhythmias, nausea, vomiting, anorexia)
Treatment: Discontinue drug; increase fluids; provide low Ca diet, supportive care

PATIENT CARE MANAGEMENT
Assessment
• Assess history of hypersensitivity to calcitriol
• Obtain baseline levels of Ca and vitamin D
• Assess for use of other medication to ensure optimum absorption and use
Interventions
• May be administered PO without regards to meals
• Provide Ca supplement as prescribed
• Provide diet to ensure adequate Ca intake
• May be administered IV as bolus dose through catheter at end of hemodialysis
• Ensure age-appropriate fluid intake

NURSING ALERT
Monitor for signs of hypercalcemia

Evaluation
• Evaluate therapeutic response (Ca 9-10 mg/dl, decreased symptoms of hypocalcemia, hypoparathyroidism)

• Evaluate serum Ca levels at least twice weekly at onset of therapy; evaluate weekly or monthly after dosage is stabilized
• Monitor for signs of hypersensitivity to drug, especially for infants (hyperthermia, nausea, vomiting, weakness, somnolence)
• Monitor for signs of hypercalcemia, hypercalcuria, hyperphosphatemia (elevated serum phosphorus)
• Monitor dietary intake to assure adequate Ca and vitamin D intake

PATIENT AND FAMILY EDUCATION
Teach/instruct
• To take as directed at prescribed intervals for prescribed length of time
• To evaluate other medications, OTC drugs for interactions
Warn/advise
• To notify care provider of hypersensitivity, side effects
• To avoid Mg-containing antacids; if necessary, take 2-3 hr before or after calcitriol

STORAGE
• Store at room temp in tightly closed container; keep protected from heat, light, moisture

---

calcium chloride, calcium gluconate

Brand Name(s): Calcium Chloride Injection✦, Calcium Gluconate Injection✦, CalPlus, Kalcinate

Classification: Calcium salt, electrolyte replacement

Pregnancy Category: C

AVAILABLE PREPARATIONS
Inj: Calcium chloride, 100 mg/ml = 1.4 mEq Ca/ml (10% sol)
Calcium gluconate, 100 mg/ml = 0.45 mEq Ca/ml (10% sol)

✦ Available in Canada.

ROUTES AND DOSAGES
Cardiac Resuscitation
Infants and children: IV calcium chloride 20 mg/kg; may repeat in 10 min
Adults: IV calcium chloride 2-4 mg/kg; may repeat in 10 min
Infants and children: IV calcium gluconate 100 mg/kg/dose
Adults: IV calcium gluconate 500-800 mg/dose
Hypocalcemia
Infants and children: IV calcium chloride 10-20 mg/kg/dose q4-6h prn
Adults: IV calcium chloride 500 mg-1 g/dose q6h
Neonates: IV calcium gluconate 200-800 mg/kg/24 hr; continuous infusion or in 4 divided doses
Infants and children: IV calcium gluconate 200-500 mg/kg/24 hr; continuous infusion or in 4 divided doses
Adults: IV calcium gluconate 2-15 g/24 hr; continuous infusion or in 4 divided doses
IV administration
• Recommended concentration: Calcium chloride, calcium gluconate, 100 mg/ml
• Maximum concentration: Calcium chloride, calcium gluconate, 100 mg/ml
• IV push rate: Calcium chloride <50-100 mg/min or 0.5-1 ml of 10% sol; calcium gluconate < 100 mg/min
• Continuous infusion rate: Total daily dose may be infused over 24 hr

MECHANISM AND INDICATIONS
Mechanism: Maintains and moderates nerve, muscle performance
Indications: For emergency treatment of hypocalcemia; hypermagnesemia; cardiac disturbances secondary to hyperkalemia; or Ca channel blocker toxicity

PHARMACOKINETICS
Absorption: Immediate, rapidly absorbed into skeletal tissue
Metabolism: No significant metabolism occurs
Excretion: Unabsorbed Ca excreted in feces

CONTRAINDICATIONS AND PRECAUTIONS
• Contraindicated with hypercalcemia, VF, renal calculi, digoxin toxicity
• Use cautiously in digitalized pts, with respiratory failure or acidosis, renal or cardiac disease
• Avoid rapid IV infusion and extravasation; may cause tissue necrosis
• Do not administer IM, SC

INTERACTIONS
Drug
• Increased arrhythmias with digitalis
• Decreased action of Ca channel blockers
• Decreased action of tetracycline
Lab
• False negatives for serum and urine Mg
• Transient increase in 17-OHCS

INCOMPATIBILITIES
• Amphotericin B, cephalothin, chlorpheniramine, carbonates, phosphates, sulfates, bicarbonate

SIDE EFFECTS
CNS: Tingling sensation
CV: Cardiac arrhythmia, bradycardia, cardiac arrest, shortened QT interval, heart block, hypotension
DERM: Burning, pain at IV site, venous thrombosis, tissue necrosis with extravasation
GI: Nausea, vomiting, abdominal pain, constipation, thirst
GU: Polyuria, nocturia, renal calculi, azotemia
METAB: Hypercalcemia, hyperphosphatemia

TOXICITY AND OVERDOSE
Clinical signs: Hypercalcemia, drowsiness, lethargy, muscle weakness, nausea and vomiting, headache, coma, elevated serum Ca levels
Treatment: Discontinue drug; IV infusion of NaCl and furosemide will cause excretion of Ca; for IV extravasation, inject 1% procaine

HCl and hyaluronidase into affected area

PATIENT CARE MANAGEMENT
Assessment
- Assess VS frequently
- Assess ECG for decreased QT interval and T-wave inversion
- Assess serum Ca levels throughout infusion
- Assess digoxin levels with digoxin
- Assess serum PO_4, Mg

Interventions
- Administer IV slowly using small bore needle into large vein; avoid scalp vein
- Avoid IM, SC administration in infants, children
- Monitor ECG continuously

> **NURSING ALERT**
> IV extravasation may cause tissue necrosis; use hyaluronidase

Evaluation
- Evaluate for symptoms of hypercalcemia (see Toxicity and Overdose)
- Evaluate IV site for signs of extravasation

PATIENT AND FAMILY EDUCATION
Teach/instruct
- About reasons for Ca infusion
Warn/advise
- To remain recumbent 30-60 min after infusion

STORAGE
- Store at room temp

---

cantharidin
Brand Name(s): Canthacur♣, Cantharone♣, Verr-Canth

Classification: Keratolytic

Pregnancy Category: C

AVAILABLE PREPARATIONS
Liquid: 0.7%

ROUTES AND DOSAGES
- *For application by care provider only, do not dispense to patient.*

Removal of Periungual and Ordinary Warts
Cover lesion completely, let dry, cover with adhesive tape (nonporous) for 24 hr; reapply if necessary

Removal of Molluscum Contagiosum
Coat each lesion, repeat in 1 wk on new or remaining lesions, cover with tape for 4-6 hr

Removal of Plantar Warts
Apply to wart and 1-3 mm around wart, let dry, cover with tape, debride in 1-3 wk, may reapply up to 3 times

MECHANISM AND INDICATIONS
Mechanism: Causes exfoliation of epithelial growths
Indications: Used for treatment of warts, molluscum contagiosum

PHARMACOKINETICS
Absorption: Limited to areas where drug applied

CONTRAINDICATIONS AND PRECAUTIONS
- Contraindicated with hypersensitivity; in areas near eyes, mucous membranes, genitalia; on birthmarks, moles, hair-growing warts
- Use cautiously with impaired circulation

INTERACTIONS
Drug
- None reported
Lab
- None reported

INCOMPATIBILITIES
- None reported

SIDE EFFECTS
Local: Irritation, tingling, burning, tenderness, erythema at site

TOXICITY AND OVERDOSE
Clinical signs: If spilled on skin, will cause breakdown

♣ Available in Canada.

Treatment: Wipe off immediately using tape remover, acetone, or alcohol; wash with soap, water

PATIENT CARE MANAGEMENT
Assessment
• Assess lesions for appropriateness of application
• Assess areas to be treated; do not apply to areas listed as contraindicated

Interventions
• Wash hands before/after application
• Apply as directed, using nonporous adhesive tape to cover area
• Do not apply to normal skin
• Use of mild antibacterial ointment recommended until skin heals

Evaluation
• Evaluate therapeutic response (gradual disappearance of lesions)
• Evaluate treated areas (signs of hypersensitivity, infection)

PATIENT AND FAMILY EDUCATION
Warn/advise
• That tingling, burning, itching, erythema at sight may develop for up to 7 days

STORAGE
• Store at room temp in light-resistant container

---

captopril

Brand Name(s): Apo-Capto✤, Capoten✤, Novo-Captoril✤, Nu-Capto✤, Syn-Captopril✤

Classification: ACE inhibitor, antihypertensive, cardiac load reducer

Pregnancy category: C

AVAILABLE PREPARATIONS
Tabs: 12.5 mg, 25 mg, 37.5 mg, 50 mg, 100 mg

ROUTES AND DOSAGES
Neonates: PO 0.05-0.1 mg/kg/dose qd-tid

Infants: PO 0.15-0.3 mg/kg/dose qd-q6h; maximum dose 6 mg/kg/24 hr
Children: PO 0.5-1 mg/kg/dose q6-12h; maximum dose 6 mg/kg/24 hr
Adult: PO 12-25 mg/dose q8-12h; increase weekly by 25 mg/dose; maximum dose of 450 mg/24 hr

MECHANISM AND INDICATIONS
Antihypertensive mechanism: Suppresses renin–angiotensin–aldosterone system, reducing Na and water retention and lowering B/P
Load-reducer mechanism: Decreases systemic vascular resistance and PCWP, increasing cardiac output with CHF
Indications: Hypertension, CHF

PHARMACOKINETICS
Onset of action: 15 min
Peak: 1 hr
Half-life: 6-7 hr
Metabolism: Liver
Excretion: Urine, feces

CONTRAINDICATIONS AND PRECAUTIONS
• Contraindicated with known hypersensitivity to medication or other ACE inhibitors, heart block
• Use with caution with hypovolemia, leukemia, scleroderma, lupus, blood dyscrasias, diabetes, renal disease, thyroid disease, COPD, asthma, dialysis

INTERACTIONS
Drug
• Increased hypotension when used with other diuretics, antihypertensives, ganglionic and adrenergic blockers
• Decreased effects of captopril with NSAIDs, antacids
• Increased risk of hyperkalemia when used with K^+-sparing diuretics, K^+ supplements, salt substitutes
Lab
• Increased BUN, creatinine, liver enzymes, and K^+
• Decreased serum Na
• False positive for urinary acetone

INCOMPATIBILITIES
• Vasodilators, hydralazine, prazosin, sympathomimetics

SIDE EFFECTS
CNS: Dizziness, syncope, fatigue, insomnia, paresthesias
CV: Tachycardia, hypotension, angina, CHF, pericarditis
DERM: Rash, urticaria, pruritus, photosensitivity
GI: Anorexia, nausea, vomiting, loss of taste, diarrhea, constipation
GU: Frequency, renal failure, impotence, dysuria, nocturia, proteinuria, nephrotic syndrome, polyuria, oliguria
RESP: Bronchospasm, dyspnea, cough
Other: Neutropenia, hyperkalemia, fever, chills, agranulocytosis, leukopenia, pancytopenia

TOXICITY AND OVERDOSE
Clinical signs: Severe hypotension
Treatment: Induce emesis or gastric lavage, use activated charcoal; supportive therapy as necessary; hemodialysis in severe cases

PATIENT CARE MANAGEMENT
Assessment
• Assess history of hypersensitivity to drug, other ACE inhibitors
• Assess baseline VS, B/P, hydration status
• Assess baseline labs (electrolytes, CBC, protein, BUN, creatinine, LFTs)
Interventions
• Administer 1 hr ac
Evaluation
• Evaluate therapeutic response (decreased B/P, diminished CHF)
• Evaluate side effects, hypersensitivity
• Evaluate labs (electrolytes, CBC, protein, BUN, creatinine, AST, ALT, bilirubin)

PATIENT AND FAMILY EDUCATION
Teach/instruct
• To take as directed at prescribed intervals; do not discontinue medication abruptly

• To take medication at least 1 hr ac
• To monitor wt regularly
Warn/advise
• To notify care provider of hypersensitivity, side effects
• To avoid hazardous activities until therapy is well-established
• Not to take OTC medications unless approved by care provider
Provide
• Emotional support as necessary
STORAGE
• Store at room temp in a tightly sealed container

---

carbamazepine

Brand Name(s): Atretol, Apo-Carbamazepine✤, Epitol, Mazepine, Novo-Carbamaz✤, Nu-Carbamazepine✤, Taro-Carbamazepine✤, Tegretol✤

Classification: Anticonvulsant, analgesic, chemically related to tricyclic antidepressants

Pregnancy Category: C

AVAILABLE PREPARATIONS
Sus: 100 mg/5 mL
Tabs: 200 mg
Tabs (chewable): 100 mg
Tabs (ext rel): 100 mg, 200 mg, 400 mg

ROUTES AND DOSAGES
Children <6 yrs: PO, initially 5 mg/kg/24 hr; increase dosage q 5-7 days to 10 mg/kg/24 hr; then up to 20 mg/kg/24 hr (if needed) divided bid to qid
Children 6 to 12 yr: PO 100 mg bid or 10 mg/kg/24 hr divided bid; increase 100 mg/24 hr at weekly intervals until therapeutic levels are achieved; usual maintenance dose 15-30 mg/kg/24 hr divided bid-qid; maximum dose 1000 mg/24 hr
Children >12 and adults: PO 200 mg bid; increase dosage 200 mg/24 hr at weekly intervals until therapeutic levels are achieved; usual

dose 600-1200 mg/24 hr divided bid-qid; some pts require up to 1.6-2.4 g/24 hr

MECHANISM AND INDICATIONS

Mechanism: Exact mechanism unknown; believed to prevent spread of seizure discharges by reducing polysynaptic responses; acts on the Na channels to create a differential inhibition of high-frequency discharges in and around the epileptic foci with little disruption of normal neural activity; has antidiuretic effect, stimulating release of ADH, which potentiates action and promotes the reabsorption of water

Indications: Used to treat clonictonic, partial (especially complex partial) and mixed partial, or generalized seizure disorders; also has anticholinergic, antineuralgic, antidiuretic, muscle relaxant, and antiarrhythmic properties; used to treat diabetic neuropathy; other uses include: treatment of bipolar disorders, control of pain and symptoms of multiple sclerosis, hemifacial spasm, dystonia, antidiuretic effects of diabetes insipidus; trigeminal neuralgia

PHARMACOKINETICS

Peak: 2-8 hr
Distribution: Widely throughout the body
Half-life: 10-20 hr
Metabolism: Liver
Excretion: Urine (primarily as glucuronides)
Therapeutic level: 4-12 mcg/ml; steady state achieved in 4-6 wk; generally 5-7 days allowed between increases in dosage to allow drug to return to steady state

CONTRAINDICATIONS AND PRECAUTIONS

• Contraindicated with known sensitivity to carbamazepine, tricyclic antidepressants; with MAOIs or within 14 days of such use; with history of bone marrow suppression
• Use cautiously with cardiovascular, hepatic, renal damage, with increased intraocular pressure, pregnancy, lactation

INTERACTIONS

Drug
• Concomitant use with MAOIs may cause hypertensive crisis; should not be used within 14 days of MAOIs
• Erythromycin, Ca channel blockers, cimetidine, isoniazid, propoxyphene inhibit metabolism of carbamazepine, cause higher serum levels
• Carbamazepine may increase metabolism of warfarin, phenytoin, valproic acid, haloperidol, ethosuximide, oral contraceptives, theophylline, corticosteroids, decreasing their effectiveness

Lab
• Increased liver enzymes
• Decreased thyroid function testing, serum Ca
• False negative for pregnancy
• May cause albuminuria, glycosuria

SIDE EFFECTS

CNS: Drowsiness, fatigue, dizziness, diplopia, ataxia, speech disturbances, involuntary movements, behavior changes (more often in children), weakness, headache, depression, trembling, hallucinations, neuritis
CV: CHF, hypertension, hypotension, thrombophlebitis, arrhythmias, chest pain, changes in HR
DERM: Rash, urticaria, erythema multiforme, Stevens-Johnson syndrome; the characteristic rash associated with carbamazepine generally appears after about 7 days of administration; rash is diffuse, erythematous, extremely itchy, uncomfortable
EENT: Conjunctivitis, dry mouth and pharynx, blurred vision, diplopia, nystagmus
GI: Nausea, vomiting, abdominal pain, diarrhea, anorexia, stomatitis, glossitis, dry mouth
GU: Urinary frequency or retention, impotence, albuminuria, glycosuria, elevated BUN
HEME: Aplastic anemia, leukopenia, thrombocytopenia, eosino-

philia, agranulocytosis, leukocytosis

Other: Fever, chills, pulmonary hypersensitivity, diaphoresis, leg cramps, joint pain, tinnitus

TOXICITY AND OVERDOSE

Clinical signs: Coma, stupor, hyperirritability, convulsions, respiratory depression, increased frequency of seizures

Treatment: Supportive care; monitor serum levels to achieve therapeutic range; discontinue drug if serious side effects occur

PATIENT CARE MANAGEMENT

Assessment

• Assess hypersensitivity to carbamazepine, tricyclic antidepressants

• Assess baseline lab studies, including CBC, differential and liver function testing (ALT, AST, bilirubin, alk phos)

• Assess seizure type, determine if appropriate anticonvulsant for this type of seizure

Interventions

• Administer with food or milk to decrease GI symptoms; chewable tabs must be chewed, not swallowed whole

• Initiate at modest dosage

• Increase the dosage/level as needed to control seizures, to point of intolerable side effects

• If drug is only partially effective, other anticonvulsants may be initiated in same way

• Gradually withdraw, initiate another anticonvulsant if not effective

• Increase frequency of administration provide more coverage if break-through seizures occur at times when serum levels are at trough or peak

Evaluation

• Evaluate therapeutic response (seizure control); initially done more frequently until seizures controlled, then q 3-6 mo, or if breakthrough seizure or side effects

• Monitor anticonvulsant levels periodically

• Monitor side effects, hypersensitivity, including significant elevation of liver function (ALT, AST, bilirubin, alk phos); abnormalities of hematologic testing or signs of bone marrow suppression, fever, sore throat, mouth ulcers, easy bruising; petechial or purpuric hemorrhages

PATIENT AND FAMILY EDUCATION

Teach/instruct

• To take medication as prescribed; not to increase or decrease dosage independently; reinforce that medication should not be stopped suddenly

• To take medication with food to decrease GI upset

• That chewable tabs need to be chewed completely, not swallowed whole

• Hard candy, frequent rinsing of mouth, chewing gum may minimize dry mouth complaints

Warn/advise

• To notify care provider of side effects; report immediately signs, symptoms of unusual bleeding, bruising, jaundice, dark urine, pale stools, abdominal pain, impotence, fever, chills, sore throat, mouth ulcers, edema, or disturbances in mood, alertness, or coordination.

• To keep record of seizure activity

• That unpleasant side effects may decrease as pt becomes more used to the drug

• That drug initially may be more sedating until pt becomes used to it; avoid hazardous activities (biking, skating, skateboarding) until stabilized on medication

• To make other health care providers aware of drug to avoid potential drug interactions, carry medical alert identification

• To alert health care provider if pregnancy occurs

STORAGE

• Store tabs at room temp

✤ Available in Canada.

carbenicillin indanyl sodium

Brand Name(s): Geocillin, Geopen♣

Classification: Antibiotic (extended-spectrum penicillin)

Pregnancy Category: B

AVAILABLE PREPARATIONS
Tabs (film-coated): 382 mg

ROUTES AND DOSAGES
Children: PO 30-50 mg/kg/24 hr divided q6h; maximum dose 2-3 g/24 hr
Adults: PO 1-2 tabs q6h

MECHANISM AND INDICATIONS
Antibiotic mechanism: Bactericidal; inhibits bacterial cell wall synthesis by adhering to bacterial penicillin-binding proteins
Indications: Effective against *Proteus mirabilis, P. vulgaris, E. coli, Pseudomonas aeruginosa, P. rettgeri, Morganella morganii, Enterobacter,* and, in large doses, *Bacteroides;* may be inactivated by penicillinase-producing staphylococci; used to treat urinary tract, respiratory tract, skin, soft tissue infections

PHARMACOKINETICS
Peak: Within 30-120 min
Distribution: Very low systemic concentrations
Half-life: Neonates <7 days, <2.5 kg, 4 hr; neonates >7 days, >2.5 kg, 2.7 hr; children 0.8-1.8 hr; adults 1-1.5 hr
Metabolism: Liver
Excretion: Urine

CONTRAINDICATIONS AND PRECAUTIONS
• Contraindicated in pts with known hypersensitivity to carbenicillin, other penicillins, or cephalosporins
• Use cautiously with impaired renal function, history of bleeding problems, and pregnancy

INTERACTIONS
Drug
• Synergistic antimicrobial activity against certain organisms with use of aminoglycosides, clavulanic acid
• Increased serum concentrations with use of probenecid
• Increased serum concentrations of methotrexate
• Decreased effectiveness with use of tetracyclines, chloramphenicol, erythromycins
• Increased risk of bleeding with use of anticoagulants
Lab
• Increased liver function tests
• Increased serum uric acid

SIDE EFFECTS
CNS: Neuromuscular irritability, seizures
ENDO/METAB: Hypokalemia, hypernatremia
GI: Nausea, vomiting, diarrhea, pseudomembranous colitis
GU: Acute interstitial nephritis
HEME: Bleeding with high doses, neutropenia, eosinophilia, leukopenia, thrombocytopenia, anemia
Other: Hypersensitivity (edema, fever, chills, rash, pruritus, urticaria, anaphylaxis), bacterial or fungal superinfection

TOXICITY AND OVERDOSE
Clinical signs: Neuromuscular hypersensitivity; seizures may result from high CNS concentrations
Treatment: Supportive care; hemodialysis

PATIENT CARE MANAGEMENT
Assessment
• Assess history of hypersensitivity to carbenicillin, penicillins, cephalosporins
• Obtain C&S; may begin therapy before obtaining results
• Assess renal function (BUN, creatinine, I&O), hepatic function (ALT, AST, bilirubin), hematologic function (CBC, differential, platelet count); K$^+$ levels with long-term therapy
Interventions
• Administer penicillins at least 1 hr before bacteriostatic antibiot-

ics (tetracyclines, erythromycins, chloramphenicol)
• Administer PO 1 hr ac or 2 hr after meals; film-coated tabs must be swallowed whole
• Maintain age-appropriate fluid intake

NURSING ALERT
Discontinue drug is signs of hypersensitivity, bleeding complications, pseudomembranous colitis develop

Evaluation
• Evaluate therapeutic response (decreased symptoms of infection)
• Monitor for signs of superinfection (perineal itching, diaper rash, fever, malaise, redness, pain, swelling, drainage, rash, diarrhea, sore throat, change in cough or sputum)
• Observe for signs of allergic reaction (wheezing, tightness in chest, urticaria), especially within 20-30 min of first dose
• Monitor bowel pattern; diarrhea may be symptomatic of pseudomembranous colitis
• Monitor renal function (BUN, creatinine, I&O), hepatic function (ALT, AST, bilirubin), electrolyte levels, particularly K^+ and Na
• Monitor for signs of bleeding (ecchymosis, bleeding gums, hematuria, daily stool guaiac); monitor PT, platelet counts

PATIENT AND FAMILY EDUCATION
Teach/instruct
• To take as directed at prescribed intervals for prescribed length of time
Warn/advise
• To notify care provider of hypersensitivity, side effects, superinfection

STORAGE
• Store tabs at room temp

carbinoxamine and pseudoephedrine
Brand Name(s): Rondec Drops, Rondec Filmtab, Rondec Syrup, Rondec-TR

Classification: Antihistamine/decongestant combination

Pregnancy Category: C

AVAILABLE PREPARATIONS
Drops: carbinoxamine maleate 2 mg, pseudoephedrine 25 mg/ml
Syr: carbinoxamine maleate 4 mg, pseudoephedrine hydrochloride 60 mg/5 ml
Tabs (film-coated): carbinoxamine maleate 4 mg, pseudoephedrine hydrochloride 60 mg
Tabs (sus rel): carbinoxamine maleate 8 mg, pseudoephedrine hydrochloride 120 mg

ROUTES AND DOSAGES
Infants 1-3 mo: PO drops 0.25 ml qid
Infants 3-6 mo: PO drops 0.5 ml qid
Infants 6-9 mo: PO drops 0.75 ml qid
Infants 9-18 mo: PO drops 1 ml qid
Children 18 mo-6 yr: PO syr 2.5 ml qid
Children 6-12 yr: PO syr or tabs 5 ml or 1 tab qid
Children >12 yr and adults: PO sus rel 1 tab bid
• Dosing in children by pseudoephedrine component: 4 mg/kg/24 hr divided qid

MECHANISM AND INDICATIONS
Antihistamine mechanism: Carbinoxamine competes with histamine for H_1-receptor sites; blocks histamine, thus decreasing allergic response; pseudoephedrine directly stimulates α-adrenergic receptors of respiratory mucosa causing vasoconstriction; directly stimulates β-adrenergic receptors causing bronchial relaxation, increased HR, contractility

Indications: Used to relieve symptoms (rhinorrhea, nasal congestion, sneezing, nose or throat itching, itchy or watery eyes) of respiratory allergies, common cold

PHARMACOKINETICS
Metabolism: Liver
Excretion: Urine

CONTRAINDICATIONS AND PRECAUTIONS
• Contraindicated with hypersensitivity to carbinoxamine or pseudoephedrine or any component, severe hypertension or CAD; MAOI therapy, GI or GU obstruction, narrow-angle glaucoma, neonates
• Use cautiously with mild-to-moderate hypertension, heart disease, diabetes, thyroid dysfunction, prostatic hypertrophy, pregnancy

INTERACTIONS
Drug
• Intensified central depressant, anticholinergic effects with use of MAOIs
• Additive sedative effects with use of alcohol, barbiturates, tranquilizers, sleeping aids, antianxiety agents
Lab
• False negative for skin allergy tests

SIDE EFFECTS
CNS: Sedation, CNS stimulation, headache, seizures, weakness
CV: Hypertension, tachycardia, arrhythmias
EENT: Diplopia
GI: Nausea, vomiting, diarrhea, anorexia, dry mouth, heartburn
GU: Dysuria

TOXICITY AND OVERDOSE
Clinical signs: CNS depression, CNS stimulation, GI symptoms, anticholinergic symptoms
Treatment: Induce vomiting, followed by activated charcoal; gastric lavage; supportive treatment; do not give stimulants

PATIENT CARE MANAGEMENT
Assessment
• Assess history of hypersensitivity to carbinoxamine, pseudoephedrine, any component
Intervention
• Administer PO with meals to reduce GI distress
• Provide sugarless hard candy, gum, frequent oral care for dry mouth
• Institute safety measures (supervise ambulation, raise bed rails) because of CNS side effects
Evaluation
• Evaluate therapeutic response (decreased allergy symptoms)
• Monitor respiratory status (change in secretions, wheezing, chest tightness)

PATIENT AND FAMILY EDUCATION
Teach/instruct
• To take as directed at prescribed intervals for prescribed length of time
Warn/advise
• To notify care provider of hypersensitivity, side effects
• Not to exceed recommended dosage
• To avoid hazardous activities if drowsiness occurs (bicycles, skateboards, skates)
• To avoid use of alcohol, medications containing alcohol, CNS depressants

STORAGE
• Store at room temp

---

carboplatin
Brand Name(s): Paraplatin❦, Paraplatin-AQ❦
Classification: Alkylating agent (heavy metal complex)
Pregnancy Category: D

AVAILABLE PREPARATIONS
Inj: 50 mg, 150 mg, 450 mg powder for inj

ROUTES AND DOSAGES

• Drug may vary in response to diagnosis, extent of disease, concurrent or previous therapy, protocol guidelines, physiologic parameters; consult current literature, protocol parameters

Genitourinary Cancers, Medulloblastoma

IV 175-560 mg/m^2 × 1 q 3-4 wk (dose is protocol driven)

Recurrent Ovarian Cancer

IV 360 mg/m^2 × 1 q 3-4 wk; should not be repeated until neutrophil count is at least 2000, platelet count is 100,000

IV administration

• Reconstitute with SW, NS, or D$_5$W; 50 mg dilute with 5 ml, 150 mg dilute with 15 ml, 450 mg dilute with 45 ml; all producing carboplatin concentration of 10 mg/ml; can further dilute for administration with D$_5$W or NS to a final concentration of 0.5-2 mg/ml

• IV infusion rate: Over at least 15 min (but usually 30-60 min); can be given by continuous infusion

• Carboplatin reacts with aluminum, causing a precipitate and loss of potency; no needles, IV sets with aluminum parts should come in contact with the drug during preparation or administration

MECHANISM AND INDICATIONS

Mechanism: Shares same mechanism of cytotoxicity as cisplatin; drug is cell cycle phase nonspecific; drug binds to nucleophilic sites on DNA causing intra- and interstrand cross-links rather than DNA–protein cross-links, resulting in non–cell cycle-dependent tumor cell lysis; these cross-links are similar to those formed with cisplatin but are formed later in the cell cycle.

Indications: Used in the treatment of ovarian cancer, genitourinary cancer (testicular, bladder, cervical), medulloblastomas

PHARMACOKINETICS

Half-life: Initial plasma half-life 1.1-2.0 hr; post-distribution plasma half-life 2.6-5.9 hr; terminal half-life 2.5-6 hr; free platinum half-life in serum 6 hr; mean half-life approximately 100 min

Excretion: About 70% excreted in urine within 24 hr; slower binding to plasma proteins compared to cisplatin; greater percentage of ultrafiltrable platinum present in urine within 4 hr of administration

CONTRAINDICATIONS AND PRECAUTIONS

• Contraindicated with history of hypersensitivity to cisplatin, platinum-containing compounds; with bleeding or severe bone marrow suppression; with compromised renal function; with pregnancy, lactation

INTERACTIONS

Drug

• Enhanced nephrotoxicity when used with other nephrotoxic agents

• Increased incidence of hematologic toxicities when used with other bone marrow depressant agents, including radiation therapy

INCOMPATIBILITIES

• Do not mix with other drugs during administration

• Incompatible with NaHCO$_3$

• Aluminum causes precipitate, loss of potency in contact with carboplatin

SIDE EFFECTS

CNS: Ototoxicity, peripheral neuropathy, central neurotoxicity, confusion, dizziness, visual disturbances, mild paresthesias, changes in taste

GI: Nausea, vomiting, diarrhea, constipation, hepatotoxicity (increased bilirubin, AST, ALT, alk phos)

HEME: Thrombocytopenia, leukopenia, neutropenia, anemia, bone marrow suppression

Other: Alopecia, anorexia, stomatitis, hypersensitivity reactions, rash, abnormal serum electrolytes (Na, K$^+$, Ca, Mg) and CrCl

---

✤ Available in Canada.

TOXICITY AND OVERDOSE
Clinical signs: Severe myelosuppression with high doses or repeated doses with poor bone marrow reserve; impaired renal function (hepatotoxicity), rising BUN, creatinine; anaphylactic reactions reported (tachycardia, wheezing, hypotension, facial edema), usually occurring within first few min of administration
Treatment: Monitor CBC, liver function (AST, ALT, alk phos, bilirubin), BUN, creatinine; before, during, after chemotherapy; provide supportive care as indicated (blood transfusions, antibiotics); steroids, epinephrine, or antihistamines used to treat anaphylaxis

PATIENT CARE MANAGEMENT
Assess
• Assess history of hypersensitivity to carboplatin, related drugs (e.g., cisplatin)
• Assess baseline VS, CBC, differential, platelet count, electrolytes (Na, K$^+$, Ca, Mg), renal function (BUN, creatinine, urine CrCl), liver function (ALT, AST, LDH, bilirubin, alk phos) before administration
• Assess hydration status (SG), urinary elimination, assess for signs of hematuria, dysuria, urinary frequency
• Assess neurologic, mental status before and during drug administration
• Assess success of previous antiemetic therapy
• Assess history of previous treatment with special attention to other therapies that might predispose pt to renal or hepatic dysfunction
Interventions
• Premedicate with antiemetics; continue periodically throughout chemotherapy treatments
• Do not use needle, IV administration sets containing aluminum parts
• Encourage small, frequent feedings of foods pt likes
• Administer IV fluids until pt

able to resume normal PO intake; check wt daily, have pt empty bladder q2h
• Provide supportive measures to maintain hemostasis, fluid and electrolyte balance, nutritional support

---

NURSING ALERT
Can cause severe bone marrow suppression; monitor blood counts regularly, provide supportive care as indicated

Carboplatin can cause severe vomiting; provide antiemetic therapy (as ordered), adequate hydration

Carboplatin reacts with aluminum, causing a precipitate and loss of potency; do not use needles, IV administration sets containing aluminum parts

---

Evaluate
• Evaluate therapeutic response (decreased tumor size, spread of malignancy)
• Evaluate CBC, differential, platelet count, electrolytes (Na, K$^+$, Ca, Mg), renal function (BUN, creatinine, urine creatinine clearance, I&O), liver function (ALT, AST, LDH, bilirubin, alk phos), at given intervals after chemotherapy; assess wt daily
• Assess for signs or symptoms of infection (fever, fatigue, sore throat), bleeding (easy bruising, nose bleeds, bleeding gums)

PATIENT AND FAMILY EDUCATION
Teach/instruct
• To have pt well-hydrated before and after chemotherapy
• About importance of follow-up visits to monitor blood counts, serum chemistry values, drug blood levels
• To take accurate temp; rectal temp contraindicated
• To notify care provider of signs of bleeding (bruising, epistaxis, bleeding gums), infection (fever, sore throat, fatigue)

Warn/advise

• About impact of body changes that may occur (hair loss, hyperpigmentation, nail ridging), how to minimize changes (wigs, caps, scarves, long sleeves)

• To avoid OTC products containing aspirin

• To report any alterations in behavior, sensation, perception; help to develop plan of care to manage side effects, stress of illness or treatment

• To monitor bowel function, call if abdominal pain, constipation noted

• To report immediately any pain, discoloration at injection site (parenteral forms)

• That good oral hygiene with very soft toothbrush is imperative

• That dental work be delayed until blood counts return to baseline, with permission of care provider

• To avoid contact with known viral, bacterial illnesses

• That household contacts of child not be immunized with live polio virus; inactivated form should be used

• That child not receive immunizations until immune system recovers sufficiently to mount needed antibody response

• To report immediately exposure to chicken pox in susceptible child

• To report immediately reactivation of zoster virus (shingles)

• If appropriate, ways to preserve reproductive patterns, sexuality (sperm banking, contraceptives)

Encourage

• Provision of nutritious food intake; consider nutritional consultation

• To comply with bowel management program

• To maintain adequate fluid intake, frequent voiding

• To use top anesthetics to control discomfort of mucositis; to avoid spicy foods, commercial mouthwashes

STORAGE

• Unopened vials stable at room temp protected from light

• Reconstituted sol stable for 8 hr at room temp

• Diluted sol stable for 24 hr at room temp

carmustine, BCNU

Brand Name(s): BiCNU✚

Classification: Antineoplastic, alkylating agent, nitrosourea; cell cycle phase nonspecific

Pregnancy Category: D

AVAILABLE PREPARATIONS
Inj: 100 mg vials

ROUTES AND DOSAGES

• Dosage may vary in response to diagnosis, extent of disease, concurrent or previous therapy, protocol guidelines, physiologic parameters; consult current literature, protocol recommendations

Lymphomas, ALL, Malignant Melanomas

IV 75-100 mg/m^2/24 hr for 2 days, repeat q 6 wk; or 40 mg/m^2/24 hr for 5 days, repeat q 6 wk; or 200 mg/m^2/dose, repeat q 6-8 wk

Myeloablative Bone Marrow Transplant

IV 300-600 mg/m^2 over 1-4 days

IV administration

• Final concentration: 0.2-1 mg/ml

• Intermittent infusion rate: Administered over 1-2 hr; drug diluent is ethanol, faster infusion may cause burning; unstable in plastic, must be in glass bottle

MECHANISM AND INDICATIONS

Mechanism: Cytotoxic to cells through action of metabolites that inhibit cellular enzymes involved with DNA formation; metabolites also intercalate, cause crosslinking of DNA base pairs leading to subsequent interference with DNA, RNA, protein synthesis

Indications: Lymphomas, malig-

✚ Available in Canada.

nant melanoma, ALL; increased lipid solubility, ability to cross blood-brain barrier also make agent useful for treating brain tumors

PHARMACOKINETICS
Half-life: 5-90 minutes
Distribution: Nitrosoureas decompose spontaneously, are cleared rapidly from plasma; drug, metabolites distribute rapidly into CSF
Metabolism: Rapid spontaneous decomposition; also metabolized in liver
Excretion: 60%-70% of drug, metabolites excreted in urine, 6%-10% excreted as CO_2 through respiration, 1% excreted in feces

CONTRAINDICATIONS AND PRECAUTIONS
• Contraindicated with known hypersensitivity, active infections (especially chicken pox and zoster lesions), history of pulmonary function impairment, pregnancy, lactation
• Use cautiously with hepatic or renal insufficiency, pts previously treated with bleomycin, chest radiation

INTERACTIONS
Drug
• Accentuated bone marrow suppression possible with cimetidine or theophylline
Lab
• Increase BUN, alk phos, AST, bilirubin

INCOMPATIBILITIES
• Drug should not be mixed with other drugs during administration
• $NaHCO_3$ causes degradation of BCNU

SIDE EFFECTS
CNS: Encephalopathy, dizziness, ataxia, neuritis, seizures
DERM: Hyperpigmentation, alopecia, local venous irritation, brown stain on skin (if cutaneous exposure occurs)
EENT: Conjunctival flushing
HEME: Causes cumulative myelosuppression with nadir of leukocytes, platelets occurring 4-5 wk after administration; recovery in 1-2 wk after nadir; myelodysplastic syndrome; acute non-lymphocytic leukemia
RESP: Pulmonary fibrosis may occur if cumulative dose > 900-1500 mg/m^2 (if treatment longer than 6 mo, or pt previously treated with bleomycin or chest radiation); process characterized by nonproductive cough, dyspnea, tachypnea, basilar crepitant rales, normal chest x-ray or radiograph showing interstitial infiltrates; can progress, becoming restrictive, causing ventilatory defects, resting hypoxemia, decreased CO_2 diffusion capacity

TOXICITY AND OVERDOSE
Clinical signs: Prolonged myelosuppression, pulmonary fibrosis, neurologic deterioration
Treatment: Supportive measures including blood transfusions, hydration, nutritional supplementation, broad-spectrum antibiotics coverage in event of fever, electrolyte replacement

PATIENT CARE MANAGEMENT
Assess
• Assess history of hypersensitivity to nitrosoureas
• Assess history of previous chemotherapy or radiation therapy, especially therapy that might predispose pt to pulmonary fibrosis, hepatic or renal dysfunction
• Assess previous history of success with antiemetic therapy
• Assess baseline VS, oximetry, pulmonary function tests, chest radiograph
• Assess baseline liver function (AST, ALT, bilirubin), renal function (BUN, creatinine)
• Assess baseline CBC, differential, platelet count
Interventions
• Administer antiemetic therapy before chemotherapy
• Monitor I&O; administer IV fluids until child able to resume oral intake
• Avoid skin contact (will cause brown staining)

✤ Available in Canada.

- Provide supportive measure to maintain hemostasis, fluid and electrolyte balance, nutritional status

> **NURSING ALERT**
> Drug causes delayed, cumulative myelosuppression

Evaluate
- Evaluate response of disease to therapy as evidenced by decreased tumor burden
- Evaluate CBC, differential, platelet count at least once weekly
- Assess breath sounds, symmetry at each visit
- Obtain chest radiographs at regular intervals
- Obtain measurements of renal function (BUN, creatinine) hepatic function (AST, ALT, bilirubin) before each subsequent course of treatment
- Assess respiratory status, including respiratory rate, oximetry, chest auscultation, chest radiographs

PATIENT AND FAMILY EDUCATION
Teach/instruct
- To have patient well hydrated before and after chemotherapy
- About the importance of follow-up visits to monitor blood counts, serum chemistry values, urinalysis
- To take an accurate temp; rectal temp contraindicated
- To notify care provider of signs of bleeding (bruising, epistaxis, bleeding gums), signs of infection (fever, sore throat, fatigue)
Warn/advise
- About impact of body changes that may occur (hair loss, hyperpigmentation, nail ridging), how to minimize changes (wigs, caps, scarves, long sleeves)
- To avoid OTC preparations containing aspirin
- To report any alterations in behavior, sensation, perception; help to develop plan of care to manage side effects, stress of illness or treatment

- To report any respiratory symptoms (such as coughing, dyspnea, fever, or chills) that occur within 3-6 hr after administration
- To report immediately any shortness of breath, persistent cough
- To report immediately any pain, discoloration at injection site
- To avoid contact with bacterial, viral illnesses
- That good oral hygiene with very soft toothbrush is imperative
- That dental work be delayed until CBC returns to normal, with permission of care provider
- That close household contacts of child not be immunized with live polio virus; use inactivated form
- That children on chemotherapy not receive immunization until immune system recovers sufficiently to mount necessary antibody response
- To report immediately exposure to chicken pox in susceptible child
- To report immediately reactivation of herpes zoster virus (shingles)
- If appropriate, ways to preserve reproductive patterns, sexuality (sperm banking, contraceptives)
Encourage
- Provision of nutritious food intake; consider nutritional consultation
- To use top anesthetics to control discomfort of mucositis; to avoid spicy foods, commercial mouthwashes

STORAGE
- Unopened vials should be refrigerated; will be stable for 2 years
- Reconstituted sol stable at room temp for 8 hr; if refrigerated, stability maintained for 24 hr

> **cefaclor**
> **Brand Name(s):** Ceclor✤
> **Classification:** Antibiotic (second-generation cephalosporin)
> **Pregnancy Category:** B

✤ Available in Canada.

AVAILABLE PREPARATIONS
Oral susp: 125 mg/5 ml, 187 mg/5 ml, 250 mg/5 ml, 375 mg/5 ml
Caps: 250 mg, 500 mg

ROUTES AND DOSAGES
Children >1 mo: PO 20-40 mg/kg/24 hr divided q8-12h; maximum dose 2 g/24 hr
Adults: PO 250-500 mg q8hr; maximum dose 4 g/24 hr

MECHANISM AND INDICATIONS
Antibiotic mechanism: Primarily bactericidal; may be bacteriostatic; inhibits bacterial protein synthesis by adhering to penicillin-binding enzymes
Indications: Active against both gram-positive and gram-negative bacteria such as staphylococci, group A β-hemolytic streptococci, *Str. pneumoniae, E. coli, Proteus mirabilis, Haemophilus influenzae,* and *Klebsiella* species; used to treat otitis media, respiratory, urinary tract, skin infections

PHARMACOKINETICS
Peak: 0.5-1 hr
Half-life: 0.5-1 hr
Metabolism: Not metabolized
Excretion: Urine

CONTRAINDICATIONS AND PRECAUTIONS
• Contraindicated with known hypersensitivity to any cephalosporin
• Use cautiously with known allergy to penicillins, impaired renal function, history of colitis or other GI disease, pregnancy, lactation

INTERACTIONS
Drug
• Increased serum concentrations with use of probenecid
• Increased nephrotoxicity possible with use of vancomycin, aminoglycosides, colistin, loop diuretics
• Decreased effectiveness with use of tetracyclines, erythromycins, chloramphenicol
Lab
• False elevation of urine creatinine using Jaffe's reaction
• False positive Coombs' test

SIDE EFFECTS
CNS: Dizziness, headache, somnolence, paresthesias, seizures
DERM: Maculopapular rash, dermatitis
GI: Nausea, vomiting, diarrhea, anorexia, pseudomembranous colitis, heartburn, glossitis, dyspepsia, abdominal cramping, tenesmus, pruritus
HEME: Transient leukopenia, lymphocytosis, anemia, eosinophilia
Other: Hypersensitivity (dyspnea, serum sickness: erythema multiforme, rashes, urticaria, polyarthritis, fever), bacterial or fungal superinfection

TOXICITY AND OVERDOSE
Clinical signs: Neuromuscular hypersensitivity; seizures may result from high CNS concentrations
Treatment: Supportive care; hemodialysis, peritoneal dialysis

PATIENT CARE MANAGEMENT
Assessment
• Assess history of hypersensitivity to cefaclor, other cephalosporins, or penicillins
• Obtain C&S; may begin therapy before obtaining results
• Assess renal function (BUN, creatinine, I&O), bowel pattern; assess liver function (ALT, AST, bilirubin) for long-term therapy
Interventions
• Administer cephalosporins at least 1 hr before bacteriostatic antibiotics (tetracyclines, erythromycins, chloramphenicol)
• May be administered PO with food to minimize GI distress; shake susp well before administering; caps may be taken apart, mixed with food or fluid
• Maintain age-appropriate fluid intake
• For group A β-hemolytic streptococcal infection, provide 10-day course of treatment to prevent risk of acute rheumatic fever, glomerulonephritis

✤ Available in Canada.

NURSING ALERT
Discontinue drug if signs of toxicity, hypersensitivity, pseudomembranous colitis develop

Evaluation
• Evaluate therapeutic response (decreased symptoms of infection)
• Monitor signs of superinfection (perineal itching, diaper rash, fever, malaise, redness, pain, swelling, drainage, rash, diarrhea, sore throat, change in cough or sputum)
• Observe for signs of allergic reaction (rash, urticaria, pruritus, chills, fever, joint pain, angioedema)
• Monitor bowel pattern; diarrhea may be symptomatic of pseudomembranous colitis
• Monitor renal function (BUN, creatinine, I&O)
• Monitor signs of bleeding (ecchymosis, bleeding gums, hematuria, daily stool guaiac) because of prolonged bleeding time

PATIENT AND FAMILY EDUCATION
Teach/instruct
• To take as directed at prescribed intervals for prescribed length of time
Warn/advise
• To notify care provider of hypersensitivity, side effects, superinfection
• To avoid use of alcohol, medications containing alcohol
Encourage
• To add live-culture yogurt or buttermilk to diet to prevent intestinal superinfection

STORAGE
• Store caps at room temp
• Reconstituted susp stable when refrigerated for 14 days or at room temp for 7 days; label date, time of reconstitution

cefadroxil
Brand Name(s): Duricef✤, Ultracef

Classification: Antibiotic (first-generation cephalosporin)

Pregnancy Category: B

AVAILABLE PREPARATIONS
Oral susp: 125 mg/5 ml, 250 mg/5 ml, 500 mg/5 ml
Tabs: 1 g
Caps: 500 mg

ROUTES AND DOSAGES
Children: PO 30 mg/kg/24 hr divided q12h; maximum dose 2 g/24 hr
Adults: PO 500 mg-2 g/24 hr qd or divided q12h; maximum dose 4 g/24 hr

MECHANISM AND INDICATIONS
Antibiotic mechanism: Primarily bactericidal; may be bacteriostatic; inhibits bacterial protein synthesis by adhering to penicillin-binding enzymes
Indications: Active against many gram-positive cocci, including *Staphylococcus aureus, S. epidermidis, Streptococcus pneumoniae,* group B streptococci, and group A β-hemolytic streptococci, and susceptible gram-negative organisms including *E. coli, Klebsiella pneumoniae, Proteus mirabilis,* and *Shigella;* used to treat lower respiratory tract, urinary tract, nasopharyngeal, skin infections

PHARMACOKINETICS
Peak: 1-2 hr
Half-life: 1-2 hr
Metabolism: Not metabolized
Excretion: Urine

CONTRAINDICATIONS AND PRECAUTIONS
• Contraindicated with known hypersensitivity to any cephalosporins
• Use cautiously with known allergy to penicillins, impaired renal

---

✤ Available in Canada.

function, history of colitis or other GI disease, pregnancy, lactation

INTERACTIONS
Drug
• Increased serum concentrations with use of probenecid
• Increased nephrotoxicity possible with use of vancomycin, aminoglycosides, colistin, loop diuretics
• Decreased effectiveness with use of tetracyclines, erythromycins, chloramphenicol
Lab
• False elevation of urine creatinine using Jaffe's reaction
• False positive Coombs' test

SIDE EFFECTS
CNS: Headache, dizziness, malaise, paresthesias, seizures
DERM: Maculopapular and erythematous rashes, urticaria
GI: Nausea, vomiting, diarrhea, anorexia, pseudomembranous colitis, glossitis, dyspepsia, abdominal cramps, anal pruritus, tenesmus
GU: Genital pruritus, moniliasis
HEME: Transient neutropenia, eosinophilia, leukopenia, anemia
Other: Dyspnea, bacterial or fungal superinfection

TOXICITY AND OVERDOSE
Clinical signs: Neuromuscular hypersensitivity; seizures may result from high CNS concentrations
Treatment: Supportive care; hemodialysis

PATIENT CARE MANAGEMENT
Assessment
• Assess history of hypersensitivity to cefadroxil, other cephalosporins, or penicillins
• Obtain C&S; may begin therapy before obtaining results
• Assess renal function (BUN, creatinine, I&O), bowel pattern; assess liver function (ALT, AST, bilirubin) for long-term therapy
Interventions
• Administer cephalosporins at least 1 hr before bacteriostatic antibiotics (tetracyclines, erythromycins, chloramphenicol)

• Shake susp well before administering; tabs may be crushed, capsules taken apart and mixed with food or fluid
• Maintain age-appropriate fluid intake
• For group A β-hemolytic streptococcal infection, provide 10-day course of treatment to prevent risk of acute rheumatic fever, glomerulonephritis

---

NURSING ALERT
Discontinue drug if signs of toxicity, hypersensitivity, pseudomembranous colitis develop

---

Evaluation
• Evaluate therapeutic response (decreased symptoms of infection)
• Monitor signs of superinfection (perineal itching, diaper rash, fever, malaise, redness, pain, swelling, drainage, rash, diarrhea, sore throat, change in cough or sputum)
• Observe for signs of allergic reaction (rash, urticaria, pruritus, chills, fever, joint pain, angioedema)
• Monitor bowel patterns; diarrhea may be symptomatic of pseudomembranous colitis
• Monitor renal function (BUN, creatinine, I&O)
• Monitor signs of bleeding (ecchymosis, bleeding gums, hematuria, daily stool guaiac) because of prolonged bleeding time

PATIENT AND FAMILY EDUCATION
Teach/instruct
• To take as directed at prescribed intervals for prescribed length of time
Warn/advise
• To notify care provider of hypersensitivity, side effects, superinfection
• To avoid use of alcohol, medications containing alcohol
Encourage
• To add live-culture yogurt or buttermilk to diet to prevent intestinal superinfection

---

🍁 Available in Canada.

STORAGE
• Store tabs and caps at room temp
• Reconstituted susp is stable refrigerated for 14 days or at room temp for 7 days; label date, time of reconstitution

---

cefamandole nafate
Brand Name(s): Mandol✤

Classification: Antibiotic (second-generation cephalosporin)

Pregnancy Category: B

AVAILABLE PREPARATIONS
Inj: 500 mg, 1 g, 2 g, 10 g

ROUTES AND DOSAGES
Infants >1 mo and children: IM/IV 50-150 mg/kg/24 hr divided q4-6h
Adults: IM/IV 4-12 g/24 hr divided q4-8h; maximum dose 12 g/24 hr, 2 g/dose
IV administration
• Recommended concentration: 100 mg/ml in D_5W, NS, SW for IV push; 10-20 mg/ml in D_5W, D_5NS, D_5 ½ NS, D_5 ¼ NS, $D_{10}W$, NS, or 50 mg/ml in SW for IV infusion
• Maximum concentration: 100 mg/ml for IV push; 50 mg/ml for IV infusion
• IV push rate: Over 3-5 min
• Intermittent infusion: Over 10-30 min

MECHANISM AND INDICATIONS
Antibiotic mechanism: Primarily bactericidal; may be bacteriostatic; inhibits bacterial protein synthesis by adhering to penicillin-binding enzymes
Indications: Active against *E. coli,* other coliform bacteria, *Staphylococcus aureus, S. epidermidis,* group A β-hemolytic streptococci, *Klebsiella, Haemophilus influenzae, Proteus mirabilis,* and *Enterobacter;* used to treat peritonitis and respiratory, GU, skin, bone, joint infections

PHARMACOKINETICS
Peak: IM 0.5-2.0 hr; IV end of infusion
Distribution: Poor CNS penetration
Half-life: 0.5-2.0 hr
Metabolism: Not metabolized
Excretion: Urine

CONTRAINDICATIONS AND PRECAUTIONS
• Contraindicated with known hypersensitivity to cefamandole, any cephalosporins, in infants <1 mo
• Use cautiously with known allergy to penicillins, impaired renal function, history of bleeding problems, pregnancy, lactation

INTERACTIONS
Drug
• Synergistic antimicrobial activity against certain organisms with use of aminoglycosides, chloramphenicol, penicillins
• Increased serum concentrations with use of probenecid
• Possible increased nephrotoxicity with use of vancomycin, aminoglycosides, colistin, loop diuretics
• Decreased effectiveness with use of tetracyclines, erythromycins, chloramphenicol
• Disulfiram-like reactions with use of alcohol
Lab
• False elevation of urine creatinine using Jaffe's reaction
• False positive Coomb's test
• Increased liver function test results
• Increased prothrombin times

INCOMPATIBILITIES
• Tetracyclines, erythromycins, calcium chloride, Mg salts, aminoglycosides, cimetidine

SIDE EFFECTS
CNS: Headache, malaise, paresthesias, dizziness, seizures
DERM: Maculopapular and erythematous rashes, urticaria
GI: Nausea, vomiting, diarrhea, anorexia, pseudomembranous colitis, glossitis, dyspepsia, abdominal cramps, tenesmus, anal pruritus

---

✤ Available in Canada.

GU: Nephrotoxicity, vaginitis
HEME: Transient neutropenia, eosinophilia, hemolytic anemia, hypoprothrombinemia, bleeding
Local: Pain, induration, sterile abscesses, tissue sloughing at injection site; phlebitis, thrombophlebitis with IV injection
Other: Hypersensitivity (dyspnea; serum sickness: erythema multiforme, rashes, polyarthritis, fever), bacterial or fungal superinfection

TOXICITY AND OVERDOSE

Clinical signs: Neuromuscular hypersensitivity; seizures may result from high CNS concentrations; hypoprothrombinemia, bleeding
Treatment: Supportive care; vitamin K or blood products, hemodialysis

PATIENT CARE MANAGEMENT

Assessment

• Assess history of hypersensitivity to cefamandole, other cephalosporins, or penicillins
• Obtain C&S; may begin therapy before obtaining results
• Assess renal function (BUN, creatinine, I&O), bowel pattern

Interventions

• Administer cephalosporins at least 1 hr before bacteriostatic antibiotics (tetracyclines, erythromycins, chloramphenicol)
• Powder discolors with exposure to light; reconstituted sol light yellow to amber; do not use if discolored or containing precipitate
• Invert vial, inject diluent above powder, quickly shake vial to avoid clumping of powder during dilution for IM; CO_2 results from mixing powder with diluent; follow manufacturer's instructions to release pressure build-up; keep needle below fluid level when withdrawing from inverted vial
• Injection not as painful as cefoxitin; no need to add lidocaine
• Administer deeply into large muscle mass; rotate injection sites
• Do not premix IV with other medications; infuse separately

• Use large vein with small-bore needle to reduce local reaction; rotate site q48-72h
• Maintain age-appropriate fluid intake
• For group A β-hemolytic streptococcal infection, provide 10-day course of treatment to prevent risk of acute rheumatic fever or glomerulonephritis

> **NURSING ALERT**
> Discontinue drug if signs of hypersensitivity, serum sickness, hypoprothrombinemia, pseudomembranous colitis develop

Evaluation

• Evaluate therapeutic response (decreased symptoms of infection)
• Monitor signs of superinfection (perineal itching, diaper rash, fever, malaise, redness, pain, swelling, drainage, rash, diarrhea, sore throat, change in cough or sputum)
• Observe for signs of allergic reaction (rash, urticaria, pruritus, chills, fever, joint pain, angioedema)
• Monitor bowel pattern; diarrhea may be symptomatic of pseudomembranous colitis
• Monitor renal function (BUN, creatinine, I&O)
• Monitor signs of bleeding (ecchymosis, bleeding gums, hematuria, daily stool guaiac) because of prolonged bleeding time
• Evaluate IM site for tissue damage, IV site for vein irritation

PATIENT AND FAMILY EDUCATION

Teach/instruct

• To take as directed at prescribed intervals for prescribed length of time

Warn/advise

• To notify care provider of hypersensitivity, side effects, superinfection
• To avoid use of alcohol, medications containing alcohol

✤ Available in Canada.

Encourage
• To add live-culture yogurt or buttermilk to diet to prevent intestinal superinfection

STORAGE
• Store powder at room temp protected from light
• Reconstituted sol stable at room temp for 24 hr; refrigerated for 96 hr

---

cefazolin sodium

Brand Name(s): Ancef✤, Kefzol✤, Zolicef

Classification: Antibiotic (first-generation cephalosporin)

Pregnancy Category: B

AVAILABLE PREPARATIONS
Inj: 250 mg, 500 mg, 1 g, 5 g, 10 g

ROUTES AND DOSAGES
Neonates <7 days: IM/IV 40 mg/kg/24 hr divided q12h (Safety and effectiveness not established. Dosage represents accepted standard practice recommendations.)
Neonates ≥7 days, <2000 g: IM/IV 40 mg/kg/24 hr divided q12h (Safety and effectiveness not established. Dosage represents accepted standard practice recommendations.)
Neonates ≥7 days, >2000 g: IM/IV 60 mg/kg/24 hr divided q8-12h (Safety and effectiveness not established. Dosage represents accepted standard practice recommendations.)
Infants >1 mo and children: IM/IV 50-100 mg/kg/24 hr divided q8-12h
Adults: IM/IV 0.5-2 g q6-8h; maximum dose 12 g/24 hr

IV administration
• Recommended concentration: 20 mg/ml in D_5W, D_5NS, $D_5\frac{1}{2}NS$, $D_5\frac{1}{4}NS$, $D_{10}W$, NS, LR, D_5LR
• Maximum concentration: 75-125 mg/ml (depending on manufacturer) in SW for slow IV push
• IV push rate: Over 3-5 min
• Intermittent infusion rate: Over 10-60 min

MECHANISM AND INDICATIONS
Antibiotic mechanism: Primarily bactericidal; may be bacteriostatic; inhibits bacterial protein synthesis by adhering to penicillin-binding enzymes
Indications: Active against *E. coli*, Enterobacteriaceae, gonococci, *Klebsiella, Proteus mirabilis, Staphylococcus aureus, Streptococcus pneumoniae,* and group A beta-hemolytic streptococci; used to treat septicemias, endocarditis, infections of respiratory, biliary, and GU tracts, skin, bone, and joint

PHARMACOKINETICS
Peak: IM 0.5-1.0 hr; IV 5-10 min after infusion
Distribution: Poor CNS penetration
Half-life: 1.0-2.0 hr
Metabolism: Not metabolized
Excretion: Urine

CONTRAINDICATIONS AND PRECAUTIONS
• Contraindicated with known sensitivity to cefazolin, any cephalosporin
• Use cautiously with known allergy to penicillin, impaired renal function, history of colitis or other GI disease, pregnancy, lactation

INTERACTIONS
Drug
• Synergistic antimicrobial activity against certain organisms with use of aminoglycosides, chloramphenicol, penicillins
• Increased serum concentrations with use of probenecid
• Possible increased nephrotoxicity with use of vancomycin, colistin, polymyxin B, aminoglycosides, loop diuretics
• Decreased effectiveness with use of tetracyclines, erythromycins, chloramphenicol
Lab
• False elevation of urine creatinine using Jaffe's reaction
• False positive Coombs' test
• Elevations in liver function test results

✤ Available in Canada.

INCOMPATIBILITIES
• Tetracyclines, erythromycins, calcium salts, magnesium salts, barbiturates, aminoglycosides, vitamin C, vitamin B with C, bleomycin, colistimethate, lidocaine

SIDE EFFECTS
CNS: Dizziness, headache, malaise, paresthesias, seizures
DERM: Maculopapular and erythematous rashes, urticaria
GI: Nausea, vomiting, diarrhea, anorexia, pseudomembranous colitis, glossitis, dyspepsia, abdominal cramps, anal pruritus, tenesmus
HEME: Transient neutropenia, leukopenia, eosinophilia, anemia
Local: Pain, induration, sterile abscesses, tissue sloughing at injection site; phlebitis and thrombophlebitis with IV injection
Other: Hypersensitivity (dyspnea, fever, chills, pruritis), bacterial or fungal superinfection

TOXICITY AND OVERDOSE
Clinical signs: Neuromuscular hypersensitivity; seizures may result from high CNS concentrations
Treatment: Supportive care; hemodialysis

PATIENT CARE MANAGEMENT
Assessment
• Assess history of hypersensitivity to cefazolin, other cephalosporins, penicillins
• Obtain C&S; may begin therapy before obtaining results
• Assess renal function (BUN, creatinine, I&O), bowel pattern

Interventions
• Administer cephalosporins at least 1 hr before bacteriostatic antibiotics (tetracyclines, erythromycins, chloramphenicol)
• Reconstituted sol pale to yellow color; if particulate matter evident after shaking, discard
• IM injection less painful than that of other cephalosporins; administer deeply into large muscle mass, rotate injection sites
• Do not premix IV with other medications, particularly aminoglycosides; infuse separately
• Use large vein with small-bore needle to reduce local reaction; rotate site q48-72h
• Maintain age-appropriate fluid intake
• For group A β-hemolytic streptococcal infection, provide 10-day course of treatment to prevent risk of acute rheumatic fever or glomerulonephritis

---

NURSING ALERT
Discontinue drug if signs of toxicity, hypersensitivity, pseudomembranous colitis develop

---

Evaluation
• Evaluate therapeutic response (decreased symptoms of infection)
• Monitor signs of superinfection (perineal itching, diaper rash, fever, malaise, redness, pain, swelling, drainage, rash, diarrhea, sore throat, change in cough or sputum)
• Observe for signs of allergic reaction (rash, urticaria, pruritus, chills, fever, joint pain, angioedema)
• Monitor bowel pattern; diarrhea may be symptomatic of pseudomembranous colitis
• Monitor renal function (BUN, creatinine, I&O)
• Monitor for signs of bleeding (ecchymosis, bleeding gums, hematuria, daily stool guaiacs) because of prolonged bleeding time
• Evaluate IM site for tissue damage; IV site for vein irritation

PATIENT AND FAMILY EDUCATION
Teach/instruct
• To take as directed at prescribed intervals for prescribed length of time
Warn/advise
• To notify care provider of hypersensitivity, side effects, superinfection
• To avoid use of alcohol, medications containing alcohol
Encourage
• To add live-culture yogurt or buttermilk to diet to prevent intestinal superinfection

---

♣ Available in Canada.

STORAGE
- Store powder at room temp protected from light
- Reconstituted sol stable at room temp for 24 hr; refrigerated for 96 hr; frozen preparation stable below −15° C for 12 wk

cefixime
Brand Name(s): Suprax✦

Classification: Antibiotic (third-generation cephalosporin)

Pregnancy Category: B

AVAILABLE PREPARATIONS
Oral susp: 100 mg/5 ml
Tabs: 200 mg, 400 mg

ROUTES AND DOSAGES
Infants >6 mo and children: PO 8 mg/kg/24 hr as single dose or divided q12h; maximum dose 400 mg/24 hr
Adults: PO 400 mg/24 hr as single dose or divided q12h
Neisseria Gonorrhoeae Infection
400 mg single dose may be as effective as ceftriaxone

MECHANISM AND INDICATIONS
Antibiotic mechanism: Primarily bactericidal; may be bacteriostatic; inhibits bacterial protein synthesis by adhering to penicillin-binding enzymes
Indications: Effective against many gram-positive and some gram-negative organisms including *E. coli, Proteus mirabilis, Streptococcus pneumoniae, Str. pyogenes,* and *Haemophilus influenzae;* used to treat respiratory, ear, GU and GI infections

PHARMACOKINETICS
Peak: 1 hr
Half-life: 3-4 hr
Metabolism: Not metabolized
Excretion: Urine

CONTRAINDICATIONS AND PRECAUTIONS
- Contraindicated with known hypersensitivity to cefixime or any cephalosporin, and in infants <6 mo
- Use cautiously with known allergy to penicillins, impaired renal function, history of colitis or other GI disease, pregnancy, lactation

INTERACTIONS
Drugs
- Increased serum concentrations with use of probenecid
- Possible increased nephrotoxicity with use of vancomycin, aminoglycosides, colistin, loop diuretics
- Decreased effectiveness with use of tetracyclines, erythromycins, chloramphenicol
Lab
- False elevation of urine creatinine using Jaffe's reaction
- False positive Coombs' test

SIDE EFFECTS
CNS: Headache, dizziness, malaise, paresthesias, seizures
DERM: Maculopapular and erythematous rashes, urticaria.
GI: Nausea, vomiting, diarrhea, anorexia, pseudomembranous colitis, tenesmus, anal pruritus
GU: Genital pruritus, vaginitis, nephrotoxicity, hematuria
HEME: Transient neutropenia, eosinophilia, anemia
Other: Hypersensitivity, dyspnea, fever, bacterial or fungal superinfection

TOXICITY AND OVERDOSE
Clinical signs: Neuromuscular hypersensitivity; seizures may result from high CNS concentrations
Treatment: Supportive care

PATIENT CARE MANAGEMENT
Assessment
- Assess history of hypersensitivity to cefixime, other cephalosporins, penicillins
- Obtain C&S; may begin therapy before obtaining results
- Assess renal function (BUN, creatinine, I&O), bowel pattern
Interventions
- Administer cephalosporins at least 1 hr before bacteriostatic

antibiotics (tetracyclines, erythro-mycins, chloramphenicol)
• May be administered PO with food to minimize GI distress; shake susp well before administering; caps may be taken apart, mixed with food or fluid
• Maintain age-appropriate fluid intake
• For group A β-hemolytic streptococcal infection, provide 10-day course of treatment to prevent risk of acute rheumatic fever or glomerulonephritis

NURSING ALERT
Discontinue drug if signs of toxicity, hypersensitivity, or pseudomembranous colitis develop

Evaluation
• Evaluate therapeutic response (decreased symptoms of infection)
• Monitor signs of superinfection (perineal itching, diaper rash, fever, malaise, redness, pain, swelling, drainage, rash, diarrhea, sore throat, change in cough or sputum)
• Observe for signs of allergic reaction (rash, urticaria, pruritus, chills, fever, joint pain, angioedema)
• Monitor bowel pattern; diarrhea may be symptomatic of pseudomembranous colitis
• Monitor renal function (BUN, creatinine, I&O)
• Monitor for signs of bleeding (ecchymosis, bleeding gums, hematuria, daily stool guaiac) because of prolonged bleeding time

PATIENT AND FAMILY EDUCATION
Teach/instruct
• To take as directed at prescribed intervals for prescribed length of time
Warn/advise
• To notify care provider of hypersensitivity, side effects, superinfection
• To avoid use of alcohol, medications containing alcohol

Encourage
• To add live-culture yogurt or buttermilk to diet to prevent intestinal superinfection

STORAGE
• Store caps at room temp
• Reconstituted susp stable for 14 days at room temp or refrigerated; label date, time of reconstitution

cefoperazone
Brand Name(s): Cefobid
Classification: Antibiotic (third-generation cephalosporin)
Pregnancy Category: B

AVAILABLE PREPARATIONS
• *Inj:* 1 g, 2 g
ROUTES AND DOSAGES
Children: IM/IV 100-150 mg/kg/24 hr divided q8-12h (Safety and effectiveness not established. Dosage represents accepted standard practice recommendations.)
Adults: 2-4 g/24 hr divided q12h; maximum dose 12 g/24 hr

IV administration
• Recommended concentration: 2-50 mg/ml in D_5W, NS, SW
• Maximum concentration: 50 mg/ml
• IV push rate: Not recommended
• Intermittent infusion: Over 15-60 min
• Continuous infusion: Must be diluted to 2-25 mg/ml

MECHANISM AND INDICATIONS
Antibiotic mechanism: Primarily bactericidal; may be bacteriostatic; inhibits bacterial protein synthesis by adhering to penicillin-binding enzymes
Indications: Active against some gram-positive and many enteric gram-negative bacilli, including *Streptococcus pneumoniae, Str. pyogenes, Staphylococcus aureus, S. epidermidis, E. coli, Klebsiella, Haemophilus influenzae, Enterobacter, Citrobacter, Proteus, Pseu-*

domonas aeruginosa, and *Bacteroides fragilis;* used to treat respiratory tract, intraabdominal, gynecologic, and skin infections, and bacteremias and septicemias

PHARMACOKINETICS
Peak: IM 1-2 hr; IV 5-20 min
Distribution: Low CNS penetration except with inflamed meninges
Half-life: 1.5-2.5 hr
Metabolism: Not substantially metabolized
Excretion: Bile, urine

CONTRAINDICATIONS AND PRECAUTIONS
• Contraindicated with known hypersensitivity to cefoperazone, any cephalosporins
• Use cautiously with known allergy to penicillins, impaired renal function, history of bleeding problems, pregnancy, lactation

INTERACTIONS
Drug
• Synergistic antimicrobial activity against certain organisms with use of aminoglycosides, clavulanic acid
• Increased serum concentrations with use of probenecid
• Increased nephrotoxicity possible with use of vancomycin, aminoglycosides, colistin, loop diuretics
• Decreased effectiveness with use of tetracyclines, erythromycins, chloramphenicol
• Disulfiram-like reactions with use of alcohol
Lab
• False elevations of urine creatinine using Jaffe's reaction
• False positive Coombs' test
• Elevations in liver function test results
• Elevations in prothrombin times

INCOMPATIBILITIES
• Aminoglycosides, labetalol, perphenazine

SIDE EFFECTS
CNS: headache, malaise, paresthesias, dizziness, seizures
DERM: Maculopapular and erythematous rashes, urticaria

GI: Nausea, vomiting, diarrhea, pseudomembranous colitis, glossitis, dyspepsia, abdominal cramps, tenesmus, anal pruritus, mildly elevated liver enzyme levels
GU: Genital pruritus
HEME: Transient neutropenia, eosinophilia, hemolytic anemia, hypoprothrombinemia, bleeding
Local: Pain, induration, sterile abscesses, tissue sloughing at injection site, phlebitis, thrombophlebitis with IV injection
Other: Hypersensitivity (serum sickness: erythema multiforme, rashes, polyarthritis, fever), dyspnea, bacterial or fungal superinfection

TOXICITY AND OVERDOSE
Clinical signs: Neuromuscular hypersensitivity; seizures may result from high CNS concentrations; hypoprothrombinemia, bleeding
Treatment: Supportive care; vitamin K or blood products; hemodialysis

PATIENT CARE MANAGEMENT
Assessment
• Assess history of hypersensitivity to cefoperazone, other cephalosporins, penicillins
• Obtain C&S; may begin therapy before obtaining results
• Assess renal function (BUN, creatinine, I&O), bowel pattern
Interventions
• Administer cephalosporins at least 1 hr before bacteriostatic antibiotics (tetracyclines, erythromycins, chloramphenicol)
• IM injection is painful; administer deeply into large muscle mass, rotate injection sites
• Do not premix IV with other medications; infuse separately
• Use large vein with small-bore needle to reduce local reaction; rotate site q48-72h
• Maintain age appropriate fluid intake
• For group A β-hemolytic streptococcal infection, provide 10-day course of treatment to prevent risk of acute rheumatic fever, glomerulonephritis

---

✦ Available in Canada.

NURSING ALERT
Discontinue drug if signs of hypersensitivity, serum sickness, hypoprothrombinemia, pseudomembranous colitis develop

cefotaxime sodium

Brand Name(s): Claforan ❦

Classification: Antibiotic (third-generation cephalosporin)

Pregnancy Category: B

Evaluation
• Evaluate therapeutic response (decreased symptoms of infection)
• Monitor signs of superinfection (perineal itching, diaper rash, fever, malaise, redness, pain, swelling, drainage, rash, diarrhea, sore throat, change in cough or sputum)
• Observe for signs of allergic reaction (rash, urticaria, pruritus, chills, fever, joint pain, angioedema)
• Monitor bowel pattern; diarrhea may be symptomatic of pseudomembranous colitis
• Monitor renal function (BUN, creatinine, I&O)
• Monitor for signs of bleeding (ecchymosis, bleeding gums, hematuria, daily stool guaiac) because of prolonged bleeding time
• Evaluate IM site for tissue damage, IV site for vein irritation

PATIENT AND FAMILY EDUCATION
Teach/instruct
• To take as directed at prescribed intervals for prescribed length of time
Warn/advise
• To notify care provider of hypersensitivity, side effects, superinfection
• To avoid use of alcohol, medications containing alcohol
Encourage
• To add live-culture yogurt or buttermilk to diet to prevent intestinal superinfection

STORAGE
• Store powder at room temp protected from light
• Reconstituted sol stable at room temp 24 hr, refrigerated for 5 days

AVAILABLE PREPARATIONS
Inj: 1 g, 2 g, 10 g

ROUTE AND DOSAGES
Neonates: Wt <1200 g, age 0-4 wk, IM/IV 50 mg/kg/dose q12h; wt 1200-2000 g, age 0-7 days, IM/IV 50 mg/kg/dose q12h; wt 1200-2000 g, age >7 days, IM/IV 50 mg/kg/dose q8h; wt >2000 g, age 0-7 days, IM/IV 50 mg/kg/dose q12h; wt >2000 g, age >7 days, IM/IV 50 mg/kg/dose q8h
Infants and children <50 kg: IM/IV 100-150 mg/kg/24 hr divided q6-8h
Children >50 kg and adults: IM/IV 1-2 g q6-8h; maximum 10-12 g/24 hr

Meningitis
Infants and children <50 kg: 200 mg/kg/24 hr divided q6-8h

IV administration
• Recommended concentration: 20-60 mg/ml in D_5NS, $D_5\frac{1}{4}NS$, $D_5\frac{1}{2}NS$, D_5W, $D_{10}W$, LR or NS
• Maximum concentration: 100-200 mg/ml in SW
• IV push rate: Over 3-5 min
• Intermittent infusion rate: Over 10-30 min

MECHANISM AND INDICATIONS
Antibiotic mechanism: Primarily bactericidal; may be bacteriostatic; inhibits bacterial protein synthesis by adhering to penicillin-binding enzymes
Indications: Active against some gram-positive organisms and many enteric gram-negative bacilli, including *Streptococcus pneumoniae, Str. pyogenes, Staphylococcus aureus, S. epidermidis, E. coli, Klebsiella, Haemophilus influenzae, Enterobacter* sp, *Proteus* sp, *Peptostreptococcus* sp, and some strains of *Pseudomonas*

aeruginosa; used to treat septicemias, gynecologic, CNS and gonococcal ophthalmic infections, infections of the lower respiratory tract, skin, GU tract, bone, and joint

PHARMACOKINETICS
Peak: IM 30 min; IV 5 min after infusion
Distribution: Penetrates CNS except with inflamed meninges
Half-life: 1 hr
Metabolism: Partially by liver
Excretion: Urine

CONTRAINDICATIONS AND PRECAUTIONS
• Contraindicated with known hypersensitivity to cefotaxime, any cephalosporin
• Use cautiously with known allergy to penicillins, impaired renal function or history of colitis or other GI disease, pregnancy, lactation

INTERACTIONS
Drug
• Synergistic antimicrobial activity against certain organisms with use of aminoglycosides, chloramphenicol, penicillins
• Increased serum concentrations with use of probenecid
• Possible increased nephrotoxicity with use of vancomycin, colistin, aminoglycosides, loop diuretics
• Decreased effectiveness with use of tetracyclines, erythromycins, chloramphenicol
Lab
• False elevation of urine creatinine using Jaffe's reaction
• Elevation in liver function test results

INCOMPATIBILITIES
• Aminoglycosides, aminophylline, erythromycins, $NaHCO_3$, alkaline solutions

SIDE EFFECTS
CNS: Headache, malaise, paresthesias, dizziness, seizures
DERM: Maculopapular and erythematous rashes, urticaria
GI: Nausea, vomiting, diarrhea, anorexia, pseudomembranous colitis, glossitis, dyspepsia, abdominal cramps, tenesmus, anal pruritus
GU: Genital pruritus
HEME: Transient neutropenia, eosinophilia, hemolytic anemia
Local: Pain, induration, sterile abscesses, tissue sloughing at injection site; phlebitis, thrombophlebitis with IV injection
Other: Hypersensitivity (dyspnea; serum sickness: erythema multiforme, rashes, urticaria, polyarthritis, fever), bacterial or fungal superinfection

TOXICITY AND OVERDOSE
Clinical signs: Neuromuscular hypersensitivity; seizures may result from high CNS concentrations
Treatment: Supportive care; hemodialysis

PATIENT CARE MANAGEMENT
Assessment
• Assess history of hypersensitivity to cefotaxime, other cephalosporins, penicillins
• Obtain C&S; may begin therapy before obtaining results
• Assess renal function (BUN, creatinine, I&O), bowel pattern
Interventions
• Administer cephalosporins at least 1 hr before bacteriostatic antibiotics (tetracyclines, erythromycins, chloramphenicol)
• Powder/sol may darken with exposure to light or heat; color other than light yellow to amber may indicate decreased potency
• IM injection painful; administer deeply into large muscle mass, rotate injection sites
• Do not premix IV with other aminoglycosides, aminophylline, $NaHCO_3$, alkaline solutions
• Use large vein with small-bore needle to reduce local reaction; rotate site q48-72h
• Maintain age-appropriate fluid intake
• For group A β-hemolytic streptococcal infection, provide 10-day course of treatment to prevent risk of acute rheumatic fever, glomerulonephritis

---

✤ Available in Canada.

NURSING ALERT
Discontinue drug if signs of toxicity, hypersensitivity, serum sickness, pseudomembranous colitis develop

C

cefotetan disodium
Brand Name(s): Cefotan ♣
Classification: Antibiotic (third-generation cephalosporin)
Pregnancy Category: B

Evaluation
• Evaluate therapeutic response (decreased symptoms of infection)
• Monitor signs of superinfection (perineal itching, diaper rash, fever, malaise, redness, pain, swelling, drainage, rash, diarrhea, sore throat, change in cough or sputum)
• Observe for signs of allergic reaction (rash, urticaria, pruritus, chills, fever, joint pain, angioedema)
• Monitor bowel pattern; diarrhea may be symptomatic of pseudomembranous colitis
• Monitor renal function (BUN, creatinine, I&O)
• Monitor for signs of bleeding (ecchymosis, bleeding gums, hematuria, daily stool guaiac) because of prolonged bleeding time
• Evaluate IM site for tissue damage, IV site for vein irritation

PATIENT AND FAMILY EDUCATION
Teach/instruct
• To take as directed at prescribed intervals for prescribed length of time
Warn/advise
• To advise care provider of hypersensitivity, side effects, superinfection
• To avoid alcohol, medications containing alcohol
Encourage
• To add live-culture yogurt or buttermilk to diet to prevent intestinal superinfection

STORAGE
• Store powder at room temp protected from heat, light
• Reconstituted sol stable at room temp for 24 hr; refrigerated for 10 days; frozen preparations reconstituted with SW, D_5W, NS stable below −15° C for 12 wk

AVAILABLE PREPARATIONS
Inj: 1 g, 2 g
ROUTES AND DOSAGES
Children: IM/IV 40-80 mg/kg/24 hr divided q12h (Safety and effectiveness not established. Dosage represents accepted standard practice recommendations.)
Adults: IM/IV 1-2 g q12h; maximum dose 6 g/24 hr
IV administration
• Recommended concentration 100 mg/ml in D_5W, NS for IV push; 10-20 mg/ml for intermittent infusion
• Maximum concentration: 100 mg/ml
• IV push rate: Over 3-5 min
• Intermittent infusion rate: Over 20-30 min

MECHANISM AND INDICATIONS
Antibiotic mechanism: Primarily bactericidal; may be bacteriostatic; inhibits bacterial protein synthesis by adhering to penicillin-binding enzymes
Indications: Effective against many gram-positive and some gram-negative organisms including *Haemophilus influenzae, E. coli, Enterobacter aerogenes, Enterobacter sp, Proteus mirabilis, Klebsiella, Citrobacter, Salmonella, Shigella, Acinetobacter, Bacteroides fragilis, Neisseria, Serratia, Streptococcus pneumoniae, Str. pyogenes,* and *Staphylococcus aureus;* used to treat septicemia, meningitis, and respiratory tract, GI, GU, skin, joint, and bone infections

PHARMACOKINETICS
Peak: 1.5-3.0 hr
Distribution: Widely distributed to

---

body tissues; poor CNS penetration

Half-life: 3-5 hr
Metabolism: Not metabolized.
Excretion: Urine

CONTRAINDICATIONS AND PRECAUTIONS

• Contraindicated with known hypersensitivity to cefotetan, any other cephalosporin
• Use cautiously with known allergy to penicillins, impaired renal function, history of colitis or other GI disease, pregnancy, lactation

INTERACTIONS
Drug
• Increased serum concentrations with use of probenecid
• Increased nephrotoxicity possible with use of aminoglycosides, loop diuretics
• Decreased effectiveness with use of tetracyclines, erythromycins, chloramphenicol
Lab
• False elevations of urine creatinine using Jaffe's reaction
• False positive Coombs' test

INCOMPATIBILITIES
• Tetracyclines, erythromycins, aminoglycosides, heparin, doxapram, any other bacteriostatic agent

SIDE EFFECTS
CNS: Headache, dizziness, weakness, paresthesias, seizures
DERM: Maculopapular and erythematous rashes, urticaria
GI: Nausea, vomiting, diarrhea, anorexia, pseudomembranous colitis, glossitis, abdominal cramps, mildly elevated liver enzyme tests
GU: Genital pruritus, vaginitis, nephrotoxicity, hematuria
HEME: Transient neutropenia, eosinophilia, hemolytic anemia, thrombocytopenia
Local: Pain, induration, sterile abscesses, tissue sloughing at injection site; phlebitis, thrombophlebitis with IV injection
Other: Hypersensitivity, dyspnea, fever, bacterial or fungal superinfection

TOXICITY AND OVERDOSE
Clinical signs: Neuromuscular hypersensitivity; seizures may result from high CNS concentrations
Treatment: Supportive care; hemodialysis

PATIENT CARE MANAGEMENT
Assessment
• Assess history of hypersensitivity to cefotetan, other cephalosporins, penicillins
• Obtain C&S; may begin therapy before obtaining results
• Assess renal function (BUN, creatinine, I&O), bowel pattern
Interventions
• Administer cephalosporins at least 1 hr before other bacteriostatic antibiotics (tetracyclines, erythromycins, chloramphenicol)
• IM injection is painful; administer deeply into large muscle mass rotate injection sites
• Do not premix IV with other medications, infuse separately
• Use large vein with small-bore needle to reduce local reaction; rotate site q48-72h
• Maintain age-appropriate fluid intake
• For group A β-hemolytic streptococcal infection, provide 10-day course of treatment to prevent risk of acute rheumatic fever or glomerulonephritis

---

NURSING ALERT
Discontinue drug if signs of toxicity, hypersensitivity, pseudomembranous colitis develop

---

Evaluation
• Evaluate therapeutic response (decreased symptoms of infection)
• Monitor signs of superinfection (perineal itching, diaper rash, fever, malaise, redness, pain, swelling, drainage, rash, diarrhea, sore throat, change in cough or sputum)
• Observe for signs of allergic reaction (rash, urticaria, pruritus, chills, fever, joint pain, angioedema)

- Monitor bowel pattern; diarrhea may be symptomatic of pseudomembranous colitis
- Monitor renal function (BUN, creatinine, I&O)
- Monitor for signs of bleeding (ecchymosis, bleeding gums, hematuria, daily stool guaiac) because of prolonged bleeding time
- Evaluate IM site for tissue damage; IV site for vein irritation

PATIENT AND FAMILY EDUCATION
Teach/instruct
- To take as directed at prescribed intervals for prescribed length of time
Warn/advise
- To notify care provider of hypersensitivity, side effects, superinfection
- To avoid use of alcohol, medications containing alcohol
Encourage
- To add live-culture yogurt or buttermilk to diet to prevent intestinal superinfection

STORAGE
- Store at room temp
- Protect from light
- Reconstituted sol stable at room temp for 24 hr, refrigerated for 96 hr
- Stable after dilution for 1 week if frozen; thaw to room temp before use

---

cefoxitin sodium
Brand Name(s): Mefoxin✤
Classification: Antibiotic (second-generation cephalosporin)
Pregnancy Category: B

AVAILABLE PREPARATIONS
Inj: 1 g, 2 g, 10 g

ROUTES AND DOSAGES
Infants <3 mo: IM/IV 90-100 mg/kg/24 hr divided q8h (Safety and effectiveness not established. Dosage represents accepted standard practice recommendations.)

Infants >3 mo and children: IM/IV 80-160 mg/kg/24 hr divided q4-6h; maximum 12 g/24 hr
Adults: IM/IV 4-12 g/24 hr divided q6-8h; maximum dose 12 g/24 hr
Surgical Prophylaxis
Children >3 mo: IM/IV 30-40 mg/kg/dose 30-60 min before surgery; then q6h for 24 hr

IV administration
- Recommended concentration: 95-180 mg/ml in SW for IV push; 10-40 mg/ml in D_5W, D_5 NS, $D_5\frac{1}{2}$NS, D_5 ¼ NS, D_5LR, D_{10}W, LR, NS, R for IV infusion
- Maximum concentration: 180 mg/ml for IV push; 40 mg/ml for IV infusion
- IV push rate: Over 3-5 min
- Intermittent infusion rate: Over 10-60 min

MECHANISM AND INDICATIONS
Antibiotic mechanism: Primarily bactericidal; may be bacteriostatic; inhibits bacterial protein synthesis by adhering to penicillin-binding enzymes
Indications: Effective against many gram-positive organisms and enteric gram-negative bacilli including *E. coli* and other coliform bacteria, *Staphylococcus aureus, S. epidermidis,* streptococci, *Klebsiella, Proteus mirabilis, Haemophilus influenzae, Salmonella, Shigella, Neisseria gonorrhoeae,* and *Bacteroides fragilis;* used to treat intra-abdominal, respiratory, GU, and skin infections

PHARMACOKINETICS
Peak: IM 1.0 hr; IV end of infusion
Distribution: Poor CNS penetration; widely distributed in body tissues
Half-life: 0.5-1.0 hr
Metabolism: Not metabolized
Excretion: Urine
Therapeutic level: 8-16 mcg/ml for most gram-positive/gram-negative bacteria; 16-32 mcg/ml for *Bacteroides*

CONTRAINDICATIONS AND PRECAUTIONS
- Contraindicated with known

sensitivity to cefoxitin, any cephalosporins
• Use cautiously with known allergy to penicillins, impaired renal function, history of colitis or other GI disease, pregnancy, lactation

INTERACTIONS
Drug
• Synergistic antimicrobial activity against certain organisms with use of aminoglycosides, chloramphenicol, penicillins
• Increased serum concentrations with use of probenecid
• Increased nephrotoxicity possible with use of vancomycin, colistin, polymyxin B, aminoglycosides, loop diuretics
• Decreased effectiveness with use of tetracyclines, erythromycins, chloramphenicol
Lab
• False elevation of urine creatinine using Jaffe's reaction
• False positive Coomb's test
• Elevations in liver function test results

INCOMPATIBILITIES
• Aminoglycosides

SIDE EFFECTS
CNS: Headache, malaise, paresthesias, dizziness, seizures
DERM: Maculopapular and erythematous rashes, urticaria
GI: Nausea, vomiting, diarrhea, anorexia, pseudomembranous colitis, glossitis, dyspepsia, abdominal cramps, tenesmus, pruritus
GU: Genital pruritus, vaginitis, hematuria, nephrotoxicity
HEME: Transient neutropenia, eosinophilia, hemolytic anemia
Local: Pain, induration, sterile abscesses, tissue sloughing at injection site; phlebitis, thrombophlebitis with IV injection
Other: Hypersensitivity (dyspnea; serum sickness: erythema multiforme, rashes, urticaria, polyarthritis, fever), bacterial or fungal superinfection

TOXICITY AND OVERDOSE
Clinical signs: Neuromuscular hypersensitivity; seizures may result from high CNS concentrations

Treatment: Supportive care; hemodialysis

PATIENT CARE MANAGEMENT
Assessment
• Assess history of hypersensitivity to cefoxitin, other cephalosporins, penicillins
• Obtain C&S; may begin therapy before obtaining results
• Assess renal function (BUN, creatinine, I&O), bowel pattern
Interventions
• Administer cephalosporins at least 1 hr before bacteriostatic antibiotics (tetracyclines, erythromycins, chloramphenicol)
• Powder/sol may darken, but potency is not altered
• Do not reconstitute with bacteriostatic water containing benzyl alcohol for use in infants because of risk of toxicity
• After reconstituting IM, shake vial, let stand until clear to ensure drug dissolution
• Administer deeply into large muscle mass, rotate injection sites
• Do not premix IV with other aminoglycosides, cephalosporins, penicillins, alkaline solutions
• Use large vein with small-bore needle to reduce local reaction; rotate site q48-72h
• Maintain age-appropriate fluid intake
• For group A β-hemolytic streptococcal infection, provide 10-day course of treatment to prevent risk of acute rheumatic fever, glomerulonephritis

> **NURSING ALERT**
> Discontinue drug if signs of toxicity, hypersensitivity, serum sickness, pseudomembranous colitis develop

Evaluation
• Evaluate therapeutic response (decreased symptoms of infection)
• Monitor signs of superinfection (perineal itching, diaper rash, fever, malaise, redness, pain, swelling, drainage, rash, diarrhea, sore

---

✤ Available in Canada.

throat, change in cough or sputum)
• Observe for signs of allergic reaction (rash, urticaria, pruritus, chills, fever, joint pain, angioedema)
• Monitor bowel pattern; diarrhea may be symptomatic of pseudomembranous colitis
• Monitor renal function (BUN, creatinine, I&O)
• Monitor for signs of bleeding (ecchymosis, bleeding gums, hematuria, daily stool guaiac) because of prolonged bleeding time
• Evaluate IM site for tissue damage, IV site for vein irritation

PATIENT AND FAMILY EDUCATION
Teach/instruct
• To take as directed at prescribed intervals for prescribed length of time
Warn/advise
• To notify care provider of hypersensitivity, side effects, superinfection
• To avoid use of alcohol, medications containing alcohol
Encourage
• To add live-culture yogurt or buttermilk to diet to prevent intestinal superinfection

STORAGE
• Store powder at room temp, protected from heat
• Reconstituted sol stable at room temp for 24 hr; refrigerated for 1 wk; frozen preparations stable below –20° C for 30 wk

---

cefpodoxime proxetil
Brand Name(s): Vantin
Classification: Antibiotic (second-generation cephalosporin)
Pregnancy Category: B

AVAILABLE PREPARATIONS
Oral susp (granules): 50 mg/5 ml, 100 mg/5 ml
Tabs (film-coated): 100 mg, 200 mg

ROUTES AND DOSAGES
Children 6 mo-12 yr: PO 10 mg/kg/24 hr divided q12h; maximum 400 mg/24 hr
Adults: 100-400 mg q12h
Uncomplicated Gonorrhea
200 mg in one dose

MECHANISM AND INDICATIONS
Antibiotic mechanism: Primarily bactericidal; may be bacteriostatic; inhibits bacterial protein synthesis by adhering to penicillin-binding enzymes
Indications: Effective against gram-negative and gram-positive organisms including *Neisseria gonorrhorae, Haemophilus influenzae, E. coli, Proteus mirabilis, Klebsiella, Streptococcus pneumoniae, St. pyogenes, Staphylococcus aureus;* used to treat upper and lower respiratory tract, urinary tract, skin infections, otitis media, sexually transmitted diseases

PHARMACOKINETICS
Peak: 2-3 hr
Distribution: Good penetration into inflammatory, pulmonary, pleural fluids; tonsils
Half-life: 2-3 hr
Metabolism: Not metabolized
Excretion: Urine

CONTRAINDICATIONS AND PRECAUTIONS
• Contraindicated with known sensitivity to cefpodoxime or any cephalosporin, infants <6 mo
• Use cautiously with known allergy to penicillins, impaired renal function, history of colitis or other GI disease, pregnancy, lactation

INTERACTIONS
Drug
• Increased serum concentrations with use of probenecid
• Increased nephrotoxicity possible with use of vancomycin, aminoglycosides, colistin, loop diuretics
• Decreased effectiveness with use of tetracyclines, erythromycins, chloramphenicol

Lab
- False elevation of urine creatinine using Jaffe's reaction
- False positive Coombs' test

SIDE EFFECTS

CNS: Dizziness, headache, paresthesias, seizures

DERM: Maculopapular and erythematous rashes, urticaria

GI: Nausea, vomiting, diarrhea, pseudomembranous colitis, abdominal cramping, glossitis, transient elevations in liver enzymes

GU: Proteinuria, increased BUN, nephrotoxicity, renal failure

HEME: Leukopenia, lymphocytosis, neutropenia, hemolytic anemia

Other: Hypersensitivity (dyspnea; serum sickness: erythema multiforme, rashes, urticaria, polyarthritis, fever), bacterial or fungal superinfection

TOXICITY AND OVERDOSE

Clinical signs: Neuromuscular hypersensitivity; seizures may result from high CNS concentrations

Treatment: Supportive care; hemodialysis or peritoneal dialysis

PATIENT CARE MANAGEMENT

Assessment
- Assess history of hypersensitivity to cefpodoxime, other cephalosporins, penicillin
- Obtain C&S; may begin therapy before obtaining results
- Assess renal function (BUN, creatinine, I&O), hepatic function (ALT, AST, bilirubin), electrolytes (K+, Na, Cl), particularly for long-term therapy, bowel pattern

Interventions
- Administer cephalosporins at least 1 hr before bacteriostatic antibiotics (tetracyclines, erythromycins, chloramphenicol)
- Increased absorption when administered PO with meals
- Shake susp well before administering each dose; tabs may be crushed, mixed with food or fluid
- Maintain age-appropriate fluid intake
- For group A β-hemolytic streptococcal infection, provide 10-day course of treatment to prevent risk of acute rheumatic fever, glomerulonephritis

> **NURSING ALERT**
> Discontinue drug if signs of toxicity, hypersensitivity, pseudomembranous colitis develop

Evaluation
- Evaluate therapeutic response (decreased symptoms of infection)
- Monitor signs of superinfection (perineal itching, diaper rash, fever, malaise, redness, pain, swelling, drainage, rash, diarrhea, sore throat, change in cough or sputum)
- Observe for signs of allergic reaction (rash, urticaria, pruritis, chills, fever, joint pain, angioedema)
- Monitor bowel patterns; diarrhea may be symptomatic of pseudomembranous colitis
- Monitor renal function (BUN, creatinine, I&O), hepatic (ALT, AST, bilirubin), electrolytes (K+, Na, Cl), particularly for long-term therapy
- Monitor for signs of bleeding (ecchymosis, bleeding gums, hematuria, daily stool guaiac) because of prolonged bleeding time

PATIENT AND FAMILY EDUCATION

Teach/instruct
- To take as directed at prescribed intervals for prescribed length of time

Warn/advise
- To notify care provider of hypersensitivity, side effects, superinfection
- To avoid use of alcohol, medications containing alcohol

Encourage
- To add live-culture yogurt or buttermilk to diet to prevent intestinal superinfection

STORAGE
- Store tablets, granules at room temp

✤ Available in Canada.

• Reconstituted susp stable for 14 days when refrigerated; label date, time of reconstitution

---

cefprozil monohydrate
Brand Name(s): Cefzil
Classification: Antibiotic (cephalosporin)
Pregnancy Category: B

AVAILABLE PREPARATIONS
Oral susp: 125 mg/5 ml, 250 mg/5 ml
Tabs: 250 mg, 500 mg

ROUTES AND DOSAGES
Infants >6 mo and children: PO 15 mg/kg/dose q12h
Adults: PO 250-500 mg q12h

MECHANISM AND INDICATIONS
Antibiotic mechanism: Primarily bactericidal; may be bacteriostatic; inhibits bacterial cell wall synthesis
Indications: Effective against many gram-positive and gram-negative organisms including *Staphylococcus aureus, S. epidermidis, Streptococcus pneumoniae, Str. pyogenes, Str. viridans, Enterococcus, Haemophilus influenzae, E. coli, Klebsiella, Neisseria gonorrhoeae, Proteus mirabilis, Salmonella, Shigella, Bacteroides;* used to treat upper respiratory tract, skin and tissue infections, otitis media, pharyngitis/tonsillitis

PHARMACOKINETICS
Peak: 6-10 hr
Half-life: 25 hr
Metabolism: Liver
Excretion: Urine

CONTRAINDICATIONS AND PRECAUTIONS
• Contraindicated with known hypersensitivity to cefprozil, any cephalosporin, infants <6 mo
• Use cautiously with known allergy to penicillins, impaired renal function, history of colitis or other GI disease, pregnancy, lactation

INTERACTIONS
Drug
• Increased serum concentrations with use of probenecid
• Increased nephrotoxicity possible with use of aminoglycosides, colistin, loop diuretics
• Decreased effectiveness with use of tetracyclines, erythromycins, chloramphenicol
Lab
• False positive Coombs' test

SIDE EFFECTS
CNS: Dizziness, headaches, paresthesias, seizures
DERM: Maculopapular and erythermatous rashes, urticaria
GI: Nausea, vomiting, diarrhea, pseudomembranous colitis, abdominal cramping, glossitis, transient elevations in liver enzymes
GU: Nephrotoxicity, proteinuria, increased BUN, hematuria, renal failure
HEME: Leukopenia, thrombocytopenia, agranulocytosis, anemia, neutropenia, lymphocytosis, eosinophilia, hemolytic anemia
Other: Hypersensitivity (dyspnea; serum sickness: erythema multiforme, rashes, urticaria, polyarthritis, fever), bacterial or fungal superinfection

TOXICITY AND OVERDOSE
Clinical signs: Neuromuscular hypersensitivity; seizures may result from high CNS concentrations
Treatment: Supportive care; hemodialysis, peritoneal dialysis

PATIENT CARE MANAGEMENT
Assessment
• Assess history of hypersensitivity to cefprozil, other cephalosporins, penicillins
• Obtain C&S; may begin therapy before obtaining results
• Assess renal function (BUN, creatinine, I&O), hepatic (ALT, AST, bilirubin), particularly for long-term therapy; bowel pattern
Interventions
• Administer cephalosporins at least 1 hr before bacteriostatic antibiotics (tetracyclines, erythromycins, chloramphenicol)

C

• May administer PO without regard to meals; shake susp well before administering each dose; tabs may crushed, mixed with food or fluid
• Maintain age-appropriate fluid intake
• For group A β-hemolytic streptococcal infection, provide a 10-day course of treatment to prevent risk of acute rheumatic fever, glomerulonephritis

---

NURSING ALERT
Discontinue drug if signs of toxicity, hypersensitivity, pseudomembranous colitis develop

---

Evaluation
• Evaluate therapeutic response (decreased symptoms of infection)
• Monitor signs of superinfection (perineal itching, diaper rash, fever, malaise, redness, pain, swelling, drainage, rash, diarrhea, sore throat, change in cough or sputum)
• Observe for signs of allergic reaction (rash, urticaria, pruritis, chills, fever, joint pain, angioedema)
• Monitor bowel pattern; diarrhea may be symptomatic of pseudomembranous colitis
• Monitor renal function (BUN, creatinine, I&O), hepatic function (ALT, AST, bilirubin), particularly for long-term therapy
• Monitor for signs of bleeding (ecchymosis, bleeding gums, hematuria, daily stool guaiac) because of prolonged bleeding time

PATIENT AND FAMILY EDUCATION
Teach/instruct
• To take as directed at prescribed intervals for prescribed length of time
Warn/advise
• To notify care provider of hypersensitivity, side effects, superinfection
• To avoid use of alcohol, medications containing alcohol

Encourage
• To add live-culture yogurt or buttermilk to diet to prevent intestinal superinfection

STORAGE
• Store tabs, powder at room temp
• Reconstituted susp stable for 14 days when refrigerated; label date, time of reconstitution

---

ceftazidime
Brand Name(s): Ceptaz✤, Fortaz, Tazicef, Tazidime✤
Classification: Antibiotic (third-generation cephalosporin)
Pregnancy Category: B

AVAILABLE PREPARATIONS
Inj: 500 mg, 1 g, 2 g, 6 g
ROUTES AND DOSAGES
Neonates: Wt <1200 g, age 0-4 wk, IM/IV 100 mg/kg/24 hr divided q12h; wt >1200 g, age 0-7 days, IM/IV 100 mg/kg/24 hr divided q12h; wt >1200 g, age >7 days, IM/IV 150 mg/kg/24 hr divided q8h
Infants and children: IM/IV 90-150 mg/kg/24 hr divided q8h
Adults: IM/IV 2-6 g/24 hr divided q8-12h; maximum 6 g/24 hr
IV administration
• Recommended concentration: 100-200 mg/ml in SW for IV push; 1-40 mg/ml in D_5W, D_5NS, $D_5\frac{1}{2}NS$, $D_5\frac{1}{4}NS$, $D_{10}W$, NS, LR, R for infusion
• Maximum concentration: 200 mg/ml for IV push
• IV push rate: Over 3-5 min
• Intermittent infusion rate: Over 10-30 min

MECHANISM AND INDICATIONS
Antibiotic mechanism: Primarily bactericidal; may be bacteriostatic; inhibits bacterial protein synthesis by adhering to penicillin-binding enzymes
Indications: Active against some gram-positive organisms and many enteric gram-negative ba-

---

✤ Available in Canada.

cilli, including *Streptococcus pneumoniae, Str. pyogenes, Staphylococcus aureus, E. coli, Klebsiella, Proteus, Enterobacter, Haemophilus influenzae,* and *Bacteroides;* more effective than any cephalosporin or penicillin derivative against *Pseudomonas;* used to treat septicemia, meningitis; infections of lower respiratory tract, skin, intraabdominal area, GU and gynecologic tracts; bone, joint

PHARMACOKINETICS
Peak: IM 1 hr; IV end of infusion
Distribution: Widely distributed throughout body including bone, bile, skin, CSF (especially with inflamed meninges), heart, pleural and lymphatic fluids
Half-life: Neonates: 2.2-4.7 hr; infants to 12 mo 2.0 hr; children/adults 1.9-2.0 hr
Metabolism: Not metabolized
Excretion: Urine

CONTRAINDICATIONS AND PRECAUTIONS
• Contraindicated with known hypersensitivity to ceftazidime, any cephalosporin
• Use cautiously with known allergy to penicillins, impaired renal function, history of colitis or other GI disease, pregnancy, lactation

INTERACTIONS
Drug
• Synergistic antimicrobial activity against certain organisms with use of aminoglycosides, clavulanic acid
• Increased serum concentrations with use of probenecid
• Increased nephrotoxicity possible with use of aminoglycosides, loop diuretics, other cephalosporins
• Decreased effectiveness with use of tetracyclines, erythromycins, chloramphenicol
Lab
• False elevation of urine creatinine using Jaffe's reaction
• False positive Coombs' test
• Elevations in liver function test results

INCOMPATIBILITIES
• Aminoglycosides

SIDE EFFECTS
CNS: Headache, dizziness, seizures
DERM: Maculopapular and erythematous rashes, urticaria
GI: Nausea, vomiting, diarrhea, pseudomembranous colitis, abdominal cramping, transient elevation in liver enzymes
GU: Hematuria, genital pruritus
HEME: Eosinophilia, thrombocytosis, neutropenia, leukopenia, anemia
Local: Pain, induration, sterile abscesses, tissue sloughing at injection site; phlebitis, thrombophlebitis with IV injection
Other: Hypersensitivity (dyspnea; serum sickness: erythema multiforme, rashes, urticaria, polyarthritis, fever), bacterial or fungal superinfection

TOXICITY AND OVERDOSE
Clinical signs: Neuromuscular hypersensitivity; seizures may result from high CNS concentrations
Treatment: Supportive care; hemodialysis, peritoneal dialysis

PATIENT CARE MANAGEMENT
Assessment
• Assess history of hypersensitivity to ceftazidime, other cephalosporins, penicillins
• Obtain C&S; may begin therapy before obtaining results
• Assess renal function (BUN, creatinine, I&O), bowel pattern
Interventions
• Administer cephalosporins at least 1 hr before bacteriostatic antibiotics (tetracyclines, erythromycins, chloramphenicol)
• CO_2 results from mixing powder with diluent; follow manufacturer's instructions to release pressure build-up; keep needle below fluid levels when withdrawing from inverted vial
• IM injection painful; administer deeply into large muscle mass, rotate injection sites
• Do not premix IV with other

aminoglycosides, bacteriostatic medications
• Use large vein with small-bore needle to reduce local reaction; rotate site q48-72h
• Maintain age-appropriate fluid intake
• For group A β-hemolytic streptococcal infection, provide 10-day course of treatment to prevent risk of acute rheumatic fever, glomerulonephritis

---

NURSING ALERT
Discontinue drug if signs of toxicity, hypersensitivity, serum sickness, pseudomembranous colitis develop

---

Evaluation
• Evaluate therapeutic response (decreased symptoms of infection)
• Monitor for signs of superinfection (perineal itching, diaper rash, fever, malaise, redness, pain, swelling, drainage, rash, diarrhea, sore throat, change in cough or sputum)
• Observe for signs of allergic reaction (rash, urticaria, pruritus, chills, fever, joint pain, angioedema)
• Monitor bowel pattern; diarrhea may be symptomatic of pseudomembranous colitis
• Monitor renal function (BUN, creatinine, I&O)
• Monitor for signs of bleeding (ecchymosis, bleeding gums, hematuria, daily stool guaiac) because of prolonged bleeding time
• Evaluate IM site for tissue damage, IV site for vein irritation

PATIENT AND FAMILY EDUCATION
Teach/instruct
• To take as directed at prescribed intervals for prescribed length of time
Warn/advise
• To notify care provider of hypersensitivity, side effects, superinfection
• To avoid use of alcohol, medications containing alcohol

Encourage
• To add live-culture yogurt or buttermilk to diet to prevent intestinal superinfection

STORAGE
• Store powder at room temp protected from light
• Reconstituted sol stable at room temp for 8 hr; refrigerated for 1 wk; frozen preparations stable below −20° C for 12 wk

---

ceftizoxime
Brand Name(s): Cefizox
Classification: Antibiotic (third-generation cephalosporin)
Pregnancy Category: B

AVAILABLE PREPARATIONS
Inj: 500 mg, 1 g, 2 g, 10 g
ROUTES AND DOSAGES
Infants >6 mo and children: IM/IV 150-200 mg/kg/24 hr divided q6-8h; maximum dose 12 g/24 hr
Adults: IM/IV 1-2 g q8-12h
IV administration
• Recommended concentration: 100 mg/ml in D_5W, NS for IV push; 10-20 mg/ml for intermittent infusion
• Maximum concentration: 100 mg/ml
• IV push rate: Over 3-5 min
• Intermittent infusion rate: Over 30 min

MECHANISM AND INDICATIONS
Antibiotic mechanism: Primarily bactericidal; may be bacteriostatic; inhibits bacterial protein synthesis by adhering to penicillin-binding enzymes
Indications: Active against some gram-positive organisms and many enteric gram-negative bacilli, including *Streptococcus pneumoniae, Str. pyogenes, Staphylococcus aureus, S. epidermidis, E. coli, Klebsiella, Haemophilus influenzae, Enterobacter, Proteus, Peptostreptococcus,* some strains

---

✤ Available in Canada.

of *Pseudomonas* and *Acineto-bacter;* used to treat septicemia, meningitis; infections of the lower respiratory tract, skin, intraabdominal area, GU, gynecologic tracts; bone, joint

PHARMACOKINETICS
Peak: IM 0.5-1.5 hr; IV 10 min after infusion
Half-life: 1.5-2.0 hr
Metabolism: Not metabolized
Excretion: Urine

CONTRAINDICATIONS AND PRECAUTIONS
• Contraindicated with known hypersensitivity to ceftizoxime, any cephalosporin
• Use cautiously with known allergy to penicillins, impaired renal function, history of colitis or other GI disease, pregnancy, lactation

INTERACTIONS
Drug
• Increased serum concentrations with use of probenecid
• Possible increased nephrotoxicity with use of aminoglycosides, loop diuretics, colistin, other cephalosporins
• Decreased effectiveness with use of tetracyclines, erythromycins, chloramphenicol
Lab
• False elevation of urine creatinine using Jaffe's reaction
• False positive Coombs' test
• Elevations in liver function test results.

INCOMPATIBILITIES
• Aminoglycosides

SIDE EFFECTS
CNS: Headache, malaise, paresthesias, dizziness, seizures
DERM: Maculopapular and erythematous rashes, urticaria
GI: Nausea, vomiting, diarrhea, anorexia, pseudomembranous colitis, glossitis, dyspepsia, abdominal cramps, tenesmus, anal pruritus, altered taste
GU: Genital pruritus, nephrotoxicity, vaginitis, hematuria
HEME: Transient neutropenia, eosinophilia, hemolytic anemia

Local: Pain, induration, sterile abscesses, tissue sloughing at injection site; phlebitis, thrombophlebitis with IV injection
Other: Hypersensitivity (dyspnea; serum sickness: erythema multiforme, rashes, urticaria, polyarthritis, fever), bacterial or fungal superinfection

TOXICITY AND OVERDOSE
Clinical signs: Neuromuscular hypersensitivity; seizures may result from high CNS concentrations
Treatment: Supportive care; hemodialysis

PATIENT CARE MANAGEMENT
Assessment
• Assess history of hypersensitivity to ceftizoxime, other cephalosporins, penicillins
• Obtain C&S; may begin therapy before obtaining results
• Assess renal function (BUN, creatinine, I&O), bowel pattern
Interventions
• Administer cephalosporins at least 1 hr before bacteriostatic antibiotics (tetracyclines, erythromycins, chloramphenicol)
• Sol clear to pale yellow when reconstituted; may darken to amber during storage without affecting potency
• IM injection painful; administer deeply into large muscle mass, rotate injection sites
• Do not premix IV with other drugs
• Use large vein with small-bore needle to reduce local reaction; rotate site q48-72h
• Maintain age-appropriate fluid intake
• For group A β-hemolytic streptococcal infection, provide 10-day course of treatment to prevent risk of acute rheumatic fever, glomerulonephritis

> **NURSING ALERT**
> Discontinue drug if signs of toxicity, hypersensitivity, serum sickness, pseudomembranous colitis develop

---

✤ Available in Canada.

Evaluation
- Evaluate therapeutic response (decreased symptoms of infection)
- Monitor signs of superinfection (perineal itching, diaper rash, fever, malaise, redness, pain, swelling, drainage, rash, diarrhea, sore throat, change in cough or sputum)
- Observe for signs of allergic reaction (rash, urticaria, pruritus, chills, fever, joint pain, angioedema)
- Monitor bowel pattern; diarrhea may be symptomatic of pseudomembranous colitis
- Monitor renal function (BUN, creatinine, I&O)
- Monitor for signs of bleeding (ecchymosis, bleeding gums, hematuria, daily stool guaiac) because of prolonged bleeding time
- Evaluate IM site for tissue damage, IV site for vein irritation

PATIENT AND FAMILY EDUCATION
Teach/instruct
- To take as directed at prescribed intervals for prescribed length of time
Warn/advise
- To notify care provider of hypersensitivity, side effects, superinfection
- To avoid use of alcohol, medication containing alcohol
Encourage
- To add live-culture yogurt or buttermilk to diet to prevent intestinal superinfection

STORAGE
- Store powder at room temp
- Protect from light
- Reconstituted sol stable at room temp for 8 hr; refrigerated for 48 days; frozen preparations stable below –20° C for 18 mo

---

ceftriaxone sodium
Brand Name(s): Rocephin✤
Classification: Antibiotic (third-generation cephalosporin)
Pregnancy Category: B

AVAILABLE PREPARATIONS
Inj: 250 mg, 500 mg, 1 g, 2 g, 10 g
ROUTES AND DOSAGES
Neonates: IM/IV 50 mg/kg/24 hr in single dose
Infants and children <12 yr: IM/IV 50-100 mg/kg/24 hr divided q12-24h; maximum dose 4 g/24 hr
Children >12 yr: IM/IV 1-2 g/24 hr divided q12-24h; maximum dose 4 g/24 hr
Meningitis
Neonates to children <12 yr: IM/IV loading dose, 75-100 mg/kg once, then 100 mg/kg/24 hr divided q12h
Children ≥12 yr: IM/IV 100 mg/kg/24 hr divided q12h; maximum dose 4 g/24 hr
Prophylaxis for Infants of Mothers with Peripartum Gonococcal Infections
50 mg/kg IM or IV as single dose at birth; maximum dose 125 mg/dose
IV administration
- Recommended concentration: 10-40 mg/ml in D_5W, D_5NS, D_5 ½NS, $D_{10}W$, NS, SW
- Maximum concentration: 40 mg/ml
- Intermittent infusion rate: Over 10-30 min

MECHANISMS AND INDICATIONS
Antibiotic mechanism: Primarily bactericidal; may be bacteriostatic; inhibits bacterial protein synthesis by adhering to penicillin-binding enzymes
Indications: Active against many gram-negative bacteria, including *Citrobacter, Neisseria meningitidis, N. gonorrhoeae, Haemophilus influenzae, Shigella, Enterobacter aerogenes, E. coli, Proteus mirabilis, Klebsiella,* and *Pseudomonas aeruginosa;* also effective against some gram-positive bacteria, in-

---

✤ Available in Canada.

cluding *Staphylococcus aureus, Streptococcus pneumoniae, Str. pygones;* used to treat infections of skin; lower respiratory tract, intra-abdominal area, bone, joint, uncomplicated gonorrhea, pelvic inflammatory disease, septicemia, meningitis

PHARMACOKINETICS
Peak: IM 2.0 hr; IV, infants: 30-60 min, children 30 min
Distribution: Widely distributed throughout body including gall bladder, lungs, bone, bile, CSF (especially with inflamed meninges)
Half-life: Neonates 16.2 hr; infants <1 mo 9.2 hr; children 6.0-9.0 hr
Metabolism: Not metabolized
Excretion: Urine, feces

CONTRAINDICATIONS AND PRECAUTIONS
• Contraindicated with known sensitivity to ceftriaxone, any cephalosporin
• Use cautiously with known allergy to penicillin, impaired renal function, history of colitis or other GI disease, history of bleeding, neonates with hyperbilirubinemia (especially prematures), pregnancy, lactation

INTERACTIONS
Drug
• Synergistic antimicrobial activity against *P. aeruginosa,* some strains of Enterobacteriaceae with use of aminoglycosides
• Increased serum concentrations with use of probenecid
• Increased nephrotoxicity possible with use of aminoglycosides, K+-depleting diuretics, other cephalosporins
• Decreased effectiveness with use of tetracyclines, erythromycins, chloramphenicol
Lab
• False elevation of urine creatinine using Jaffe's reaction
• False positive Coombs' test
• Elevations in liver functions test results

INCOMPATIBILITIES
• Erythromycin, aminoglycosides

SIDE EFFECTS
CNS: Headache, dizziness, seizures
DERM: Maculopapular and erythematous rashes, urticaria
GI: Nausea, vomiting, diarrhea, pseudomembranous colitis, abdominal cramps
GU: Genital pruritus, hematuria, cysts
HEME: Eosinophilia, neutropenia, thrombocytosis, leukopenia, anemia, thrombocytopenia
Local: Pain, induration, sterile abscesses, tissue sloughing at injection site; phlebitis, thrombophlebitis with IV injection
Other: Hypersensitivity (dyspnea; serum sickness: erythema multiforme, rashes, polyarthritis, fever), bacterial or fungal superinfection

TOXICITY AND OVERDOSE
Clinical signs: Neuromuscular hypersensitivity; seizures, may result from high CNS concentrations
Treatment: Supportive care

PATIENT CARE MANAGEMENT
Assessment
• Assess history of hypersensitivity to ceftriaxone, penicillins, other cephalosporins
• Obtain C&S; may begin therapy before obtaining results
• Assess renal function (BUN, creatinine, I&O), bowel pattern
Interventions
• Administer cephalosporins at least 1 hr before bacteriostatic antibiotics (tetracyclines, erythromycins, chloramphenicol)
• Do not reconstitute IM with bacteriostatic water with benzyl alcohol for neonates
• Injection painful; administer deeply into large muscle mass, rotate injection site
• Do not premix IV with other aminoglycosides, other bacteriostatic agents
• Use large vein with small-bore needle to reduce local reaction; rotate site q48-72h

• Maintain age-appropriate fluid intake
• For group A β-hemolytic streptococcal infection, provide 10-day course of treatment to prevent risk of acute rheumatic fever, glomerulonephritis

Evaluation
• Evaluate therapeutic response (decreased symptoms of infection)
• Monitor for signs of superinfection (perineal itching, diaper rash, fever, malaise, redness, pain, swelling, drainage, rash, diarrhea, sore throat, change in cough or sputum)
• Observe for signs of allergic reaction (rash, urticaria, pruritus, chills, fever)
• Monitor bowel pattern; diarrhea may be symptomatic of pseudomembranous colitis
• Monitor for signs of bleeding (ecchymosis, bleeding gums, hematuria, daily stool guaiac) because of prolonged bleeding time
• Monitor renal function (BUN, creatinine, I&O)
• Evaluate IM site for tissue damage, IV site for vein irritation

PATIENT AND FAMILY EDUCATION
Teach/instruct
• To take as directed at prescribed intervals for prescribed length of time
Warn/advise
• To notify care provider of hypersensitivity, side effects, superinfection
• To avoid use of alcohol, medications containing alcohol
Encourage
• To add live-culture yogurt or buttermilk to diet to prevent intestinal superinfection

STORAGE
• Store powder at room temp protected from light
• Stability of reconstituted sol depends on diluent used; check package insert

---

cefuroxime axetil
Brand Name(s): Ceftin❧
Classification: Antibiotic (second-generation cephalosporin)
Pregnancy Category: B

AVAILABLE PREPARATIONS
Tabs: 125 mg, 250 mg, 500 mg

ROUTES AND DOSAGES
Infants and children: PO 30 mg/kg/24 hr divided bid
Adults: PO 250 mg q12h; for severe infections 500 mg q12h
Otitis Media
Infants and children: PO 40 mg/kg/24 hr divided bid

MECHANISM AND INDICATIONS
Antibiotic mechanism: Primarily bactericidal, may be bacteriostatic; inhibits bacterial protein synthesis by adhering to penicillin-binding enzymes
Indications: Active against gram-negative bacilli, including *Haemophilus influenzae, E. coli, Neisseria, Proteus mirabilis, Klebsiella,* and some gram-positive organisms including *Streptococcus pneumoniae, Str. pyogenes,* and *Staphylococcus aureus;* used to treat otitis media; lower respiratory tract, GU, skin infections

PHARMACOKINETICS
Peak: 2 hr
Distribution: Widely distributed throughout body tissues or fluids; penetrates inflamed meninges
Half-life: 1-2 hr
Metabolism: Not metabolized
Excretion: Urine

CONTRAINDICATIONS AND PRECAUTIONS
• Contraindicated with known hypersensitivity to cefuroxime axetil, any cephalosporin, in infants <1 mo
• Use cautiously with known allergy to penicillins, impaired renal function, history of colitis or other GI disease, pregnancy, lactation

---

INTERACTIONS
Drugs
• Increased serum concentrations with use of probenecid
• Increased nephrotoxicity possible with use of vancomycin, aminoglycosides, colistin, loop diuretics
• Decreased effectiveness with use of tetracyclines, erythromycins, chloramphenicol
Lab
• False elevation of urine creatinine using Jaffe's reaction
• False positive Coombs' test

SIDE EFFECTS
CNS: Dizziness, headache, paresthesias, seizures
DERM: Maculopapular and erythematous rashes, urticaria
GI: Nausea, vomiting, diarrhea, pseudomembranous colitis, abdominal cramping, glossitis, transient elevations in liver enzymes
HEME: Leukopenia, lymphocytosis, neutropenia, hemolytic anemia
Other: Hypersensitivity (dyspnea; serum sickness: erythema multiforme, rashes, urticaria, polyarthritis, fever), bacterial or fungal superinfection

TOXICITY AND OVERDOSE
Clinical signs: Neuromuscular hypersensitivity; seizures may result from high CNS concentrations
Treatment: Supportive care; hemodialysis, peritoneal dialysis

PATIENT CARE MANAGEMENT
Assessment
• Assess history of hypersensitivity to cefuroxime axetil, other cephalosporins, penicillins
• Obtain C&S; may begin therapy before obtaining results
• Assess renal function (BUN, creatinine, I&O), bowel pattern
Interventions
• Administer cephalosporins at least 1 hr before bacteriostatic antibiotics (tetracyclines, erythromycins, chloramphenicol)
• Increased PO absorption when administered with meals; tab may be crushed, mixed with food or fluid, but drug has a very bitter taste
• If child cannot swallow tab whole, provide flavored ice or fluids before/after administration
• Maintain age-appropriate fluid intake
• For group A β-hemolytic streptococcal infection, provide 10-day course of treatment to prevent risk of acute rheumatic fever, glomerulonephritis

> **NURSING ALERT**
> Discontinue drug if signs of hypersensitivity, pseudomembranous colitis develop

Evaluation
• Evaluate therapeutic response (decreased symptoms of infection)
• Monitor for signs of superinfection (perineal itching, diaper rash, fever, malaise, redness, pain, swelling, drainage, rash, diarrhea, sore throat, change in cough or sputum)
• Observe for signs of allergic reaction (rash, urticaria, pruritus, chills, fever, joint pain, angioedema)
• Monitor bowel pattern; diarrhea may be symptomatic of pseudomembranous colitis
• Monitor for signs of bleeding (ecchymosis, bleeding gums, hematuria, daily stool guaiac) because of prolonged bleeding time

PATIENT AND FAMILY EDUCATION
Teach/instruct
• To take as directed at prescribed intervals for prescribed length of time
Warn/advise
• To notify care provider of hypersensitivity, side effects, superinfection
• To avoid use of alcohol, medications containing alcohol
Encourage
• To add live-culture yogurt or buttermilk to diet to prevent intestinal superinfection

---

✤ Available in Canada.

STORAGE

• Store tabs at room temp protected from moisture

---

cefuroxime sodium

Brand Name(s): Kefurox✤, Zinacef✤

Classification: Antibiotic (second-generation cephalosporin)

Pregnancy Category: B

AVAILABLE PREPARATION

Inj: 750 mg, 1.5 g, 7.5 g

ROUTES AND DOSAGES

Neonates: IM/IV 20-50 mg/kg/24 hr divided q12h (Safety and effectiveness not established. Dosage represents accepted standard practice recommendations.)

Infants >3 mo and children: IM/IV 100-150 mg/kg/24 hr divided q8h; maximum dose 6 g/24 hr

Adults: IM/IV 750 mg-1.5 g q8h; maximum dose 9 g/24 hr

Meningitis

Infants >3 mo and children: IM/IV 200-240 mg/kg/24 hr divided q6-8h; maximum dose 3 g/8 hr

IV administration

• Recommended concentration: 50-100 mg/ml in SW for IV push; 1-30 mg/ml in D_5W, D_5NS, D_5 ½NS, D_5 ¼NS, $D_{10}W$, NS, LR, R for IV infusion

• Maximum concentration: 100 mg/ml for IV push

• IV push rate: Over 3-5 min

• Intermittent infusion rate: Over 15-60 min

MECHANISM AND INDICATIONS

Antibiotic mechanism: Primarily bactericidal; may be bacteriostatic; inhibits bacterial protein synthesis by adhering to penicillin-binding enzymes

Indications: Active against many gram-positive organisms and enteric gram-negative bacilli, including *Streptococcus pneumoniae, Str. pyogenes, Haemophilus influenzae, Klebsiella, Staphylococcus au-*

reus, E. coli, Enterobacter, and *Neisseria gonorrhoeae;* used to treat septicemias, meningitis; lower respiratory, skin, GU tract, bone, joint infections

PHARMACOKINETICS

Peak: IM 15-60 min; IV 15 min after end of infusion

Distribution: Widely distributed throughout body tissues and fluids including CSF (especially with inflamed meninges)

Half-life: 1-2 hr

Metabolism: Not metabolized

Excretion: Urine

CONTRAINDICATIONS AND PRECAUTIONS

• Contraindicated with known hypersensitivity to cefuroxime, any cephalosporins

• Use cautiously with known allergy to penicillins, impaired renal function, history of colitis or other GI disease, pregnancy, lactation

INTERACTIONS

Drug

• Synergistic antimicrobial activity against certain organisms with use of aminoglycosides, chloramphenicol, penicillins

• Increased serum concentrations with use of probenecid

• Increased nephrotoxicity possible with use of vancomycin, aminoglycosides, colistin, loop diuretics

• Decreased effectiveness with use of tetracyclines, erythromycins, chloramphenicol

Lab

• False elevations of urine creatinine using Jaffe's reaction

• False positive Coombs' test

• Elevations in liver function test results

INCOMPATIBILITIES

• Aminoglycosides, calcium chloride, Mg salts

SIDE EFFECTS

CNS: Headache, malaise, paresthesias, dizziness, seizures

DERM: Maculopapular and erythematous rashes, urticaria

GI: Nausea, vomiting, diarrhea, anorexia, pseudomembranous co-

---

✤ Available in Canada.

litis, glossitis, dyspepsia, abdominal cramps, tenesmus, anal pruritus
GU: Genital pruritus, hematuria, nephrotoxicity
HEME: Transient neutropenia, eosinophilia, hemolytic anemia, decrease in Hct, Hgb
Local: Pain, induration, sterile abscesses, tissue sloughing at injection site; phlebitis, thrombophlebitis with IV injection
Other: Hypersensitivity (dyspnea; serum sickness: erythema multiforme, rashes, polyarthritis, fever), bacterial or fungal superinfection

TOXICITY AND OVERDOSE
Clinical signs: Neuromuscular hypersensitivity; seizures may result from high CNS concentrations
Treatments: Supportive care; hemodialysis, peritoneal dialysis

PATIENT CARE MANAGEMENT
Assessment
• Assess history of hypersensitivity to cefuroxime, other cephalosporins, penicillins
• Obtain C&S; may begin therapy before obtaining results
• Assess renal function (BUN, creatinine, I&O), bowel pattern
Interventions
• Administer cephalosporins at least 1 hr before bacteriostatic antibiotics (tetracyclines, erythromycins, chloramphenicol)
• Reconstituted sol light yellow to amber; powder and sol may darken with storage without affecting potency
• IM injection is painful; administer deeply into large muscle mass, rotate injection sites
• Do not premix IV with other medications; infuse separately
• Use large vein with small-bore needle to reduce local irritation; rotate site q48-72h
• Maintain age-appropriate fluid intake
• For group A β-hemolytic streptococcal infection, provide 10-day course of treatment to prevent risk

of acute rheumatic fever, glomerulonephritis

> **NURSING ALERT**
> Discontinue drug if signs of hypersensitivity, serum sickness, pseudomembranous colitis develop

Evaluation
• Evaluate therapeutic response (decreased symptoms of infection)
• Monitor for signs of superinfection (perineal itching, diaper rash, fever, malaise, redness, pain, swelling, drainage, rash, diarrhea, sore throat, change in cough or sputum)
• Observe for signs of allergic reaction (rash, urticaria, pruritus, chills, fever, joint pain, angioedema)
• Monitor bowel pattern; diarrhea may be symptomatic of pseudomembranous colitis
• Monitor renal function (BUN, creatinine, I&O)
• Monitor for signs of bleeding (ecchymosis, bleeding gums, hematuria, daily stool guaiac) because of prolonged bleeding time
• Evaluate IM site for tissue damage, IV site for vein irritation

PATIENT AND FAMILY EDUCATION
Teach/instruct
• To take as directed at prescribed intervals for prescribed length of time
Warn/advise
• To notify care provider of hypersensitivity, side effects, superinfection
• To avoid use of alcohol, medications containing alcohol
Encourage
• To add live-culture yogurt or buttermilk to diet to prevent intestinal superinfection

STORAGE
• Store powder at room temp protected from light
• Reconstituted sol stable at room temp for 24 hr; refrigerated for 48 hr

cephalexin monohydrate/cephalexin hydrochloride

Brand Name(s): Cefanex, Keflex, Cephalexin, Keftab

Classification: antibiotic (first-generation cephalosporin)

Pregnancy Category: B

AVAILABLE PREPARATIONS
Drops: 100 mg/ml
Oral susp: 125 mg/5 ml, 250 mg/5 ml
Tabs: 250 mg, 500 mg, 1 g
Caps: 250 mg, 500 mg

ROUTES AND DOSAGES
Children: PO 25-50 mg/kg/24 hr divided q6-12h; maximum dose 4 g/24 hr
Adults: PO 250 mg-1 g q6h; maximum dose 4 g/24 hr

MECHANISM AND INDICATIONS
Antibiotic mechanism: Primarily bactericidal; may be bacteriostatic; inhibits bacterial protein synthesis by adhering to penicillin-binding enzymes
Indications: Effective against many gram-positive organisms including *Staphylococcus aureus, S. epidermis, Streptococcus pneumoniae,* group B streptococci, group A β-hemolytic streptococci, and gram-negative organisms including *Klebsiella pneumoniae, E. coli, Proteus mirabilis, Shigella;* used to treat middle ear, respiratory and GU tract, skin and bone infections

PHARMACOKINETICS
Peak: Infants <6 mo 3 hr; infants 9-12 mo 2 hr; infants >1 yr 1 hr
Distribution: Widely distributed in body fluids
Half-life: Infants <3 mo 5 hr; infants 3-12 mo 2.5 hr; children >1 yr 0.5-1.5 hr
Metabolism: Not metabolized
Excretion: Urine
Therapeutic level: 2-9 mcg/ml

CONTRAINDICATIONS AND PRECAUTIONS
• Contraindicated with known hypersensitivity to cephalexin, any cephalosporin
• Use cautiously with known allergy to penicillins, impaired renal function, or history of colitis or other GI disease, pregnancy, lactation

INTERACTIONS
Drug
• Increased serum concentrations with use of probenecid
• Possible increased nephrotoxicity with use of vancomycin, aminoglycosides, colistin, loop diuretics
• Decreased effectiveness with use of tetracyclines, erythromycins, chloramphenicol
Lab
• False elevation of urine creatinine using Jaffe's reaction
• False positive Coombs' test

SIDE EFFECTS
CNS: Dizziness, headache, malaise, paresthesias, seizures
DERM: Maculopapular and erythematous rashes, urticaria
GI: Nausea, vomiting, diarrhea, anorexia, pseudomembranous colitis, glossitis, dyspepsia, abdominal cramps, anal pruritus, tenesmus
GU: Genital pruritus, vaginitis, hematuria, nephrotoxicity
HEME: Transient neutropenia, eosinophilia, anemia
Other: Hypersensitivity (dyspnea; serum sickness: erythema multiforme, rashes, polyarthritis, fever) bacterial or fungal superinfection

TOXICITY AND OVERDOSE
Clinical signs: Neuromuscular hypersensitivity; seizures may result from high CNS concentrations
Treatment: Supportive care; peritoneal dialysis, hemodialysis

PATIENT CARE MANAGEMENT
Assessment
• Assess history of hypersensitivity to cephalexin, other cephalosporins, penicillins

---

✤ Available in Canada.

- Obtain C&S; may begin therapy before obtaining results
- Assess renal function (BUN, creatinine, I&O), bowel pattern; liver function (ALT, AST, bilirubin) for long-term therapy

Interventions
- Administer cephalosporins at least 1 hr before bacteriostatic antibiotics (tetracyclines, erythromycins, chloramphenicol)
- May be administered PO with food to minimize GI distress; shake susp well before administering; tabs may be crushed, caps taken apart and mixed with food or fluid
- Maintain age-appropriate fluid intake
- For group A β-hemolytic streptococcal infection, provide 10-day course of treatment to prevent risk of acute rheumatic fever, glomerulonephritis

---

NURSING ALERT
Discontinue drug if signs of toxicity, hypersensitivity, pseudomembranous colitis develop

---

Evaluation
- Evaluate therapeutic response (decreased symptoms of infection)
- Monitor signs of superinfection (perineal itching, diaper rash, fever, malaise, redness, pain, swelling, drainage, rash, diarrhea, sore throat, change in cough or sputum)
- Observe for signs of allergic reaction (rash, urticaria, pruritus, chills, fever, joint pain, angioedema)
- Monitor bowel pattern; diarrhea may be symptomatic of pseudomembranous colitis
- Monitor renal function (BUN, creatinine, I&O)
- Monitor for signs of bleeding (ecchymosis, bleeding gums, hematuria, daily stool guaiac) because of prolonged bleeding time

PATIENT AND FAMILY EDUCATION
Teach/instruct
- To take as directed at prescribed

intervals for prescribed length of time

Warn/advise
- To notify care provider of hypersensitivity, side effects, superinfection
- To avoid use of alcohol, medications containing alcohol

Encourage
- To add live-culture yogurt or buttermilk to diet to prevent intestinal superinfection

STORAGE
- Store caps, tabs, powder at room temp
- Reconstituted susp stable when refrigerated for 14 days or when kept at room temp for 7 days; label date, time of reconstitution

---

cephalothin sodium
Brand Name(s): Ceporacin✤, Keflin✤, Seffin
Classification: Antibiotic (first-generation cephalosporin)
Pregnancy Category: B

AVAILABLE PREPARATIONS
Inj: 1 g, 2 g, 4 g
ROUTES AND DOSAGES
Infants and children: IM/IV 75-125 mg/kg/24 hr divided q4-6h
Adults: IM/IV 500 mg-2 g q4-6h; maximum dose 12 g/24 hr
IV administration
- Recommended concentration: ≤100 mg/ml in D_5W, NS, SW
- Maximum concentration: 100 mg/ml
- IV push rate: Over 3-5 min
- Intermittent infusion rate: Over 30-60 min

MECHANISM AND INDICATIONS
Antibiotic mechanism: Primarily bactericidal; may be bacteriostatic; inhibits bacterial protein synthesis by adhering to penicillin-binding enzymes
Indications: Effective against many gram-positive and some

✤ Available in Canada.

gram-negative organisms including *E. coli* and other coliform bacteria, Enterobacteriaceae, enterococci, gonococci, group A β-hemolytic streptococci, *Klebsiella, Proteus mirabilis, Salmonella, Staphylococcus aureus, Shigella, Streptococcus pneumoniae, Str. veridans;* used to treat septicemia, endocarditis, meningitis, and respiratory, GU, GI, skin, soft tissue, bone, joint infections

PHARMACOKINETICS
Peak: IM 30 min; IV end of infusion
Distribution: Poor CNS penetration
Half-life: 0.5-1.0 hr
Metabolism: Liver, kidneys
Excretion: Urine

CONTRAINDICATIONS AND PRECAUTIONS
• Contraindicated with known hypersensitivity to cephalothin, any cephalosporin
• Use cautiously with known allergy to penicillins, impaired renal failure, history of colitis or other GI disease, pregnancy, lactation

INTERACTIONS
Drug
• Increased serum concentrations with use of probenecid
• Increased nephrotoxicity possible with use of vancomycin, aminoglycosides, colistin, loop diuretics
• Decreased effectiveness with use of tetracyclines, erythromycins, chloramphenicol
Lab
• False elevation of urine creatinine using Jaffe's reaction
• False positive Coombs' test

INCOMPATIBILITIES
• Tetracyclines, erythromycins, CaCl, Mg salts, aminoglycosides, barbiturates, aminophylline, heparin, levarterenol, metaraminol, methylprednisolone, metoclopramide, penicillin G, phenytoin, phytonadione, polymyxin B, prochlorperazine, succinylcholine, thiopental, warfarin.

SIDE EFFECTS
CNS: Headache, malaise, paresthesias, dizziness, seizures
DERM: Maculopapular and erythematous rashes, urticaria
GI: Nausea, vomiting, diarrhea, anorexia, pseudomembranous colitis, glossitis, dyspepsia, abdominal cramps, tenesmus, anal pruritus
GU: Nephrotoxicity, genital pruritus, hematuria
HEME: Transient neutropenia, eosinophilia, hemolytic anemia
Local: Pain, induration, sterile abscesses, tissue sloughing at injection site; phlebitis, thrombophlebitis with IV injection
Other: Hypersensitivity, dyspnea, fever, bacterial or fungal superinfection

TOXICITY AND OVERDOSE
Clinical signs: Neuromuscular hypersensitivity; seizures may result from high CNS concentrations
Treatment: Supportive care; hemodialysis, peritoneal dialysis

PATIENT CARE MANAGEMENT
Assessment
• Assess history of hypersensitivity to cephalothin, other cephalosporins, penicillins
• Obtain C&S; may begin therapy before obtaining results
• Assess renal function (BUN, creatinine, I&O), bowel patterns
Interventions
• Administer cephalosporins at least 1 hr before bacteriostatic antibiotics (tetracyclines, erythromycins, chloramphenicol)
• Discoloration in sol stored at room temperature does not indicate loss of potency
• IM injection painful; administer deeply into large muscle mass, rotate injection sites
• Do not premix IV with other medications; infuse separately
• Use large vein with small-bore needle to reduce local reaction; rotate site q48-72h
• Maintain age-appropriate fluid intake

- For group A β-hemolytic streptococcal infection, provide 10-day course of treatment to prevent risk of acute rheumatic fever, glomerulonephritis

> **NURSING ALERT**
> Discontinue drug if signs of toxicity, hypersensitivity, pseudomembranous colitis develop

Evaluation
- Evaluate therapeutic response (decreased symptoms of infection)
- Monitor for signs of superinfection (perineal itching, diaper rash, fever, malaise, redness, pain, swelling, drainage, rash, diarrhea, sore throat, change in cough or sputum)
- Observe for signs of allergic reaction (rash, urticaria, pruritus, chills, fever, joint pain, angioedema)
- Monitor bowel pattern; diarrhea may be symptomatic of pseudomembranous colitis
- Monitor renal function (BUN, creatinine, I&O)
- Monitor for signs of bleeding (ecchymosis, bleeding gums, hematuria, daily stool guaiac) because of prolonged bleeding time
- Evaluate IM site for tissue damage, IV site for vein irritation

PATIENT AND FAMILY EDUCATION
Teach/instruct
- To take as directed at prescribed intervals for prescribed length of time
Warn/advise
- To notify care provider of hypersensitivity, side effects, superinfection
- To avoid use of alcohol, medications containing alcohol
Encourage
- To add live-culture yogurt or buttermilk to diet to prevent intestinal superinfection

STORAGE
- Store powder at room temp
- Protect from light

- Reconstituted sol stable at room temp 24 hr; refrigerated 96 hr
- Warm to body temp if precipitate forms on refrigeration; gently agitate to dissolve

> **cephapirin sodium**
> **Brand Name(s):** Cefadyl
> **Classification:** Antibiotic (first-generation cephalosporin)
> **Pregnancy Category:** B

AVAILABLE PREPARATIONS
Inj: 500 mg, 1 g, 2 g, 4 g

ROUTES AND DOSAGES
Infants >3 mo and children: IM/IV 40-80 mg/kg/24 hr divided q6h
Adults: IM/IV 500 mg-1 g q6h; maximum dose 12 g/24 hr
IV administration
- Recommended concentration: 100 mg/ml in D₅W, NS for IV push; 10-20 mg/ml for intermittent infusion
- Maximum concentration: 100 mg/ml
- IV push rate: Over 5 min
- Intermittent infusion rate: Over 30-60 min

MECHANISM AND INDICATIONS
Antibiotic mechanism: Primarily bactericidal; may be bacteriostatic; inhibits bacterial protein synthesis adhering to penicillin-binding enzyme
Indications: Effective against many gram-positive and some gram-negative organisms including *Streptococcus pneumoniae, Str. viridans; E. coli,* group A β-hemolytic streptococci, *Haemophilus influenzae, Klebsiella, Proteus mirabilis* and *Staphylococcus aureus;* used to treat serious infections of the respiratory, GI, GU tracts; skin, bone, joint infections; septicemia, endocarditis

PHARMACOKINETICS
Peak: IM 30 min; IV at end of infusion

Distribution: Widely distributed in body fluids
Half-life: 30-60 min
Metabolism: Liver
Excretion: Urine

CONTRAINDICATIONS AND PRECAUTIONS

• Contraindicated with known hypersensitivity to cephapirin, any cephalosporin, in infants <3 mo
• Use cautiously with known allergy to penicillins, impaired renal function, history of colitis or other GI distress, pregnancy, lactation

INTERACTIONS
Drug
• Increased serum concentrations with use of probenecid
• Increased nephrotoxicity possible with use of vancomycin, aminoglycosides, colistin, loop diuretics
• Decreased effectiveness with use of tetracyclines, erythromycins, chloramphenicol
Lab
• False elevation of urine creatinine using Jaffe's reaction
• False positive Coombs' test
• Elevation in liver function test results

INCOMPATIBILITIES
• Tetracyclines, aminoglycosides, aminophylline, epinephrine, levarterenol, mannitol, phenytoin, thiopental

SIDE EFFECTS
CNS: Dizziness, headache, malaise, paresthesias, seizures
DERM: Maculopapular and erythematous rashes, urticaria
GI: Nausea, vomiting, diarrhea, anorexia, pseudomembranous colitis, glossitis, dyspepsia, abdominal cramps, tenesmus, anal pruritus
GU: Genital pruritus, vaginitis, nephrotoxicity, hematuria
HEME: Transient neutropenia, eosinophilia, anemia
Local: Pain, induration, sterile abscesses, tissue sloughing at injection site; phlebitis, thrombophlebitis with IV injection
Other: Hypersensitivity, dyspnea, bacterial or fungal superinfections

TOXICITY AND OVERDOSE
Clinical signs: Neuromuscular hypersensitivity; seizures may result from high CNS concentrations
Treatment: Supportive care; hemodialysis

PATIENT CARE MANAGEMENT
Assessment
• Assess history of hypersensitivity to cephapirin, other cephalosporins, penicillins
• Obtain C&S; may begin therapy before obtaining results
• Assess renal function (BUN, creatinine, I&O), bowel pattern
Interventions
• Administer cephalosporins at least 1 hr before bacteriostatic antibiotics (tetracyclines, erythromycins, chloramphenicol)
• Discoloration of sol to slightly yellow does not indicate loss of potency
• IM injection painful; administer deeply into large muscle mass, rotate injection sites.
• Do not premix IV with other medications; infuse separately
• Use large vein with small-bore needle to reduce local reaction; rotate site q48-72h
• Maintain age-appropriate fluid intake
• For group A β-hemolytic streptococcal infection, provide 10-day course of treatment to prevent risk of acute rheumatic fever, glomerulonephritis

---

NURSING ALERT
Discontinue drug if signs of toxicity, hypersensitivity, pseudomembranous colitis develop

---

Evaluation
• Evaluate therapeutic response (decreased symptoms of infection)
• Monitor signs of superinfection (perineal itching, diaper rash, fever, malaise, redness, pain, swelling, drainage, rash, diarrhea, sore throat, change in cough or sputum)

✤ Available in Canada.

• Observe for signs of allergic reaction (rash, urticaria, pruritus, chills, fever, joint pain, angioedema)
• Monitor bowel pattern; diarrhea may be symptomatic of pseudomembranous colitis
• Monitor renal function (BUN, creatinine, I&O)
• Monitor for signs of bleeding (ecchymosis, bleeding gums, hematuria, daily stool guaiac) because of prolonged bleeding time
• Evaluate IM site for tissue damage, IV site for vein irritation

PATIENT AND FAMILY EDUCATION
Teach/instruct
• To take as directed at prescribed intervals for prescribed length of time
Warn/advise
• To notify care provider of hypersensitivity, side effects, superinfection
• To avoid use of alcohol, medications containing alcohol
Encourage
• To add live-culture yogurt or buttermilk to diet to prevent intestinal superinfection

STORAGE
• Store powder at room temp
• Protect from light
• Reconstituted sol stable at room temp for 24 hr; refrigerated for 10 days

cephradine
Brand Name(s): Anspor, Velosef

Classification: Antibiotic (first-generation cephalosporin)

Pregnancy Category: B

AVAILABLE PREPARATIONS
Oral susp: 125 mg/5 ml, 250 mg/5 ml
Caps: 250 mg, 500 mg
Inj: 250 mg, 500 mg, 1 g, 2 g, 4 g

ROUTES AND DOSAGES
Children >9 mo: PO 25-50 mg/kg/24 hr divided q6h; maximum dose 4 g/24 hr; IM/IV 50-100 mg/kg/24 hr divided q6h; maximum dose 4 g/24hr
Adults: PO 1-4 g/24hr divided q6h; maximum dose 4 g/24hr; IM/IV 2-8 g/24 hr divided q6h; maximum dose 8 g/24 hr

IV administration
• Recommended concentration: 50-100 mg/ml in D_5W, D_5NS, D_5 ½NS, $D_{10}W$, NS for IV push; 30-50 mg/ml in D_5W, D_5NS, D_5 ½NS, $D_{10}W$, NS for IV infusion
• Maximum concentration: 100 mg/ml for IV push
• IV push rate: Over 3-5 min
• Intermittent infusion rate: Over 30-60 min

MECHANISM AND INDICATIONS
Antibiotic mechanism: Primarily bactericidal; may be bacteriostatic; inhibits bacterial protein synthesis by adhering to penicillin-binding enzymes
Indications: Effective against many gram-positive and some gram-negative organisms including *E. coli* and other coliform bacteria, group A β-hemolytic streptococci, *Haemophilus influenzae*, *Klebsiella, Proteus mirabilis, Staphylococcus aureus, Streptococcus pneumoniae, Str. viridans;* used to treat septicemias, endocarditis, respiratory, ear, GU, GI, skin, soft tissue, bone, joint infections

PHARMACOKINETICS
Peak: PO 1 hr; IM 1-2 hr; IV 5 min
Distribution: Widely distributed in body fluids
Half-life: 0.5-2.0 hr
Metabolism: Not metabolized
Excretion: Urine

CONTRAINDICATIONS AND PRECAUTIONS
• Contraindicated with known hypersensitivity to cephradine, any other cephalosporins
• Use cautiously with known allergy to penicillins, impaired renal

function, history of colitis or other GI disease, pregnancy, lactation

INTERACTIONS
Drug
• Increased serum concentrations with use of probenecid
• Possible increased nephrotoxicity with use of vancomycin, aminoglycosides, colistin, loop diuretics
• Decreased effectiveness with use of tetracyclines, erythromycins, chloramphenicol
Lab
• False elevations of urine creatinine using Jaffe's reaction
• False positive Coombs' test
• Elevations in liver function test results

INCOMPATIBILITIES
• Tetracyclines, erythromycins, Ca salts, Mg salts, aminoglycosides, epinephrine, lidocaine, Ringer's solution, all antibiotics

SIDE EFFECTS
CNS: Dizziness, headache, malaise, paresthesias, seizures
DERM: Maculopapular and erythematous rashes, urticaria
GI: Nausea, vomiting, diarrhea, anorexia, pseudomembranous colitis, tenesmus, anal pruritus
GU: Genital pruritus, vaginitis, nephrotoxicity, hematuria
HEME: Transient neutropenia, eosinophilia
Local: Pain, induration, sterile abscesses, tissue sloughing at injection site; phlebitis, thrombophlebitis with IV injection
Other: Hypersensitivity, dyspnea, fever, bacterial or fungal superinfection

TOXICITY AND OVERDOSE
Clinical signs: Neuromuscular hypersensitivity; seizures may result from high CNS concentrations
Treatment: Supportive care; hemodialysis

PATIENT CARE MANAGEMENT
Assessment
• Assess history of hypersensitivity to cephradine, other cephalosporins, penicillins
• Obtain C&S; may begin therapy before obtaining results
• Assess renal function (BUN, creatinine, I&O), bowel pattern
Interventions
• Administer cephalosporins at least 1 hr before bacteriostatic antibiotics (tetracyclines, erythromycins, chloramphenicol)
• May be administered PO with food to minimize GI distress; shake susp well before each dose; cap may be taken apart, mixed with food or fluid
• IM injection painful; administer deeply into large muscle mass, rotate injection sites
• Do not premix IV with other medications; infuse separately
• Use large vein with small-bore needle to reduce local reaction; rotate site q48-72h
• Maintain age-appropriate fluid intake
• For group A β-hemolytic streptococcal infection, provide 10-day course of treatment to prevent risk of acute rheumatic fever, glomerulonephritis

---
NURSING ALERT
Discontinue drug is signs of toxicity, hypersensitivity, pseudomembranous colitis develop

---

Evaluation
• Evaluate therapeutic response (decreased symptoms of infections)
• Monitor for signs of superinfection (perineal itching, diaper rash, fever, malaise, redness, pain, swelling, drainage, rash, diarrhea, sore throat, change in cough or sputum)
• Observe for signs of allergic reactions (rash, urticaria, pruritus, chills, fever, joint pain, angioedema)
• Monitor bowel pattern; diarrhea may be symptomatic of pseudomembranous colitis
• Monitor renal function (BUN, creatinine, I&O)
• Monitor for signs of bleeding

✤ Available in Canada.

(ecchymosis, bleeding gums, hematuria, daily stool guaiac) because of prolonged bleeding time
• Evaluate IM site for tissue damage, IV site for vein irritation

PATIENT AND FAMILY EDUCATION
Teach/instruct
• To take as directed at prescribed intervals for prescribed length of time
Warn/advise
• To notify care provider of hypersensitivity, side effects, superinfection
• To avoid use of alcohol, medications containing alcohol
Encourage
• To add live-culture yogurt or buttermilk to diet to prevent intestinal superinfection

STORAGE
• Store cap, powder at room temp
• Reconstituted susp stable when refrigerated for 14 days or at room temp for 7 days; label date, time of reconstitution
• Reconstituted IM and direct IV sol stable at room temp for 2 hr; refrigerated 24 hr
• Reconstituted sol for IV infusion stable at room temp 10 hr, refrigerated 48 hr

---

charcoal (activated)
Brand Name(s): Arm-a-char, Liqui-Char, SuperChar, Charcoaide, Charcocaps

Classification: Antidote (adsorbent)

Pregnancy Category: C

AVAILABLE PREPARATIONS
Liq: 12.5 g, 15 g, 25 g, 30 g, 50 g
Powder for oral susp: 30 g, 50 g
Tabs: 325 mg
Caps: 250 mg

ROUTES AND DOSAGES
Acute Poisoning
Single dose, charcoal with sorbitol
• The use of repeated oral doses of charcoal with sorbitol is not recommended
Children 1-12 yr: PO 1-2 g/kg or 15-30 g, or approximately 10× the weight of ingested poison
Adults: 30-100 g
Single dose, charcoal in water
Infants <1 yr: 1 g/kg
Children 1-12 yr: 1-2 g/kg or 15-30 g
Adults: 30-100 g or 1-2 g/kg
Multiple dose, charcoal in water
• Doses are repeated until clinical status and serum drug concentrations are in subtherapeutic range
Infants <1 yr: 1 g/kg q4-6h
Children 1-12 yr: 1-2 g/kg or 15-30 g q2-6h
Adults: 25-50 g or 1-2 g/kg q2-6h

MECHANISM AND INDICATIONS
Antidote mechanism: Adsorbs toxic substances or irritants, resulting in inhibited GI absorption
Indications: Used to treat drug overdoses, poisonings

PHARMACOKINETICS
Metabolism: Not metabolized
Excretion: Feces

CONTRAINDICATIONS AND PRECAUTIONS
• Contraindicated in poisonings involving cyanide, mineral acids, caustic alkalis, organic solvents, iron, ethanol, methanol, or lithium, with hypersensitivity to charcoal or any component, or with unconscious or semiconscious patients; charcoal with sorbitol contraindicated with fructose intolerance, in children <1 yr

INTERACTIONS
Drug
• Decreased effectiveness of both drugs with use of ipecac syr, laxatives; administer charcoal after induced emesis from ipecac syr has occurred
Nutrition
• Decreased effectiveness with milk, dairy products, sherbet

SIDE EFFECTS
GI: Emesis, nausea, constipation, diarrhea with sorbitol, black stools

---

PATIENT CARE MANAGEMENT
Assessment
• Obtain complete history of ingestion, treatment initiated
• Assess LOC, contraindications for use of activated charcoal
• Assess VS
Interventions
• Administer PO after induced vomiting unless contraindicated; activated charcoal negates effect of ipecac syr; if possible, administer within 30 min of poison ingestion for binding of poison to occur
• Powder most absorbent form; mix with water (20-30 g/240 ml water); add fruit juice, corn syrup, powdered chocolate flavoring to aid palatability
• To make more appealing to children, administer sol in opaque covered container with straw, provide sips of juice or flavored ices between swallows
• Do not administer with milk, dairy products, sherbet
• Repeat dose if vomiting occurs soon after dose
• Provide laxative to promote elimination as ordered
• Provide gastric lavage, emergency equipment if poisoning is not reversed
• Maintain age-appropriate fluid intake
Evaluation
• Evaluate therapeutic response (LOC, no side effects of poison)
• Monitor VS
• Do not use for more than 72 hr to prevent interference with nutrient absorption

PATIENT AND FAMILY EDUCATION
Teach/instruct
• About how to prevent poisonings, what to do in the event of ingestion
• Provide ipecac syr for home, telephone number for poison control center
Warn/advise
• That stools will be black, constipation may develop

STORAGE
• Store at room temp in tightly closed glass or metal container to prevent absorption of gases

chloral hydrate
Brand Name(s): Aquachoral Supprettes, Chloral Hydrate, Noctec, PMS-Chloral Hydrate✤

Classification: Premedication for procedures; sedative; hypnotic

Controlled Substance Schedule IV

Pregnancy Category: C

AVAILABLE PREPARATIONS
Syrup: 250 mg/5 ml, 500 mg/5 ml
Caps: 250 mg, 500 mg
PR: 324 mg, 500 mg, 648 mg suppositories

ROUTES AND DOSAGES
Premedication
Children: PO/PR 50-100 mg/kg 30 min before procedure
Sedative
Neonates: PO/PR 25 mg/kg/dose
Children: PO/PR 25-50 mg/kg q6-8h; maximum dose 500 mg
Adults: PO/PR 250 mg tid
Hypnotic
Children: PO/PR 50 mg/kg; maximum dose 1 g
Adults: PO/PR 500 mg-1 g hs; maximum dose 2 g/24 hr

MECHANISM AND INDICATIONS
Mechanism: Trichloroethanol, the active metabolite of chloral hydrate, produces CNS depression
Indications: For use in short-term relief of symptoms of mild-to-moderate anxiety and insomnia; also used as a premedication for procedures

PHARMACOKINETICS
Onset of action: PO 15 min
Peak: PO 30-60 min
Half-life: Neonates 8.5-66 hr; children and adults: 8-11 hr

✤ Available in Canada.

Metabolism: Liver
Elimination: Urine

CONTRAINDICATIONS AND PRECAUTIONS

• Contraindicated with hypersensitivity to chloral derivatives, severe heart disease, liver or renal disease; do not use with esophagitis, gastritis, colitis
• Use cautiously with depression, suicidal ideation; in pts performing hazardous activities; with lactation

INTERACTIONS
Drug

• Increased sedative effects with alcohol, tricyclic antidepressants, antihistamines, barbiturates, CNS depressants
• Use of chloral hydrate with warfarin may increase the tendency for bleeding
• Use of chloral hydrate with IV furosemide may result in flushing, tachycardia, diaphoresis, B/P changes

Nutrition
• Do not drink alcohol

Lab
• False positive urine glucose test when using Clinitest tabs
• Interferes with fluorometric urine catecholamine and 17-OHCS
• Urine screening tests for drug abuse may be positive (depending on amount of drug taken, testing method used)

INCOMPATIBILITIES
• No information available

SIDE EFFECTS
CNS: Dizziness, drowsiness, anxiety, ataxia, confusion, headache, paradoxical excitement, psychological and physical dependence with long term use
CVS: Hypotension
DERM: Rash, urticaria
GI: Gastric irritation, nausea, vomiting, diarrhea
HEME: Leukopenia, eosinophilia

TOXICITY AND OVERDOSE
Clinical signs: Respiratory depression, stupor, pinpoint pupils, hypotension, hypothermia; esophageal stricture, gastric necrosis with perforation and GI hemorrhage, and hepatic damage have been reported
Treatment: Support B/P and respiration, treat hypotension with norepinephrine, phenylephrine, or dopamine; induce vomiting if is conscious; use gastric lavage with ET tube in place to prevent aspiration if pt is comatose; support respiration with mechanical ventilation if necessary; support body temp with blankets, warming bed, or hyperthermia unit; hemodialysis will remove chloral hydrate and its metabolite, trichloroethanol

PATIENT CARE MANAGEMENT
Assessment

• Assess history of hypersensitivity to drug
• Assess ability to function in daily activities
• Assess ability to sleep throughout night
• Assess mental status (mood, sensorium, affect, impulsiveness, suicidal ideation)
• Assess baseline physical assessment (including orthostatic blood pressure)
• Assess for previous history of gastritis
• Assess for previous history of drug abuse

Interventions
• Limit continual use to 1-3 wks with PO administration
• Provide small amount of water or juice with PO administration to reduce GI distress
• Notify provider if gastrointestinal symptoms occur with PO administration
• Maintain safe environment with side or crib rails up; provide assistance with ambulation
• Do not allow pt to drink alcohol

NURSING ALERT
Monitor patient for respiratory depression

Evaluation
• Evaluate therapeutic response (sedation, ability to sleep throughout night)
• Evaluate mental status (sensorium, suicidal ideation, thoughts)
• For long-term therapy, monitor alk phos, AST, ALT, bilirubin, CBC, creatinine, BUN
• Monitor for physical dependency and withdrawal symptoms with long-term use (headache, nausea, vomiting, muscle pain, weakness)
• Evaluate respiratory status
• Evaluate INR if pt is taking warfarin
• Evaluate pt for signs or symptoms of esophagitis or gastritis

PATIENT AND FAMILY EDUCATION
Teach/instruct
• To take as directed at prescribed intervals for prescribed length of time
• To make sure medication is swallowed
• That chloral hydrate may be habit forming
• Not to discontinue this drug abruptly if taken for >4 wks; withdrawal symptoms include confusion, depression, hallucinations, muscle cramping, seizures, sweating, tremor, vomiting
• To take with water or juice
Warn/advise
• That chloral hydrate can produce psychologic or physical dependence if used in large doses for an extended period of time
• To avoid ingesting alcohol, other CNS depressants
• To avoid OTC preparations unless approved by prescriber
• That this medication may cause drowsiness; to be careful on bicycles, skates, skateboards, while driving, or with other activities requiring alertness
• That impairment of intellectual and physical skills may persist the following day if chloral hydrate is taken at bedtime
• That marijuana smoking may increase sedation and significant impairment of intellectual and physical performance

STORAGE
• Store at room temp in tightly sealed containers

---

chloramphenicol, chloramphenicol palitate, chloramphenicol sodium succinate
Brand Name(s): AK-Chlor, Chloromycetin, Chloromycetin Injection✤, Chloromycetin Ophthalmic Preparation✤, Chloroptic✤, Chloroptic SOP✤, Ophthochlor, Ophthochloram✤, Pentamycetin✤, Sopamycetin✤
Classification: Antibiotic (dichloroacetic acid derivative)
Pregnancy Category: C

AVAILABLE PREPARATIONS
Oral susp: 150 mg/5 ml
Caps: 250 mg, 500 mg
Inj: 1 g
Ophthal: 0.5% sol; 1% oint
Top Cream: 1%
Otic sol: 0.5%

ROUTES AND DOSAGES
• For all pts, PO, IV loading dose 20 mg/kg; first maintenance dose given 12 hr after loading dose
Neonates ≤7 days: 25 mg/kg/24 hr qd
Neonates >7 days, ≤2000 g: 25 mg/kg/24 hr qd
Neonates >7 days, >2000 g: PO, IV maintenance 50 mg/kg/24 hr divided q12h
Infants, children, and adults: PO, IV maintenance dose 50-100 mg/kg/24 hr divided q6h, maximum dose 4 g/24 hr; ophthal sol, instill 1-2 gtt into conjunctival sac q3-6h; oint, instill 1 cm strip into conjunctival sac q3-6h; top, apply sparingly to affected are tid-qid; otic, instill 2-3 gtt into ear canal tid-qid

---

IV administration
- Recommended concentration: 20 mg/ml in D-LR, D-R, D-S, D_5LR, D_5NS, D_5W, D_{10}W, LR, NS, ½NS, or R for intermittent infusion; 100 mg/ml in D_5W or SW for IV push
- Maximum concentration: 100 mg/ml for IV push
- IV push rate: Over ≥1 min
- Intermittent infusion rate: Over 30-60 min

MECHANISM AND INDICATIONS

Antibiotic mechanism: Bacteriostatic; inhibits bacterial protein synthesis by binding to ribosome's 50S subunit; chloramphenicol palmitate, chloramphenicol sodium succinate must be hydrolyzed to chloramphenicol before becoming effective

Indications: Effective against most gram-positive and gram-negative organisms, *Rickettsia, Chlamydia, Mycoplasma, Salmonella typhi;* used to treat *Haemophilus influenzae, Neisseria,* Rocky Mountain spotted fever, lymphogranuloma, psittacosis, severe meningitis, bacteremia when less-toxic drugs are ineffective

PHARMACOKINETICS

Peak: PO 1-3 hr; IV variable
Distribution: Widely distributed into most body tissues including ascitic, pleural, synovial fluids; penetrates CNS; concentrates in liver, kidneys
Half-life: Neonates 1-2 days, 24 hr; neonates 10-16 days, 10 hr; adults, 1.6-3.3 hr
Metabolism: Liver
Excretion: Urine, feces
Therapeutic levels: Meningitis peak 5-25 mcg/ml, trough 5-15 mcg/ml, other infections peak 10-20 mcg/ml, trough 5-10 mcg/ml

CONTRAINDICATIONS AND PRECAUTIONS

- Contraindicated with known hypersensitivity to chloramphenicol, with minor infections, for prophylaxis against infections
- Use cautiously with neonates, impaired renal or hepatic function, acute intermittent porphyria, G-6-PD deficiency; pregnancy, lactation; with drugs that cause bone marrow suppression

INTERACTIONS

Drug
- Increased risk of toxicity from phenytoin, dicumarol, tolbutamide, chlorpropamide, phenobarbital, cyclophosphamide
- Decreased effectiveness of iron salts, vitamin B_{12}, folic acid, penicillins
- Increased serum chloramphenicol level with use of acetaminophen

Lab
- Decreased erythrocyte, platelet, leukocyte counts in blood (and possibly bone marrow)

Nutrition
- Reduced absorption when given with food

INCOMPATIBILITIES
- Ampicillin, amobarbital, carbenicillin, chlorpromazine, digitoxin, erythromycins, glycopyrrolate, hydrocortisone, hydroxyzine, metoclopramide, oxacillin, pentobarbital, phenytoin, polymyxin B, procaine, prochlorperazine, promazine, promethazine, thiopental, tripelennamine, vancomycin, warfarin

SIDE EFFECTS

CNS: Headache, mild depression, confusion, delirium, peripheral neuropathy with prolonged use
CV: Gray syndrome in newborns (failure to feed, pallor, cyanosis, abdominal distention, irregular respiration, vasomotor collapse, death within a few hours of symptom onset)
DERM: Possible contact sensitivity, itching, burning, urticaria, angioneurotic edema with hypersensitivity to topical application
EENT: Itching or burning ears, vesicular or maculopapular dermatitis with otic application; optic neuritis with cystic fibrosis; decreased visual acuity; optic atrophy in children; stinging, burning, or itching eyes with ophthal application
GI: Nausea, vomiting, glossitis,

stomatitis, diarrhea, enterocolitis, jaundice

HEME: Granulocytopenia, aplastic anemia, hypoplastic anemia, thrombocytopenia

Other: Infection by nonsusceptible organisms; hypersensitivity reaction (fever, rash, urticaria, anaphylaxis), angioedema

TOXICITY AND OVERDOSE

Clinical signs: Parenteral overdose (anemia, metabolic acidosis followed by hypotension, hypothermia, abdominal distention, possible death); oral overdose: nausea, vomiting, diarrhea

Treatment: Supportive care; charcoal hemoperfusion

PATIENT CARE MANAGEMENT

Assessment

• Assess history of hypersensitivity to chloramphenicol

• Obtain C&S; may begin therapy before obtaining results

• Assess renal function (BUN, creatinine, I&O), hepatic function (ALT, AST, bilirubin), hematologic function (CBC, differential, platelet count)

• Assess wound or eye if using top or ophthal forms

Interventions

• Administer penicillin 1 hr or more before chloramphenicol if administering drug concomitantly with penicillins

• Administer PO 1 hr ac or 2 hr after meals

• Shake susp well before administering; cap may be taken apart, mixed with food or fluid

• Do not premix IV with other medications; infuse separately

• Use large vein with small-bore needle to reduce local reaction; rotate site q48-72h

• Wash hands before, after ophthal instillation; cleanse crusts or discharge from eye before instillation; apply gentle pressure to lacrimal sac for 1 min after instillation to minimize systemic absorption; wipe excess medication from eye; do not flush medication from eye

• Wash hands before, after top application; cleanse wound; apply sparingly

• See Chapter 2 regarding otic instillation

• Maintain age-appropriate fluid intake

NURSING ALERT

Discontinue if signs of hypersensitivity, Gray syndrome, optic or peripheral neuritis, blood dyscrasias develop

Potential exists for severe toxicity

Evaluation

• Evaluate therapeutic response (decreased symptoms of infection)

• Evaluate renal function (BUN, creatinine, I&O), hepatic function (ALT, AST, bilirubin), hematologic function (CBC, differential, platelet count); monitor for bone marrow depression

• Monitor children <2 yr for Gray syndrome; if neonate's mother received chloramphenicol during labor or delivery, monitor infant for side effects

• Observe for signs of superinfection (perineal itching, diaper rash, fever, malaise, redness, pain, swelling, drainage, rash, diarrhea, sore throat, change in cough or sputum).

• Evaluate IV site for vein irritation; evaluate eye, ear canal, skin for rash, itching, swelling

PATIENT AND FAMILY EDUCATION

Teach/instruct

• To take as directed at prescribed intervals for prescribed length of time

Warn/advise

• To notify care provider of hypersensitivity, side effects, superinfection

STORAGE

• Store powder, cap, susp, top, and otic forms at room temp in airtight container

• Protect from heat

✤ Available in Canada.

• Reconstituted sol of 100 mg/ml stable at room temp for 30 days
• Store ophthal forms per package insert

chlordiazepoxide

Brand Name(s): Librium♣, Mitran, Reposans, Libritabs

Classification: mild tranquilizer, benzodiazepine

Controlled Substance Schedule IV

Pregnancy Category: D

AVAILABLE PREPARATIONS
Tabs: 5 mg, 10 mg, 25 mg
Caps: 5 mg, 10 mg, 25 mg
Inj: 100 mg/ampule

ROUTES AND DOSAGES
Mild Anxiety
Child >6 yr: PO 5 mg bid-qid, maximum dose 10 mg bid-tid
Adult: PO 5-10 mg tid-qid
Severe Anxiety
Adult: PO 20-25 mg tid-qid, maximum dose 150 mg/24 hr
Adolescent and adult: IM/IV 50-100 mg, then 25-50 mg tid-qid prn
Alcohol Withdrawal
Adult: PO 50-100 mg, maximum dose 300 mg/24 hr
Preoperative
Adult: PO 5-10 mg tid-qid on day before surgery
• Should not be used in hyperactive or psychotic child of any age
• Children may be more sensitive to benzodiazepine; use smallest dose possible
• Oral not recommended in children <6 yr
• Inj not recommended in children <12 yr
IV administration
• Recommended concentration: Dilute 100 mg powder in 5 ml NS
• IV push rate: 100 mg or less over 1 min

MECHANISM AND INDICATIONS
Mechanism: Produces calming effect by enhancing action of nerve transmitter γ-aminobutyric acid (GABA); blocks arousal of limbic system and reticular formation
Indications: Used in short-term relief of anxiety disorders, for treating acute alcohol withdrawal, and preoperatively for relaxation; unlabeled use for irritable bowel syndrome

PHARMACOKINETICS
Onset of action: PO 30 min; continual use on a regular schedule for 3 to 5 days usually necessary to determine effectiveness in relieving anxiety
Peak: PO ½ hr
Duration: 4-6 hr
Half-life: 5-30 hr
Metabolism: Liver
Excretion: Urine

CONTRAINDICATIONS AND PRECAUTIONS
• Contraindicated with hypersensitivity to this or any component of this medication or hypersensitivity to benzodiazepines, tartrazine (FD&C Yellow No. 5, in some preparations of chlordiazepoxide); with history of alcoholism or drug addiction, hyperactivity, narrow-angle glaucoma, psychosis
• Use cautiously with asthma, depression, emphysema, kidney disease, liver disease, myasthenia gravis, porphyria, seizures, elderly, or very ill pts, pregnancy, lactation

INTERACTIONS
Drug
• Increased effects of chlordiazepoxide with alcohol, cimetidine, CNS depressants, disulfiram, isoniazid
• Decreased effects of chlordiazepoxide with rifampin, scopolamine
• Increased risk of digoxin toxicity with digoxin
• Decreased effects of levodopa
• Increased sedation with antihistamines
Lab
• Increased ALT, AST, alk phos, serum bilirubin
• Decreased RAIU, RBCs, Hgb, WBCs, platelets
• Falsely elevated 17-OHCS

♣ Available in Canada.

- False positive for urine pregnancy test with Gravindex
- Urine screening tests for drug abuse may be positive
- Liver reaction with jaundice may be mistaken for viral hepatitis

Nutrition
- Avoid excessive intake of caffeine-containing beverages (coffee, tea, cola)
- Ingestion of antacids with chlordiazepoxide may impair absorption of chlordiazepoxide
- Do not drink alcohol
- Some forms of chlordiazepoxide contain the dye tartrazine (FD&C Yellow No. 5), which can cause allergic reactions in certain individuals

INCOMPATIBILITIES
- Vitamin C, benzquinamide, heparin, pentobarbital, phenytoin, promethazine, R, NS

SIDE EFFECTS
CNS: Dizziness, drowsiness, decreased activity, anxiety, apathy, behavior changes, confusion, crying, delirium, depression, disorientation, vivid dreams, euphoria, fatigue, hallucinations, hangover, headache, acute hyperexcited state, uncoordination, insomnia, lethargy, memory loss, muscle spasms, nervousness, restlessness, seizures, sleep disturbances, stimulation, tremors, vertigo, weakness, unsteadiness
CV: Orthostatic hypotension, ECG changes, hypotension, palpitations, tachycardia
DERM: Bruising, dermatitis, fixed skin eruptions, excessive hair growth, hair loss, hives, itching, rash, yellowing of skin or eyes
EENT: Blurred vision, decreased hearing, nasal congestion, sore gums, dry mouth, mydriasis, increased salivation, difficulty swallowing, coated tongue, slurred speech, tinnitus, visual disturbances, double vision, loss of voice
GI: Anorexia, constipation, diarrhea, dry mouth, liver damage, nausea, stomach upset, vomiting, abnormal liver function

GU: Incontinence, changes in sex drive, menstrual problems, urine retention
HEME: Blood dyscrasias
Other: Balance problems, breathing problems, edema, excitement, galactorrhea, gynecomastia, hiccups, joint pain, swollen lymph nodes, uncontrollable muscle movement, acute rage, stimulation, sweating, ankle and facial swelling, wt gain or loss

TOXICITY AND OVERDOSE
Clinical signs: Marked drowsiness, feeling of drunkenness, staggering gait, tremor, weakness, stupor progressing to deep sleep or coma
Treatment: Lavage, vital signs, supportive care

PATIENT CARE MANAGEMENT
Assessment
- Assess history of hypersensitivity to drug
- Assess ability to function in daily activities, ability to sleep throughout the night, anxiety
- Assess mental status (mood, sensorium, affect, impulsiveness, suicidal ideation, thoughts)
- Obtain baseline B/P, AST, ALT, bilirubin, creatinine, LDH, alk phos
- If use is long-term, obtain CBC counts

Interventions
- Caps may be opened, tab may be crushed for PO administration
- Limit continual use to 1 to 3 wk; avoid prolonged, uninterrupted use
- Administer with food, milk if GI symptoms occur
- Rinse with water, take sips of fluid, sugarless gum, or hard candy for dry mouth
- Increase fluids, fiber in diet if constipation occurs
- Do not drink alcohol
- Avoid heavy smoking; may reduce calming action of drug
- Avoid marijuana smoking; leads to increased sedation, significant impairment of intellectual and

physical performance with chlordiazepoxide

NURSING ALERT
Drug can produce psychologic or physical dependence if used in large doses for an extended period of time

---

Evaluation
• Evaluate therapeutic response (decreased anxiety, ability to function in daily activities, ability to sleep throughout night)
• Evaluate mental status (mood, sensorium, affect, impulsiveness, suicidal ideation, thoughts)
• Monitor for ataxia, oversedation, excitement, stimulation, acute rage
• Monitor CBC, AST, ALT, bilirubin, creatinine, LDH, alk phos regularly during long-term therapy
• Monitor for physical dependency, withdrawal symptoms (headache, nausea, vomiting, muscle pain, weakness)
• Monitor orthostatic B/P; If systolic B/P drops 20 mm Hg, hold drug, notify prescriber

PATIENT AND FAMILY EDUCATION
Teach/instruct
• To take as directed at prescribed intervals for prescribed length of time
• To ensure that PO medication is swallowed
• Not to discontinue medication without approval of care provider
• Not to stop drug abruptly if taken for more than 4 wk; withdrawal symptoms could include depression, confusion, hallucinations, tremor, seizures, muscle cramping, sweating, vomiting
Warn/advise
• That chlordiazepoxide can be addictive if used in large doses or for a long time
• To avoid ingesting alcohol, other CNS depressants, other psychotropic medications

• That medication may cause drowsiness
• To be careful on bicycles, skates, skateboards, while driving, with other activities requiring alertness

STORAGE
• Store at room temp

---

chlorothiazide
Brand Name(s): Diachlor, Diuril, Diurigen
Classification: Diuretic, antihypertensive
Pregnancy Category: D

AVAILABLE PREPARATIONS
Tabs: 250 mg, 500 mg
Oral susp: 250 mg/5 ml
Inj: 500 mg vial

ROUTES AND DOSAGES
Infants <6 mo: PO 20-40 mg/kg/24 hr divided bid
Infants >6 mo and children: PO 20 mg/kg/24 hr divided bid
Adults: PO 0.5-2 g qd or divided bid; IV 500 mg-1 g/24 hr
IV administration
• Recommended concentration: 28 mg/ml
• Maximum concentration: 28 mg/ml
• IV push rate: Over 5 min

MECHANISM AND INDICATIONS
Diuretic mechanism: Inhibits Na reabsorption in distal tubules, promoting more excretion of water, Na^+, K^+, Cl^-, Mg
Antihypertensive mechanism: Exact mechanism unclear; may decrease total peripheral resistance by vasodilating arterioles
Indications: Edema, hypertension, CHF

PHARMACOKINETICS
Onset of action: 1.5 to 2 hr
Peak: 4 hr
Half-life: 13 hr
Metabolism: None, remains unchanged

Excretion: Urine

CONTRAINDICATIONS AND PRECAUTIONS
- Contraindicated with hypersensitivity to thiazides or sulfonamides, anuria, neonatal jaundice
- Use cautiously with severe renal disease, hypokalemia, hepatic disease, gout, COPD, lupus, diabetes, pts taking digoxin, pregnancy, lactation

INTERACTIONS
Drug
- Increased toxicity of lithium, digoxin, non-depolarizing skeletal muscle relaxants
- Potentiated hyperglycemia, hypotension, hyperuricemic effects of diazoxide possible
- Increased insulin requirements in diabetic pts possible
- Increased antihypertensive effect when used in conjunction with other antihypertensives
- Decreased urinary excretion of amphetamines, quinidine possible
- Decreased therapeutic effects of methenamine compounds, antidiabetics, sulfonylureas possible
- Decreased absorption of chlorothiazide when administered in conjunction with cholestyramine, colestipol

Lab
- Altered serum electrolyte levels, urine steroid tests possible
- Increased serum urate, BG, cholesterol, triglycerides, BSP retention, Ca, amylase, parathyroid tests
- False negative phentolamine, tyramine tests
- Decreased PBI, PSP

INCOMPATIBILITIES
- Amikacin, chlorpromazine, codeine, hydralazine, insulin, ionosol sol, levarterenol, levorphanol, methadone, morphine, polymyxin B, procaine, prochlorperazine, promazine, promethazine, streptomycin, tetracycline, triflupromazine, vancomycin, vitamin C, vitamin B with C, warfarin

SIDE EFFECTS
CNS: Fatigue, headache, drowsiness, weakness, mood change, paresthesia, anxiety, depression
CV: Orthostatic hypotension, irregular pulse, dehydration, hypercholesterolemia, hypertriglyceridemia
DERM: Dermatitis, rash, photosensitivity, purpura
EENT: Blurred vision
GI: Anorexia, nausea, pancreatitis, vomiting, constipation, diarrhea, cramps, hepatitis, heartburn
GU: Polyuria, frequency, glucosuria, uremia
Other: Fever, aplastic anemia, hemolytic anemia, leukopenia, agranulocytosis, thrombocytopenia, neutropenia, hyperglycemia, hyperuricemia, hypomagnesemia, hypokalemia, hypercalcemia, hyponatremia, hypochloremia, hypophosphatemia

TOXICITY AND OVERDOSE
Clinical signs: GI irritation, hypermotility, diuresis, lethargy, progression to coma
Treatment: Induce vomiting with ipecac in conscious pt, gastric lavage if pt is unconscious; supportive therapy include monitoring CV and renal status, electrolytes

PATIENT CARE MANAGEMENT
Assessment
- Assess hypersensitivity to drug, sulfonamides
- Assess baseline wt, respiratory and hydration status
- Assess B/P in standing, lying position
- Obtain baseline labs (electrolytes, BUN, glucose, CBC, creatinine pH, ABG, uric acid, Ca, Mg)

Interventions
- Administer PO medication in AM to avoid interference with sleep
- Administer with food if nausea occurs
- Do not administer IV with blood products

> **NURSING ALERT**
> Chlorothiazide should not be administered IV to pediatric pts

Evaluation
• Evaluate therapeutic response (decreased dependent edema, improvement in CVP)
• Evaluate for hypersensitivity, side effects
• Monitor for signs of metabolic alkalosis (drowsiness, restlessness)
• Evaluate for signs of hypokalemia (postural hypotension, malaise, fatigue, tachycardia, leg cramps, weakness)
• Monitor daily temp
• Evaluate signs of confusion, especially in the elderly
• Evaluate wt, B/P daily
• Evaluate labs regularly (electrolytes, creatinine, BUN, uric acid levels)

PATIENT AND FAMILY EDUCATION
Teach/instruct
• To take as directed at prescribed intervals for prescribed length of time
• To monitor daily wt
Warn/advise
• To notify care provider of hypersensitivity, side effects
• To identify and report signs of electrolyte imbalance (weakness, fatigue, muscle cramps, paresthesias, confusion, nausea, vomiting, diarrhea, headache, dizziness, palpitations)
• To avoid hazardous activities until treatment is well established
• To wear protective clothing in sunlight, avoid sunscreens (especially those containing PABA)
Encourage
• To increase intake of K⁺-rich foods such as bananas, citrus fruits, potatoes, dates, raisins
• To avoid high Na foods
Provide
• Emotional support as indicated

STORAGE
• Store at room temp in a tightly closed container

---

chlortetracycline hydrochloride
Brand Name(s): Aureomycin✤
Classification: Antibiotic, anti-infective (tetracycline)
Pregnancy Category: D

AVAILABLE PREPARATIONS
Ophthal oint: 10 mg/g in 3.75 g tube
Ophthal susp: 1%

ROUTES AND DOSAGES
Ophthalmic Neonatorum Prophylaxis
1-2 cm ribbon of ophthal oint or 1-2 gtt of ophthal susp to conjunctival sac within 1 hr of delivery
Superficial Ophthalmic Bacterial Infection
Children and adults: Small amount of ophthal oint to conjunctival sac every 2-12 hr or 1-2 gtt ophthal susp bid-qid
Ophthalmic Chlamydia Infections
Children and adults: Small amount of ophthal oint to conjunctival sac or 2 gtt of ophthal susp OU bid-qid

MECHANISM AND INDICATIONS
Antibiotic and antiinfective mechanism: Bacteriostatic; inhibits bacterial protein synthesis by inhibiting binding of transfer RNA to messenger RNA complex at the 30S subunit
Indications: Broad antimicrobial spectrum; used to treat ophthal bacterial infections, ophthal chlamydia infections, prophylaxis of gonorrheal ophthalmia neonatorum

CONTRAINDICATIONS AND PRECAUTIONS
• Contraindicated with known hypersensitivity to any tetracyclines, pregnancy (second and third trimester), lactation.
• Use cautiously to avoid overgrowth of nonsusceptible organ-

---

isms during long-term therapy and in early pregnancy

SIDE EFFECTS
EENT: Foreign body sensation, transient stinging or burning sensation, increased tearing

TOXICITY AND OVERDOSE
Clinical signs: Nausea, vomiting, abdominal discomfort, headache may occur if entire tube of ophthal oint is accidentally ingested; severe toxicity unlikely
Treatment: Supportive care; antacids to reduce gastric irritation; induced emesis for substantial ingestion

PATIENT CARE MANAGEMENT
Assessment
• Assess history of hypersensitivity to tetracyclines
• Obtain C&S; may begin therapy before obtaining results
• Assess eye for redness, discharge, swelling
Interventions
• Wash hands before, after application; cleanse crusts or discharge from eye before application; wipe excess medication from eye; do not flush medication from eye
• For prophylaxis of ophthalmia neonatorum, use new or single unit tube for each neonate; gently massage eyelids to distribute medication
• Administer an oral antibiotic to patients with chlamydial ophthalmic infections
Evaluation
• Evaluate therapeutic response (decreased symptoms of infection)
• Monitor for signs of overgrowth of nonsusceptible organisms with prolonged use
• Monitor for signs of eye sensitivity (constant burning, itching eyelids)

PATIENT AND FAMILY EDUCATION
Teach/instruct
• To take as directed at prescribed intervals for prescribed length of time

Warn/advise
• To notify care provider of hypersensitivity, side effects, superinfection
• Not to share towels, wash cloths, linens, eye make-up with family member being treated

STORAGE
• Store at room temp

---

cholestyramine
Brand Name(s): Cholybar, Questran, Questran Light

Classification: Antilipemic agent, antipruritic, antidiarrheal

Pregnancy Category: C

AVAILABLE PREPARATIONS
Powder: 4 g cholestyramine resin/9 g packet of powder

ROUTES AND DOSAGES
Children 6-12 yr: PO 240 mg/kg/24 hr divided tid
Adults: PO 3-4 g tid; maximum 32 g/24 hr

MECHANISM AND INDICATIONS
Mechanism: In intestine, cholestryramine forms insoluble complex with bile acids; complex is excreted in feces, thereby making bile acids less available to support absorption of lipids and cholesterol; may decrease pruritus as it decreases bile acids available for deposit in skin
Indications: Used as adjunct therapy in management of primary hypercholesterolemia, diarrhea, pruritis

PHARMACOKINETICS
Peak: 21 days
Metabolism: Not absorbed
Excretion: Feces

CONTRAINDICATIONS AND PRECAUTIONS
• Contraindicated in pts with complete biliary obstruction, with drug hypersensitivity; Questran contains tartrazine (yellow dye

---

✤ Available in Canada.

#5), should not be used in allergic persons
• Use cautiously with constipation, malabsorption, renal dysfunction, CAD, gallstones, pregnancy, lactation

INTERACTIONS
Drug
• Delayed or reduced absorption of warfarin possible
• Binds to digoxin, thus decreases absorption
• Decreased absorption of thiazide diuretics, penicillin G, tetracycline, vancomycin possible
• Decreased plasma levels of acetaminophen
• Interferes with absorption of oral phosphate supplement
• Interferes with absorption of fat-soluble medications
Lab
• Increased alk phos, AST, Cl, PO_4
• Decreased Ca, K, Na, serum cholesterol, triglycerides

NUTRITION
• Interferes with absorption of fat-soluble vitamins, folic acid; vitamin K synthesis

SIDE EFFECTS
DERM: Rash; irritation to skin, tongue, perianal area
GI: Nausea, GI bleed, vomiting, constipation, flatulence, steatorrhea, abdominal distention and pain, malabsorption of fat-soluble vitamins
GU: Increased urinary Ca excretion
HEME: Bleeding tendency because of possible vitamin K deficiency
Other: Hyperchloremic acidosis, especially in children

TOXICITY AND OVERDOSE
Clinical signs: Vomiting, abdominal pain and distention, constipation, nausea, GI obstruction
Treatment: Discontinue medication; supportive care

PATIENT CARE MANAGEMENT
Assessment
• Assess history of hypersensitivity to cholestyramine
• Assess hypersensitivity to yellow dye #5
• Obtain baseline serum cholesterol, triglyceride levels
• Assess other medication being taken to ensure optimal absorption, use
• Assess history of constipation
Interventions
• Reconstitute PO powder in 2-6 oz water, noncarbonated beverage, applesauce; mix before administering; do not administer as a powder
• Administer medications with meals
• Administer other medications 1 hr before or 4-6 hr after cholestyramine
• Discontinue if constipation continues despite reduction in dose
• Maintain age-appropriate fluid intake
Evaluation
• Evaluate therapeutic response (decreased cholesterol, triglyceride levels)
• Monitor serum cholesterol, triglyceride q 3-6 mo
• Monitor INR if taking anticoagulants
• Monitor for signs, symptoms of fat-soluble vitamin deficiency
• Monitor bowel function; treat constipation appropriately; decrease dosage if necessary
• Check therapeutic levels of other medications; may need to adjust dosage of other medication

PATIENT AND FAMILY EDUCATION
Teach/instruct
• To take as directed at prescribed intervals for prescribed length of time
• To evaluate other medications, OTC drugs for interactions
• To schedule regular monitoring of blood cholesterol, triglyceride levels
• To monitor serial wt, linear growth of children; plot on appropriate growth grid
Warn/advise
• To notify care provider of hypersensitivity, side effects

- To increase fluid, fiber in diet to prevent constipation

Encourage
- Encourage daily intake of balanced diet, foods low in cholesterol and total fats
- To consider consulting dietitian for dietary guidance for low cholesterol diet, wt control
- To consider vitamin, mineral supplement
- To exercise regularly per care provider

STORAGE
- Store at room temp in tightly sealed container
- Protect from moisture, direct light

---

choline magnesium trisalicylate

Brand Name(s): Trilisate

Classification: Non-narcotic analgesic

Pregnancy Category: C

AVAILABLE PREPARATIONS
Tabs: 500 mg, 750 mg, 1000 mg
Liq: 500 mg

ROUTES AND DOSAGES
Children: PO 12-13 kg, 500 mg/24 hr divided bid; 14-17 kg, 750 mg/24 hr divided bid; 18-22 kg, 1000 mg/24 hr divided bid; 23-27 kg, 1250 mg/24 hr divided bid; 28-32 kg, 1500 mg/24 hr divided bid; 33-37 kg, 1750 mg/24 hr divided bid
- Dosages are calculated as total daily dose of 50 mg/kg/24 hr for child ≤37 kg and 2250 mg/24 hr for child >37 kg; or 30-60 mg/kg/24 hr divided tid-qid
Adults: PO 500-1500 mg qd-tid

MECHANISM AND INDICATIONS
Mechanism: Blocks pain impulses in CNS that occur in response to inhibition of prostaglandin synthesis; antipyretic action results from inhibition of hypothalamic heat-regulating center to produce vasodilation to allow heat dissipation
Indications: Used to treat mild-to-moderate pain, fever, arthritis (including juvenile rheumatoid arthritis)

PHARMACOKINETICS
Onset: 15-30 min
Peak: 1-2 hr
Half-life: 9-17 hr
Metabolism: Liver
Excretion: Urine
Therapeutic level: 15-30 mg/100 ml

CONTRAINDICATIONS AND PRECAUTIONS
- Contraindicated with hypersensitivity to non-acetylated salicylates, GI bleeding, bleeding disorders, children <3 yr, vitamin K deficiency, children with influenza, flu-like symptoms, or chicken pox (no reported cases of Reyes syndrome with choline, but there should be concern about the possibility)
- Use cautiously with anemia, hepatic disease, renal disease, Hodgkins disease, pregnancy, lactation, gastritis, peptic ulcer disease

INTERACTIONS
Drug
- Decreased effects with antacids, steroids, urinary alkalizers
- Increased blood loss with alcohol, heparin
- Increased effects of anticoagulants, insulin, methotrexate
- Decreased effects of probenecid, spironolactone, sulfinpyrazone, sulfonylamides
- Possible toxic effects with PABA, furosemide, carbonic anhydrase inhibitors
- Decreased BG levels with other salicylates
- Increased risk of GI bleeding with steroids, other antiinflammatory agents
- Increased plasma salicylate concentration (potentially toxic salicylate levels) with other salicylate-containing products

Lab
- Increase in coagulation studies, liver function studies, serum uric

---

✢ Available in Canada.

acid, amylase, CO_2, urinary protein
• Decreased serum K^+, PBI, cholesterol
• Interferes with urine catecholamines, pregnancy test

SIDE EFFECTS
CNS: Stimulation, drowsiness, dizziness, confusion, convulsion, headache, flushing, hallucinations, coma, lethargy
CV: Rapid pulse, pulmonary edema
DERM: Rash, urticaria, bruising, pruritis
ENDO: Hypoglycemia, hyponatremia, hypokalemia
EENT: Tinnitus, hearing loss, epistaxis
GI: Nausea, vomiting, GI bleeding, gastric upset, diarrhea, heartburn, constipation, gastric pain, anorexia, hepatitis
GU: Increased BUN, creatinine
HEME: Thrombocytopenia, agranulocytosis, leukopenia, neutropenia, hemolytic anemia, increased pro-time
RESP: Wheezing, hyperpnea

TOXICITY AND OVERDOSE
Clinical signs: Headache, dizziness, tinnitus, hearing impairment, confusion, drowsiness, sweating, vomiting, diarrhea, hyperventilation, CNS disturbances, alteration in electrolyte balance, respiratory and metabolic acidosis, hyperthermia, dehydration
Treatment: Supportive care; lavage, activated charcoal; IV fluids; forced diuresis with alkalinizing sol recommended to accelerate salicylate excretion; peritoneal dialysis, hemodialysis in extreme cases

PATIENT CARE MANAGEMENT
Assessment
• Assess history of hypersensitivity to choline magnesium trisalicylate-related medications
• Assess current medication regime to determine any possible drug interactions
• Assess liver function (ALT, AST,

bilirubin), renal function, (BUN, creatinine, I&O), and CBC, Hct, Hgb, and pro-time before implementation of long-term therapy
• Perform audiometric tests before implementation of long-term therapy; test periodically thereafter

Interventions
• Tab may be crushed, mixed with fruit juice, carbonated beverage, or water

> **NURSING ALERT**
> Death has been reported in adults following ingestion of doses from 10-30 g of salicylate; however, larger doses have been taken without resulting in fatality
>
> Do not use for children with active chicken pox, influenza, flu-like symptoms

Evaluation
• Evaluate therapeutic response (decreased pain, fever, stiffness in joints)
• Evaluate labs, I&O, audiometric tests
• Evaluate side effects, hypersensitivity

PATIENT AND FAMILY EDUCATION
Teach/instruct
• To take as directed at prescribed intervals for prescribed length of time
• To avoid alcohol
• That therapeutic response for treatment of arthritis may not be seen for up to 2 wk
Warn/advise
• To notify care provider of hypersensitivity, side effects
• Never to exceed recommended dosage because acute poisoning can occur
• Do not take with any other aspirin product
• That choline magnesium trisalicylate should be decreased 2 wk before surgery (discuss with health care provider) if also taking anticoagulants

STORAGE
- Store at room temp

---

cimetidine

Brand Name(s): Tagamet, Apo-Cimetidine✤, Novo-cimetine✤, Nu-Cimet✤, Peptol✤, Tagamet✤

Classification: Antihistamine, H_2-receptor antagonist

Pregnancy Category: B

AVAILABLE PREPARATIONS
Liq: 300 mg/5 ml
Tabs: 200 mg, 300 mg, 400 mg, 800 mg
Inj: 300 mg/2 ml

ROUTES AND DOSAGES
Gastroesophageal Reflux
Neonates: PO 10-20 mg/kg/24 hr divided q6-12h
Infants and children: PO 10-40 mg/kg/24 hr divided qid
Adults: PO 800-1600 mg/24 hr divided qid for 12 wk
Duodenal or Peptic Ulcer
Infants and children: PO 20-40 mg/kg/24 hr divided qid
Duodenal Ulcer
Adults: PO 300 mg qid; or 400-600 mg bid; or 800 mg qhs (1600 mg qhs more effective in selected pts)
Gastric Ulcer
Adults: PO 300 mg qid with meals and hs; or 400 mg bid and 400 mg hs
Duodenal or Gastric Ulcer
Infants and children: IV 5-10 mg/kg q6-8h
Adults: IV 300 mg q6-8h
Gastric Hypersecretory Conditions
Adults: PO 300 mg qid with meals and hs; IV 300 mg q6-8h
Upper GI Bleeding
Adults: PO 300 mg qid; or 600 mg bid
Prophylaxis of Aspiration Pneumonitis
Adults: IM 300 mg before induction of anesthesia followed by 300 mg IM or IV q4h until pt responds to verbal commands

Urticaria Therapy Adjunct
Adults: IV 300 mg
IV administration
- Recommended concentration: 6 mg/ml in D_5LR, D_5NS, $D_5\frac{1}{4}NS$, $D_5\frac{1}{2}NS$, $D_{10}NS$, D_5W, $D_{10}W$, LR, NS, or R
- Maximum concentration: 15 mg/ml for IV push; 6 mg/ml for IV infusion
- IV push rate: Over ≥5 min.
- Intermittent infusion rate: Over 15-30 min
- Continuous infusion: Adults with upper GI bleeding, 37.5 mg/hr; prophylaxis of stress-related mucosal bleeding, 50 mg/hr for up to 7 days; a loading dose of 150-300 mg infused over ≥5 min can be given before continuous infusion; total daily dose has been added to compatible fluid, infused over 24 hr

MECHANISM AND INDICATIONS
Mechanism: Reversible competitive antagonist of the actions of histamine on H_2 receptor resulting in decrease of histamine-mediated basal and nocturnal gastric acid secretion by parietal cell
Indications: Used as therapy for gastric or duodenal ulcer, gastroesophageal reflux, pathological hypersecretory conditions, prevention of duodenal ulcer, prevention and treatment of upper GI bleeding in critically ill pts; investigational use for treatment of acute upper GI bleed; prophylaxis of pulmonary aspiration of acid during anesthesia; enhanced absorption of orally administered pancreatic enzymes with pancreatic insufficiency; in combination with antihistamine to treat acute urticaria

PHARMACOKINETICS
Peak: 45-90 min after oral dose
Half-life: 2 hr
Metabolism: Liver
Excretion: Urine, bile

CONTRAINDICATIONS AND PRECAUTIONS
- Contraindicated with hypersensitivity to cimetidine, any other

---

✤ Available in Canada.

histamine H_2-receptor antagonists
- Use cautiously with renal or hepatic impairment, pregnancy, lactation

INTERACTIONS
Drug
- Potential effect on bioavailability of drug, dosage forms (e.g., enteric-coated) with pH-dependent absorption
- Prevention of degradation of acid-labile drugs possible
- Impaired elimination of drugs requiring hepatic metabolism possible
- Impaired absorption with use of antacids, sucralfate
- Increased risk of neutropenia or other blood dyscrasias possible when administered with bone marrow depressants
- Impaired absorption of ketoconazole
- Increased toxicity with use of alcohol, anticonvulsants, antidepressants, glipizide, glyburide, metoprolol, metronidazole, phenytoin, propranolol, aminophylline, caffeine, theophylline, Ca channel blocking agents, cyclosporine, lidocaine, procainamide, quinine

Lab
- Interference possible with interpretation of Hemoccult and Gastroccult tests on gastric content aspirate; wait fifteen minutes after oral administration before drawing sample
- Increased serum prolactin, creatinine, serum transaminase
- Decreased parathyroid hormone possible
- False negative allergy skin test possible
- Antagonism of pentagastrin and histamine in evaluation of gastric acid secretory function possible

Nutrition
- Vitamin B_{12} deficiency possible with long-term therapy for pts likely to have impaired secretion of intrinsic factor (severe fundic gastritis)

INCOMPATIBILITIES
- Aminophylline, amphotericin B, barbiturates, cefamandole, cefazolin, cephalothin

SIDE EFFECTS
CNS: Headaches (about 1%), dizziness, somnolence; reversible confusion states, predominantly in very ill patients
CV: Bradycardia, hypotension, tachycardia (rare)
DERM: Rash
ENDO/METAB: Gynecomastia
GI: Jaundice, diarrhea
GU: Reversible impotence with treatment for hypersecretory syndromes
HEME: Decrease in WBC count, agranulocytosis (rare)
Other: Rare cases of fever, allergic reactions

TOXICITY AND OVERDOSE
Clinical signs: CNS symptoms (unresponsiveness); respiratory failure, tachycardia
Treatment: Supportive care; induce emesis or perform gastric lavage followed by activated charcoal; propranolol if necessary for tachycardia

PATIENT CARE MANAGEMENT
Assessment
- Assess hypersensitivity to cimetidine, other histamine H_2-receptor antagonists
- Assess baseline renal function (BUN, creatinine), hepatic function (ALT, AST, bilirubin), gastric pH (therapeutic goal ≥5), abdominal symptoms

Interventions
- May administer PO without regard to meals; tab may be crushed, mixed with food or fluid
- Do not administer within 1 hr of antacids
- Do not administer within 2 hr of sucralfate, ketoconazole
- Do not use if IM sol is discolored or contains precipitate
- Injection painful

NURSING ALERT
Do not administer rapid IV (<5 min); may result in arrhythmias, hypotension, cardiac arrest

Evaluation
• Evaluate therapeutic response (decreased abdominal pain)
• Evaluate gastric pH (>5), hematologic function (CBC), signs of GI bleeding (melena, brown-tinged or coffee-ground emesis); VS with IV push administration
• Evaluate renal function (BUN, creatinine), hepatic function (ALT, AST, bilirubin)

PATIENT AND FAMILY EDUCATION
Teach/instruct
• To take as directed at prescribed intervals for prescribed length of time
• To continue taking even after symptoms subside
Warn/advise
• To notify care provider of hypersensitivity, side effects
• To avoid smoking, caffeine, alcohol; may exacerbate symptoms
• To avoid OTC drugs unless directed by care provider

STORAGE
• Store all forms at room temp, protected from light
• Diluted sol stable at room temp for 18 hr

ciprofloxacin
Brand Name(s): Cipro, Cipro IV❧

Classification: Antibiotic (fluoroquinolone)

Pregnancy Category: C

AVAILABLE PREPARATIONS
Tabs: 250 mg, 500 mg, 750 mg
Inj: 200 mg, 400 mg

ROUTES AND DOSAGES
Children: PO 20-30 mg/kg/24 hr divided q12h; maximum dose 1.5 g/24 hr
Adults: PO 250-500 mg q12h
Cystic Fibrosis
Children: IV 3.2-12.5 mg/kg/24 hr divided q12h
Adults: IV 200-400 mg q12h
IV administration
• Recommended concentration: 1-2 mg/ml in D₅W or NS
• Maximum concentration: 2 mg/ml (available commercially)
• IV push rate: Not recommended
• Intermittent infusion rate: Over 60 min

MECHANISM AND INDICATIONS
Antibiotic mechanism: Bactericidal; alters bacterial DNA by interfering with DNA gyrase, possibly by direct interaction with DNA staff
Indications: Effective against gram-positive and gram-negative organisms including *E. coli, Enterobacter cloacae, Proteus mirabilis, Klebsiella pneumoniae, Proteus vulgaris, Citrobacter freundii,* group D streptococcus; used to treat urinary tract, skin, bone, joint infections

PHARMACOKINETICS
Peak: 1-2 hr
Half-life: 3-4 hr
Metabolism: Liver
Excretion: Urine

CONTRAINDICATIONS AND PRECAUTIONS
• Contraindicated with known hypersensitivity to ciprofloxacin, other quinolones
• Use cautiously with children <18, with impaired renal or hepatic functions, known CNS disorders, pregnancy, lactation

INTERACTIONS
Drug
• Increased risk of toxicity from theophylline
• Increased serum levels with use of probenecid
• Decreased absorption with use of Mg antacids, aluminum hydroxide

---

- Increased anticoagulant effect of oral anticoagulants
- Increased nephrotoxic effects from cyclosporine
- Increased serum levels with use of cimetidine

Lab

- Increased liver function tests
- Increased serum creatinine, BUN

INCOMPATIBILITIES

- Do not give with other medications in syringe or sol

SIDE EFFECTS

CNS: Headache, dizziness, fatigue, insomnia, depression, restlessness, increased intracranial pressure, seizures

CV: Cardiac toxicity (atrial flutter, ventricular ectopy, angina pectoris, syncope)

DERM: Rash, pruritus, urticaria, photosensitivity

EENT: Photosensitivity, blurred vision, tinnitus

GI: Nausea, vomiting, constipation, diarrhea, flatulence, pseudomembranous colitis, dysphagia, elevated liver function tests, jaundice, hepatic necrosis

GU: Interstitial nephritis, renal impairment, polyuria, urinary retention, crystalluria

HEME: Eosinophilia, anemia, neutropenia

Local: Vein irritation, phlebitis at IV injection site

Other: Hypersensitivity reaction (anaphylaxis, cardiovascular collapse, dyspnea, facial or pharyngeal edema), fever, bacterial or fungal superinfection

TOXICITY AND OVERDOSE

Clinical signs: No information available

Treatment: Oral: empty stomach by induced vomiting or gastric lavage; hydration supportive care; parenteral: supportive care

PATIENT CARE MANAGEMENT

Assessment

- Assess history of hypersensitivity to ciprofloxacin, other quinolones

- Obtain C&S; may begin therapy before obtaining results
- Assess renal function (BUN, creatinine, I&O), hepatic function (ALT, AST, bilirubin), hematologic function (CBC, differential, platelet count), bowel pattern

Interventions

- Administer PO 1 hr ac or two hr after meals; may administer with food or milk to decrease GI irritation
- Tab may be crushed, mixed with food or fluid; administer PO with generous amount of water to prevent crystalluria
- Do not administer antacids containing Mg or Al with or within 2 hr of medication
- Do not premix IV with other medications; infuse separately
- Use large vein with small-bore needle to reduce local reaction; rotate IV site q48-72h
- Maintain age-appropriate fluid intake

NURSING ALERT

Discontinue if signs of hypersensitivity, crystalluria or renal abnormalities, pseudomembranous colitis develop

Do not give IV push

Evaluation

- Evaluate therapeutic response (decreased symptoms of infection)
- Evaluate hematologic function (CBC, differential, platelet count), renal function (BUN, creatinine, I&O), hepatic function (ALT, AST, bilirubin), maintain alkaline urine to prevent crystalluria
- Observe for allergic reaction (fever, flushing, rash, urticaria, pruritus)
- Observe for signs of superinfection (perineal itching, diaper rash, fever, malaise, redness, pain, swelling, drainage, rash, diarrhea, sore throat, change in cough or sputum)
- Evaluate IV site for vein irritation

PATIENT AND FAMILY EDUCATION
Teach/instruct
• To take as directed at prescribed intervals for prescribed length of time
Warn/advise
• To notify care provider of hypersensitivity, side effects, superinfection
• To avoid direct exposure to sunlight

STORAGE
• Store powder, tabs at room temp, protected from light
• Reconstituted sol stable for 14 days refrigerated or at room temp

---

cisapride
Brand Name(s): Propulsid
Classification: Cholinergic enhancer, GI emptying (delayed) adjunct
Pregnancy Category: C

AVAILABLE PREPARATIONS
Tabs: 10 mg
• Susp not commercially available, instructions for formulation of susp are available from manufacturer for use by pharmacists

ROUTES AND DOSAGES
Gastroesophageal Reflux/Gastroparesis
Infants and children: PO 0.15-0.3 mg/kg/dose tid or qid 30 min ac and hs
Adults: PO 5-10 mg tid or qid 30 min ac and hs

MECHANISM AND INDICATIONS
Mechanism: Causes release of acetylcholine from postganglionic nerve endings of myenteric plexus; results in increased esophageal activity, increased lower esophageal sphincter tone, enhanced gastric and duodenal emptying; transit is improved in both small, large intestines
Indications: Accepted use in prophylaxis, treatment of gastroesophageal reflux; experimental use in treatment of gastroparesis, intestinal pseudo-obstruction

PHARMACOKINETICS
Onset: 30-60 min
Peak: 1-2 hr
Half-life: 7-10 hr
Metabolism: Liver
Excretion: Urine, feces

CONTRAINDICATIONS AND PRECAUTIONS
• Contraindicated with hypersensitivity to cisapride, GI hemorrhage, mechanical obstruction, perforation
• Use cautiously with epilepsy, history of seizures, hepatic or renal impairment, pregnancy, lactation

INTERACTIONS
Drug
• Increased sedative effects of alcohol and benzodiazepines possible
• Increased plasma concentration of diazepam
• Administration of anticholinergic medications would theoretically be expected to compromise effectiveness of cisapride
• Accelerated absorption of cimetidine and ranitidine

SIDE EFFECTS
CNS: Headache; fatigue; rare reports of seizures with history of seizures
GI: Abdominal cramping, diarrhea, constipation, flatulence, nausea

TOXICITY AND OVERDOSE
Clinical signs: Retching, borborygmi, flatulence, stool frequency, urinary frequency (few reports of overdose)
Treatment: Gastric lavage or activated charcoal; supportive measures

PATIENT CARE MANAGEMENT
Assessment
• Assess hypersensitivity to cisapride
• Assess baseline renal function (BUN, creatinine), hepatic func-

---

✤ Available in Canada.

tion (ALT, AST, bilirubin) mechanical obstruction, perforation
• Assess baseline symptoms of GERD (frequency and volume of emesis)
• Assess baseline symptoms of gastroparesis (abdominal distention, nausea, belching, early satiety)

Interventions
• Administer 30 min ac; tab may not be crushed, chewed, broken apart
• Smaller, more frequent meals sometimes better tolerated by individuals with gastroesophageal reflux, gastroparesis
• Upright positioning following feedings may diminish gastroesophageal reflux
• Elevation of HOB may improve nighttime comfort, diminish nighttime gastroesophageal reflux
• Care provider may recommend thickening of infant feedings

Evaluation
• Evaluate therapeutic response (decreased postprandial discomfort)
• Evaluate for side effects, hypersensitivity
• Monitor I&O
• Monitor renal function (BUN, creatinine), hepatic function (ALT, AST, bilirubin)

PATIENT AND FAMILY EDUCATION
Teach/instruct
• To take as directed at prescribed intervals for prescribed length of time
• Reinforce care provider recommendations regarding size and frequency of meals, modification of feedings, positioning

Warn/advise
• To notify care provider of side effects

STORAGE
• Store at room temp
• Protect from light, moisture

cisplatin

Brand Name(s): Platinol, Platinol-Aq❦

Classification: Heavy metal, acts as an alkylating agent

Pregnancy Category: D

AVAILABLE PREPARATIONS
Inj: 10 mg, 50 mg powder

ROUTES AND DOSAGES
• Drug may vary in response to diagnosis, extent of disease, concurrent or previous therapy, protocol guidelines, physiologic parameters; consult current literature, protocol recommendations
• IV 40-120 mg/m^2 single dose or 20-33 mg/m^2/24 hr for 3-5 days; repeat in 1-4 wk depending on tolerance and bone marrow reserve/recovery

Testicular Cancer
IV 20 mg/m^2 × 5 days q 3 wk or 120 mg/m^2 × 1 q 3 wk

Cervical Cancer
IV 50 or 100 mg/m^2 × 1 q 3-4 wk

Bladder Cancer
IV 50-70 mg/m^2 × 1 q 3-4 wk

Ovarian Cancer
IV 50 mg/m^2 × 1 q 3-4 wk in combination with doxorubicin or IV 50-70 mg/m^2 × 1 q 3 wk as single agent therapy

Neuroblastoma, Osteosarcoma, Brain Tumor
Children: IV 30 mg/m^2 q wk; or 60 mg/m^2/24 hr × 2 days q 3-4 wk; or 90 mg/m^2 × 1 q 3-4 wk

IV administration
• Recommended concentration: 1 mg/ml (dilute 10 mg with 10 ml SW, 50 mg with 50 ml); should be clear and colorless; further dilute with NS to final concentration of 0.1-1.0 mg; add mannitol to facilitate urine flow
• IV infusion rate: Over at least 1 hr, up to 24 hr (per protocol)
• Do not use needles, IV sets with any aluminum parts; causes precipitation, decreases potency of cisplatin

❦ Available in Canada.

MECHANISM AND INDICATIONS

Mechanism: Cell cycle phase non-specific; primary mode of action is cisplatin interaction with DNA; inhibits DNA synthesis by forming inter- and intrastrand cross-links and denaturing the double helix, thereby preventing cell replication
Indications: Used to treat osteogenic sarcoma; pediatric brain tumors; neuroblastoma, bladder, cervical, lung, ovarian, metastatic testicular cancer

PHARMACOKINETICS

Peak: Plasma drug, platinum concentrations occur immediately when administered via IV infusion
Absorption: Rapid after IV injection
Distribution: Body fluids, kidneys, liver, prostate
Half-life: Triphasic kinetics with half-lives of 0.3 hr, 1.0 hr, and 24 hr; with renal insufficiency or ascites, clearance can be considerably longer
Metabolism: Cleared rapidly from plasma during 1st 2 hr after IV administration, slowly due to binding to plasma proteins and erythrocytes; clearance prolonged in pts with renal insufficiency or ascites; exact mechanisms of action not conclusively determined
Excretion: In urine, 23%-70% recovered within 24 hr and 90% recovered within 5 days

CONTRAINDICATIONS AND PRECAUTIONS

• Contraindicated with known hypersensitivity to this drug, other platinum-containing compounds, with severe renal disease, hearing impairment, myelosuppression, pregnancy, lactation
• Use cautiously with mild-to-moderate renal problems, myelosuppression, hearing difficulties (may need dosage modifications)

INTERACTIONS

Drug
• Increased nephrotoxicity possible with use of aminoglycosides
• Increased ototoxicity possible with use of furosemide

• Decreased serum phenytoin levels possible

INCOMPATIBILITIES

• 5FU, metoclopramide
• Inactivated by alkaline sols (e.g., $NaHCO_3$), sodium bisulfite, sodium thiosulfate
• Do not use aluminum or aluminum-containing products

SIDE EFFECTS

CNS: Peripheral neuropathy or neuritis, seizures, headache, sensory paresthesias, loss of taste
EENT: Hearing loss, tinnitus, papilledema, deafness
ENDO/METAB: Hypomagnesemia, hypocalcemia, hypokalemia, hypophosphatemia, hypouricemia
GI: Nausea, vomiting, diarrhea, constipation, anorexia, metallic taste
GU: With repeated course of cisplatin, prolonged and severe renal toxicity may occur, decreased CrCl, azoospermia, infertility
HEME: Leukopenia, thrombocytopenia, anemia, neutropenia
Other: Facial flushing, urticaria, angioneurotic edema

TOXICITY AND OVERDOSE

Clinical signs: Anaphylactoid reaction (facial edema, wheezing, tachycardia, hypotension)
Treatment: Usually responds immediately when treated with epinephrine, corticosteroids, antihistamines; supportive care

PATIENT CARE MANAGEMENT

Assessment
• Assess history of hypersensitivity to cisplatin, other platinum-containing drugs
• Assess baseline VS, CBC, differential, platelet count, renal function (BUN, creatinine, urine CrCl), liver function (ALT, AST, LDH, bilirubin, alk phos), serum electrolytes (Mg, Ca, K^+, PO_4), audiology status
• Assess urinary elimination, hydration status (SG), presence of hematuria including RBCs in urine, dysuria, urinary frequency

C

• Assess neurologic and mental status before, during drug administration, on follow-up visits
• Assess success of previous antiemetic therapy
• Assess history of previous treatment, with special attention to other therapies that might predispose pt to renal, hepatic, or audiologic dysfunction

Interventions
• Premedicate with antiemetics, continue for at least 24 hr after drug is administered
• Prehydrate with NS several hr before, for 24 hr after drug administration to ensure good urine output, decrease potential nephrotoxicity
• Do not use needles, IV administration sets containing aluminum parts; causes precipitate, decreases potency
• Encourage small, frequent feedings of foods pt likes
• Monitor I&O; administer IV fluids until pt able to resume normal PO intake
• Provide supportive measures to maintain hemostasis, fluid and electrolyte balance, nutritional support

NURSING ALERT
Patient must be well-hydrated, have adequate urine output per protocol guidelines (specific gravities ≤1.010)

High levels of repeated dosing with cisplatin can cause hearing loss; periodic audiology exams must be done

Do not use needles, IV administration sets containing aluminum; platinol may react with aluminum, causing precipitate, loss of potency

Evaluate
• Evaluate therapeutic response (decreased tumor size, spread of malignancy)
• Evaluate CBC, differential, platelet count, electrolytes (Mg, Ca, K^+, PO_4), renal function (BUN,

creatinine, urine CrCl) liver function (ALT, AST, LDH, bilirubin, alk phos), audiology status at given intervals after chemotherapy
• Evaluate for signs of infection (fever, fatigue, sore throat), bleeding (easy bruising, nose bleeds, bleeding gums)
• Evaluate I&O carefully, check wt daily, have pt empty bladder at least q2h

PATIENT AND FAMILY EDUCATION
Teach/instruct
• To have pt well-hydrated before, after chemotherapy
• About importance of follow-up to monitor blood counts, serum chemistry values, drug blood levels
• To take an accurate temp; rectal temp contraindicated
• To notify care provider of signs of bleeding (bruising, epistaxis, bleeding gums), infection (fever, sore throat, fatigue)
• To take antiemetic before receiving cisplatin; continue for at least 24 hr following up to 3-5 days after to manage delayed nausea or vomiting
• To take prescribed supplements to prevent hypokalemia, hypomagnesemia, hypocalcemia, hypophosphatemia
• To report any tinnitus

Warn/advise
• About impact of body changes that may occur (hair loss, hyperpigmentation, nail ridging) and how to minimize changes (wigs, caps, scarves, long sleeves)
• To avoid OTC products containing aspirin
• To report any alterations in behavior, sensation, perception; help to develop a plan of care to manage side effects, stress of illness or treatment
• To monitor bowel function, call if abdominal pain, constipation noted
• To report immediately any pain, discoloration at injection site (parenteral forms)

• That good oral hygiene with very soft toothbrush is imperative
• That dental work be delayed until blood counts return to baseline, with permission of care provider
• To avoid contact with known viral or bacterial illnesses
• That household contacts of child not be immunized with live polio virus; inactivated form should be used
• That child not receive immunizations until immune system recovers sufficiently to mount needed antibody response
• To report immediately exposure to chicken pox in susceptible child
• To report immediately reactivation of herpes zoster virus (shingles)
• If appropriate, ways to preserve reproductive patterns and sexuality (sperm banking, contraceptives)

Encourage
• Provision of nutritional food intake; consider nutritional consultation
• To comply with bowel management program
• To drink plenty of fluids, void frequently
• To use top anesthetics to control discomfort of mucositis; avoid spicy foods, commercial mouthwashes

STORAGE
• Store at room temp
• Protect from light
• Do not refrigerate; precipitate may form
• Reconstituted sol stable for 20 hr at room temp, protected from light
• Multi-use vials stable for 28 days following initial entry if protected from light or 7 days under fluorescent room lighting

---

clarithromycin
Brand Name(s): Biaxin✤
Classification: Antibiotic (macrolide)
Pregnancy Category: C

AVAILABLE PREPARATIONS
Oral susp: 125 mg/5 ml, 250 mg/5 ml
Tabs (film-coated): 250 mg, 500 mg

ROUTES AND DOSAGES
Children: Not currently FDA-approved for use in children <12 yr; PO dosages of 15 mg/kg/24 hr divided q12h have been used in clinical trials; maximum dose 1 g/24 hr
Adults: PO 250-500 mg bid for 7-14 days

MECHANISM AND INDICATIONS
Antibiotic mechanism: Binds to ribosome's 50S subunit, thus inhibiting bacterial protein synthesis
Indications: Effective against *Streptococcus pneumoniae, Str. pyogenes, Mycoplasma pneumoniae, Corynebacterium diphtheriae, Bordatella pertussis, Listeria monocytogenes, Haemophilus influenzae, Staphylococcus aureus;* used to treat mild-to-moderate upper and lower respiratory tract infections, otitis media, skin and soft tissue infections

PHARMACOKINETICS
Peak: 2 hr
Distribution: Distributed widely throughout body except CNS
Half-life: 4-6 hr
Metabolism: Liver
Excretion: Bile, feces

CONTRAINDICATIONS AND PRECAUTIONS
• Contraindicated with known hypersensitivity to clarithromycin, erythromycin, any macrolide antibiotic
• Use cautiously with impaired renal or hepatic function, pregnancy, lactation

---

INTERACTIONS
Drug
- Increased effects of oral anticoagulants, digoxin, theophylline, methylprednisolone, cyclosporine, bromocriptine, disopyramide
- Increased toxicity of carbamazepine
- Decreased action of clindamycin
- Increased or decreased action of penicillins

Lab
- False elevations of liver function tests, urinary catecholamines, steroids
- Decreased folate assay

SIDE EFFECTS
DERM: Rash, urticaria, pruritus
GI: Nausea, vomiting, diarrhea, abdominal pain, stomatitis, anorexia, altered sense of taste, hepatotoxicity
GU: Vaginitis
Other: Bacterial or fungal superinfection, headache

PATIENT CARE MANAGEMENT
Assessment
- Assess history of hypersensitivity to clarithromycin, erythromycin, other macrolide antibiotics
- Obtain C&S; may begin therapy before obtaining results
- Assess renal function (BUN, creatinine, I&O), hepatic function (ALT, AST, bilirubin)

Interventions
- Administer without regard to meals; shake susp well before administering; film-coated tab must be swallowed whole; administer with full glass of water
- Maintain age-appropriate fluid intake
- For group A β-hemolytic streptococcal infections, provide 10-day course to prevent acute rheumatic fever, glomerulonephritis.

> **NURSING ALERT**
> Discontinue drug if signs of toxicity, hypersensitivity develop

Evaluation
- Evaluate therapeutic response (decreased symptoms of infection)
- Monitor renal function (BUN, creatinine, I&O), hepatic function (ALT, AST, bilirubin); bowel pattern
- Observe for signs of allergic reactions (rash, pruritus, wheezing, tightness in chest)
- Observe for signs of superinfection (perineal itching, diaper rash, fever, malaise, redness, pain, swelling, drainage, rash, diarrhea, sore throat, change in cough or sputum)

PATIENT AND FAMILY EDUCATION
Teach/instruct
- To take as directed at prescribed intervals for prescribed length of time

Warn/advise
- To notify provider of hypersensitivity, side effects, superinfection

STORAGE
- Store tab, susp at room temp in tight container
- Protect from light

---

clindamycin hydrochloride, clindamycin palmitate hydrochloride, clindamycin phosphate

Brand Name(s): Cleocin, Dalacin C✤, (clindamycin hydrochloride); Cleocin Pediatric (clindamycin palmitate hydrochloride); Cleocin Phosphate, Cleocin T (clindamycin phosphate)

Classification: Antibiotic (lincomycin derivative)

Pregnancy Category: B

AVAILABLE PREPARATIONS
Oral susp: 75 mg/5 ml
Caps: 75 mg, 150 mg
Inj: 150 mg/ml
Top gel, sol, lotion: 1%

ROUTES AND DOSAGES
Neonates: ≤7 days, ≤2000 g: IM/IV 10 mg/kg/24 hr divided q12h; ≤7 days, >2000 g: IM/IV 15 mg/kg/24 hr divided q8h; >7 days, <1200 g: IM/IV 10 mg/kg/24 hr divided q12h; >7 days, 1200-2000 g: IM/IV 15 mg/kg/24 hr divided q8h; >7 days, >2000 g: IM/IV 20 mg/kg/24 hr divided q6-8h
Infants and children: PO 10-30 mg/kg/24 hr divided q6h; IM/IV 25-40 mg/kg/24 hr divided q6-8h
Adults: PO 150-450 mg/dose q6-8h (maximum dose 1.8 g/24 hr); IM/IV 1.2-1.8 g/24 hr divided q6-12h (maximum 4.8 g/24 hr)
Acne Vulgaris
Adolescents and adults: TOP, apply thin film to affected areas bid
IV administration
• Recommended concentration: 6-12 mg/ml in D_5W, LR, or NS or 18 mg/ml in D_5W
• Maximum concentration: 18 mg/ml
• Intermittent infusion rate: Over 10-60 min; infusion rate should not exceed 30 mg/min; too rapid infusion may cause hypotension, cardiac arrest

MECHANISM AND INDICATIONS
Antibiotic mechanism: Bactericidal or bacteriostatic; inhibits bacterial protein synthesis by binding to ribosome's 50S subunit
Indications: Effective against most aerobic gram-positive cocci and several anaerobic gram-negative and gram-positive organisms, including staphylococci, pneumococci, streptococci, *Bacteroides;* also effective against *Mycoplasma pneumoniae, Leptotrichia buccalis, Actinomyces, Clostridium;* used to treat sepsis and respiratory tract, GU tract, intraabdominal, skin, and soft tissue infections; topic forms used to treat acne

PHARMACOKINETICS
Peak: PO 1 hr; IM 1-3 hr; IV end of infusion
Distribution: Widely throughout body except CNS
Half-life: Neonates, premature 8.7 hr, full term 3.6 hr; infants 3 hr; children 2-3 hr
Metabolism: Liver
Excretion: Urine, bile, feces

CONTRAINDICATIONS AND PRECAUTIONS
• Contraindicated with known hypersensitivity to clindamycin or lincomycin, with history of inflammatory bowel disease or antibiotic-induced colitis
• Use cautiously with renal or hepatic impairment, GI disorders, asthma or significant allergies, tartrazine sensitivity, newborns, pregnancy, lactation; top forms should be used cautiously in atopic pts

INTERACTIONS
Drug
• Increased risk of neuromuscular blockade with use of neuromuscular blocking agents such as tubocurarine or pancuronium
• Decreased GI absorption of clindamycin with use of kaolin products
• Increased clindamycin-induced diarrhea with use of antidiarrheals such as diphenoxylate or opiates
• Decreased effectiveness of clindamycin with use of erythromycin
• In vitro inactivation of aminoglycosides
• Increased irritation or dryness with use of top forms, other acne preparations (e.g., benzoyl peroxide, tretinoin)
Lab
• Increased liver function tests
Nutrition
• Slightly decreased absorption if given with food

INCOMPATIBILITIES
• Aminophylline, ampicillin, all barbiturates, calcium gluconate, magnesium sulfate, phenytoin, ranitidine, tobramycin, Ringer's sol

SIDE EFFECTS
DERM: Maculopapular rash, urticaria, erythema multiforme, con-

---

✤ Available in Canada.

tact dermatitis, dryness with top forms

EENT: Stinging in eyes with top form

GI: Nausea, vomiting, abdominal pain, diarrhea, pseudomembranous colitis, esophagitis, flatulence, anorexia, bloody or tarry stools, dysphagia, elevated liver function tests, elevated bilirubin, jaundice

HEME: Transient leukopenia, eosinophilia, thrombocytopenia

Local: Pain, induration, sterile abscess with IM injection, thrombophlebitis, pain with IV injection

Other: Unpleasant taste, anaphylaxis, sensitization and systemic adverse effects with top sol, hypersensitivity reaction, hypotension with rapid IV infusion, bacterial or fungal superinfection

PATIENT CARE MANAGEMENT
Assessment
• Assess history or hypersensitivity to clindamycin, lincomycin
• Obtain C&S; may begin therapy before obtaining results
• Assess renal function (BUN, creatinine, I&O), hepatic function (ALT, AST, bilirubin), hematologic function (CBC, differential, platelet count), bowel pattern; with top use, assess skin

Interventions
• May administer PO without regard to meals (possible delay in peak levels if given with meals); decreased GI upset if administered with food
• Administer with as much fluid as possible to reduce eosphageal irritation
• Do not refrigerate oral susp (thickens); shake well before administering each dose; caps may be taken apart, mixed with food or fluid
• IM injection painful; administer deeply and rotate injection sites; do not administer >600 mg per injection site
• Do not premix IV with other medications; infuse separately
• Use large vein with small-bore needle to reduce local reaction; rotate site q48-72h
• Wash hands before, after top application; cleanse face; apply sparingly to affected areas; avoid eyes or mucous membranes
• Maintain age-appropriate fluid intake

> **NURSING ALERT**
> Discontinue drug if signs of hypersensitivity, pseudomembranous colitis develop
>
> Do not administer IV push

Evaluation
• Evaluate therapeutic response (decreased symptoms of infection)
• Evaluate renal function (BUN, creatinine, I&O), hepatic function (ALT, AST, bilirubin), hematologic function (CBC, differential, platelet count)
• Monitor for signs of pseudomembranous colitis (severe diarrhea, abdominal cramps, blood or mucus in stools); discontinue drug, notify care provider if these symptoms develop; symptoms may develop just after therapy begins or several wk after therapy has ended
• Observe for signs of superinfection (perineal itching, diaper rash, fever, malaise, redness, pain, swelling, drainage, rash, diarrhea, sore throat, change in cough or sputum)
• Evaluate IM site for tissue damage; IV site for vein irritation
• Discontinue top forms if rash, itching, swelling develop; systemic symptoms may develop with top applications

PATIENT AND FAMILY EDUCATION
Teach/instruct
• To take as directed at prescribed intervals for prescribed length of time
Warn/advise
• To notify care provider of hypersensitivity, side effects, superinfection
• To avoid use of OTC antidiarrheals if diarrhea develops

STORAGE

• Store all forms at room temp reconstituted oral susp stable at room temp for 14 days

---

clomipramine hydrochloride

Brand Name(s): Anafranil✤, Apo-Clomipromine✤, Gen-Clomipromine✤, Novo-Clomipromine✤

Classification: Tricyclic antidepressant

Pregnancy Category: C

AVAILABLE PREPARATIONS

Caps: 25 mg, 50 mg, 75 mg

DOSAGES AND ROUTES

• Safety and effectiveness have not been established in children <age 10. Dosage represents accepted standard practice recommendations

Depression

Children 10 yr to adolescent: Daily doses are given bid; initial daily dose of 1 mg/kg/24 hr is increased gradually to target dose of approximately 3 mg/kg/24 hr; maximum dose 200 mg/24 hr

Obsessive Compulsive Disorder

Children 10 yr to adolescent: Initial daily dose of 1 mg/kg/24 hr is increased gradually to target dose of 50 mg/24 hr; maximum dose 200 mg/24 hr

Adults: Initially 25 mg daily, taken in PM; at intervals of 3 to 4 days, dose may be increased cautiously prn by 25 mg/24 hr until a dose of 100 mg/24 hr is reached in about two wk; this larger dose should be divided and taken after meals, but may be given at hs in a single dose; usual maintenance dose is 50-150 mg/24 hr; maximum dose 250 mg/24 hr

MECHANISM AND INDICATIONS

Mechanism: Not completely known; thought that clomipramine inhib-

its serotonin uptake, increases dopamine metabolism

Indications: For use in treatment of depression, obsessive compulsive disorder; unlabeled uses include agoraphobia, anxiety, panic disorder, phobia; also helps to reduce the repetitive, ritualized behaviors of some autistic children

PHARMACOKINETICS

Onset of action: Therapeutic blood levels not yet established; therapeutic effects may take 2-4 wk; optimal response in treatment of obsessive compulsive behavior may require 3 or more mo of use

Half-life: 21 hr parent compound, 36 hr metabolite

Metabolism: Liver

Excretion: Urine

CONTRAINDICATIONS AND PRECAUTIONS

• Contraindicated with hypersensitivity to drug or any tricyclic antidepressant; arrhythmia, recent MI, undiagnosed syncope; active bone marrow depression or a current blood cell disorder; pts who have taken an MAOI within past 14 days; pregnancy

• Use cautiously with adrenalin-producing tumor; history of alcoholism; angina; asthma; history of bone marrow or blood cell disorder; cardiac disease, arrhythmia, heart failure; family history of sudden cardiac death or cardiomyopathy; known electrolyte abnormality with binging and purging; electroshock therapy; hyperthyroid or thyroid medication; narrow-angle glaucoma, increased intraocular pressure; kidney disease, impaired kidney function; liver disease, impaired liver function; paranoia; enlarged prostate; schizophrenia; seizure disorder; at risk for suicide; spasms of ureter or urethra; urinary retention; lactation; surgery under general anesthesia

INTERACTIONS

Drug

• Increased effects of all drugs with atropine-like or sedative effects, warfarin

---

✤ Available in Canada.

• Decreased effects of clonidine, guanadrel, guanethidine, possible
• Increased effects of clomipramine possible with cimetidine, estrogens, fluoxetine, methylphenidate, oral contraceptives, phenothiazines, ranitidine
• Decreased effects of clomipramine possible with barbiturates, carbamazepine, chloral hydrate, lithium, reserpine
• Increased sedation with alcohol, antihistamines, antipsychotics, barbiturates, glutethimide, chloral hydrate, sedatives, benzodiazepines
• Increased hypotension with methyldopa, β-adrenergic blockers, bethanidine, clonidine, diuretics
• Increased cardiotoxicity with quinidine, mesoridazine, thioridazine, thyroid preparations, phenothiazines
• Increased anticholinergic toxicity with antihistamines, antiparkinsonians, GI antispasmodics and antidiarrheals, thioridazine, OTC sleeping medications
• Decreased seizure threshold possible; dosage of anticonvulsant may need to be adjusted
• Increased hypertensive crisis, high fever, seizures possible when taken at same time as or within 14 days of MAOI type A drugs
• Hypertension or high fever with stimulant drugs (e.g., amphetamine, cocaine, epinephrine, phenylpropanolamine)
Lab
• Increased prolactin, TBG, liver enzymes (ALT, AST); liver toxicity may appear to be viral hepatitis
• Decreased serum thyroid hormone, RBCs, hemoglobin, WBCs, and platelets
Nutrition
• Avoid drinking alcohol

SIDE EFFECTS
CNS: Dizziness, tremors, aggressiveness, confusion, delirium, delusions, disorientation, drowsiness, hallucinations, headache, insomnia, light-headedness, mania, conversion of depression to mania in manic-depressive disorders, impaired memory, nervousness, aggravation of paranoid psychoses and schizophrenia, drug-induced seizures ($\approx 1\%$), weakness
CV: Arrhythmias, cardiac arrest, hypotension, tachycardia
DERM: Flushing, itching, photosensitivity, rash, sweating
EENT: Altered taste, blurred vision
GI: Constipation, dry mouth, appetite increase, diarrhea, hepatitis with or without jaundice, indigestion, liver toxicity, nausea, vomiting, weight gain
GU: Anorgasmy, delayed ejaculation, galactorrhea, hyperprolactinemia, impotence, urinary retention
HEME: Agranulocytosis, neutropenia, pancytopenia
Other: Drug fever, hyponatremia, muscle cramps, neuroleptic malignant syndrome

TOXICITY AND OVERDOSE
Clinical signs: Agitation, arrhythmias, confusion, delirium, drowsiness, fever, hallucinations, urinary retention, hypothermia, hypotension, seizures, stupor, sweating, tachycardia, tremors, unsteadiness
Treatment: Monitor vital signs, ECG, induce emesis, lavage, administer activated charcoal, anticonvulsant

PATIENT CARE MANAGEMENT
Assessment
• Assess history of hypersensitivity to drug
• Review family history for sudden cardiac death, patient's history for cardiac disease, arrhythmias, syncope, congenital hearing loss (associated with prolonged QT syndrome), schizophrenia, seizure disorder
• Obtain baseline studies (B/P, CBC counts, cardiac examination, baseline ECG, measurement of internal eye pressure, kidney function tests, liver function tests, pulse, serum electrolytes)
• Obtain BUN for patients with eating disorders

Interventions
• May be administered without regard to meals; administer with food or milk if GI upset occurs
• Increase fluids and bulk in diet if constipation occurs
• Offer sips of fluids, rinse with water, sugarless gum, or hard candy for dry mouth

---

NURSING ALERT

A possible effect of clomipramine is neuroleptic malignant syndrome; symptoms include fever, fast or irregular heartbeat, fast breathing, sweating, weakness, muscle stiffness, seizures, loss of bladder control; if these occur, obtain medical intervention immediately; monitor vital signs, ECG, urine output, renal function; symptom management with medications, hydration, cooling blankets

---

Evaluation
• Evaluate therapeutic response (ability to function in daily activities, ability to sleep throughout night; if taken for obsessive compulsive disorder, evaluate for relief of anxiety; obtain parent and teacher reports about status of OCD behaviors; if taken for depression, evaluate for symptoms of depression
• Evaluate mental status (affect, impulsiveness, mood, panic, psychiatric symptoms, sensorium, suicidal ideation)
• Obtain serial B/P readings and ECGs; if systolic B/P drops 20 mm Hg, withhold drug, notify physician
• Monitor and document pulse, B/P, and repeat ECG with each dose increase >3 mg/kg/24 hr
• Upper limits of cardiovascular parameters: Heart rate >130/min, systolic B/P >130 mm Hg, diastolic B/P >85 mm Hg, PR interval >0.20 sec, QRS interval >0.12 sec, or no more than 30% over baseline, QT corrected >0.45 sec; if readings exceed these limits, clomipramine should be discontinued
• Monitor and document height, wt, pulse, B/P, ECG when dose reaches a steady state, q 3-4 mo
• Monitor leukocytes, differential
• Monitor cardiac enzymes, periodically evaluate response and adjust dosage as necessary if pt is receiving long-term therapy
• Observe for any change in the frequency or severity of seizures if pt has history of seizures
• Evaluate bowel and bladder patterns for signs of constipation, urinary retention
• Observe for early indications of toxicity or overdose (confusion, agitation, rapid heart rate, heart irregularity); measurement of blood level of the drug may clarify the situation
• Taper dosage down when discontinuing this medication over a period of 3-4 wk; stopping this medication suddenly may cause irritability, insomnia, headache, dizziness, nausea, vomiting, diarrhea, muscle pain, weakness, malaise
• Obsessive-compulsive behavior may worsen when this drug is stopped
• Adjust the dosages of other drugs taken concurrently as necessary when discontinuing clomipramine

PATIENT AND FAMILY EDUCATION
Teach/instruct
• To take as directed at prescribed intervals for prescribed length of time
• That medication is most helpful when used as part of a comprehensive multimodal treatment program
• That therapeutic effects may take 2-4 wk
• To increase fluids, fiber in diet if constipation occurs
• That neuroleptic malignant syndrome is a possible effect; symptoms include fever, fast or irregular heartbeat, fast breathing, sweating, weakness, muscle stiff-

ness, seizures, loss of bladder control; if these occur, obtain medical help immediately
• To make sure medication is swallowed
• That drug may be taken without regard to meals; if GI symptoms occur, take with food or milk
• To rinse with water, take sips of fluid, sugarless gum, hard candy for dry mouth
Warn/advise
• That medication may cause drowsiness; be careful on bicycles, skates, skateboards, while driving, or with other activities requiring alertness
• To avoid consuming alcohol, other CNS depressants while taking clomipramine
• To limit food intake to avoid excessive wt gain if necessary
• To monitor for constipation; it is more likely to occur in children than adults taking clomipramine
• That drug may cause seizures, or impair mental alertness, judgment, physical coordination, and reaction time; restrict activities as necessary
• That medicine may cause skin to be more sensitive to sunlight than usual; stay out of direct sunlight, especially between 10 AM and 3 PM, if possible; if pt must be outside, protective clothing, a hat, and sunglasses should be worn; put on sun block with a skin protection factor (SPF) of ≥15
• To use caution when exposed to heat; clomipramine may impair the body's adaptation to hot environments, increasing risk of heat stroke; avoid saunas
• That tobacco smoking may delay elimination of drug and necessitate dosage adjustment
• That marijuana smoking may increase drowsiness, mouth dryness; it may also reduce effectiveness of clomipramine
• That clomipramine may mask the symptoms of poisoning caused by handling organophosphorus insecticides; read labels of such insecticides carefully

• Not to stop taking medication quickly after long-term use; stopping suddenly may cause headache, nausea, vomiting, muscle pain, weakness
STORAGE
• Store at room temp in tightly closed container
• Do not freeze

clonazepam

Brand Name(s): Klonopin♣, PMS-Clonazepam♣, Rivotril♣, Syn-Clomazepam♣

Classification: Anticonvulsant, benzodiazepine

Controlled Substance Schedule IV

Pregnancy Category: C

AVAILABLE PREPARATIONS
Tabs: 0.5 mg, 1 mg, 2 mg
ROUTES AND DOSAGES
Children <10 yr or <30 kg: PO 0.01-0.03 mg/kg/24 hr; initially divided bid-tid; increase by 0.25-0.5 mg/kg/24 hr q 3 days, until seizures are controlled or adverse effects are seen; to a usual dose of 0.1-0.2 mg/kg/24 hr divided bid-tid
Children ≥10 and adults: Initial daily dose not to exceed 1.5 mg divided tid; may increase by 0.5-1 mg until seizures are controlled; usual maintenance dose 0.05-0.2 mg/kg, not to exceed 20 mg/24 hr
MECHANISM AND INDICATIONS
Mechanism: Suppresses seizure activity in the cortex, thalamus, limbic systems, probably through potentiation of neural inhibition mediated by γ-aminobutyric acid (GABA)
Indications: Used to treat myoclonic, atonic, absence seizures; to suppress or eliminate attacks of sleep-related nocturnal myoclonus (restless leg syndrome); to treat tonic–clonic psychomotor, infantile spasm seizures

♣ Available in Canada.

PHARMACOKINETICS
Onset of action: 20-60 min
Peak: 2 hr
Distribution: Widely throughout the body
Duration: Children 6-8 hr; adults up to 12 hr
Half-life: 18-50 hr
Metabolism: Liver, metabolized to glucuronide or sulfate conjugates
Excretion: Urine
Therapeutic level: 20-80 ng/ml

CONTRAINDICATIONS AND PRECAUTIONS
• Contraindicated with known hypersensitivity to clonazepam, other benzodiazepines; with hepatic disease, chronic respiratory problems, acute narrow angle glaucoma
• Use with caution with renal dysfunction, pregnancy

INTERACTIONS
Drug
• Additive effect with use of other CNS depressants (alcohol, narcotics, tranquilizers, anxiolytics, barbiturates, other anticonvulsants)
• Increased phenytoin levels when taken together
• Increased serum levels may occur when taken with cimetidine or disulfiram
• Decreased levels of both carbamazepine, clonazepam when taken together
• May induce absence seizures when used with valproic acid

SIDE EFFECTS
CNS: Drowsiness, sedation, behavioral changes (particularly in pts with brain damage, mental retardation, or mental illness), aggression, irritability, hyperactivity, confusion, depression, dizziness, tremor, vertigo, headache, insomnia, choreiform movements (most related to CNS depression)
CV: Palpitations, thrombophlebitis
DERM: Skin rash, hirsutism or hair loss (alopecia)
EENT: Hypersalivation, diplopia, nystagmus, abnormal eye movement, rhinorrhea, difficulty swallowing

GI: Dry mouth, thirst, sore gums, nausea, changes in appetite, anorexia, gastritis, constipation
GU: Dysuria, enuresis, urinary retention, nocturia
HEME: Anemia, leukopenia, thrombocytopenia, eosinophilia
RESP: Respiratory depression, increased bronchial secretion, dyspnea, chest congestion
Other: Metabolic hypercalcemia, hepatomegaly, liver enzyme changes

TOXICITY AND OVERDOSE
Clinical signs: Ataxia, confusion, coma, decreased reflexes and hypotension
Treatment: Gastric lavage, supportive care; vasopressors should be used to treat hypotension; clonazepam not dialyzable

PATIENT CARE MANAGEMENT
Assessment
• Assess history of hypersensitivity to clonazepam, other benzodiazepines
• Assess baseline laboratory studies including CBC, differential, liver function (ALT, AST, bilirubin, alk phos), renal function (BUN, creatinine, I&O)
• Assess seizure type, determine if clonazepam is appropriate anticonvulsant for this type of seizure
Interventions
• Administer with food or milk to reduce GI symptoms if necessary; antacids may retard absorption, if used should be administered about 1 hr before or after medication dose
• Initiate at modest dose
• Increase dosage level to the point of intolerable side effects as needed to control seizures
• Initiate another anticonvulsant in the same way if drug is only partially effective
• Gradually withdraw the drug if not effective, initiate another anticonvulsant if necessary
• Increase dosage frequency if break-through seizures occur at times when serum levels are at

---

trough or peak to provide more even coverage

Evaluation
• Evaluate therapeutic response (seizure control); initially done more frequently until seizures controlled then q 3-6 mo, or if seizure break-throughs or side effects
• Monitor anticonvulsant levels periodically
• Monitor side effects including significant elevation of liver function (ALT, AST, bilirubin, alk phos), abnormalities in hematologic testing or signs of bone marrow suppression, with fever, sore throat, mouth ulcers, easy bruising, petechial or purpuric hemorrhages

PATIENT AND FAMILY EDUCATION
Teach/instruct
• To take medication as prescribed, not to increase or decrease dosage independently; also reinforce that medication should not be stopped suddenly
• Take with food to decrease GI upset; note that antacids may retard absorption; if used, antacids should be taken approximately 1 hr before or after medication dose
Warn/advise
• To notify care provider of side effects; report immediately signs or symptoms of unusual bleeding, bruising, jaundice, dark urine, pale stools, abdominal pain, impotence, fever, chills, sore throat, mouth ulcers, edema, disturbances in mood, alertness, or coordination
• To keep a record of seizure activity
• That unpleasant side effects may decrease as the pt becomes more used to drug
• That drug may initially be more sedating; avoid hazardous tasks (biking, skating, skateboarding) until stabilized on medication
• To make other health care providers aware of drug usage to avoid potential interactions with

other drugs; carry medical alert identification
• To alert health care provider immediately should pregnancy occur

STORAGE
• Store tabs at room temp

---

clonidine

Brand Name(s): Apo-Clonidine✤, Catapres✤, Catapres-TTS✤, Clonidine HCL, Dixarit✤, Novo-Clonidine✤, Nu-Clonidine✤

Classification: Antihypertensive, α-adrenergic agonist

Pregnancy Category: C

AVAILABLE PREPARATIONS
Tabs: (clonidine hydrochloride) 0.1 mg, 0.2 mg, 0.3 mg; *transDERMal-1 patch:* 0.1 mg/24 hr; *transDERMal-2 patch:* 0.2 mg/24 hr; *transDERMal-3 patch:* 0.3 mg/24 hr

DOSAGES AND ROUTES
Antihypertensive
Children <6 yr: PO 5-10 mcg/kg/24 hr divided q6h; may increase gradually at 5-7 day intervals to maximum of 25 mcg/kg/24 hr divided q6h; maximum dose 0.9 mg/24 hr
Children >6 yr: PO 0.05 mg bid, increase 0.1-0.2 mg until desired effect is achieved
Adults: PO 0.1 mg bid; usual maintenance dose 0.2-1.2 mg/24 hr divided bid-qid
Narcotic Withdrawal
Neonate: PO 3-4 mcg/kg/24 hr divided q4-6h
Management of ADD/ADHD
Initial dose of clonidine 0.05 mg at hs; after 3-5 days add 0.05 mg in the AM; additional dosage increases are made by adding 0.05 mg alternating in the AM at noon, or in the PM every 3-5 days; maximum dose 0.3 mg (3-5 mcg/kg/24 hr) in 3 divided doses.

✤ Available in Canada.

Tourette Syndrome

Children >12 yr and adults: PO, begin at very low dosages, 0.05 mg/24 hr with gradual increases over several wk to the range of 0.15-0.2 mg/24 hr given in 2 divided doses; transDERMal patch, 0.1 mg/24 hr, apply once every 7 days; may gradually increase up to 0.3 mg/24 hr

Adult: 0.1 mg bid

• Patches should not be used on children <age 12

• Dosages >0.5 mg/24 hr often produce a significant degree of side effects, which often outweighs the benefit

• Dosage modification may be required with renal impairment

• Therapeutic dosages of methylphenidate can frequently be decreased by 30%-50% when used in conjunction with clonidine

MECHANISM AND INDICATIONS

Mechanism: Clonidine stimulates α_2-adrenoreceptors in the brain stem, thus activating an inhibitory neuron, decreasing activity of vasomotor center in brain; this reduces impulses in sympathetic nervous system, resulting in decreases in B/P, pulse rate, cardiac output

Indications: Clonidine is used to treat high B/P; opioid withdrawal; to decrease states of hyperarousal and panic, specifically anxiety disorders, mania, posttraumatic stress disorder, social phobia; for highly aroused, overactive children who respond poorly to or have persistent side effects from stimulants; useful as an adjunct to methylphenidate in children with ADHD who have a history of very early onset of hyperactivity, aggression, explosiveness, oppositional behavior; effective in treatment of ADHD and ADD, but does not alleviate symptoms of distractibility, inattentiveness; clonidine has been clinically useful in treating overfocused children, adolescents who are compulsive, rigid, excessively deliberate, have difficulty changing activities; tics and obsessive compulsive disorder associated with Tourette syndrome, children who develop tics or Tourette syndrome with the use of stimulants; ADHD-like symptoms in some autistic children; in the management of neuroleptic-induced akathisia

• Clonidine is used as an aid in diagnosis of pheochromocytoma, growth hormone deficiency

PHARMACOKINETICS

Onset of action: Clinical response may become apparent in about 4 wk, but may take 2-3 mo to be optimally effective; PO onset of effects 30-60 min

Peak: Within 1-5 hr

Duration: 6-10 hr

Half-life: Neonates 44-72 hr, adults with normal renal function 6-20 hr, with renal impairment 18-41 hr

Metabolism: Liver, to inactive metabolites

Excretion: 65% in urine (32% unchanged), 22% in feces; in breast milk

CONTRAINDICATIONS AND PRECAUTIONS

• Contraindicated with hypersensitivity to clonidine hydrochloride or any component; family or personal history of depression; cardiovascular and renal disease

• Use cautiously with asthma, cerebrovascular disease, recent MI, coronary insufficiency, sinus node dysfunction, COPD, DM, Raynaud's disease, renal impairment, thyroid disease, lactation

INTERACTIONS

Drug

• Decreased effects of levodopa possible, causing an increase in Parkinson symptoms

• Increased sedation possible with CNS depressants (e.g., narcotics, sedatives, alcohol, anesthetics)

• Increased bradycardia possible with β blockers, cardiac glycosides

• β blockers may increase rebound hypertension seen with clonidine withdrawal; discontinue β blocker

---

several days before clonidine is tapered off
• Increased hypotensive effects with diuretics
• Decreased effectiveness possible with tricyclic antidepressants, MAOIs, appetite suppressants, other antihypertensives
• Increase cardiotoxicity possible with cocaine

Lab
• Increased BG
• Decreased VMA, catecholamines, aldosterone

Nutrition
• Avoid excessive salt
• No beverage restrictions; may be taken with milk
• Combined effects with alcohol can cause marked drowsiness, exaggerated reduction in B/P

SIDE EFFECTS
CNS: Drowsiness, fatigue, headache, sedation, anxiety, delirium, depression, dizziness, vivid dreams, hallucinations, insomnia, malaise, nightmares, restlessness
CV: Hypotension, palpitations, arrhythmia, bradycardia, lowered cardiac output, CHF, ECG abnormalities, mild Raynaud's phenomenon, tachycardia, decreased peripheral vascular resistance
DERM: Rash, alopecia, edema, excoriation with transDERMal patch, facial pallor, hives, itching, burning papules, or local skin reactions with patch (transDERMal administration of clonidine can be quite effective but may result in significant skin irritation in 40% of cases)
EENT: Dry eyes, parotid pain, taste change
GI: Nausea, vomiting, anorexia, increased appetite, constipation, dry mouth, GI distress, wt gain
GU: Impotence, nocturia, dysuria, gynecomastia
Other: Hyperglycemia, leg cramps, muscle or joint pain, Na and water retention

TOXICITY AND OVERDOSE
Clinical signs: Decreased B/P, heart rate, respiratory rate; pts may appear to have opioid overdose (stuporous or comatose with small pupils)
Treatment: Provide ventilatory support, IV fluids or pressors for hypotension and atropine for bradycardia

PATIENT CARE MANAGEMENT
Assessment
• Assess history of hypersensitivity to drug
• Obtain baseline studies (pulse, B/P, baseline ECG); blood studies (neutrophils, platelets), renal studies (protein, BUN, creatinine), liver studies (ALT, AST, bilirubin)

Interventions
• Tab form is most therapeutic if administered in divided doses tid-qid
• Administer 1 hr ac
• TransDERMal patch is effective for 5-7 days; an advantage in situations where compliance is a problem
• Pay close attention to titration of this medication since sedative effects, which may occur for several wk, can be detrimental to the child's overall academic, social, emotional adjustment
• Assess B/P 2-3 hrs after dose
• Infuse 0.9% NaCl IV, as ordered, to expand fluid volume if severe hypotension occurs
• Sudden withdrawal of clonidine may precipitate a hypertensive crisis that could be life-threatening; hypertensive rebound begins 18-20 hr after last dose; treatment includes combined α- and β-adrenergic blockers or sodium nitroprusside

> **NURSING ALERT**
> Do not stop this medication abruptly; B/P could rapidly increase; other symptoms include agitation, anxiety, increased heart rate, tremor, insomnia, sweating, palpitations; to discontinue, taper dose gradually over >1 wk

210 • clonidine

Evaluation
- Evaluate therapeutic response (ability to function in daily activities, to sleep throughout the night); activity level, impulsivity, distractibility, attending; obtain parent and teacher reports about anxiety, panic, tics, attention, behavioral performance
- Evaluate mental status (mood, sensorium, affect, impulsiveness, suicidal ideation, psychiatric symptoms)
- Pulse and B/P should be monitored and recorded q 2 wk for 2 mo, then q 3 mo; a slight decrease in systolic B/P is often detected, but generally produces no significant symptoms or discomfort
- Monitor renal studies (protein, BUN, creatinine); watch for increased levels indicating nephrotic syndrome
- Monitor for edema in feet, legs; dipstick of urine for protein; if protein is increased, collect 24 hr urinary protein; monitor for renal symptoms (polyuria, oliguria, frequency)
- Monitor K⁺ levels, although hyperkalemia rarely occurs
- Monitor for allergic reaction (rash, fever, pruritus, urticaria); clonidine should be discontinued if antihistamines fail to help; if allergic reaction is in response to patch, switch to oral form
- Monitor for symptoms of CHF (edema, dyspnea, wet rales)
- Schedule a periodic eye exam to look for retinal degeneration
- Taper pt from drug when discontinuing rather than stop it suddenly in any pt who has received high dosages for more than 2-3 wk; dosage should be reduced gradually over 3-4 days, with periodic monitoring of B/P

PATIENT AND FAMILY EDUCATION
Teach/instruct
- To take as directed at prescribed intervals for prescribed length of time
- That medication is most helpful when used as part of a comprehensive multimodal treatment program
- To rinse with water, take sips of fluid, sugarless gum, hard candy for dry mouth
- Not to stop taking this medication without prescriber approval
- To increase fluids, fiber in diet if constipation occurs

Warn/advise
- Not to discontinue medication quickly after long-term use; stopping suddenly may cause withdrawal symptoms (anxiety, increased B/P, headache, insomnia, increased pulse, tremors, nausea, sweating); a severe withdrawal reaction with very high B/P can occur within 12-48 hr after last dose; if need to discontinue, taper dose gradually over >1 wk
- To make sure PO medication is swallowed
- To use caution on exposure to heat; drug may impair perspiration; hot environments may reduce B/P significantly
- To use caution with exposure to cold; drug may cause painful blanching, numbness of hands, feet when exposed to cold air, water (Raynaud's phenomenon)
- To use caution with heavy exercise, exertion; drug may intensify hypertensive response to isometric exercise
- May cause drowsiness; be careful on bicycles, skates, skateboards, while driving, with other activities requiring alertness
- Not to use OTC cold, cough, or allergy products unless directed by prescriber
- To avoid sunlight, wear sunscreen if in sunlight; photosensitivity may occur
- To notify prescriber if any of the following occur: mouth sores, sore throat, fever, swelling of hands or feet, irregular heart beat, chest pain, signs of angioedema

STORAGE
- Store patches in cool environment
- Store tabs in tight containers

clorazepate dipotassium

Brand Name(s): Apo-Clorazepate✤, Gen-Xene, Novo-Clopate✤, Tranxene✤, Tranxene-SD, Tranxene-SD Half Strength

Classification: Mild tranquilizer, benzodiazepine

Pregnancy Category: D

AVAILABLE PREPARATIONS

Caps: 3.75 mg, 7.5 mg, 15 mg (clorazepate dipotassium)
Tabs: 3.75 mg, 7.5 mg, 15 mg (Gen-Xene, Tranxene)
Single dose tabs: 11.25 mg, 22.5 mg (Tranxene-SD, Tranxene-SD Half Strength)

DOSAGES AND ROUTES

• Therapeutic range: 0.12-1 mcg/ml
• Safety and effectiveness have notbeen established in children <9 yr
• Give smallest dose possible, children may be sensitive to benzodiazepines

Anticonvulsant

Children 9-12 yr: PO initial 3.75-7.5 mg/dose bid; increase by 3.75 mg at weekly intervals; maximum 60 mg/24 hr divided bid-tid

Children >12 and adults: PO initial up to 7.5 mg/dose bid-tid; increase by 7.5 mg at weekly intervals; usual dose 0.5-1 mg/kg/24 hr; maximum dose 90 mg/24 hr; up to 3 mg/kg/24 hr has been used

Anxiety

Adults: PO 15-60 mg/24 hr divided bid-qid, or as single dose of 15-22.5 mg at hs; continuous use on a regular schedule for 5-7 days usually necessary to determine effectiveness

Alcohol Withdrawal

Adults: PO initial dose 30 mg, then 30-60 mg in divided doses on first day; second day 45-90 mg in divided doses; third day 22.5-45 mg in divided doses; fourth day 15-30 mg in divided doses; then reduce daily dose to 7.5-15 mg; maximum dose 90 mg/24 hr

MECHANISM AND INDICATIONS

Mechanism: Potentiates the action of γ aminobutyric acid (GABA) in the limbic system and reticular formation

Indications: For use in short-term relief of symptoms of mild-to-moderate anxiety, for symptomatic relief in alcohol withdrawal, and with other drugs to manage partial seizures; unlabeled use for irritable bowel syndrome

PHARMACOKINETICS

Onset of action: PO 15 min; continual use on a regular schedule for 5-7 days is usually necessary to determine effectiveness in relieving moderate anxiety

Peak: PO 1-2 hr
Duration: 4-6 hr
Half-life: Adults 30-100 hr
Metabolism: Liver
Excretion: Urine

CONTRAINDICATIONS AND PRECAUTIONS

• Contraindicated in pts with hypersensitivity to benzodiazepines, clorazepate, or any component of this medication; history of drug addiction, pre-existing CNS depression, hyperactive children; narrow-angle glaucoma; psychosis; severe uncontrolled pain, pregnancy, lactation

• Use cautiously with asthma, depression, emphysema, epilepsy, kidney disease, liver disease, myasthenia gravis, psychiatric disorders, history of alcoholism or drug abuse, allergy to tartrazine (FD&C Yellow No. 5), elderly, very ill, planning pregnancy

INTERACTIONS

Drug

• Increased effects with alcohol, antidepressants, antihistamines, barbiturates, cimetidine, oral contraceptives, CNS depressants, disulfiram, isoniazid
• Decreased effects with rifampin, theophylline

✤ Available in Canada.

- Increased effects of digoxin, and may cause digoxin toxicity
- Decreased effects of levodopa

Lab
- Increased AST/ALT, serum bilirubin
- Decreased RAIU
- Falsely elevated 17-OHCS
- False positive urine screening tests for drug abuse, depending on amount of drug taken and testing method used

Nutrition
- Do not drink alcohol
- Some preparations contain tartrazine (FD&C Yellow No. 5)

SIDE EFFECTS

CNS: Dizziness, drowsiness, decreased activity, amnesia, anxiety, apathy, ataxia, behavior changes, confusion, crying, delirium, depression, disorientation, vivid dreams, euphoria, fatigue, hallucinations, hangover, headache, insomnia, lethargy, nervousness, restlessness, seizures, stimulation, tremors, vertigo, weakness

CV: Orthostatic hypotension, ECG changes, hypotension, palpitations, tachycardia

EENT: Blurred vision, yellowing of eyes, glassy-eyed appearance, sore gums, decreased hearing, dry mouth, mydriasis, nasal congestion, increased salivation, slurred speech, difficulty swallowing, tinnitus, coated tongue, double vision, loss of voice

DERM: Dermatitis, excessive hair growth, hair loss, hives, itching, rash, yellowing of skin

GI: Anorexia, constipation, diarrhea, dry mouth, nausea, vomiting, dehydration, hiccups, abnormal liver function

GU: Incontinence, changes in sex drive, menstrual problems, urine retention

HEME: Abnormal blood counts (CBC)

Other: Balance problems, edema, fainting, fever, galactorrhea, gynecomastia, joint pain, swollen lymph nodes, uncontrollable muscle movement, sweating, ankle and facial swelling, wt gain or loss; with long-term use, physical and psychological dependence, liver or kidney injury, reduced Hct; unusual reactions are anxiety, excitement, hallucinations, insomnia, increased muscle spasms, stimulation, acute rage

TOXICITY AND OVERDOSE

Clinical signs: Apnea, marked drowsiness, feeling of drunkenness, unsteady gait, hypoactive reflexes, hypotension, respiratory depression, slurred speech, stupor progressing to deep sleep or coma, tremor, weakness

Treatment: Support B/P and respiration; treat hypotension with norepinephrine, phenylephrine, or dopamine; if comatose, use gastric lavage with endotracheal tube to prevent aspiration; flumazenil, a benzodiazepine antagonist, can reverse the effects of clorazepate; action of flumazenil may be shorter than duration of benzodiazepine; repeat doses as needed; dialysis is of limited value

PATIENT CARE MANAGEMENT

Assessment
- Assess history of hypersensitivity to drug
- Assess ability to function in daily activities, to sleep throughout the night
- Assess mental status (mood, sensorium, affect, impulsiveness, suicidal ideation)
- Assess baseline physical assessment, including orthostatic B/P
- Assess baseline alk phos, AST, ALT, bilirubin, CBC, creatinine, LDH

Interventions
- Limit continual PO use to 1-3 wk
- May be given PO on an empty stomach; if GI symptoms occur, take with food or milk
- Cap may be opened, regular tab may be crushed for administration; ext rel tabs should not be crushed
- Increase fluids, fiber in diet if constipation occurs
- Take sips of fluid, sugarless

gum, hard candy for dry mouth; rinse with water
• Avoid excessive intake of caffeine, such as in coffee, tea, or cola
• Do not drink alcohol

Evaluation
• Evaluate therapeutic response (anxiety, restlessness, ability to function in daily activities, to sleep throughout the night)
• Evaluate mental status (mood, sensorium, affect, impulsiveness, suicidal ideation, thoughts)
• Monitor orthostatic B/P; if systolic B/P drops 20 mm Hg, hold drug and notify prescriber
• Monitor alk phos AST, ALT, bilirubin, CBC, creatinine, I&O, LDH for long term therapy
• Monitor for physical dependency and withdrawal symptoms with long-term use (headache, nausea, vomiting, muscle pain, weakness)

PATIENT AND FAMILY EDUCATION
Teach/instruct
• To take as directed at prescribed intervals for prescribed length of time
• To make sure medication is swallowed
• That medication is most helpful when used as part of a comprehensive multimodal treatment program
• Not to discontinue this drug abruptly if taken for more than 4 wk; (withdrawal symptoms include confusion, depression, hallucinations, muscle cramping, seizures, sweating, tremor, vomiting)

Warn/advise
• That clorazepate can produce psychological or physical dependence if used in large doses for an extended period of time
• To avoid ingesting alcohol, other CNS depressants
• To avoid OTC preparations unless approved by prescriber
• That medication may cause drowsiness; be careful on bicycles, skates, skateboards, while driving, with other activities requiring alertness
• If taken at hs, significant impairment of intellectual and physical skills may persist the following day
• That heavy smoking may reduce calming action
• That marijuana smoking may increase sedation and significant impairment of intellectual and physical performance

STORAGE
• Store at room temp

---

clotrimazole

Brand Name(s): Mycelex troches, Lotrimin AF, Mycelex, Mycelex OTC, FemCare, Gyne-Lotrimin, Mycelex G, Mycelex F

Classification: Antifungal agent

Pregnancy Category: B

AVAILABLE PREPARATIONS
Vaginal tabs: 100 mg, 500 mg
Vaginal cream: 1%
Top cream, lotion, sol: 1%
Troches: 10 mg

ROUTES AND DOSAGES
PO (troches): 10 mg troche dissolved slowly over 15-30 min 5 × per 24 hr for 15 days
TOP (cream lotion, solution): Apply to lesions bid for up to 8 wk
Vulvovaginal Candidiasis
Tabs: Insert vaginally one 500 mg tab at bedtime; or insert one 100 mg tab at bedtime for 7 days; or insert one 200 mg tab at bedtime for 3 days
Cream: Insert vaginally with applicator at bedtime for 7-14 days

MECHANISM AND INDICATIONS
Antifungal mechanism: Alters fungal cell membrane permeability; inhibits or kills many fungi, including yeast and dermatophytes
Indications: For use in tinea pedis, tinea cruris, tinea corporis, tinea versicolor; cutaneous, vulvovaginal, oropharyngeal candidiasis

---

♣ Available in Canada.

PHARMACOKINETICS
Absorption: Negligible through intact skin
Distribution: Minimal with local application

CONTRAINDICATIONS AND PRECAUTIONS
• Contraindicated with known hypersensitivity
• Use cautiously (vaginally) during first trimester of pregnancy, with hepatic dysfunction

INTERACTIONS
Drug
None reported
Lab
LFTs (AST, ALT, bilirubin) may be abnormal with use of troches

SIDE EFFECTS
GI: Abdominal cramps
GU: Vaginal burning, urinary frequency
Local: Blistering, pruritus, erythema, burning, irritation

TOXICITY AND OVERDOSE
Clinical signs: Severe side effects
Treatment: Discontinue drug

PATIENT CARE MANAGEMENT
Assessment
• Assess history of hypersensitivity to drug
• Assess mouth, skin, vulvovaginal area for appropriateness of treatment
Interventions
• Insert tabs and vaginal cream high into vagina; use sanitary napkin to absorb discharge
• Wash hands well before, after treatment
• Troches not recommended in children <3 yr
• Troches must dissolve slowly in mouth for maximum effect; do not chew
• Completely cover lesions with top application
Evaluation
• Evaluate therapeutic response (relief of signs and symptoms)

PATIENT AND FAMILY EDUCATION
Teach/instruct
• To take as directed at prescribed intervals for prescribed length of time
Warn/advise
• To call care provider if irritation develops
• To wash hands well before, after treatment
• To complete full course of treatment; call care provider if no improvement noted in 4 wk

STORAGE
• Store all forms at room temp

---

cloxacillin
Brand Name(s): Cloxapen, Tegopen
Classification: Antibiotic (penicillinase-resistant penicillin)
Pregnancy Category: B

AVAILABLE PREPARATIONS
Oral susp: 125 mg/5 ml
Caps: 250 mg, 500 mg

ROUTES AND DOSAGES
Children >1 mo, wt <20 kg: PO 50-100 mg/kg/24 hr divided q6h
Children >20kg and adults: 250-1000 mg q6h; maximum dose 4 g/24 hr

MECHANISM AND INDICATIONS
Antibiotic mechanism: Bactericidal; inhibits bacterial cell wall synthesis by adhering to bacterial penicillin-binding proteins
Indications: Effective against gram-positive cocci including *Staphylococcus aureus, S. epidermidis, Streptococcus pyogenes, Str. faecalis, Str. pneumoniae,* and infections caused by penicillinase-producing *Staphylococcus;* used to treat respiratory tract, skin, soft tissue, bone, joint infections

PHARMACOKINETICS
Peak: 0.5-1.0 hr
Distribution: Throughout body; highest concentrations in liver, spleen, kidney, bile, bone
Half-life: Neonates 0.8-1.5 hr; children 0.4-0.8 hr

✤ Available in Canada.

Metabolism: Liver
Excretion: Urine, bile

CONTRAINDICATIONS AND PRECAUTIONS

• Contraindicated with known hypersensitivity to cloxacillin, penicillins, cephalosporins; in neonates
• Use cautiously with impaired renal or hepatic function; history of colitis or other GI distress; pregnancy

INTERACTIONS

Drug
• Synergistic antimicrobial activity against certain organisms with use of aminoglycosides
• Increased serum concentrations with use of probenecid
• Decreased effectiveness with use of erythromycins, tetracyclines, chloramphenicol

Lab
• False positive for urine protein
• Increased liver function tests
• Decreased uric acid

Nutrition
• Decreased absorption if given with meals, acidic fruit juices, citrus fruits, acidic beverages such as cola drinks

SIDE EFFECTS

GI: Nausea, vomiting, epigastric distress, diarrhea, pseudomembranous colitis, intrahepatic cholestasis
GU: Acute interstitial nephritis
HEME: Eosinophilia, leukopenia, granulocytopenia, thrombocytopenia, agranulocytosis
Other: Hypersensitivity (rash, urticaria, chills, fever, wheezing, anaphylaxis), bacterial or fungal superinfection

TOXICITY AND OVERDOSE

Clinical signs: Neuromuscular irritability; seizures
Treatment: Supportive care; if ingested within 4 hr, empty the stomach by induced emesis or gastric lavage, followed by activated charcoal to reduce absorption

PATIENT CARE MANAGEMENT

Assessment
• Assess history of hypersensitivity to cloxacillin, penicillins, cephalosporins
• Obtain C&S; may begin therapy before obtaining results
• Assess renal function (BUN, creatinine, I&O), hepatic function (ALT, AST, bilirubin), hematologic function (CBC, differential, platelet count), particularly for long-term therapy

Interventions
• Administer penicillins at least 1 hr before bacteriostatic antibiotics (tetracyclines, erythromycins, chloramphenicol)
• Administer PO 1 hr ac or 2 hr after meals; give with water; avoid acidic beverages; shake susp well before administering; caps may be taken apart, mixed with food or fluid
• Maintain age-appropriate fluid intake
• For group A β-hemolytic streptococcal infection, provide 10-day course to prevent risk of acute rheumatic fever, glomerulonephritis

> **NURSING ALERT**
> Discontinue drug if signs of hypersensitivity, interstitial nephritis, pseudomembranous colitis develop

Evaluation
• Evaluate therapeutic response (decreased symptoms of infection)
• Monitor for signs of superinfection (perineal itching, diaper rash, fever, malaise, redness, pain, swelling, drainage, rash, diarrhea, sore throat, change in cough or sputum)
• Observe for signs of allergic reaction (wheezing, tightness in chest, urticaria), especially within 20-30 min of first dose
• Monitor bowel pattern; diarrhea may be symptomatic of pseudomembranous colitis

C

• Monitor renal function (BUN, creatinine, I&O), hepatic function (ALT, AST, bilirubin), electrolyte levels, especially K⁺ and Na
• Monitor for signs of bleeding (ecchymosis, bleeding gums, hematuria, daily stool guaiac); monitor pro-times and platelet counts

PATIENT AND FAMILY EDUCATION
Teach/instruct
• To take as directed at prescribed intervals for prescribed length of time
Warn/advise
• To notify care provider of hypersensitivity, side effects, superinfection

STORAGE
• Store powder, caps at room temp
• Reconstituted susp stable when refrigerated for 14 days; label date and time of reconstitution

---

codeine
Classification: Narcotic analgesic, opiate agonist, antipyretic
Controlled Substance Schedule II
Pregnancy Category: C

AVAILABLE PREPARATIONS
Syr: 10 mg/5 ml, 60 mg/5 ml (codeine sulfate)
Tab: 15 mg, 30 mg, 60 mg (codeine sulfate)
Inj: 30 mg/ml, 60 mg/ml (codeine phosphate)

ROUTES AND DOSAGES
Antitussive
Children 2-5 yr: PO 2.5-5 mg q4-6h, not to exceed 30 mg/24 hr
Children 6-11 yr: PO 5-10 mg q4-6h; not to exceed 60 mg/24 hr
Children >12 yr and adults: PO 10-20 mg q4-6h; not to exceed 120 mg/24 hr
Analgesia
Children: PO/IM/SC 0.5-1 mg/kg/dose q4-6hr; maximum dose 60 mg/dose

Adults: PO/IM/SC 15-60 mg/dose q4-6h

MECHANISM AND INDICATIONS
Mechanism: Suppresses cough by action on the medulla cough center; acts on CNS by using neurotransmitters to create analgesia; binds to opiate receptors in CNS; alters perception of and response to painful stimuli
Indications: Used to treat mild-to-moderate pain and to suppress cough

PHARMACOKINETICS
Onset: PO 30-45 min, IM/SC 10-30 min
Peak: PO 60-120 min, IM 30-60 min, SC: not known
Duration: 4-6 hr
Half-life: 2.5-4 hr
Metabolism: Liver
Excretion: Kidneys
Absorption: Moderately absorbed (50%) from GI tract; completely absorbed from IM sites; PO and parenteral doses are not equal

CONTRAINDICATIONS AND PRECAUTIONS
• Contraindicated with known hypersensitivities, pregnancy, lactation; not used as antitussive in children <2 yr; ext rel oral susp not used in children <6 yr; preparations with sulfite not to be given to those with sulfite allergy
• Use cautiously with head trauma; increased ICP; severe renal, hepatic, and pulmonary disease; hypothyroidism; adrenal insufficiency; alcoholism; undiagnosed abdominal pain; respiratory depression, altered mental status, anemia

INTERACTIONS
Drug
• Additive CNS effects with alcohol, antihistamines, sedative/hypnotics
• Increased metabolism and possible decreased analgesic effectiveness when smoking
• Precipitates narcotic withdrawal when administered with partial

antagonist (buprenorphine, butorphanol, nalbuphine, or pentazocine)
• Antagonized action possible with phenothiazines
• Increased effects if given with dextroamphetamine
• Increased effects of neuromuscular-blocking agents possible
• Decreased effects of diuretics in CHF possible

Lab
• Increased serum amylase and lipase; wait 24 hr after last dose of codeine
• Decreased serum and urine 17-KS, 17-OHCS

INCOMPATIBILITIES
• When administered IM/SC, incompatible with aminophylline, heparin, methicillin, nitrofurantoin, phenobarbital, $NaHCO_3$ (consult with pharmacist before mixing with any sol)

SIDE EFFECTS
CNS: Sedation, confusion, behavior changes, dizziness, depression, coma, euphoria, restlessness, insomnia, floating feeling, unusual dreams, hallucinations, dysphoria, agitation, lethargy
CV: Circulatory depression, orthostatic hypotension, palpitation, bradycardia, tachycardia
DERM: Rash, erythema, urticaria, pruritus, facial flushing (indicates hypersensitivity reaction), sweating
EENT: Miosis, diplopia, blurred vision
GI: Nausea, vomiting, constipation, anorexia
GU: Urinary retention, oliguria, impotence
RESP: Respiratory depression, respiratory paralysis
Other: Tolerance, physical dependence, psychologic dependence

TOXICITY AND OVERDOSE
Clinical signs: Respiratory and circulatory depression
Treatment: Supportive care; naloxone hydrochloride

PATIENT CARE MANAGEMENT
Assessment
• Assess history of hypersensitivity to codeine and related drugs
• Assess pain (type, location, severity) or cough characteristics
• Assess baseline VS, I&O

Interventions
• Administer with food or milk to decrease GI irritation
• Determine dosing interval based on pt response
• Administer when pain is not too severe to enhance its effectiveness
• Institute safety measures (supervise ambulation, raise side rails, place call light within reach)

> **NURSING ALERT**
> Physical dependency may result if used for extended periods of time
>
> Parenteral doses not recommended for children <50 kg (by the U.S. Department of Health and Human Services, 1992)

Evaluation
• Evaluate therapeutic response (decreased pain without significant alteration in LOC or respiratory status; suppression of cough)
• Evaluate VS and CNS changes, bowel function
• Evaluate side effects, hypersensitivity

PATIENT AND FAMILY EDUCATION
Teach/instruct
• To take as directed at prescribed intervals for prescribed length of time
• To take with food or milk to decrease GI irritation
• About best time to take medication if ordered prn

Warn/advise
• To notify care provider of hypersensitivity, side effects
• That drug may cause drowsiness, dizziness, orthostatic hypertension; make position changes slowly, seek assistance with ambu-

lation until effects of medication are known
• To avoid hazardous activities
• To avoid alcohol, other CNS depressants (unless prescribed), smoking

STORAGE
• Store at room temp, protect from light

---

colfosceril palmitate

Brand Name(s): Exosurf, Exosurf Neonatal✤

Classification: Lung surfactant

Pregnancy Category: X

AVAILABLE PREPARATIONS
Susp: 108 mg/10 ml must be reconstituted with 8 ml preservative-free SW for injection (only use accompanying diluent)

ROUTES AND DOSAGES
Prophylactic treatment: Intratracheal 5 ml/kg as soon as possible; second and third doses given 12-24 hr after first dose to infants who remain ventilated
Rescue treatment: Intratracheal 5 ml/kg as soon as diagnosis of respiratory distress syndrome made, second 5 ml/kg given 12 hr after first dose to infants who remain ventilated

MECHANISM AND INDICATIONS
Mechanism: Replaces deficient endogenous lung surfactant, prevents alveoli from collapsing during expiration by lowering surface tension between air and alveolar surfaces
Indications: Indicated for use in prevention and treatment of RDS in neonates

PHARMACOKINETICS
Absorption: Following intratracheal administration, drug is absorbed from alveoli, catabolized, and reused for further synthesis and secretion in lung tissue

CONTRAINDICATIONS AND PRECAUTIONS
• Contraindications, none known
• Use cautiously with bradycardia, rales, infections; give only in highly supervised areas with trained clinicians experienced in intubation and mechanical ventilation of premature infants, neonates; arterial measurement of PO_2 and PCO_2 should be performed before, during, after treatment
• Warning: drug can rapidly affect oxygenation, lung compliance; if chest expansion improves significantly, ventilator peak inspiratory pressure settings should be reduced immediately; change ventilator settings based on O_2 saturation

SIDE EFFECTS
CV: Transient bradycardia
RESP: Apnea; ET tube reflux or blockage; transient rales; moist breath sounds after administration; pulmonary air leak

TOXICITY AND OVERDOSE
• Has not been reported in humans

PATIENT CARE MANAGEMENT
Assessment
• Assess respiratory rate, rhythm, ABGs, color
• Assess ET tube placement before administration
• Assess for apnea after administration
• Assess for reflux of drug into ET tube; if reflux occurs, stop drug administration, increase peak inspiratory ventilation pressure until tube is clear
Interventions
• Suction infant before administration
• Reconstitute immediately before use with accompanying dilu-

---

ent; swirl vial gently before administration
• Administer via a 5F Ng tube cut to length of ET tube; 4 equal aliquots are given with infant in 4 different positions (order does not matter)
• Head and body down, head turned to right; head and body down, head turned to left; head and body up, head turned to right; head and body up, head turned to left; bed can be adjusted to place infant in "up" or "down" position
• During dosing, infant should be mechanically ventilated (not hand-bagged) after each aliquot; duration of ventilation between aliquots should be ≥30 sec until infant stable
• Infant should not be suctioned for at least 1 hr unless ET tube occlusion is suspected

Evaluation
• Evaluate therapeutic response (improvement in respiratory status)
• Monitor VS, ECG, and O_2 saturation continuously
• Evaluate infant for necessity of repeat dosing using chest x-ray results, clinical status, monitoring parameters

PATIENT AND FAMILY EDUCATION
Teach/instruct
• About rationale for treatment and treatment protocol
Provide
• Support to family

STORAGE
• Store at room temp
• Reconstituted susp stable for 12 hr at room temp

---

corticotropin (adreno-corticotropic hormone [ACTH])

Brand Name(s): ACTH, Acthar, Corticotropin, ACTH-40, ACTH-80, HP Acthar Gel, ACTH Gel, Cortigel-40, Cortigel-80, Cortrophin Gel, Cortrophin-Zinc

Classification: Pituitary hormone

Pregnancy Category: C

AVAILABLE PREPARATIONS
Inj: 25 U/vial, 40 U/vial
Repository inj: 40 U/ml 80 U/ml

ROUTES AND DOSAGES
Diagnosis of adrenocortical function: IM/SC up to 80 U in divided doses or single dose of repository form; IV 10-25 U in 500 ml D_5W over 8 hr between blood samples
Antiinflammatory: IM, IV, SC 1.6 U/kg/24 hr or 50 U/m²/24 hr divided tid-qid or repository form 0.8 U/kg/24 hr or 25 U/m²/24 hr divided qd or bid (Safety and effectiveness not established. Dosage represents accepted standard practice recommendations.)
Infantile spasms: IM 40 U qd or 80 U qod using IM ACTH gel until seizures subside or toxicity develops, then taper gradually (Safety and effectiveness not established. Dosage represents accepted standard practice recommendations.)

MECHANISM AND INDICATIONS
Mechanism: Binds with receptor in adrenal gland stimulating adrenal hormone synthesis (androgens, mineralocorticoids, glucocorticoids)
Indications: Used to assess adrenal function; to treat infantile spasms; as an antiinflammatory

PHARMACOKINETICS
Onset: <6 hr
Peak: 1 hr (IM or rapid IV); 3-12 hr repository; 7-24 hr zinc
Half-life: 15 min

✦ Available in Canada.

Metabolism: Liver
Excretion: Urine

CONTRAINDICATIONS AND PRECAUTIONS

• Contraindicated with known hypersensitivity, primary adrenal insufficiency, adrenal hyperfunction, CHF, hypertension, scleroderma, osteoporosis, ocular herpes simplex, peptic ulcer disease, recent surgery, systemic fungal disease
• Use cautiously with sensitivity to porcine proteins, AIDS, latent TB, hepatic disease, hypothyroidism, pregnancy, lactation, women of childbearing age, psychiatric disorders, myasthenia gravis, gouty arthritis

INTERACTIONS

Drug

• Increased electrolyte loss with diuretics, amphotericin B, carbonic anhydrase inhibitors
• Increased risk of arrhythmias or digitalis toxicity and hypokalemia with digitalis
• Elevated cortisol levels possible with corticosteroids, estrogen
• Higher doses of insulin may be required.
• Decreased adrenal responsiveness to corticotropin with amphotericin B

Lab

• Alters glucose, Na, PO_4, iodine, total protein, serum amylase, urine amino acid, serotonin, uric acid, Ca, 17-KS levels, WBC counts

INCOMPATIBILITIES

• Aminophylline, $NaHCO_3$

SIDE EFFECTS

CNS: Convulsions, dizziness, euphoria, insomnia, headache, mood swings, behavior changes, depression, psychosis, papilledema
CV: Hypertension, CHF, necrotizing angiitis
DERM: Impaired wound healing, thinned skin, petechiae, ecchymoses, hirsutism, facial erythema, sweating, hyperpigmentation, acne, urticaria, rash
EENT: Cataracts, glaucoma, exophthalmos
GI: Peptic ulcer perforation, pancreatitis, distention, nausea, vomiting, ulcerative esophagitis
GU: Menstrual irregularities
METAB: Na and water retention, K^+ and Ca loss, negative nitrogen balance, hyperglycemia
Other: Suppression of linear growth in children, osteoporosis, muscle weakness, steroid myopathy, decreased muscle mass, DM, hypersensitivity, cushingoid state, increased antibody formation

TOXICITY AND OVERDOSE

Clinical signs: Hypothalamic–pituitary–adrenal axis suppression
Treatment: Supportive care

PATIENT CARE MANAGEMENT

Assessment

• Assess history of hypersensitivity to corticotropin or porcine products; skin test pts with suspected porcine sensitivity
• Assess baseline VS, wt, linear growth, signs of infection, fluid balance, electrolytes (Na, K^+, Ca)

Interventions

• Warm IM gel to room temp, give slowly, deep in large muscle mass with 22G needle
• Provide low Na/high K^+ diet to decrease edema, hypokalemia; high protein diet if nitrogen loss
• Increased stress may require increased dose
• Pts receiving insulin/hypoglycemic agents may require higher doses of antidiabetic medications

Evaluation

• Evaluate therapeutic response (decreased seizures, inflammation)
• Evaluate diagnostic response (adrenal steroid levels pre- and post-infusion)
• Evaluate side effects, hypersensitivity

PATIENT/FAMILY EDUCATION

Teach/instruct

• To take as directed at prescribed intervals for prescribed length of time

---

✤ Available in Canada.

Warn/advise
- To notify care provider of hypersensitivity, side effects (edema, wt gain, weakness, abdominal pain, headaches)
- Not to discontinue medication abruptly
- To notify care provider if child is ill or otherwise stressed
- To notify all medical, dental providers of therapy
- Not to receive vaccinations during therapy

Encourage
- To carry medical alert identification with chronic therapy

STORAGE
- Reconstituted forms stable in refrigerator for 24 hr

---

cortisone acetate

Brand Name(s): Cortone, Cortone Suspension♣, Cortone Tablets♣

Classification: Anti-inflammatory, replacement therapy for adrenal insufficiency

Pregnancy Category: D

AVAILABLE PREPARATIONS
Tabs: 5 mg, 10 mg, 25 mg
Inj: 25 mg/ml, 50 mg/ml

ROUTES AND DOSAGES
Antiinflammatory or Immunosuppressive
Adults and children: PO 2.5-10 mg/kg/24 hr divided q6-8h; IM 1-5 mg/kg/24 hr qd or divided bid
Physiologic Replacement
Adults and children: PO 0.5-0.75 mg/kg/24 hr divided q8h; IM 0.25-0.35 mg/kg/24 hr qd

MECHANISM AND INDICATIONS
Mechanism: Decreases inflammation by reducing migration of PMN leukocytes and reversing increased capillary permeability; suppresses immune system by decreasing activity of lymphatic system
Indications: For use in inflammation, severe allergy, adrenal insufficiency, collagen vascular disorders, respiratory and dermatologic disorders

PHARMACOKINETICS
Peak: 1-2 hr
Half-life: 8-12 hr
Metabolism: Liver
Excretion: Urine
Absorption: Readily absorbed PO

CONTRAINDICATIONS AND PRECAUTIONS
- Contraindicated with known hypersensitivity to adrenocorticoid preparations; fungal infections AIDS, TB, psychosis, ITP; receiving live virus vaccines
- Use cautiously with GI ulcer, renal disease, hypertension, osteoporosis, DM, CHF, cirrhosis, hypothyroidism, emotional instability, psychotic tendencies, hyperlipidemia, glaucoma or cataracts, pregnancy, lactation

INTERACTIONS
Drug
- Decreased cortisone action with colestipol, cholestyramine, barbiturates, rifampin, phenytoin, theophylline
- Decreased effects of anticoagulants, anticonvulsants, antidiabetic agents, vaccines, salicylates, isoniazid
- Increased side effects with alcohol, salicylates, indomethacin, amphotericin B, digitalis, cyclosporine, diuretics
- Increased cortisone action with salicylates, estrogens, indomethacin, oral contraceptive pills, ketoconazole, macrolide antibiotics

Lab
- Suppressed skin test response
- Decreased iodine uptake and protein-bound iodine in thyroid function tests
- Increased glucose, cholesterol possible
- Decreased serum K^+, Ca, thyroxine possible

SIDE EFFECTS
CNS: Fatigue, depression, flushing, sweating, headache, mood changes

---

CV: Facial edema, hypertension, thrombophlebitis, embolism, tachycardia
DERM: Pruritis, hypertrichosis, skin atrophy, hyper- and hypopigmentation, acne
EENT: Increased intraocular pressure, blurred vision, cataracts, fungal infections
GI: Oral candidiasis, diarrhea, nausea, increased appetite, peptic ulcer, pancreatitis
HEME: Thrombocytopenia
MS: Osteoporosis, fractures

TOXICITY AND OVERDOSE

Clinical signs: Acute ingestion is rarely a clinical problem; chronic use causes suppression of the hypothalamic−pituitary−adrenal axis, cushingoid appearance, muscle weakness, osteoporosis
Treatment: Decrease drug gradually if possible
Warning: Sudden withdrawal may exacerbate underlying disease, may be fatal; chronic use in children may delay growth, maturation

PATIENT CARE MANAGEMENT

Assessment

• Assess for hyperglycemia, hypokalemia
• Assess wt qd
• Assess B/P, HR q4h
• Assess I&O, looking for decreased urinary output, increased fluid retention (edema)
• Assess baseline behavior
• Assess during time of physiologic stress; additional dose may be required

Interventions

• Administer PO with food or milk
• Administer IM deeply into large muscle mass, rotate sites, avoid deltoid
• Administer once in AM, avoid SC administration

NURSING ALERT

In children, limit top application to least effective amount

Do not abruptly decrease or withdraw drug

Evaluation

• Evaluate therapeutic response (decreased inflammatory response)
• Evaluate for signs, symptoms of infection
• Evaluate for K^+, Ca depletion
• Evaluate for edema, hypertension
• Evaluate mental status changes
• Evaluate need for continued therapy; withdraw drug very gradually

PATIENT/FAMILY EDUCATION

Teach/instruct

• To take as directed at prescribed intervals for prescribed length of time
• Not to decrease, discontinue drug abruptly
• About top, inhaled administration
• About side effects; to notify care provider
• To carry medical alert identification
• To avoid OTC products unless directed by care provider
• To report sudden wt gain to care provider
• To have regular opthalmologic exams if on long term therapy

STORAGE

• Store at room temp

---

co-trimoxazole

Brand Name(s): Apo-Sulfatrim✦, Bactrim, Bactrim Roche✦, Bethaprim, Cotrim, Comoxal, Septra✦, Septrads✦, Septra Injection✦, Sulfatrim

Classification: Antibiotic (sulfonamide)

Pregnancy Category: C

AVAILABLE PREPARATIONS

Oral susp: Trimethoprim 40 mg, sulfamethoxazole 200 mg/5 ml
Tabs: Trimethoprim 80 mg, sulfamethoxazole 400 mg; trimethoprim 160 mg, sulfamethoxazole 800 mg

---

✦ Available in Canada.

Inj: Trimethoprim 16 mg/ml, sulfamethoxazole 80 mg/ml

ROUTES AND DOSAGES
• Dosage based on trimethoprim component
• Do not use in infants <2 mo

Minor Infections
Children <40 kg: PO, IV 6-10 mg/kg/24 hr divided q12h
Children >40 kg and adults: PO, IV 320 mg/24 hr divided q12h

UTI Prophylaxis
PO, IV 2 mg/kg/24 hr qd

Severe Infections, *Pneumocystis carinii* Pneumonia
PO, IV 15-20 mg/kg/24 hr divided q6-8h

***Pneumocystis carinii* Prophylaxis**
PO, IV 5-10 mg/kg/24 hr divided q12h or 150 mg/m^2/24 hr divided q12h, 3 consecutive days/wk; maximum dose 320 mg/24 hr

IV administration
• Recommended concentration: Dilute each 1 ml of drug with 20 or 25 ml D$_5$W and use within 4 or 6 hr, respectively
• Maximum concentration: Dilute 1 ml of drug with 15 ml D$_5$W and use within 2 hr
• IV push rate: Not recommended
• Intermittent infusion rate: Over 60-90 min

MECHANISM AND INDICATIONS
Antibiotic mechanism: Bactericidal; combination of trimethoprim and sulfamethoxazole prevents bacterial cell synthesis of essential nucleic acids by blocking folic acid synthesis
Indications: Effective against *E. coli, Klebsiella, Enterobacter, Proteus mirabilis, Haemophilus influenzae, Streptococcus pneumoniae, Staphylococcus aureus, Acinetobacter, Salmonella, Shigella,* and *Pneumocystis carinii;* used to treat otitis media, shigellosis, *Pneumocystis carinii* pneumonia, and UTIs

PHARMACOKINETICS
Peak: 1-4 hr
Distribution: Widely distributed, including CNS

Half-life: Trimethoprim 11 hr, sulfamethoxazole 14.5 hr
Metabolism: Liver
Excretion: Urine
Therapeutic Level: Ratio of 1:20 (trimethoprim 0.1-1.0 mcg/ml, sulfamethoxazole 1.0-50.0 mcg/ml)

CONTRAINDICATIONS AND PRECAUTIONS
• Contraindicated in infants <2 mo because of risk of kernicterus; with known hypersensitivity to sulfonamides, to any drug containing sulfur, or to trimethoprim; in children with severe renal or hepatic dysfunction or porphyria; pregnancy at term
• Use cautiously in children with AIDS; mild-to-moderate renal or hepatic impairment; urinary obstruction; severe allergies; asthma; blood dyscrasias or folate or G-6-PD deficiency; early pregnancy

INTERACTIONS
Drug
• Increased pro-time with use of oral anticoagulants
• Increased sulfinpyrazone toxicity with use of probenecid
• Increased hypoglycemic response with use of sulfonylurea agents
• Increased nephrotoxicity with use of cyclosporine
• Increased bone marrow depressant effects with use of methotrexate
• Decreased hepatic clearance of phenytoin with use of co-trimoxazole
Lab
• Elevated liver function tests
• Decreased serum concentrations of erythrocytes, platelets, leukocytes

SIDE EFFECTS
CNS: Headache, mental depression, seizures, hallucinations
DERM: Erythema multiforme, generalized skin eruption, epidermal necrolysis, exfoliative dermatitis, photosensitivity, urticaria, pruritus, petechiae
GI: Nausea, vomiting, diarrhea, abdominal pain, anorexia, stomatitis, jaundice

♣ Available in Canada.

GU: Toxic nephrosis with oliguria and anuria, crystalluria, hematuria

HEME: Agranulocytosis, aplastic anemia, megaloblastic anemia, thrombocytopenia, leukopenia, hemolytic anemia

Other: Hypersensitivity, serum sickness, drug fever, anaphylaxis

TOXICITY AND OVERDOSE

Clinical signs: Mental depression, confusion, headache, nausea, vomiting, diarrhea, facial swelling, slight elevations in liver function tests, bone marrow depression

Treatment: Empty stomach by induced vomiting or gastric lavage; supportive care; hemodialysis has limited ability to remove co-trimoxazole

PATIENT CARE MANAGEMENT

Assessment

• Assess history of hypersensitivity to co-trimoxazole, sulfonamides
• Obtain C&S; may begin therapy before obtaining results
• Assess renal (BUN, creatinine, I&O) function status, baseline CBC, UA

Interventions

• Administer PO 1 hr ac or 2 hr after meals; shake susp well before administering; tabs may be crushed, mixed with food or fluid
• Do not premix IV with other medications or sols
• Use large vein with small-bore needle to reduce local reaction; rotate site q48-72h
• Maintain age-appropriate fluid intake

NURSING ALERT

Discontinue drug if signs of hypersensitivity, toxicity, hematologic abnormalities, nephrotoxicity, pseudomembranous colitis develop

Do not administer IV push, rapid infusion

Evaluation

• Evaluate therapeutic response (decreased symptoms of infection)
• Monitor signs of superinfection (perineal itching, diaper rash, fever, malaise, redness, pain, swelling, drainage, rash, diarrhea, sore throat, change in cough or sputum)
• Observe for allergic reactions (rash, dermatitis, urticaria, pruritus, dyspnea, bronchospasm)
• Observe for blood dyscrasias (rash, fever, sore throat, bruising, bleeding, fatigue, joint pain)
• Monitor hematologic function (CBC, differential, platelet count), renal function (BUN, creatinine, I&O)
• Observe IV site for vein irritation

PATIENT AND FAMILY EDUCATION

Teach/instruct

• To take as directed at prescribed intervals for prescribed length of time

Warn/advise

• To notify care provider of hypersensitivity, side effects, superinfection
• To avoid sunlight, use sunscreen during treatment
• To avoid OTC medications (particularly aspirin, vitamin C) unless prescribed by care provider
• To use alternative contraception (females only) since medication may decrease effectiveness of oral contraceptives

STORAGE

• Store at room temp in light-resistant container
• Check package insert for storage information after dilution

---

cromolyn sodium

Brand Name(s): Intal, Nasalcrom, Gastrocrom

Classification: Anti-allergic, antiasthmatic

Pregnancy Category: B

AVAILABLE PREPARATIONS
Caps: PO 100 mg
Caps (inhalation by "spinhaler"): 20 mg
Aerosol inhaler: 800 mcg/spray
Nebulizer sol: 10 mg/ml
Nasal spray: 5.2 mg/metered spray

ROUTES AND DOSAGES
Asthma
Children >2 yr and adults: Inhalation, aerosol inhaler 2 inhalations qid; nebulization 20 mg q6-8h
Children >5 yr and adults: Inhalation 20 mg caps via "spinhaler" q6h

Exercise Induced Asthma
Children >5 yr and adults: Aerosol inhaler 2 inhalations no more than 1 hr before exercise
Inhalant caps: 20 mg cap inhaled no more than 1 hr before exercise

Allergic Rhinitis
Nasal spray, 1 spray in each nostril tid-qid; may use 1 spray in each nostril up to 6 ×/24 hr if needed

Food Allergy and Inflammatory Bowel Disease
Children 2-14 yr: PO 100 mg qid 15-20 min ac; maximum dose 40 mg/kg/24 hr
Adults: PO 200 mg qid 15-20 min ac; maximum dose PO 400 mg qid

Systemic Mastocytosis
Children <2 yr: PO 20 mg/kg/24 hr divided qid at least 30 min ac; maximum dose 30 mg/kg/24 hr
Children 2-12 yr: PO 100 mg qid at least 30 min ac; maximum dose 40 mg/kg/24 hr
Adults: PO 200 mg qid at least 30 min ac

MECHANISM AND INDICATIONS
Antiallergic, antiasthma mechanisms: Inhibits release of chemical mediators of allergic reaction from sensitized mast cells by indirectly blocking Ca ions from entering the mast cell; acts locally on the mucosa of the nose, lung, gut; inhibits bronchoconstriction, rhinitis from inhaled antigen; has no intrinsic bronchodilator, antihistamine, or antiinflammatory activity
Indications: Used to prevent and treat allergic rhinitis symptoms, GI allergy symptoms; bronchial hyperactivity in response to activity, cold air, aspirin, some environmental pollutants, sulfur dioxide, toluene, diisocyanate; to manage pts with mastocytosis; as prophylactic in management of bronchial asthma, to decrease severity of asthma symptoms and need for bronchodilators

PHARMACOKINETICS
Onset: 2-4 wk until full benefit is achieved; some therapeutic effect may be seen in several days; no effect seen in 30%-40% of cases
Peak: 15 min
Half-life: 80 min
Metabolism: Not metabolized, excreted unchanged
Excretion: Urine, bile

CONTRAINDICATIONS AND PRECAUTIONS
• Contraindicated with hypersensitivity to cromolyn sodium, other ingredients (lactose); do not use for treatment of acute asthma
• Use cautiously with decreased renal or hepatic function because of routes of excretion (decreased dosages may be indicated); history of CAD or cardiac arrhythmias because of aerosol propellants; lactation

INTERACTIONS
Drug
• Use of with isoproterenol in pregnancy increases resorption by fetus, fetal malformations

SIDE EFFECTS
CNS: Headache, dizziness, malaise, peripheral neuritis, irritability
CV: Pericarditis, anemia
DERM: Rash, urticaria, angioedema, exfoliative dermatitis
EENT: Swelling of parotid gland, nasal congestion, stinging, burning; pharyngeal irritation, hoarseness, epistaxis
GI: Nausea, diarrhea, abdominal pain, vomiting, esophagitis, bad taste
GU: Dysuria, frequency, urgency, nephrosis

RESP: Cough, bronchospasm, wheezing, hemoptysis, eosinophilic pneumonia, laryngeal edema, tracheal irritation, possible inhalation of gelatin capsules with spinhaler system
Other: Anaphylaxis, myalgia, joint pain or swelling

TOXICITY AND OVERDOSE
Clinical signs: There is no clinical syndrome associated with overdose of cromolyn sodium
Treatment: None needed

PATIENT CARE MANAGEMENT
Assessment
• Assess history of hypersensitivity to cromolyn sodium, related drugs
• Assess history of lactose intolerance
• Assess respiratory status
Interventions
• Administer PO as a solution in water (see manufacturer's directions)
• Shake aerosol inhaler well before use (see Chapter 3 for discussion of inhaler and nebulizer use)
• See manufacturer's instructions for assembly, loading of Spinhaler
• Offer sips of fluids, gum, oral hygiene after inhaler, Spinhaler, or nebulized cromolyn to reduce irritation, dryness
• Administer bronchodilator (if prescribed) 5-15 min before inhaled cromolyn sodium dose to lessen adverse effects of inhaled cromolyn
• Notify care provider if no improvement seen after 3-4 wk of treatment
• Reduce bronchodilators or corticosteroid therapy only gradually as condition and response to cromolyn allow and only under close supervision of prescriber
• Reduce cromolyn to the lowest effective dose (from qid to tid or bid)
• Follow manufacturer's instructions for priming, assembly of nasal inhaler; shake well before use
• Have pt clear nose of secretions before intranasal dose is administered

---

NURSING ALERT

Cromolyn sodium has no role in treatment of status asthmaticus; it is a prophylactic drug of no benefit in acute situations

Cromolyn sodium caps contraindicated in those with lactose intolerance

Cromolyn sodium caps provide no benefit for asthma treatment when swallowed since they are poorly absorbed

---

Evaluation
• Evaluate for PO therapeutic effect (lessened GI distress)
• Evaluate for possible reduction to minimum PO dosage for symptom control
• Evaluate therapeutic response to inhaled drug (decreased asthma attacks, cough, sputum production)
• Evaluate pulmonary function tests
• Evaluate adverse effects or hypersensitivity
• Evaluate eosinophil count for increase (can indicate hypersensitivity)
• Evaluate compliance with regime
• Evaluate status closely when cromolyn sodium is discontinued if it has allowed reduction of maintenance doses of corticosteroids or bronchodilators, since severe asthma may recur; this may require reintroduction or increase of discontinued or decreased medications

PATIENT AND FAMILY EDUCATION
Teach/instruct
• About correct use of inhaler, "spinhaler," nebulizer; each preparation comes with specific manufacturer's instructions
• To maintain concurrent therapies during first 4 wk of treatment or until full benefit achieved, then

---

consult prescriber for modifications to regime
• To use only as prescribed
• To administered 5-15 min before inhaled cromolyn if using a bronchodilator inhaler
• To report to care provider if no improvement after 4 wk
• To avoid contact with eyes (aerosol forms)
• To rinse and gargle after administration of inhaled forms
• To relieve mouth and throat irritation, dryness, aftertaste
• To administer the drug at regular intervals to yield maximum clinical effectiveness in the case of seasonal asthma or rhinitis
• About manufacturer's recommendation for PO administration
• About specifics of dose, route, and indication since numerous preparations exist and pt may be confused

Warn/advise
• That drug benefit may not be achieved until 4 wk; reinforce compliance; stress that drug is a *preventive* medication, that it may not be effective in 30%-40% of cases
• That drug will provide no benefit in cases of acute asthma; may worsen symptoms
• That post-administration cough, wheeze, any worsening symptoms should be reported
• That caps for inhalation should *not* be swallowed; excessive handling of caps should be avoided
• That nasal spray may cause transient nasal stinging or sneezing immediately after instillation

STORAGE
• Store caps at room temp in tightly closed container
• Store aerosol inhaler at room temp, do not puncture, incinerate, place near heat sources since contents are under pressure
• Store nebulizer sol at room temp, protect from light
• Do not use if nebulizer sol contains precipitate
• Store nasal spray at room temp; protect from light
• Keep out of the reach of children

crotamiton
Brand Name(s): Eurax✤
Classification: Scabicide; antipruritic
Pregnancy Category: C

AVAILABLE PREPARATIONS
Top: Cream 10%, lotion 10%

ROUTES AND DOSAGES
Scabicide
Top, wash thoroughly, scrub away loose scales, towel dry; shake lotion well; massage into skin of entire body from neck to toes; give special attention to skin folds, creases, interdigital spaces; repeat application in 24 hr; take a cleansing bath 24 hr after final application; repeat treatment in 7-10 days if mites appear

MECHANISMS AND INDICATIONS
Mechanism: Unknown; eradicates parasitic mite *Sarcoptes scabiei*
Indications: Used to treat scabies in infants, children

CONTRAINDICATIONS AND PRECAUTIONS
• Contraindicated with a history of hypersensitivity to crotamiton, other components, and pts who exhibit irritation after application
• Use cautiously in children; avoid contact with face, eyes, mucous membranes, urethral meatus; safety in pregnancy, lactation have not been established; do not apply to raw, acutely inflamed skin

SIDE EFFECTS
DERM: Pruritis, contact dermatitis
Local: Irritation

TOXICITY AND OVERDOSE
Clinical signs: Local irritation
Treatment: Wash thoroughly with soap, water; discontinue treatment

PATIENT CARE MANAGEMENT
Assessment
• Assess history of hypersensitiv-

ity to crotamiton, other components
• Inspect carefully and note extent, amount of infestation
Interventions
• Take proper isolation precautions if child is hospitalized during infestation

---

NURSING ALERT
Avoid applying to face, eyes, mucous membranes, urethral meatus

---

Evaluation
• Evaluate therapeutic response (decreased itching after several wk, decreased redness)
• Evaluate skin (crusts, trails, papules)
• Evaluate spread of infection to other household members

PATIENT AND FAMILY EDUCATION
Teach/instruct
• To use as directed at prescribed intervals for prescribed length of time
Warn/advise
• To notify care provider of hypersensitivity, side effects
• That all contaminated clothing, bed linens should be machine washed in hot water, dried in hot dryer, or dry cleaned
• That thick applications will not hasten healing, may cause skin irritation; to reapply if accidentally washed off, but avoid overuse
• That pruritus may persist after treatment
• That partner needs treatment if sexually active
• That child should be kept home from school or day care until treatment is rendered; notify agencies of infestation
• That scabies is contagious; teach how to prevent reinfestation, spread

STORAGE
• Store at room temp in light-resistant containers

---

cyanocobalamin (vitamin B₁₂)

Brand Name(s): Redisol, Rubramin♣, Rubramin PC

Classification: Water-soluble vitamin

Pregnancy Category: A
(C if dose exceeds RDA)

AVAILABLE PREPARATIONS
Tabs: 25 mcg, 50 mcg, 100 mcg, 250 mcg, 500 mcg, 1000 mcg
Inj: 30 mcg/ml, 100 mcg/ml, 1000 mcg/ml

ROUTES AND DOSAGES
Dietary Supplement
(See Appendix F Table of Recommended Daily Dietary Allowances)
Vitamin Deficiency (not caused by malabsorption)
Children: SC/IM 10-100 mcg/24 hr × 10-15 days; maintenance dose 60 mcg q mo
Adults: SC/IM 30-100 mcg for 5-10 days; maintenance dose 100-200 mcg q mo
Vitamin Deficiency (caused by malabsorption)
Children: SC/IM initial 1000-5000 mcg, over 2 wk in 100-500 mcg doses; maintenance dose 60-100 mcg q mo
Adults: IM initial 100-1000 mcg/24 hr × 2 wk; maintenance dose 100-1000 mcg IM q mo
Methylmalonic Acidemia
Neonates: IM/Deep SC 1000 mcg/24 hr qd × 11 days
Schilling Test *Children and adults:* IM/Deep SC 1000 mcg × 1

MECHANISM AND INDICATIONS
Mechanism: Acts as a coenzyme in DNA synthesis and carbohydrate, fat, protein metabolism; involved in conversion of methylmalonate to succinate, synthesis of methionine from homocysteine; Essential for hematopoietic, neurologic function; deficiency causes megaloblastic anemia, decreased myelin, nerve damage; absorption depends on adequate intrinsic factor and Ca

---

♣ Available in Canada.

Indications: Treatment and prevention of vitamin B$_{12}$ deficiency, pernicious anemia, thyrotoxicosis, hemorrhage, malignancy, liver or kidney disease; supplementation may be necessary for strict vegetarians

PHARMACOKINETICS
Peak: Oral 8-10 hr; IM 1 hr
Half-life: 6 days
Metabolism: Liver, bone marrow
Excretion: Urine
Absorption: In terminal ileum, in presence of Ca; intrinsic factor needed to transfer across intestinal mucosa

CONTRAINDICATIONS AND PRECAUTIONS
• Contraindicated with Leber's disease (optic nerve atrophy), allergy to vitamin or cobalt
• Use cautiously for pts susceptible to gout, heart disease; with pregnancy, lactation; doses exceeding 10 mcg/24 hr may mask hematologic response with folate deficiency

INTERACTIONS
Drug
• Decreased absorption with use of aminoglycosides, anticonvulsants, cholestyramine, neomycin
• Interference of metabolism when used with large doses of vitamin C
• Lowered drug levels with use of folic acid
Lab
• Interference with serum measurements of vitamin B$_{12}$ possible with methotrexate, pyrimethamine, and antibiotics
• False and intrinsic factor antibodies
Nutrition
• Decreased absorption of vitamin B$_{12}$ possible with excess alcohol consumption

INCOMPATIBILITIES
• Warfarin, ascorbic acid, dextrose, strong acid solutions

SIDE EFFECTS
CV: Pulmonary edema, CHF, peripheral vascular thrombosis
DERM: Itching, urticaria, swelling

EENT: Severe optic nerve atrophy in patients with Leber's disease
GI: Diarrhea
LOCAL: Pain at injection site
RESP: Wheezing, anaphylaxis
Other: Hypokalemia

TOXICITY AND OVERDOSE
Clinical signs: Vitamin B$_{12}$ is a water-soluble vitamin, has a wide margin of safety; usually nontoxic even in large doses

PATIENT CARE MANAGEMENT
Assessment
• Assess history of hypersensitivity to vitamin B$_{12}$
• Assess diet; single vitamin deficiencies rare
• Assess serum folic acid, reticulocyte count, vitamin B$_{12}$ levels to evaluate folic acid deficiency
• Determine history drug, alcohol use
Interventions
• Administer PO in those with normal GI tract or those without neurologic symptoms
• Administer higher doses for those with malabsorption; preferred route is IM or SC
• Administer IM for those with pernicious anemia
• ID test dose is recommended
• Obtain serum K$^+$ levels within 8 hours because of possibility of hypokalemia; K$^+$ supplement may be necessary

> **NURSING ALERT**
> Assess serum folic acid levels before vitamin B$_{12}$ therapy to evaluate folic acid deficiency
>
> ID test dose recommended before IM/SC dosing

Evaluation
• Evaluate therapeutic response (decreased fatigue, improved appetite)
• Monitor folic acid, vitamin B$_{12}$; reticulocyte count 5-7 days after initiation of therapy; therapeutic response expected within 48 hr

♣ Available in Canada.

PATIENT AND FAMILY EDUCATION
Teach/instruct
- To take as directed at prescribed intervals for prescribed length of time
- To take with meals to improve absorption
- To take immediately if oral sols are mixed with fruit juice since ascorbic acid can destabilize vitamin B_{12}

Warn/advise
- To notify care provider of hypersensitivity, side effects
- To avoid megadosing

Encourage
- To eat balanced diet; foods high in vitamin B_{12} are meats, fish, eggs, cheese

STORAGE
- Store at room temp in a tightly sealed container
- Protect from light, heat, and moisture

---

cyclacillin
Brand Name: Cyclapen-W
Classification: Antibiotic (aminopenicillin)
Pregnancy Category: B

AVAILABLE PREPARATIONS
Oral susp: 125 mg/5 ml, 250 mg/5 ml
Tabs: 250 mg, 500 mg

ROUTES AND DOSAGES
Children: PO 50-100 mg/kg/24 hr divided q6-8h
Adults: PO 250-500 mg qid
Tonsillitis/Pharyngitis
Children >2 mo, <20 kg: PO 125 mg q8h
Children >2 months, >20 kg: PO 250 mg q8h

MECHANISM AND INDICATIONS
Antibiotic mechanism: Bactericidal; inhibits bacterial cell wall synthesis by adhering to bacterial penicillin-binding proteins
Indications: Effective against non–penicillinase-producing gram-positive bacteria including *Neisseria gonorrhoeae, N. meningitidis, Haemophilus influenzae, E. coli, Proteus mirabilis, Salmonella,* and *Shigella;* used to treat septicemia, urinary tract, otitis media, skin, soft tissue infections; tonsillitis, pharyngitis

PHARMACOKINETICS
Peak: 0.5-1.0 hr
Half-life: 0.5-1.0 hr
Metabolism: Liver
Excretion: Urine

CONTRAINDICATIONS AND PRECAUTIONS
- Contraindicated with known hypersensitivity to cyclacillin, penicillins, cephalosporins
- Use cautiously with impaired renal function, pregnancy

INTERACTIONS
Drug
- Increased serum concentrations with use of probenecid
- Decreased effectiveness with use of tetracyclines, erythromycins, chloramphenicol

Nutrition
- Reduced absorption with meals, acidic fruit juices, citrus fruits, acidic beverages (such as cola drinks)

SIDE EFFECTS
GI: Nausea, vomiting, diarrhea
GU: Acute interstitial nephritis
HEME: Anemia, thrombocytopenia, thrombocytopenic purpura, leukopenia, neutropenia, eosinophilia
Other: Hypersensitivity reaction (edema, fever, chills, rash, pruritus, urticaria, anaphylaxis), bacterial or fungal superinfection

TOXICITY/OVERDOSE
Clinical signs: Neuromuscular hypersensitivity, seizures
Treatment: If ingested within 4 hr, empty stomach by induced vomiting or gastric lavage, followed with activated charcoal; supportive care; hemodialysis

---

✤ Available in Canada.

PATIENT CARE MANAGEMENT
Assessment
• Assess history of hypersensitivity to cyclacillin, penicillins, cephalosporins
• Obtain C&S; may begin therapy before obtaining results
• Assess renal function (BUN, creatinine, I&O), bowel pattern
Interventions
• Administer penicillins at least 1 hr before bacteriostatic antibiotics (tetracyclines, erythromycins, chloramphenicol)
• Administer PO 1 hr before or 2 hr after meals; provide with water; avoid acidic beverages; shake susp well before administering; tabs may be crushed, mixed with food or fluid
• Maintain age-appropriate fluid intake

NURSING ALERT
Discontinue drug if signs of hypersensitivity, bone marrow toxicity, acute interstitial nephritis develop

---

Evaluation
• Evaluate therapeutic response (decreased symptoms of infection)
• Monitor signs of superinfection (perineal itching, diaper rash, fever, malaise, redness, pain, swelling, drainage, rash, diarrhea, sore throat, change in cough, sputum)
• Monitor bowel pattern
• Observe for hypersensitivity (wheezing, tightness in chest, urticaria) especially within 15-30 min of first dose
• Monitor renal function (BUN, creatinine, I&O), hepatic function (ALT, AST, bilirubin), hematologic function (CBC, differential, platelet count)
• Monitor for signs of bleeding (ecchymosis, bleeding gums, hematuria, daily stool guaiac); monitor pro-times, platelet counts
PATIENT AND FAMILY EDUCATION
Teach/instruct
• To take as directed at prescribed intervals for prescribed length of time
Warn/advise
• To notify care provider of hypersensitivity, side effects, superinfection

STORAGE
• Store powder, tabs at room temp
• Reconstituted susp stable refrigerated for 14 days, at room temp for 7 days; label date and time of reconstitution

---

cyclophosphamide
Brand Name(s): Cytoxan❦, Procytox❦
Classification: Alkylating Agent
Pregnancy Category: D

AVAILABLE PREPARATIONS
Tabs: 25 mg, 50 mg
Oral elixir: Liquid preparation can be made by dissolving injectable Cytoxan in aromatic elixir and refrigerating; concentration should be 1 mg/ml or 5 mg/ml
Inj: 100 mg, 200 mg, 500 mg, 1 g, 2 g vials

ROUTES AND DOSAGES
• Drug dosages may vary in response to diagnosis, extent of disease, concurrent or previous therapy, protocol guidelines, physiologic parameters; consult current literature, protocol recommendations
Pediatric Induction
PO 2-8 mg/kg/24 hr; IV 10-20 mg/kg/24 hr
Pediatric Maintenance
PO 2-5 mg/kg twice weekly
Adult Induction
PO 1-5 mg/kg/24 hr; IV 40-50 mg/kg in divided doses over 2-5 days
Adult Maintenance
PO 1-5 mg/kg/24 hr; IV 10-15 mg/kg q 7-10 days or 3-5 mg/kg twice weekly

---

❦ Available in Canada.

IV administration

- Recommended concentration: 20 mg/ml in SW or bacteriostatic water; can be further diluted with D_5W, NS, D_5NS, D_5LR, LR; (dilute 100 mg with 5 ml, 200 mg with 10 ml, 500 mg with 25 ml, 1 g with 50 ml, 2 g with 100 ml for concentration of 20 mg/ml)
- Injectable form may be given IV, IM, intraperitoneally, or intrapleurally

MECHANISMS AND INDICATIONS

Mechanism: Prevents cell division primarily by cross-linking DNA strands and interfering with RNA transcription causing imbalance of growth that leads to cell death; cell cycle nonspecific with major activity against rapidly proliferating cells

Indications: Used in Hodgkin's lymphoma, non-Hodgkin's lymphoma (Burkitt's lymphoma), neuroblastoma, CLL (chronic lymphocytic leukemia), CML (chronic myelocytic leukemia), ALL (acute lympoblastic leukemia), AML (acute myelocytic leukemia), multiple myeloma, retinoblastoma, Ewing's sarcoma

PHARMACOKINETICS

Peak: Within 1 hr after IV dose, metabolites in about 2-3 hr

Distribution: Throughout the body including brain, CSF

Half-life: Unchanged drug 3-12 hr; drug or metabolites can be detected in serum up to 72 hr after drug administration

Metabolism: Must be activated by liver enzymes (hepatic microsomal enzymes) to get direct cytotoxic metabolites

Excretion: Urine; 36%-99% of dose eliminated within 48 hr; of amount excreted, about 5%-30% is unchanged drug

Absorption: Well absorbed after oral administration

CONTRAINDICATIONS AND PRECAUTIONS

- Contraindicated with known hypersensitivity to drug, pregnancy, lactation pts with repeated courses who have developed hemorrhagic cystitis
- Use cautiously with recent radiation or other chemotherapy, with severe leukopenia, thrombocytopenia, malignant cell infiltration of bone marrow, severely suppressed bone marrow function, hepatic or renal disease

INTERACTIONS

Drug

- Increased toxicity of cyclophosphamide, increased sedative effects possible with use of barbiturates
- Increased cardiotoxicity possible with use of digoxin, other cardiac drugs
- Decreased serum digoxin levels possible
- Reduced activity of cyclophosphamide possible with use of chloramphenical, corticosteroids
- Increased leukopenia possible with use of phenobarbital
- Prolonged neuromuscular blockade possible with use of succinylcholine
- Increased rate of hepatic conversion of cytoxan to its metabolites possible with use of phenytoin, chloral hydrate

INCOMPATIBILITIES

- Should not be mixed with other drugs during administration

SIDE EFFECTS

CV: Cardiotoxic with very high doses, when given with doxorubicin

GI: Nausea, vomiting, anorexia, stomatitis, mucositis, diarrhea, abdominal pain

GU: Hemorrhagic cystitis, bladder fibrosis, nephrotoxicity, gonadal suppression (may be irreversible), oogenesis, spermatogenesis, amenorrhea

HEME: Myelosuppression including leukopenia, thrombocytopenia, anemia

RESP: Pulmonary fibrosis with high doses

Other: Alopecia, secondary malignancies, hyperuricemia, anaphylaxis, SIADH (water intoxication), impaired hepatic function, skin rashes, pigmentation changes in skin, changes in nails

TOXICITY AND OVERDOSE

Clinical signs: Secondary malignancies (bladder cancer, lymphoma, leukemia) have occurred; hemorrhagic cystitis may develop from repeated courses; bladder irrigation may be needed, possibly discontinuance of drug

Treatment: No specific antidote; manage with supportive measures (antibiotics, blood products)

PATIENT CARE MANAGEMENT

Assessment

• Assess history of hypersensitivity to cyclophosphamide, related drugs (Ifosfamide)

• Assess baseline VS, CBC, differential, platelet count, serum electrolytes (Na, K⁺), renal function (BUN, creatinine, urine CrCl), liver function (ALT, AST, LDH, bilirubin, alk phos), pulmonary and cardiac functions

• Assess hydration status (SG), hematuria, urinary frequency, dysuria

• Assess urinary elimination before each course of chemotherapy containing cyclophosphamide

• Assess neurologic and mental status before, during, and after drug administration

• Assess success of previous antiemetic therapy

• Assess history of previous treatment with special attention to other therapies that might predispose pt to renal, cardiac, or pulmonary dysfunction

Interventions

• Premedicate with antiemetics, continue periodically throughout chemotherapy

• Encourage small, frequent feedings of foods pt likes

• Monitor I&O; administer IV fluids until pt is able to resume normal PO intake

• Provide supportive measures to maintain hemostasis, fluid and electrolyte balance, nutritional support

NURSING ALERT

To minimize risk of hemorrhagic cystitis, encourage pts to drink plenty of fluids; if unable to drink, IV fluids may be needed; SG should be ≤1.010; cystitis can occur months after cessation of therapy; mesna may be used to lower incidence and severity of bladder toxicity

When administering oral cyclophosphamide, give in AM with plenty of fluids throughout day to prevent drug accumulation in bladder

Evaluation

• Evaluate therapeutic response (decreased tumor size, spread of malignancy)

• Evaluate CBC, differential, platelet count, serum electrolytes (Na, K⁺), renal function (BUN, creatinine, urine, CrCl), liver function (ALT, AST, LDH, bilirubin, alk phos), pulmonary and cardiac functions at given intervals after chemotherapy

• Evaluate for signs or symptoms of infection (fever, fatigue, sore throat), bleeding (easy bruising, nose bleeds, bleeding gums)

• Evaluate I&O carefully, dip urine with every urinary void for SG and blood; check wt daily; have pt empty bladder every 2-3 hr

• Evaluate side effects, response to antiemetic regimen

PATIENT AND FAMILY EDUCATION

Teach/instruct

• To have pt well-hydrated before and after chemotherapy

• About importance of follow-up to monitor blood counts, serum chemistry values, drug blood levels

• To take an accurate temp; rectal temp contraindicated

• To notify care provider of signs of bleeding (bruising, epistaxis, bleeding gums), infection (fever, sore throat, fatigue)

- To take oral cyclophosphamide early in day, drink plenty of fluids after oral administration
- To report any persistent cough, dyspnea

Warn/advise
- About impact of body changes that may occur (hair loss, hyperpigmentation, nail ridging), how to minimize changes (wigs, caps, scarves, long sleeves)
- To avoid OTC products containing aspirin
- To immediately report any pain, discoloration at injection site (parenteral forms)
- That good oral hygiene with very soft toothbrush is imperative
- That dental work be delayed until blood counts return to baseline, with permission of care provider
- To avoid contact with known viral, bacterial illnesses
- That household contacts of child not be immunized with live polio virus; inactivated form should be used
- That child not receive immunizations until immune system recovers sufficiently to mount needed antibody response
- To report exposure to chicken pox in susceptible child immediately
- To report reactivation of herpes zoster virus (shingles) immediately
- If appropriate, ways to preserve reproductive patterns, sexuality (sperm banking, contraceptives)
- To drink plenty of fluids, void frequently; avoid giving drug at hs because of increased risk of cystitis developing when bladder is not emptied regularly
- To report any alterations in behavior, sensation, perception; help to develop a plan of care to manage side effects, stress of illness or treatment
- To monitor bowel function, call if abdominal pain, constipation noted

Encourage
- Provision of nutritious food intake; consider nutritional consultation
- To comply with bowel management program
- To use top anesthetics to control discomfort of mucositis; avoid spicy foods, commercial mouthwashes

STORAGE
- Store tabs at room temp in airtight container
- Liquid preparation stored in refrigerator in glass container, used within 14 days
- Reconstituted injectable cyclophosphamide stable for 24 hr at room temp or 6 days in refrigerator

---

cyclosporine (cyclosporin)

Brand Name(s): Sandimmune♣, Sandimmune Neoral♣

Classification: Immunosuppressive agent (A nonpolar, cyclic, polypeptide antibiotic)

Pregnancy Category: C

AVAILABLE PREPARATIONS
Oral sol: 100 mg/ml
Caps: 25 mg, 100 mg
Inj: 50 mg/ml

ROUTES AND DOSAGES
- Dosage individualized per pt based on cyclosporine levels, serum creatinine concentrations
- Drug may vary in response to diagnosis, extent of disease, concurrent or previous therapy, protocol guidelines, physiologic parameters; consult current literature, protocol recommendations

Organ Transplants
PO 14-18 mg/kg/dose 4-12 hr before transplantation then continue daily dosage post-transplantation for wks to mos; gradually reduce

---

dosage by 5% each week to maintenance level of 5-10 mg/kg/24 hr; administer on a consistent schedule with regard to time of day, in relation to meals; IV 5-6 mg/kg 4-12 hr before transplantation then continue daily until pt is able to tolerate PO; maintenance dose 2-10 mg/kg/24 hr divided q8-12h

IV administration
• Recommended concentration: 1 ml concentrate in 20-100 ml NS or D₅W immediately before administration
• Maximum concentration: 2.5 mg/ml
• Infusion rate: Administer over 2-6 hr or as continuous infusion

MECHANISMS AND INDICATIONS
Mechanism: Inhibits proliferation of T lymphocytes
Indications: Used prophylactically against organ rejection in kidney, liver, bone marrow, heart transplantation; used also in high doses in multiply-drug resistant pts to enable cell wall to admit and retain chemotherapy

PHARMACOKINETICS
• Appears to be biologic fluid-dependent blood vs plasma vs serum; therefore, pharmacokinetics are difficult to interpret
Peak: PO 3-4 hr
Absorption: Variable
Distribution: Widely distributed in body fluids, tissue; approximately 90% in plasma, protein bound
Half-life: Initial phase 1.2 hr; terminal phase 19-27 hr
Metabolism: Liver
Excretion: Bile, urine

CONTRAINDICATIONS AND PRECAUTIONS
• Contraindicated with known hypersensitivity to the drug or to polyoxylethylated caster oil (if receiving injectable form); pregnancy, lactation

INTERACTIONS
Drug
• Increased incidence of nephrotoxicity with aminoglycosides, amphotericin B, cotrimoxazole, NSAIDs
• Increased blood levels of cyclosporine possible with amphotericin B, cimetidine, diltiazem, erythromycin, imipenem-cilastatin, ketoconazole, metoclopramide, and prednisolone
• Increased immunosuppression in combination with azathioprine, corticosteroids, cyclophosphamide, verapamil
• Decreased immunosuppressant effect of cyclosporine possible with carbamazepine, isoniazid, phenobarbital, phenytoin, and rifampin
• Decreased immune system response to routine immunizations

INCOMPATIBILITIES
• Do not use with K⁺-sparing diuretics
• Do not mix with other drugs during administration

SIDE EFFECTS
CNS: Tremor, headache, convulsions, amnesia, visual hallucinations
CV: Hypertension
EENT: Oral thrush, gum hyperplasia, sore throat, hearing loss
GI: Nausea, vomiting, diarrhea, anorexia, hepatotoxicity
GU: Nephrotoxicity, urinary retention
HEME: Anemia, leukopenia, thrombocytopenia
Other: Sinusitis, flushing, infections, hirsutism, increased LDL, hyperkalemia, hyperuricemia, acne

TOXICITY AND OVERDOSE
Clinical signs: Overdose mainly produces symptoms that are common adverse reactions; transient hepatotoxicity, nephrotoxicity
Treatment: Stop drug; monitor serum chemistries, liver functions

PATIENT CARE MANAGEMENT
Assessment
• Assess history of hypersensitivity to cyclosporine
• Assess baseline renal function (BUN, creatinine) and liver function (ALT, AST, bilirubin, alk phos)

- Assess baseline VS, CBC, differential, platelet count
- Assess neurologic and mental status before administration
- Assess urinary elimination pattern before each course of chemotherapy
- Assess success of previous antiemetic regimen
- Assess history of previous treatment with special attention to other therapies that might predispose pt to renal or hepatic dysfunction

Interventions
- Measure oral doses carefully in syringe; increase palatability by mixing with chocolate milk or fruit juice; use a glass container to decrease adherence of drug to container wall
- Administer daily dose in AM; may administer with meals if pt is experiencing anorexia, nausea, vomiting
- Premedicate with antiemetics, continue periodically through chemotherapy
- Offer small, frequent feedings of foods pt likes
- Administer IV fluids until pt is able to resume normal PO fluid intake
- Provide supportive measures to maintain hemostasis, fluid and electrolyte balance, nutritional support

> **NURSING ALERT**
> Administer medication at same time each day, preferably in AM; be sure to measure oral doses carefully, mix with fruit juice or chocolate milk to increase palatability
>
> Mix oral sol in glass container, not plastic or styrofoam (because these are porous and may absorb the drug)
>
> Absorption of cyclosporine can be erratic; levels should be monitored regularly

Evaluation
- Evaluate therapeutic response (absence of rejection)
- Evaluate serum electrolytes (SMA-6), BUN, creatinine, and liver function (ALT, AST, bilirubin, alk phos)
- Evaluate CBC, differential, platelet count at given intervals after chemotherapy
- Evaluate cyclosporine levels, make appropriate adjustments in dose as needed
- Evaluate for signs or symptoms of infection (fever, fatigue, sore throat), bleeding (easy bruising, nose bleeds, bleeding gums)
- Evaluate side effects, response to antiemetic regimen

PATIENT AND FAMILY EDUCATION
Teach/instruct
- To take as directed at prescribed intervals for prescribed length of time; measure doses carefully, give at consistent times; give with meals if nausea, vomiting, or anorexia occur
- About importance of follow-up to monitor blood counts, serum chemistry values, drug blood levels
- To take accurate temp; rectal temp contraindicated
- To notify care provider of signs of bleeding (bruising, epistaxis, bleeding gums), infection (fever, sore throat, fatigue)

Warn/advise
- To avoid OTC products containing aspirin
- To report any alterations in behavior, sensation, perception; help to develop plan of care to manage side effects, stress of illness or treatment
- To monitor bowel function, call care provider if abdominal pain, constipation noted
- That good oral hygiene with very soft toothbrush is imperative

♣ Available in Canada.

• That dental work be delayed until blood counts return to baseline, with permission of care provider
• To avoid contact with known viral, bacterial illnesses
• That household contacts of child not be immunized with live polio virus; inactivated form should be used
• That child not receive immunizations until immune system recovers sufficiently to mount needed antibody response
• To report exposure to chicken pox in susceptible child immediately
• To report reactivation of herpes zoster virus (shingles) immediately

Encourage
• Provision of nutritious food intake; consider nutritional consultation

STORAGE
• Store oral sol and caps at room temp
• Do not place oral sol in heated liquid for administration or in refrigerator; store oral sol in original container, use within 2 mo of opening
• IV forms reconstituted with NS stable in polyvinyl chloride for 6 hr or 12 hr in glass container; if diluted in D_5W, stable 24 hr in polyvinyl chloride or glass containers

---

cyproheptadine hydrochloride

Brand Name(s): Periactin✤, PMS-Cyproheptadine✤

Classification: Antihistamine

Pregnancy Category: B

AVAILABLE PREPARATIONS
Syr: 2 mg/5 ml
Tabs: 4 mg

ROUTES AND DOSAGES
Children over 2 yr: 0.25 mg/kg/24 hr divided bid-tid
OR
Children 2-6 yr: PO 2 mg q8-12h; maximum dose 12 mg/24 hr
Children 7-14 yr: PO 4 mg q8-12h; maximum dose 16 mg/24 hr
Adults: PO 4 mg q8h; maximum dose 0.5 mg/kg/24 hr

MECHANISM AND INDICATIONS
Antihistamine mechanism: Competes with histamine for H_1-receptor sites; blocks histamine, thus decreasing allergic response
Indications: Used to treat seasonal and perennial allergic rhinitis, other allergic symptoms

PHARMACOKINETICS
Metabolism: Liver
Excretion: Urine, feces

CONTRAINDICATIONS AND PRECAUTIONS
• Contraindicated with hypersensitivity to cyproheptadine, any component; in newborns or premature infants; with lactation; with MAOIs, angle-closure glaucoma, stenosing peptic ulcer, symptomatic prostatic hypertrophy, bladder neck obstruction, pyloroduodenal obstruction
• Use cautiously with bronchial asthma, increased intraocular pressure, hyperthyroidism, cardiovascular disease, hypertension, pregnancy

INTERACTIONS
Drug
• Intensified central depressant, anticholinergic effects with use of MAOIs
• Additive sedative effects with use of alcohol, barbiturates, tranquilizers, sleeping aids, antianxiety agents
Lab
• False negative skin allergy tests

SIDE EFFECTS
CNS: Sedation, CNS stimulation, seizures, headache

✤ Available in Canada.

CV: Tachycardia, hypotension
DERM: Urticaria, photosensitivity
EENT: Blurred vision, tinnitus, dry nose, throat
GI: Dry mouth, constipation, increased appetite, jaundice
GU: Dysuria, retention
HEME: Hemolytic anemia, leukopenia, thrombocytopenia
Other: Fatigue, chills

TOXICITY AND OVERDOSE
Clinical signs: CNS depression, CNS stimulation, GI symptoms, anticholinergic symptoms
Treatment: Induce vomiting, followed by activated charcoal; gastric lavage; supportive treatment; do not give stimulants

PATIENT CARE MANAGEMENT
Assessment
• Assess history of hypersensitivity to cyproheptadine, any component
Interventions
• Administer PO with meals to reduce GI distress
• Provide sugarless hard candy, gum, frequent oral care for dry mouth
• Institute safety measures (supervise ambulation, raise bed rails) because of CNS side effects
Evaluation
• Evaluate therapeutic response (decreased allergy symptoms)
• Monitor respiratory status (change in secretions, wheezing, chest tightness)
• Monitor cardiac status (palpitations, tachycardia, hypotension)

PATIENT AND FAMILY EDUCATION
Teach/instruct
• To take as directed at prescribed intervals for prescribed length of time
Warn/advise
• To notify care provider of hypersensitivity, side effects
• Not to exceed recommended dosage

• To avoid hazardous activities if drowsiness occurs (bicycles, skateboards, skates)
• To avoid use of alcohol, medications containing alcohol, CNS depressants

STORAGE
• Store at room temp in tight container

---

cytosine arabinoside (cytarabine)
Brand Name(s): Cytosar-U (ARA-C)

Classification: Antimetabolite

Pregnancy Category: D

AVAILABLE PREPARATIONS
Inj: 100 mg, 500 mg, 1 g, 2 g powder vials

ROUTES AND DOSAGES
• Drug may vary in response to diagnosis, extent of disease, concurrent or previous therapy, protocol guidelines, physiological parameters; consult current literature, protocol recommendations
Induction Remission
IV, children and adults: 200 mg/m^2/24 hr for 5 days; repeat q2wk as single agent; in combination therapy, 100-200 mg/m^2/24 hr for 5-10 days or qd until remission; given as IV continuous drip or in 2 divided doses/24 hr
IT, children and adults: 5-75 mg/m^2 q2-7 days until CNS signs and symptoms normalize
Maintenance Remission
IV, children and adults: 70-200 mg/m^2/24 hr for 2-5 days; repeat q mo
IM/SC, children and adults: 1-1.5 mg/m^2 in single dose for maintenance q 1-4 wk
IT, children and adults: 5-75 mg/m^2 q 2-7 days until CNS signs and symptoms normalize

---

Ara-C
Children < 1 yr: 20 mg
Children 1-2 yr: 30 mg
Children 2-3 yr: 50 mg
Children > 3 yr and adults: 70 mg
Refractory Leukemia, Secondary Leukemia, Refractory Non–Hodgkin's Lymphoma
Children and adults: IV 3 g/m^2 q12h for 4-12 doses (as single agent or in combination chemotherapy); repeat q 2-3 wk
IV administration
• Recommended concentration for administration: ≤100 mg/ml
• IV infusion rate: 1-3 hr
• IT: Reconstitute with preservative-free NS or preservative-free LR

**MECHANISM
AND INDICATIONS**
Mechanism: Inhibits DNA synthesis; the antimetabolite (pyrimidine analogue) incorporates into DNA, slowing DNA synthesis and causing defects in the linkages of new DNA fragments; cells in the S phase exposed to ARA-C reinitiate DNA synthesis when the drug is removed, resulting in erroneous duplication in the early portions of DNA strands; most effective in cells undergoing rapid DNA synthesis
Indications: Used in treatment of AML and other acute lymphocytic and non-lymphocytic leukemias; non-Hodgkin's lymphoma; in blast phase of CML; intrathecally in meningeal leukemia

PHARMACOKINETICS
Peak: 8-24 hr constant plasma concentrations with IV administration; with SC or IV, within 20-60 min
Absorption: Not effective if given orally, < 20% absorbed from GI tract
Distribution: Rapid and widely into tissues and fluid, including liver, plasma, peripheral granulocytes; crosses blood–brain barrier to a limited extent during continuous infusion, with IV or SC injection; CSF concentration higher with IV infusion
Half-life: IV, 10-15 min during initial phase, and 1-3 hr in terminal phase; IT, about 2 hr
Metabolism: Rapidly and extensively in liver, but also kidneys, GI mucosa, granulocytes
Excretion: 70%-80% in urine as metabolites in 24 hr

**CONTRAINDICATIONS
AND PRECAUTIONS**
• Contraindicated with known hypersensitivity, active infections, chicken pox or herpes zoster lesions, pregnancy, lactation
• Use cautiously with thrombocytopenia, leukopenia, renal or hepatic disease, after other chemotherapy or radiation therapy

**INTERACTIONS
Drug**
• Decreased serum digoxin levels possible
• Decreased therapeutic levels of aminoglycosides, flucytosine
• Possible acute pancreatitis in pts who previously received asparaginase

INCOMPATIBILITIES
• Fluorouracil, methylprednisolone, solumedrol

SIDE EFFECTS
CNS: Neurotoxicity including ataxia, cerebellar dysfunction, especially with high doses; lethargy, somnolence, personality changes, peripheral neuropathies
EENT: Keratitis, nystagmus, conjunctivitis
GI: Nausea, vomiting, diarrhea, dysphagia, mouth sores or oral ulcers, stomatitis, anal inflammation or ulceration, hepatotoxicity (usually mild and reversible; jaundice)
HEME: Leukopenia, anemia, thrombocytopenia, reticulocytopenia, megaloblastosis, bleeding at any site
Other: Skin rash, flu-like symptoms, hyperuricemia, urate neuropathy, anorexia, alopecia, weight loss, anorexia, thrombophlebitis

---

♣ Available in Canada.

TOXICITY AND OVERDOSE

Clinical signs: Too-rapid IV infusion may cause dizziness; infusion should be stopped, restarted at a slower rate once symptoms have resolved

Treatment: Cerebellar toxicity indicates for immediate cessation of therapy; continue dexamethasone ophthal sol in eyes; consult ophthalmologist if severe keratitis develops

PATIENT CARE MANAGEMENT
Assessment
- Assess history hypersensitivity to ARA-C, related drugs
- Assess baseline VS, CBC, differential, platelet count, serum electrolytes (Mg, K^+, Ca, PO_4), renal function (BUN, creatinine, urine CrCl), liver function (ALT, AST, LDH, bilirubin, alk phos)
- Assess neurologic and mental status before, during drug administration
- Assess success of previous antiemetic therapy
- Assess history of previous treatment with special attention to other therapies that may predispose to hepatic or renal dysfunction

Interventions
- Premedicate with antiemetics, continue periodically through chemotherapy
- Administer dexamethasone ophthal drops as ordered before chemotherapy administration, continuing for 24-48 hr after to prevent keratitis
- Encourage small, frequent feedings of foods pt likes
- Monitor I&O; administer IV fluids until pt able to resume normal PO intake
- Provide supportive measures to maintain hemostasis, fluid electrolyte balance, nutritional support

NURSING ALERT
Stop drug immediately if cerebellar symptoms or toxicity occur (personality changes, somnolence, coma which is usually reversible)

Be sure to provide dexamethasone ophthalmic drops to pt as ordered, starting before and continuing for 24-48 hr after drug administration is complete; explain importance to pt and family to prevent keratitis

Evaluation
- Evaluate therapeutic response (decreased tumor size, spread of malignancy)
- Evaluate CBC, differential, platelet count, serum electrolytes (Mg, K^+, Ca, PO_4), renal function (BUN, creatinine, urine CrCl), liver function (ALT, AST, LDH, bilirubin, alk phos) at given intervals after chemotherapy
- Evaluate for signs or symptoms of bleeding (easy bruising, nosebleeds, bleeding gums), infection (fever, fatigue, sore throat)
- Evaluate I&O carefully, check regularly
- Evaluate side effects, response to antiemetic regimen
- Evaluate for any symptoms of keratitis (burning or itchy eyes, intolerance for bright lights, pain)
- Monitor during drug infusion for lethargy, somnolence, any cerebellar changes; neurologic status at given intervals after chemotherapy

PATIENT AND FAMILY EDUCATION
Teach/instruct
- To have pt well-hydrated before, after chemotherapy
- About importance of follow-up to monitor blood counts, serum chemistry values, drug blood levels
- To take accurate temp; rectal temp contraindicated
- To notify care provider of signs of bleeding (bruising, epistaxis,

---

bleeding gums), infection (fever, sore throat, fatigue)
• To give dexamethasone ophthal drops as ordered to prevent keratitis

Warn/advise
• About impact of body changes that may occur (hair loss, hyperpigmentation, nail ridging), how to minimize changes (wigs, caps, scarves, long sleeves)
• To avoid OTC products containing aspirin
• To report any alterations in behavior, sensation, perception; help to develop plan of care to manage side effects, stress of illness or treatment
• To monitor bowel function, call care provider if abdominal pain, constipation noted
• To immediately report any pain, discoloration at injection site (parenteral forms)
• That good oral hygiene with very soft toothbrush is imperative
• That dental work be delayed until blood counts return to baseline, with permission of care provider
• To avoid contact with known viral, bacterial illnesses
• That household contacts of child not be immunized with live polio virus; inactivated form should be used
• That child not receive immunizations until immune system recovers sufficiently to mount needed antibody response
• To report exposure to chicken pox in susceptible child immediately
• To report reactivation of herpes zoster virus (shingles) immediately
• If appropriate, ways to preserve reproductive patterns, sexuality (sperm banking, contraceptives)

Encourage
• Provision of nutritious food intake; consider nutritional consultation
• To comply with bowel management program
• To use top anesthetics to control discomfort of mucositis; avoid spicy foods, commercial mouthwashes

STORAGE
• Sterile powder, injectable at room temp
• Reconstituted sol for injection stable for 8 days at room temp
• IT sol of Elliott's B stable for 7 days at room temp

---

dacarbazine

Brand Name(s): DTIC✤

Classification: Antineoplastic, alkylating agent cell cycle phase nonspecific

Pregnancy Category: C

AVAILABLE PREPARATIONS
Inj: 100 mg, 200 mg, 500 mg

ROUTES AND DOSAGES
• Dosage may vary in response to diagnosis, extent of disease, concurrent or previous therapy, protocol guidelines, physiological parameters; consult current literature, protocol recommendations
• May be given according to single dose schedule every 3-4 wk or as consecutive daily dosing schedule

Neuroblastoma
Children: IV 850 mg/m^2/dose repeated at 3-4 wk intervals

Solid Tumors
Children: IV 200-470 mg/m^2/24 hr over 5 days q 21-28 days

Hodgkin's Disease
Adolescents and adults: IV 375 mg/m^2/dose on days 1 and 15 in 28 day cycle

Malignant Melanoma
Adolescents and adults: IV 2-4.5 mg/kg/24 hr for 10 days q 28 days

IV administration
• Recommended concentration: 10 mg/ml
• Maximum concentration: 10 mg/ml
• IV push: Over several min
• Intermittent infusion rate: Over 15-30 min; pH low, may cause less burning if infused over 15-30 min

MECHANISM AND INDICATIONS
Mechanism: Exact mechanism of cytotoxicity not clear; inhibits syn-

thesis of DNA, RNA, protein through role as alkylating agent, antimetabolite, and bonding to protein sulfhydryl group

Indications: Hodgkin's Disease, neuroblastoma, rhabdomyosarcoma, malignant melanoma, abdominal neuroendocrine tumor, brain tumors

PHARMACOKINETICS

Half-life: Biphasic, with terminal half-life of about 5 hr

Distribution: Disappears rapidly from plasma with little distribution into CSF

Metabolism: Liver

Excretion: 30%-45% excreted in urine (50% unchanged 50% inactive metabolite); renal tubular secretion rather than glomerular filtration facilitates urinary excretion of drug

CONTRAINDICATIONS AND PRECAUTIONS

• Contraindicated in known hypersensitivity, pregnancy, lactation

• Use cautiously with hepatic or renal dysfunction

INTERACTIONS

Drug

• Increased metabolism of drug possible with phenytoin, phenobarbital

• Addictive effects possible with allopurinol (drug inhibits xanthine oxidase action)

• Increased toxicity possible with 6-mercaptopurine

• Increased cardiotoxicity of doxorubicin possible

• Compatible with heparin, doxorubicin, actinomycin, cyclophosphamide, methotrexate, 5-FU, cytarabine, carmustine, ondansetron

Lab

• Increased AST, ALT, BUN, alk phos (transient)

INCOMPATIBILITIES

• Heparin, lidocaine, hydrocortisone sodium phosphate

SIDE EFFECTS

CNS: Neurotoxicity manifested by confusion, headache, seizures, paresthesias (especially in facial area)

CV: Burning along injection route; thrombophlebitis, hypotension with high doses (possibly secondary to Ca chelation by citric acid preservative in commercial product); may enhance doxorubicin cardiotoxicity

DERM: Alopecia, facial flushing, photosensitivity causing intense burning and pain on head, hands when exposed to sunlight (most often with higher dosages), urticaria at injection site

EENT: Blurred vision, photosensitivity

GI: Severe nausea, vomiting (90%) that characteristically lessens with each dose and lasts for 1-12 hr after dose, requiring aggressive antiemetic therapy; anorexia, hepatic toxicity with elevated AST, BUN, ALT (ranges from delayed hepatic dysfunction to acute failure, believed to be caused by thrombosis from allergic vasculitis)

HEME: Moderately myelosuppressive with nadir of leukocytes and platelets at 21-25 days after administration

Other: Mildly immunosuppressive; may cause transient metallic taste in mouth; flu-like syndrome in pts receiving higher doses (fever, myalgia, malaise, with onset by 7 days after dose and lasting 1-3 wk)

TOXICITY AND OVERDOSE

Clinical signs: Prolonged myelosuppression

Treatment: Supportive measures including blood transfusions, hydration, nutritional supplementation, broad-spectrum antibiotic coverage in event of fever, electrolyte replacement

PATIENT CARE MANAGEMENT

Assessment

• Assess history of hypersensitivity to dacarbazine

• Assess history of previous chemotherapy, radiation therapy that

---

might predispose pt to prolonged myelosuppression
• Assess baseline CBC, differential, platelet count
• Assess baseline renal function (BUN, creatinine), liver function (alk phos, AST, ALT)
• Assess baseline neurologic examination
• Assess success of previous antiemetic therapy

Interventions
• Administer antiemetic therapy before chemotherapy
• Monitor I&O, wt
• Provide IV hydration until pt is able to resume normal intake
• Provide nutritional supplementation as needed
• Provide appropriate supportive therapy including blood products, fluid and electrolyte replacement, nutritional supplementation

---

NURSING ALERT

Drug must be protected from light if administered as infusion over several hr; if administered via IV push method, drug causes intense burning along injection route

---

Evaluation
• Evaluate therapeutic response through radiologic or clinical demonstration of tumor regression
• Evaluate CBC, differential, platelet count weekly
• Evaluate renal function (BUN, creatinine), liver function (alk phos, AST, ALT) regularly

PATIENT AND FAMILY EDUCATION
Teach/instruct
• To have patient well hydrated before, after chemotherapy
• About importance of follow-up to monitor blood counts, serum chemistry values
• To take accurate temp; rectal temp contraindicated
• To notify care provider of signs of bleeding (bruising, epistaxis, bleeding gums), infection (fever, sore throat, fatigue)

Warn/advise
• About impact of body changes that may occur (hair loss, hyperpigmentation, nail ridging), how to minimize changes (wigs, caps, scarves, long sleeves)
• To avoid OTC preparations containing aspirin
• To report any alterations in behavior, sensation, perception; help to develop plan of care to manage side effects, stress of illness or treatment
• That good oral hygiene with very soft toothbrush is imperative
• That dental work be delayed until blood counts return to baseline, with permission of care provider
• To avoid contact with known viral, bacterial illnesses
• That close household contacts of child not be immunized with live polio virus; use inactivated form
• That children on chemotherapy not receive immunization until immune system recovers sufficiently to mount necessary antibody response
• To report exposure to chicken pox in susceptible child immediately
• To report reactivation of herpes zoster virus (shingles) immediately
• If appropriate, ways to preserve reproductive patterns, sexuality (sperm banking, contraceptives)

Encourage
• Provision of nutritious food intake; consider nutrition consultation
• To use top anesthetics to control the discomfort of mucositis; avoid spicy foods, commercial mouthwashes

STORAGE
• Intact vials stable under refrigeration for 4 yr, at room temp for several mo
• Drug extremely light sensitive, must be protected during storage
• Reconstituted sol stable for 8 hr at room temp, 72 hr under refrigeration
• Change in sol color from pale

yellow to pink denotes decomposition of drug
• Drug suffers 50% loss of potency in 4 hr if diluted for IV administration and not protected from light

---

dactinomycin

Brand Name(s): Cosmegen✤, actinomycin-D

Classification: Antineoplastic, antibiotic cell cycle phase nonspecific

Pregnancy Category: C

AVAILABLE PREPARATIONS
Inj: 0.5 mg powder

ROUTES AND DOSAGES
• Dosages may vary in response to diagnosis, extent of disease, concurrent or previous therapy, protocol guidelines, physiological parameters; consult current literature, protocol recommendations
• The National Wilms' Tumor Study advises that doses above 45 mcg/kg may predispose to hepato–veno–occlusive disease
• Generally given as part of combination chemotherapy in a variety of doses and at a variety of intervals; doses are generally written as mcg/kg or mcg/m^2

All Indications
Children >6 and adults: IV 10-15 mcg/kg or 400-600 mcg/m^2 qd for 5 days at intervals of q 3-8 wk or 2.5 mg/m^2 over 1 wk in divided doses; adult dose not to exceed 500 mcg (0.5 mg) daily for maximum of 5 days; dosage for children not to exceed 15 mcg/kg and 400-600 mcg/m^2 daily for 5 days

IV administration
• Recommended concentration: 500 mcg/ml in preservative-free SW
• Maximum concentration: 500 mcg/ml
• IV push rate: Over several min, followed by flush to ensure delivery; may also be injected IV push into tubing of free-flowing IV, followed with 10-15 ml flush
• Use of cellulose ester membrane filter in IV may remove part of drug

MECHANISM AND INDICATIONS
Mechanism: Cytotoxic effect exerted from capacity to bind or intercalate between guanine and cytosine base pairs of DNA helix; this blocks DNA transcription, inhibiting DNA and DNA-dependent RNA synthesis; can also cause single strand breaks in DNA
Indications: Pediatric usage includes rhabdomyosarcoma, Wilms' tumor, Ewing's sarcoma, neuroblastoma, retinoblastoma, embryonal or germ cell tumors; malignant melanoma, testicular tumors, Kaposi's sarcoma; occasionally for Hodgkin's and non-Hodgkin's lymphoma

PHARMACOKINETICS
Distribution: Rapid after IV injection; highest levels found in bone marrow, nucleated cells; does not cross blood–brain barrier.
Half-life: Terminal half-life approximately 36 hr as significant drug retention occurs in granulocytes, lymphocytes; this has led to the recent recommendation that dactinomycin be administered by single, intermittent interval injections rather than daily divided doses
Metabolism: Liver
Excretion: 50% unchanged in bile; small fraction in urine

CONTRAINDICATIONS AND PRECAUTIONS
• Contraindicated with active infections, especially chicken pox or active herpes zoster; hypersensitivity; pregnancy, lactation
• Use cautiously in infants <12 mo, in peripheral IV line as drug is severe vesicant; pts receiving recent radiation therapy as treatments potentiate each other (radiation recall phenomenon)

INTERACTIONS
Drug
• Radiation recall (syndrome of erythema progressing to desquamation noted in areas of skin and mucous membrane previously exposed to radiation)
• Increased myelosuppression possible with other antineoplastic agents
Lab
• Increased blood and urine concentrations of uric acid possible
• Interference with vitamin K effects possible

INCOMPATIBILITIES
• Reconstitution with diluent containing preservative may cause precipitation of drug

SIDE EFFECTS
CNS: Fatigue, malaise
DERM: Alopecia, acneiform changes on face and trunk, hyperpigmentation, maculopapular rash, radiation recall phenomena
GU: Hyperuricemia
GI: Nausea; vomiting beginning several hr after administration and lasting for 24 hr; proctitis; diarrhea; glossitis; ulceration of oral mucosa; hepato–veno–occlusive disease evidenced by increase in liver function tests; ascites; hepatomegaly
HEME: Pancytopenia within first 7-10 days, primarily affecting platelets, leukocytes; recovery generally occurs within 21 days
MS: Inhibits osteoclast growth; has hypocalcemic effect
Local: Extravasation causes local inflammation, erythema that can progress to necrosis, sloughing, contractures
Other: Potent immunosuppressant, allergic reactions including anaphylaxis, fever; secondary malignancies reported (more evident in pts receiving radiation in close temporal relation to drug administration)

TOXICITY AND OVERDOSE
Clinical signs: Prolonged myelosuppression, severe and extensive mucositis; inadvertent overdose has been reported, causing seizure; hyponatremia; hypokalemia; hypocalcemia; hypomagnesemia; intense erythema with desquamation and bullae; GI ulceration with profuse diarrhea; mucositis; febrile neutropenia (resolution in 3 wk)
Treatment: Supportive measures including blood products, hydration, nutritional supplementation, broad spectrum antibiotics, electrolyte replacement

PATIENT CARE MANAGEMENT
Assessment
• Assess history of hypersensitivity to dactinomycin
• Assess history of previous treatment, including chemotherapy or radiation therapy
• Assess baseline VS, abdominal girth
• Assess baseline CBC, differential, platelet count
• Assess baseline renal function (BUN, creatinine), liver function (alk phos, AST, ALT, bilirubin, LDH)
• Assess baseline Na, K^+, Ca, Mg
• Assess success of previous antiemetic therapy
Interventions
• Ensure correct dosage (dosed in mcg/kg)
• Ensure absolute patency of IV before administration
• Do not place IV over joint; if extravasation occurs, joint may become immobilized
• Administer antiemetic before administering drug
• Provide supportive measures to maintain hemostasis, fluid, electrolyte and nutritional balance

---

NURSING ALERT

Drug is potent vesicant; ensure patency of IV line just before administration; if infiltration occurs, apply cool compresses

Single dose must not exceed 500 mcg (0.5 mg)

Evaluation
• Evaluate therapeutic response to treatment through radiologic or clinical demonstration of tumor regression
• Evaluate CBC, differential, platelet count at least once a week
• Evaluate renal function (BUN, creatinine), liver function (alk phos, LDH, AST, ALT), electrolytes (Na, K$^+$, Ca, Mg) regularly

PATIENT AND FAMILY EDUCATION
Teach/instruct
• To have patient well hydrated before, after chemotherapy
• About the importance of follow-up to monitor blood counts, serum chemistry values
• To take accurate temp; rectal temp contraindicated
• About likelihood of radiation recall phenomenon
• To notify care provider of signs of bleeding (bruising, epistaxis, bleeding gums), infection (fever, sore throat, fatigue)

Warn/advise
• About impact of body changes that may occur (hair loss, hyperpigmentation, nail ridging), how to minimize changes (wigs, caps, scarves, long sleeves)
• To avoid OTC preparations containing aspirin
• To report any alterations in behavior, sensation, perception; help to develop a plan of care to manage side effects, stress of illness or treatment
• That good oral hygiene with very soft toothbrush is imperative
• That dental work be delayed until blood counts return to baseline, with permission of care provider
• To avoid contact with known viral, bacterial illnesses
• That close household contacts of child not be immunized with live polio virus; use inactivated form
• That children on chemotherapy not receive immunization until immune system recovers sufficiently to mount necessary antibody response

• To report exposure to chicken pox in susceptible child immediately
• To report reactivation of herpes zoster virus (shingles) immediately
• About ways to provide meticulous skin care in event of radiation recall
• If appropriate, ways to preserve reproductive patterns, sexuality (sperm banking, contraceptives)

Encourage
• Provision of nutritious food intake; consider nutrition consultation
• To use top anesthetics to control discomfort of mucositis; avoid spicy foods, commercial mouthwashes

STORAGE
• Reconstituted sol stable at room temp for prolonged period but must be discarded after 24 hr to minimize bacterial growth
• Reconstituted sol should be protected from light

---

dantrolene
Brand Name(s): Dantrium
Classification: Skeletal muscle relaxant
Pregnancy Category: C

AVAILABLE PREPARATIONS
Caps: 25 mg, 50 mg, 100 mg
Inj: 20 mg

ROUTES AND DOSAGES
Spasticity
Children: PO, initial 0.5 mg/kg/dose bid, increase by 0.5 mg/kg to maximum of 3 mg/kg/dose; maximum 400 mg/24 hr
Adult: PO 25 mg/24 hr to start, increase frequency to tid-qid, then increase by 25 mg q 4-7 days, maximum 400 mg/24 hr

Hyperthermia
Children and adults: PO 4-8 mg/kg/24 hr divided qid 1-2 days before surgery for patients at risk, and for up to 3 days after crisis; IV 1 mg/kg,

---

✦ Available in Canada.

may repeat to cumulative dose of 10 mg/kg

IV administration
- Recommended concentration for administration: Dilute 20 mg in 60 ml sterile water (not bacteriostatic)
- IV push rate: Rapid
- Continuous infusion rate: Over 1 hr

MECHANISM AND INDICATIONS
Mechanism: Interferes with release of Ca, resulting in decreased muscle contraction; prevents catabolic processes associated with malignant hyperthermia
Indications: For use in spasticity, prevention and treatment of malignant hyperthermia

PHARMACOKINETICS
Half-life: 7-8 hr
Absorption: GI tract
Peak: 5 hr
Metabolism: Liver
Excretion: Urine

CONTRAINDICATIONS AND PRECAUTIONS
- Contraindicated with active hepatic disease, upper motor neuron disorders, pulmonary or myocardial dysfunction
- Use cautiously with peptic ulcer disease, renal or hepatic disease, stroke, DM, seizure disorder, elderly, pregnancy, lactation

INTERACTIONS
Drug
- Increased CNS depression with alcohol, narcotics, antipsychotics, anxiolytics, tricyclic antidepressants
- Ventricular fibrillation with verapamil

Lab
- Increased ALT, AST, alk phos, LDH, BUN, total bilirubin

INCOMPATIBILITIES
- Incompatible with dextrose, NS, bacteriostatic water; precipitates when placed in glass containers for infusion

SIDE EFFECTS
CNS: Seizures, drowsiness, dizziness, confusion, fatigue, depression, headache, speech disturbances, hallucinations
CV: Tachycardia, phlebitis, pericarditis
DERM: Rash
EENT: Visual, auditory disturbances, excessive tearing
GI: Hepatitis, nausea, vomiting, anorexia, diarrhea, constipation, dysphagia, abdominal cramps
GU: Urinary retention, hematuria, incontinence
RESP: Pleural effusion
Other: Chills, fever, drooling

TOXICITY AND OVERDOSE
Clinical signs: Exaggeration of side effects especially CNS depression, nausea, vomiting
Treatment: Supportive care, gastric lavage, monitor VS, ECG

PATIENT CARE MANAGEMENT
Assessment
- Assess history of hypersensitivity to dantrolene
- Assess baseline neuromuscular function (gait, coordination, posture, ROM, muscle strength and tone, spasticity, reflexes)
- Assess baseline liver function tests (ALT, AST, bilirubin)
- Assess I&O
- Assess pt for potential for falls

Interventions
- Administer PO with meals
- Reconstitute IV by adding 60 ml sterile water; do not use bacteriostatic water
- Administer diluted drug by rapid IV infusion in malignant hyperthermia crisis
- Provide assistance with ambulation

NURSING ALERT

Not recommended for long term use in children under 5 yr

Do not reconstitute with bacteriostatic water

Evaluation
- Evaluate therapeutic response (decreased pain, spasticity)
- Evaluate CNS depression
- Monitor for signs of hepatic dys-

✤ Available in Canada.

function (jaundice, abdominal pain, nausea, fever)
• Evaluate liver function (AST, ALT, bilirubin) regularly
• Evaluate pt for weakness

PATIENT AND FAMILY EDUCATION
Teach/instruct
• To take as directed at prescribed intervals for prescribed length of time
• To report signs of hepatotoxicity (jaundice, dark urine, abdominal discomfort)
Warn/advise
• To carry medical alert identification for malignant hyperthermia
• That drug causes dizziness, and drowsiness, to be alert to safety hazards
• Not to take drug with alcohol, other CNS depressants

STORAGE
• Room temp in light-resistant containers

---

daunorubicin hydrochloride

Brand Name(s): Cerubidine

Classification: Antineoplastic, anthracycline antibiotic cell cycle phase nonspecific

Pregnancy Category: D

AVAILABLE PREPARATIONS
Inj: 20 mg powder

ROUTES AND DOSAGES
• Dosages may vary in response to diagnosis, extent of disease, concurrent or previous therapy, protocol guidelines, physiological parameters; consult current literature, protocol recommendations
• Cumulative lifetime dose of 550 mg/m^2 should not be exceeded since potential exists for cardiotoxicity; this maximum must be reduced if child has received radiation involving the heart or has received previous treatment with

another anthracycline preparation
• If child is <2 yr or 0.5 m^2, dosage calculated in mg/kg
Pediatric Acute Lymphocytic Leukemia (ALL) *Children:* IV induction therapy 25 mg/m^2/wk
Children <2 yr or <0.5 m^2: IV 1 mg/kg per protocol
Pediatric Solid Tumor Range 15-30 mg/m^2/24 hr for 5 days
Acute Non-Lymphocytic Leukemia
Adults: 45-60 mg/m^2/24 hr for 3 days (represents 50% higher dosage than with doxorubicin because of increased rate of renal clearance for daunorubicin)
IV administration
• IV push rate: Over several min followed by 5-10 ml flush to ensure administration well into venous system; potent vesicant
• Recommended concentration: Reconstitute 20 mg in 4 ml SW; dilute reconstituted dose in 10-15 ml/NS

MECHANISM AND INDICATIONS
Mechanism: Cytotoxic effect from capacity to intercalate between base pairs in DNA causing uncoiling of DNA helix with subsequent interruption of DNA synthesis and DNA-dependent RNA synthesis; also generates oxygen free radical, capable of damage to cell membranes; cytotoxic action greatest, but not limited to S phase
Indications: Preferred anthracycline in acute non-lymphocytic leukemias in adults; pediatric use limited but may be effective in relapsed ALL, Hodgkin's disease, non-Hodgkin's lymphoma, Ewing's sarcoma, rhabdomyosarcoma, neuroblastoma

PHARMACOKINETICS
Distribution: Does not cross blood–brain barrier; rapid uptake in heart, kidney, lungs, liver, spleen
Metabolism: Liver (to slightly less active metabolite daunorubicinol)
Half-life: Long terminal half-life (18.5 hr) secondary to extensive tissue binding

---

✚ Available in Canada.

Excretion: 40% hepatobiliary; 25% in urine

CONTRAINDICATIONS AND PRECAUTIONS

• Contraindicated with pregnancy, lactation; in children with preexisting cardiac disease, CHF; with active infections, especially chicken pox or herpes zoster; single high-dose bolus delivery (associated with high mortality)

• Use cautiously with hepatobiliary or renal dysfunction; children with cumulative doses >300 mg/m^2 (increased cardiomyopathy); previous chemotherapy, radiation therapy, disease response, current cardiac status must be carefully evaluated before exceeding cumulative dose of 300 mg/m^2

INTERACTIONS

Drug

• Decreased efficacy of methotrexate

• Affected by multiple drug resistance phenomena

• Increased risk of hepatotoxicity possible with other hepatotoxic drugs

Lab

• Increased uric acid in blood, urine

• Increased alk phos, AST, bilirubin

INCOMPATIBILITIES

• NaHCO$_3$, 5-FU, hydrocortisone, aminophylline, cephalexin; dexamethasone and heparin may cause precipitation

SIDE EFFECTS

CV: Cardiomyopathy evidenced by fatigue; dyspnea on exertion; tachycardia; arrhythmias, hypotension; progressing to pericardial effusion; CHF unresponsive to digoxin; pericarditis; myocarditis; early ECG changes include ST-T wave changes, low voltage QRS, flattened T-waves; early arrhythmias include transient sinus tachycardia, heart block, premature ventricular contractions; cardiomyopathy may have long latency period

DERM: Alopecia; hyperpigmented areas in nail beds; contact dermatitis; generalized skin rash; urticaria; erythema along venous administration route (believed secondary to release of histamine from mast cells); radiation recall phenomena; severe vesicant

EENT: Conjunctivitis; mucositis characterized by erythema, burning of oral mucosa followed by ulceration in 2-3 days

GI: Stomatitis, nausea, vomiting (rarely persisting beyond 48 hrs), diarrhea

GU: Hyperuricemia; urine pink to red up to 48 hr after dose; nephrotoxicity

HEME: Leukopenia and thrombocytopenia with nadir 10-14 days, recovery 21 days; anemia

Other: Transient chills; fever during or shortly after administration; anaphylactoid reaction

TOXICITY AND OVERDOSE

Clinical signs: Prolonged myelosuppression, severe extensive mucositis

Treatment: Supportive measures including blood products; hydration; nutritional supplementation; broad spectrum antibiotic coverage for febrile neutropenia; electrolyte replacement

PATIENT CARE MANAGEMENT

Assessment

• Assess history of hypersensitivity

• Assess history of previous treatment, including chemotherapy and radiation therapy; ascertain cumulative anthracycline dose

• Assess baseline VS, oximetry

• Assess baseline ECG, echocardiogram

• Assess baseline CBC, differential, platelet count

• Assess baseline renal function (BUN, creatinine), liver function (bilirubin, alk phos, LDH, AST)

Interventions

• Administer antiemetic therapy before chemotherapy

• Ensure patent IV access not located over joint area

D

• Top dimethylsulfoxide (DMSO) in the event of extravasation for 14 days may be helpful
• Monitor I&O; administer IV fluids until child is able to resume adequate oral intake
• Provide supportive measures to maintain hemostasis, fluid, electrolyte, nutritional status

---

NURSING ALERT

Drug is a potent vesicant; ensure patency of IV line just before administration; if infiltration occurs, cool compresses may be applied

Drug can cause progressive, potentially fatal cardiomyopathy; resting HR, B/P, oximetry should be assessed regularly; ECG, echocardiography should be performed on routine basis

---

Evaluation
• Evaluate therapeutic response through radiologic or clinical demonstration of tumor regression
• Evaluate CBC, differential, platelet counts at least q wk
• Evaluate baseline renal function (BUN, creatinine), liver function (bilirubin, alk phos, LDH, AST)

PATIENT AND FAMILY EDUCATION
Teach/instruct
• To have patient well-hydrated before, and after chemotherapy
• That urine may be pink or red for 48 hr
• About importance of follow-up to monitor blood counts, serum chemistry values
• To take accurate temp; rectal temp contraindicated
• About likelihood of radiation recall phenomenon
• To notify care provider of signs of bleeding (bruising, epistaxis, bleeding gums), infection (fever, sore throat, fatigue)
Warn/advise
• About impact of body changes that may occur (hair loss, hyperpigmentation, nail ridging), how to minimize (wigs, caps, scarves, long sleeves)
• To avoid OTC preparations containing aspirin
• To report any alterations in behavior, sensation, perception; help to develop a plan of care to manage side effects, stress of illness or treatment
• To immediately report any signs of pain, irritation at injection site
• That good oral hygiene with very soft toothbrush is imperative
• That dental work be delayed until blood counts return to baseline, with permission of care provider
• To avoid contact with known viral and bacterial illnesses
• That close household contacts of child not be immunized with live polio virus; use inactivated form
• That children on chemotherapy not receive immunization until immune system recovers sufficiently to mount necessary antibody response
• To report exposure to chicken pox in susceptible child immediately
• To report reactivation of herpes zoster virus (shingles) immediately
• About ways to provide meticulous skin care in event of radiation recall
• To report fatigue, shortness of breath for evaluation as may be early signs of cardiotoxicity
• If appropriate, ways to preserve reproductive patterns, sexuality (sperm banking, contraceptives)
Encourage
• Provision of nutritious food intake; consider nutrition consultation
• To use top anesthetics to control discomfort of mucositis; avoid spicy foods, commercial mouthwashes
STORAGE
• Powder may be stored at room temp, protected from light
• Reconstituted sol may be stored at room temp for 24 hr or refrigerated for 48 hr

---

✤ Available in Canada.

demeclocycline hydrochloride

Brand Name(s): Declomycin✤, Ledermycin

Classification: Antibiotic (tetracycline)

Pregnancy Category: D

AVAILABLE PREPARATIONS
Caps: 150 mg
Tabs: 150 mg, 300 mg

ROUTES AND DOSAGES
Children >8 yr: PO 6-12 mg/kg/24 hr divided q6-12h
Adults: PO 150 mg q6h or 300 mg q12h

Gonnorhea
Adults: PO 600 mg once, then 300 mg q12h for 4 days (total 3 g)
• Not recommended for children <8 yr

MECHANISM AND INDICATIONS
Antibiotic mechanism: Bacteriostatic; inhibits bacterial protein synthesis by binding reversibly to ribosomal subunits
Indications: Effective against gram-positive and gram-negative organisms including *Mycoplasma, Rickettsia, Chlamydia,* and spirochetes; used to treat *Chlamydia trachomatis,* mycoplasma pneumonia, rickettsial infections

PHARMACOKINETICS
Peak: 3-6 hr
Distribution: Concentrates in liver
Half-life: 10-17 hr
Metabolism: Partially metabolized in liver
Excretion: Urine

CONTRAINDICATIONS
• Contraindicated in second half of pregnancy, lactation, children <8 yr (risk of permanent discoloration of teeth, enamel defects, retardation of bone growth); known hypersensitivity to any tetracycline
• Use cautiously with impaired renal or hepatic function

INTERACTIONS
Drug
• Decreased bactericidal effects of penicillins
• Increased effects of oral anticoagulants
• Decreased absorption with use of antacids containing aluminum, Ca, or Mg, laxatives containing Mg, oral iron, zinc, $NaHCO_3$
• Increased effects of digoxin
• Increased risk of nephrotoxicity from methoxyflurane
Lab
• False-positive for urine catecholamines
Nutrition
• Decreased oral absorption if given with food or dairy products

SIDE EFFECTS
CNS: Dizziness, headache, increased intracranial pressure
CV: Pericarditis
DERM: Maculopapular and erythematous rashes, photosensitivity, increased pigmentation, discolored nails and teeth
GI: Anorexia, nausea, vomiting, diarrhea, glossitis, dysphagia, enterocolitis, inflammatory anogenital lesions
GU: Reversible nephrotoxicity with outdated tetracycline
HEME: Neutropenia, eosinophilia
METAB: Elevated BUN, diabetes insipidus syndrome (polyuria, polydipsia, weakness)
Other: Hypersensitivity, bacterial or fungal superinfection

TOXICITY AND OVERDOSE
Clinical signs: GI disturbance
Treatment: Antacids; if ingested within 4 hr, empty stomach by gastric lavage; supportive care

PATIENT CARE MANAGEMENT
Assessment
• Assess history of hypersensitivity to tetracyclines
• Obtain C&S; may begin therapy before obtaining results
• Assess renal function (BUN, creatinine, I&O), hepatic function

D

(ALT, AST, bilirubin), hematologic function (CBC, differential, platelet count) (particularly for long-term therapy), bowel pattern

Interventions
• Check expiration dates; nephrotoxicity may result from outdated tetracycline
• Administer penicillins at least 1 hr before tetracycline if pt is receiving concurrent penicillins
• Administer PO 1 hr ac or 2 hr after meals; administer with water to prevent esophageal irritation; do not administer within 1 hr of hs to prevent esophageal irritation; do not administer with milk or dairy products, $NaHCO_3$, oral iron, zinc, antacids
• Tabs may be crushed, caps taken apart, mixed with food or fluid
• Maintain age-appropriate fluid intake

NURSING ALERT
Discontinue drug if signs of toxicity, hypersensitivity, renal dysfunction, superinfection, erythema from sun or ultraviolet exposure, pseudomembranous colitis develop

Evaluation
• Evaluate therapeutic response (decreased symptoms of infection)
• Monitor for signs of superinfection (perineal itching, diaper rash, fever, malaise, redness, pain, swelling, drainage, rash, diarrhea, sore throat, change in cough or sputum)
• Observe for signs of allergic reaction (rash, pruritus, angioedema)
• Monitor bowel pattern; diarrhea may be symptomatic of pseudomembranous colitis
• Monitor renal function (BUN, creatinine, I&O), hepatic function (ALT, AST, bilirubin), hematologic function (CBC, differential, platelet count)

PATIENT AND FAMILY EDUCATION
Teach/instruct
• To take as directed at prescribed intervals for prescribed length of time
Warn/advise
• To notify care provider of hypersensitivity, side effects, superinfection
• Not to use outdated medication
• To avoid sun or UV light

STORAGE
• Store at room temp in airtight, light-resistant containers

---

desipramine, desipramine hydrochloride

Brand Name(s): Desipramine✤, Norpramin (tabs)✤, Pertofrane✤, Pertofrane (caps), PMS-Desipramine✤

Classification: Tricyclic antidepressant

Pregnancy Category: C

AVAILABLE PREPARATIONS
Tabs: 10 mg, 25 mg, 50 mg, 75 mg, 100 mg, 150 mg (available as generic)
Caps: 25 mg, 50 mg (no generic available)

ROUTES AND DOSAGES
Major Depressive Disorder, Anxiety Disorders
Children and adolescents: PO 3-5 mg/kg/24 hr divided bid
Attention Deficit Hyperactivity Disorder (ADHD)
Children 6-12 yr: PO 1-3 mg/kg/24 hr divided bid; maximum dose up to 5 mg/kg/24 hr
Adolescents: PO starting dose 25-50 mg/24 hr; gradually increase to 100 mg/24 in single or divided doses; maximum dose 150 mg/24 hr
Adult: Starting dose 75 mg/24 hr; gradually increase to 150-200 mg/

---

24 hr qd or divided bid; do not exceed 300 mg/24 hr

Other Indications

Children 6-12 yr: PO starting dose 1 mg/kg/24 hr; increase by 25% q 4-5 days as tolerated, up to 3-5 mg/kg/24 hr; may go as high as 1-5 mg/kg/24 hr in divided doses

MECHANISM
AND INDICATIONS

Mechanism: Desipramine hydrochloride is the active metabolite of imipramine; desipramine blocks reuptake of norepinephrine or serotonin into nerve endings, increasing their concentration and action at the synapse

Indications: For use in treating depression and ADHD, impulsivity, hyperactivity, distractibility, panic attacks, anxiety-based school refusal, separation anxiety disorder, bulimia, primary nocturnal enuresis, night terrors, sleepwalking; often preferred over imipramine because it causes fewer anticholinergic side effects

PHARMACOKINETICS

Onset of action: Steady state achieved in 2-11 days; therapeutic antidepressant effects may take 2-3 wk

Absorption: Well absorbed from GI tract

Half-life: 14-62 hr in adults

Metabolism: Liver; rate of metabolism varies greatly among individuals; up to a 36-fold difference in plasma level has been found in individuals taking equivalent doses of medication

Excretion: Urine

Therapeutic levels: For best clinical antidepressant response, steady state plasma levels should be between 125 and 300 ng/ml; levels established for depression are not directly applicable for treatment of attention disorders, dose should be determined by clinical response rather than blood levels; therapeutic range 150-300 ng/ml; plasma levels above 300 ng/ml should be avoided

CONTRAINDICATIONS
AND PRECAUTIONS

• Contraindicated with hypersensitivity to this or any component of this medication; potential for alcohol abuse, cardiac disease or arrhythmia or recent MI; in pts receiving MAOIs within past 14 days; with narrow-angle glaucoma, prostatic hypertrophy, undiagnosed syncope, history of urinary retention

• Use cautiously with children <12 yr (cardiac toxicity is a significant risk); with family history of sudden cardiac death or cardiomyopathy; with known electrolyte abnormality associated with binging and purging; with increased intraocular pressure, hyperthyroidism or pts receiving thyroid replacement; with seizure disorder; urinary retention; with suicidal tendencies; with pregnancy (crosses placenta)

INTERACTIONS
Drug

• With MAOIs may lead to hyperpyretic crisis, hypertensive episode, tachycardia, seizures, death

• Increased effects of alcohol, barbiturates, benzodiazepines, CNS depressants, epinephrine, warfarin

• Decreased effects of guanethidine, clonidine, ephedrine

• Increased sedation with alcohol, antihistamines, antipsychotics, barbiturates, benzodiazepines, chloral hydrate, glutethimide, sedatives

• Increased hypotension with α methyldopa, β-adrenergic blockers, diuretics

• Increased cardiotoxicity with quinidine, thioridazine, mesoridazine

• Additive anticholinergic toxicity with antihistamines, antiparkinsonian, GI antispasmodics and antidiarrheals, OTC sleeping medications, thioridazine

• Tachycardia may be more pronounced with marijuana

• Decrease plasma levels and effectiveness of desipramine pos-

sible with barbiturates, cigarette smoking
• Increased effects of desipramine with methylphenidate, oral contraceptives, phenothiazines

Lab
• Increased serum bilirubin, BG, alk phos
• Falsely elevated urinary catecholamines
• Decreased VMA, 5-HIAA

Nutrition
• Some formulations contain tartrazine (yellow dye #5) which may cause an allergic reaction
• If alcohol is consumed, hold dose until morning

SIDE EFFECTS
• Desipramine produces less sedation and anticholinergic adverse effects than amitriptyline or imipramine
CNS: Dizziness, drowsiness, anxiety, confusion, headache, insomnia, nightmares, paresthesia, increased psychiatric symptoms, sedation, stimulation, tremors, weakness
CV: ECG changes, hypotension, tachycardia, arrhythmias, hypertension, palpitations
DERM: Hives, photosensitivity, pruritus, rash, sweating
EENT: Blurred vision, increased intraocular pressure, mydriasis, ophthalmoplegia, tinnitus
GI: Diarrhea, dry mouth, increased appetite, constipation, cramps, epigastric distress, hepatitis, paralytic ileus, jaundice, nausea, stomatitis, vomiting, wt gain
GU: Urinary retention, acute renal failure
HEME: Agranulocytosis, eosinophilia, leukopenia, thrombocytopenia
Other: SIADH

TOXICITY AND OVERDOSE
Clinical signs: Possible toxicity at >300 ng/ml; toxic at >1000 ng/ml; agitation, confusion, hallucinations, hypotension, hypothermia, tachycardia, urinary retention
Treatment: Monitor ECG, induce emesis; administer lavage, activated charcoal, and anticonvulsant; maintain normal temp; correct acidosis with $NaHCO_3$ to increase protein binding, decrease free fraction; correction of acidosis may decrease cardiovascular toxicities; avoid disopyramide, procainamide, quinidine; lidocaine, phenytoin, or propranolol may be necessary; reserve physostigmine for refractory life-threatening anticholinergic toxicities

PATIENT CARE MANAGEMENT
Assessment
• Assess history of hypersensitivity to drug
• Assess family history, especially for sudden cardiac death
• Assess pt's history for cardiac disease, arrhythmias, syncope, seizure disorder, congenital hearing loss (associated with prolonged QT interval)
• Obtain baseline ECG with specific emphasis on QT (corrected); cardiac examination; CBC, leukocytes, differential; AST, ALT, bilirubin; serum electrolytes; BUN in pts with eating disorders; B/P lying and standing, pulse

Interventions
• Crush tab if pt cannot swallow it whole
• Ensure that medication is swallowed
• Administer with food or milk if GI symptoms occur
• When used for ADD or ADHD, drug is clinically most effective administered in divided doses in AM and later in day; some adolescents and adults respond better to evening administration
• Administer at hs if oversedation occurs
• Take sips of fluid, sugarless gum, hard candy for dry mouth rinse with water
• Increase fluids, fiber in diet if constipation occurs

> **NURSING ALERT**
> Do not discontinue abruptly in pts receiving long-term high-dose therapy

Evaluation

• Monitor pulse, B/P lying and standing and repeat ECGs carefully with each dose increase above 3 mg/kg/24 hr; if systolic B/P drops 20 mm Hg, hold drug and notify prescriber

• Monitor cardiac enzymes of pts receiving long-term therapy

• Monitor ECGs for flattening of T-wave, bundle branch block, AV block, arrhythmias

• Monitor and document height, pulse, B/P, ECG q 3-4 mo when dose has reached a steady state

• Evaluate therapeutic response (ability to function in daily activities, to sleep throughout the night) evaluate the symptoms for which desipramine was prescribed (depression, panic attacks, anxiety, bulimia, disturbances at night); if taken for attention deficit, obtain parent and teacher reports about attention, behavioral performance

• Evaluate mental status (mood, sensorium, affect, impulsiveness, panic, suicidal ideation, psychiatric symptoms)

• Evaluate for signs and symptoms of EPS (rigidity, dystonia, akathisia)

• Monitor for urinary retention, constipation

• Upper limits of cardiovascular parameters: Heart rate >130/min, systolic B/P >130 mm Hg, diastolic B/P >85 mm Hg, PR interval >0.20 sec, QRS interval >0.12 sec, or no more than 30% above baseline, QT corrected >0.45 sec

• Desipramine should not be discontinued abruptly, but tapered over 10-14 days

• If medication is discontinued abruptly, withdrawal symptoms include headache, nausea, vomiting, muscle pain, weakness

PATIENT AND FAMILY EDUCATION
Teach/instruct

• To take as directed as prescribed intervals for prescribed length of time

• That medication is most helpful when used as part of a comprehensive multimodal treatment program

• Not to stop taking this medication without prescriber approval

• That therapeutic effects may take 2-4 wk

• To increase fluids, fiber in diet if constipation occurs

Warn/advise

• To ensure that medication is swallowed

• To avoid ingesting alcohol, other CNS depressants while taking desipramine

• That medication may cause drowsiness; be careful on bicycles, skates, skateboards, while driving, or with other activities requiring alertness

• To stay out of direct sunlight (especially between 10 AM and 3 PM) if possible; if pt must be outside, wear protective clothing, hat, and sunglasses; put on sun block with a skin protection factor (SPF) of at least 15

• Not to discontinue medication quickly after long-term use; sudden discontinuation may cause headache, nausea, vomiting, muscle pain, weakness

STORAGE

• Store at room temp

---

desmopressin

Brand Name(s): DDAVP

Classification: Pituitary hormone, antidiuretic, hemostatic agent

Pregnancy Category: B

AVAILABLE PREPARATIONS
Nasal sol: 0.1 mg/ml
Inj: 4 mcg/ml
Rhinal tube: 0.1 mg/ml

ROUTES AND DOSAGES
Nocturnal Enuresis
Children ≥6 yr: Intranasal, initial 20 mcg hs; range 10-40 mcg
Diabetes Insipidus
Children 3 mo-12 yr: Intranasal, initial 5 mcg/24 hr qd or divided

bid; range 5-30 mcg/24 hr qd or divided bid
Children >12 yr and adults: SC/IV 2-4 mcg/24 hr divided bid or ¹⁄₁₀ of maintenance intranasal dose; intranasal 5-40 mcg/24 hr qd or divided tid

Hemophilia and von Willebrand's Disease

Children > 3 mo-12 yr: IV 0.3 mcg/kg; may repeat dose if needed; begin 30 min before procedure
Children > 12 yr and adults: IV 0.3 mcg/kg by slow infusion; begin 30 min before procedure

IV administration

• Maximum concentration: 0.5 mcg/ml in NS for von Willebrand's disease
• IV infusion: Over 15-30 min for von Willebrand's disease
• Direct IV: Undiluted over 30 sec for diabetes insipidus

MECHANISM AND INDICATIONS

Antidiuretic mechanism: Increases reabsorption of water at the renal tubule, increases urine osmolality
Hemostatic mechanism: Increases plasma levels of Factor VIII, which increases platelet aggregation
Indications: Diabetes insipidus, von Willebrand's disease, hemophilia A, primary nocturnal enuresis

PHARMACOKINETICS

Onset: 1 hr
Peak: 1-5 hr

CONTRAINDICATIONS AND PRECAUTIONS

• Contraindicated with history of hypersensitivity to this drug
• Use cautiously with CAD, hypertension, pregnancy, lactation

INTERACTIONS

Drug
• Increased effect with carbamazepine, chlorpropamide, clofibrate
• Decreased effect with lithium, epinephrine, norepinephrine, demeclocycline, heparin, alcohol

SIDE EFFECTS

CNS: Headache, drowsiness, confusion, seizures, coma
CV: Slight increase in B/P, hypotension with rapid IV administration
GI: Nausea, heartburn, abdominal cramps
GU: Anuria, vulval pain
EENT: Nasal irritation, congestion, rhinitis
Local: Pain, redness at injection site
Other: Wt gain, flushing, anaphylaxis

TOXICITY AND OVERDOSE

Clinical signs: Signs of water intoxication (e.g., drowsiness, headache, confusion, anuria, weight gain)
Treatment: Restriction of water and temporary withdrawal of drug until polyuria returns; severe cases may require osmotic diuresis (possibly in conjunction with furosemide)

PATIENT CARE MANAGEMENT

Assessment
• Assess history of hypersensitivity to desmopressin
• Assess I&O, wt, edema, irritation of nares, signs of water intoxication

Interventions
• Do not use outdated, discolored, or cloudy nasal sol
• Position pt in upright sitting position; administer onto nasal mucosa by measuring dose into the flexible catheter provided by the manufacturer, inserting one end of catheter into pt's nose, and having patient blow into the other end of the catheter; for infants or young children, use an air-filled syringe on the oral end of catheter instead of having the pt blow into it.
• If nasal therapy is ineffective or inappropriate because of rhinorrhea, may administer ¹⁄₁₀ of maintenance intranasal dose SC or IV
• Provide appropriate fluid intake especially in young children or those with impaired thirst mechanism

Evaluation
• Evaluate therapeutic response (appropriate I&O, absence of polyuria or anuria)

- Monitor pulse, B/P during infusion
- Monitor wt (appropriate for age; use same scale at same time of day); urine osmolality (appropriate for age); serum and urine electrolytes
- Monitor for signs of water intoxication (behavioral changes, lethargy, disorientation, neuromuscular excitability)
- Evaluate nasal irritation, rhinorrhea (nasal inflammation will impair absorption)
- Evaluate appropriate laboratory test: hemophilia A (factor VIII concentration) von Willebrand's disease (bleeding times, factor VIII, ristocetin factor, Willebrand's factor)

PATIENT AND FAMILY EDUCATION
Teach/instruct
- To take as directed at prescribed intervals for prescribed length of time
- To notify care provider of hypersensitivity, side effects (hyponatremia, water intoxication)
- To notify care provider of cold, allergy symptoms
- To avoid use of OTC medications, especially cough, allergy products which may contain epinephrine
- To carry medical alert identification

STORAGE
- Store at 4° C (40° F)

---

desonide
Brand Name(s): Desocort✢, DesOwen, Tridesilon✢
Classification: Topical anti-inflammatory
Pregnancy Category: C

AVAILABLE PREPARATIONS
Cream, oint: 0.05%

ROUTES AND DOSAGES
Children: Top apply cream or oint sparingly to affected area qd

Adults: Top, apply cream or oint sparingly to affected area bid-qid

MECHANISM AND INDICATIONS
Mechanism: Stimulates production of enzymes needed to reduce inflammatory response; decreases all proliferation
Indications: For use in treatment of inflammatory and pruritic dermatoses (psoriasis, eczema, pruritus, contact dermatitis)

PHARMACOKINETICS
Absorption: Amount absorbed depends on amount applied and on nature of skin at site of application; on thick skin (palms, soles, elbows, knees) absorption is minimal; on thin skin (face, eyelids, genitals) absorption is high
Distribution: Primarily in the skin; any absorbed drug removed rapidly from circulation, distributed into muscle, skin, liver, intestine, kidneys
Metabolism: Liver
Excretion: Urine, feces

CONTRAINDICATIONS AND PRECAUTIONS
- Contraindicated with known hypersensitivity to drug or its components; with viral, fungal, or tubercular lesions
- Use cautiously with impaired circulation (because of the risk of skin ulceration); in children because of increased systemic absorption (which could lead to Cushing syndrome, intracranial hypertension, and hypothalamic–pituitary–adrenal axis suppression); use the least amount of drug for as short a time as possible

INTERACTIONS
None significant

INCOMPATIBILITIES
None significant

SIDE EFFECTS
Significant systemic absorption may cause the following:
CNS: Euphoria, insomnia, headache, pseudotumor cerebri, mental changes, restlessness
CV: Edema, hypertension

ENDO: Adrenal suppression
DERM: Acneiform eruptions, delayed healing
GI: Increased appetite, peptic ulcer and irritation
Local: Burning pruritus, hypopigmentation, atrophy, striae, allergic contact dermatitis

TOXICITY AND OVERDOSE
Clinical signs: No information available
Treatment: No information available

PATIENT CARE MANAGEMENT
Assessment
• Assess skin for appropriateness of application; do not apply to skin with skin ulcerations or viral, fungal, or tubercular lesions
Interventions
• Apply small amount sparingly to clean, dry skin lesion(s) for shortest time as possible; stop drug if signs of systemic absorption appear; do not apply occlusive dressings over drug unless severe or resistant dermatoses; occlusive dressing will increase absorption

NURSING ALERT
In children, limit top application to least effective amount

Evaluation
• Evaluate therapeutic response (decreased skin inflammation)
• Assess skin for side effects after application (especially striae, increased inflammation, atrophy, infection)

PATIENT/FAMILY EDUCATION
Teach/instruct
• To use as directed at prescribed intervals for prescribed length of time; *do not over-apply*
• To apply sparingly using a light film, to rub into affected area(s) gently
• Not to use occlusive dressing over area of application; diapers may be used if changed regularly, not in place >8 hr

• To call provider if side effects occur or if skin not improved in 1 wk
• About side effects, especially if over-applied
• To wash, dry hands before, after application
• To avoid prolonged application on face, skin folds, genital area; to notify care provider of hypersensitivity reactions
• Not to apply to ulcerated skin

STORAGE
• Store at room temp

desoximetasone
Brand Name(s): Topicort❧
Classification: Topical anti-inflammatory
Pregnancy Category: C

AVAILABLE PREPARATIONS
Cream: 0.05%, 0.25%
Oint: 0.25%
Gel: 0.05%

ROUTES AND DOSAGES
Children: Top, apply sparingly qd
Adults: Top, apply sparingly qd-bid

MECHANISM AND INDICATION
Mechanism: Stimulates synthesis of enzymes, which decrease inflammatory response
Indications: For treatment of inflammatory and pruritic dermatoses (psoriasis, eczema, pruritis, contact dermatitis)

PHARMACOKINETICS
Absorption: Amount absorbed depends on amount applied, on nature of skin at site of application; on thick skin (palms, soles, elbows, knees) absorption is minimal, on thin skin (face, eyelids, genitals) absorption is high
Distribution: Primarily in the skin; any absorbed drug is removed rapidly from circulation, distributed into muscle, skin, liver, intestine, kidneys

Metabolism: Liver
Excretion: Urine, feces

CONTRAINDICATIONS AND PRECAUTIONS

• Contraindicated with known hypersensitivity to drug or its components; with viral, fungal, or tubercular lesions

• Use cautiously with impaired circulation because of the risk of skin ulceration; in children because of increased systemic absorption (which could lead to Cushing syndrome, intracranial hypertension, and hypothalamic–pituitary–adrenal axis suppression); use least amount of drug for shortest time possible

INTERACTIONS

None reported

INCOMPATIBILITIES

None reported

SIDE EFFECTS

Significant systemic absorption may cause the following:
CNS: Euphoria, insomnia, headache, pseudotumor cerebri, mental changes, restlessness
CV: Edema, hypertension
DERM: Acneiform eruptions, delayed healing
ENDO: Adrenal suppression
GI: Increased appetite, peptic irritation, ulcer
Local: Burning, pruritus, hypopigmentation, atrophy, striae, allergic contact dermatitis

TOXICITY AND OVERDOSE

Clinical signs: No information available
Treatment: No information available

PATIENT CARE MANAGEMENT

Assessment

• Assess skin for appropriateness of application, do not apply to skin with ulcerations or viral, fungal, or tubercular lesions

Interventions

• Apply small amount sparingly to clean, dry skin lesion(s) for shortest time possible; stop drug if signs of systemic absorption appear; do not apply occlusive dressings over drug, unless severe or resistant dermatoses; occlusive dressing will increase absorption

> **NURSING ALERT**
> In children, limit top application to least effective amount

D

Evaluation

• Evaluate therapeutic response (decreased skin inflammation)

• After application, assess skin for side effects (especially striae, increased inflammation, atrophy, infection)

PATIENT/FAMILY EDUCATION

Teach/instruct

• To use as directed at prescribed intervals for prescribed length of time; *do not over-apply*

• To apply sparingly using a light film, to rub into affected area(s) gently

• Not to use occlusive dressing over area of application; diapers may be used if changed regularly, not in place >8 hr

• To call provider if side effects occur or if skin not improved in 1 wk

• About side effects, especially if over applied

• To wash, dry hands before, after application

• To avoid prolonged application on face, skin folds, genital area, to notify care provider of hypersensitivity reactions

• Not to apply to ulcerated skin

STORAGE

• Store at room temp

❖ Available in Canada.

dexamethasone, dexamethasone acetate, dexamethasone sodium phosphate

Brand Name(s): Aeroseb-Dex, AKDex, Baldex, Dalalone LA, Decadron, Decadron Eye-Ear Solution✤, Decadron LA, Decadron Tablets✤, Dexasone✤, Dexone LA, Hexadrol, Maxidex✤, PMS-Dexamethasone✤, Turbinaire

Classification: Glucocorticoid

Pregnancy Category: C

AVAILABLE PREPARATIONS
Oral elixir: 0.5 mg/5 ml
Sol: 0.5 mg/5 ml, 1 mg/ml
Sol, concentrate: 0.5 mg/0.5 ml
Tabs: 0.25 mg, 0.5 mg, 0.75 mg, 1 mg, 1.5 mg, 2 mg, 4 mg, 6 mg
Inj: Dexamethasone sodium phosphate 4 mg/ml, 10 mg/ml, 20 mg/ml, 24 mg/ml (20 mg/ml 24 mg/ml for IV use only); dexamethasone acetate 8 mg/ml, 16 mg/ml (freely soluble in water

ROUTES AND DOSAGES
Cerebral Edema
Children and adults: IM/IV 0.5-1.5 mg/kg initially, then 0.2-0.5 mg/kg/24 hr divided q6h×5 days, then gradually taper
Airway Edema
Children and adults: IV 0.25-0.5 mg/kg/dose q6h prn for croup or beginning 24‍ hr before elective extubation and continuing for 4-6 doses
Antiemetic
Children and adult: IV 4-8 mg/m² loading dose, then 2-4 mg/m²/dose q6h
Antiinflammatory
Children: PO/IM/IV 0.03-0.15 mg/kg/24 hr divided q6-12h
Adults: PO/IM/IV 0.75-9 mg/24 hr divided q6-12h

Meningitis
Children and adult: IV 0.15 mg/kg/dose q6h × 4 days
• Dexamethasone is insoluble in water, sparingly soluble in alcohol; may mix tabs, elixir, sol, concentrated sol in juices or semi-solids foods (applesauce)
IV administration
• Recommended concentration: 24 mg/ml or dilute in D₅W or NS for IV infusion
• Maximum concentration: 24 mg/ml
• IV push rate: Over 1-4 min if dose is <10 mg
• Intermittent infusion: High dose therapy over 15-30 min

MECHANISM AND INDICATIONS
Mechanism: Decreases inflammation by stabilizing leukocyte lysosomal membranes and suppressing immune response; helps stimulate bone marrow, influences protein, fat, and carbohydrate metabolism
Indications: Used for antiinflammatory or immunosuppressive effects in treatment of cerebral edema, inflammatory conditions, allergic reactions, neoplasias, shock, and to prevent chemotherapy-induced nausea or vomiting

PHARMACOKINETICS
Onset of action: PO 1-2 hr; IM/IV after administration
Absorption: Readily absorbed
Distribution: Into muscle, liver, skin, intestines, kidneys
Peak: IM/IV within 1 hr; PO within 1-2 hr; plasma peak concentration (dexamethasone acetate) 8 hr
Half-life: 36-54 hr
Duration: PO 2.5 days; IM 6 days (dexamethasone acetate)
Metabolism: Liver (primarily)
Excretion: Inactive metabolites in urine; small amounts of unmetabolized drugs in urine, negligible amounts in bile

---

CONTRAINDICATIONS AND PRECAUTIONS

• Contraindicated with hypersensitivity to any component of the drug (sulfites); with systemic fungal infections, acute or active infections, chicken pox, herpes zoster, or known viral illnesses (because adrenocorticoids increase suspectibility, mask symptoms of infection)

• Use cautiously with GI ulcerations, renal disease, hypertension, osteoporosis, varicella, DM, seizures, emotional instability, psychotic tendencies, CHF, glaucoma, cataracts, cirrhosis, tuberculosis, thromboembolytic disorders, hyperlipidemias, hypoalbuminemia, hypothyroidism, pregnancy; in pts receiving anticoagulants

INTERACTIONS
Drug

• Increased risk of GI bleeding or distress with use of aspirin, indomethacin, other NSAIDs

• Decreased action of dexamethasone possible with use of barbiturates, phenytoin, rifampin

• Decreased effects of oral anticoagulants possible

• Enhanced K^+-wasting effects of dexamethasone with K^+-depleting drugs such as thiazide diuretics

• Decreased response of skin-test antigens

• Decreased antibody response, increased risk of neurologic complications with use of toxoids, vaccines

Lab

• Increased glucose, cholesterol possible

• Decreased serum K^+, Ca, thyroxine possible

INCOMPATIBILITIES

• Should not be mixed with other drugs during administration

SIDE EFFECTS

Most adverse reactions to corticosteroids are dependent upon dose and duration

CNS: Euphoria, insomnia, psychotic behavior, pseudotumor cerebri, transient increase in intracranial pressure, headache, mental changes, nervousness, restlessness

CV: CHF, hypertension, edema

EENT: Cataracts, glaucoma, increase intraocular pressure

ENDO/METAB: Hypokalemia, hyperglycemia, glucose intolerance, growth suppression; cushingoid state

DERM: Delayed wound healing, acne, various skin eruptions, atrophy at IM injection sites, striae

GI: Peptic ulcer, GI irritation, increased appetite, pancreatitis

Other: Muscle weakness, osteoporosis, hirsutism, suspectibility to infection; acute adrenal insufficiency may follow increased stress (infection, surgery, trauma) or abrupt withdrawal after long therapy; rebound inflammation, fatigue, weakness, arthralgia, fever, dizziness, lethargy, depression, fainting, orthostatic hypotension, dyspnea, anorexia, hypoglycemia may occur after abrupt withdrawal: after prolonged use, sudden withdrawal may be fatal

TOXICITY AND OVERDOSE

Clinical signs: Acute ingestion is rarely a clinical problem

Treatment: Decrease drug gradually if possible

PATIENT CARE MANAGEMENT
Assessment

• Assess history of hypersensitivity to drug, related drugs

• Assess baseline VS (especially B/P), serum electrolytes (K^+, Ca, BG), cardiac function, renal function (BUN, creatinine, urine CrCl), liver function (ALT, AST, LDH, bilirubin, alk phos)

• Assess baseline wt, accurate I&O, hydration status (SG)

- Assess baseline growth and development status
- Assess baseline neurologic and mental status before starting therapy
- Assess history of previous treatment with special attention to other therapies that may predispose to renal, cardiac, psychologic dysfunction

Interventions

- Give oral medication with food whenever possible to decrease chance of GI upset; may be mixed with food, fluid
- Administer IM deeply in large muscle mass; rotate injection sites
- Monitor pt's wt, VS (especially B/P), I&O
- Provide supportive measures to maintain fluid and electrolyte balance, nutritional support
- Administer K⁺ supplements as indicated
- Provide low Na, high K⁺, high protein diet

NURSING ALERT

Administer with food to decrease chances of GI irritation

Provide low Na diet high in K⁺, protein

Do not stop drug abruptly if pt has been on long-term therapy; must be tapered over time

Avoid SC injection; atrophy and abscesses may develop

Evaluation

- Evaluate therapeutic response (decreased inflammation)
- Monitor serum electrolytes (K⁺, BG, Ca), VS (especially B/P)
- Monitor I&O, check wt regularly
- Evaluate for any signs of depression or psychotic episodes, especially with high-dose therapy
- Assess skin for petechiae, bruising
- Assess growth and development in children on prolonged therapy

- Assess for signs or symptoms of infection (fever, fatigue, sore throat), bleeding (easy bruising, nose bleeds, bleeding gums)
- Assess BG in pts with a history of diabetes

PATIENT/FAMILY EDUCATION

Teach/instruct

- About importance of follow-up to monitor serum chemistry values
- To notify care provider of signs of infection (fever, sore throat, fatigue), delayed healing
- About possibility of weakening bones (osteoporosis) and the need for proper exercise, diet, and limitations for pts on prolonged therapy
- Not to stop drug abruptly or without care provider's consent because of possible side effects associated with abrupt withdrawal
- To take medication in AM with breakfast for best results and less GI distress
- About cushingoid syndromes and to report sudden wt gain or swelling, especially for pts on long-term therapy

Warn/advise

- To avoid OTC products containing aspirin, NSAIDs
- To report any alterations in behavior; help to develop a plan of care to manage side effects, stress of illness or treatment
- To immediately report any pain, discoloration at injection site (parenteral forms)
- To avoid contact with known viral or bacterial illnesses
- That household contacts of child not be immunized with live polio virus; inactivated form should be used
- That child not receive immunizations until immune system recovers sufficiently to mount needed antibody response
- To report exposure to chicken

---

pox in susceptible child immediately
• To report reactivation of herpes zoster virus (shingles) immediately
• To notify care provider of signs or symptoms of adrenal insufficiency (fatigue, muscle weakness, joint pain, fever, anorexia, nausea, dyspnea, dizziness, fainting)
• To have periodic ophthalmic examinations (for pts on long-term therapy)
• That pts with diabetes may need more insulin while on steroids; monitor blood glucose carefully
• To limit the amount of salt or salty foods when on steroids; use low Na, high K+, high protein diet
• About impact of body changes that may occur (wt gain, cushingoid syndrome), how to minimize (loose clothing, decrease salt intake)

Encourage
• Pts experiencing excessive wt gain to decrease salt intake; to eat a high protein, high K+ diet; nutritional consult may be needed
• To carry medical alert identification indicating steroid use

STORAGE
• Store oral preparations at room temp in tight containers
• Parenteral dexamethasone sodium phosphate and dexamethasone acetate should be protected from light, freezing; use diluted sol within 24 hr

---

dextroamphetamine sulfate

Brand Name(s): Dexedrine♣, Dexedrine Spansules

Classification: CNS stimulant

Controlled Substance Schedule II

Pregnancy Category: C

D

AVAILABLE PREPARATIONS
Elixir: 5 mg/ml
Tabs: 5 mg, 10 mg
Sus rel caps: 5 mg, 10 mg, 15 mg; 6.25 mg with 6.25 mg amphetamine, 10 mg with 10 mg amphetamine

DOSAGES AND ROUTES
• Tolerance may develop, requiring dosage adjustment over time
Attention Deficit Hyperactivity Disorder (ADHD)
• Do not use in children <3 yr
Children 3-6 yr: PO, initial 2.5 mg/24 hr qd in AM, increase by 2.5 mg/24 hr at weekly intervals until optimal response is reached; usual range 0.1-0.5 mg/kg/dose qd; maximum dose 40 mg/24 hr
Children >6 yr: PO, initial 5 mg qd-bid, increase in increments of 5 mg/24 hr at weekly intervals until optimal response is reached; usual range 0.1-0.5 mg/kg/dose, or 2.5-10 mg/dose, or 5-20 mg/24 hr administered bid before school and at noon; another dose may be administered at 4 PM if needed; maximum dose 40 mg/24 hr
Exogenous Obesity
Children >12 yr and adults: PO 5-30 mg/24 hr in divided doses of 5-10 mg given 30-60 min ac; ext rel caps qd in AM
• Do not use in children <12 yr
Narcolepsy
Children 6-12 yr: PO, initial 5 mg/24 hr; may increase in 5 mg increments at weekly intervals until side effects appear; maximum dose 60 mg/24 hr

---

Children >12 yr and adults: 10 mg/24 hr; may increase in 10 mg increments at weekly intervals until side effects appear; maximum dose 60 mg/24 hr

MECHANISM AND INDICATIONS

Mechanism: Blocks reuptake of dopamine and norepinephrine from the synapse, increasing amounts circulating in the cerebral cortex to the reticular activating system; causes CNS and respiratory stimulation, improving attention span, task performance

Indications: For use in treating attention deficit disorder with hyperactivity (ADHD), narcolepsy, exogenous obesity; effective for many adolescents who were responsive to methylphenidate as children, but have become unresponsive as they matured

PHARMACOKINETICS

Onset of action: 30-60 min

Peak: 1-3 hr

Duration: Tabs 4-20 hr. sus rel caps: 8-12 hr, depending on the individual

Half-life: 10-30 hr pH dependent

Metabolism: Liver

Excretion: Urine, breast milk; crosses placenta

CONTRAINDICATIONS AND PRECAUTIONS

• Contraindicated with hypersensitivity to sympathomimetic amines, dextroamphetamine or any component of this medication; agitation, anxiety, severe arteriosclerosis, bipolar disorder, cardiovascular disease, history of drug abuse, glaucoma, hypertension, hyperthyroidism; within 14 days of MAOIs; pregnancy, psychosis, Tourette syndrome

• Use cautiously with aspirin sensitivity, general anesthetics, psychopathic personalities, lactation, <3 yr old

INTERACTIONS

Drug

• Increased effects of dextroamphetamine with acetazolamide, antacids, haloperidol, phenothiazines, NaHCO$_3$

• Decreased effect of dextroamphetamine with ammonium chloride, ascorbic acid, barbiturates, tricyclic antidepressants

• May precipitate hypertensive crisis if given within 14 days of MAOIs

• Decreases effects of guanethidine, methyldopa, and sedative effects of antihistamines

• May precipitate arrhythmias with general anesthetics

• Increases serum concentration of tricyclic antidepressants

Lab

• Increased serum corticosteroids, urinary epinephrine

Nutrition

• 5 mg tabs and sus rel 5 mg, 10 mg, and 15 mg Dexedrine Spansule caps contain tartrazine (yellow dye #5)

• Elimination of dextroamphetamine enhanced by ≥1 g vitamin C (ascorbic acid)

• GI acidifying agents (orange juice, gastric secretions) decrease absorption of dextroamphetamine

• Antacids containing NaHCO$_3$ (Alka-Seltzer) extend the action of dextroamphetamine by reducing its elimination.

• Do not take with alcohol

SIDE EFFECTS

CNS: Hyperactivity, insomnia, restlessness, talkativeness, addiction, aggressiveness, chills, dependence, depression, dysphoria, dizziness, euphoria, headache, irritability, nervousness, psychosis, stimulation, tremor

CV: Increased heart rate, palpitations, arrhythmias, decreased heart rate, increased or decreased B/P

DERM: Hives

EENT: Dry mouth, metallic taste, mydriasis

GI: Abdominal cramps, anorexia, constipation, diarrhea, dry mouth, nausea, vomiting, wt loss

GU: Impotence, change in libido

Other: Growth suppression, movement disorders

✦ Available in Canada.

TOXICITY AND OVERDOSE
Clinical signs: Dehydration, fever, hyperactivity, insomnia, pain
Treatment: Administer fluids, hemodialysis, or peritoneal dialysis; administer antihypertensive for increased B/P, ammonium chloride for increased elimination

PATIENT CARE MANAGEMENT
Assessment
• Assess history of hypersensitivity to drug (including yellow dye #5)
• Obtain baseline pulse, B/P, CBC, UA
Interventions
• Administer the single daily dose after breakfast or as early in the day as possible when prescribed qd
• Empty contents for administration if the sus rel cap cannot be swallowed whole; do not crush or chew
• Dextroamphetamine is most helpful when used as part of a comprehensive multimodal treatment program
• Administer daily dose in one to three divided doses/24 hr for ADHD; last daily dose should be administered at least six hr before hs, to avoid insomnia
• May be given after eating if given for ADHD and appetite is suppressed
• Sus rel caps should be administered once a day
• Treatment for ADHD should include a drug holiday or periodic discontinuation; this allows time to decrease tolerance and limit suppression of linear growth, wt; assess the pt's requirements and determine if the drug is still necessary
• Spansules have been observed to build up sometimes, which can result in irritability, tension, and other overdose effects after several wk of administration; those taking the Spansule do much better with at least 1 drug holiday per week
• Take sips of fluid, sugarless gum, hard candy for dry mouth rinse with water

• When dextroamphetamine is stopped, there may be a withdrawal depression with tearfulness for no apparent reason
• Treatment includes dietary changes and exercise when given for obesity; administer 30-60 min ac

> **NURSING ALERT**
> Dextroamphetamine has a high potential for abuse; prolonged administration may lead to drug dependence; use in wt reduction programs only when alternative therapy has been ineffective

Evaluation
• Evaluate therapeutic response (ability to function in daily activities, to sleep throughout the night, increased CNS stimulation, decreased drowsiness); if taken for attention deficit, obtain parent and teacher reports about attention and behavioral performance
• Evaluate mental status (affect, mood, sensorium, impulsiveness, irritability, psychiatric symptoms, stimulation, suicidal ideation)
• Evaluate q 3-4 mo and at times of dose increases, monitor and record pulse, B/P; plot height and wt on growth grids
• Assess for abnormal movements at each visit
• Check BG if pt has diabetes; insulin changes may be needed because eating will decrease
• Assess tolerance or dependency with long-term use; an increased amount may be needed to get same effect

PATIENT AND FAMILY EDUCATION
Teach/instruct
• To take as directed at prescribed intervals for prescribed length of time
• That this medication is most helpful when used as part of a comprehensive multimodal treatment program

---

✦ Available in Canada.

• Not to stop taking this medication without prescriber approval
• That therapeutic effects may take 2-4 wk
• To increase fluids, fiber in diet if constipation occurs
• About the purpose of drug holidays
• To report drowsiness, other side effects; drug or dosage may be adjusted
• That medication use is short-term and must be accompanied by emotional support, exercise, and diet management if the medication is given for obesity

Warn/advise
• To work with teachers, health care provider, school nurse to apply consistent behavior therapies and monitor child's therapeutic response to medication
• To report to prescriber improvement or worsening of behavioral symptoms at home and school
• To make sure medication is swallowed
• Not to crush or chew sus rel forms
• To decrease caffeine consumption (e.g., coffee, tea, cola, chocolate), which may increase stimulation, irritability
• To avoid ingesting alcohol, other CNS depressants
• To avoid OTC medications unless approved by prescriber
• That this medication may cause dizziness; be careful on bicycles, skates, skateboards, while driving, or with other activities
• That Spansules have been observed clinically to sometimes cause a build-up which can result in irritability, tension, other overdose effects after several wk of administration
• To taper off drug over several wk under prescriber's supervision; depression, increased sleeping, lethargy may be experienced

STORAGE
• Store at room temp in a tightly covered, light-resistant container
• Protect elixir from freezing.

dextrose

Classification: Fluid replacement, carbohydrate supplement

Pregnancy Category: B

AVAILABLE PREPARATIONS
Inj: 2.5%, 5%, 10%, 20%, 25%, 30%, 40%, 50%, 60%, 70% sol

ROUTES AND DOSAGES
Children and adults: IV dose is dependent on fluid and calorie needs and BG concentration peripheral IV, do not use >12.5% sol; central IV as needed, to maximum of 25% sol
• If hypoglycemic during arrest: 2-4 ml/kg/dose of 25% sol as IV bolus

IV administration
• Recommended concentration: ≤25% dextrose, depending on indication and venous access
• Maximum concentration: 25% dextrose
• IV push rate: 200 mg/kg over 1 min
• Continuous infusion rate: 4.5-15 mg/kg/min

MECHANISM AND INDICATIONS
Mechanism: Rapidly metabolized, increasing BG levels to provide a source of energy; may also decrease protein and N losses, promote glycogen storage, and reduce or prevent ketosis
Indications: Used as a fluid replacement or calorie supplement in pts unable to maintain adequate oral or enteral intake

PHARMACOKINETICS
Absorption: Rapid
Peak: 40 min
Excretion: Urine

CONTRAINDICATIONS AND PRECAUTIONS
• Contraindicated with diabetic coma while BG levels are excessively high, in pts with delirium tremens, dehydrated pts with

glucose-galactose malabsorption syndrome, hypertonic sol contraindicated in presence of intracranial or intraspinal hemorrhage or with known corn allergy
• Use cautiously with DM or carbohydrate intolerance, rapid administration of hypertonic sol may lead to hyperglycemia and hyperosmolar syndrome; caution in infants of diabetic mothers, vitamin B complex deficiency may occur with dextrose use

INTERACTIONS
Drug
• Administer dextrose with Na^+ ions cautiously with corticosteroid, corticotropin
Lab
• May cause hyperglycemia, hypomagnesemia, hypokalemia, hypophosphatemia
Nutrition
• May cause vitamin B_6 deficiency
• May require increased PO_4 for glucose metabolism

SIDE EFFECTS
CNS: Confusion, unconsciousness, hyperosmolar syndrome
CV: Fluid overload, pulmonary edema, hypertension, CHF, phlebitis, sclerosis of vein
DERM: Sloughing, tissue necrosis
GU: Glycosuria, osmotic diuresis
Local: Irritation and redness at site
Other: Hyperglycemia, hypervolemia, hyperosmolarity, rebound hypoglycemia, fever

TOXICITY AND OVERDOSE
Clinical signs: Signs of fluid overload or hyperglycemia
Treatment: Decrease infusion rate, decrease concentration, provide appropriate corrective treatment and supportive care

PATIENT CARE MANAGEMENT
Assessment
• Assess history of hypersensitivity to dextrose
• Obtain baseline BG levels
• Assess appropriateness of concentration in peripheral and central vein

• Assess infusion rate; maximum dosage of 6-8 mg/kg/min for peripheral vein
Interventions
• Avoid rapid IV administration; hypertonic sol should be administered to central vein only; may need insulin secondary to decreased pancreatic production and secretion
• Ensure age-appropriate fluid intake
• Institute safety measures, such as safety restraints

> **NURSING ALERT**
> Evaluate appropriateness of sol concentration; may cause thrombosis if hypertonic sol administered via peripheral vein
>
> Discontinue or decrease if signs of fluid overload; monitor site hourly
>
> Rapid termination of long-term infusion may result in hypoglycemia from rebound hyperinsulinemia

Evaluation
• Evaluate therapeutic response (hydration status and energy requirements)
• Evaluate side effects and injection site for signs of irritation, redness, necrosis, phlebitis
• Monitor VS, I&O, wt, especially in pts with cardiac or renal dysfunction
• Evaluate fluid status, electrolyte and acid–base balance; make appropriate changes in fluid, electrolytes based on laboratory values

PATIENT AND FAMILY EDUCATION
Teach/instruct
• To take as directed at prescribed intervals for prescribed length of time
• About need for IV therapy, importance of following infusion directions

Warn/advise
• To notify care provider of hypersensitivity, side effects
• To watch for signs of infection at site (erythema, edema, blanching, exudate)

Encourage
• Parents to hold, comfort children during IV therapy

STORAGE
• Store at room temp, protected from freezing, extreme heat

---

diazepam

Brand Name(s): Apo-Diazepam✤, Diazemuls (Diazepam Injectable Emulsion)✤, Diazepam, Diazepam Intensol, Valium, Valium Roche Injection✤, Valium Roche Oral✤, Valrelease, Vivol✤, Zetran

Classification: Antianxiety agent, anticonvulsant, benzodiazepine, sedative

Controlled Substance Schedule IV

Pregnancy Category: D

AVAILABLE PREPARATIONS
Sol: Wintergreen-spice flavor 5 mg/5ml (Diazepam, Diazepam Intensol)
Concentrate: 5 mg/ml
Tabs: 2 mg, 5 mg, 10 mg
Caps (ext rel): 15 mg (Valrelease)
Inj: 5 mg/ml

DOSAGES AND ROUTES
• Do not use PO form in children <6 mo
• Use smallest PO dose possible; children may be more sensitive to benzodiazepines

Conscious Sedation for Procedures
Children 6 mo-12 yr: 0.2-0.3 mg/kg 45 min before procedure; maximum 10 mg
Adolescents and adults: PO 10 mg, may repeat with ½ dose if needed; IV 5 mg, may repeat with ½ dose if needed

Sedation or Muscle Relaxation or Anxiety
Children 6 mo-12 yr: PO 0.12-0.8 mg/kg/24 hr divided q6-8h; IM/IV 0.04-0.2 mg/kg/24 hr in divided doses q2-4h; maximum 0.6 mg/kg within an 8 hr period, if needed
Adolescents and adults: 2-10 mg tid-qid; extended release 15-30 mg qd; dosage may be increased cautiously as needed and tolerated
• Safety and effectiveness of injectable forms have not been established in newborns

Tetanic Muscle Spasms
Infants >30 days: IM/IV 1-2 mg q3-4h prn
Children >5 years: IM/IV 5-10 mg q3-4h prn

Status Epilepticus
Children: IV bolus 0.05-0.3 mg/kg administered 1 mg/min over 3 min; may repeat q 15-30 min × 2 doses; maximum 5 mg/dose in children ≤5 yr, 10 mg/dose in children >5 yrs
Adolescents and adults: IV 5-10 mg q 10-20 min; maximum 30 mg/dose q8h

Prophylaxis of Febrile Seizures
Children >6 mo: 1 mg/kg/24 hr divided q8h beginning with onset of fever and continuing until afebrile for 24 hr

Anxiety
Children 6 mo-12 yr: IM/IV 0.04-0.3 mg/kg/dose q2-4h; maximum 0.6 mg/kg within 8 hrs
Adolescents and adults: PO 2-10 mg bid-qid; IM/IV 2-10 mg; may repeat in 3-4 hrs if needed; maximum 60 mg/24 hr

IV administration
• Recommended concentration: Do not dilute
• IV push rate: Administer total dose over 3 min minimum for infants and children; 5 mg/min for adolescents and adults

MECHANISM AND INDICATIONS
Mechanism: Increases action of γ-aminobutyric acid (GABA), a major inhibitory neurotransmitter in the brain; depresses all levels of

---

✤ Available in Canada.

CNS, especially the limbic system and reticular formation

Indications: For use in treating muscle spasms, acute alcohol withdrawal (acute agitation, tremor, delirium tremens), as adjunct in seizure disorders; short-term treatment of anxiety; used preoperatively to reduce anxiety, as light anesthesia, and for amnesia; unlabeled use for panic attacks

PHARMACOKINETICS

• Continuous use on a regular schedule for 3-5 days is usually necessary to determine effectiveness in relieving moderate anxiety

Onset of action: PO, ½ hr; IM, 15-30 min; IV, 1-5 min (in status epilepticus, onset is almost immediate)

Duration: PO, 2-3 hr; IM, 1-1½ hr; IV, 15 min (in status epilepticus, 20 to 30 min)

Half life: In adults, 20-50 hr; increased half-life in neonates, elderly, those with severe liver disorders

Metabolism: Liver
Elimination: Urine

CONTRAINDICATIONS AND PRECAUTIONS

• Contraindicated with hypersensitivity to this or any component of this medication, hypersensitivity to benzodiazepines, CNS depression, history of drug addiction, hyperactive or psychotic children of any age, narrow-angle glaucoma, uncontrolled pain, psychoses, respiratory depression, coma, pregnancy, lactation, pts planning pregnancy

• Use cautiously with neonates, elderly; low albumin, asthma, depression, emphysema, epilepsy, history of serious depression or mental disorder, history of alcoholism or drug abuse, serious illness, kidney or liver disease, myasthenia gravis, psychiatric disorders, with other CNS depressants

INTERACTIONS

Drug

• Increased effects of diazepam with alcohol, barbiturates, cimetidine, CNS depressants, disulfiram, isoniazid, ketoconazole, opioids

• Decreased effects of diazepam with rifampin, theophylline

• Increased effects of digoxin, phenytoin; can cause toxicity

• Decreased effects of levodopa; can reduce its effectiveness in treating Parkinson's disease

• Interacts with antacids, antihistamines, fluoxetine, metoprolol, neuromuscular blocking agents, oral contraceptives, probenecid, propoxyphene, ranitidine, scopolamine, valproic acid

Lab

• Increased alk phos, ALT, AST, serum bilirubin

• Decreased WBC counts, blood thyroxine (T^4), RAIU

• False increase for 17-OHCS

• Liver reaction with jaundice may be confused with viral hepatitis

• Urine screening tests for drug abuse may be positive; depends upon amount of drug taken and testing method used

Nutrition

• Do not drink alcohol

• Some preparations contain the dye tartrazine (FD&C Yellow No. 5) which can cause allergic reactions in certain individuals

INCOMPATIBILITIES

• With all drugs in sol or syringe

SIDE EFFECTS

CNS: Dizziness, drowsiness, decreased activity, amnesia, anxiety, apathy, ataxia, behavior changes, confusion, impaired coordination, crying, delirium, depression, disorientation, vivid dreams, euphoria, excitement, fatigue, hallucinations, hangover, headache, insomnia, lethargy, nervousness, acute rage, restlessness, seizures, stimulation, tremors, unsteadiness, vertigo, weakness

CV: Orthostatic hypotension, bradycardia, cardiac arrest, cardiovascular collapse, ECG changes, fainting, hypotension, palpitations, tachycardia

DERM: Dermatitis, excessive hair growth, hair loss, hives, itching, rash, sweating, yellowing of skin or eyes

EENT: Blurred vision, glassy-eyed, decreased hearing, sore gums, dry mouth, mydriasis, nasal congestion, increased salivation, slurred speech, difficulty swallowing, tinnitus, coated tongue, double vision, loss of voice

GI: Anorexia, constipation, diarrhea, dry mouth, nausea, stomach upset, vomiting, abnormal liver function, hiccups

GU: Incontinence, menstrual problems, changes in sex drive, urine retention

HEME: Bone marrow depression

RESP: Apnea, laryngospasm, decrease in respiratory rate

Local: Pain with injection, phlebitis

Other: Physical and psychological dependence with prolonged use, balance problems, dehydration, fever, galactorrhea, gynecomastia, joint pain, swollen lymph nodes, uncontrollable muscle movement, muscle spasms, ankle and facial swelling, tremors, wt gain or loss

TOXICITY AND OVERDOSE

Clinical signs: Apnea, coma, marked drowsiness, feeling of drunkenness, unsteady gait, hypoactive reflexes, hypotension, respiratory depression, slurred speech, stupor, tremor, weakness

Treatment: Monitor VS; support B/P and respiration; for comatose pt, administer gastric lavage with ET tube in place to prevent aspiration; flumazenil can be used to reverse effects of diazepam; treat hypotension with norepinephrine, phenylephrine, or dopamine

PATIENT CARE MANAGEMENT

Assessment

• Assess history of hypersensitivity to drug

• Assess ability to function in daily activities, ability to sleep throughout night

• Assess mental status (mood, sensorium, affect, impulsiveness, suicidal ideation, thoughts)

• Obtain baseline AST, ALT, alk phos, bilirubin, creatinine, LDH

• Obtain baseline history and physical exam

• Obtain baseline CBC if therapy will be long-term

Interventions

• Tab may be crushed if pt cannot swallow it whole

• Ext rel caps should not be opened

• May be given on an empty stomach; if GI symptoms occur, give with food or milk

• Administer IV into large vein

• Inj faster than 1-2 mg/min may cause respiratory depression or hypotension

• Monitor HR, respiratory rate, O_2 saturation, B/P if giving IV

• Limit continual use to 1 to 3 wk

• Reduce narcotic dosage by ⅓ if giving narcotic at the same time as diazepam

• Rinse with water, take sips of fluid, sugarless gum, or hard candy for dry mouth.

• Avoid excessive intake of caffeine-containing beverages (e.g., coffee, tea, cola)

• Do not drink alcohol, smoke tobacco or marijuana

• Do not stop diazepam suddenly if it has been taken for over 4 wk without interruption; dosage should be tapered gradually to prevent a withdrawal syndrome that could include depression, confusion, hallucinations, tremor, seizures, muscle cramping, sweating, vomiting

• Use caution until the effect of excessive perspiration is determined; this may be sufficient to reduce urine volume, and diazepam may accumulate in the body

> **NURSING ALERT**
> Do not administer rapid IV push; may cause apnea, hypotension, sudden respiratory depression

✚ Available in Canada.

Evaluation

- Evaluate therapeutic response (decreased anxiety, decreased ability to function in daily activities, decreased ability to sleep through-out the night)
- Evaluate mental status (mood, sensorium, affect, impulsiveness, restlessness, suicidal ideation, thoughts)
- Monitor AST, ALT, alk phos, bilirubin, creatinine, LDH
- Monitor orthostatic B/P, pulse; if systolic B/P drops 20 mm Hg, hold diazepam, notify prescriber
- Monitor for dizziness, drowsiness, excessive sedation, incoordination
- Monitor CBC periodically during long-term therapy
- After long term use, signs of physical dependence and withdrawal symptoms include headache, nausea, vomiting, muscle pain, weakness

PATIENT AND FAMILY EDUCATION

Teach/instruct

- To take as directed at prescribed intervals for prescribed length of time
- That diazepam can be habit forming if used in large doses or for a long time
- That sometimes this medicine must be taken for 3-5 days before improvement is noticed
- That signs of physical dependence and withdrawal symptoms include headache, nausea, vomiting, muscle pain, weakness
- Not to discontinue medication without prescriber approval

Warn/advise

- To avoid ingesting alcohol, antacids, antihistamines, CNS depressants.
- That this medication may cause drowsiness; be careful on bicycles, skates, skateboards, while driving, or with other activities requiring alertness
- To carry medical alert identification if diazepam is being used for epilepsy

STORAGE

- Store at room temp
- Protect IV form from light

---

diazoxide

Brand Name(s): Hyperstat IV Injection✹, Proglycem✹

Classification: Antihypertensive, antihypoglycemic

Pregnancy Category: C

AVAILABLE PREPARATIONS

Inj: 300 mg/20 ml
Caps: 50 mg
Susp: 50 mg/ml

ROUTES AND DOSAGES

Antihypertensive

Children and adults: IV 1-3 mg/kg IV push every 5-15 min until B/P satisfactory; maximum dose 150 mg

Antihypoglycemic

Infants and neonates: PO 8-15 mg/kg/24 hr divided bid-tid
Children and adults: PO 3-8 mg/kg/24 hr divided bid-tid

IV administration

- Recommended concentration: 15 mg/ml
- Maximum concentration: 15 mg/ml
- IV push rate: Over 15-30 sec; rapid IV injection preferred over IV infusion
- Intermittent infusion rate: Over 20-60 min

MECHANISM AND INDICATIONS

Mechanisms: Antihypertensive, produces smooth muscle relaxation of peripheral arterioles; antihypoglycemic, inhibits insulin secretion from pancreas
Indications: For use in hypertensive crises and for hypoglycemia caused by insulin-producing tumors

PHARMACOKINETICS

Onset of action: IV immediate, PO 1 hr
Peak: IV 5 min, PO 2 hr

Half-life: Children 9-24 hr; adults 20-36 hr
Metabolism: Liver

CONTRAINDICATIONS AND PRECAUTIONS
• Contraindicated with known hypersensitivity to diazoxide, thiazides, other sulfonamide diuretics; coarctation of the aorta; A-V shunts; aortic aneurysm
• Use cautiously with DM, renal or hepatic disease, CAD, cerebral vascular insufficiency, pregnancy, lactation

INTERACTIONS
Drug
• Increased antihypertensive effects with other antihypertensive drugs, diuretics
• Increased anticoagulant effects of warfarin
• Decreased clinical response of phenytoin
Lab
• False negative for insulin response to glucagon

INCOMPATIBILITIES
• Do not mix in syringe with any drug

SIDE EFFECTS
CNS: Dizziness, headache, weakness, seizures
CV: Hypotension, tachycardia flushing, angina, arrhythmias, ECG changes
DERM: Rash, hirsutism
GI: Nausea, vomiting, anorexia, constipation
GU: Hyperuricemia
METAB: Hyperglycemia, hyponatremia, ketoacidosis, Na and water retention (diuresis may be required)
Local: Pain, burning, cellulitis, phlebitis if extravasated

TOXICITY AND OVERDOSE
Clinical signs: Severe hypotension
Treatment: Administer dopamine, norepinephrine or levarterenol, dialysis

PATIENT CARE MANAGEMENT
Assessment
• Assess history of hypersensitivity to diazoxide, related drugs
• Assess baseline VS, B/P
• Assess baseline wt
Interventions
• Shake PO susp well before use
• Keep pt recumbent during IV infusion
• Administer in peripheral vein; avoid extravasation
• Do not administer IM or SC
• Discontinue drug if severe hypotension develops
Evaluation
• Evaluate B/P q 5 min until stable and q1h thereafter
• Evaluate IV site for extravasation or infiltration
• Monitor I&O, BG
• Monitor urine glucose, ketone levels

PATIENT AND FAMILY EDUCATION
Teach/instruct
• To take as directed at prescribed intervals for prescribed length of time
Warn/advise
• That drug can cause orthostatic hypotension; rise slowly from sitting or lying position
• To report side effects immediately, especially burning at IV site
• To monitor wt (with PO use at home) because of Na and water retention

STORAGE
• Store in light resistant containers
• Avoid heat or freezing
• Do not use darkened sol

---

dicloxacillin sodium
Brand Name(s): Dycill, Dynapen, Pathocil

Classification: Antibiotic (penicillinase-resistant penicillin)

Pregnancy Category: B

AVAILABLE PREPARATIONS
Oral susp: 62.5 mg/5 ml
Caps: 125 mg, 250 mg, 500 mg

✦ Available in Canada.

ROUTES AND DOSAGES

Neonates: PO 4-8 mg/kg q6h (Safety and effectiveness not established. Dosage represents accepted standard practice recommendations.)

Children >1 mo <40 kg: PO for mild or moderate infections 12.5-25 mg/kg/24 hr divided q6h; for severe infections 50-100 mg/kg/24 hr divided q6h

Children >40 kg and adults: 125-500 mg q6h; maximum 4 g/24 hr

MECHANISM AND INDICATIONS

Antibiotic mechanism: Bactericidal; inhibits bacterial cell wall synthesis by adhering to bacterial penicillin-binding proteins

Indications: Effective against gram-positive cocci including *Staphylococcus aureus, S. epidermidis, Streptococcus pyogenes, Str. faecalis, Str. pneumoniae,* and infections caused by penicillinase-producing *Staphylococcus;* used to treat respiratory tract, skin, soft tissue, bone, joint infections

PHARMACOKINETICS

Peak: 1 hr

Distribution: Throughout body; highest concentrations in liver, kidney; low CSF penetration

Half-life: 0.5-1.0 hr

Metabolism: Liver

Excretion: Urine, bile

Therapeutic level (for Staphylococci infections): 0.1-0.3 mcg/ml

CONTRAINDICATIONS AND PRECAUTIONS

• Contraindicated with known hypersensitivity to dicloxacillin, penicillins, cephalosporins

• Use cautiously with impaired renal function, history of colitis or other GI disorders, pregnancy

INTERACTIONS

Drug

• Synergistic antimicrobial activity against certain organisms with use of aminoglycosides

• Increased serum concentrations with use of probenecid

• Decreased effectiveness with use of erythromycins, tetracyclines, chloramphenicol

Lab

• False positive for urine protein

• Increased liver function tests

Nutrition

• Decreased absorption if given with meals, acidic fruit juices, citrus fruits, or acidic beverages (such as cola drinks)

SIDE EFFECTS

CNS: Neuromuscular irritability, seizures

GI: Nausea, vomiting, epigastric distress, flatulence, diarrhea, pseudomembranous colitis, intrahepatic cholestasis

GU: Acute interstitial nephritis

HEME: Eosinophilia, leukopenia, granulocytopenia, thrombocytopenia, agranulocytosis

Other: Hypersensitivity reaction (pruritis, urticaria, rash, anaphylaxis), bacterial or fungal superinfection

TOXICITY AND OVERDOSE

Clinical signs: Neuromuscular irritability, seizures

Treatment: Supportive care; if ingested within 4 hr, empty stomach by induced emesis or gastric lavage, followed by activated charcoal to reduce absorption

PATIENT CARE MANAGEMENT

Assessment

• Assess history of hypersensitivity to dicloxacillin, penicillins, cephalosporins

• Obtain C&S; may begin therapy before obtaining results

• Assess renal function (BUN, creatinine, I&O), hepatic function (ALT, AST, bilirubin), hematologic function (CBC, differential, platelet count), bowel pattern, particularly for long-term therapy

Interventions

• Administer penicillins at least 1 hr before bacteriostatic antibiotics (tetracyclines, erythromycins, chloramphenicol)

• Administer PO 1 hr ac or 2 hr after meals; give with water; avoid acidic beverages; shake susp well

before administering; caps may be taken apart, mixed with food or fluid
• Maintain age-appropriate fluid intake
• Provide 10-day course for group A β-hemolytic streptococcal infection to prevent risk of acute rheumatic fever or glomerulonephritis

> **NURSING ALERT**
> Discontinue drug if signs of hypersensitivity, interstitial nephritis, pseudomembranous colitis develop

Evaluation
• Evaluate therapeutic response (decreased symptoms of infection)
• Monitor for signs of superinfection (perineal itching, diaper rash, fever, malaise, redness, pain, swelling, drainage, rash, diarrhea, sore throat, change in cough or sputum)
• Observe for signs of allergic reaction (wheezing, tightness in chest, urticaria), especially within 20-30 min of first dose
• Monitor bowel pattern; diarrhea may be symptomatic of pseudomembranous colitis
• Monitor renal function (BUN, creatinine, I&O), hepatic function (ALT, AST, bilirubin), electrolyte levels
• Monitor for signs of bleeding (ecchymosis, bleeding gums, hematuria, daily stool guaiac); monitor pro-times, platelet counts

PATIENT AND FAMILY EDUCATION
Teach/instruct
• To take as directed at prescribed intervals for prescribed length of time
Warn/advise
• To notify care provider of hypersensitivity, side effects, superinfection

STORAGE
• Store powder, caps at room temp
• Reconstituted susp stable refrigerated for 14 days; label date, time of reconstitution

---

> # dicyclomine hydrochloride
> **Brand Name(s):** Antispas, A-spas, Bentyl, Bentylol✚, Di-Spaz, Formulex✚, Lomine, Neoquess, Or-Tyl, Spasmoban, Spasmoject
> **Classification:** Anticholinergic/antispasmodic
> **Pregnancy Category:** B

AVAILABLE PREPARATIONS
Syr: 10 mg/5 ml
Tabs: 20 mg
Caps: 10 mg
Inj: 10 mg/ml

ROUTES AND DOSAGES
Infants 6 mo-2 yr: PO 5 mg tid-qid
Children 2-6 yr: PO 10 mg tid-qid
Adults: PO 20 mg tid-qid prn; may increase up to 160 mg/24 hr; IM 20 mg q4-6h
• Not recommended for infants <6 mo
• IM route not recommended for infants or children
• For all routes and ages, adjust dose prn and as tolerated

MECHANISM AND INDICATIONS
Mechanism: It has been suggested that dicyclomine hydrochloride exerts a local and direct action upon the smooth muscles in the GI tract resulting in reduced tone, motility
Indications: Used in irritable bowel syndrome

PHARMACOKINETICS
Onset: 1-2 hr
Half life: 1-8 hr initial phase, 9-10 hr secondary phase
Metabolism: Liver
Excretion: Urine, feces

CONTRAINDICATIONS AND PRECAUTIONS
• Contraindicated in infants <6 mo; hypersensitivity to drug, obstruction of bladder or GI tract, paralytic ileus, intestinal atony, unstable cardiac conditions, in acute hemorrhage, toxic megacolon, narrow-angle glaucoma

• Use cautiously with infants, Down Syndrome, children with spastic paralysis, pts with brain damage who may show an increased response to anticholinergics, in autonomic neuropathy, hepatic or renal impairment, hyperthyroidism, CAD, CHF, hypertension, arrhythmias, biliary tract disease, with extreme caution in pts at risk for toxic megacolon (severe inflammatory bowel disease, acute colitis), pregnancy, lactation

INTERACTIONS
Drug
• Drugs which cause alkalinization of urine (e.g., antacids) may delay urinary secretion of anticholinergics thereby potentiating their effects.
• Decreased absorption possible with simultaneous use of antacids or adsorbent diarrheals.
• Intensified anticholinergic effects possible with other anticholinergics
Lab
• Interference with gastric emptying studies
• Antagonism effect of pentagastrin and histamine in evaluation of gastric acid secretory function

SIDE EFFECTS
CNS: Seizures, syncope, and coma have been reported in infants <3 mo; dizziness, light-headedness, drowsiness, weakness, headache, insomnia, confusion, hyperexcitability
CV: Pulse rate fluctuations, palpitations
DERM: Urticaria, pruritus, decreased sweating
GI: Delayed gastric emptying, dry mouth, decreased lower esophageal sphincter tone, suppression of intestinal motility, paralytic ileus
GU: Urinary retention
RESP: Anaphylaxis; in infants <3 mo, difficulty breathing, shortness of breath, respiratory collapse, apnea
Other: Fever, allergic reaction

TOXICITY AND OVERDOSE
Clinical signs: Headache, nausea, vomiting, blurred vision, dilated pupils, hot, dry skin, dizziness, dry mouth, difficulty swallowing, CNS stimulation, respiratory depression, hypotension, seizures
Treatment: Induce emesis or perform gastric lavage with 4% tannic acid sol; give aqueous slurry of activated charcoal; to reverse severe anticholinergic symptoms, IV administration of physostigmine; equipment should be available to support pt experiencing respiratory depression, including O_2 and artificial respiration equipment

PATIENT CARE MANAGEMENT
Assessment
• Assess for history of hypersensitivity to dicyclomine hydrochloride
• Assess baseline VS, GI symptoms
Interventions
• Do not administer to infants <6 mo
• Do not administer PO within 2-3 hr of antacids or adsorbent-diarrheals
• IM not recommended for infants, children
• Care provider may recommend a high fiber diet or fiber supplementation for treatment of irritable bowel syndrome
• Institute safety measures (raise bed rails, ambulate with supervision)

NURSING ALERT

Pts taking this medication during hot weather are at increased risk for heat stroke

Pts with Down syndrome, spastic paralysis, brain damage are at increased risk for developing side effects

---

Evaluation
• Evaluate therapeutic response (absence of epigastric pain, bleeding, nausea, vomiting)
• Evaluate for hypersensitivity, side effects

• During therapy monitor VS, I&O, bowel function; assess for signs of toxic megacolon, paralytic ileus

PATIENT AND FAMILY EDUCATION

Teach/instruct
• To take as directed at prescribed intervals for prescribed length of time
• Pt with irritable bowel syndrome regarding high fiber diet, stress management, other non-pharmacologic approaches to management of irritable bowel syndrome

Warn/advise
• To notify care provider of hypersensitivity, side effects
• To use drug with care in hot weather; drug inhibits sweating, increasing risk for heat stroke
• May cause dizziness or drowsiness; hazardous activities such as bikes, skates, skateboards, and driving should be avoided

STORAGE

• Store at room temp
• Protect from heat and light

---

didanosine

Brand Name(s): Videx✤

Classification: Antiviral (synthetic purine nucleoside of deoxyadenosine)

Pregnancy Category: B

AVAILABLE PREPARATIONS

Powder for oral sol: Buffered, 100 mg, 167 mg, 250 mg, 375 mg; pediatric, 2 g, 4 g
Tabs, buffered, chewable: 25 mg, 50 mg, 100 mg, 150 mg

ROUTES AND DOSAGESS

Children: PO dosage based on body surface area (m^2), <1 yr or <0.4 m^2, 100-300 mg/m^2/24 hr divided q12h (single tab/dose bid)
Children ≥1 yr: 100-300 mg/m^2/24 hr divided q12h (2 tabs/dose bid)
Children ≥35 kg and adults: Dosing based on wt; initial recommended dose 5-10 mg/kg/24 hr divided q12h; 35-49 kg, 125 mg q12h using 2 tabs/dose, buffered oral sol 167 mg q12h; 50-74 kg, 200 mg q12h using 2 tabs/dose, buffered oral sol 250 mg q12h; ≥75 kg: 300 mg q12h using 2 tabs/dose, buffered oral sol 375 mg q12h

MECHANISM AND INDICATIONS

Antiviral mechanism: Inhibits HIV by conversion of didanosine by cellular enzymes to active metabolite dideoxyadenosine triphosphate
Indications: Used to treat pts with advanced HIV infection who are resistant to or intolerant of zidovudine therapy

PHARMACOKINETICS

Half-life: Children/adolescents 0.8 hr; adults 1.3-1.6 hr
Distribution: Into CSF
Excretion: Urine

CONTRAINDICATIONS AND PRECAUTIONS

• Contraindicated with known hypersensitivity to didanosine
• Use cautiously with renal or hepatic impairment, PKU, K^+-restricted diets, pregnancy, lactation

INTERACTIONS

Drug
• Decreased absorption of ketoconazole, dapsone, ciprofloxacin, tetracyclines
• Decreased plasma concentrations of quinolone antibiotics

Nutrition
• Decreased absorption if given with food; do not give with fruit juices or acidic beverages (e.g., cola drinks)

SIDE EFFECTS

CNS: Peripheral neuropathy, headache, seizures, asthma, insomnia, malaise, CNS depression, fever
DERM: Rash, pruritus, alopecia
EENT: Retinal depigmentation
ENDO/METAB: Hypokalemia, hyperuricemia
GI: Diarrhea, nausea, vomiting, anorexia, stomatitis, pancreatitis,

---

✤ Available in Canada.

abdominal pain, elevated liver function tests, hepatic failure
HEME: Leukopenia, granulocytopenia, thrombocytopenia, anemia
RESP: Cough, dyspnea

TOXICITY AND OVERDOSE
Clinical signs: Pancreatitis, peripheral neuropathy, diarrhea, hyperuricemia
Treatment: Supportive care

PATIENT CARE MANAGEMENT
Assessment
• Assess history of hypersensitivity to didanosine
• Assess hematologic function (CBC, differential, platelet count), renal function (BUN, creatinine, I&O), hepatic function (ALT, AST, bilirubin) dilated retinal exam

Interventions
• Administer PO 1 hr ac or 2 hr after meals
• Tabs should be chewed, crushed, or dispersed in water; do not mix with fruit juices or acidic beverages such as cola drinks
• Administer ketoconazole, dapsone, tetracyclines, quinolone antibiotics at least 2 hr before didanosine
• Maintain age-appropriate fluid intake
• Administer antibiotics, antivirals as ordered to prevent opportunistic infections

> **NURSING ALERT**
> Discontinue drug if signs of pancreatitis develop
>
> Withhold drug if WBC is <4000 or platelet count is <75,000

Evaluation
• Evaluate therapeutic response (control of symptoms, decreased incidence of opportunistic infections)
• Monitor hematologic (CBC, differential, platelet count) function; treatment may need to be discontinued and restarted after hematologic recovery

• Monitor renal function (BUN, creatinine, I&O), hepatic function (ALT, AST, bilirubin), dilated retinal exam q6mo
• Monitor for signs of neuropathy (tingling or pain in hands and feet, distal numbness)
• Monitor for signs of pancreatitis (abdominal pain, nausea, vomiting, elevated liver function tests); treatment may need to be discontinued because condition can be fatal
• Monitor for signs of opportunistic infection such as pneumonia, meningitis, sepsis

PATIENT AND FAMILY EDUCATION
Teach/instruct
• To take as directed at prescribed intervals for prescribed length of time
• About HIV disease measures to prevent transmission, reasons for medication therapy, including concomitant use of antibiotic or antiviral medications; include information that pt is still infective during didanosine therapy and that didanosine will not cure the illness but will control symptoms

Warn/advise
• To notify care provider of hypersensitivity, side effects, opportunistic infection
• To notify care provider if signs of infection (fever, sore throat, flu-like symptoms), anemia (fatigue, headache, faintness, shortness of breath, irritability), or bruising, bleeding develop
• That hair loss may occur during therapy; pt may choose to wear a wig or hairpiece

STORAGE
• Store at room temp
• Tabs dispersed in water stable at room temp for 1 hr
• Reconstituted buffered sol stable at room temp for 4 hr
• Reconstituted unbuffered sol stable refrigerated for 30 days

digoxin

Brand Name(s): Digoxin, Lanoxin♣, Lanoxicaps

Classification: Antiarrhythmic, inotropic

Pregnancy Category: A

AVAILABLE PREPARATIONS

Elixir: 50 mcg/ml
Tabs: 0.125 mg, 0.25 mg, 0.5 mg
Caps (Lanoxicaps): 0.05 mg, 0.10 mg, 0.20 mg
Inj: 100 mcg/ml, 250 mcg/ml

ROUTES AND DOSAGESS

• Lanoxicaps have greater bioavailability than tabs; 0.05 mg cap = 0.0625 mg tab, 0.1 mg cap = 0.125 mg tab, 0.2 mg cap = 0.25 mg tab

Total Digitalizing Dose (TDD)

PO route

Premature neonates: 20 mcg/kg/24 hr qd
Neonates: 30 mcg/kg/24 hr qd
Infants <2 yr: 40-50 mcg/kg/24 hr qd
Children 2-10 yr: 30-40 mcg/kg/24 hr qd
Children >10 yr: 750-1250 mcg/24 hr qd

IV route

Premature neonates: 15 mcg/kg/24 hr qd
Neonates: 20 mcg/kg/24 hr qd
Infants <2 yr: 30-40 mcg/kg/24 hr qd
Children 2-10 yr: 20-30 mcg/kg/24 hr qd
Children >10 yr: 750-1250 mcg/24 hr qd

• Administer ½ of TDD initially, then two doses of ¼ TDD at 8 hr intervals; assess clinical response, monitor for toxicity before each dose (since this dose is very variable)

• Administer digoxin PO as soon as pt is able to take oral medication

Maintenance Dosages

PO route

Premature neonates: 5 mcg/kg/24 hr divided bid
Neonates: 8-10 mcg/kg/24 hr divided bid
Infants <2 yr: 10-12 mcg/kg/24 hr divided bid
Children 2-10 yr: 8-10 mcg/kg/24 hr divided bid
Children >10 yr: 0.125-0.250 mg/24 hr qd

IV route

Premature neonates: 3-4 mcg/kg/24 hr divided bid
Neonates: 6-8 mcg/kg/24 hr divided bid
Infants <2 yr: 7-9 mcg/kg/24 hr divided bid
Children 2-10 yr: 6-8 mcg/kg/24 hr divided bid
Children >10 yr: 0.125-0.250 mg/24 hr qd

• Administer digoxin PO as soon as pt is able to take oral medication

IV administration

• Recommended concentration: 1:10 dilution with D_5W, $D_{10}W$, NS, SW

• Maximum concentration: 100 mcg/ml for pediatric pts

• IV push rate: Over >5-10 min (rapid IV infusion may cause systemic and coronary artery vasoconstriction)

• Intermittent infusion rate: Over >5-10 min

MECHANISM AND INDICATIONS

Inotropic mechanism: Acts on heart by inhibiting action of ATPase to increase myocardial contractility, cardiac output
Antiarrhythmic mechanism: Reduces myocardial excitability and conduction velocity, prolongs refractory period
Indications: Used in treatment of CHF, atrial fibrillation and flutter, supra-ventricular tachycardia, and for ventricular rate control

PHARMACOKINETICS

Onset of action: PO 30-120 min; IV 5-30 min
Peak: PO 2-6 hr; IV 1-5 hr
Half-life: 32-48 hr, premature 61-170 hr
Metabolism: Liver and intestines
Excretion: Urine

♣ Available in Canada.

Therapeutic level: 0.7-2.0 ng/ml; serum concentration must be used in conjunction with clinical symptoms and ECG to confirm diagnosis of digoxin toxicity

CONTRAINDICATIONS AND PRECAUTIONS

• Contraindicated with hypersensitivity to digitalis, ventricular tachycardia (VT) and ventricular fibrillation not caused by CHF, bradycardia, AV heart block, hypertrophic cardiomyopathy, constrictive pericarditis
• Use cautiously with premature infants, hypokalemia, hypothyroidism, acute myocarditis, renal impairment

INTERACTIONS
Drug
• Increased drug levels with use of quinidine, verapamil, aminoglycosides, spironolactone, indomethacin, anticholinergics, amiodarone
• Decreased absorption with use of thyroid agents, antacids, kaolin-pectin, radiation, chemotherapy, metoclopramide
• Increased the toxicity of digoxin with drugs that cause hypokalemia, including diuretics, amphotericin B, carbenicillin, ticarcillin, corticosteroids
Lab
• Increased CPK
• Falsely elevated 17-KS

INCOMPATIBILITIES
• With other drugs in IV sol

SIDE EFFECTS
CNS: Headache, drowsiness, depression, fainting, weakness, vertigo, disorientation
CV: Bradycardia, arrhythmias, hypotension, tachycardia, AV block, SA block
EENT: Blurred vision, yellow halos, photophobia, diplopia, flashing lights
GI: Nausea, vomiting, diarrhea, anorexia, stomach pain, feeding intolerance, wt loss

TOXICITY AND OVERDOSE
Clinical signs: Anorexia, nausea, vomiting, arrhythmias, conduction disturbances

Treatment: Withhold drug, obtain serum digoxin levels, administer antiarrhythmic drugs, consider treatment with digoxin immune fab

PATIENT CARE MANAGEMENT
Assessment
• Assess history of hypersensitivity to drug
• Assess baseline VS and ECG, I&O, daily wts, apical heart rate and rhythm
• Assess serum electrolytes, especially K^+; if low, be alert for signs of digoxin toxicity
Interventions
• Compatible with D_5W, $D_{10}W$, NS, SW for IV injection; do not mix with other drugs
• With PO elixir, use calibrated syringe or dropper; administer at same time daily with or without food
• Administer in PO form as soon as pt stable

> **NURSING ALERT**
> Digitalizing doses should be given only in hospital where pt can be cardiac monitored
>
> If pt hypokalemic, monitor for signs of digoxin toxicity
>
> Keep medication out of reach: overdose can be fatal

Evaluation
• Monitor digoxin levels if pt has clinical symptoms or hypokalemia
• Monitor wt, edema, apical heart rate and rhythm, periodic ECG
• Evaluate therapeutic response (normal heart rate and rhythm, improvement of CHF)
• Evaluate for signs and symptoms of early toxicity (tachycardia, stomach upset)
• Evaluate serum K^+ if indicated (pt on diuretics); if <3.5 notify provider; monitor for signs and symptoms of digoxin toxicity

♣ Available in Canada.

PATIENT AND FAMILY EDUCATION
Teach/instruct
- To take as directed at prescribed intervals for prescribed length of time
- About drawing up elixir dose in calibrated syringe or dropper
- To administer drug at same time(s) daily
- About signs and symptoms of CHF; call provider if symptoms present
- About signs and symptoms of toxicity; withhold drug, call provider
- To keep medication out of reach, since overdose can be fatal, and to have ipecac and poison control number on hand
- To have child carry medical alert identification
- Not to discontinue drug without provider approval

STORAGE
- Store at room temp
- Reconstituted IV sol stable for 4 hr in refrigerator

---

digoxin immune fab
Brand Name(s): Digibind✤
Classification: Digoxin antidote
Pregnancy Category: C

AVAILABLE PREPARATIONS
Inj: 40 mg/vial (binds 0.6 mg digoxin or digitoxin)

ROUTES AND DOSAGES
Children and adults: Determine total body digoxin load (TBL); TBL (mg) = serum digoxin level (ng/ml) $\times 5.6 \times$ wt (kg) $\div 1000$; then calculate dose of digoxin immune fab; fab (mg) = TBL $\times 66.7$; infuse IV over 15-30 min

IV administration
- Recommended concentration: Reconstitute with 4 ml SW or NS for concentration of 10 mg/ml; for very small doses, a reconstituted vial can be diluted to 1 mg/ml by adding 36 ml sterile isotonic saline

- Maximum concentration 10 mg/ml
- IV push rate: Over 5 min using filter (0.22 micron)
- Intermittent infusion rate: Over 15-30 min through filter (0.22 micron)

MECHANISM AND INDICATIONS
Mechanism: Contains antibodies which bind digoxin, digitoxin molecules, which are excreted in urine
Indications: For use in life-threatening digoxin toxicity

PHARMACOKINETICS
Peak: After infusion complete
Absorption: Binds rapidly, within 2-20 min
Half-life: 14-20 hr
Excretion: Urine

CONTRAINDICATIONS AND PRECAUTIONS
- Contraindicated with mild digoxin toxicity, renal failure, cardiac failure
- Use cautiously with children (limited experience), renal disease (anaphylactoid, hypersensitivity, and febrile reactions have occurred)

INTERACTIONS
Drug
- Increased total serum digoxin (although most bound)
- Interference with digitalis immuno-assay fragments
- Arrhythmias with catecholamine use
Lab
- Decreased K^+ levels once therapy is begun

INCOMPATIBILITIES
- Incompatible with all drugs in syringe

SIDE EFFECTS
CV: Worsening of low cardiac output or CHF, ventricular rate increase, atrial fibrillation
DERM: Urticarial rash with hypersensitivity
METAB: Hypokalemia
RESP: Increased respiratory rate, decreased respiratory function

---

✤ Available in Canada.

TOXICITY AND OVERDOSE
Clinical signs: Hypersensitivity possible; therapeutic effects of digoxin may be lost
Treatment: Treat anaphylaxis prn, support exacerbated cardiac conditions prn

PATIENT CARE MANAGEMENT
Assessment
• Assess history of hypersensitivity to drug
• Assess serum digoxin levels before treatment
• Assess VS, B/P
• Assess ECG
• Assess electrolytes, especially K^+
• If suicide attempt, assess pt for other drug ingestion(s)

Interventions
• Place pt on cardiac monitor

NURSING ALERT
Use with caution in children; anaphylactoid reactions have occurred

---

Evaluation
• Monitor for hypersensitivity reaction, treat with steroids, antihistamines, vasopressors prn
• Monitor VS, B/P, ECG
• Monitor electrolytes especially K^+
• Monitor digoxin levels during, after treatment

PATIENT AND FAMILY EDUCATION
Provide
• Support to pt, family during treatment

STORAGE
• Use reconstituted sol promptly or store in refrigerator up to 4 hr

---

dihydrotachysterol
Brand Name(s): DHT, Hytakerol♣

Classification: Antihypocalcemic or vitamin D analog

Pregnancy Category: A (D if dosage exceeds RDA)

AVAILABLE PREPARATIONS
Oral sol: 0.2 mg/ml
Tabs/caps: 0.125 mg, 0.2 mg, 0.4 mg

ROUTES AND DOSAGES
• 1 mg dihydrotachysterol = 3 mg (120,000 IU) of vitamin D_2
• Goal is to achieve and maintain normal serum calcium levels.

Hypoparathyroidism
Neonates: PO 0.05-0.1 mg/24 hr
Infants and young children: PO Initial 1-5 mg for 4 days; maintenance 0.5-1.5 mg/24 hr
Older children and adults: PO Initial 0.8-2.4 mg for 4 days; maintenance 0.2-1 mg/24 hr; maximum 1.5 mg/24 hr

Nutritional Rickets
PO 0.5 mg as single dose or 13-50 mcg/24 hr until healed

Renal Osteodystrophy
Children and adolescents: PO 0.1-0.5 mg/24 hr
Adults: PO 0.1-0.6 mg/24 hr

MECHANISM AND INDICATIONS
Mechanism: Works with parathyroid hormone to stimulate Ca and PO_4 absorption from the small intestine; promotes Ca bone resorption; increases renal phosphate excretion
Indications: Used in the treatment of hypocalcemia associated with hypoparathyroidism or prophylaxis of hypocalcemic tetany following thyroid surgery; its use is faster acting than pharmacologic doses of vitamin D and it is less available after administration, thereby decreasing risk of hypercalcemia

PHARMACOKINETICS
Peak: Within 2 wk
Metabolism: Liver
Excretion: Urine and bile

CONTRAINDICATIONS AND PRECAUTIONS
• Contraindicated with hypercalcemia, abnormal sensitivity to vitamin D and hypervitaminosis D
• Use cautiously with renal osteodystrophy and hyperphosphatemia; dosage should be ti-

D

trated based on pt needs with regular assessments of Ca levels

INTERACTIONS
Drug
• Decreased absorption with use of thiazide diuretics, cholestyramine, antacids
• Altered metabolism with use of corticosteroids
• Increase Ca levels and risk of cardiac arrhythmias possible with use of cardiac glycosides
• Altered metabolism, reduced drug activity with use of barbiturates
Lab
• Altered serum alk phos
• Altered cholesterol
• Altered electrolytes

SIDE EFFECTS
(related to hypercalcemia)
CNS: Convulsions, headaches, lethargy, depression, disorientation, hallucinations
CV: Hypertension
EENT: Vertigo, tinnitus
GI: Nausea, vomiting, anorexia, weight loss, constipation
GU: Polyuria, polydipsia, renal damage
HEME: Anemia
Other: Weakness, metastatic calcification

TOXICITY AND OVERDOSE
Clinical signs: Signs of hypercalcemia (nausea, vomiting, headaches, convulsions, depression, disorientation, weakness, hypertension, polyuria)
Treatment: Crisis should be treated with hydration; discontinue medication, increase fluid intake, give low Ca diet and laxative, supportive care

PATIENT CARE MANAGEMENT
Assessment
• Assess history of hypersensitivity to dihydrotachysterol
• Obtain baseline levels of Ca and PO_4
• Assess for use of other medications to ensure optimal absorption and use

Interventions
• Discontinue drug, increase fluids if signs of hypercalcemia noted; give low Ca diet, laxatives if necessary
• Maintain age-appropriate fluid intake

NURSING ALERT
Monitor Ca and PO_4 levels closely, evaluate for symptoms of hypercalcemia (convulsions, disorientation, depression, nausea, vomiting, anorexia, or weakness)

Evaluation
• Evaluate therapeutic response (decreased symptoms of hypercalcemia, normal serum Ca [9-10 mg/dl] and normal PO_4 levels)
• Monitor infants for possibilities of drug reaction
• Monitor Ca, PO_4 levels for signs of hypercalcemia (discontinue drug, increase fluids if needed)

PATIENT AND FAMILY EDUCATION
Teach/instruct
• To take as directed at prescribed intervals for prescribed length of time
• To evaluate other medications, OTC drugs for interactions
Warn/advise
• To notify care provider of hypersensitivity, side effects
• Avoid Mg-containing antacids; if necessary, take 2-3 hr before or after medication
• PO_4 intake should be moderated to decrease risk of metastatic calcification
Encourage
• Diet should be balanced to ensure sufficient intake of Ca to meet the RDA (see Appendix F, Table of Recommended Daily Dietary Allowances); if diet is inadequate, use a supplement

STORAGE
• Store at room temp
• Protect from heat, direct light, moisture
• Do not refrigerate or freeze

✤ Available in Canada.

diltiazem hydrochloride

Brand Name(s): Apo-Diltiaz♣, Cardizem♣, Cardizem SR♣, Cardizem CD♣, Diltiazem

Classification: Calcium channel blocker

Pregnancy Category: C

AVAILABLE PREPARATIONS
Tabs: 30 mg, 60 mg, 90 mg, 120 mg
SR tabs: 60 mg, 90 mg, 120 mg, 150 mg
Inj: 25 mg/5 ml, 50 mg/10 ml (5 mg/ml)

ROUTES AND DOSAGESS
Infants and children: Not approved for use in infants and children; dosages not standardized but have been extrapolated from adult dosages
Adult: PO tabs, 30 mg qid (initial) then adjust per pt response (average optimal dose 180-360 mg/24 hr); SR tabs; 60-120 mg bid (initial), then adjust per pt response (average optimal dose 240-360 mg/kg/24 hr); IV bolus, initial 0.25 mg/kg over 2 min; second dose can be administered after 15 min, 0.35 mg/kg over 2 min; subsequent IV doses individualized per pt response; continuous IV, initial infusion rate of 10 mg/hr; may increase to 15 mg/hr for 24 hr only
IV administration
• Recommended concentration: Dilute in D_5W or ½ NS, titrate to desired dose
• Maximum concentration: May be administered undiluted
• IV push rate: Direct IV bolus
• Contiunous infusion rate: 5 mg/hr, may be increased by 5 mg/hr to maximum dose of 15 mg/hr; discontinue infusion in 24 hr

MECHANISM AND INDICATIONS
Mechanism: Inhibits movement of Ca across myocardium; relaxes coronary vascular smooth muscle; dilates coronary arteries; slows SA/AV node conduction; dilates peripheral arteries
Indications: For use in angina, hypertension, atrial fibrillation or flutter, and supraventricular tachycardia in pts without accessory conduction pathway or preexcitation syndrome

PHARMACOKINETICS
Onset: PO 30-60 min; PO (SR) 30-60 min; IV immediate
Peak: PO 2-3 hr; PO(SR) 6-11 hr; IV 15 min
Duration: PO 3-4 hr; PO(SR) 8-12 hr
Metabolism: Liver
Excretion: Urine, bile

CONTRAINDICATIONS AND PRECAUTIONS
• Contraindicated with known hypersensitivity, acute MI, CHF, accessory conduction pathways or preexcitation syndrome, severe hypotension, cardiogenic shock, 2nd- or 3rd-degree heart block (unless ventricular cardiac pacemaker is in place or available)
• Use cautiously with cardiac pacemakers, severe bradycardia, liver or renal insufficiency, older adults, pregnancy, lactation

INTERACTIONS
Drug
• Increased effects of digitalis, β-blockers, carbamazepine, quinidine, vasodilators, neuromuscular blocking agents, fentanyl
• Increased diltiazem effects with cimetidine
• Decreased diltiazem effects with Ca, barbiturates
Lab
• Elevated AST, ALT, LDH, CPK (mild)

INCOMPATIBILITIES
• Furosemide

SIDE EFFECTS
CNS: Dizziness, muscle weakness, headache paresthesias, tremor
CV: Peripheral edema, AV heart block, hypotension, bradycardia, syncope, palpitations, CHF
DERM: Rash, pruritus, flushing, sweating

♣ Available in Canada.

GI: Nausea, vomiting, diarrhea, gastric upset, thirst
GU: Nocturia, polyuria, acute renal failure
HEME: Thrombocytopenia, anemia, leukopenia (rare)
RESP: SOB, dyspnea

TOXICITY AND OVERDOSE
Clinical signs: Profound hypotension, arrhythmias, drowsiness, confusion
Treatment: If PO, induce emesis, gastric lavage, activated charcoal; if IV, supportive care, treat symptomatically; vasopressors, atropine, lidocaine, Ca cardioversion

PATIENT CARE MANAGEMENT
Assessment
• Assess history of hypersensitivity to drug
• Assess HR, B/P, monitor continuous ECG and IV dose
• Assess for evidence of pulmonary edema
• Assess heart rhythm; check for presence of gallops
• Assess for perfusion or oxygenation deficit
Interventions
• Administer IV bolus doses undiluted over 2 min, dilute for continuous infusion
• If pt on IV diltiazem, must be cardiac-monitored
• Monitor diltiazem levels (normal = 50-200 ng/ml)
• If pt taking digoxin, monitor digoxin serum level

> **NURSING ALERT**
> Do not use calcium channel blockers together with β-blockers

Evaluation
• Evaluate therapeutic response (decreased angina, B/P, arrhythmias)
• Evaluate cardiac status (HR, B/P, ECG, PR, QRS, and QT intervals)
• Evaluate cardiac monitoring if on IV dose

PATIENT AND FAMILY EDUCATION
Teach/instruct
• To take as directed at prescribed intervals for prescribed length of time
• About rationale for drug use
Warn/advise
• About side effects
• About importance of regular follow-up care

STORAGE
• Store in tight container at room temp

---

dimercaprol
Brand Name(s): BAL in Oil
Classification: Antidote (arsenic, gold, lead, mercury toxicity)
Pregnancy Category: C

AVAILABLE PREPARATIONS
Inj: 100 mg/ml

ROUTES AND DOSAGES
Mild Arsenic and Gold Poisoning
Children and adults: IM 2.5 mg/kg/dose q6h for 2 days, then q12h on the 3rd day, qd thereafter for 10 days
Severe Arsenic and Gold Poisoning
Children and adults: IM 3 mg/kg/dose q4h for 2 days, then q6h on the 3rd day, then q12h thereafter for 10 days
Mercury Poisoning
Children and adults: IM 5 mg/kg initially, followed by 2.5 mg/kg/dose qd-bid for 10 days
Lead Poisoning (Use with Edetate Calcium Disodium)
Children and adults: IM Mild, 4 mg/kg/dose once, then 3 mg/kg/dose q4h for 2-5 days; severe, 4 mg/kg/dose q4h in combination with edetate calcium disodium for 2-7 days

MECHANISM AND INDICATIONS
Antidote mechanism: Binds ions from arsenic, gold, lead, and mer-

---

✤ Available in Canada.

cury, forming a soluble complex that is excreted in urine.

Indications: Used to treat arsenic, gold, and mercury poisoning and as an adjunct to edetate calcium disodium in lead poisoning

PHARMACOKINETICS

Peak: 30-60 min
Distribution: Distributes to all tissues (including brain)
Metabolism: Plasma enzymes
Excretion: Urine, feces

CONTRAINDICATIONS AND PRECAUTIONS

• Contraindicated with hypersensitivity to dimercaprol, hepatic insufficiency, or anuria; do not use for iron, cadmium, or selenium poisoning
• Use cautiously with renal impairment, hypertension, pregnancy, lactation; produces hemolysis with G-6-PD deficiency

INTERACTIONS

Drug
• Increased toxicity with iron, cadmium, selenium

INCOMPATIBILITIES

• Do not mix in syringe with edetate calcium disodium

SIDE EFFECTS

CNS: Nervousness, headache
CV: Hypertension, tachycardia
DERM: Urticaria, erythema, pruritus
EENT: Nasal congestion, throat pain, lacrimation, blepharospasm
ENDO/METAB: Metabolic acidosis
GI: Nausea, vomiting
GU: Nephrotoxicity
HEME: Transient neutropenia
Local: Pain at injection site
Other: Anaphylaxis, fever

PATIENT CARE MANAGEMENT

Assessment
• Assess history of hypersensitivity to dimercaprol
• Assess renal function (BUN, creatinine, I&O), specific heavy metal level status
• Identify lead sources in child's environment
• Assess VS

Interventions
• Do not use if particulate matter or discoloration present
• Administer IM deeply into large muscle mass, rotate injection sites; if administering edetate calcium disodium also, use separate sites
• Administer edetate calcium disodium as ordered
• Provide emergency equipment
• Maintain alkaline urine
• Maintain age-appropriate fluid intake

Evaluation
• Evaluate therapeutic response (decreased specific heavy metal blood level)
• Monitor renal function (BUN, creatinine, I&O), heavy metal level, VS status
• Monitor allergic reaction (rash, urticaria)
• Evaluate IM site for tissue damage

PATIENT AND FAMILY EDUCATION

Teach/instruct
• To take as directed at prescribed intervals for prescribed length of time
• About sources of heavy metal poisoning, ways to prevent further exposure or poisoning (particularly lead)

Warn/advise
• To notify care provider of hypersensitivity, side effects
• To comply with follow-up care to monitor heavy metal blood concentrations, neurologic and developmental status

STORAGE

• Store at room temp

♣ Available in Canada.

diphenoxylate hydro-chloride (with atropine)

Brand Name(s): Diphenatol, Latropine, Lofene, Logen, Lomocot, Lomotil, Lonox, Nor-Mil Vi-Atro

Classification: Antidiarrheal (opiate)

Controlled Substance Schedule V

Pregnancy Category: C

AVAILABLE PREPARATIONS

Oral sol: 2.5 mg diphenoxylate hydrochloride and 25 mcg atropine sulfate/5 ml
Tabs: 2.5 mg diphenoxylate hydrochloride and 25 mcg atropine sulfate

ROUTES AND DOSAGES

• Not recommended for children <2 yrs
Children >2 yr: PO 0.3-0.4 mg/kg/24 hr of diphenoxylate component divided qid
Adult: PO initially 1-2 tabs or teaspoons tid-qid; maintenance, decrease to 1 tab or teaspoon bid-tid

MECHANISM AND INDICATIONS

Mechanism: Diphenoxylate is believed to act both locally and centrally to reduce intestinal motility and diminish secretions; chemically related to meperidine, but does not have its analgesic properties; high doses over a prolonged period of time may cause euphoria, physical dependence; atropine is added below therapeutic levels in an attempt to prevent deliberate overdose or abuse
Indications: Diarrhea

PHARMACOKINETICS

Onset: 45-60 min
Duration: 3-4 hr
Half-life: Atropine 2.5 hr; diphenoxylate 2.5 hr; diphenoxylic acid (major metabolite) 4.5 hr
Metabolism: Hepatic
Excretion: Atropine, urine; diphenoxylate, feces/urine

CONTRAINDICATIONS AND PRECAUTIONS

• Contraindicated with known hypersensitivity to this drug, atropine, meperidine
• Use cautiously with infants and young children, pregnancy, lactation, hepatic insufficiency, severe colitis, pseudomembranous colitis, infectious diarrhea, hepatic disease, Down syndrome, dehydrated pts, retention of fluid in bowel lumen may worsen dehydration and predispose pt to delayed diphenoxylate toxicity

INTERACTIONS

Drug
• Increased risk of habituation when taken with alcohol or addictive medications (especially CNS depressants)
• Potentiation of either diphenoxylate, alcohol, or CNS depression-producing medications possible when taken concurrently
• Intensified anticholinergic effects of tricyclic antidepressants possible
• Increased risk for hypertensive crisis potentiation of atropine when taken with MAOIs
• Potentiation of atropine possible with concurrent use of anticholinergics or medications with anticholinergic effects
• Risk of severe constipation and additive CNS effects with concurrent use of opiod narcotics
Lab
• Elevated serum amylase

SIDE EFFECTS

CNS: Sedation, dizziness, headache, drowsiness, lethargy, restlessness, depression, euphoria
CV: Tachycardia
DERM: Pruritus, urticaria, rash, dryness
GI: Dry mouth, nausea, vomiting, abdominal discomfort or distention, paralytic ileus, anorexia, fluid retention in bowel, abdominal cramps, toxic megacolon, constipation
GU: Urinary retention
EENT: Dilated pupils

RESP: Respiratory depression
Other: Risk for physical dependence with long term use; flushing, fever

TOXICITY AND OVERDOSE
Clinical signs: Those of severe anticholinergic effects including continuing blurred vision or change in near vision; tachycardia; severe drowsiness; severe dryness in mouth, nose, throat; unusual warmth, dryness, flushing; coma; respiratory depression; unusual excitement, nervousness, restlessness, irritability
Treatment: Gastric lavage, supportive treatment to maintain airway and respiratory function; narcotic antagonist may be given to reverse respiratory depressive effects

PATIENT CARE MANAGEMENT
Assessment
• Assess history of hypersensitivity to diphenoxylate hydrochloride, atropine, meperidine
• Obtain baseline VS, GI function, hydration, hepatic function (ALT, AST, bilirubin)
Interventions
• Tab may be crushed
• Drug should be withheld in the presence of severe dehydration or electrolyte imbalance
• Maintain age-appropriate fluid intake

NURSING ALERT

Not recommended for children <2 yr

Use with extreme caution with severe inflammatory bowel disease, acute colitis, infectious diarrhea

---

Evaluation
• Evaluate therapeutic response (decreased diarrhea)
• Evaluate for hypersensitivity, side effects
• Evaluate VS, I&O, hepatic function (ALT, AST, bilirubin), electrolyte balance, observe for signs of dehydration
• Monitor bowel function, assess for signs of toxic megacolon and paralytic ileus

PATIENT AND FAMILY EDUCATION
Teach/instruct
• To take as directed at prescribed intervals for prescribed length of time
• About signs, symptoms of dehydration and fluid and electrolyte imbalance
• To ensure adequate fluid intake
Warn/advise
• To notify care provider if hypersensitivity or side effects occur
• That drug should be discontinued if signs of toxicity or toxic megacolon develop
• That drug should be discontinued if no improvement in symptoms occurs after 48 hr of therapy

STORAGE
• Store at room temp in a light resistant container

---

disopyramide phosphate
Brand Name(s): Napamide, Norpace✚, Norpace CR✚

Classification: Antiarrhythmic

Pregnancy Category: C

AVAILABLE PREPARATIONS
Caps: 100 mg, 150 mg
Caps (ext rel): 100 mg, 150 mg

ROUTES AND DOSAGES
• Start with lowest dose
Children <1 yr: PO tabs 10-30 mg/kg/24 hr in 4 divided doses
Children 1-4 yr: PO tabs 10-20 mg/kg/24 hr in 4 divided doses
Children 4-12 yr: PO tabs 10-15 mg/kg/24 hr in 4 divided doses
Children 12-18 yr: PO tabs 6-15 mg/kg/24 hr in 4 divided doses
Adults <50 kg: PO 100 mg q6h or 200 mg q12h (ext rel)

✚ Available in Canada.

Adults >50 kg: PO 150 mg q6h or 300 mg q12h (ext rel)

MECHANISM AND INDICATIONS

Mechanism: Decreases myocardial excitability; prolongs action potential duration and effective refractory period; anticholinergic action increases AV node conductivity

Indications: Use in PVCs, ventricular tachycardia, supraventricular tachycardia

PHARMACOKINETICS

Peak: 30 min-3 hr, duration 6-12 hr
Half-life: 4-10 hr
Metabolism: Liver
Excretion: Urine, feces

CONTRAINDICATIONS AND PRECAUTIONS

• Contraindicated with hypersensitivity, 2nd- or 3rd-degree heart block, myasthenia gravis, glaucoma, CHF, cardiogenic shock, prolonged QT syndrome
• Use cautiously with children DM, renal and liver disease, sick sinus syndrome, Wolf–Parkinson–White syndrome, pregnancy, lactation

INTERACTIONS

Drug
• Increased hypoglycemia with insulin
• Increased effects with quinidine, procainamide, propranolol, lidocaine, atenolol, other antiarrhythmics
• Increased side effects with anticholinergics
• Decreased effects with phenytoin, rifampin

Lab
• Increased liver enzymes (AST, ALT), lipids, BUN, creatinine
• Decreased Hgb, Hct, BG

INCOMPATIBILITIES

• Do not administer within 48 hrs of verapamil

SIDE EFFECTS

CNS: Fatigue, headache, malaise, nervousness, acute psychosis, depression, dizziness, weakness
CV: CHF, edema, dyspnea, wt gain, chest pain, syncope, conduction disturbances, hypotension
DERM: Rash
EENT: Blurred vision, dry eyes, nose and throat
GI: Dry mouth, constipation, nausea, vomiting, diarrhea, pain, gas, anorexia
GU: Urinary retention, hesitancy
METAB: Hypoglycemia, elevated cholesterol; hyperkalemia may enhance toxicity

TOXICITY AND OVERDOSE

Clinical signs: Anticholinergic effects, severe hypotension, ventricular arrhythmias, asystole, seizures, respiratory arrest
Treatment: Supportive measures, induce emesis, gastric lavage, activated charcoal

PATIENT CARE MANAGEMENT

Assessment
• Assess history of hypersensitivity to drug
• Assess VS, B/P
• Assess ECG
• Assess daily wt, edema
• Assess electrolytes, liver function (AST, ALT, bilirubin), kidney function, BG

Interventions
• Administer PO at regular dosing intervals
• Have pharmacist prepare disopyramide susp when necessary

Evaluation
• Monitor blood levels during treatment (therapeutic level 2-8 mcg/ml)
• Evaluate clinical response (decrease arrhythmias)
• Evaluate for side effects
• Evaluate ECG; if increase in QRS, QT intervals, discontinue drug
• Evaluate, report wt gain

PATIENT AND FAMILY EDUCATION

Teach/instruct
• To take as directed at prescribed intervals for prescribed length of time

---

❦ Available in Canada.

Warn/advise
• To use gum, hard candy, or frequent sips of water to alleviate dry mouth
• Not to make sudden position changes
• To avoid hazardous activities if dizzy or if vision is blurred

STORAGE
• Store at room temp

---

dobutamine hydrochloride

Brand Name(s): Dobutrex✤

Classification: Catecholamine, adrenergic agonist

Pregnancy Category: C

AVAILABLE PREPARATIONS
Inj: 12.5 mg/ml in 20 ml vial

ROUTES AND DOSAGES
Adults and children: IV 2.5-15 mcg/kg/min; maximum dose 40 mcg/kg/min
IV administration
• Recommended concentration: 1 mg/ml in D_5W
• Maximum concentration (minimum dilution): 5 mg/ml
• Continuous infusion rate: 2.5-15 mcg/kg/min

MECHANISM AND INDICATIONS
Inotropic: Selectively stimulates β_1-adrenergic receptors to increase myocardial contractility and stroke volume, thereby increasing cardiac output; decreases afterload by decreasing peripheral resistance and decreases preload by reducing ventricular filling pressure; may increase urine flow because of increased cardiac output
Indications: Short-term support for cardiac failure secondary to decreased contractility or cardiac surgery

PHARMACOKINETICS
Onset of action: 2 min
Peak: 10 min
Half-life: 2 min

Metabolism: Liver, conjugation
Excretion: Urine, feces (metabolites and conjugates)

CONTRAINDICATIONS AND PRECAUTIONS
• Contraindicated with known hypersensitivity to medication, hypertrophic obstructive cardiomyopathy
• Use with caution with hypertension, acute MI

INTERACTIONS
Drug
• Ventricular arrhythmias possible when used with halothane, cyclopropane
• Decreased action when used with other β-blockers
• Decreased hypotensive effects of guanadrel, guanethidine; may cause hypertension
• Increased cardiac output and lower wedge pressure with nitroprusside
• Increased pressor effects with tricyclic antidepressants, MAOIs, reserpine

INCOMPATIBILITIES
• Acyclovir, aminophylline, alteplase, bretylium, bumetanide, calcium chloride, calcium gluconate, cefamandole, cefazolin, cephalothin, diazepam, digoxin, furosemide, heparin, hydrocortisone, insulin, magnesium sulfate, penicillin, phenytoin, phytonadione, potassium phosphate, sodium chloride, sodium ethacrynate

SIDE EFFECTS
CNS: Anxiety, headache, dizziness, paresthesias
CV: Tachycardia, angina, chest pain, palpitations, hypertension, arrhythmias
GI: Nausea, vomiting, heartburn
RESP: Dyspnea
Other: Muscle cramps, hypokalemia

TOXICITY AND OVERDOSE
Clinical signs: Nervousness, fatigue, anorexia, nausea, vomiting, tremors, palpitations, headache, shortness of breath, hypertension, hypotension, tachyarrhythmias

---

✤ Available in Canada.

Treatment: Discontinue medication, supportive therapy as necessary; may treat tachyarrhythmias with propranolol or lidocaine

PATIENT CARE MANAGEMENT

Assessment
• Assess history of hypersensitivity to drug, catecholamines
• Assess baseline ECG, B/P, VS, cardiac output, LOC, pulmonary wedge pressure
• Assess baseline wt, hydration status

Interventions
• Administer IV digoxin before starting dobutamine if pt has atrial fibrillation
• Adjust dosage to meet individual pt needs
• Administer blood products for hypovolemia.

> **NURSING ALERT**
> Monitor IV site carefully; extravasation can cause serious tissue damage and necrosis

Evaluation
• Evaluate therapeutic effects (stabilization of cardiac status, increased B/P)
• Monitor ECG, B/P continually
• Monitor IV site continually

PATIENT AND FAMILY EDUCATION

Teach/instruct
• About need for medication
• That VS need to be monitored frequently

Warn/advise
• To notify care provider of hypersensitivity, side effects

Provide
• Emotional support as indicated

STORAGE
• Store at room temp

---

dopamine hydrochloride

Brand Name(s): Dopastat, Inotropin✤, Revimine

Classification: Inotropic, vasopressor

Pregnancy Category: C

AVAILABLE PREPARATIONS
Inj: 40 mg/ml, 80 mg/ml, 160 mg/ml; in D_5W sol 0.8 mg/ml, 1.6 mg/ml, 3.2 mg/ml

ROUTES AND DOSAGES
Children and adults: IV 2-5 mcg/kg/min maximum dose 20-50 mcg/kg/min

IV administration
• Recommended concentration: 400-800 mcg/ml in D_5W
• Maximum concentration (minimum dilution): 3.2 mg/ml
• IV push rate: Not recommended
• Continuous infusion rate: 2-5 mcg/kg/min; titrate dose 1-5 mcg/kg/min at 10-30 min intervals

MECHANISM AND INDICATIONS
Mechanism: Inotropic, stimulates β_1-adrenergic and α-adrenergic receptors, increases myocardial contractility and stroke volume, thereby increasing cardiac output; vasopressor, vasodilates renal, mesenteric, coronary, and cerebral arteries, thereby increasing systolic B/P and pulse pressure
Indications: Shock, hypotension, cardiac failure, decreased renal blood flow

PHARMACOKINETICS
Onset of action: 5 min
Peak: 8 min
Half-life: 2 min
Metabolism: Liver, kidney, plasma
Excretion: Urine (metabolites)

CONTRAINDICATIONS AND PRECAUTIONS
• Contraindicated with known hypersensitivity to medication, ventricular fibrillation, tachyarrhythmias, pheochromocytoma, sulfite allergies

---

✤ Available in Canada.

- Use cautiously with asthma, myocardial ischemia, peripheral vascular disease, acidosis, hypoxia

INTERACTIONS
Drug
- Increased effects of dopamine when used with MAOIs and thyroid medications
- Decreased effects with β-adrenergic blockers and α-adrenergic blockers
- Arrhythmias possible with digoxin, guanethidine, levodopa, sympathomimetics
- Additive effect with diuretics
- Hypotension and bradycardia possible with IV phenytoin
- Increased B/P with oxytocics
Lab
- Increases BG
Incompatibilities
- Acyclovir, amphotericin B, alkaline solutions, aminophylline, cephalothin, gentamycin, $NaHCO_3$

SIDE EFFECTS
CNS: Headache, numbness, tingling, nervousness, paresthesias
CV: Tachycardia, palpitations, hypertension, angina, peripheral vasoconstriction, hypotension, bradycardia, arrhythmias, widened QRS complex
DERM: Color changes, tissue necrosis with extravasation, piloerection
GI: Nausea, vomiting, diarrhea
RESP: Dyspnea

TOXICITY AND OVERDOSE
Clinical signs: Severe hypertension
Treatment: Discontinue medication; supportive therapy as necessary; may administer β_1-adrenergic blocker

PATIENT CARE MANAGEMENT
Assessment
- Assess history of hypersensitivity to drug, sulfites
- Assess baseline VS, ECG, CVP, B/P, hydration status
Interventions
- Administer IV into large vein; monitor site carefully

- Treat with 10-15 ml sodium chloride injection with 5-10 mg phentolamine injection into site if extravasation occurs.
- Correct hypovolemia before administration

> **NURSING ALERT**
> Monitor IV site carefully; extravasation can cause serious tissue necrosis, sloughing

Evaluation
- Evaluate therapeutic response (stabilization, increased B/P)
- Evaluate side effects, hypersensitivity
- Evaluate VS, B/P continuously
- Monitor I&O
- Evaluate electrolytes
- Monitor ECG regularly

PATIENT AND FAMILY EDUCATION
Teach/instruct
- About need for medication
Warn/advise
- To notify care provider of hypersensitivity, side effects
- About need for frequent VS
Encourage
- To provide emotional support as indicated

STORAGE
- Store at room temp
- Protect from light

doxapram hydrochloride
Brand Name(s): Dopram ♣
Classification: CNS and respiratory stimulant; analeptic; sympathomimetic agent
Pregnancy Category: B

AVAILABLE PREPARATIONS
Inj: 20 mg/ml (benzyl alcohol 0.9%)

ROUTES AND DOSAGES
Neonatal Apnea (Apnea of Prematurity)
Premature infants: IV initial dose 2.5-3 mg/kg; maintenance dose 1

mg/kg/hr, titrated to the lowest rate at which apnea is controlled; maximum 2.5 mg/kg/hr

Respiratory Depression Following Anesthesia

Adults: IV initial dose 0.5-1 mg/kg; may repeat q 15 min; maximum total dose 2 mg/kg; IV infusion, initial 5 mg/min until adequate response or adverse effects evident; decrease to 1-3 mg/min; usual dose 0.5-4 mg/kg or 300 mg

IV administration

• Loading dose: Dilute to maximum concentration of 2 mg/ml; infuse over 15-30 min

• IV infusion: Dilute to 1 mg/ml (maximum 2 mg/ml) in NS or D_5W

MECHANISM AND INDICATIONS

Mechanism: Acts in low doses to directly stimulate medullary respiratory center and activate peripheral carotid chemoreceptors, thereby stimulating respiration and increasing tidal volume; with higher dosages drug loses selectivity and stimulates both respiratory and non-respiratory neurons in the medulla

Indications: Used to treat neonatal apnea and to alleviate postanesthesia and drug-induced respiratory depression

PHARMACOKINETICS

Onset of action: 20-40 sec

Peak: 1-2 min

Half-life: 2-4 hr in adults; 7-10 hr in premature neonates

Metabolism: Liver

Excretion: Urine within 24-48 hr

CONTRAINDICATIONS AND PRECAUTIONS

• Use cautiously in newborns (reserved for neonates who are unresponsive to treatment of apnea with therapeutic serum concentrations of theophylline or caffeine); preparations with benzyl alcohol have been associated with fatal gasping syndrome

INTERACTIONS

Drug

• Significantly increased B/P possible with MAO inhibitors or sympathomimetic drugs

• Anesthetics should be discontinued at least 10 min before administration of doxapram, because these agents sensitize the myocardium to catecholamines

• Doxapram may temporarily mask residual effects of neuromuscular blockers used after anesthesia

• Use with halothane, cycloprane, or enflurane may cause cardiac arrhythmias

Lab

• Decreased erythrocyte and leukocyte counts; reduced Hgb and Hct

• Increased BUN; albuminuria

• Depression of T-wave on ECG

INCOMPATIBILITIES

• Aminophylline, alkaline solutions carbenicillin, cefaperazone, cefotaxime, cefotetan, cefuroxime, dexamethasone, diazepam, digoxin, dobutamine, furosemide, hydrocortisone, ketamine, methylprednisolone, minocycline, pentobarbital, phenobarbital, secobarbital, thiopental, ticarcillin

SIDE EFFECTS

CNS: Seizures, headache, dizziness, apprehension, disorientation, pupillary dilation, hyperreflexia, flushing, sweating, paresthesias

CV: Chest pain and tightness, arrhythmias, hypertension, sweating, flushing, feeling of warmth, hemolysis, phlebitis

DERM: Pruritis

GI: Nausea, vomiting, retching, diarrhea, urge to defecate

GU: Urinary retention, stimulation of bladder, incontinence

RESP: Cough, sneezing, hiccups, bronchospasm, rebound hypoventilation

TOXICITY AND OVERDOSE

Clinical signs: Hypertension, tachycardia, arrhythmias, skeletal muscle hyperactivity, dyspnea

Treatment: Supportive care, however O_2 should be used cautiously because the rapid increase of par-

---

tial pressure may result in suppression of carotid chemoreceptors activity; anticonvulsants may be administered to control excessive CNS stimulation

PATIENT CARE MANAGEMENT
Assessment
• Assess history of hypersensitivity to doxapram hydrochloride, respiratory stimulants, sympathomimetic drugs
• B/P, HR, deep tendon reflexes, ABGs before administration and q 30 min

Interventions
• Drug should be administered only by experienced clinicians
• Establish adequate airway before administering drug
• Prevent aspiration of vomitus by placing patient on side
• B/P, HR, deep tendon reflexes, and ABGs should be monitored q 30 min
• Monitor PO_2, PCO_2, O_2 saturation during treatment
• Do not infuse doxapram faster than recommended rate because it may result in hemolysis; should be used only on an intermittent basis with maximum infusion period of 2 hr
• Avoid repeated injections in the same site because of risk of thrombophlebitis or local skin irritation
• Do not combine with alkaline sols (doxapram is acidic); it is compatible with D_5W, $D_{10}W$, NS
• Give concomitant O_2 cautiously to pts who have just undergone surgery because doxapram stimulates respiration and increases demand for O_2
• Monitor (particularly hypertensive pts) for signs of toxicity, including tachycardia, muscle tremor, spasticity, hyperactive reflexes, and B/P changes

---

NURSING ALERT

Injectable sol may contain benzyl alcohol, which as been associated with fatal gasping syndrome in neonates

Anesthetics should be discontinued at least 10 min before administering doxapram because these agents sensitize the myocardium to catecholamines

Doxapram may temporarily mask residual effects of neuromuscular blockers used after anesthesia

---

Evaluation
• Evaluate therapeutic response (increase in breathing capacity; respiratory stimulation, such as increased respiratory rate, abnormal rhythm)
• Observe for hypertension, arrhythmias, tachycardia, dyspnea, skeletal muscle hyperactivity (may indicate overdose); discontinue should any of these occur
• Monitor IV site for any evidence of extravasation

PATIENT AND FAMILY EDUCATION
Teach/instruct
• About the purpose of therapy, the potential benefits, and adverse effects

STORAGE
• Store at room temp

---

doxorubicin hydrochloride

Brand Name(s): Adriamycin, Adriamycin PFS✤, Adriamycin RDF✤

Classification: Antineoplastic, anthracycline antibiotic, cell cycle phase nonspecific

Pregnancy Category: D

AVAILABLE PREPARATIONS
Inj: 2 mg/ml

✤ Available in Canada.

ROUTES AND DOSAGES

- Doses may vary in response to diagnosis, extent of disease, concurrent or previous therapy, protocol guidelines, physiological parameters; consult current literature, protocol recommendations

Children and adults: IV Interval dosing, 30-75 mg/m^2/dose, repeat q 21 days; consecutive daily dosing, 25-30 mg/m^2/24 hr for 3 days, repeat q 3-4 wk; weekly dosing, 15-30 mg/m^2/dose q wk; continuous infusion dosing, 9-20 mg/m^2/24 hr infused over 48-144 hr

- Maximum lifetime cumulative doxorubicin dose is $\approx$ 450 mg/m^2; if used in conjunction with chest radiation, maximum cumulative dose should be decreased; must also take into account other anthracycline agents administered
- Dosage adjustments are required for hepatic dysfunction but generally not necessary for renal dysfunction

IV administration

- Maximum concentration: 2 mg/ml
- IV push: Slowly over 5 min
- Continuous infusion: Over 24-96 hr through central venous line

MECHANISM AND INDICATIONS

Mechanism: Exerts several biochemical effects on cell, any or all may play part in cytotoxicity; drug intercalates between DNA base pairs causing DNA strand breaks, interruption of DNA synthesis, and DNA-dependent RNA synthesis; also produces hydrogen peroxide and hydroxyl radicals that are highly destructive; can also interact with cell membranes, altering cell function; maximally cytotoxic in S phase of cell cycle

Indications: Used in wide variety of pediatric tumors, including ALL, Hodgkin's and non-Hodgkin's lymphoma, Wilm's tumor, neuroblastoma, soft tissue sarcomas, Ewing's sarcoma, osteogenic sarcoma, germ cell tumors of the ovary and testis, melanoma, hepatocellular carcinoma

PHARMACOKINETICS

Distribution: Rapid uptake by heart, kidneys, lungs, liver, spleen; does not cross blood–brain barrier

Half-life: Multiphasic with prolonged terminal half-life (16-32 hr) related to tight binding of drug to DNA

Metabolism: To less active metabolite, doxorubinicol, that may actually have increased potential for cardiac toxicity but decreased effect on tumor

Excretion: Feces; urine (small amount)

CONTRAINDICATIONS AND PRECAUTIONS

- Contraindicated with hypersensitivity, pregnancy, lactation, preexisting cardiac defects, CHF, children with active infections (especially chicken pox or herpes zoster virus), children who have reached lifetime cumulative dose
- Use cautiously with hepatic dysfunction (demonstrated by increased bilirubin); dosage adjustments may not be necessary if renal dysfunction present because biliary excretion will increase to compensate; children who have received doses of 450 mg/m^2 as they demonstrate increased incidence of cardiomyopathy; previous chemotherapy, specifically with another anthracycline, radiation therapy, and current cardiac status, must be carefully evaluated before approaching this cumulative dose

INTERACTIONS

Drug

- Substantial dosage decrease required if doxorubicin is administered with interferon alfa
- Increased toxicity of doxorubicin possible with histamine$_2$ antagonists (ranitidine and cimetidine)
- Affected by multiple drug resistance phenomena
- Increased incidence of cardiotoxicity and cystitis possible if used concurrently with cyclophosphamide

---

❦ Available in Canada.

• Increased possibility of hepatotoxicity if used with other hepatotoxic drugs
Lab
• Increased serum concentration of hepatocellular enzymes (LDH and AST); may also cause hyperbilirubinemia

INCOMPATIBILITIES
• Cephalothin, dexamethasone, and furosemide may cause a precipitate; aminophylline, 5-FU, and $NaHCO_3$ cause pH degradation of solution

SIDE EFFECTS
CV: Dose-limiting effect is cardiotoxicity; acute phase characterized by abnormal ECG changes (T-wave changes, ST depression, SVT, extrasystole, premature contraction); more chronic phase characterized by CHF not responsive to digoxin and carrying greater than 50% mortality rate
DERM: Reversible alopecia, erythema at injection site, facial flushing, radiation recall phenomena (intense erythema, desquamation in areas previously exposed to radiation; evident externally but can also occur internally in esophagus, heart, lungs, GI mucosa)
EENT: Mucositis (beginning in sublingual and lateral tongue region as burning sensation progressing to ulceration within a few days), photosensitivity, conjunctivitis, lacrimation
GI: Nausea, vomiting beginning 1-4 hr after administration, lasting about 24 hrs; diarrhea, esophagitis, anorexia
GU: Hyperuricemia, red-orange urine up to 48 hr after administration
HEME: Myelosuppression with nadir for leukopenia at 10-14 days; recovery in 21 days; thrombocytopenia and anemia less pronounced
Other: Fever, chills; anaphylactoid reaction

TOXICITY AND OVERDOSE
Clinical signs: Prolonged myelosuppression; severe, extensive mucositis
Treatment: Supportive measures (including blood products, hydration, nutritional supplementation, broad spectrum antibiotic coverage in event of febrile neutropenia and electrolyte replacement)

PATIENT CARE MANAGEMENT
Assessment
• Assess history of hypersensitivity to doxorubicin
• Assess history of previous treatment with attention to anthracycline chemotherapy, radiation therapy
• Assess cumulative anthracycline therapy
• Assess baseline VS, oximetry
• Assess CBC, differential, platelet count
• Assess success of previous antiemetic therapy
• Assess baseline ECG, echocardiogram
• Assess baseline renal function (BUN, creatinine), liver function (bilirubin, alk phos, LDH, AST, ALT)
Interventions
• Administer antiemetic therapy before chemotherapy
• Ensure absolute patency of IV before administration
• Do not place IV over joint; if extravasation occurs, joint may become immobilized
• Provide supportive measures to maintain hemostasis, fluid, electrolyte, nutritional balance
• Apply top dimethysulfoxide (DMSO) for 14 days if extravasation occurs; application of ice after initial discovery may also be helpful
• Monitor I&O; administer IV fluids until child is able to resume normal oral intake

NURSING ALERT

Drug is potent vesicant; ensure patency of IV line just before administration; if infiltration occurs, apply cool compresses

Doxorubicin can cause progressive, potentially fatal cardiomyopathy; assess resting HR, B/P, and oximetry at regular intervals; ECG and echocardiograms routinely to evaluate cardiac function

Evaluation
• Evaluate therapeutic response (radiologic or clinical demonstration of tumor regression)
• Evaluate CBC, differential, platelet count at least q wk
• Evaluate renal function (BUN, creatinine), liver function (alk phos, LDH, AST, ALT, bilirubin) regularly
• Evaluate cardiac status using periodic ECG, echocardiogram

PATIENT AND FAMILY EDUCATION
Teach/instruct
• To have patient well hydrated before and after chemotherapy
• That urine may be pink or red for 48 hr
• About the importance of follow-up to monitor blood counts, serum chemistry values
• To take accurate temp; rectal temp contraindicated
• About likelihood of radiation recall phenomenon
• To notify care provider of signs of bleeding (bruising, epistaxis, bleeding gums), infection (fever, sore throat, fatigue)
Warn/advise
• About impact of body changes that may occur (hair loss, hyperpigmentation, nail ridging), how to minimize changes (wigs, caps, scarves, long sleeves)
• To avoid OTC preparations containing aspirin
• To report any alterations in behavior, sensation, perception; help to develop a plan of care to manage side effects, stress of illness or treatment
• To immediately report any signs of pain or irritation at injection site
• That good oral hygiene with very soft toothbrush is imperative
• That dental work be delayed until blood counts return to baseline, with permission of care provider
• To avoid contact with known viral and bacterial illnesses
• That close household contacts of child not be immunized with live polio virus; use inactivated form
• That children receiving chemotherapy not receive immunizations until immune system recovers sufficiently to mount necessary antibody response
• To report exposure to chicken pox in susceptible child immediately
• To report reactivation of herpes zoster virus (shingles) immediately
• About ways to provide meticulous skin care in event of radiation recall
• To report fatigue, SOB for evaluation; may be early signs of cardiotoxicity
• If appropriate, ways to preserve reproductive patterns, sexuality (sperm banking, contraceptives)
Encourage
• Provision of nutritious food intake; consider nutrition consultation
• To use top anesthetics to control the discomfort of mucositis; avoid spicy foods, commercial mouthwashes

STORAGE
• Intact vials of sol may be stored for 2 yr at room temp if protected from light
• Diluted sol should be protected from light; stable at room temp for 24 hr, 48 hr refrigerated

---

✦ Available in Canada.

doxycycline hyclate, doxycycline monohydrate

Brand Name(s): Apo-Doxy✤, Apo-Doxy Tabs✤, Doryx✤, Doxy-100, Doxy-200, Doxy-Caps, Doxychel, Doxy-Lemmon, Doxycin✤, Doxy-Tabs, Doxytec✤, Novo-Doxylin✤, Nu-Doxycicline✤, Rho-Doxycin✤, Rho-Doxycin Tabs✤, Vibramycin✤, Vibra-Tabs✤, Vivox

Classification: Antibiotic (tetracycline)

Pregnancy Category: D

AVAILABLE PREPARATIONS
Oral susp: 25 mg/5 ml /50 mg/5ml
Caps: 50 mg, 100 mg
Caps (ext rel): 100 mg
Tabs: 50 mg, 100 mg
Inj: 100 mg, 200 mg

ROUTES AND DOSAGES
Children ≥8 yr, <45 kg: PO/IV 4.4 mg/kg divided q12h first 24 hr, then 2.2 mg/kg/24 hr divided q12-24h
Children >45 kg and adults: PO 100 mg q12h first 24 hr, then 100 mg/24 hr divided q12-24h; IV 200 mg divided q12-24h first 24 hr, then 100-200 mg/24 hr divided q12-24h

Chlamydia Trachomatis
Children >45 kg and adults (both not pregnant): PO 100 mg bid for 7 days; not recommended for children <8 yr

IV administration
• Recommended concentration: 0.1-1 mg/ml in D_5LR, D_5W, LR, NS, or R
• Maximum concentration: 1 mg/ml
• IV push rate: Not recommended
• Intermittent infusion rate: 0.1-1 mg/ml over 1-4 hr or longer

MECHANISM AND INDICATIONS
Antibiotic mechanism: Bacteriostatic; inhibits bacterial protein synthesis by binding reversibly to ribosomal units
Indications: Effective against gram-positive and gram-negative organisms, *Mycoplasma, Chlamydia, Rickettsia,* and spirochetes; used to treat syphilis, *C. trachomatis,* gonorrhea, lymphogranuloma venereum

PHARMACOKINETICS
Peak: 1.5-4 hr
Distribution: Penetrates CSF, prostate, eye
Half-life: 12-14 hr
Metabolism: Not metabolized
Excretion: Urine, feces

CONTRAINDICATIONS AND PRECAUTIONS
• Contraindicated with pregnancy, lactation, in children <8 yr (because of risk of permanent discoloration of teeth, enamel defects, and retardation of bone growth, with known hypersensitivity to any tetracycline
• Use cautiously with impaired renal or hepatic function

INTERACTIONS
Drug
• Decreased bactericidal effects of penicillins
• Increased effects of oral anticoagulants
• Decreased absorption with use of antacids containing aluminum, Ca, or Mg, laxatives containing Mg, oral iron, zinc, $NaHCO_3$
• Increased effects of digoxin
• Decreased serum half-life with use of barbiturates, carbamazepine, phenytoin, cimetidine
Lab
• False positive urine catecholamines
Nutrition
• Decreased oral absorption if given with food or dairy products

INCOMPATIBILITIES
• Cephalothin; D_5LR, LR may present compatibility problems with some drugs

SIDE EFFECTS
CNS: Increased intracranial pressure

✤ Available in Canada.

CV: Pericarditis
DERM: Maculopapular and erythematous rashes, photosensitivity, increased pigmentation, urticaria, discolored nails
EENT: Sore throat
GI: Anorexia, epigastric distress, nausea, vomiting, diarrhea, glossitis, dysphagia, enterocolitis, inflammatory anogenital lesions
GU: Reversible nephrotoxicity with outdated tetracyclines
HEME: Neutropenia, eosinophilia
LOCAL: Thrombophlebitis with IV injection
Other: Hypersensitivity, bacterial or fungal superinfection, discolored teeth

TOXICITY AND OVERDOSE
Clinical signs: GI disturbance
Treatment: Antacids; if ingested within 4 hr, empty stomach by gastric lavage; supportive care

PATIENT CARE MANAGEMENT
Assessment
• Assess history of hypersensitivity to tetracyclines
• Obtain C&S; may begin therapy before obtaining results
• Assess renal function (BUN, creatinine, I&O), hepatic function (ALT, AST, bilirubin), hematologic function (CBC, differential, platelet count—particularly for long-term therapy), bowel pattern
Interventions
• Check expiration dates; nephrotoxicity may result from outdated doxycycline
• Administer penicillins at least 1 hr before doxycycline if pt is receiving concurrent penicillins
• Administer PO 1 hr ac or 2 hr after meals; give with water to prevent esophageal irritation; do not administer within 1 hr of hs to prevent esophageal reflux; do not give with milk or dairy products, $NaHCO_3$, oral iron, zinc, antacids
• Shake susp well before administering; tab may be crushed, capsules taken apart and mixed with food or fluid; ext rel caps may be taken apart; particles should not be chewed; give water after administration to wash particles from mouth
• Do not mix IV with other medications; infuse separately
• Use large vein with small-bore needle to reduce local reaction; rotate site q48-72h
• Maintain age-appropriate fluid intake

> **NURSING ALERT**
> Discontinue drug if signs of toxicity, hypersensitivity, renal dysfunction, superinfection, erythema from sun or ultraviolet exposure, or pseudomembranous colitis develop
>
> Do not administer IV push

Evaluation
• Evaluate therapeutic response (decreased symptoms of infection)
• Monitor signs of superinfection (perineal itching, diaper rash, fever, malaise, redness, pain, swelling, drainage, rash, diarrhea, sore throat, change in cough or sputum)
• Observe for signs of allergic reaction (rash, pruritus, angioedema)
• Monitor bowel pattern; diarrhea may be symptomatic of pseudomembranous colitis
• Monitor renal function (BUN, creatinine, I&O), hepatic function (ALT, AST, bilirubin), hematologic function (CBC, differential, platelet count)
• Evaluate IV site for vein irritation; replace IV route with oral therapy as soon as possible to prevent thrombophlebitis

PATIENT AND FAMILY EDUCATION
Teach/instruct
• To take as directed at prescribed intervals for prescribed length of time
Warn/advise
• To notify care provider of hypersensitivity, side effects, superinfection
• Not to use outdated medication

- To avoid sun or ultraviolet light exposure

STORAGE
- Store powder, tabs, caps at room temp in airtight, light-resistant containers
- Reconstituted oral susp stable at room temp for 2 wk; label date and time of reconstitution; reconstituted IV sol stable refrigerated 72 hr

---

droperidol

Brand Name(s): Droperidol, Inapsine✤

Classification: Analgesic, narcotic, neuroleptic

Controlled Substance Schedule II

Pregnancy Category: C

AVAILABLE PREPARATIONS
Inj: 2.5 mg

DOSAGES AND ROUTES
Premedication
Children 2-12 yr: IM 0.088-0.165 ml/kg 30-60 min before procedure; 0.088-0.165 mg/kg titrated to response needed
Nausea and Vomiting
Children 2-12 yr: IM/IV 0.05-0.06 mg/kg/dose q4-6h prn
- Do not give to children <2 yr
IV administration
- Recommended concentration: May dilute as desired in D₅W, NS, or LR
- Maximum concentration: May be given undiluted
- IV push rate: Over 2-5 min
- Continuous infusion rate: Titrate per patient response

MECHANISM AND INDICATIONS
Mechanism: Acts on CNS at subcortical levels, producing tranquilization, sleep, antiemetic effects
Indications: For use in preparation for surgery to reduce anxiety; for induction and maintenance of general anesthesia; also used as an antipsychotic and antiemetic

PHARMACOKINETICS
Onset of action: IM, IV 3-10 min
Peak: IM, IV ½ hr
Duration: IM, IV 3-6 hr
Metabolism: Liver
Excretion: Urine

CONTRAINDICATIONS AND PRECAUTIONS
- Contraindicated with hypersensitivity to this or any component of this medication; with MAOIs taken within 14 days
- Use cautiously with bradyarrhythmias, cardiovascular disease, hypotension, kidney disease, liver disease, Parkinson's disease, pregnancy, elderly pts

INTERACTIONS
Drug
- Increased CNS depression with alcohol, antipsychotics, barbiturates, CNS depressants, narcotics
- Decreased effects of amphetamines, anticonvulsants, anticoagulants
- Increased side effects of lithium
- Hypertensive crisis, high fever, seizures within 14 days of MAOIs
Nutrition
- Do not drink alcohol

INCOMPATIBILITIES
- Incompatible with epinephrine, barbiturates, foscarnet

SIDE EFFECTS
CNS: Akathisia, anxiety, depression, disorientation, dizziness, drowsiness, dystonia, hallucination, fine tremors, flexion of arms, restlessness, delirium, dysphoria, EPS
CV: Hypotension, tachycardia, bradycardia, hypertension
DERM: Chills, shivering, facial sweating
EENT: Miosis, oculogyric crisis
GI: Nausea, vomiting
RESP: Apnea, bronchospasm, laryngospasm, respiratory depression
Other: Hyperglycemia, hypothermia, muscular rigidity

D

PATIENT CARE MANAGEMENT
Assessment
- Assess history of hypersensitivity to drug
- Obtain baseline medical history and physical examination
- Assess history of MAOI use; droperidol should not be taken concurrently or within 14 days; may cause hypertensive crisis, high fever, seizures
- Assess VS (including B/P, O_2 saturation) q 10 min during IV administration
- Assess VS q 30 min after IM dose

Interventions
- Administer only with emergency cart nearby, and an opioid antagonist, resuscitative and intubation equipment, and O_2 available
- Administer benztropine or diphenhydramine if extrapyramidal reaction occurs
- Move pt slowly to avoid orthostatic hypotension

> **NURSING ALERT**
> Rapid IV injection can cause muscle rigidity, especially of the muscles of respiration

Evaluation
- Evaluate therapeutic response (decreased anxiety, absence of vomiting during, after surgery)
- Monitor for increasing HR or decreasing B/P; do not place pt in Trendelenburg position because sympathetic blockade may occur, causing respiratory arrest
- Evaluate for EPS (dystonia, akathisia)

PATIENT/FAMILY EDUCATION
Teach/instruct
- Not to rise quickly from a recumbent position

STORAGE
- Store in light resistant container at room temp

---

edetate calcium disodium
Brand Name(s): Calcium Disodium Versenate✤

Classification: Antidote (lead toxicity)

Pregnancy Category: C

AVAILABLE PREPARATIONS
Inj: 200 mg/ml

ROUTES AND DOSAGES
Diagnosis of Lead Poisoning, Mobilization Test
Children: IM 500 mg/m²/dose as single dose or divided into 2 doses (maximum 1 g/dose); IV 500 mg/m² in D_5W infused over 1 hr
Adults: IM 500 mg/m²/dose

Asymptomatic Lead Poisoning
Children, blood lead concentration 45-69 mcg/dl: IV 1000 mg/m²/24 hr for 5 days as an 8-24 hr infusion or divided into 2 doses given q12h
Children, blood lead concentration >70 mcg/dl: IM 167 mg/m² q4h for 3-5 days with dimercaprol; IV 1000 mg/m²/24 hr for 5 days as an 8-24 hr infusion or divided into 2 doses administered q12h with dimercaprol

Symptomatic Lead Poisoning
Children: IM 250 mg/m² dose administered q4h for 5 days given with dimercaprol; IV 1500 mg/m²/24 hr for 5 days as an 8-24 hr infusion or divided into 2 doses administered q12h with dimercaprol; after a 2-day drug-free period, another course of treatment (with or without dimercaprol) may be administered based on blood lead concentration and symptoms

IV administration
- Recommended concentration: 2-4 mg/ml in D_5W or NS
- Maximum concentration: ≤5 mg/ml
- IV push rate: Not recommended
- Intermittent infusion rate: 15-30 min to 2 hr, depending on dosage
- Continuous infusion rate: 1000-

✤ Available in Canada.

1500 mg/m^2/24 hr for 5 days; preferred method of administration

MECHANISM AND INDICATIONS

Antidote mechanism: Binds ions of lead, forming a non-ionizing soluble complex that is excreted in urine

Indications: Used to treat acute and chronic lead poisoning; used as an agent in mobilization tests to diagnose lead poisoning

PHARMACOKINETICS

Half-life: IM 1.5 hr; IV 20 min
Distribution: Distributed to extracellular fluid; does not penetrate CSF
Metabolism: Not metabolized
Excretion: Urine

CONTRAINDICATIONS AND PRECAUTIONS

• Contraindicated with hypersensitivity to edetate calcium disodium, severe renal or hepatic impairment, anuria
• Use cautiously with hypertension, gout, active tuberculosis, pregnancy, lactation

INTERACTIONS

Drug
• Chelation effect with use of zinc insulin preparations; do not use concomitantly

Lab
• Decreased cholesterol/triglycerides, K$^+$

INCOMPATIBILITIES

• Do not mix in same syringe with dimercaprol; incompatible with D$_{10}$W, LR, R

SIDE EFFECTS

CNS: Numbness, tingling headache
CV: Hypotension, arrhythmias, ECG changes
DERM: Urticaria, erythema, pruritus
EENT: Nasal congestion, lacrimation, sneezing
ENDO / METAB: Hypercalcemia
GI: Vomiting, diarrhea, abdominal cramps, anorexia
GU: Renal tubular necrosis, proteinuria, microscopic hematuria

HEME: Transient bone marrow suppression
Local: Pain at IM injection site; thrombophlebitis with IV infusion (>5 mg/ml sol)
MS: Leg cramps, myalgia, arthralgia
Other: Fever, chills

TOXICITY AND OVERDOSE

Clinical signs: Aggravated symptoms of lead poisoning (cerebral edema, renal tubular necrosis); severe zinc deficiency
Treatment: Supportive care; mannitol for cerebral edema

PATIENT CARE MANAGEMENT

Assessment
• Assess history of hypersensitivity to edetate calcium disodium
• Assess renal function (BUN, creatinine, I&O), hepatic function (ALT, AST, bilirubin), hematologic blood lead concentration (CBC, differential, platelet count), neurologic status
• Identify lead sources in child's environment

Interventions
• Never use edetate disodium to treat lead poisoning; chelation of calcium induces tetany, possibly fatal hypocalcemia
• IM injection is very painful; add 1 ml 1% lidocaine or procaine hydrochloride/ml EDTA calcium to minimize pain at injection site
• Administer deeply into large muscle mass, rotate injection sites
• Administer IV dimercaprol separately as ordered
• Provide emergency equipment
• Maintain age-appropriate fluid intake

NURSING ALERT

Never use edetate disodium to treat lead poisoning; tetany and fatal hypocalcemia may result

For IM administration, add 1% lidocaine or procaine hydrochloride to minimize pain at injection site

---

Evaluation
- Evaluate therapeutic response (decreased symptoms of lead poisoning, decreased blood lead concentrations)
- Monitor renal function (BUN, creatinine, I&O), hepatic function (ALT, AST, bilirubin), hematologic function (CBC, differential, platelet count), blood lead concentration, neurologic status
- Monitor for cardiac abnormalities (arrhythmias, hypotension, tachycardia)
- Monitor allergic reaction (rash, urticaria)
- Evaluate IM site for tissue damage, IV site for vein irritation

PATIENT AND FAMILY EDUCATION
Teach/instruct
- About sources of lead poisoning, ways to prevent further exposure or poisoning
Warn/advise
- To notify care provider of hypersensitivity, side effects
- To comply with follow-up to monitor blood lead concentrations, neurologic or developmental status

STORAGE
- Store at room temp

EMLA cream (eutectic mixture of lidocaine and prilocaine)
Classification: Local anesthetic
Pregnancy Category: B

AVAILABLE PREPARATIONS
Cream: 5 g tube with occlusive dressing; 30 g tube without dressing

ROUTES AND DOSAGES
Minor Dermal Procedures (Venipunctures)
Top 2.5 g (½ of 5 g tube) over 20-25 cm^2 of skin surface for at least 1 hr

Major Dermal Procedures (Split Thickness Skin Graft Harvesting)
Top 2 g/10 cm^2 of skin for at least 2 hrs; maximum application area, up to 10 kg, 100 cm^2; 10-20 kg 600 cm^2; >20 kg, 2000 cm^2

MECHANISM AND INDICATIONS
Mechanism: Releases lidocaine and prilocaine from the cream into epidermal and dermal layers of skin; lidocaine and prilocaine accumulate in the vicinity of dermal pain receptors, nerve endings
Indications: Used to provide topical anesthesia during invasive procedures such as venipuncture, lumbar puncture, bone marrow aspirates, split-thickness skin graft harvesting

PHARMACOKINETICS
Onset of action: Variable, depends on duration of application and extent of area applied
Peak: Variable
Half-life: Lidocaine, 65-150 min; prilocaine, 10-150 min
Duration: Variable
Metabolism: Lidocaine, liver; prilocaine, liver and kidneys; unknown if both are metabolized by the skin

CONTRAINDICATIONS AND PRECAUTIONS
- Contraindicated with known sensitivity to local anesthetics of the amide type, or to any other component; with congenital or idiopathic methemoglobinemia, infants <12 mo receiving treatment with methemoglobin-inducing agents; lactation; do not use near eyes or ears or on open wounds
- Use cautiously with severe hepatic disease, pregnancy

INTERACTIONS
Drug
- Increased risk of methemoglobinemia with drugs associated with drug-induced methemoglobinemia (sulfonamides, acetaminophen, acetamilid, aniline dyes, benzocaine, chloroquine, dapsone, naphthalene, nitrates and ni-

trites, nitrofurantoin, nitroglycerin, pamaquine, paraaminosali-
cylic acid, phenacetin, phenobarbital, phenytoin, primaquine,
quinine)
• Additive and synergistic potential of toxic side effects possible
when given with Class I antiarrhythmic drugs (such as tocainide
and mexiletine)

SIDE EFFECTS
• Systemic adverse effects unlikely to be caused by the small
dose absorbed
CNS: Lightheadedness, nervousness, apprehension, euphoria, confusion, dizziness, drowsiness,
twitching, tremors, convulsions,
unconsciousness
CV: Bradycardia, hypotension,
cardiovascular collapse (all rare)
DERM: Erythema, edema, pale-
ness (pallor or blanching), alteration in temperature sensations,
pruritus, rash
EENT: Tinnitus, blurred vision,
diplopia
GI: Vomiting
Local: Sensations of heat, cold, or
numbness
Other: Allergic and anaphylactoid
reactions characterized by urticaria, angioedema, bronchospasm,
shock

TOXICITY AND OVERDOSE
Clinical signs: Decrease in cardiac
output, total peripheral resistance, mean arterial pressure
Treatment: Supportive care

**PATIENT CARE
MANAGEMENT**
Assessment
• Assess history of hypersensitivity to EMLA, related drugs
• Assess skin to ensure intactness
before application
• Assess extent of skin that needs
to be anesthetized; ensure that
area per wt is not larger than
maximum allowed
• Assess previous history of methemoglobinemia or use of any
drugs that may increase risk of
developing methemoglobinemia
Interventions
• Apply cream to identified area at

least 1 hr before minor procedure
or 2 hr before major procedure; for
young children, try to disguise the
cream and dressing once applied
(e.g., with clothing) so anxiety
about procedure won't be prolonged as they stare at the cream
and dressing
• Place an occlusive dressing (e.g.,
Tegaderm) over the cream (ensure
that a thick layer of cream is
underneath)
• Secure dressing edges carefully
to avoid leakage
• Remove dressing after time
limit, wipe off cream, clean entire
area with an antiseptic solution,
prepare pt for the procedure

NURSING ALERT
Not to be used in infants <1 mo
or in infants <12 mo who are
receiving treatment with methemoglobin-inducing agents
Use on intact skin only

Evaluation
• Evaluate therapeutic response
(effective anesthesia for procedure)
• Evaluate for side effects, hypersensitivity

**PATIENT AND FAMILY
EDUCATION**
Teach/instruct
• About importance of not touch-
ing the cream or dressing once it
has been applied
• About duration of application for
effective anesthesia
• That it may be necessary to
cover more than one site with
cream or dressing if more than one
procedure needs to be done (such
as more than one venipuncture
because of failed attempt)
Warn/advise
• That local reaction of erythema,
blanching, or pallor of skin is
temporary and will only last for
approximately 1 hr

STORAGE
• Store at room temp
• Protect from light

enalapril

Brand Name(s): Vasotec

Classification: ACE inhibitor, antihypertensive, cardiac afterload reducer

Pregnancy Category: D

AVAILABLE PREPARATIONS
Tabs: 2.5 mg, 5 mg, 10 mg, 20 mg
Inj: Enalaprilat, 1.25 mg/ml

ROUTES AND DOSAGES
Infants and children: PO 0.1 mg/kg/24 hr qd, increase prn over 2 wk to maximum of 0.5 mg/kg/24 hr qd; IV (as Enalaprilat) 5-10 mcg/kg/dose q8-24h based on B/P readings (certain patients may require higher dosages)
Adults: PO 2.5-5 mg/24 hr qd or divided bid, increase prn to 10-40 mg/24 hr qd or divided bid; IV (as Enalaprilat) 0.625-1.25 mg/dose q6h

IV administration
• Recommended concentration: May administer undiluted, or dilute in small amount of D_5W, NS, or LR
• Maximum concentration: May administer undiluted
• Intermittent infusion rate: Over 5 min

MECHANISM AND INDICATIONS
Mechanisms: Antihypertensive, suppress renin–angiotensin–aldosterone system, reducing Na and water retention and lowering B/P; load reducer, decreases systemic vascular resistance and pulmonary capillary wedge pressure, increasing cardiac output in pts with congestive heart failure or left ventricular dysfunction
Indications: Hypertension, congestive heart failure, left ventricular dysfunction

PHARMACOKINETICS
Onset of action: IV 5-15 min; PO 15 min
Peak: Enalapril 0.5-1.5 hr; enalaprilat: 3-4.5 hr
Half-life: Enalapril 2 hr; enalaprilat, infants 6-10 hrs, adults 35-38 hrs
Metabolism: Enalapril undergoes biotransformation in liver to enalaprilat
Elimination: Urine, feces

CONTRAINDICATIONS AND PRECAUTIONS
• Contraindicated with known hypersensitivity to drug, other ACE inhibitors
• Use cautiously with renal dysfunction, hyponatremia, hypovolemia, severe CHF, diuretics, lactation

INTERACTIONS
Drug
• Increased hypotensive effects with phenothiazines, phenytoin, quinidine, nifedipine, diuretics, other antihypertensive drugs
• Decreased hypotensive effects with indomethacin
• Hyperkalemia with K^+-sparing diuretics (e.g., spironalactone), salt substitutes
• Hypokalemia with thiazide-type diuretics (e.g., furosemide, hydrochlorothiazide)
• Increased effects of neuromuscular blocking agent, barbiturates, hypoglycemics with use of enalapril
Lab
• Increased BUN, creatinine, AST, ALT, bilirubin

INCOMPATIBILITIES
• None reported

SIDE EFFECTS
CNS: Dizziness, syncope, fatigue, headache, insomnia
CV: Hypotension, tachycardia, arrhythmias
DERM: Rash, purpura, alopecia, hyperhidrosis
EENT: Tinnitus, visual changes
GI: Diarrhea, nausea, dry mouth, cramps, colitis
GU: Decrease in renal function, male impotence
HEME: Agranulocytosis, neutropenia, anemia
RESP: Cough, rales, angioedema
Other: Hypokalemia, hyperkalemia

✣ Available in Canada.

TOXICITY AND OVERDOSE
Clinical signs: Hypotension, bradycardia, bronchospasm
Treatment: Discontinue drug; provide supportive care; hemodialysis in severe cases

PATIENT CARE MANAGEMENT
Assessment
• Assess history of hypersensitivity to enalapril, other ACE inhibitors
• Assess baseline VS, B/P, wt, hydration status
• Assess baseline renal function (BUN, creatinine), liver function (AST, ALT, bilirubin)
• Assess baseline CBC, differential, electrolytes
Interventions
• Administer PO 1 hour ac
• Monitor for side effects
• Monitor I&O
• Monitor B/P after administering drug

> **NURSING ALERT**
> Severe hypotension may result in sodium- or volume-depleted pts

Evaluation
• Evaluate therapeutic response (decreased B/P, CHF)
• Evaluate side effects
• Evaluate hydration status; withhold drug, notify care provider if patient is volume depleted
• Evaluate renal function (BUN, creatinine), liver function (AST, ALT, bilirubin)
• Evaluate wt

PATIENT AND FAMILY EDUCATION
Teach/instruct
• To take as directed at prescribed intervals for prescribed length of time
• To monitor wt regularly
• To notify care provider if excessive perspiration, vomiting, diarrhea occur
• To notify care provider if side effects occur

Warn/advise
• To avoid direct sunlight or wear sunscreen; photosensitivity reactions may occur
• That drug may cause dizziness, fainting, lightheadedness; avoid hazardous activities
• To rise slowly to sitting or standing positions to avoid orthostatic hypotension
• Not to take other medications unless approved by care provider

STORAGE
• Store at room temp in tightly sealed container

---

epinephrine, epinephrine bitartrate, epinephrine hydrochloride, racemic epinephrine

Brand Name(s): Epinephrine: Adrenalin, Bronkaid, EpiPen, EpiPen Jr, Primatene
Epinephrine bitartrate: AsthmaHaler, Bronitin Mist, Bronkaid, Epitrate, Medihaler-Epi, Primatene
Epinephrine hydrochloride: Adrenalin Chloride, Epifrin, Glaucon, SusPhrine
Racemic epinephrine: AsthmaNefrin, MicroNefrin, S-2 Inhalant, Vaponefrin

Classification: Bronchodilator; α- and β-adrenergic agonist agent; vasopressor; cardiac stimulant; local anesthetic, mydriatic, topical antihemorrhagic

Pregnancy Category: C

AVAILABLE PREPARATIONS
Many dosage forms, including combination preparations exist
Inj: 1:200 susp; 1:1000, 1:2000, 1:10,000, 1:100,000 ampules
AutoInjection syringes: 0.15 mg (1:2000); 0.30 mg (1:1000)
Inhal spray: 160 mcg, 200 mcg, 250 mcg metered spray

Nebulization sol: 2.25%, 1%
Top sol: 0.1%
Nasal sol: 1:1000
Ophthal sol: 0.1%, 0.25%, 0.5%, 1%, 2%

ROUTES AND DOSAGES
Anaphylaxis
Children: SC 0.01 ml/kg of 1:1000 q 10-15 min prn, maximum single dose 0.3 ml; IV 0.01 ml/kg of 1:1000 q 10-15 min
Adults: SC/IM 0.1-0.5 ml of 1:1000 q 10-15 min prn; IV 0.1-0.25 ml of 1:1000 q 10-15 min prn

Cardiac Arrest
Neonates: IV 0.01-0.03 mg/kg (0.1-0.3 ml/kg of 1:10,000 q 5 min prn)
Children: IV 0.01 mg/kg (0.1 ml/kg of 1:10,000) × 1, then 0.1 mg/kg q 5 min prn (0.1 ml/kg of 1:1000); intracardiac 0.05-0.1 mg/kg
Adults: IV 0.1-1 mg (1-10 ml of 1:10,000) q 5 min prn; intracardiac 0.1-1 mg

Asthma
Children: SC 0.01 ml/kg of 1:1000 q 20 min-4 hr, maximum single dose 0.3 ml; inhal, 1-2 inhalations q4h prn
Adults: SC/IM 0.1-0.5 ml of 1:1000 q 20 min-4 hr; inhal, 1-2 inhalations q4h prn

Croup
Children: Inhal, 0.05 ml/kg/dose (racemic epinephrine) diluted to 3 ml with NS, via nebulizer over 15 min prn, not more frequently than q2h; maximum dose 0.5 ml

Glaucoma
Children and adults: Top 1-2 gtt 0.25%-2% sol qd or bid

Ocular Mydriasis, Hemostasis
Children and adults: Top 1-2 gtt 0.1% ophthal or 0.1% nasal sol

Topical Hemostatic
Children and adults: Top 1:50,000-1:1000 applied topically; or 1:500,000-1:50,000 mixed with a local anesthetic

Prolongation of Local Anesthetic Effect
Children and adults: Top 1:500,000-1:50,000 mixed with local anesthetic

IV administration
• Recommended concentration: 100 mcg/ml (1:10,000 sol) in NS for IV push; do not use undiluted sol (1:1000) for IV administration; 5 or 10 mcg/ml (1:200,000 or 1:100,000 respectively) in D-LR, D-R, D-S, D_5LR, D_5NS, D_5W, $D_{10}W$, LR, NS, or R for continuous infusion
• The AAP recommends the following formula for preparation of the infusion: $0.6 \times wt$ (kg) = mg of drug to be added to IV sol for a total volume of 100 ml; an infusion rate of 1 ml/hr provides 0.1 mcg/kg/min
• Maximum concentration: 100 mcg/ml for IV push
• IV push rate: Over 5-10 min
• Continuous infusion rate: 0.1-1 mcg/kg/min

MECHANISM AND INDICATIONS
• Acts by directly stimulating α- and β-adrenergic receptors in the sympathetic nervous system, resulting in relaxation of bronchial smooth muscle, cardiac stimulation, and dilation of skeletal muscle vasculature; potent activator of α receptors
Bronchodilator mechanism: Relaxes bronchial smooth muscle by stimulating β_2-adrenergic receptors; constricts bronchial arterioles by stimulating α-adrenergic receptors, resulting in relief of bronchospasm, reduced congestion and edema, increased tidal volume and vital capacity; possibly reverses bronchiolar constriction, vasodilation, and edema through inhibition of histamine release
Cardiovascular and vasopressor mechanism: Produces positive chronotropic and inotropic effects as a cardiac stimulant by action on β_1 receptors in heart, increasing cardiac output, myocardial O_2 consumption, and force of contraction, decreasing cardiac efficiency; vasodilation results from its effect on β_2 receptors; vasoconstriction results from α-adrenergic effects
Local anesthetic action: Acts as an adjunct via effect of α receptors in skin, mucous membranes, viscera; produces vasoconstriction, reduc-

---

ing absorption of local anesthetic, prolonging its duration of action, localizing effects of anesthesia, and decreasing risk of anesthetic toxicity

Local vasoconstricting mechanism: Acts via action on α receptors in skin, mucous membranes, viscera, producing vasoconstriction and hemostasis in small vessels

Ophthalmic mechanism: Lowers intraocular pressure by decreasing aqueous humor formation and increasing ease of aqueous outflow; produces brief mydriasis and slight relaxation of ciliary muscle; has only slight effect on normal eye

Indications: Used in cardiac arrest to treat asystole; in acute asthma attack, croup, hypersensitivity reactions, anaphylaxis; treatment of open-angle glaucoma, as ophthalmic decongestant; used in small amounts in local anesthetics to decrease their systemic absorption; top preparation used to control superficial bleeding

PHARMACOKINETICS

Onset of action: Inhaled, within 1 min; SC 5-10 min (bronchodilation); IM variable

Peak: SC 20 min (bronchodilation); IM variable; IV 1-2 min

Half-life: Short; doses repeated in 3-5 min

Metabolism: Sympathetic nerve endings, liver, tissues

Excretion: Urine

CONTRAINDICATIONS AND PRECAUTIONS

• There are no absolute contraindications to the use of epinephrine in life-threatening situations

• Contraindicated with hypersensitivity to epinephrine or any component, shock (except anaphylaxis), narrow-angle glaucoma, organic brain damage, cerebral arteriosclerosis, general anesthesia with halogenated hydrocarbons, cardiac arrhythmia, acute coronary disease, cardiac dilatation; in conjunction with local anesthetics in fingers, toes, ears, nose, genitalia (vasoconstriction can cause necrosis of these tissues); labor (delays the second stages)

• Use cautiously with hypertension hyperthyroidism, diabetes, cardiovascular disease, sensitivity to sympathomimetics, asthma, emphysema, psychoneurotic disorders, sulfite sensitivity, thyrotoxicosis, infants and children, elderly, lactation

INTERACTIONS

Drug

• Increased risk of arrhythmias or cardiac irritability with halogenated inhalational anesthetics; digitalis, mercurial diuretics

• Antagonism of cardiac and bronchodilating effects of epinephrine with β blockers

• Antagonized vasoconstriction and hypertension with α blockers

• Increased risk of fluorocarbon toxicity with multiple inhalers; wait 5 minutes between inhalers

• Increased adverse cardiac effects of epinephrine possible with tricyclic antidepressants, cocaine, antihistamines, thyroid hormones

• Severe hypertension possible with oxytocics or ergot alkaloids

• Additive effects and toxicity with other sympathomimetics

Lab

• Increased serum lactic acid, BG, BUN

• Altered urinary catecholamines

INCOMPATIBILITIES

• Do not mix with alkalies, halogens, permanganates, chromates, nitrates

SIDE EFFECTS

CNS: Anxiety, headache, restlessness, tremor, dizziness, nervousness, insomnia

CV: Tachycardia, hypotension, palpitations, syncope, hypertension, angina, vasoconstriction, pulmonary edema, ECG changes, arrhythmias, chest pain

DERM: Pallor, sweating; necrosis at injection site with repeated injections; contact dermatitis

EENT: Eye discomfort, transient stinging, burning, irritation; tear-

---

ing, vision disturbances (ophthal preparations); rebound nasal congestion, burning, stinging, dryness, sneezing (nasal preparations); dry mouth or throat (inhaled preparations)
GI: Nausea, vomiting
GU: Difficulty with urination, retention
RESP: Dyspnea, rebound bronchospasm, respiratory weakness, apnea
Other: Altered state of perception and thought, psychosis

TOXICITY AND OVERDOSE
Clinical signs: Increased systolic and diastolic B/P, rise in venous pressure, severe anxiety, hallucinations, mood changes, irregular heartbeat, chest pain or pressure, severe nausea or vomiting, severe headache, severe respiratory distress, dizziness, unusually large pupils, pale or cold skin, pulmonary edema, metabolic acidosis, renal failure, seizure
Treatment: Symptomatic and supportive measures are indicated because epinephrine is rapidly inactivated in the body; monitor VS closely; β blockers may be indicated for arrhythmias, or trimethaphan or phentolamine for hypotension

PATIENT CARE MANAGEMENT
Assessment
• Assess history of hypersensitivity to epinephrine, related drugs
• Assess VS; respiratory status, ECG, PCO_2, $NaHCO_3$, pH, CVP, urine output
• Assess medical, medication, allergy history
Interventions
• See Chapter 3 for discussion of the use of nebulizers or inhalers
• Start treatment at first sign of bronchospasm; administer fewest number of inhalations to provide relief; allow 1-2 min to elapse before additional inhalations
• Alternate inhal with other adrenergics if necessary; do not administer simultaneously with isoproterenol

• Offer oral hygiene, sips of fluids to prevent dry, irritated throat or mouth
• Pt should be in upright position for administration
• Keep spray away from eyes
• Remove contact lenses before eye drops are instilled
• Miotic eye drops (if prescribed) should be administered 2-10 min before epinephrine eye drops
• Instruct pt to apply gentle finger pressure against nasolacrimal duct immediately after drug is instilled for 1-2 min
• Instill nose drops with pt's head in lateral, head low position to prevent entry of drug into throat
• Do not remove IM ampules or syringes from carton until ready to use
• Before drawing susp into syringe, shake vial or ampule to disperse particles, inject promptly; do not use sol if discolored or contains a precipitate
• TB syringe may most accurately measure parenteral doses
• After SC or IM injection, massage site if needed to hasten absorption
• Rotate injection sites to prevent tissue necrosis
• Avoid IM injection to buttocks
• When IV route is used, monitor B/P repeatedly during first 5 min, then every 3-5 min until stable
• Correct fluid depletion before administration if used as a pressor agent
• Tolerance may develop after prolonged use
• Bradycardia, tachycardia, arrhythmias, myocardial ischemia, syncope, weakness, renal failure, and hypertension have occurred with IV administration
• Central route is preferred, or secured peripheral catheter; extravasation causes tissue necrosis
• Maintain age-appropriate fluid balance
• Check preparation, concentration dilution, dosage, and route carefully before administration

NURSING ALERT
Extravasation may cause local ischemia, tissue necrosis; monitor IV site closely

Check concentration or dilution, dosage, route carefully before administration

Inadvertent IV injection may result in cerebral hemorrhage

If administered IM do not inject into buttock

Evaluation
• Evaluate therapeutic response based on indication
• Evaluate VS, ECG, PCO_2, $NaHCO_3$ pH, CVP, urine I&O; monitor B/P closely for first 5 min after IV administration then q 3-5 min until stable
• Evaluate respiratory status
• Evaluate BG for diabetic pts
• Evaluate injection site for blanching or extravasation
• Evaluate with cardiac monitor with IV epinephrine; keep resuscitation equipment available
• Evaluate amount, color, consistency of sputum; respiratory effort
• Evaluate for signs of systemic absorption (nasal, conjunctival routes)
• Evaluate for rebound bronchospasm (inhaled routes)

PATIENT AND FAMILY EDUCATION
Teach/instruct
• About use of nebulizer or inhaler; proper techniques for instillation of eye, nasal drops; proper injection technique, specific indications
• About how to facilitate expectoration after inhaler
• To rinse mouth, gargle after after use of inhaler
• To use inhaler at first sign of bronchospasm
• To allow 1-2 min between inhalations
• To maintain age-appropriate fluid balance

Warn/advise
• About risks of excessive use of inhaler (cardiac arrest, rebound bronchospasm, decreased effect); advise to use only as often as prescribed
• To call provider if pt requires more than 3 treatments with inhaler in 24 hr, or if dizziness, chest pain, or lack of therapeutic response to usual dose occurs
• To keep spray away from eyes
• To avoid other adrenergic drugs unless prescribed
• Not to inject IM into buttocks
• If administered SC, aspirate before injecting to ensure that needle is not in vein
• About transient stinging, headache, browache, which usually subside with continued use of ophthal form
• To report persistent ophthal side effects
• To administer ophthal at hs or after prescribed miotic to minimize blurred vision, sensitivity to light
• That slight stinging may occur with intranasal drops
• That rebound congestion may occur; to report persistent or worsening symptoms
• That rinsing nose dropper or spray tip with hot water after use avoids contamination of sol

STORAGE
• Store susp under refrigeration, do not freeze, do not expose to temp above 30° C (86° F)
• Store other forms at controlled room temp, protect sol from light, freezing, and heat
• Keep out of reach of children

epoetin alfa
Brand Name(s): Epogen, Eprex, Eprex Sterile Solution✤, Erythropoietin, Procrit
Classification: Antianemic
Pregnancy Category: C

AVAILABLE PREPARATIONS
Inj: 2000 U/ml, 4000 U/ml, 10,000 U/ml

ROUTES AND DOSAGES
Renal Dysfunction
Initiation, pts on dialysis, IV 3 ×/wk 50-100 U/kg; not on dialysis, IV/SC 3 ×/wk 50-100 U/kg; increase dosage if Hct does not increase 5-6 points in 8 wks; decrease if Hct increases >4 points/2 wk; goal is to maintain Hct at 30%-33%; general maintenance dosage is 25 U/kg 3 ×/wk

Cancer Chemotherapy or AZT-Treated Patients
IV/SC initial 100 U/kg/dose 3 ×/wk for 8 wk; adjust in 50-100 U/kg increments, 3 ×/wk to maximum of 300 U/kg 3 ×/wk; Hct not exceed 40%

Anemia of Prematurity
SC 25-100 U/kg/dose 3 ×/wk

IV administration
• Recommended concentration: Dilute with equal volume of NS
• IV push rate: Over 1-3 min
• May be administered into venous line at end of dialysis

MECHANISM AND INDICATIONS
Mechanism: Glycoprotein that stimulates the division and differentiation of committed erythroid progenitors in bone marrow; releases reticulocytes from the marrow into bloodstream where they mature into erythrocytes
Indications: Treatment of anemia for pts with chronic renal failure, those on dialysis and those who do not require regular dialysis; used to elevate or maintain RBC level and decrease need for transfusions; antianemic for cancer chemotherapy and AZT-treated HIV pts; anemia of prematurity

PHARMACOKINETICS
Peak: 5-24 hr after SC infusion, immediate after IV infusion
Half-life: 4-13 hr for chronic renal failure; 20% less in pts with normal renal function
Excretion: Urine

CONTRAINDICATIONS AND PRECAUTIONS
• Contraindicated with sensitivity to human albumin, uncontrolled hypertension, neutropenia of newborns, pregnancy, lactation
• Use cautiously with porphyria

INCOMPATIBILITIES
• Should not be mixed with other drugs during administration

SIDE EFFECTS
CNS: Fatigue, dizziness, headache, seizures
CV: Hypertension, edema, chest pain
DERM: Rash
GI: Nausea, vomiting, diarrhea, abdominal cramps
HEME: Clotting with thrombi formation; iron deficiency anemia; polycythemia, elevated platelet count
GU: Pelvic pain
Other: Arthralgia, pyrexia, chills, diaphoresis, clotting of AV fistula

TOXICITY AND OVERDOSE
Clinical signs: Hypertension, seizures, thrombotic events
Treatment: Reduce dosage or discontinue, supportive care

PATIENT CARE MANAGEMENT
Assessment
• Assess history of hypersensitivity to epoetin alfa and related drugs
• Assess baseline VS
• Assess baseline erythropoietin and Hct, platelet count
• Assess pre-therapy iron status; assess iron stores, including transferrin saturation and serum ferritin; transferrin should be at least 20%, ferritin at least 100 ng/ml; supplemental iron may be needed to support erythropoiesis
• Assess history of previous treatment with special attention to other therapies that may predispose patient to cardiac dysfunction
• Assess baseline neurologic or mental status before drug administration

---

Interventions
• May be administered into venous line at the end of dialysis to decrease need for additional access; can also be administered IV or SC for pts with chronic renal failure not on dialysis
• Rotate injection sites
• Because of the length of time for erythropoiesis, an increase in Hct may not be seen for 2-6 wk
• Increase or decrease medication depending on Hct response over time; reduce dosage if response is >4 points in any 2 wk period; maintenance dosage must be individualized; rate of increase in Hct is dependent on dosage rate, availability of iron stores, baseline Hct and concurrent health issues
• When Hct reaches normal levels, achieve maintenance dosage to avoid exceeding target range
• B/P should be adequately controlled; may need dietary restrictions or drug therapy to control B/P
• Administer supplemental iron as needed
• Do not shake vial (may denature the drug)
• Provide supportive measures to maintain homeostasis and nutritional status

NURSING ALERT
Therapy can result in polycythemia if Hct is not carefully monitored and dosage adjusted appropriately

Monitor B/P carefully; diet restrictions or drug therapy may be needed to control B/P

Evaluation
• Evaluate therapeutic response (increase in Hct)
• Check Hct regularly, adjust medication as needed
• Monitor B/P, serum iron stores
• Monitor renal function (BUN, creatinine, I&O), fluid balance, electrolyte status
• Monitor for signs of excessive clotting

• Monitor cardiac function
• Monitor for signs, symptoms of infection

PATIENT AND FAMILY EDUCATION
Teach/instruct
• To take as directed at prescribed intervals for prescribed length of time; follow dose administration guidelines precisely to avoid reaching the target Hct too quickly or exceeding the target
• About the importance of follow-up to monitor blood values
• About the need to take supplemental iron
Warn/advise
• To notify care provider of hypersensitivity, side effects
• That responsiveness may decrease with concurrent illness or inflammatory process
• That weekly blood values will be checked and that dosage needs to be based on individual erythropoietin response of Hct levels
• To avoid hazardous activities such as contact sports
• That patient may feel pain or discomfort, coldness or sweating in limbs, pelvis; symptoms may persist for up to 12 hr and then disappear

STORAGE
• Store in refrigerator
• Protect from direct light
• Do not shake vial

---

ergocalciferol
Brand Name(s): Calciferol, Deltalin Gelseals, Drisdol, Ostoforte✢, Vitamin D Capsules

Classification: Vitamin, antihypocalcemic

Pregnancy Category: C

AVAILABLE PREPARATIONS
Liquid: 200 mcg/ml (8000 IU/ml)
Caps: 0.625 mg (25,000 IU), 1.25 mg (50,000 IU)
Tabs: 1.25 mg (50,000 IU)
Inj: 12.5 mg (500,000 IU)/ml

✢ Available in Canada.

ROUTES AND DOSAGES

PO route preferred; IM used only when disease is associated with malabsorption of vitamin D

Dietary Supplementation

Preterm infants: 10-20 mcg/24 hr (400-800 IU)

Infants, children, and adults: 10 mcg/24 hr (400 IU)

Hypoparathyroidism

Children: 1.25-5 mg/24 hr (50,000-200,000 IU) with Ca supplements

Adults: 625 mcg-5 mg/24 hr (25,000-200,000 IU) with Ca supplements

Vitamin D-Dependent Rickets

Children: 75-125 mcg/24 hr (3000-5000 IU); maximum 1500 mcg/24 hr

Adults: 250 mcg-1.5 mg/24 hr (10,000-60,000 IU)

Nutritional Rickets and Osteomalacia

Children and adults (with normal absorption): 25-125 mcg/24 hr (1000-5000 IU)

Children with malabsorption: 250-625 mcg/24 hr (10,000-25,000 IU)

Adults with malabsorption: 250-7500 mcg/24 hr (10,000-300,000 IU)

MECHANISM AND INDICATIONS

Antihypocalcemic: Regulates Ca absorption from GI tract and bone resorption

Indications: Nutritional rickets, osteomalacia, familial hypophosphatemia, vitamin D-dependent rickets, hypoparathyroidism, pseudohypoparathyroidism

PHARMACOKINETICS

Onset of action: 10-24 hr

Half-life: 24 hr

Metabolism: Liver, kidneys

Excretion: Feces

CONTRAINDICATIONS AND PRECAUTIONS

• Contraindicated with hypercalcemia, vitamin D toxicity, malabsorption syndrome, abnormal sensitivity to vitamin D effects

• Use cautiously with impaired renal function, heart disease, renal stones, arteriosclerosis, cardiac glycosides, pregnancy, lactation, infants (may be hyperreactive)

INTERACTIONS

Drug

• Use with cardiac glycosides may cause arrhythmias

• Thiazide diuretics can cause hypercalcemia in pts with hypoparathyroidism

• Mg antacids can cause hypermagnesemia

• Verapamil can cause atrial fibrillation with hypercalcemia

• Decreased effects with corticosteroids

• Increased metabolism to inactive metabolites with phenytoin, phenobarbital

• Interference with absorption with cholestyramine, colestipol, mineral oil

Lab

• Elevated AST, ALT

• Falsely elevated cholesterol

INCOMPATIBILITIES

None reported

SIDE EFFECTS

• Generally seen with vitamin D toxicity only

CNS: Headache, fatigue, mood changes, seizures

CV: Hypertension, arrhythmias

DERM: Pruritus, calcification of soft tissues

EENT: Dry mouth, metallic taste, rhinorrhea, calcific conjunctivitis, photophobia, tinnitus

GI: Constipation, anorexia, nausea, vomiting, diarrhea, abdominal pain

GU: Renal stones, polyuria, albuminuria, hypercalciuria, impaired renal function

Other: Hypercalcemia, hyperphosphatemia, bone and muscle pain, bone demineralization

TOXICITY AND OVERDOSE

Clinical signs: Hypercalcemia, hyperphosphatemia, hypercalciuria

Treatment: Stop therapy, low Ca diet, increased fluid intake; loop diuretics with saline infusion can be used to increase Ca excretion;

✦ Available in Canada.

calcitonin may decrease hypercalcemia

PATIENT CARE MANAGEMENT
Assessment
• Assess history of hypersensitivity to ergocalciferol
• Assess baseline Ca and PO_4 as indicated by diagnosis
Interventions
• Tab should be swallowed whole, not crushed or chewed
• Inject IM deeply, slowly; rotate injection sites
• Provide PO_4 restriction and binding agents for pts with hyperphosphatemia to decrease risk of renal stones and calcifications
Evaluation
• Evaluate therapeutic response (Ca and PO_4 within target range)
• Monitor serum and urine Ca, K^+, urea
• Monitor for signs of toxicity (dry mouth, nausea, vomiting, metallic taste, constipation)

PATIENT AND FAMILY EDUCATION
Teach/instruct
• To take as directed at prescribed intervals for prescribed length of time
Warn/advise
• To notify care provider of hypersensitivity, side effects
• To restrict use of Mg-containing antacids
• Not to increase dosage without consulting with provider
Encourage
• High Ca diet

STORAGE
• Store at room temperature in light resistant container

---

ergotamine tartrate
Brand Names(s): Cafergot, Ercaf, Ergomar✤, Ergostat, Medihaler-Ergotamine
Classification: Vasoconstrictor
Pregnancy Category: X

AVAILABLE PREPARATIONS
Tab: 2 mg SL
Aerosol inh: 360 mcg/metered spray

ROUTES AND DOSAGES
Older children and adolescents: PO/SL 1 mg may repeat q 30 min to maximum of 3 mg/attack
Adults: PO/SL 2 mg, then 1-2 mg SL q 30 min; 6 mg maximum/24 hr; do not exceed 10 mg/wk
Inhal: One puff, may repeat q 5 min; maximum 6 inhalations/24 hr or 15 inhalations/wk

MECHANISM AND INDICATIONS
Mechanism: Stimulates vascular smooth muscle to vasoconstrict peripheral and cerebral blood vessels
Indications: Prevention or abortion of vascular, migraine, or cluster headaches

PHARMACOKINETICS
Peak: 0.5-3 hr
Absorption: Rapid with inhalation; variable with oral
Metabolism: Liver
Elimination: Bile, feces

CONTRAINDICATIONS AND PRECAUTIONS
• Contraindicated with hypersensitivity, peripheral vascular disease, hypertension, hepatic or renal disease, sepsis, peptic ulcer disease, pregnancy
• Use cautiously with children

INTERACTIONS
Drug
• Increased vasoconstriction with propranolol, other β blockers.
• Increased effects of ergotamine with erythromycin, troleandomycin

---

✤ Available in Canada.

Lab
• None reported

INCOMPATIBILITIES
None reported

SIDE EFFECTS
CV: Numbness or tingling in fingers, toes, tachycardia, bradycardia, arterial spasm, coronary insufficiency, angina-like precordial pain
GI: Nausea, vomiting, diarrhea, abdominal pain, ischemic colitis
MS: Paresthesias of extremities, leg weakness, myalgia, muscle cramps

TOXICITY AND OVERDOSE
Clinical signs: Hypertension, rapid weak pulse, lassitude, impaired mental function, delirium, seizures, shock, unquenchable thirst
Treatment: Emesis or gastric lavage; provide respiratory support, warmth to ischemic extremities, vasodilators, dialysis; administer vasodilators; nitroprusside, tolazoline

PATIENT CARE MANAGEMENT
Assessment
• Assess history of hypersensitivity to drug or caffeine
• Assess VS (especially B/P)
• Assess for coldness, tingling in extremities
• Assess frequency, intensity of headaches
Interventions
• Administer during prodromal stage of headaches for best results; titrate drug to pt response
• Administer PO with food to avoid GI symptoms
• Provide quiet, low-light environment for pt after drug administration
Evaluation
• Evaluate therapeutic response (decrease frequency, severity of headaches)
• Evaluate pt for headache triggers; assist pt in making lifestyle changes

• Evaluate pt for side effects
• Evaluate for signs and symptoms of toxicity (dyspnea, hypotension, hypertension, delirium, rapid or weak pulse, nausea, vomiting)

PATIENT AND FAMILY EDUCATION
Teach/instruct
• To take as directed at prescribed intervals for prescribed length of time
• To report side effects (especially numbness), chest pain, irregular HR
• About how to use inhaler (if necessary)
• Not to give with other prescription or OTC drugs
• That rebound headache may occur when drug withdrawn
• To avoid prolonged exposure to cold temp
Warn/advise
• To avoid alcohol use
• That ergotamine is a vasoconstrictor and may increase response to heat and cold
• To keep record of frequency, duration, and intensity of headaches

STORAGE
• Store at room temperature in light-resistant containers

✤ Available in Canada.

**erythromycin base,
erythromycin estolate,
erythromycin
ethylsuccinate,
erythromycin
gluceptate,
erythromycin
lactobionate,
erythromycin stearate,
erythromycin
(ophthalmic),
erythromycin (topical)**

Brand Name(s): erythromycin base: Apo-Erythro Base✿, Diomycin✿, E-Mycin, Erybid✿, Eryc✿, Erythrocin, Erythromycin Base Filmtabs, Novo-Rythro Encap✿, PMS-Erithromycin, Robimycin, Ethril 500, PCE✿
erythromycin estolate: Ilosone✿
erythromycin ethylsuccinate: Apo-Erythro-ES✿, E.E.S., EES-200✿, EES-400✿, EES-600✿, EryPed, Pediamycin, Wyamycin E
erythromycin gluceptate: Ilotycin Gluceptate, Ilotycin Gluceptate IV✿
erythromycin lactobionate: Erythrocin Lactobionate-IV, Erythromucin IV✿
erythromycin stearate: Apo-Erythro-S✿, Eramycin, Erypar, Ethril, Erythrocin Stearate, Nu-Erythromycin-S✿, SK-Erythromycin, Wyamycin S
erythromycin (ophthalmic): AK-Mycin, Erythromycin, Ilotycin
erythromycin (topical): Akne-Mycin, A/T/S, Erycette, Eryderm, Erymax, Staticin, T-Stat

Classification: Antibiotic (macrolide)

Pregnancy Category: B

AVAILABLE PREPARATIONS
Oral susp: 100 mg/5 ml, 125 mg/5 ml, 200 mg/5 ml, 250 mg/5 ml, 400 mg/5 ml
Tabs (chewable): 125 mg, 200 mg, 250 mg
Tabs: 500 mg
Tabs (film-coated): 250 mg, 400 mg, 500 mg
Tabs (ext-rel): 250 mg, 333 mg, 500 mg
Caps: 250 mg
Caps (ext-rel): 125 mg, 250 mg
Inj: 250 mg, 500 mg, 1 g
Ophthal oint: 0.5%
Top: 1.5%, 2% sol, 2% oint, 2% gel, 2% pledgets

ROUTES AND DOSAGES
Neonates 1-7 days, <1200 g: PO 20 mg/kg/24 hr divided q12h
Neonates 1-7 days, >1200 g: PO 20 mg/kg/24 hr divided q12h
Neonates >7 days, >1200 g: PO 30 mg/kg/24 hr divided q8h
Children: PO 30-50 mg/kg/24 hr divided q6-8h; maximum dose 2 g/24 hr; IV 15-20 mg/kg/24 hr divided q6h; top, apply to affected area bid
Adults: PO 1-4 g/24 hr divided q6h; maximum dose 4 g/24 hr; IV 15-20 mg/kg/24 hr divided q6h; top, apply to affected area bid
Bacterial Endocarditis Prophylaxis
Children and adults: PO 20 mg/kg (maximum 800 mg ethylsuccinate, 1.0 g stearate) 2 hr before procedure, then ½ of initial dose 6 hr after initial dose
Neonatal Gonococcal Ophthalmia Prophylaxis
Ophthal 0.5-2.0 cm oint strip instilled into conjunctival sac within 1 hr after delivery
Ophthalmic Infections
Ophthal 0.2-2.0 cm oint strip instilled into conjunctival sac bid-qid
Top
Apply to affected area bid.
IV administration (erythromycin gluceptate/lactobionate)
• Recommended concentration: 1-2.5 mg/ml

- Maximum concentration: 5 mg/ml
- IV push rate: Not recommended
- Intermittent infusion rate: Over 20-60 min
- Continuous infusion: To minimize vein irritation, slow continuous infusion of ≤1 mg/ml is recommended

MECHANISM AND INDICATIONS

Antibiotic mechanism: Binds to ribosome's 50S subunit, thus inhibiting bacterial protein synthesis

Indications: Effective against *Haemophilus influenzae, Entamoeba histolytica, Mycoplasma pneumoniae, Corynebacterium diptheriae, Legionella pneumophila,* and *Bordetella pertussis;* may be used as an alternative to penicillins and tetracyclines in treatment of *Streptococcus pneumoniae, Str. viridans, Listeria monocytogenes, Staphylococcus aureus, Chlamydia trachomatis, Neisseria gonorrhoeae, Treponema pallidum;* used to treat infections of lower and upper respiratory tract, otitis media, skin, soft tissue, and Lyme disease; ophthal oint used for prophylaxis of ophthalmia neonatorum and neonatal conjunctivitis and for ocular infections; top forms used to treat acne vulgaris, superficial skin infections

PHARMACOKINETICS

Peak: PO 1-2 hr; IV at end of infusion

Distribution: Into body tissues, fluids; poor penetration into CSF; concentrates in liver

Half-life: 1-1.5 hr

Metabolism: Liver

Excretion: Bile, urine

CONTRAINDICATIONS AND PRECAUTIONS

- Contraindicated with known hypersensitivity to erythromycin, hepatic disease
- Use cautiously with preexisting hepatic diseases, pregnancy, lactation

INTERACTIONS

Drug

- Increased action and potential toxicity of theophylline, warfarin, digoxin, carbamazepine, cyclosporine
- Decreased action of clindamycin, penicillins
- Increased irritation with use of topical desquamating or abrasive acne preparations (top)

Lab

- Falsely elevated ALT, AST, urinary catecholamines, steroids

Nutrition

- Decreased absorption if given with food, acidic fruit juices, citrus fruits, acidic beverages such as cola drinks (erythromycin base and stearate)

Incompatibilities

- Do not mix in sol or syringe with amikacin, aminophylline, vitamin C, carbenicillin, cephalothin, cephapirin, chloramphenicol, colistimethate, heparin, lincomycin, metaraminol, metoclopramide, pentobarbital, phenobarbital, phenytoin, prochlorperazine, secobarbital, Na salts, tetracycline, thiopental, vancomycin, vitamin B complex with C, warfarin

SIDE EFFECTS

DERM: Urticaria, rashes, erythema, burning, dryness, pruritus

EENT: Eye irritation (top), hearing loss (high IV dosages, especially in pts with renal failure)

GI: Abdominal pain, nausea, vomiting, diarrhea, cholestatic jaundice (estolate)

Local: Venous irritation, thrombophlebitis (IV)

Other: Anaphylaxis, fever, sensitivity reaction (top), bacterial or fungal superinfection

PATIENT CARE MANAGEMENT

Assessment

- Assess history of hypersensitivity to erythromycin
- Obtain C&S; may begin therapy before obtaining results
- Assess renal function (BUN, creatinine, I&O), hepatic function

---

LT, AST, bilirubin), bowel pattern
• Assess eye and skin for redness, drainage, swelling
Interventions
• Administer PO erythromycin base and stearate 1 hr ac or 2 hr after meals; estolate without regard to meals; ethylsuccinate 1 hr ac or 2 hr after meals in pts <2 yr; without regard to meals ≥2 yr
• Shake susp well
• Regular tabs can be crushed, caps taken apart and mixed with food-fluid; film-coated or enteric-coated tablets must be swallowed whole; ext rel caps can be taken apart; do not chew particles; provide water to ensure particles are swallowed; chewable tablets must be chewed
• Do not premix IV with other medications; infuse separately
• Use large vein with small-bore needle to reduce local reaction; rotate site q48-72h
• Unstable in acid sol (pH <5.5); NaHCO$_3$ buffer may be needed if pH <5.5
• See Chapter 2 for instructions on ophthal instillation; when using for ophthalmia neonatorum prophylaxis, wipe away excess medication; do not flush from eye; use single unit or new tube for each neonate
• Wash hands before, after top application
• Cleanse skin; apply thin film to affected area
• Maintain age-appropriate fluid intake
• For group A β-hemolytic streptococcal infection, provide 10-day course to prevent risk of acute rheumatic fever or glomerulonephritis

NURSING ALERT
Discontinue drug if signs of hypersensitivity reaction develop
Do not administer IV push

Evaluation
• Evaluate therapeutic response (decreased symptoms of infection)
• Observe for signs of allergic reaction (rash, pruritus, dyspnea, bronchospasm)
• Monitor bowel pattern
• Monitor renal function (BUN, creatinine, I&O), hepatic function (ALT, AST, bilirubin), hematologic function (CBC, differential, platelet count)
• Monitor for signs of hearing loss during and up to 3 wk after use of stearate, ethylsuccinate, lactobionate
• Observe for signs of superinfection (perineal itching, diaper rash, fever, malaise, redness, pain, swelling, drainage, rash, diarrhea, sore throat, change in cough or sputum)
• Monitor IV sites for irritation or thrombophlebitis; replace IV route with oral therapy as soon as possible to minimize discomfort

PATIENT AND FAMILY EDUCATION
Teach/instruct
• To take as directed at prescribed intervals for prescribed length of time
Warn/advise
• To notify care provider of hypersensitivity, side effects, superinfection
• Not to share towels, wash clothes, linens, eye make-up with family member being treated with ophthal forms
STORAGE
• Store tabs, caps, ophth, and top at room temp
• Store susp and reconstituted sol according to manufacturer's recommendation

erythromycin and sulfisoxazole

Brand Names(s): Eryzole, Pediazole✤

Classification: Antibiotic (macrolide and sulfonamide derivative combination)

Pregnancy Category: C

AVAILABLE PREPARATIONS
Oral susp: 200 mg erythromycin ethylsuccinate, 600 mg sulfisoxazole acetyl/5 ml

ROUTES AND DOSAGES
Infants >2 mo and children: PO 50 mg erythromycin/150 mg sulfisoxazole/kg/24 hr divided q6h; maximum dose 2 g erythromycin or 6 g sulfisoxazole/24 hr
Adults: PO 400 mg erythromycin/ 1200 mg sulfisoxazole q6h

MECHANISM AND INDICATIONS
Antibiotic mechanism: Erythromycin binds to ribosome's 50S subunit, thus inhibiting bacterial protein synthesis; sulfisoxazole prevents bacterial cell wall synthesis of essential nucleic acids by inhibiting the formation of dihydrofolic acid from paraaminobenzoic acid (PABA)
Indications: Effective against *Haemophilus influenzae, Streptococcus, Staphylococcus, Chlamydia trachomatis;* used to treat upper and lower respiratory tract infections and otitis media

PHARMACOKINETICS
Peak: Erythromycin 1-2 hr; sulfisoxazole 2-4 hr
Distribution: Erythromycin concentrates in liver; sulfisoxazole into intracellular space, crosses blood–brain barrier
Half-life: Erythromycin 1-1.5 hr; sulfisoxazole 6 hr
Metabolism: Liver
Excretion: Erythromycin, bile, urine; sulfisoxazole, urine

CONTRAINDICATIONS AND PRECAUTIONS
• Contraindicated with infants <2 mo, known hypersensitivity to erythromycin, sulfisoxazole, sulfonamides, drugs containing sulfur; with hepatic impairment, porphyria, concomitant astemizole or terfenadine
• Use cautiously with impaired renal or hepatic function, pregnancy, lactation

INTERACTIONS
Drug
• Increased action and potential toxicity of theophylline, warfarin, carbamazepine, cyclosporine with erythromycin
• Decreased action of clindamycin, penicillins with erythromycin
• Increased anticoagulant effect with use of oral anticoagulants and sulfisoxazole
• Increased hypoglycemic response with use of sulfonylurea agents, sulfisoxazole
• Decreased renal excretion of methotrexate with sulfisoxazole
• Decreased hepatic clearance of phenytoin with sulfisoxazole
• Decreased effectiveness of oral contraceptives with sulfisoxazole
• Synergistic antibacterial effects with use of trimethoprim or pyrimethamine and sulfisoxazole
• Decreased antibacterial effectiveness with use of PABA derivatives and sulfisoxazole
• Increased risk of crystalluria with use of urine acidifying agents and sulfisoxazole
Lab
• Falsely elevated ALT, AST, urinary catecholamines, steroids with erythromycin
Nutrition
• Decreased absorption if given with food

SIDE EFFECTS
CNS: Headache, dizziness
DERM: Rash, photosensitivity, Stevens-Johnson syndrome, toxic epidermal necrolysis
GI: Nausea, vomiting, diarrhea, abdominal pain, hepatic necrosis
GU: Toxic nephrosis, crystalluria

✤ Available in Canada.

HEME: Agranulocytosis, aplastic anemia
Other: Hypersensitivity, anaphylaxis, fever, bacterial or fungal superinfection

TOXICITY AND OVERDOSE
Clinical signs: Sulfisoxazole may cause nausea, vomiting, dizziness, headache, drowsiness, unconsciousness
Treatment: If ingested within 4 hrs, perform gastric lavage, followed by correction of acidosis, forced fluids, urinary alkalinization to increase excretion; supportive care

PATIENT CARE MANAGEMENT
Assessment
• Assess history of hypersensitivity to erythromycin, sulfonamides, any drug containing sulfur
• Obtain C&S; may begin therapy before obtaining results
• Assess renal function (BUN, creatinine, I&O), hepatic function (ALT, AST, bilirubin), hematologic function (CBC, differential, platelet count), bowel pattern
Interventions
• May be administered PO without regard to meals; give with a full glass of water; shake susp well before administering
• Maintain age-appropriate fluid intake

NURSING ALERT
Discontinue drug if signs of toxicity, hypersensitivity, blood dyscrasias, crystalluria, renal abnormalities develop

---

Evaluation
• Evaluate therapeutic response (decreased symptoms of infection)
• Evaluate renal function (BUN, creatinine, I&O), hepatic function (ALT, AST, bilirubin), hematologic function (CBC, differential, platelet count)
• Monitor bowel pattern
• Observe for allergic reaction (rash, pruritus, dyspnea, bronchospasm)

• Monitor signs of hearing loss during and up to 3 wk after therapy
• Observe for signs of superinfection (perineal itching, diaper rash, fever, malaise, redness, pain, swelling, drainage, rash, diarrhea, sore throat, change in cough or sputum)

PATIENT AND FAMILY EDUCATION
Teach/instruct
• To take as directed at prescribed intervals for prescribed length of time
Warn/advise
• To notify care provider of hypersensitivity, side effects, superinfection
• To use alternate method of contraception if using oral contraceptives
• To avoid OTC medications (particularly aspirin, vitamin C) unless directed by care provider
• To avoid direct sunlight exposure

STORAGE
• Store granules at room temp
• Reconstituted susp stable refrigerated for 14 days; label date and time of reconstitution

---

esmolol hydrochloride
Brand Names(s): Brevibloc✤
Classification: β-blocker, antiarrhythmic; antihypertensive
Pregnancy Category: C

AVAILABLE PREPARATIONS
Inj: 10 mg/ml in 10 ml vial; 250 mg/ml ampule

ROUTES AND DOSAGES
Children and adults: IV loading dose 500 mcg/kg/min × 1 min; maintenance 50 mcg/kg/min × 4 min, may repeat q 5 min, increasing maintenance by 50 mcg/kg/min; maximum dose 200 mcg/kg/min

---

✤ Available in Canada.

IV administratión
- Recommended concentration: 10 mg/ml
- Maximum concentration: 10 mg/ml
- Continuous infusion rate: 50-200 mcg/kg/min

MECHANISM AND INDICATIONS
β-*blocker mechanism:* Blocks stimulation of β_1-adrenergic receptors in myocardium, thereby decreasing rate of SA node discharge; increases recovery time; slows conduction of AV node; decreases HR; decreases myocardial O_2 consumption; may decrease renin–aldosterone–angiotensin system at high dosages; inhibits β_2 receptors in bronchial system

Indications: Short-term management of supraventricular tachycardia, noncompensatory sinus tachycardia, atrial flutter, atrial fibrillation; perioperative and postoperative hypertension

PHARMACOKINETICS
Onset of action: Immediate
Peak: 1 min
Half-life: 9 min
Metabolism: Hydrolysis of ester linkage
Excretion: Urine

CONTRAINDICATIONS AND PRECAUTIONS
- Contraindicated with known hypersensitivity, sinus bradycardia, 2nd- or 3rd-degree heart block, cardiogenic shock, cardiac failure
- Use cautiously with hypotension, peripheral vascular disease, diabetes, hypoglycemia, thyrotoxicosis, renal disease

INTERACTIONS
Drug
- Increased digoxin levels with digoxin
- Increased effects of lidocaine, disopyramide
- Increased esmolol levels and effects with morphine, disopyramide
- Reversal of esmolol effects with isoproterenol, norepinephrine, dopamine, dobutamine

Lab
- Interferes with glucose/insulin tolerance test

INCOMPATIBILITIES
Furosemide, $NaHCO_3$

SIDE EFFECTS
CNS: Dizziness, somnolence, confusion, headache, agitation, fatigue, paresthesias, depression, abnormal thinking, anxiety, lightheadedness
CV: Hypotension, diaphoresis, pallor, flushing, chest pain, bradycardia, syncope, pulmonary edema, heart block, peripheral ischemia, CHF, conduction disturbances
DERM: Induration and inflammation at infusion site, edema, erythema, discoloration, thrombophlebitis, rash, pruritis, dry skin, alopecia
EENT: Speech disorder, blurred vision
GI: Nausea, vomiting, anorexia, constipation, dry mouth, taste aversion, gastric pain, flatulence, heartburn, bloating
GU: Urinary retention, impotence, dysuria
RESP: Bronchospasm, dyspnea, cough, wheeziness, nasal stuffiness

TOXICITY AND OVERDOSE
Clinical signs: Hypotension, bradycardia, drowsiness, LOC
Treatment: Discontinue medication, administer atropine or other anticholinergic, intravenous β_2-stimulating agent or theophylline; administer fluids, pressor agents, dopamine, dobutamine, isoproteronol, or amrinone

PATIENT CARE MANAGEMENT
Assessment
- Assess history of hypersensitivity to drug
- Assess baseline VS, apical and radial pulse before administration
- Obtain baseline labs (BUN, creatinine, ALT, AST)

Interventions
- Dilute 2.5 g ampule before IV injection

✤ Available in Canada.

Evaluation
• Evaluate therapeutic response (immediate decrease in B/P)
• Evaluate labs (BUN, creatinine, ALT, AST, electrolytes)
• Evaluate hydration, respiratory status

PATIENT AND FAMILY EDUCATION
Teach/instruct
• About need for medication
Warn/advise
• Notify care provider of hypersensitivity, side effects
Provide
• Emotional support as indicated

STORAGE
• Store in cool environment in a tightly sealed, light-resistant container

---

ethacrynate sodium, ethacrynic acid
Brand Names(s): Edecrin, Sodium Edecrin ✤

Classification: Loop diuretic

Pregnancy Category: D

AVAILABLE PREPARATIONS
Tabs: 25 mg, 50 mg
Inj: 50 mg

ROUTES AND DOSAGES
Children: PO 1 mg/kg/dose qd, increase q 2-3 days to maximum of 3 mg/kg/24 hr as needed IV; 0.5-1 mg/kg/dose, repeat with caution q8-12 hr as needed
Adults: PO 50-400 mg/24 hr in 1-2 divided doses; IV 0.5-1 mg/kg/dose (maximum of 100 mg/dose), repeat with caution q8-12 hr as needed
IV administration
• Recommended concentration: Dilute with 50 ml NS or D_5W for 1 mg/ml
• IV push rate: ≤10 mg/min
• Intermittent infusion rate: Over 30 min

MECHANISM AND INDICATIONS
Mechanism: Inhibits reabsorption of Na, Ca in the loop of Henle and renal tubule causing increased excretion of water, Na, Cl, Mg, Ca
Indications: For use in pulmonary edema, edema in CHF, hepatic or renal disease

PHARMACOKINETICS
Onset of action: PO <30 min; IV 5 min
Peak: PO 2 hr; IV 30 min
Duration: PO 6-8 hr; IV 2 hr
Metabolism: Liver
Excretion: Bile, urine

CONTRAINDICATIONS AND PRECAUTIONS
• Contraindicated with hypersensitivity, hypotension, anuria, hyponatremic dehydration, metabolic alkalosis with hypokalemia
• Use cautiously with renal dysfunction, liver dysfunction, diabetes, cardiac glycosides (digoxin)

INTERACTIONS
Drug
• Increased hypotension with antihypertensives
• Increased ototoxicity with aminoglycosides
• Increased diuretic effects with other diuretics
• Decreased K^+ loss with K^+-sparing diuretics
Lab
• Altered electrolyte balance, liver function (AST, ALT, bilirubin), renal function (BUN, creatinine)

INCOMPATIBILITIES
• Hydralazine, procainamide, reserpine, tolazoline, blood, blood products

SIDE EFFECTS
CNS: Vertigo, headache, fatigue, weakness
CV: Circulatory volume depletion, dehydration, hypotension
DERM: Dermatitis, Stevens-Johnson syndrome
EENT: Transient deafness, ototoxicity, blurred vision, tinnitus
GI: Abdominal discomfort, pain, diarrhea, GI bleeding, acute pancreatitis
GU: Polyuria, renal failure, glycosuria
HEME: Thrombocytopenia, neutropenia, agranulocytosis

✤ Available in Canada.

METAB: Hypochloremic alkalosis, fluid and electrolyte imbalance (hypokalemia, hypocalcemia, hypomagnesemia, hyponatremia, hyperglycemia)

TOXICITY AND OVERDOSE
Clinical signs: Profound electrolyte and volume depletion, circulatory collapse
Treatment: Supportive care, replace fluids and electrolytes

PATIENT CARE MANAGEMENT
Assessment
• Assess history of hypersensitivity to drug
• Assess wt, I&O, B/P lying and standing, HR, respiratory rate
• Assess electrolytes, BUN, CBC, creatinine (baseline and ongoing)
• Assess hearing when administering IV
Interventions
• Administer IV or PO only; do not administer IM or SC
• Administer PO with food
• Have urinal, commode readily available
Evaluation
• Evaluate therapeutic response (decreased edema)
• Monitor serum K^+; provide K^+ supplement prn
• Evaluate signs and symptoms of electrolyte imbalance
• Evaluate risk for falls caused by orthostatic hypotension

PATIENT AND FAMILY EDUCATION
Teach/instruct
• To take as directed at prescribed intervals for prescribed length of time
Warn/advise
• To take in AM to avoid nocturia
• About side effects; report to care provider
• To eat K^+-rich foods
• To comply with drug therapy, follow-up care
• To avoid rapid changes in position

STORAGE
• Store at room temp

---

ethambutol hydrochloride
Brand Name(s): Etibi✤, Myambutol✤
Classification: Antitubercular (semisynthetic antitubercular)
Pregnancy Category: B

AVAILABLE PREPARATIONS
Tabs: 100 mg, 400 mg

ROUTES AND DOSAGES
Children >13 yr and adults: PO 15-25 mg/kg/24 hr qd (maximum dose 2.5 g/24 hr) or 50 mg/kg/dose twice weekly (maximum dose 2.5 g/dose)

MECHANISM AND INDICATIONS
Antitubercular mechanism: Bacteriostatic; inhibits protein metabolism and cell replication by interfering with RNA synthesis
Indications: Effective against *Mycobacterium tuberculosis, M. bovis, M. marinum,* and some strains of *M. kansasii, M. avium, M. fortuitum,* and *M. intracellulare;* used as adjunct therapy in tuberculosis

PHARMACOKINETICS
Peak: 2-4 hr
Distribution: Throughout body; high concentrations in kidneys, lungs, saliva, erythrocytes
Half-life: 2.5-3.5 hr
Metabolism: Liver
Excretion: Urine, feces

CONTRAINDICATIONS AND PRECAUTIONS
• Contraindicated with children <13 yr, known hypersensitivity to ethambutol, optic neuritis
• Use cautiously with renal or hepatic impairment, ocular defects, pregnancy

INTERACTIONS
Drug
• Increased risk of neurotoxicity from neurotoxic medications such as aminoglycosides, penicillins, anticonvulsants

---

✤ Available in Canada.

Lab
- Elevated serum urate levels, liver function tests

SIDE EFFECTS

CNS: Headache, dizziness, confusion, hallucinations, peripheral neuritis

EENT: Optic neuritis, decreased visual acuity, decreased color discrimination

ENDO / METAB: Elevated uric acid levels

GI: Anorexia, nausea, vomiting, abdominal pain, hepatic impairment

Other: Anaphylaxis, fever, malaise, joint pain

TOXICITY AND OVERDOSE

Clinical signs: No information available

Treatment: Supportive care; if ingested within 4 hr, induce emesis or perform gastric lavage followed by activated charcoal

PATIENT CARE MANAGEMENT

Assessment
- Assess history of hypersensitivity to ethambutol
- Obtain C&S; may begin therapy before obtaining results
- Assess hepatic function (ALT, AST, bilirubin), renal function (BUN, creatinine, I&O), hematologic function (CBC, differential, platelet count), ophthal function (visual acuity and color discrimination)

Interventions
- May be administered PO with food to reduce GI distress; tab may be crushed, mixed with food or fluid
- Maintain age-appropriate fluid intake

NURSING ALERT
Discontinue drug if signs of hypersensitivity or significant visual changes occur

Evaluation
- Evaluate therapeutic response (decreased TB symptoms, negative culture)

- Monitor hepatic function (ALT, AST, bilirubin), renal function (BUN, creatinine, I&O), hematologic function (CBC, differential, platelet count), ophthalmologic function (visual acuity, visual fields, red–green discrimination)
- Monitor for hepatic impairment (anorexia, jaundice, dark urine, malaise, fatigue, liver tenderness)
- Monitor CNS toxicity (affect, behavioral changes)

PATIENT AND FAMILY EDUCATION

Teach/instruct
- To take as directed at prescribed intervals for prescribed length of time

Warn/advise
- To notify care provider of hypersensitivity, side effects
- To comply with follow-up care
- To avoid use of alcohol, medications containing alcohol

STORAGE
- Store at room temp
- Protect from light, air

---

ethionamide

Brand Name(s): Trecator-SC

Classification: Antitubercular (isonicotinic acid derivative)

Pregnancy Category: D

AVAILABLE PREPARATIONS

Tabs: 250 mg

ROUTES AND DOSAGES

Children: PO 15-20 mg/kg/24 hr divided bid; maximum dose 1 g/24 hr

Adults: 500-1000 mg/24 hr qd or divided tid

MECHANISM AND INDICATIONS

Antitubercular mechanism: Bacteriostatic or bactericidal; inhibits bacterial peptide synthesis

Indications: Effective against *Mycobacterium tuberculosis, M. bovis, M. kansasii,* and some strains of *M. avium* and *M. intracellulare;*

---

used as adjunct therapy in tuberculosis

PHARMACOKINETICS
Peak: 3 hr
Distribution: Widely into body fluids and tissues
Half-life: 2-3 hr
Metabolism: Liver
Excretion: Urine

CONTRAINDICATIONS AND PRECAUTIONS
• Contraindicated with known hypersensitivity to ethionamide; severe hepatic impairment
• Use cautiously with known hypersensitivity to chemically related medications (such as isoniazid and pyrazinamide); diabetes, pregnancy

INTERACTIONS
Drug
• Increased adverse reactions from concomitant antitubercular medications
• Increased risk of neurotoxicity with use of alcohol, cycloserine
Lab
• Transient elevation of liver function tests
• Decreased serum protein-bound iodine, T_4

SIDE EFFECTS
CNS: Peripheral neuritis, depression, tremors, paresthesias, seizures, dizziness
CV: Postural hypotension, ganglionic blockade
DERM: Rash, photosensitivity
EENT: Blurred vision, optic neuritis
GI: Anorexia, nausea, vomiting, diarrhea, abdominal pain, stomatitis, metallic taste, jaundice, hepatitis, elevated liver function tests
HEME: Thrombocytopenia
Other: Gynecomastia, impotence, hypoglycemia

TOXICITY AND OVERDOSE
Clinical signs: No information available
Treatment: Supportive care; if ingested within 4 hr, induce emesis or perform gastric lavage followed by activated charcoal

PATIENT CARE MANAGEMENT
Assessment
• Assess history of hypersensitivity to ethionamide, other chemically related antitubercular medications
• Assess hepatic function (ALT, AST, bilirubin), renal function (BUN, creatinine, I&O), hematologic function (CBC, differential, platelet count)
Interventions
• Administer PO with food to reduce GI distress; tab may be crushed, mixed with food or fluid
• Pyridoxine may be prescribed to prevent peripheral neuropathy
• Maintain age-appropriate fluid intake

> **NURSING ALERT**
> Discontinue drug if signs of hypersensitivity, hepatic impairment, acute bleeding disorder develop

Evaluation
• Evaluate therapeutic response (decreased TB symptoms, negative culture)
• Monitor hepatic function (ALT, AST, bilirubin), renal function (BUN, creatinine, I&O), hematologic function (CBC, differential, platelet count)
• Monitor for hepatic impairment (anorexia, jaundice, dark urine, malaise, fatigue, liver tenderness)
• Monitor DM control
• Monitor CNS toxicity (affect, behavioral changes)
• Monitor safety in case of postural hypotension

PATIENT AND FAMILY EDUCATION
Teach/instruct
• To take as directed at prescribed intervals for prescribed length of time
Warn/advise
• To notify care provider of hypersensitivity, side effects
• To comply with follow-up care

- To avoid use of alcohol, medications containing alcohol

STORAGE
- Store at room temp
- Protect from light, air

---

ethosuximide
Brand Name(s): Zarontin ✤
Classification: Anticonvulsant, succinimide derivative
Pregnancy Category: C

AVAILABLE PREPARATIONS
Caps: 250 mg
Syr: 250 mg/5 ml

ROUTES AND DOSAGES
Children 3-6 yr: Initially 15 mg/kg/24 hr divided bid to maximum 250 mg/dose; may increase 250 mg q 4-7 days, building up to 20-30 mg/kg/24 hr; maximum dose 1.5 g/24 hr divided bid
Children >6 yr and adults: PO initial dose of 250 mg bid; may increase by 250 mg/24 hr q 4-7 days up to a maximum dose of 1.5 g/24 hr divided bid
- Ethosuximide historically has been given by starting with 250 mg/24 hr, increasing dosage q wk by one cap until seizures are controlled, usually to maximum of 5 caps/24 hr

**MECHANISM
AND INDICATIONS**
Mechanism: Acts to suppress neuronal transmission in the motor cortex and basal ganglia which results in suppression of the characteristic spike-and-wave pattern seen on EEG with absence seizures
Indications: Used primarily to treat absence seizures; also used in combination with other anticonvulsants to treat mixed seizure disorders

PHARMACOKINETICS
Peak: Caps 2-4 hr; syr <2-4 hr
Half-life: Children 30 hr; adults 40-50 hr
Metabolism: Liver (80%)
Excretion: Urine (as metabolites and unchanged drug); small amount in feces
Therapeutic level: 40-100 mcg/ml

**CONTRAINDICATIONS
AND PRECAUTIONS**
- Contraindicated with known hypersensitivity to succinimides
- Use cautiously with liver and renal disease, pregnancy, lactation; if prescribed for treatment of mixed seizure disorders alone, may increase seizure frequency; if withdrawn suddenly, may precipitate absence seizures

INTERACTIONS
Drug
- Additive CNS depression and sedation possible with other anticonvulsants, alcohol, anxiolytics, narcotics, antidepressants, antipsychotics
- Decreased effectiveness of oral contraceptives
- Decreased anticonvulsant effects possible with phenothiazines, antipsychotics
- Decreased haloperidol level possible
- Inhibited metabolism and higher ethosuximide levels possible with isoniazid
Lab
- Elevated liver enzymes, false positive Coombs' test
- Altered renal function tests

SIDE EFFECTS
CNS: Drowsiness, fatigue, lethargy, dizziness, headache, ataxia, hyperactivity, irritability, hiccups, behavioral changes
DERM: Urticaria, pruritic and erythematous rashes, Stevens-Johnson syndrome, hirsutism, lupus-like syndromes
EENT: Myopia
GI: Nausea, vomiting, diarrhea, gum hypertrophy, tongue swelling, anorexia, epigastric and abdominal pain

E

✤ Available in Canada.

GU: Vaginal bleeding
HEME: Leukopenia, eosinophilia, agranulocytosis, pancytopenia, thrombocytopenia, aplastic anemia

TOXICITY AND OVERDOSE

Clinical signs: CNS depression, ataxia, stupor, coma
Treatment: Supportive symptomatic care with careful monitoring of VS, fluids and electrolytes (Na, K$^+$)

PATIENT CARE MANAGEMENT

Assessment

• Assess for history of hypersensitivity to ethosuximide or succinimides
• Assess baseline laboratory studies including CBC, differential and liver function (ALT, AST, bilirubin, alk phos)
• Assess seizure type; determine (if ethosuximide is appropriate) anticonvulsant for this type of seizure

Interventions

• Administer with food or milk to decrease GI symptoms
• Initiate at modest dosage
• Increase dosage as needed to control seizures (to the point of intolerable side effects)
• Initiate another anticonvulsant in same way if drug is only partially effective
• Gradually withdraw and initiate another anticonvulsant if drug is not effective
• If breakthrough seizures occur at times when serum levels are at trough or peak, frequency of administration may be increased to provide more even coverage

Evaluation

• Evaluate therapeutic response (seizure control); this should initially be done more frequently until seizures are controlled; then q 3-6 mo or if seizure breakthrough or side effects occur
• Monitor anticonvulsant levels periodically

PATIENT AND FAMILY EDUCATION

Teach/instruct

• To take drug as prescribed; not to change dosage or withdraw the drug suddenly without notifying provider
• That the medication should be taken with food or milk to decrease GI irritation
• About process for initiating anticonvulsant drugs and about the need for frequent visits (especially initial visits)
• About rationale for measuring serum levels, how these should be obtained (peak/trough)
• That unpleasant side effects may decrease as pt becomes more used to drug; initially may be more sedating; avoid hazardous tasks (bike, skates, skateboards) that require mental alertness until stabilized on the drug

Warn/advise

• That some pts have shown a tolerance to medications after 3 mo and may require adjustment in dosage
• About potential for increased CNS depression if given with other CNS depressants (alcohol, antihistamines, analgesics, MAOIs, antidepressants, barbiturates)
• About potential side effects; to report serious side effects immediately (any signs of unusual bleeding, bruising, jaundice, dark urine, pale stools, abdominal pain, fever, chills, sore throat, mouth ulcers, edema; disturbances in mood, alertness, coordination)
• To inform other health care providers of their medications in order to avoid drug interactions
• To inform care provider if pregnancy should occur while taking drug

Encourage

• To keep a record of any seizures (seizure calendar)

STORAGE

• Store at room temp

✣ Available in Canada.

etoposide
Brand Name(s): VP-16✤,
Vepesid✤

Classification: Antineoplastic; vinca alkaloids

Pregnancy Category: D

AVAILABLE PREPARATIONS
Caps: 50 mg, 100 mg
Inj: 20 mg/ml

ROUTES AND DOSAGES
• Drug may vary in response to diagnosis, extent of disease, concurrent or previous therapy, protocol guidelines, physiologic parameters; consult current literature, protocol recommendations
Children and adults: IV 50-150 mg/m²/24 hr for 3-5 days q 3-4 wk or 100-125 mg/m²/24 hr alternating day schedule q 3-4 wk or 125-150 mg/m²/24 hr continuous infusion over 3-5 days q 3-4 wk; PO twice the IV dosage (round to nearest 50 mg)
IV administration
• Recommended concentration: Dilute with NS or D_5W to concentration of 0.2 or 0.4 mg/ml; at 1 mg/ml, crystallization occurs; therefore concentrations above 0.4 mg/ml are not recommended
• Continuous infusion rate: Over at least 30 min to prevent hypotension

MECHANISM AND INDICATIONS
Mechanism: Is cell cycle phase specific, inhibiting DNA synthesis in the S and G_2 phase so cells cannot enter cell mitosis; causes single-strand breaks in DNA by inhibiting DNA topoisomerase II enzymes; drug-induced inhibition of TOPO-II is an energy-requiring process dependent on both dosage and duration of drug exposure; Mg also required as an enzymatic cofactor
Indications: Used in the treatment of AML, Hodgkin's disease, non-Hodgkin's lymphoma, Ewing's sarcoma, refractory testicular cancer, small cell carcinoma of the lung; in some treatments for neuroblastoma, rhabdomyosarcoma, brain tumors, refractory advanced breast cancer, but role is not fully determined; used in high dosages for some autologous bone marrow transplant regimens

PHARMACOKINETICS
Peak: PO 1-1.5 hr; IV at end of infusion
Absorption: Variable after PO administration, not affected by food
Distribution: Undergoes rapid distribution after IV administration
Half-life: Initial phase 0.6-2 hr; terminal phase 5.3-10.8 hr
Metabolism: Not completely determined
Excretion: Rapidly excreted in urine, to a lesser extent in bile

CONTRAINDICATIONS AND PRECAUTIONS
• Contraindicated with known hypersensitivity to drug, active infection, chicken pox or herpes zoster, pregnancy, lactation
• Use cautiously with impaired renal or hepatic functions; cytotoxic or radiation therapy

INTERACTIONS
Drug
• Prolonged PT possible with use of warfarin

INCOMPATIBILITIES
• Cisplatin with mannitol, potassium chloride in NS, idarubicin; hydrolysis may occur in alkaline sol

SIDE EFFECTS
CNS: Occasional headache, fever, fatigue, somnolence, peripheral neuropathy, weakness
CV: Hypotension with too rapid infusion
GI: Nausea, vomiting, anorexia, abdominal pain, stomatitis, aftertaste, constipation, hepatotoxicity
GU: Nephrotoxicity
HEME: Leukopenia, myelosuppression (dose-limiting); anemia; thrombocytopenia
RESP: Bronchospasm, severe wheezing
Other: Alopecia, anaphylaxis

✤ Available in Canada.

(rare), phlebitis at injection site (infrequent), fever, rash, pigmentation changes

TOXICITY AND OVERDOSE

Hepatotoxicity has been reported in pts receiving VP-16; generally occurs in pts receiving high dosages

Treatment: Withhold drug

PATIENT CARE MANAGEMENT
Assessment

• Assess history of hypersensitivity to VP-16, related drugs
• Assess baseline VS, CBC, differential, platelet count, renal function (BUN, creatinine, urine CrCl), liver function (ALT, AST, LDH, bilirubin, alk phos), serum electrolytes, pulmonary function
• Assess hydration status, urine output, SG, adequate fluid intake (IV, PO)
• Assess motor and sensory function before therapy
• Assess neurologic and mental status before and during drug administration and on follow-up visits
• Assess success of previous antiemetic therapy
• Assess history of previous treatment with special attention to other therapies that may predispose to renal or pulmonary dysfunction

Interventions

• Premedicate with antiemetics, continue periodically through therapy
• Have diphenhydramine, hydrocortisone, epinephrine, and necessary emergency equipment available to establish an airway in case of anaphylaxis
• Monitor VS (especially B/P) during etoposide infusion
• Encourage small, frequent feedings of foods pt likes
• Monitor I&O; administer IV fluids until pt is able to resume normal PO intake
• Provide supportive measures to maintain hemostasis, fluid and electrolyte balance, nutritional support

> **NURSING ALERT**
> Infuse over at least 30 min; too-rapid infusion may cause hypotension
>
> Inspect oral mucosa daily for evidence of ulcerations or bleeding

Evaluation

• Evaluate therapeutic response (decreased tumor size, spread of malignancy)
• Evaluate CBC, differential, platelet count, serum electrolytes, renal function (BUN, creatinine, urine CrCl), liver function (ALT, AST, LDH, bilirubin, alk phos) at given intervals after chemotherapy
• Evaluate for signs or symptoms of infection (fever fatigue, sore throat), bleeding (easy bruising, nose bleeds, bleeding gums)
• Inspect oral mucosa daily for ulcerations, bleeding
• Evaluate I&O, check wt daily
• Evaluate for side effects, and response to antiemetic regimen

PATIENT AND FAMILY EDUCATION
Teach/instruct

• To have pt well-hydrated before and after chemotherapy
• About importance of follow-up to monitor blood counts, serum chemistry values, drug blood levels
• To take accurate temp; rectal temp contraindicated
• To notify care provider of signs of bleeding (bruising, epistaxis, bleeding gums), infection (fever, sore throat, fatigue)

Warn/advise

• About impact of body changes that may occur (hair loss, hyperpigmentation, nail ridging), how to minimize changes (wigs, caps, scarves, long sleeves)
• To avoid OTC products containing aspirin
• To report any alterations in behavior, sensation, perception; help

---

♣ Available in Canada.

to develop a plan of care to manage side effects, stress of illness or treatment
• To monitor bowel function, call care provider if abdominal pain or constipation are noted
• To immediately report any pain, discoloration at injection site (parenteral forms)
• That good oral hygiene with very soft toothbrush is imperative
• That dental work be delayed until blood counts return to baseline, with permission of care provider
• To avoid contact with known viral or bacterial illnesses
• That household contacts of child not be immunized with live polio virus; inactivated form should be used
• That child not receive immunizations until immune system recovers sufficiently to mount needed antibody response
• To report exposure to chicken pox in susceptible child immediately
• To report reactivation of herpes zoster virus (shingles) immediately
• If appropriate, ways to preserve reproductive patterns, sexuality (sperm banking, contraceptives)
Encourage
• Provision of nutritional food intake; consider nutritional consultation
• To comply with bowel management program
• To use top anesthetics to control discomfort of mucositis; avoid spicy foods, commercial mouthwashes
STORAGE
• Store caps in refrigerator
• Stability of injection is concentration-dependent; 0.2 mg/ml stable at room temp for 96 hr; 0.4 mg/ml stable at room temp for 48 hr; crystallization can occur within 30 min at higher concentrations (1 mg/ml)

factor IX complex
Brand Name(s): Konyne, Profilnine, Proplex
Classification: Hemostatic (blood derivative)
Pregnancy Category: C

F

AVAILABLE PREPARATION
Inj: Vials with diluents (number of units specified on label)

ROUTES AND DOSAGES
Children and adults: IV, slow IVP or IV infusion; dosage individualized based on degree of deficiency, desired level of factor IX, wt, degree of bleeding

MECHANISM AND INDICATIONS
Mechanism: Increases blood clotting factors II, VII, IX, X
Indications: For use in factor IX deficiency (hemophilia B) and anticoagulant overdose

PHARMACOKINETICS
Half-life: Approximately 24 hr
Excretion: Rapidly cleared by plasma

CONTRAINDICATIONS AND PRECAUTIONS
• Contraindicated with hepatic disease, disseminated intravascular clotting, fibrinolysis
• Use cautiously in infants and neonates (increased risk of hepatitis)

INTERACTIONS
Drug
• Increased hemostatic effect with other anticoagulants
Lab
• None significant

INCOMPATIBILITIES
• Protein products

SIDE EFFECTS
CNS: Headache, paresthesia, dizziness
CV: Tachycardia, hypotension, thromboembolic reactions
DERM: Rash, flushing urticaria

GI: Nausea, vomiting, jaundice, abdominal cramping
RESP: Bronchospasm
Other: Risk of acquiring HIV and hepatitis B

TOXICITY AND OVERDOSE
Clinical signs: Disseminated intravascular clotting
Treatment: Discontinue drug, supportive care

PATIENT CARE MANAGEMENT
Assessment
• Assess history of hypersensitivity to drug
• Assess blood coagulation studies (PT, PTT, levels of blood factors)
• Assess for bleeding
• Assess VS, B/P; for shock

Interventions
• Warm diluent to room temp, add to powder slowly for IV
• Administer through filtered needle; administer slow IVP ≈ 100 U/min, not to exceed 3 ml/min
• Discontinue if anaphylaxis occurs

> **NURSING ALERT**
> Monitor for signs of allergic reaction during administration

Evaluation
• Evaluate therapeutic response (decreased bleeding)
• Evaluate for reaction (fever, chills, rash; slow infusion)
• Monitor for signs of disseminated intravascular clotting (ecchymosis, changes in blood coagulation studies)

PATIENT AND FAMILY EDUCATION
Teach/instruct
• To take as directed at prescribed intervals for prescribed length of time
• About in-home use of drug (if appropriate)
• To report any side effects or reactions
• About risk of hepatitis B or HIV
• That hepatitis B immunization series be given before treatment when possible

STORAGE
• Store powder up to 2 yr (check expiration date)
• Store reconstituted sol for 3 hr at room temp

---

famotidine

Brand Name(s): Apo-Famotidine✤, Novo-Famotidine✤, Nu-Famotidine✤, Pepcid✤, Pepcid IV✤

Classification: Antihistamine, H_2-receptor antagonist

Pregnancy Category: B

AVAILABLE PREPARATIONS
Oral susp: 40 mg/5 ml
Tabs: 20 mg, 40 mg
Inj: 10 mg/ml, 20 mg/50 ml (premixed)

ROUTES AND DOSAGES
PO
Infants and children: For GERD <10 kg: 1-2 mg/kg/24 hr divided tid; >10 kg: 1-2 mg/kg/24 hr divided bid; maximum 40 mg/24 hr
Adults: For duodenal ulcer: 40 mg qhs or 20 mg bid; for prophylaxis of recurrent duodenal ulcer: 20 mg qhs; for gastric ulcer: 40 mg qhs; for hypersecretory conditions: 20 mg q6h; for gastroesophageal reflux: 20 mg bid for up to 6 wk; for prophylaxis of aspiration pneumonitis: 40 mg either night before or morning of surgery
IM
Adult: For prophylaxis of aspiration pneumonitis: 20 mg either night before or morning of surgery
IV
Infants and children: For GERD 0.3-0.4 mg/kg/dose q8h; maximum 40 mg/24 hr
Adults: For duodenal ulcer, gastric ulcer and gastric hypersecretory conditions: 20 mg q12h
IV administration
• Recommended concentration: IV push 20 mg in 5-10 ml NS; intermittent infusion 20 mg in 100

---

ml D_5W, $D_{10}W$, LR, NS, 5% $NaHCO_3$
• Maximum concentration: 4 mg/ml
• IV push rate: Over ≥ 2 min
• Intermittent infusion rate: Over 15-30 min

MECHANISM AND INDICATIONS

Mechanism: Reversible competitive antagonist of the actions of histamine on H_2 receptors resulting in a decrease of the histamine-mediated basal and nocturnal gastric acid secretion by the parietal cell

Indications: Used as therapy for gastric or duodenal ulcer, GERD, pathological hypersecretory conditions, prevention of GI bleeding in critically ill pts; investigational use in treatment of acute upper GI bleeding, prophylaxis of pulmonary aspiration of acid during anesthesia

PHARMACOKINETICS

Peak: 1-3 hr after oral dose; 30 min after parenteral dose
Half-life: 2.5-3.5 hours after both oral and parenteral doses
Metabolism: Hepatic
Excretion: Urine

CONTRAINDICATIONS AND PRECAUTIONS

• Contraindicated with hypersensitivity to famotidine or any other H_2-receptor antagonists
• Use cautiously with renal or hepatic impairment, pregnancy, lactation

INTERACTIONS

Drug
• Potential effect on bioavailability of drug, dosage forms (e.g., enteric-coated) with pH dependent absorption
• Possible prevention of degradation of acid-labile drugs
• Possible impaired elimination of drugs requiring hepatic metabolism
• Impaired absorption with use of antacids and possibly sucralfate
• Increased risk of neutropenia or other blood dyscrasias possible with bone marrow depressants

Lab
• Elevated serum transaminase levels
• False negative allergy skin test possible
• Antagonism of pentagastrin and histamine in evaluation of gastric acid secretory function possible

Nutrition
• Vitamin B_{12} deficiency possible with long-term therapy in pts likely to have impaired secretion of intrinsic factor (severe fundic gastritis)

INCOMPATIBILITIES

• None reported

SIDE EFFECTS

CNS: Headache, dizziness; rarely, weakness, fatigue, seizures
CV: Cardiac arrhythmias, palpitations, AV block (all rare)
DERM: Rash (hypersensitivity), pruritus, urticaria, dry skin
GI: Constipation, diarrhea, nausea, vomiting, abdominal discomfort, flatulence, belching, anorexia, dry mouth, heartburn, jaundice
HEME: Leukocytosis, leukopenia, neutropenia, pancytopenia, agranulocytosis, thrombocytopenia (all rare)
Other: Hypersensitivity: (anaphylaxis, angioedema, bronchospasm, orbital or facial edema, conjunctival congestion)

TOXICITY AND OVERDOSE

Treatment: No experience to date with acute overdosage of famotidine; if it should occur induce vomiting or perform gastric lavage; supportive and symptomatic treatment should be initiated

PATIENT CARE MANAGEMENT

Assessment
• Assess for hypersensitivity to famotidine, other H_2-receptor antagonists
• Assess baseline renal function (BUN, creatinine), hepatic function (ALT, AST, bilirubin), gastric pH, abdominal symptoms

Interventions

- May administer PO without regard to meals; tab may be crushed, mixed with food or fluid
- Shake susp well before administering each dose
- Do not administer within 1 hr of antacids
- Do not administer within 2 hr of sucralfate
- Do not administer within 2 hr of ketoconazole
- Do not administer IM/IV if discolored or if precipitate is present
- Administer IV over ≥ 2 min

Evaluation

- Evaluate therapeutic response (decreased abdominal pain)
- Evaluate for history of hypersensitivity, side effects
- Evaluate gastric pH (>5), hematologic function (CBC), signs of GI bleeding (melena, brown-tinged or coffee-ground emesis)
- Evaluate renal function (BUN, creatinine), hepatic function (ALT, AST, bilirubin)

PATIENT AND FAMILY EDUCATION

Teach/instruct

- To take as directed at prescribed intervals for prescribed length of time
- To continue taking even after symptoms subside
- To shake oral susp well

Warn/advise

- To notify care provider of history of hypersensitivity, side effects
- To avoid smoking, caffeine, alcohol; these may exacerbate symptoms
- To avoid OTC drugs unless directed by care provider

STORAGE

- Store all forms at room temp, protect tabs from light
- Unused oral susp should be discarded after 30 days
- Diluted injectable sol stable for 48 hr at room temp

---

fentanyl citrate

Brand Name(s): Fentanyl, Sublimaze✤

Classification: Narcotic analgesic

Controlled Substance Schedule II

Pregnancy Category: C

AVAILABLE PREPARATIONS

Inj: 50 mcg/ml (in 2 ml, 5 ml containers)

DOSAGES AND ROUTES

Sedation for Procedures/Analgesia

Children 1-12 yr: IM/IV 1-2 mcg/kg/dose; may repeat q 30-60 min
Children >12 yr and adults: IM/IV 0.5-1 mcg/kg/dose; may repeat after 30-60 min

Continuous Sedation/Analgesia

Children 1-12 yr: IV bolus, initial 1-2 mcg/kg/dose, then 1 mcg/kg/hr; titrate upward; usual dosage 1-3 mcg/kg/hr; may increase to 5 mcg/kg/hr

Adjunct to General Anesthesia

Children >12 yr and adults: IV 2-50 mcg/kg as slow infusion (1 ml over 1-2 min) until sleep occurs

Post-Operative Pain

Children >12 yr and adults: IM/IV 50-100 mcg/dose

IV administration

- Recommended concentration: Dilute with 5 ml or more SW or NS
- Maximum concentration: May be given undiluted
- IV push rate: 0.1 mg (maximum) of diluted drug over 3-5 min
- Continuous infusion rate: 1-3 mcg/kg/hr (may increase to 5 mcg/kg/hr)

MECHANISM AND INDICATIONS

Mechanism: Inhibits ascending pain pathways in CNS
Indications: For use preoperatively, postoperatively for pain control as an adjunct to general anesthesia

---

✤ Available in Canada.

PHARMACOKINETICS
Onset of action: IM 7-15 min; IV immediate
Peak: IM 30 min; IV 3-5 min
Duration: IM 1-2 hr; IV ½-1 hr
Half-life: 2½ to 4 hr
Metabolism: Liver
Excretion: Urine

CONTRAINDICATIONS AND PRECAUTIONS
• Contraindicated with hypersensitivity to this or any component of this medication; hypersensitivity to droperidol or opiates; myasthenia gravis; MAOIs (taken within 14 days)
• Use cautiously with cardiac arrhythmias, increased intracranial pressure, impaired kidney function or liver function, respiratory depression, severe respiratory disorders, seizures

INTERACTIONS
Drug
• Additive effects with alcohol, antipsychotics, CNS depressants, hypnotics, narcotics, sedatives, skeletal muscle relaxants
• Administration within 14 days of administration of MAOIs may cause a hypertensive crisis, high fever, seizures
Nutrition
• Do not drink alcohol

INCOMPATIBILITIES
• Incompatible in sol or syringe with diazepam, methohexital, pentobarbital, phenytoin, $NaHCO_3$, thiopental

SIDE EFFECTS
CNS: Delirium, disorientation, dizziness, drowsiness, dysphoria, euphoria, EPS, restlessness
CV: Arrest, bradycardia, hypertension, hypotension
EENT: Miosis, blurred vision
GI: Nausea, vomiting
RESP: Apnea, laryngospasm, respiratory depression
Other: Hyperglycemia, hypothermia, muscular rigidity, shivering

PATIENT CARE MANAGEMENT
Assessment
• Assess history of hypersensitivity to drug
• Assess medical history; screen for use of MAOIs within past 14 days
• Assess baseline liver (ALT, AST) and kidney functions (BUN, creatinine)
Interventions
• Administer only if an opioid antagonist, resuscitative equipment, and O_2 are available
• Administer IM and IV slowly to prevent rigidity
• Maintain safety precautions upon recovery (siderails up, night light, call bell within reach)

> **NURSING ALERT**
> Avoid rapid IV injection; can cause muscle rigidity (particularly involving muscles of respiration)
>
> Avoid administering within 14 days of administration of MAOIs; may cause a hypertensive crisis, high fever, seizures

Evaluation
• Evaluate therapeutic response (induction of anesthesia, pain relief)
• Monitor respiratory status; if respirations are <10 per min, notify care provider
• Monitor VS, O_2 saturation, B/P
• Monitor for rash, hives, muscle rigidity
• Monitor for dizziness, drowsiness, euphoria, hallucinations, LOC, pupil reaction

PATIENT AND FAMILY EDUCATION
Warn/advise
• To avoid ingesting alcohol, other CNS depressants
• That medication may cause dizziness, drowsiness until recovery is complete

STORAGE
• Store at room temp in light-resistant container

✣ Available in Canada.

ferrous salts (ferrous gluconate, ferrous sulfate)

Brand Name(s): ferrous gluconate: Apo-Ferrous Gluconate♣, Fergon, Ferralet, Simron
Ferrous sulfate: Apo-Ferrous Sulfate♣, Feosol, Fer-In-Sol♣, Ferodan♣, Fero-Gradumet, Mol-Iron, PMS-Ferrous Sulfate♣, Slo-Fe♣

Classification: Iron supplement and antianemic

Pregnancy Category: C

AVAILABLE PREPARATIONS
Ferrous gluconate (12% elemental iron)
Elixir: 300 mg (34 mg Fe)/5 ml
Tabs: 300 mg (34 mg Fe), 320 mg (37 mg Fe), 325 mg (38 mg Fe)
Ext rel caps: 320 mg (37 mg Fe), 435 mg (50 mg Fe)
Caps: 86 mg (10 mg Fe), 325 mg (38 mg Fe), 435 mg (50 mg Fe)
Ferrous sulfate (20% elemental iron)
Drops: 75 mg (15 mg Fe)/0.6 ml
Syrup: 90 mg (18 mg Fe)/5 ml
Elixir: 220 mg (44 mg Fe)/5 ml
Caps: 250 mg (50 mg Fe)
Tabs: 195 mg (39 mg Fe), 300 mg (60 mg Fe), 324 mg (65 mg Fe)

ROUTES AND DOSAGES
PO
Dietary supplement (see Appendix F, Table of Recommended Daily Dietary Allowances)
Iron Deficiency Anemia (in terms of elemental iron)
Children: PO 3-6 mg/kg/24 hr in 1-2 divided doses
Adults: PO 60-100 mg/24 hr in divided doses qd-bid

MECHANISM AND INDICATIONS
Mechanism: Replaces iron, a mineral essential in the formation of Hgb, which is the major component of RBCs and carries O_2 throughout the body

Indications: Used in prevention, treatment of iron deficiency anemia

PHARMACOKINETICS
Metabolism: Bone marrow, liberated by destruction of hemoglobin
Excretion: Blood losses, hair, feces, nails, urine

CONTRAINDICATIONS AND PRECAUTIONS
• Contraindicated with hemochromatosis, hemosiderosis, hemolytic anemias, iron overload, hypersensitivity to iron
• Use cautiously with peptic ulcer, regional enteritis, ulcerative colitis, non-iron deficient anemias, pregnancy; avoid use for >6 mo

INTERACTIONS
Drug
• Decreased absorption with antacids, cholestyramine, penicillamine
• Altered absorption with doxycycline
• Inhibited absorption with tetracycline
Lab
• Altered occult blood tests in stool
• Altered skeletal imaging
Nutrition
• Increased absorption with vitamin C
• Decreased absorption with dairy products, vitamin E

SIDE EFFECTS
CNS: Fatigue
CV: Rapid pulse, decreased B/P
GI: Nausea, vomiting, black tarry stools, appetite loss, constipation, diarrhea, epigastric pain
HEME: Hemosiderosis
Other: Liquid preparation may stain teeth

TOXICITY AND OVERDOSE
• Dose of 180-300 mg/kg taken within ½-8 hr may be lethal
Clinical signs: Lethargy, vomiting, nausea, green (and then tarry) stools, hypotension, weakness, rapid pulse, dehydration, acidosis, coma, pulmonary edema, shock convulsions, anuria, hyperthermia

♣ Available in Canada.

Treatment: Maintain airway, respiration, and circulation; induce vomiting with ipecac and gastric lavage using a 1%-5% sol of $NaHCO_3$; deferoxamine sol may be necessary for systemic chelation for pts with serum iron levels >300 mg/dl; supportive care

PATIENT CARE MANAGEMENT

Assessment

• Assess history of hypersensitivity to ferrous salts
• Obtain baseline hematologic status (CBC, reticulocyte count, serum Fe, TIBC, ferritin levels)
• Assess for other medication use to ensure optimal absorption (salicylates, sulfonamides, antimalarials, quinidine may cause anemia)

Interventions

• Administer PO between meals for optimal absorption; after meals if GI upset occurs; enhanced absorption if given with orange juice (>200 mg vitamin C/30 mg elemental iron enhances absorption); decreased absorption if given with eggs, milk products, chocolate, caffeine; do not give with antacids
• Administer liquid forms through straw to avoid discoloration of tooth enamel; only chewable tabs should be chewed

---

NURSING ALERT

Keep medication away from children; overdose can be lethal

Check dosage to ensure safe levels

Evaluation

• Evaluate therapeutic response (improved Hct, Hgb, reticulocyte, serum ferritin levels, decreased fatigue, weakness)
• Monitor for signs of hypersensitivity, toxicity (nausea, vomiting, diarrhea, hematemesis, pallor)
• Monitor stools (may turn black); if constipation occurs, increase water and fiber in diet; exercise
• Monitor dietary intake; pt should consume adequate amounts of iron (see Appendix F)

PATIENT AND FAMILY EDUCATION

Teach/instruct

• To take as directed at prescribed intervals for prescribed length of time
• To evaluate other medications, OTC drugs for interactions

Warn/advise

• To notify care provider of hypersensitivity, side effects
• About concern of iron toxicity, emphasize need to keep supplements out of the reach of children
• About separate timing of medications and OTC supplements; if necessary, take 2-3 hr before or after iron supplement
• To report changes in stools because dosage may need to be adjusted

Encourage

• Explain importance of a balanced diet; common sources of iron include meat, eggs, vegetables, fortified or enriched foods

STORAGE

• Store at room temp in an airtight, light-resistant container
• Protect from heat, light, moisture

---

filgrastim, G-CSF

Brand Name(s): Neupogen ✤

Classification: Human granulocyte colony-stimulating factor

Pregnancy Category: C

AVAILABLE PREPARATIONS

Inj: 300 mcg/ml or 480 mg/1.6 ml

ROUTES AND DOSAGES

Children and adults: IV/SC 5 mcg/kg/24 hr as single daily dose until WBC counts recover; may be increased to 10 mcg/kg/24 hr; often administered at home via SC inj

IV administration

• IV push: 15-30 min
• Continuous infusion rate: If final concentration of G-CSF in D_5W is <15 mcg/ml, add 2 mg

---

✤ Available in Canada.

albumin/ml of IV fluids (albumin prevents adsorption of G-CSF by IV tubing); may run over ≤24 hr

MECHANISM AND INDICATIONS

Mechanism: Produced through recombinant DNA technology; binds to specific cell surface receptors and causes a proliferative stimulus of immature neutrophils in marrow, induces release of neutrophils from marrow, and increases phagocytic potential of leukocytes

Indications: To decrease length of time a pt is severely neutropenic and at risk for contracting infections (febrile neutropenia) while undergoing chemotherapy with myelosuppressive agents; may also be used to accelerate bone marrow recovery following bone marrow transplantation, increase blood counts in primary neutropenia and aplastic anemia, treating neutropenia in HIV-infected patients treated with zidovudine

PHARMACOKINETICS

Peak: Immediately after IV injection, 2-8 hr after SC

Half-life: 3.5 hr

Excretion: Urine; unaffected by renal or hepatic dysfunction

CONTRAINDICATIONS AND PRECAUTIONS

• Contraindicated with history of hypersensitivity to *E. coli*-derived products; for use within 24 hr immediately before or after cytotoxic chemotherapy; could act as growth factor for underlying malignancy, particularly myeloid tumors, discontinue if disease progression is noted

• Use cautiously with pregnancy, lactation; in septic pts (since an increased risk of developing adult respiratory distress syndrome exists because of influx of increased numbers of activated neutrophils invading site of inflammation); theoretical possibility exists that drug could serve as a growth factor for *any* tumor type

INTERACTIONS

Drugs

• Synergistic action with other growth factors to stimulate cell lines possible

Lab

• Increased LDH, alk phos, uric acid; increased number and appearance of earlier granulocyte progenitor cells (including immature cells not often seen in peripheral blood)

SIDE EFFECTS

CV: Vasculitis

DERM: Flaring of preexisting eczema

GI: Splenomegaly

HEME: Peripheral circulation appearance of more immature granulocyte progenitor cells (left shift) including promyelocytes and myeloblasts; potential for receiving increased doses of chemotherapy at shorter intervals may cause pt to be at increased risk for anemia, thrombocytopenia

RESP: ARDS (if pt becomes septic while on G-CSF)

Other: Mild-to-moderate medullary bone pain in 20% of pts (less of a problem in SC administration); fever

PATIENT CARE MANAGEMENT

Assessment

• Assess history of hypersensitivity to G-CSF, proteins derived from *E. coli*

• Assess baseline CBC, differential, platelet counts

• Assess history of response to growth factors (including side-effects, route of administration, efficacy)

Interventions

• Transfuse with RBCs, platelets as appropriate

Evaluation

• Evaluate therapeutic response (decrease in length of neutropenic state; absence of infection)

• Monitor CBC counts at least twice weekly to avoid leukocytosis

PATIENT AND FAMILY EDUCATION
Teach/instruct
- About importance of follow-up to monitor blood counts, chemistry values
- To take accurate temp; rectal temp contraindicated
- To notify care provider of signs of bleeding (bruising, epistaxis, bleeding gums), infection (fever, sore throat, fatigue)

Warn/advise
- To immediately report any pain or inflammation at injection site
- That good oral hygiene with very soft toothbrush is imperative
- That dental care be delayed until blood counts return to baseline levels
- To avoid contact with known viral or bacterial illnesses

STORAGE
- Unopened vials should be stored in refrigerator but may be warmed to room temp for not more than 6 hr before administration

---

fluconazole
Brand Name(s): Diflucan✤, Diflucan-150✤

Classification: Antifungal agent

Pregnancy Category: C

AVAILABLE PREPARATIONS
Tabs: 50 mg, 100 mg, 200 mg
Inj: 2 mg/ml

ROUTES AND DOSAGES
Children 3-13 yr: PO, IV loading dose 10 mg/kg; administer maintenance 24 hr after loading dose 3-6 mg/kg/24 hr qd. (Safety and effectiveness not established. Dosage represents accepted standard practice recommendations.)

Systemic Candidiasis
Adults: PO, IV loading dose 400 mg; administer maintenance dose 24 hr after loading dose, 200 mg qd

Cryptococcal Meningitis
Adults: PO, IV loading dose 400 mg; administer maintenance dose 24 hr after loading dose, 200-400 mg qd

Oropharyngeal and Esophageal Candidiasis
Adults: PO, IV loading dose 200 mg; administer maintenance dose 24 hr after loading dose 100 mg qd; maximum dose 400 mg/24 hr for esophageal candidiasis

IV administration
- Recommended concentration: 2 mg/ml
- Maximum concentration: 2 mg/ml
- IV push rate: Not recommended
- Intermittent infusion rate: Over 2 hr in children; do not exceed 200 mg/hr in adults

MECHANISM AND INDICATIONS
Mechanism: Decreases ergosterol synthesis, inhibits cell membrane function by interfering with cytochrome P-450 activity
Indications: Used to treat fungal infections including oropharyngeal, esophageal, systemic (UTI, peritonitis, pneumonia) candidiasis, and cryptococcal meningitis

PHARMACOKINETICS
Peak: PO 2-4 hr
Distribution: Distributes widely into body tissues and fluids (including CSF)
Half-life: 25-30 hr
Metabolism: Partially by liver
Excretion: Urine

CONTRAINDICATIONS AND PRECAUTIONS
- Contraindicated with known hypersensitivity to fluconazole or other azoles
- Use cautiously with children <3 yr, impaired renal or hepatic function, pregnancy

INTERACTIONS
Drug
- Increased PT with use of warfarin
- Increased serum concentration of phenytoin, cyclosporine
- Increased risk of hypoglycemia reactions with oral sulfonylureas
- Decreased fluconazole levels with use of rifampin, cimetidine

F

✤ Available in Canada.

INCOMPATIBILITIES
• With other drugs in syringe or sol

SIDE EFFECTS
CNS: Vertigo, seizures, headache
CV: Pallor
DERM: Rash, exfoliation
ENDO/METAB: Hypokalemia
GI: Nausea, abdominal pain, vomiting, diarrhea, elevated ALT, AST, alk phos
HEME: Eosinophilia

PATIENT CARE MANAGEMENT
Assessment
• Assess history of hypersensitivity to fluconazole, other azoles
• Assess baseline hematologic function (CBC, differential, platelet count), renal function (BUN, creatinine, I&O), hepatic function (ALT, AST, bilirubin), baseline wt
Interventions
• Use distal veins for IV
• Do not premix with other medications; infuse separately
• Obtain VS q 15-30 min during first infusion
• Maintain age-appropriate fluid intake

NURSING ALERT
Monitor closely for abnormal liver or renal function tests; discontinue if symptoms of liver or renal dysfunction develop

Do not administer IV push

Evaluation
• Evaluate therapeutic response (decreasing oral candidiasis, fever, malaise, rash, negative C&S)
• Evaluate hematologic function (CBC, differential, platelet count), renal function (BUN, creatinine, I&O), hepatic function (ALT, AST, bilirubin); weekly wt

PATIENT AND FAMILY EDUCATION
Teach/instruct
• To take as directed at prescribed intervals for prescribed length of time

Warn/advise
• To notify care provider of hypersensitivity, side effects
• That treatment may require wks or mos

STORAGE
• Store at room temp

---

flucytosine
Brand Name(s): Ancobon
Classification: Antifungal agent
Pregnancy Category: C

AVAILABLE PREPARATIONS
Cap: 250 mg, 500 mg

ROUTES AND DOSAGES
Children and adults: 50-150 mg/kg/24 hr divided q6h

MECHANISM AND INDICATIONS
Mechanism: Penetrates fungal cells, is converted to fluorouracil, interferes with fungal RNA and protein synthesis
Indications: Treatment of fungal infections including *Candida, Cryptococcus, Torulopsis*

PHARMACOKINETICS
Peak: 2-6 hr
Distribution: CSF, aqueous humor, joints
Half-life: 3-6 hr
Metabolism: Minimal
Excretion: Urine
Therapeutic level: 25-100 mcg/ml

CONTRAINDICATIONS AND PRECAUTIONS
• Contraindicated with hypersensitivity to flucytosine or any component
• Use cautiously with renal impairment, bone marrow depression, AIDS, blood dyscrasias, radiation or chemotherapy, pregnancy

INTERACTIONS
Drug
• Synergistic with amphotericin B
Lab
• False increase, creatinine

✦ Available in Canada.

SIDE EFFECTS

CNS: Confusion, sedation, headache, ataxia, hallucinations, vertigo

DERM: Rash

GI: Nausea, vomiting, diarrhea, enterocolitis, anorexia, cramps, increased AST, ALT, alk phos

GU: Increased serum creatinine, BUN

HEME: Thrombocytopenia, agranulocytosis, anemia, leukopenia, pancytopenia

Other: Anaphylaxis, growth failure

TOXICITY AND OVERDOSE

Clinical signs: May affect cardiovascular and pulmonary function

Treatment: Emesis and lavage within 4 hr of ingestion; supportive care; readily removed by dialysis

PATIENT CARE MANAGEMENT

Assessment

• Assess history of hypersensitivity to flucytosine

• Obtain baseline CBC, platelets, renal function (BUN, creatinine, I&O), liver function (ALT, AST, bilirubin) function tests

• Assess C&S before therapy

Interventions

• Caps may be taken apart, mixed with small amounts of food or fluid

• Nausea and vomiting may be decreased by administering caps over 15 min

---

NURSING ALERT

Do not confuse this drug with 5-FU

Evaluation

• Evaluate therapeutic response (decreased fever, malaise, rash, negative C&S for organism)

• Monitor for therapeutic levels of drug (25-100 mcg/ml)

• Evaluate side effects (hypersensitivity, dermatitis, nausea, vomiting, diarrhea, headache, decreased urine output, bruising)

• Monitor CBC, platelets, renal function (BUN, creatinine, I&O), liver function (ALT, AST, bilirubin) tests

• Monitor I&O wt

PATIENT AND FAMILY EDUCATION

Teach/instruct

• To take as directed at prescribed intervals for prescribed length of time

Warn/advise

• To notify care provider of hypersensitivity

• That therapy may need to be continued for months to clear infection

Encourage

• To comply with therapeutic regimen

STORAGE

• Store at room temp in light-resistant containers

---

fludrocortisone acetate

Brand Name(s): Florinef♣

Classification: Mineralocorticoid

Pregnancy Category: C

AVAILABLE PREPARATIONS

Tabs: 0.1 mg

ROUTES AND DOSAGES

Replacement Therapy

Infants and children: PO 0.05-0.1 mg qd

Adults: 0.05-0.2 mg qd

Neurally Mediated Syncope

Adolescents: 0.1 mg qd

MECHANISM AND INDICATIONS

Mechanism: Increases Na reabsorption and K^+ excretion from renal tubules; has a moderate glucocorticoid effect

---

♣ Available in Canada.

Indications: Replacement mineralocorticoid used as partial replacement therapy in adrenocortical insufficiency and salt-losing forms of congenital adrenal hyperplasia (CAH); also used to treat neurally mediated syncope.

PHARMACOKINETICS
Onset: Readily absorbed from GI tract
Peak: 1½ hr
Half-life: 3½ hr
Metabolism: Liver
Excretion: Urine

CONTRAINDICATIONS AND PRECAUTIONS
• Contraindicated with hypersensitivity, systemic fungal infections
• Use cautiously with hypertension, CHF or cardiac disease, renal disease, hepatic disease, amebiasis, Addison's disease, pregnancy

INTERACTIONS
Drug
• Increased metabolic clearance of fludrocortisone acetate with barbiturates, phenytoin, rifampin
• Hypokalemia with amphotericin B, diuretics
• Arrhythmias and toxicity associated with hypokalemia with digitalis
• Decreased pro-time with oral anticoagulants
• Diminished effect of insulin and oral hypoglycemics
Lab
• Increased Na, BG
• Decreased K^+

SIDE EFFECTS
CNS: Headaches, dizziness
CV: Edema, hypertension, CHF, cardiac arrhythmias, cardiomegaly
METAB: Wt gain, hypokalemia
MS: weakness, fractures, osteoporosis

TOXICITY AND OVERDOSE
Clinical signs: Disturbances in fluid and electrolytes, hypokalemia, edema, hypertension, cardiac insufficiency

Treatment: Discontinue drug, supportive treatment; correct fluid and electrolyte imbalance

PATIENT CARE MANAGEMENT
Assessment
• Assess history of hypersensitivity to fludrocortisone acetate
• Assess B/P, I&O, wt, Na, K^+, plasma renin
Interventions
• Tab may be crushed, mixed with food or fluids; administer with meals to decrease GI symptoms
• Supplemental doses may be necessary with increased physiologic stress
• Check B/P weekly for one mo to observe for hypertension during neurally mediated syncope treatment.
Evaluation
• Evaluate therapeutic response (Na, K, wt); adjust dosage based on plasma renin level
• Monitor B/P q1-6h with initial dose
• Monitor for hypokalemia (paresthesias, fatigue, nausea, vomiting, depression, polyuria, arrhythmias, weakness)
• Monitor edema, hypertension, cardiac symptoms

PATIENT AND FAMILY EDUCATION
Teach/instruct
• To take as directed at prescribed intervals for prescribed length of time
• Signs of hypokalemia, edema, Na imbalance
Warn/advise
• To notify care provider of hypersensitivity, side effects
• Not to discontinue medication suddenly
• To notify all medical or dental providers of therapy
Encourage
• Carry medical alert identification

STORAGE
- Store at room temp in airtight container
- Protect from light

---

flumazenil

Brand Name(s): Anexate✤, Mazicon, Romazicon

Classification: Benzodiazepine receptor antagonist

Pregnancy Category: C

AVAILABLE PREPARATIONS
Inj: 0.1 mg/ml

ROUTES AND DOSAGES
Reversal of Conscious Sedation, General Anesthesia
Infants and children: IV 0.01 mg/kg; then 0.005 mg/kg q1 min (Safety and effectiveness not established. Dosage represents accepted standard practice recommendations.)
Adults: IV, initial dose 0.2 mg (2 ml) administered over 15 sec; if desired LOC not obtained, wait 45 sec, administer another dose of 0.2 mg, and repeat at 60 sec intervals where necessary (maximum 4 additional times) to a maximum total dose of 1 mg (10 ml); if resedation occurs, repeated doses may be administered at 20 min intervals prn; for repeat treatment, maximum 1 mg/dose (at 0.2 mg/min), 3 mg/hr
Management of Suspected Benzodiazepine Overdose
Infants and children: IV 0.01-0.02 mg/kg, then 0.01 mg/kg (Safety and effectiveness not established. Dosage represents accepted standard practice recommendations.)
Adults: IV initial 0.2 mg (2 ml) over 30 sec; if desired LOC not obtained after waiting 30 sec, give 0.3-0.5 mg (3-5 ml) over 30 sec at 1 min intervals, to maximum total dose of 1-3 mg; if pt has not responded 5 min after receiving cumulative dose, major cause of

the sedation is likely not caused by benzodiazepines
IV administration
- Recommended concentration: Administer undiluted into IV; sol is compatible with D_5W, LR and NS
- IV push rate: 15-30 sec

MECHANISM AND INDICATIONS
Mechanism: Antagonizes actions of benzodiazepines on the CNS, competitively inhibits activity at the benzodiazepine recognition site on the GABA/benzodiazepine receptor complex
Indications: Used to reverse sedative effects of benzodiazepines; can be used to reverse conscious sedation or anesthesia or in the case of benzodiazepine overdose

PHARMACOKINETICS
Onset: 1-2 min
Peak: 6-10 min
Half-life: 41-79 min (terminal)
Duration: Related to dosage and plasma concentration
Metabolism: Liver
Excretion: Urine
Therapeutic level: 3-6 ng/ml produces partial antagonism; 12-28 ng/ml produces complete antagonism

CONTRAINDICATIONS AND PRECAUTIONS
- Contraindicated with known hypersensitivity to this drug or benzodiazepines; serious cyclic antidepressant overdose; in pts given benzodiazepines for control of life-threatening condition (e.g., increased ICP, status epilepticus)
- Use cautiously with lactation, renal and hepatic disease, seizure disorders, head injury, labor and delivery, hypoventilation, panic disorder, drug and alcohol dependency, ambulatory pts

INTERACTIONS
Drug
- Increased risk of toxic effects (convulsion, cardiac arrhythmias)

✤ Available in Canada.

of other drugs taken in overdose (especially cyclic antidepressants) may emerge with reversal of benzodiazepines effected by flumazenil, in cases of mixed drug overdose

Lab
• Has not been evaluated

Nutrition
• Ingestion of food during IV infusion increases flumazenil clearance

SIDE EFFECTS

CNS: Dizziness, agitation, emotional lability, fatigue, confusion, convulsions, somnolence, anxiety, nervousness, headache, insomnia
CV: Hypertension, palpitations, cutaneous vasodilation, arrhythmias, bradycardia, tachycardia, chest pain
DERM: Increased sweating
EENT: Abnormal vision, blurred vision, tinnitus
GI: Nausea, vomiting, hiccups
RESP: Hyperventilation
Local: Pain at injection site
Other: Rigors

TOXICITY AND OVERDOSE

Clinical signs: Anxiety, agitation, increased muscle tone, hyperesthesia, possibly seizures (rare)
Treatment: Supportive care; treat seizures with barbiturates, benzodiazepines, and phenytoin with prompt resuscitation

PATIENT CARE MANAGEMENT

Assessment
• Assess history of hypersensitivity to flumazenil or related drugs
• Assess baseline VS, cardiac status, patency of airway

Interventions
• Administer through free-flowing IV into large vein
• Protect from injury, respiratory compromise if seizures occur
• Place in side-lying position if vomiting occurs
• In treatment of reversal of sedation or anesthesia, administer as a series of small injections to allow the practitioner to control reversal of sedation to the approximate endpoint desired and to minimize possibility of adverse effects
• In treatment of suspected benzodiazepine overdose, secure airway and IV access before administration of the drug; awaken patient gradually

> **NURSING ALERT**
> Not generally recommended for use in children (either for the reversal of sedation, the management of overdose, or the resuscitation of the newborns), as no clinical studies have been performed to determine the risks, benefits, and dosages
>
> Deaths have occurred with pts who received flumazenil in a variety of clinical settings; the majority occurred in pts with serious underlying disease or who had ingested large amounts of non-benzodiazepines (usually cyclic antidepressants) as part of the overdose

Evaluation
• Evaluate therapeutic response (decreased sedation)
• Evaluate for side effects, hypersensitivity
• Evaluate VS, cardiac status; monitor continuously
• Monitor for any development of seizures

PATIENT AND FAMILY EDUCATION

Teach/instruct
• About rationale for medication

Warn/advise
• To avoid alcohol or nonprescription drugs for 18-24 hr after medication
• To avoid hazardous activities for 18-24 hr after administration

STORAGE

• Discard mixed sol after 24 hr; store at room temp

---

flunisolide

Brand Name(s): Aerobid, AeroBid-M, Bronalide✿, Nasalide, Rhinalar (Flunisolide Nasal Mist)✿, Rhinaris-F✿, Syn-Flunisolide✿

Classification: Antiinflammatory corticosteroid; antiasthma

Pregnancy Category: C

AVAILABLE PREPARATIONS
Aerosol inhaler: 250 mcg/dose
Nasal spray: 25 mcg/spray

ROUTES AND DOSAGES
Asthma
Children > 4 yr: Aerosol inhaler, 2 inhalation bid; maximum of 4 inhalations/24 hr
Adults: 2 inhalations bid; maximum of 8 inhalations/24 hr
Allergic Rhinitis
Children > 4 yr: Nasal spray, 1 spray per nostril tid or 2 sprays per nostril bid; maximum of 4 sprays per nostril/24 hr
Adults: 2 sprays per nostril bid; maximum of 8 sprays per nostril/24 hr

MECHANISM AND INDICATIONS
Antiinflammatory: Precise mechanisms unclear, but likely inhibits activation of and mediator release from inflammatory cells associated with asthma; increases responsiveness of β receptors in airway smooth muscle; decreases bronchial activity with chronic use
Indications: Used in bronchial asthma in pts receiving systemic corticosteroids and pts who are poorly controlled on a non-steroid regimen; used increasingly for mild-to-moderate asthma as a first-line drug; used in seasonal or perennial rhinitis when conventional therapy has been unsatisfactory or not well tolerated

PHARMACOKINETICS
Onset of action: 1-2 wk (nasal spray); 1-4 wk (inhaler)
Peak: 10-30 min
Half-life: 1-2 hr
Metabolism: Liver
Excretion: Urine, feces

CONTRAINDICATIONS AND PRECAUTIONS
• Contraindicated as primary treatment of acute bronchospasm and status asthmaticus when intensive measures are required; hypersensitivity to any of the ingredients; recent nasal surgery, nasal injury, nasal ulcers (nasal spray)
• Use cautiously with pulmonary tuberculosis; untreated fungal, bacterial or systemic viral infections of the nose or respiratory tract, or ocular herpes simplex; in pts transferring from systemic steroids to flunisolide (deaths caused by adrenal insufficiency have occurred during and after transfer from systemic corticosteroids to flunisolide, as well as rebound bronchospasm; systemic steroids may be indicated in severe asthma, periods of stress, or emergency situations); with long term treatment; with lactation; in children < 4 yr (because safety has not been established)

SIDE EFFECTS
CNS: Irritability, nervousness, shakiness, restlessness, headache, dizziness, anxiety
CV: Flushing, tachycardia, palpitations
DERM: Rash
EENT: Nasal spray: nasal congestion, nasal itching, dryness, burning and irritation, sneezing, bloody mucus, epistaxis, nasal septal perforation (rare); aerosol: altered taste, dry mouth, hoarseness, irritation of tongue, throat, fungal infection of mouth or throat
GI: Nausea, vomiting, diarrhea, anorexia
RESP: Wheezing, dyspnea, cough
Other: Hypersensitivity reactions (urticaria, angioedema, rash)

F

TOXICITY AND OVERDOSAGE

• Acute overdosage is unlikely
Clinical signs: Hypercorticism (bruising, weight gain, mental disturbances, cushingoid features, acneiform lesions, menstrual irregularities) and hypothalamic–pituitary–adrenal suppression (decreased height, wt) may occur when used at excessive dosages
Treatment: Discontinue slowly (consistent with accepted procedures for discontinuing oral steroid therapy)

PATIENT CARE MANAGEMENT
Assessment

• Assess history of hypersensitivity to flunisolide, related drugs
• Assess respiratory status, HEENT
• Assess baseline VS
• Review other medications used
• Measure baseline height and wt

Interventions

• Follow manufacturer's instructions; see Chapter 3 for information regarding inhaler use
• Shake inhaler before use
• Administer bronchodilator (if prescribed) 5-15 min before flunisolide
• Administer 2nd inhalation of flunisolide (if prescribed) 1 min after 1st inhalation
• Have pt rinse mouth, offer oral care; do not allow pt to swallow water used for rinsing
• Follow manufacturer's instructions for intranasal use
• Have pt clear nose before intranasal use

NURSING ALERT

Deaths caused by adrenal insufficiency have occurred in asthma pts during and after transfer from systemic corticosteroids to aerosol

Not recommended for children <4 yr

Not for rapid relief of bronchospasm

Evaluation

• Evaluate therapeutic response (lessened respiratory or nasal symptoms; decreased need for systemic steroids; decreased need for bronchodilators, decongestants)
• Evaluate for side effects, hypersensitivity
• Evaluate respiratory status during treatment
• Evaluate compliance with regime
• Evaluate height, wt, development for any signs of growth retardation
• Evaluate oropharynx daily for symptoms of fungal infection
• Evaluate response, reduce dosage to smallest amount necessary to control symptoms after consulting prescriber
• Evaluate need for oral steroids, reduce oral steroid gradually (if transferring from oral to aerosol or inhaler), only under the care of the prescriber
• Evaluate pt for symptoms of systemic steroid withdrawal (if transferred from oral to inhaled steroid)
• Evaluate pts receiving treatment several mo or more for possible changes in nasal mucosa
• Evaluate for any diminished response to medication, report to provider for possible dosage change
• Evaluate pt for systemic effects of flunisolide (steroid effects) such as mental disturbance, wt gain, bruising, cushingoid features, decreased growth velocity; report to prescriber for possible dosage change or slow discontinuation

PATIENT AND FAMILY EDUCATION
Teach/instruct

• Shake aerosol inhaler or nasal spray before use
• About proper use of aerosol inhaler or nasal sprays
• To rinse, dry inhaler between uses
• That mild transient nasal stinging, burning common with intranasal use

---

• That local fungal infections of oropharynx, larynx, esophagus are possible; to check nose, mouth, throat daily and report symptoms to provider
• That rinsing mouth, using good oral hygiene can prevent infections of mouth; not to swallow water used for rinsing mouth
• That therapeutic effect of medication may be diminished if the canister is cold

Warn/advise

• To contact provider if no clinical improvement is seen by 3 wk (nasal spray) or 4 wk (aerosol inhaler), and drug will gradually be discontinued
• To comply with regime, that regular use is required to achieve full benefit
• About need to work closely with provider to titrate drug to lowest maintenance dosage needed to control symptoms
• That drug is *not* a bronchodilator, is not indicated for rapid relief of bronchospasm
• Not to exceed recommended dosage to prevent systemic effects, hypothalamic–pituitary–adrenal axis suppression
• That symptoms of steroid withdrawal may occur (lassitude, muscle joint pain, depression, nausea or vomiting, low B/P) with previous use of oral steroids by pt; hypothalamic–pituitary–adrenal axis suppression may last up to 1 yr; to carry a card indicating potential need for supplemental systemic steroids (because of hypothalamic–pituitary–adrenal axis suppression) in stress, acute asthma, trauma, surgery, infection (especially gastroenteritis); provider should be notified immediately; transfer from oral to inhaled steroids may unmask symptoms suppressed by oral dose (e.g., eczema)
• To administer bronchodilator (if prescribed) *before* use of this drug for maximum penetration into bronchial tree, to allow several min to elapse between inhalation of the 2 drugs

• That administration of an oral decongestant or nasal vasoconstrictor may be indicated if pt's nasal passages are blocked; to contact provider
• To avoid chicken pox or measles exposure; to report any exposure to care provider
• That wheezing that does not respond to treatment with bronchodilators and flunisolide should be reported immediately as systemic steroids may be indicated
• About symptoms of hypercorticism and hypothalamic–pituitary–adrenal axis suppression; notify provider if these occur
• That long-term effects of drug are unknown

STORAGE

• Store nasal spray, aerosol at room temp
• Do not puncture; do not use or store aerosol near heat or open flame; temp >120° may cause aerosol canister to explode
• Discard open containers after 3 mo
• Keep out of reach of children

---

fluocinonide

Brand Name(s): FAPct, Lidex✤, Lidex-E, Lyderm✤, Tiamol✤, Trisyn✤

Classification: Topical antiinflammatory

Pregnancy Category: C

AVAILABLE PREPARATIONS:
Cream, gel, oint, sol: 0.05%

ROUTES AND DOSAGES
Children and adults: Top, apply sparingly to affected areas bid-qid

MECHANISM AND INDICATIONS
Mechanism: Stimulates production of enzymes needed to reduce inflammatory response; decreases cell proliferation
Indications: Used for treatment of inflammatory and pruritic derma-

---

✤ Available in Canada.

toses (psoriasis, eczema, pruritus, contact dermatitis)

PHARMACOKINETICS

Absorption: Amount absorbed depends on amount applied; effectiveness depends on vehicle used, highest to lowest effectiveness oint, gel, cream, sol, amount absorbed depends on nature of skin at site of application—on thick skin (palms, soles, elbows, knees) absorption is minimal, on thin skin (face, eyelids, genitals) absorption is high; any absorbed drug is removed rapidly from circulation, distributed into muscle, skin, liver, intestines, kidney
Distribution: Distributed and metabolized primarily in skin
Metabolism: Liver
Excretion: Urine, feces

CONTRAINDICATIONS AND PRECAUTIONS

• Contraindicated with known hypersensitivity to drug or its components; with viral, fungal, or tubercular lesions
• Use cautiously with impaired circulation (risk of skin ulceration); in children (increased systemic absorption could lead to Cushing syndrome, intracranial hypertension, and hypothalamic–pituitary–adrenal axis suppression); use the least amount of drug needed for as short a time as possible

SIDE EFFECTS

Local: Burning, pruritus, hypopigmentation, atrophy, striae, allergic contact dermatitis

Significant systemic absorption may cause the following:

CNS: Euphoria, insomnia, headache, pseudotumor cerebri, mental changes, restlessness
CV: Edema, hypertension
DERM: Acneiform eruptions, delayed healing
ENDO: Adrenal suppression
GI: Increased appetite, peptic irritation and ulcer

TOXICITY AND OVERDOSE

Clinical signs: No information available

Treatment: No information available

PATIENT CARE MANAGEMENT

Assessment

• Assess skin for appropriateness of application; do not apply to skin with skin ulcerations or viral, fungal, or tubercular lesions
• Assess for side effects after application, especially striae, increased inflammation, atrophy, infection

Interventions

• Apply small amount sparingly to clean, dry skin lesion(s) for as short a period as possible; stop drug if signs of systemic absorption appear; do not apply occlusive dressings over drug unless severe or resistant dermatoses; occlusive dressings will increase absorption

---

NURSING ALERT
In children, limit topical application to smallest effective dosage

---

Evaluation

• Evaluate therapeutic response (decreased inflammation, pruritus)
• Inspect skin for infection, striae, atrophy

PATIENT AND FAMILY TEACHING

Teach/instruct

• To use as directed at prescribed intervals for prescribed length of time; *do not over-apply*
• To apply sparingly in a light film, to rub into affected area(s) gently
• Not to use occlusive dressing over area of application; a diaper may be used if changed regularly and not in place >8 hr
• To call provider if side effects occur or if skin not improved in 1 wk
• About side effects, especially if over-applied
• To wash and dry hands before, after application
• To avoid prolonged application

✤ Available in Canada.

on face, skin folds, genital area; to notify care provider of hypersensitivity reactions

STORAGE
• Store at room temp

---

fluoride
Brand Name(s): Fluorigard, Fluoritab, Luride, Pediaflor
Classification: Mineral, antimicrobial
Pregnancy Category: C

AVAILABLE PREPARATIONS
Drops: 0.5 mg/ml
Rinse: 0.09%
Tabs: 1.1 mg (0.5 mg fluoride ion), 2.2 mg (1 mg fluoride ion)
Gel: 1.1%

ROUTES AND DOSAGES
<0.3 ppm Fluoride in Water Supply
Birth-6 mo: None
6 mo-3 yr: 0.25 mg/24 hr
3-6 yr: 0.5 mg/24 hr
6-16 yr: 1 mg/24 hr
0.3-0.6 ppm Fluoride in Water Supply
Birth-6 mo: None
6 mo-3 yr: None
3-6 yr: 0.25 mg/24 hr
6-16 yr: 0.5 mg/24 hr
>0.6 ppm Fluoride in Water Supply
Birth-6 mo: None
6 mo-3 yr: None
3-6 yr: None
6-16 yr: None
Dental Rinse
6-12 yr: 5-10 ml
Adults: 10 ml

MECHANISM AND INDICATIONS
Mechanism: Reduces acid production of bacteria and increases tooth resistance to acid dissolution; acts on teeth before and after eruption to provide a resistance to bacteria and decay
Indications: Used to control cavities when water supply is low in fluoride content; can also be used to treat osteoporosis and decrease bone pain in some neoplastic diseases; for tooth hypersensitivity to mechanical, electrical, or temperature stimuli

PHARMACOKINETICS
Metabolism: 50% deposited in teeth and bone
Excretion: Urine, feces

CONTRAINDICATIONS AND PRECAUTIONS
• Contraindicated with low Na diet, hypersensitivity to fluoride, or if drinking water has fluoride content >0.6 ppm
• Use cautiously as rinse for children <3 yr or tabs for children <6 yr; some products may contain tartrazine and should not be administered to those sensitive to yellow dye # 5; do not exceed recommended dosage

INTERACTIONS
Drug
• Monitor use with other OTC or prescription medications containing fluoride
• Decreased absorption with use of Ca, aluminum, or Mg
Nutrition
• Absorption may be decreased with use of dairy products, Ca supplements

SIDE EFFECTS
DERM: Rash
GI: Nausea, vomiting
Other: Stained teeth

TOXICITY AND OVERDOSE
• Lethal dose for children is 500 mg; for adults it is 70-140 mg/kg
Clinical signs: Hypersalivation, salty or soapy taste, epigastric pain, nausea, vomiting, diarrhea, rash, muscle weakness, tremor, seizures, cardiac failure, respiratory distress, shock
Treatment: Administer gastric lavage with calcium chloride, calcium hydroxide solution, or aluminum hydroxide to bind fluoride; administer large quantities of mild solution at frequent intervals; provide supportive care

PATIENT CARE MANAGEMENT
Assessment
• Assess history of hypersensitivity to fluoride, yellow dye # 5
• Assess for use of other medications or other forms of fluoride to assure optimal absorption, use
• Assess fluoride content of water supply

Interventions
• Administer PO supplement as prescribed with food, not dairy products

> **NURSING ALERT**
> Do not exceed recommended dosage; overdose can be lethal

Evaluation
• Monitor for signs of hypersensitivity, side effects, signs of overdosing (see toxicity information)

PATIENT AND FAMILY EDUCATION
Teach/instruct
• To take as directed at prescribed intervals for prescribed length of time
• To evaluate water supply, other medications or OTC drugs, and multiple vitamin or mineral supplements for overdosing

Warn/advise
• To notify dentist if teeth become stained
• Not to use 1 mg tabs for children <6 yr or rinse for children <3 yr
• To keep medication away from children to avoid potential overdose

STORAGE
• Store in tightly covered container at room temp
• Protect from freezing

> **fluorometholone**
>
> **Brand Name(s):** Fluor-Op Ophthalmic, FML Liquifilm Ophthalmic, FML Ointment
>
> **Classification:** Ophthalmic antiinflammatory agent (corticosteroid)
>
> **Pregnancy Category:** C

AVAILABLE PREPARATIONS
Ophthal sol: 0.1%, 0.25%
Ophthal oint: 0.1%

ROUTES AND DOSAGES
Ophthalmic
Children > 2 yr and adults: Ophthal sol, instill 1-2 gtt of 0.1% or 0.25% sol into conjunctival sac bid-qid; may use q1h during first 1-2 days if necessary; oint, instill 1 cm strip into conjunctival sac q4h in severe cases or bid-tid in mild-moderate cases

MECHANISM AND INDICATIONS
Antiinflammatory mechanism: Inhibits inflammatory response by suppression of migration of leukocytes and reversal of increased capillary permeability
Indications: Used to treat inflammatory conditions of the eye including keratitis, iritis, cyclitis, conjunctivitis

PHARMACOKINETICS
Metabolism: Liver
Excretion: Urine, feces

CONTRAINDICATIONS AND PRECAUTIONS
• Contraindicated with known hypersensitivity to any component (some products contain sulfites); with ocular fungal, viral, tubercular, or acute untreated purulent bacterial infections
• Use cautiously with children < 2 yr because of increased risk of systemic effects; with corneal abrasions, glaucoma, cataracts, DM, pregnancy

SIDE EFFECTS
EENT: Transient stinging, burning, corneal thinning, increased intraocular pressure, glaucoma,

---

damage to optic nerve, defects in visual acuity, cataracts
Other: Adrenal suppression with excessive dosages or long-term use

PATIENT CARE MANAGEMENT

Assessment

- Assess history of hypersensitivity to any component (some products contain sulfites)
- Assess eye inflammation

Interventions

- Shake sol well before instillation; wash hands before, after application; cleanse crusts, discharge from eye before application; after instillation, apply gentle pressure to lacrimal sac for 1 min to minimize systemic absorption; wipe excess medication from eye; do not flush medication from eye
- Gradually taper drug if used for long-term therapy to prevent disease exacerbation

> **NURSING ALERT**
> Discontinue drug if signs of local irritation, infection, systemic absorption, hypersensitivity, or visual changes develop

Evaluation

- Evaluate therapeutic response (decreased inflammation); discontinue if no improvement after several days of treatment
- Monitor for symptoms of adrenal suppression
- Monitor for signs of skin irritation or ulceration, hypersensitivity, infection

PATIENT AND FAMILY EDUCATION

Teach/instruct

- To use as directed at prescribed intervals for prescribed length of time

Warn/advise

- To notify care provider of hypersensitivity, side effects
- To notify care provider if no improvement after 1 wk of treatment, if condition worsens, or if

eye pain, itching, or swelling develops
- To wear dark glasses to reduce photophobia
- To taper medication after long-term therapy
- Not to use ophthal preparations unless prescribed by care provider
- Not to use this medication for any new eye inflammation

STORAGE

- Store at room temp in tightly closed container
- Protect from light
- Do not freeze

5-fluorouracil

Brand Name(s): Adrucil✤, Efudex (5-Fluororacil)✤, Fluoroplex✤, Fluorouracil Injection, 5-FU

Classification: Antineoplastic, antimetabolite

Pregnancy Category: D

AVAILABLE PREPARATIONS

Inj: 500 mg powder

ROUTES AND DOSAGES

- Dosage may vary in response to diagnosis, extent of disease, concurrent or previous therapy, protocol guidelines, physiological parameters; consult current literature, protocol recommendations
- Multiple dosing regimens have been developed including weekly IV bolus dosing with or without a loading dose, continuous infusions over 4-5 days or up to 6 wk
Children and Adults: IV conventional bolus dose (based on lean body weight) 400-500 mg/m^2 (12 mg/kg) qd for 4 days as daily bolus (or up to 1000 mg/m^2/24 hr for 4-5 days as continuous infusion), followed by weekly maintenance dosage 200-250 mg/m^2 (6 mg/kg) qod for 4 doses, repeating cycle in 4 wk or 500-600 mg/m^2 (15 mg/kg) weekly as bolus injection or continuous infusion; maximum daily dose 800 mg (per manufacturer);

with continuous infusion, amounts as high as 1-2 g/24 hr have been administered without increased adverse effects; prolonged infusion may maximize effectiveness

• An additional series of dosing regimens have been developed around the belief that leucovorin has a synergistic effect with this drug

IV administration

• Recommended concentration: Dilute in convenient volume of D_5W

• IV push rate: Over 1-2 min

MECHANISM AND INDICATIONS

Mechanism: Acts as false pyrimidine base-inhibiting formation of DNA-specific nucleotide base thymidine, action ultimately interferes with synthesis of both DNA and RNA

Indications: Used in a wide variety of adult solid tumors that are not amenable to surgical resection; not used often in children

PHARMACOKINETICS

Distribution: Widely to all areas of body water (including CNS) by passive diffusion

Metabolism: Liver; clearance lower in females than in males

Excretion: 15% of dose excreted intact in urine within 6 hr; 60%-80% excreted through lungs as respiratory CO_2

CONTRAINDICATIONS AND PRECAUTIONS

• Contraindicated with pregnancy, lactation; hypersensitivity to drug; poor nutritional state; familial history of dihydropyrimidine dehydrogenase (familial pyrimidinemia) because it may cause severe neurotoxicity; intrathecal administration

INTERACTIONS

Drug

• Increased efficacy, side effects of 5-FU possible with leucovorin

• Altered 5-FU catabolism with prednisolone (uncertain clinical relevance)

• Decreased toxicity to normal tissue with allopurinol (uncertain clinical relevance)

• Mutual antagonism between 5-FU and methotrexate

• Potentiates action of anticoagulants

Lab

• Transient increase in AST, bilirubin, LDH possible

INCOMPATIBILITIES

• Drugs with acidic formulation; methotrexate, diazepam, doxorubicin, cisplatin, cytarabine, droperidol; drug is compatible with heparin and stable over 7 day-period in ambulatory infusion pump

SIDE EFFECTS

CNS: Headache, visual disturbances, dizziness, euphoria, aphasia, acute cerebellar syndrome that may persist beyond time of treatment

CV: Discoloration of venous tract, MI, angina, arrhythmias, ECG changes, cardiogenic shock, sudden death

DERM: Reversible alopecia, partial loss of nails, hyperpigmentation, pruritus, burning, swelling, maculopapular rash on extremities and trunk, palmar-plantar erythrodysesthesia

EENT: Lacrimation

GI: Nausea and vomiting (moderately emetogenic), stomatitis approximately 5-8 days after therapy, diarrhea, proctitis, esophagitis, gastric ulceration

HEME: Leukopenia with nadir at 9-14 days, thrombocytopenia with nadir at 7-14 days

TOXICITIES AND OVERDOSE

Clinical signs: Prolonged myelosuppression, intractable vomiting/or diarrhea

Treatment: Supportive measures including blood transfusions, hydration, nutritional supplementation, broad-spectrum antibiotic therapy in event of febrile neutropenia, electrolyte replacement

---

PATIENT CARE MANAGEMENT
Assessment
- Assess history of hypersensitivity to 5-fluorouracil
- Assess history of previous treatment with antineoplastics or radiation therapy (especially those that may predispose pt to increased risk of hepatic toxicity)
- Assess baseline VS
- Assess baseline CBC, differential, platelet count
- Assess baseline renal function (BUN, creatinine), liver function (alk phos, LDH, AST, ALT, bilirubin)
- Assess success of previous antiemetic therapy

Interventions
- Administer antiemetic therapy before chemotherapy
- Ensure absolute patency of IV before administration
- Do not place IV over joint; if extravasation occurs, joint may become immobilized
- Provide supportive measures to maintain hemostasis, fluid, electrolyte, nutritional balance

> **NURSING ALERT**
>
> Drug is potent vesicant; should only be administered into an unquestionably patent IV that is not over a joint; if extravasation occurs, area may be infiltrated with hyaluronidase.
>
> Inadvertent intrathecal administration of drug has been fatal

Evaluate
- Evaluate therapeutic response (radiologic or clinical demonstration of tumor regression)
- Evaluate efficacy of antiemetic therapy
- Monitor baseline renal function (BUN, creatinine), liver function (alk phos, LDH, AST, ALT, bilirubin) before each course
- Monitor CBC, differential, platelet count weekly (at least)

PATIENT AND FAMILY EDUCATION
Teach/instruct
- To have pt well hydrated before, after chemotherapy
- About importance of follow-up visits to monitor blood counts, serum chemistry values
- To take accurate temp; rectal temp contraindicated
- To notify care provider of signs of bleeding (bruising, epistaxis, bleeding gums), infection (fever, sore throat, fatigue)

Warn/advise
- About impact of body changes that may occur (hair loss, hyperpigmentation, nail ridging), how to minimize changes (wigs, caps, scarves, long sleeves)
- To avoid OTC preparations containing aspirin
- To report any alterations in behavior, sensation, perception; help to develop a plan of care to manage side effects, stress of illness or treatment
- To immediately report any signs of pain or irritation at injection site
- That good oral hygiene with very soft toothbrush is imperative
- That dental work be delayed until blood counts returns to baseline, with permission of caretaker
- To avoid contact with known viral, bacterial illnesses
- That close household contacts of child not be immunized with live polio virus; use inactivated form
- That children on chemotherapy not receive immunization until immune system recovers sufficiently to mount necessary antibody response
- To report exposure to chicken pox in susceptible child immediately
- To report reactivation of herpes zoster virus (shingles) immediately
- If appropriate, ways to preserve reproductive patterns, sexuality (sperm banking, contraceptives)

F

Encourage
• Provision of nutritious food intake; consider nutrition consultation
• To use top anesthetics to control the discomfort of mucositis; avoid spicy foods, commercial mouthwashes

STORAGE
• Store at room temp
• Protect from light

---

fluoxetine, fluoxetine hydrochloride

Brand Name(s): Prozac❦

Classification: Selective serotonin reuptake inhibitor; antidepressant

Pregnancy Category: B

AVAILABLE PREPARATIONS
Caps: 10 mg, 20 mg
Pulvules: 10 mg, 20 mg
Liquid: (mint flavor) 20 mg/5 ml

DOSAGES AND ROUTES
Adolescents: PO initial dosage of 5-10 mg/24 hr is increased by 5-10 mg every 1-2 wk as tolerated; maximum 40 mg/24 hr
Adults: PO initial 20 mg/24 hr q 1-3 days as a single AM dose; may increase after several wk by 10 mg/24 hr increments; doses of 5 mg/24 hr have been used for initial treatment; maximum 80 mg/24 hr
• Safety and effectiveness for use in children <18 yr have not been established
• Preliminary experience in children 6-17 yrs has been reported, using initial dosage of 10 mg/24 hr
• Dosages >20 mg should be divided and given in AM and at noon

MECHANISM AND INDICATIONS
Mechanism: Fluoxetine is a non-tricyclic selective serotonin reuptake inhibitor; inhibits CNS neuron uptake of serotonin, but not of norepinephrine or dopamine
Indications: For use in treating depression (especially when there is a greater risk of drug overdose); unlabeled uses, addictive disorders, anorexia, anxiety, undifferentiated attention deficit disorder (ADD), bulimia, obsessive-compulsive disorders (especially those associated with Tourette syndrome); obesity

PHARMACOKINETICS
Onset of action: Continuous use on a regular schedule for 6 wk is usually necessary to determine effectiveness in relieving depression, side effects
Peak: Within 4-8 hr
Absorption: Oral, well absorbed
Half-life: 2-7 days
Metabolism: Liver
Excretion: Urine

CONTRAINDICATIONS AND PRECAUTIONS
• Contraindicated with hypersensitivity to fluoxetine or any component of this medication; within 14 days of any MAOI
• Use cautiously with anxiety, changes in appetite and wt, cardiac dysfunction, DM, history of drug abuse, electroconvulsive therapy, recent heart attack, unstable heart disease, concomitant illness, insomnia, impaired kidney or liver function, mania, Parkinson's disease, history of seizures, history of attempted suicide or at high risk for suicide, pregnancy or planning pregnancy, add or initiate other antidepressants with caution for up to 5 wk after stopping fluoxetine

INTERACTIONS
Drug
• Increased effects of diazepam and digitalis preparations, tricyclic antidepressants, trazodone, warfarin
• Do not use within 14 days of MAOIs; could lead to dangerous elevations of B/P and agitation, confusion, hyperpyrexia, tremor, seizures, delirium, coma, death
• Psychomotor agitation and GI distress with L-tryptophan
• Decreased effects of buspirone

possible; may displace highly protein-bound drugs
• Interacts with isocarboxazid, lithium, phenelzine, selegiline
• Increased the risk of hypoglycemic reactions with insulin or oral hypoglycemics; monitor BG and urine sugar levels carefully

Lab
• Increased serum bilirubin, BG, alk phos
• Decreased BG, Na, VMA, 5-HIAA
• Falsely elevated urinary catecholamines
• Abnormal blood counts

Nutrition
• The 20 mg pulvules contain FD&C Blue No. 1
• Do not drink alcohol

SIDE EFFECTS
CNS: Psychomotor agitation, anxiety, impaired concentration, dizziness, abnormal dreams, drowsiness, fatigue, headache, insomnia, nervousness, sedation, tremors, euphoria, excitability, EPS, hallucinations, lightheadedness, mania, psychosis, restlessness, seizures, sensation disturbances, suicidal ideation, weakness, apathy, delusions; behavioral disinhibition; impulsivity
CV: Hot flashes, palpitations, 1st-degree AV block, bradycardia, chest pain, hemorrhage, hypertension, MI, tachycardia, thrombophlebitis
DERM: Itching, rash, sweating, acne, flushing, hair loss, hives (approximately 4% of pts develop a rash or hives; most improve promptly with discontinuation of fluoxetine or with treatment with antihistamines or steroids)
EENT: Ear or eye pain, dry mouth, photophobia, taste changes, tinnitus, vision disturbances
GI: Anorexia, constipation, cramps, diarrhea, gas, dry mouth, nausea, upset stomach, vomiting, indigestion, wt loss
GU: Painful menstruation, changes in sex drive, frequent urination, UTIs, amenorrhea, impotence, sexual dysfunction; proteinuria
RESP: Bronchitis, cough, dyspnea, nasal congestion, pharyngitis, pneumonia, upper respiratory tract infections (cold, flu, sore throat); sinus headache, sinus infection, hyperventilation, asthma; respiratory distress
Other: Allergy, chills, joint and muscle pain, viral infections, anaphylactoid reactions, arthritis, back pain, carpal tunnel syndrome, hypoglycemia, hyponatremia, leg and arm pain, serum sickness-like syndrome (fever, weakness, joint pain and swelling, swollen lymph glands, fluid retention, rash/hives), twitching

TOXICITY AND OVERDOSE
Clinical signs: Agitation, excitement, nausea, restlessness, seizures, vomiting
Treatment: Supportive care

PATIENT CARE MANAGEMENT
Assessment
• Assess history of hypersensitivity to drug
• Obtain general physical examination
• Assess for risk factors, diabetes mellitus, history of drug abuse, risk for suicide, pregnancy, use of other antidepressants within 5 wk
• Assess ECG for flattening of T-wave, bundle branch, AV block, arrhythmias in cardiac pts
Interventions
• Usually administered PO as a single AM dose, but if there are side effects, it may be divided and administered in AM and noon
• Tab may be crushed if unable to swallow medication whole
• Cap may be opened for administration, contents may be mixed with food
• Doses of 5-10 mg may prove effective and better-tolerated; if smaller doses are needed than are available, cap contents may be mixed well with orange juice or apple juice and refrigerated
• May be given without regard to food

- Give with food or milk if GI symptoms occur
- Increase fluids and fiber in diet if constipation occurs
- Rinse with water, take sips of fluid, sugarless gum, or hard candy for dry mouth
- Diabetic pts should monitor BG levels daily; prescriber should be notified if hypoglycemia or hyperglycemia occur
- Withhold drug if electroconvulsive therapy (ECT) is to be used to treat depression

NURSING ALERT

Do not use within 14 days of MAOIs; could lead to dangerous elevations of B/P and agitation, confusion, hyperpyrexia, tremor, seizures, delirium, coma, death

Evaluation
- Evaluate therapeutic response (ability to function in daily activities, to sleep throughout the night; symptoms of depression, mania); maximum therapeutic antidepressant effects usually occur after more than 4 wk
- Evaluate mental status (mood, sensorium, affect, impulsiveness, suicidal ideation, psychiatric symptoms)
- Assess B/P and pulse; if systolic B/P drops 20 mm Hg hold drug, notify prescriber
- Obtain cardiac enzymes and evaluate ECG for flattening of T-wave, bundle branch, AV block, and arrhythmias if pt is receiving long-term therapy
- Monitor and document wt, blood Na, BG
- Therapeutic reference range: fluoxetine 100-800 ng/ml, norfluoxetine 100-600 ng/ml
- In diabetes, hypoglycemia has occurred during therapy, and hyperglycemia has developed following discontinuation; dosage of insulin or other BG-lowering drug may need to be adjusted when fluoxetine is started or discontinued

- Resolution of adverse reactions after discontinuation may be slow because of long half-life
- Continue periodic evaluation of response and dosage adjustment if fluoxetine is used over months to years
- Add or initiate other antidepressants with caution for up to 5 wk after stopping fluoxetine

PATIENT AND FAMILY EDUCATION
Teach/instruct
- To take as directed at prescribed intervals for prescribed length of time
- That medication is most helpful when used as part of a comprehensive multimodal treatment program
- Not to stop taking this medication without prescriber approval
- That therapeutic effects may take 3-4 wk
- To increase fluids and fiber in diet if constipation occurs
- To ensure that medication is swallowed
- To take missed doses as soon as possible; if several hr have passed or if it is nearing time for the next dose, do not double dose in order to catch up (unless advised to do so by provider); if more than one dose is missed or it is necessary to establish a new dosage schedule, contact prescriber or pharmacist
Warn/advise
- To notify prescriber immediately if rash or hives develop, if anxiety or nervousness becomes troublesome, or if extreme appetite loss develops
- To tell prescriber or pharmacist if taking or planning to take any OTC or prescription medications with fluoxetine; dosages of one or both of the drugs may need to be modified, or a different drug prescribed
- That fluoxetine may cause dizziness or drowsiness; be careful on bicycles, skates, skateboards, while driving, or with other activities requiring alertness

- To avoid ingesting alcohol, other CNS depressants
- To notify prescriber if pregnant, breastfeeding, or planning to become pregnant

STORAGE
- Store at room temp
- Do not freeze

---

fluoxymesterone

Brand Name(s): Android-F, Halotestin✤, Hysterone, Ora-Testryl

Classification: Androgen

Controlled Substance Schedule III

Pregnancy Category: X

AVAILABLE PREPARATIONS
Tabs: 2 mg, 5 mg, 10 mg

ROUTES AND DOSAGES
Treatment of Delayed Puberty
PO 2.5-10 mg qd for up to 6 mo

MECHANISM AND INDICATIONS
Mechanism: Stimulates receptors in androgen-responsive organs; accelerates linear growth rate in children
Indications: Replacement therapy in conditions associated with insufficient edogenous testosterone, delayed puberty in males, Turner syndrome

PHARMACOKINETICS
Half-life: 9.2 hr
Metabolism: Liver

CONTRAINDICATIONS AND PRECAUTIONS
- Contraindicated with pregnancy, lactation, hypersensitivity to fluoxymesterone, severe renal, cardiac, or hepatic disease, males with breast or prostatic cancer, undiagnosed genital bleeding, tartrazine sensitivity (contained in brands Halotestin and Ora-Testryl)
- Use cautiously with children (can accelerate bone age without concomitant linear growth, leading to premature fusion of the epiphysis)

INTERACTIONS
Drug
- Increased sensitivity to oral anticoagulants
- Increased serum levels of oxyphenbutazone when used concurrently
Lab
- Altered thyroid function tests

SIDE EFFECTS
CNS: Headache, anxiety, depression, generalized paresthesia, altered libido
CV: Edema
DERM: Hirsutism, male pattern baldness, seborrhea, acne, flushing, sweating, oily skin
GI: Gastroenteritis, nausea, vomiting, diarrhea, constipation, change in appetite, wt gain, cholestatic jaundice, cholestatic hepatitis
GU: Bladder irritability, priapism, virilization in females, vaginitis, menstrual irregularity
HEME: Polycythemia, suppression of clotting factors II, V, VII, X
Other: Hypercalcemia, hepatocellular cancer (long term use)

PATIENT CARE MANAGEMENT
Assessment
- Assess history of hypersensitivity to fluoxymesterone
- Assess growth rate, bone age, pubertal status (Tanner stage), wt, K^+, Na, Cl, Ca, ALT, AST, bilirubin
Interventions
- Administer with food to decrease GI upset
Evaluation
- Evaluate therapeutic response (monitor pubertal status/bone age for appropriate progression, increased growth velocity may occur as puberty progresses)
- Evaluate for signs of virilization in females (increased libido, deepening of voice, breast tissue, enlarged clitoris, menstrual irregularities), in males evaluate for gynecomastia, impotence, testicular atrophy

---

✤ Available in Canada.

- Monitor for signs of hypoglycemia in diabetics
- Monitor for edema, hypertension, cardiac symptoms, jaundice
- Monitor bone age q 6 mo (bone age advancement should not exceed increase in linear growth)
- Monitor for priapism (may need to decrease dosage)
- Monitor K$^+$, Na, Cl, Ca, ALT, AST, bilirubin
- Monitor for signs of hypercalcemia (lethargy, polyuria, polydipsia, nausea, vomiting, constipation)

PATIENT AND FAMILY EDUCATION
Teach/instruct
- To take as directed at prescribed intervals for prescribed length of time
- Anticipated changes in body image with adolescents

Warn/advise
- To notify care provider of hypersensitivity, side effects (GI distress, diarrhea, jaundice, priapism, menstrual irregularities)
- Not to discontinue medication suddenly
- That excess hair growth in females and acne are reversible with discontinuation of medication
- That sexually active pts should practice contraception when taking this medication
- About dangers of steroid use to improve athletic performance

STORAGE
- Store at room temp

---

folic acid (vitamin B$_9$)
Brand Name(s): Apo-Folic✿, Folvite✿

Classification: Water soluble vitamin, antianemic

Pregnancy Category: A (C if dosage exceeds RDA)

AVAILABLE PREPARATIONS
Tabs: 0.1 mg, 0.4 mg, 0.8 mg, 1.0 mg
Inj: 5 mg/ml, 10 mg/ml

ROUTES AND DOSAGE
Dietary Supplement
See Appendix F, Table of Recommended Daily Dietary Allowances

PO
Deficiency
Infants: PO/IM/SC/IV 15 mcg/kg/dose or 50 mcg/24 hr
Children: PO/IM/SC/IV initial 1 mg/24 hr; maintenance 0.1-0.3 mg/24 hr
Children >11 yr and adults: PO/IM/SC/IV initial 1 mg/24 hr; maintenance 0.5 mg/24 hr
Women of childbearing age, pregnancy: PO/IM/SC/IV 0.4 mg/24 hr; with personal history or immediate family history of neural tube defect, 4 mg/24 hr

IV administration
- Recommended concentration: Undiluted
- Direct infusion rate: Over 30-60 sec; may be added to continuous infusion

MECHANISM AND INDICATIONS
Mechanism: Acts as a coenzyme important for normal erythropoiesis; also involved in pyrimidine nucleotide and purine synthesis and amino acid transaminations
Indications: Used in the treatment and prevention of megaloblastic and macrocytic anemias caused by folate deficiency; during prepregnancy and pregnancy to reduce risk of neural tube defect

PHARMACOKINETICS
Peak: 0.5-1 hr
Metabolism: Liver
Excretion: Urine

CONTRAINDICATIONS AND PRECAUTIONS
- Contraindicated in pts with allergy to folic acid or leucovorin; not effective for pernicious, aplastic, or normocytic anemias; monitor use because large doses may mask vitamin B$_{12}$ deficiency
- Use cautiously in pts with alcoholism or taking antimetabolite drugs

---

✿ Available in Canada.

INTERACTIONS
Drug
• Decreased phenytoin concentration possible
• Decreased response possible with chloramphenicol
• Methotrexate, pyrimethamine, trimethoprim are folic acid antagonists and prevent formation of the active metabolite
• Increased need with phenytoin, barbiturates, and primidone
• Impaired folate metabolism with oral contraceptives
Lab
• False decrease with *Lactobacillus casei* assay on antiinfectives

SIDE EFFECTS
DERM: Pruritis, skin redness
RESP: Difficulty breathing
Other: General malaise

PATIENT CARE MANAGEMENT
Assessment
• Assess history of hypersensitivity to folic acid
• Obtain baseline vitamin B_{12} by using blood level tests and Schilling test to rule out pernicious anemia
• Assess for other medication use to ensure optimal absorption and use
• Assess for other vitamin deficiencies
• Assess medical history as persons with bowel disease, malignant disease, burns, chronic hemolytic anemia, decreased hepatic stores, alcoholism, liver disease, and pregnant women have increased requirements for folic acid
Interventions
• Administer PO unless pt has severe malabsorption
• Provide nutritional counseling to ensure adequate folic acid intake

> **NURSING ALERT**
> Evaluate for pernicious anemia before therapy because folic acid can mask this diagnosis and cause irreversible neurologic damage to result

Evaluation
• Evaluate therapeutic response (serum folate levels 6-15 mcg/ml, wt gain, decreased fatigability)
• Monitor Hgb, Hct, reticulocyte count

PATIENT AND FAMILY EDUCATION
Teach/instruct
• To take as directed at prescribed intervals for prescribed length of time
Warn/advise
• To notify care provider of hypersensitivity, side effects
Encourage
• A well-balanced diet should contain adequate amounts of folic acid; good sources of folic acid are green vegetables, potatoes, cereal, cereal products, fruit, organ meats; see Appendix F, Table of Recommended Daily Dietary Allowances

STORAGE
• Store at room temp in a tightly closed container
• Protect from light, heat, and moisture

---

foscarnet sodium
Brand Name(s): Foscavir
Classification: Antiviral (inorganic pyrophosphate organic analog)
Pregnancy Category: C

AVAILABLE PREPARATIONS
Inj: 24 mg/ml

ROUTES AND DOSAGES
CMV Retinitis
Adolescents and adults: IV induction 180 mg/kg/24 hr divided q8h

for 14-21 days; maintenance dose 90-120 mg/kg/24 hr qd

Acyclovir-resistant HSV Infection

Adolescents and adults: 40 mg/kg/dose q8h or 40-60 mg/kg/dose q12h for up to 3 wk or until lesions heal

IV administration

• Recommended concentration: Central venous catheter 24 mg/ml; peripheral vein, must be further diluted with D_5W or NS to maximum concentration 12 mg/ml

• Maximum concentration: Continuous infusion, over 1 hr at maximum rate 60 mg/kg/dose or over 2 hr at maximum rate 120 mg/kg/dose

MECHANISM AND INDICATIONS

Antiviral mechanism: Inhibits DNA synthesis by interfering with viral DNA polymerase

Indications: Treatment of CMV retinitis in patients with AIDS, acyclovir-resistant herpes simplex virus, and herpes zoster infections

PHARMACOKINETICS

Distribution: Minimal penetration across blood–brain barrier

Half-life: 3-4.5 hr

Excretion: Urine

Therapeutic level: CMV 150 mcg/ml

CONTRAINDICATIONS AND PRECAUTIONS

• Contraindicated with known hypersensitivity to foscarnet

• Use cautiously with renal impairment, electrolyte imbalance, neurologic or cardiac abnormalities, anemia, pregnancy, lactation

INTERACTIONS

Drug

• Additive hypocalcemia with use of IV pentamidine

• Increased nephrotoxicity with use of aminoglycosides, amphotericin B, IV pentamidine

• Increased anemia with use of zidovudine

INCOMPATIBILITIES

• Any other drug in sol or syringe

SIDE EFFECTS

CNS: Peripheral neuropathy, fatigue, fever, headache, seizures, hallucinations

ENDO/METAB: Hypocalcemia, hypomagnesemia, hypokalemia, change in serum phosphorus

GI: Nausea, vomiting, diarrhea, elevated liver function tests

GU: Acute renal failure, glomerulonephritis, nephrosis, hematuria, proteinuria

HEME: Anemia, granulocytopenia, leukopenia, thrombocytopenia

Local: Thrombophlebitis with IV injection

TOXICITY AND OVERDOSE

Clinical signs: Seizures, renal impairment, electrolyte imbalance

Treatment: Supportive care; hydration; hemodialysis

PATIENT CARE MANAGEMENT

Assessment

• Assess history of hypersensitivity to foscarnet

• Obtain cultures, ophthalmologic exam to confirm diagnosis

• Assess hematologic function (CBC, differential, platelet count), renal function (BUN, creatinine, I&O), hepatic function (ALT, AST, bilirubin), electrolyte function (Ca, PO_4, Mg, K), ophthalmologic exam

Interventions

• Provide adequate hydration with IV NS before and during treatment to minimize nephrotoxicity

• Do not administer by rapid or bolus IV

• Use large vein with small-bore needle to reduce local reaction; rotate site q48-72h

• Maintain age-appropriate fluid intake

NURSING ALERT
Discontinue drug if signs of electrolyte imbalance, severe GI distress, or granulocytopenia develop

Do not administer by rapid or bolus IV

furazolidone
Brand Name(s): Furoxone
Classification: Antibacterial, antiprotozoal
Pregnancy Category: C

F

Evaluation
• Evaluate therapeutic response (decreased symptoms of CMV)
• Monitor hematologic function (CBC, differential, platelet count), renal function (BUN, creatinine, I&O), hepatic function (ALT, AST, bilirubin), electrolyte function (Ca, PO_4, Mg, K^+), ophthalmologic exams
• Monitor for blood dyscrasias including anemia, granulocytopenia (bruising, fatigue, bleeding, poor healing)
• Monitor for allergic reactions (flushing, rash, urticaria, pruritis)
• Evaluate IV site for vein irritation

PATIENT AND FAMILY EDUCATION
Teach/instruct
• To take as directed at prescribed intervals for prescribed length of time
• That medication will not cure infection but will control symptoms
Warn/advise
• To notify care provider of hypersensitivity, side effects
• That regular ophthalmologic examinations are necessary
• To notify care provider if any symptoms of infection (sore throat, fever, malaise, swollen lymph nodes), or if perioral tingling, numbness in extremities, paresthesias develop
• To maintain adequate hydration
• To check with care provider before using any OTC medications

STORAGE
• Store at room temp
• Do not refrigerate

AVAILABLE PREPARATIONS
Liquid: 50 mg/15 ml
Tabs: 100 mg

ROUTES AND DOSAGES
Children >1 mo: PO 5-8.8 mg/kg/24 hr divided q6h; maximum 400 mg/24 hr
Adults: PO 100 mg qid

MECHANISM AND INDICATIONS
Mechanism: Interferes with bacterial enzyme systems, causing antibacterial and antiprotozoal action; has MAOI activities
Indications: Used to treat bacterial and protozoal diarrhea, caused by *Giardia lamblia, Vibrio cholerae, E. coli, Salmonella, Shigella*

PHARMACOKINETICS
Metabolism: Inactivated in the intestine
Excretion: Mainly in feces; 5% in urine

CONTRAINDICATIONS AND PRECAUTIONS
• Contraindicated in infants <1 mo (may induce hemolytic anemia), with hypersensitivity
• Use cautiously with G-6-PD deficiency; pregnancy, lactation

INTERACTIONS
Drug
• Disulfiram-like effect with alcohol (flushing, nausea, vomiting, hypotension, sweating, tachycardia)
• Hypertensive reaction with sympathomimetic drugs
• Toxic psychosis with use of tricyclic antidepressants
Nutrition
• Flushing, tachycardia, hypertensive crisis with tyramine-containing foods

♣ Available in Canada.

SIDE EFFECTS

CNS: Headache, malaise, vertigo, partial deafness
CV: Hypotension, angioedema
DERM: Urticaria, rash, erythema multiforme
ENDO/METAB: Hypoglycemia
GI: Nausea, vomiting, abdominal pain, diarrhea
HEME: Agranulocytosis, hemolysis
Other: Fever, arthralgia

PATIENT CARE MANAGEMENT

Assessment

• Assess history of hypersensitivity to furazolidone
• Obtain history of diarrhea, assess hydration status
• Assess C&S before initiating therapy

Interventions

• Tab may be crushed, mixed with small amount food or fluid
• Decrease dosage as needed if nausea or vomiting occurs

NURSING ALERT

Use with caution in neonates

May cause hypokalemia which increases risk of digitalis toxicity

---

Evaluation

• Evaluate therapeutic response (decrease in diarrhea)
• Evaluate for side effects (hypoglycemia, headache, GI distress, rash, hypotension, fever)
• Evaluate and monitor blood and urine tests with G-6-PD deficiency
• Monitor wt during treatment
• Evaluate for number and character of stools
• Evaluate I&O

PATIENT AND FAMILY EDUCATION

Teach/instruct

• To take as directed at prescribed intervals for prescribed length of time
• Parent how to assess for dehydration, to keep track of number and character of stools
• That diarrhea should resolve in 2-5 days from initiation of therapy

Warn/advise

• To notify care provider of hypersensitivity, side effects
• That drug may turn urine brown
• To take no OTC drugs without consulting health care provider
• To avoid foods high in tyramine (yeast extracts, beer, wine, cheese, fermented products)
• To notify care provider if diarrhea worsens
• That no alcohol or alcohol products should be consumed for at least 4 days after drug is stopped (read labels of all foods and OTC medications)

STORAGE

• Store at room temp in light-resistant container

---

furosemide

Brand Name(s): Apo-Furosemide❧, Furosemide Injection❧, Lasix❧, Lasix Special❧

Classification: Loop diuretic, antihypertensive

Pregnancy Category: C

AVAILABLE PREPARATIONS

Sol: 10 mg/ml, 40 mg/5 ml
Tabs: 20 mg, 40 mg, 80 mg
Inj: 10 mg/ml

ROUTES AND DOSAGES

Infants and children: PO 2 mg/kg/dose qd-bid; may increase by 1-2 mg/kg/dose to maximum of 6 mg/kg/24 hr; IM/IV 1 mg/kg/dose q6-12h, may increase by 1 mg/kg/dose
Adult: 20-80 mg/24 hr qd or divided bid; may increase 20 or 40 mg up to total of 600 mg/24 hr; IM/IV 20-80 mg/dose, maximum single dose (PO/IM/IV) 6 mg/kg

IV administration

• Recommended concentration: 10 mg/ml
• Maximum concentration: 10 mg/ml
• IV push rate: Over 1-2 min
• Intermittent infusion rate: 1-2

❧ Available in Canada.

mg/kg q4-12h; dosage may be increased by 1 mg/kg/dose to achieve desired response
• Continuous infusion rate: 0.1-0.4 mg/kg/hr

MECHANISM AND INDICATIONS

Diuretic mechanism: Inhibits reabsorption of Na and Cl in the ascending loop of Henle, promoting the excretion of Na, water, Cl, K^+
Antihypertensive mechanism: Causes renal and peripheral vasodilatation with a temporary increase in glomerular filtration rate; decreases peripheral vascular resistance
Indications: Used in treatment of hypertension in adults and edema caused by CHF, pulmonary edema, renal failure, cerebral edema, and nephrotic syndrome

PHARMACOKINETICS

Onset of action: PO 30-60 min, IV 5 min
Peak: PO 1-2 hr; IV 20-60 min
Half-life: 2-10 hr
Metabolism: Liver
Excretion: Urine

CONTRAINDICATIONS AND PRECAUTIONS

• Contraindicated with known hypersensitivity to furosemide, anuria, liver disease, increasing BUN and creatinine levels
• Use cautiously in neonates (because of long half-life) with digoxin (may predispose pts to digitalis toxicity); with hearing difficulties, hepatic or renal dysfunction, pregnancy, lactation

INTERACTIONS

Drugs

• Increased risk of ototoxicity with other ototoxic drugs (aminoglycosides, amphotericin B)
• Increased hypotensive effects with other antihypertensives and other diuretics
• Increased neuromuscular blockade when used with neuromuscular blockers
• Increased K^+ loss with steroids and amphotericin B
• Decreased diuretic and antihypertensive effect with indomethacin
• Decreased furosemide-induced K^+ loss with use of K^+-sparing diuretics (spironolactone, triamterene, amiloride)

Lab

• Increased BG, urine glucose, BUN, uric acid
• Decreased serum Ca, Mg, K^+, Na

SIDE EFFECTS

CNS: Vertigo, headache, fatigue, confusion
CV: Volume depletion, dehydration, orthostatic hypotension, irregular pulse
DERM: With IV use, local pain, irritation, thrombophlebitis
EENT: Ototoxicity (associated with administration at >4 mg/min IV)
GI: Nausea, vomiting, dry mouth, diarrhea (with oral sol), stomach pain
HEME: Thrombocytopenia, neutropenia, leukopenia, agranulocytosis
METAB: Hypokalemia, hypocalcemia, hyponatremia, hyperglycemia, metabolic acidosis, hypochloremic alkalosis

TOXICITY AND OVERDOSAGE

Clinical signs: Volume and electrolyte depletion leading to circulatory collapse
Treatment: Supportive care, fluid and electrolyte replacement

PATIENT CARE MANAGEMENT

Assessment

• Assess history of hypersensitivity to drug
• Assess baseline VS, B/P
• Assess baseline electrolytes, CBC, differential, BUN, creatinine and liver function tests (AST, ALT, bilirubin)
• Assess hydration status
• Assess baseline wt

Interventions

• Monitor B/P and heart rate, especially during rapid diuresis
• Administer IV slowly, not to exceed 4 mg/min

F

🍁 Available in Canada.

- Administer PO dose with meals to decrease GI upset
- Administer in AM when possible to avoid nocturnal diuresis
- Weigh pt q AM
- Measure I&O

Evaluation
- Evaluate therapeutic response (diuresis, decreased wt)
- Evaluate for edema, ascites
- Evaluate blood work over time, especially electrolytes, BUN, liver function tests (ALT, AST, bilirubin), CBC, and differential
- Report abnormal results
- Monitor I&O

PATIENT AND FAMILY EDUCATION
Teach/instruct
- To take as directed at prescribed intervals for prescribed length of time
- About rationale for drug, expected response, and common side effects (weakness, fatigue, cramping, nausea, vomiting, diarrhea); advise family to promptly call care provider if these occur

Warn/advise
- To eat K$^+$-rich foods (bananas, citrus fruits, dates, raisins, potatoes)
- Not to eat foods with high Na content
- Not to change positions rapidly to prevent dizziness from orthostatic hypotension
- To report rapid wt loss or gain

STORAGE
- Store all preparations in light-resistant, tightly closed containers at room temp
- Protect sol from freezing

---

ganciclovir

Brand Name(s): Cytovene

Classification: Antiviral (synthetic nucleoside analog)

Pregnancy Category: C

AVAILABLE PREPARATIONS
Inj: 500 mg/vial

ROUTES AND DOSAGES
CMV Retinitis
Infants over 3 mo, children, and adults: IV induction 10 mg/kg/24 hr divided q12h as 1-2 hr infusion for 14-21 days; maintenance dose 5 mg/kg/24 hr qd for 7 days/wk or 6 mg/kg/24 hr qd for 5 days/wk

Other CMV Infections
Infants over 3 mo, children, and adults: IV induction 10 mg/kg/24 hr divided q12h for 14-21 days or 7.5 mg/kg/24 hr divided q8h maintenance dose 5 mg/kg/24 hr qd for 7 days/wk or 6 mg/kg/24 hr qd for 5 days/wk

IV administration
- Recommended concentration: 1-10 mg/ml in D$_5$W, NS, LR
- Maximum concentration: 10 mg/ml
- Continuous infusion rate: Over at least 1 hr using infusion pump

MECHANISM AND INDICATIONS
Antiviral mechanism: Inhibits replication of herpes virus in vitro; in vivo by selective inhibition of human CMV DNA polymerase and by direct incorporation into viral DNA
Indications: Treatment of CMV retinitis, CMV GI infections, and pneumonitis in immunocompromised pts; prevention of CMV disease in transplant patients with latent or active CMV

PHARMACOKINETICS
Half-life: 1.7-5.8 hr
Excretion: Urine

CONTRAINDICATIONS AND PRECAUTIONS
- Contraindicated with known hypersensitivity to ganciclovir or acyclovir and those with absolute neutrophil count <500/mm^3 or platelet count <25,000/mm^3
- Use cautiously with children; with neutropenia, thrombocytopenia, or impaired renal function; pregnancy, lactation

---

✤ Available in Canada.

INTERACTIONS
Drug
• Decreased renal clearance with use of probenecid
• Increased toxicity with use of dapsone, pentamidine, flucytosine, vincristine, vinblastine, adriamycin, doxorubicin, amphotericin B, trimethoprim/sulfa combinations, other nucleoside analogs
• Severe granulocytopenia with use of zidovudine; do not give concomitantly
• Increased seizures with use of imipenem-cilastatin

INCOMPATIBILITIES
• Any other drug in sol or syringe

SIDE EFFECTS
CNS: Headaches, seizures, confusion, tremor, dizziness, hallucinations, coma, fever, encephalopathy, malaise
CV: Edema, arrhythmias, hypertension, hypotension
DERM: Rash, urticaria
EENT: Retinal detachment in CMV retinitis
GI: Nausea, vomiting, diarrhea, elevated liver function tests
GU: Hematuria, elevated BUN, serum creatinine
HEME: Granulocytopenia, thrombocytopenia, neutropenia, anemia, eosinophilia
Local: Phlebitis with IV injection
Other: Hypersensitivity (dyspnea)

TOXICITY AND OVERDOSE
Clinical signs: Pancytopenia, neutropenia, abdominal pain, vomiting, lethargy
Treatment: Supportive care; hydration; hemodialysis

PATIENT CARE MANAGEMENT
Assessment
• Assess history of hypersensitivity to ganciclovir, acyclovir
• Obtain cultures and ophthalmologic exam to confirm diagnosis
• Assess hematologic function (CBC, differential, platelet count), renal function (BUN, creatinine, I&O), hepatic function (ALT, AST, bilirubin), ophthalmologic exam

Interventions
• Handle and dispose IV per agency guidelines issued for cytotoxic drugs
• Do not administer IM, SC, or IV bolus
• Use large vein with small-bore needle to reduce local reaction; rotate site q48-72h
• Maintain age-appropriate fluid intake

NURSING ALERT

Discontinue drug if signs of granulocytopenia, thrombocytopenia, or hypersensitivity develop

Do not administer by IV bolus, IM, or SC

Evaluation
• Evaluate therapeutic response (decreased symptoms of CMV)
• Monitor hematologic function (CBC, differential, platelet count), renal function (BUN, creatinine, I&O), hepatic function (ALT, AST, bilirubin), ophthalmologic exams
• Monitor for CNS effects (tremor, confusion, seizures)
• Evaluate IV site for vein irritation

PATIENT AND FAMILY EDUCATION
Teach/instruct
• To take as directed at prescribed intervals for prescribed length of time
• That medication will not cure infection, but will control symptoms
Warn/advise
• To notify care provider of hypersensitivity, side effects
• That regular ophthalmologic examinations are necessary
• To use contraception during treatment because of risk of reproductive toxicity; men should continue barrier contraception for at least 90 days

STORAGE
• Store powder at room temp
• Reconstituted sol stable at room temp for 12 hr

---

gentamicin sulfate

Brand Name(s): Alcomicin✢, Diogent✢, Garamycin, Ophthalmic/Otic Preparations✢, Garamycin Parenteral✢, Garamycin Topical Preparations✢, Garatec✢, Genoptic, Gentacidin✢, Jenamicin, Lydomycin✢, Ocugram✢, PMS-Gentamicin Sulfate✢

Classification: Antibiotic (aminoglycoside)

Pregnancy Category: C

AVAILABLE PREPARATIONS

Inj: 10 mg/ml, 40 mg/ml
Intrathecal/intraventricular: 2 mg/ml
Ophthal oint/sol: 0.3%
Top cream/oint: 0.1%

ROUTES AND DOSAGES

• Treatment limited to 7-10 days
IM, IV
Premature infants ≤7 days, gestation <28 wk: 2.5 mg/kg/dose q24h
Premature infants ≤7 days, gestation 28-34 wk: 2.5 mg/kg/dose q18h
Premature infants >7 days, gestation <28 wk: 2.5 mg/kg/dose q18h
Premature infants >7 days, gestation 28-34 wk: 2.5 mg/kg/dose q12h
Full term neonates ≤7 days: 2.5 mg/kg/dose q12h
Full term neonates/infants >7 days: 2.5 mg/kg/dose q8h
Children: 6-7.5 mg/kg/24 hr divided q8h
Adults: 3-5 mg/kg/24 hr divided q8h
Intrathecal/Intraventricular
Children and infants >3 months: 1-2 mg qd
Adult: 4-8 mg qd
Ophthalmic
Drops: Instill 1-2 gtts into conjunctival sac q4-8h
Ointment: Instill 1 cm strip into conjunctival sac q6-12h
Topical
Children and adults: Apply sparingly to affected areas tid-qid

IV administration

• Recommended concentration: 10 or 40 mg/ml (both available commercially) or dilute dose in appropriate volume of D_5W or NS
• Maximum concentration: 40 mg/ml
• IV push rate: Not recommended
• Intermittent infusion rate: Over 20-30 min using constant-rate volumetric infusion device
• Continuous infusion rate: Not recommended

MECHANISM AND INDICATIONS

Antibiotic mechanism: Bactericidal; inhibits bacterial protein synthesis by binding directly to the 30S ribosomal subunit
Indications: Effective against gram-positive and gram-negative bacteria including staphylococci, enterococci, *E. coli, Proteus, Klebsiella, Serratia, Enterobacter,* and *Pseudomonas;* used to treat septicemia, meningitis, severe systemic infections of CNS, respiratory, GI, urinary tracts, bone, skin, and soft tissue

PHARMACOKINETICS

Peak: IM 30-90 min; IV up to 30 min after a 30-min infusion
Distribution: Widely distributed in body fluids; poor CNS penetration
Half-life: Neonates 3-11.5 hr; infants and children 2-3.5 hr; intrathecal 5.5 hr
Metabolism: Not metabolized
Excretion: Urine, bile
Therapeutic levels: Peak 4-10 mcg/ml; trough 0.5-2 mcg/ml

CONTRAINDICATIONS AND PRECAUTIONS

• Contraindicated with known hypersensitivity to gentamicin or any other aminoglycoside
• Use cautiously in neonates and infants (because of renal immaturity); with impaired renal function, dehydration, 8th cranial nerve impairment, myasthenia gravis, parkinsonism, hypocalcemia, pregnancy, lactation

---

✢ Available in Canada.

INTERACTIONS
Drug
• Increased risk of nephrotoxicity, ototoxicity, and neurotoxicity with use of methoxyflurane, polymyxin B, vancomycin, capreomycin, cisplatin, cephalosporins, amphotericin B, other aminoglycosides
• Increased risk of ototoxicity with use of ethacrynic acid, furosemide, bumetanide, urea, mannitol
• Masked symptoms of ototoxicity with use of dimenhydrinate and other antiemetic or antivertigo drugs
• Synergistic antimicrobial activity against certain organisms with use of penicillins
• Increased risk of neuromuscular blockade with use of general anesthetics or neuromuscular blocking agents such as succinylcholine and tubocurarine
• Increased respiratory depression with use of opioids and analgesics
• Inactivated when administered with parenteral carbenicillin, ticarcillin
Lab
• Increased LDH, BUN, nonprotein nitrogen, serum creatine levels
• Increased urinary excretion of casts
• Decreased serum Na

INCOMPATIBILITIES
• Amphotericin B, ampicillin, cefamandole, cephalothin, cephapirin, dopamine, furosemide, heparin; inactivated in sol with carbenicillin, other penicillins, most cephalosporins

SIDE EFFECTS
CNS: Headache, lethargy, neuromuscular blockade with respiratory depression, muscle twitching, arachnoiditis
DERM: Minor skin irritation, photosensitivity, allergic contact dermatitis
EENT: Ototoxicity (tinnitus, vertigo, hearing loss), burning, stinging, transient irritation from ophthal oint/sol

GI: Diarrhea, elevated AST
GU: Nephrotoxicity (cells or casts in urine, oliguria, proteinuria, decreased CrCl; increased BUN, nonprotein nitrogen, serum creatinine levels)
HEME: Blood dyscrasias
Local: Pain or irritation at IM injection site
Other: Hypersensitivity reactions (eosinophilia, fever, rash, urticaria, pruritus), bacterial or fungal, superinfection, phlebitis

TOXICITY AND OVERDOSE
Clinical signs: Ototoxicity, nephrotoxicity, neuromuscular toxicity
Treatment: Supportive care, hemodialysis, or peritoneal dialysis; neuromuscular blockade reversed with Ca salts or anticholinesterases

PATIENT CARE MANAGEMENT
Assessment
• Assess history of hypersensitivity to gentamicin, other aminoglycosides
• Obtain C&S; may begin therapy before obtaining results
• Assess eye, skin for redness, drainage, swelling
• Assess renal function (BUN, creatinine, I&O), baseline wt, and hearing tests before beginning therapy
Interventions
• Administer gentamicin at least 1 hr before or 2 hr after other antibiotics (penicillins, cephalosporins)
• Sol should be colorless and clear to very pale yellow; do not use if dark yellow, cloudy, or containing precipitates
• Administer IM deeply into large muscle mass and rotate injection sites; do not inject more than 2 g per injection site
• Do not premix IV with other medications; infuse separately and flush line with D_5W or NS
• Use large vein with small-bore needle to reduce local reaction; rotate site q48-72h
• Use IT preparation only for IT; discard unused portion

G

• After lumbar puncture, provider may dilute gentamicin with CSF, then inject over 3-5 min; can be diluted with NS if CSF is purulent
• See Chapter 2 regarding ophthal instillation; wash hands before, after application; cleanse crusts or discharge from eye before application; wipe excess medication from eye; do not flush medication from eye
• Wash hands before, after top application; cleanse area with soap and water and dry well before application; do not apply to large denuded areas because of risk of increased systemic absorption; cream used for oozing wounds; oint used for dry areas
• Maintain age-appropriate fluid intake; keep patient well-hydrated to reduce renal toxicity
• Supervise ambulation, other safety measures with vestibular dysfunction
• Obtain drug levels after 3rd dose; sooner in neonates or pts with rapidly changing renal function; peak levels drawn 30 min after end of 30-min IV infusion, 1 hr after IM injection; trough levels drawn within 30 min before next dose

---

NURSING ALERT

Discontinue if signs of ototoxicity, nephrotoxicity, hypersensitivity develop

Do not administer IV push

Evaluation
• Evaluate therapeutic response (decreased symptoms of infection)
• Evaluate renal function (BUN, creatinine, I&O), daily wt and hearing evaluations
• Monitor signs of respiratory depression with IV infusion
• Observe for signs of superinfection (perineal itching, diaper rash, fever, malaise, redness, pain, swelling, drainage, rash, diarrhea, sore throat, change in cough or sputum)

• Evaluate IM site for tissue damage, IV site for vein irritation

PATIENT AND FAMILY EDUCATION
Teach/instruct
• To take as directed at prescribed intervals for prescribed length of time
Warn/advise
• To notify care provider of hypersensitivity, side effects, superinfection
• Not to share towels, washcloths, bed linens, eye makeup with family member being treated with ophthal forms

STORAGE
• Store at room temp
• Parenteral forms without preservatives should be discarded after opening

---

gentian violet
Brand Name(s): Genapax
Classification: Topical antibacterial, antifungal
Pregnancy Category: C

AVAILABLE PREPARATIONS
Sol: 1%, 2%

ROUTES AND DOSAGES
Children and adults: Top, apply sol to lesions with cotton swab bid or tid for 3 days; do not swallow

MECHANISM AND INDICATIONS
Mechanism: Inhibits growth of many fungi and some gram-positive organisms
Indications: For use in treatment of mucocutaneous infections caused by *Candida albicans* and other superficial skin infections

PHARMACOKINETICS
Unknown

CONTRAINDICATIONS AND PRECAUTIONS
• Contraindicated with known hypersensitivity to gentian violet; for use on ulcerated or granulated

---

areas (permanent discoloration may result)
• Use cautiously, drug turns clothing and skin purple

INTERACTIONS
None reported

INCOMPATIBILITES
None reported

SIDE EFFECTS
DERM: Local burning, irritation, vesicle formation

TOXICITY AND OVERDOSE
Clinical signs: Laryngeal obstruction may develop after prolonged treatment with drug
Treatment: Discontinue drug; specific treatment information not available

PATIENT CARE MANAGEMENT
Assessment
• Assess history of hypersensitivity to gentian violet
• Assess lesions for appropriateness of treatment, skin for areas of granulation tissue; do not apply drug in these areas
Interventions
• Apply sol to lesion with cotton or cotton swabs bid or tid for 3 days
Evaluation
• Evaluate therapeutic response (decreased lesions)
• Evaluate need for continued treatment

PATIENT AND FAMILY EDUCATION
Teach/instruct
• To use as directed at prescribed intervals for prescribed length of time
• About proper way to administer drug
Warn/advise
• About staining which can occur with application of drug
• To call care provider if side effects occur or if lesions do not respond to treatment

STORAGE
• Store in a light-resistant container at room temp

---

glucagon
Classification: Antihypoglycemic
Pregnancy Category: B

AVAILABLE PREPARATIONS
Inj: 1 mg, 10 mg (1 unit = 1 mg)

ROUTES AND DOSAGES
Hypoglycemia
Neonates: SC/IV/IM 0.3 mg/kg/dose, maximum 1 mg/dose
Children: SC/IV/IM 0.025-0.1 mg/kg/dose, maximum 1 mg/dose; may be repeated after 20 min for a total of 2-3 doses
Adults: SC/IV/IM 0.5-1 mg, repeat in 20 min prn
Diagnostic Aid
IM/IV 0.25-2 mg 10 min before procedure
IV administration
• Recommended concentration: 1 mg/ml
• Maximum concentration: 1 mg/ml
• IV push rate: Over 1 min

MECHANISM AND INDICATIONS
Mechanism: As a polypeptide hormone that is normally released from the pancreas, increases plasma glucose by promoting hepatic glycogenolysis and gluconeogenesis; increases BG levels only if hepatic stores are available and therefore does not help with chronic hypoglycemia, starvation, or adrenal insufficiency; when given parenterally, also relaxes smooth muscle of the GI tract; decreases gastric and pancreatic secretions and increases myocardial contractility
Indications: Used for the emergency treatment of hypoglycemia in patients with DM and before diagnostic procedures of the gut (such as endoscopy)

PHARMACOKINETICS
Peak: 5-30 min
Half-life: 3-10 min
Duration: 1-1.5 hr
Metabolism: Liver
Excretion: Urine

CONTRAINDICATIONS AND PRECAUTIONS
- Contraindicated with known hypersensitivity to drug or protein compounds; birth asphyxia, infants with intrauterine growth retardation, with hypoglycemia of premature infants
- Use cautiously with history of insulinoma, hypoglycemia, pregnancy, lactation

INTERACTIONS
Drug
- Prolonged effects with use of epinephrine
- Inhibited insulin release with phenytoin
- Increased hypoprothrombinemic effect possible with oral anticoagulants

Lab
- Altered cholesterol and serum K⁺ levels

INCOMPATIBILITIES
- Any other drug in solution or syringe; NS

SIDE EFFECTS
CV: Hypotension
DERM: Rash
GI: Nausea, vomiting
Other: Allergic reaction, dizziness, light-headedness, breathing difficulties, rebound hypoglycemia

TOXICITY AND OVERDOSE
Clinical signs: Nausea, vomiting, hypokalemia
Treatment: Supportive care

PATIENT CARE MANAGEMENT
Assessment
- Assess history of hypersensitivity to glucagon
- Obtain history of event precipitant (increased exercise, illness, diet, insulin dosing)
- Assess concurrent use of other medications or OTC drugs to assure maximum effectiveness
- Check PT/INR of patients on oral anticoagulants

Interventions
- Use diluent provided to reconstitute IM/SC; medication may precipitate in NS or sol with pH of 3-9.5
- Can be administered as IV push or with drip infusions; compatible with dextrose
- Have IV glucose available if child has nausea or vomiting and cannot retain some form of sugar for 1 hr
- Have IV glucose available if child does not respond to glucagon
- Turn unconscious child on side to decrease risk of vomiting; emesis may occur as child awakens; give food after pt is awake

> **NURSING ALERT**
> Observe for nausea, vomiting, or non-responsiveness

Evaluation
- Evaluate therapeutic response (normalization of blood glucose); expect response in 5-20 min; repeat dose if child does not awaken after 20 min
- Document patterns; report if hypoglycemia is a recurring event
- Evaluate side effects and hypersensitivity

PATIENT AND FAMILY EDUCATION
Teach/instruct
- To take as directed at prescribed time
- That family must recognize signs and symptoms of hypoglycemia (nervous, sweating, behavior changes, headache, difficulties in concentration, tiredness, chill, cool, pale, nausea, weakness, unconsciousness, coma)
- That all patients with DM should carry a glucagon kit; read instructions and understand how to use, reconstitute, and inject medication properly before it is actually needed; check expiration dates on vial
- To evaluate other medications or OTC drugs for interactions

Warn/advise
- To notify care provider of hypersensitivity, side effects
- To repeat and obtain medical

---

assistance if no response to injection in 20 min

• To avoid the risk of aspiration, turn child to side; anticipate possible vomiting as the child awakens

• To administer sugar or protein after recovery to prevent rebound hypoglycemia; inform care provider to evaluate cause for event; child may need evaluation of insulin dosage

STORAGE

• Store reconstituted medication in refrigerator for up to 3 mo

• Store unreconstituted medication at room temp

• Protect from light, heat, and humidity

---

granisetron

Brand Name(s): Kytril

Classification: Antiemetic, selective 5HT$_3$ receptor antagonist

Pregnancy Category: B

AVAILABLE PREPARATIONS

Tab: 1 mg
Inj: Single use vials, 1 mg/ml

ROUTES AND DOSAGES

• Oral dosing has not yet been established; clinical trials will compare efficacy of 2 mg PO dose to standard IV dose

Children and adults: IV 10 mcg/kg/24 hr, 30 min before chemotherapy

IV administration

• Recommended concentration: Dilute in 20-50 ml of NS or D$_5$W

• Intermittent infusion rate: Over 5 min

MECHANISM AND INDICATIONS

Mechanism: Binds to 5-HT$_3$ serotonin receptors located on vagal nerve terminals and in chemoreceptor trigger zone in CNS (in response to chemotherapy, mucosal cells secrete serotonin which affects 5-HT$_3$ receptors, evoking vagal discharge and causing vomiting)

Indications: Prevention of chemotherapy-induced nausea and vomiting

PHARMACOKINETICS

Onset of action: Immediate with IV
Peak: 30 min
Half-life: 9-31 hr
Metabolism: Liver
Excretion: 12% unchanged in urine; remainder as metabolites, 49% in urine, 34% in feces

CONTRAINDICATIONS AND PRECAUTIONS

• Contraindicated with known hypersensitivity to drug

INTERACTIONS

Drug

• Does not induce or inhibit cytochrome P-450 drug-metabolizing enzyme system of liver

Lab

• Increased AST, ALT possible (transient)

INCOMPATIBILITIES

• Not to be mixed with other medications

SIDE EFFECTS

CNS: Headache, asthenia, somnolence, agitation, anxiety, CNS stimulation, insomnia; EPS reported only rarely and in concomitant therapy with drugs having extrapyramidal effects

CV: Hypertension, arrhythmias, ECG changes infrequently noted

EENT: Taste disorder

GI: Diarrhea, constipation

Other: Fever

TOXICITY AND OVERDOSE

Clinical signs: Overdose of up to 38.5 mg of drug reported with only occasional slight headaches reported

Treatment: No known antidote to drug, supportive therapy administered as needed

PATIENT CARE MANAGEMENT

Assessment

• Assess history of hypersensitivity to granisetron

G

• Assess efficacy of previous anti-emetic regimen

Interventions

• Administer 30 minutes before initiating chemotherapy

Evaluation

• Evaluate therapeutic response (control of chemotherapy-associated nausea and vomiting)

PATIENT AND FAMILY EDUCATION

Teach/instruct

• To take medication as ordered

Warn/advise

• To report perceived effectiveness of drug

• To report side effects, especially involuntary movements of eyes, face, limbs

STORAGE

• Vials should be protected from light, stored at room temp

• Do not freeze

---

griseofulvin microsize/ultramicrosize

Brand Name(s): Microsize: Grifulvin V, Fulvin-U/F✤, Grisactin; ultramicrosize: Fulvin P/G, Grisactin-Ultra

Classification: Antifungal

Pregnancy Category: C

AVAILABLE PREPARATIONS

Oral susp: 125 mg/5 ml
Caps: 125 mg, 250 mg (Microsize)
Tabs: 250 mg, 500 mg (Microsize)
Tabs: 125 mg, 165 mg, 250 mg, 330 mg (Ultramicrosize)

ROUTES AND DOSAGES

Children >2 yr: PO microsize 10-15 mg/kg/24 hr divided qd or bid; ultramicrosize 5.5-7 mg/kg/24 hr divided qd or bid
Adults: PO microsize 500-1000 mg/24 hr divided qd or bid; ultramicrosize 330-750 mg/24 hr divided qd or bid

• Duration of therapy: For tinea corporis 2-4 wk, tinea pedis 4-8 wk, tinea capitis 4-6 wk, infected fingernails 3-6 mo

MECHANISM AND INDICATIONS

Antifungal mechanism: Arrests cell division at metaphase; binds to human keratin making it resistant to fungal invasion
Indications: Used to treat fungal infections of skin, hair, and nails caused by *Trichophyton, Epidermophyton,* and *Microsporum*

PHARMACOKINETICS

Peak: 4-8 hr
Distribution: Concentrates in hair, skin, nails, fat, and skeletal muscle
Half-life: 9-24 hr
Excretion: Urine, feces, perspiration
Absorption: Microsize, variable 25%-70%; ultramicrosize, complete

CONTRAINDICATIONS AND PRECAUTIONS

• Contraindicated with hypersensitivity to griseofulvin or any component, porphyria, or hepatic disease; safety in children < 2 yr has not been established

• Use cautiously with sensitivity to penicillin (drug is a penicillin derivative); pregnancy

INTERACTIONS

Drug

• Flushing, tachycardia with use of alcohol

• Decreased drug concentration with use of phenobarbital

• Decreased pro-time with use of warfarin

• Increased risk of breakthrough bleeding and possible decreased effectiveness with use of oral contraceptives

Lab

• False positive urinary VMA levels

Nutrition

• Enhanced action with high fat meal

SIDE EFFECTS

CNS: Fatigue, confusion, impaired judgment, insomnia, paresthesia, headache
DERM: Rash, urticaria, photosensitivity

✤ Available in Canada.

GI: Nausea, vomiting, diarrhea, hepatotoxicity

GU: Proteinuria

HEME: Leukopenia, granulocytopenia

Other: Lupus-like symptoms

TOXICITY AND OVERDOSE

Clinical signs: Headache, lethargy, confusion, nausea, vomiting

Treatment: Emesis or gastric lavage followed by activated charcoal; supportive care

PATIENT CARE MANAGEMENT

Assessment

• Assess history of hypersensitivity to griseofulvin, penicillins

• Obtain fungal culture to confirm diagnosis

• Assess baseline renal function (BUN, creatinine, I&O), hepatic function (ALT, AST, bilirubin), hematologic function (CBC, differential, platelet count)

Interventions

• Administer PO with food to decrease GI distress; shake susp well before administering each dose; tabs may be crushed, mixed with food or fluid

• Maintain age-appropriate fluid intake

Evaluation

• Evaluate therapeutic response (decreased fever, malaise, rash, negative fungal culture)

• Monitor renal function (BUN, creatinine, I&O), hepatic function (ALT, AST, bilirubin), hematologic function (CBC, differential, platelet count)

PATIENT AND FAMILY EDUCATION

Teach/instruct

• To take as directed at prescribed intervals for prescribed length of time

Warn/advise

• To notify care provider of hypersensitivity, side effects

• To take with a high fat meal to enhance drug absorption

• To avoid intense sunlight to prevent photosensitivity reaction

• Avoid use of alcohol or medications containing alcohol

• That female patient should use another form of birth control if using oral contraceptives

• To use proper skin, nail care; skin should be kept dry

STORAGE

• Store at room temp in a tight container

---

halcinonide

Brand Name(s): Halog preparations✤

Classification: Antiinflammatory agent

Pregnancy Category: C

AVAILABLE PREPARATIONS

Cream: 0.025%, 0.1%

Oint: 0.17%

Sol: 0.1%

ROUTES AND DOSAGES

Children and adults: Top apply to affected area bid-tid

MECHANISM AND INDICATIONS

Mechanism: Stimulates synthesis of enzymes which decreases inflammatory response

Indications: For use in corticosteroid-responsive dermatoses

PHARMACOKINETICS

Absorption: Amount absorbed depends on strength and amount applied, nature of skin at site of application; on thick skin absorption is minimal, on thin skin absorption is high

Distribution/metabolism: Primarily in skin

Excretion: Urine and feces

CONTRAINDICATIONS AND PRECAUTIONS

• Contraindicated with known hypersensitivity; viral, fungal, or tubercular lesions

• Use cautiously with impaired circulation (risk of skin ulceration)

INTERACTIONS

None significant

INCOMPATIBILITIES

None significant

✤ Available in Canada.

SIDE EFFECTS

Local: Burning, itching, hypopigmentation, atrophy, striae

Significant systemic absorption may cause the following:

CNS: Euphoria, insomnia, headache, mental changes, pseudotumor cerebri
CV: Edema, hypertension
DERM: Delayed healing, acneiform eruptions
ENDO: Adrenal suppression
GI: Increased appetite, peptic ulcer, irritation

TOXICITY AND OVERDOSE

Clinical signs: No information available
Treatment: No information available

PATIENT CARE MANAGEMENT

Assessment

• Assess skin for appropriateness of application, do not apply to skin with skin ulcerations, viral, fungal, or tubercular lesions

Interventions

• Apply small amount sparingly to clean, dry skin lesion(s) for shortest time possible, stop drug if signs of systemic absorption appear, do not apply occlusive dressings unless severe or resistant dermatoses; occlusive dressings will increase absorption

> **NURSING ALERT**
> In children, limit TOP application to least effective amount

Evaluation

• Evaluate therapeutic response (decreased skin inflammation)
• After application, assess skin for side effects especially striae, increased inflammation, atrophy, infection

PATIENT/FAMILY EDUCATION

Teach/instruct

• To use as directed at prescribed intervals for prescribed length of time; *do not over-apply*

• To apply sparingly using a light film, rub into affected area(s) gently
• Not to use occlusive dressing; a diaper may be used if changed regularly and not in place >8 hr
• To call provider if side effects occur or if skin not improved in 1 wk
• About side effects, especially if over-applied
• To wash and dry hands before, after application
• To avoid prolonged application on face, skin folds, genital area; to notify care provider of hypersensitivity reactions
• Not to apply to ulcerated skin

STORAGE

• Store at room temp

---

haloperidol, haloperidol decanoate, haloperidol lactate

Brand Name(s): Apo-Haloperidol❧, Haldol, Haldol Decanoate, Haldol-LA❧, Haloperidol, Novo-Peridol❧, Peridol❧, PMS-Haloperidol

Classification: Antipsychotic agent, neuroleptic

Pregnancy Category: C

AVAILABLE PREPARATIONS

Elixir (lactate): 2 mg/ml
Tabs: 0.5 mg, 1 mg, 2 mg, 5 mg, 10 mg, 20 mg
Inj (lactate): 5 mg/ml
Inj (decanoate): 50 mg/ml, 100 mg/ml

DOSAGES AND ROUTES

• For long-term treatment, use the smallest dose that is effective
• Do not use in children <3 years old or <15 kg in wt; safety and effectiveness have not been established

PO
Children 3-12 yr (15-40 kg): 0.25-0.5 mg/24 hr divided bid-tid, in-

crease by 0.25-0.5 mg every 3-7 days to clinical effect, side effects, or maximum daily dose (0.15 mg/kg/24 hr or 4 mg; daily doses of 4-6 mg should be reserved for the most disturbed and refractory pts); maintenance, agitation or hyperkinesia 0.01-0.03 mg/kg/24 hr qd; psychotic disorders 0.05-0.15 mg/kg/24 hr divided bid-tid; Tourette syndrome, tics, vocal utterances 0.05-0.075 mg/kg/24 hr divided bid-tid; some children benefit from as little as 1 mg/24 hr

Adult: Initially 0.5-2 mg bid-tid; increase by 0.5 mg/24 hr at 3-4 day intervals as needed and tolerated; maximum daily dosage should not exceed 100 mg; usual maintenance dosage for psychosis 0.5-30 mg/24 hr; usual maintenance dosage for Tourette syndrome, tics, vocal utterances 0.5-5 mg bid or tid, increase until desired response occurs

IM (as Lactate)

• IM not approved for young children

Children 6 to 12 years: 1-3 mg/dose every 4-8 hrs to maximum dose of 0.15 mg/kg/24 hr; change to oral therapy as soon as pt is able

IM (as Decanoate)

• Not approved for children; doses are too concentrated

Adult: For chronic schizophrenia, 10-15 times the pt's PO dose q 4 wk

MECHANISM AND INDICATIONS

Mechanism: Interferes with action of dopamine in the brain, depresses the cerebral cortex, hypothalamus, and limbic system; this improves coherence and organization of thinking; controls activity and aggression; reduces anxiety, agitation, delusions, hallucinations

Indications: For use in treating psychotic symptoms of schizophrenia and acute mania (disorganized thinking, delusions, hallucinations, paranoia, abnormal behavior, psychotic depression); effective in controlling tics and vocal utterances in Gilles de la Tourette syndrome; for short-term treatment of hyperactive children showing excessive motor activity and severe behavioral problems; also used to treat specific target symptoms in autistic disorder; because of the risk of tardive dyskinesia, should be reserved for children and adolescents for whom less harmful treatments are not effective

PHARMACOKINETICS

Onset of action: PO erratic; IM lactate 15-30 min

Peak: PO 2-6 hr; IM lactate 15-20 min; IM decanoate 4-11 days

Half-life: PO 12-38 hr; IM lactate 21 hr; IM decanoate 3 wk

Duration: PO 2-3 days

Metabolism: Liver

Excretion: Urine, feces

Therapeutic level: 3-10 ng/ml; therapeutic antipsychotic effects may take 2-3 wk of continued treatment; if not significantly beneficial within 6 wk, discontinue drug

CONTRAINDICATIONS AND PRECAUTIONS

• Contraindicated with hypersensitivity to this or any component of this medication, alcohol and barbiturate withdrawal states, angina, arrhythmias, blood dyscrasias, bone marrow depression, brain damage, breast cancer, lactation, CNS depression, coma, mental depression, narrow-angle glaucoma, active liver disease, history of neuroleptic malignant syndrome, any form of Parkinson's disease, pregnancy, poorly controlled seizures, history of tardive dyskinesia, urinary depression

• Use cautiously with cardiovascular disorders, history of mental depression, hypertension, hypotension, kidney dysfunction, liver dysfunction, seizures; planning surgery under general or spinal anesthesia in the near future; overactive thyroid, thyrotoxicosis; pts allergic or abnormally sensitive to phenothiazines; pts with lupus erythematosus or taking prednisone are more susceptible to CNS reactions

INTERACTIONS
Drug
• Increased effects of alcohol, antidepressants, β-adrenergic blockers
• Decreased effects of amoxapine, guanethidine, levodopa, lithium, metoclopramide, metyrosine, pemoline, pimozide
• Decreased effects of haloperidol with antacids containing aluminum or magnesium, barbiturates, benztropine, carbamazepine, phenobarbital, phenytoin, trihexyphenidyl
• Neurotoxicity and brain damage possible with lithium
• Serious dementia possible with methyldopa
• Increased susceptibility to nervous system reactions with prednisone
• Oversedation possible with alcohol, anesthetics, barbiturate, CNS depressants
• Hypotension possible with epinephrine
• Increased intraocular pressure possible with anticholinergic agents
• Concurrent use with marijuana smoking may moderately increase drowsiness, accentuate orthostatic hypotension, increase risk of precipitating psychosis and confuse the interpretation of mental status and of drug response

Lab
• Increased ALT, AST, alk phos, bilirubin, cardiac enzymes, cholinesterase, eosinophils, BG, prolactin, PBI
• Decreased hormones in blood and urine, RBCs, Hgb, WBCs, protime, Na
• Increased or decreased cholesterol
• False positive pregnancy tests, PKU
• False negative urinary steroids
• Liver reaction may mimic viral hepatitis; CNS reactions may mimic Parkinson's disease or Reye syndrome

Nutrition
• Avoid alcohol completely; haloperidol can increase sedation and intoxicating effects
• Allergic reactions possible with 1, 5, 10 mg tabs, which contain tartrazine (yellow dye #5)

INCOMPATIBILITIES
• Haloperidol lactate inj should not be mixed with other drugs
• Haloperidol decanoate inj incompatible with SW for inj and NS

SIDE EFFECTS
CNS: Drowsiness, headache, seizures, agitation, cognitive slowing, confusion, depression, dizziness, insomnia, intellectual dulling, weakness; EPS (spasm of neck muscles; eye rolling; tonic muscle spasms, often of the tongue, jaw, or neck, which may result in such dramatically distressing symptoms as oculogyric crisis, torticollis, and even opisthotonos), onset usually occurs within days after a dosage change, may occur in up to 25% of children treated with haloperidol; dystonia (pseudoparkinsonism, bradykinesia, cogwheel rigidity, drooling, masked facies, muscle stiffness, pill-rolling tremor), usually manifested 1-4 wk after start of treatment, acute neuroleptic-induced dystonias are quickly relieved by diphenhydramine; akathisia (constant movement, dysphoric agitation with frantic pacing, ague, muscular discomfort, restlessness), usually manifested after 1-6 wk of treatment, anticholinergic agents or β-blockers are sometimes helpful; neuroleptic malignant syndrome (severe muscular rigidity, altered sensorium, hyperpyrexia, autonomic lability and myoglobinemia—a medical emergency with mortality rates as high as 30% have been reported); rabbit syndrome (rapid chewing-like movements), a rare parkinsonian-like tremor that develops late; withdrawal symptoms (dyskine-

---

sias), after withdrawal, reversible dyskinetic movements develop within 1-4 wk and may persist for mos before resolving; occur in up to 25% of children exposed to neuroleptics for 1 yr and in about 50% of those exposed for 2½ yr; tardive dyskinesia (choreoathetoid movements of tongue and mouth, facial grimacing, movements of extremities and trunk), late-developing, irreversible movement disorders that appear after long-term use of neuroleptic medications, there is no effective treatment, and risk of tardive dyskinesia is thought to be small in pts exposed to neuroleptics for <6 mo

CV: Hypotension, arrhythmias, cardiac arrest, ECG changes, hypertension, tachycardia
DERM: Rash, contact dermatitis, hives, photosensitivity
EENT: Cataracts, eye damage, dry eyes, glaucoma, retinopathy, visual changes, blurred vision
GI: Anorexia, constipation, nausea, vomiting, diarrhea, dry mouth, hepatitis, hypersalivation, ileus, indigestion, jaundice, liver dysfunction, wt gain
GU: Amenorrhea, painful ejaculation, enuresis, galactorrhea, gynecomastia, impotence, irregular menses, priapism, sexual dysfunction, urinary frequency, urinary retention
HEME: Anemia, leukocytosis, leukopenia
RESP: Dyspnea, asthma, laryngospasm, respiratory depression
Other: Hyperglycemia, hypoglycemia, hyperpyrexia

TOXICITY AND OVERDOSE

Clinical signs: Agitation, difficulty breathing, coma, convulsions, dizziness, marked drowsiness, stupor, tremor, unsteadiness, weakness
Treatment: If ingested orally, activated charcoal lavage; do not induce vomiting; provide an airway

PATIENT CARE MANAGEMENT

Assessment

• Assess history of hypersensitivity to drug
• Obtain baseline ECG, CBC, AST, ALT, bilirubin, UA
• Obtain baseline orthostatic B/P, pulse
• Obtain physical assessment
• Review history for neuroleptic malignant syndrome, arrhythmia, cardiac disease

Interventions

• Tab may be crushed for administration; do not crush film-coated tabs
• If GI symptoms occur, give with or following food or milk
• Make sure oral med is swallowed
• Concentrate may be diluted in 2 oz water or fruit juice; do not add to coffee or tea
• Usually administered in 2 daily doses
• Administer more at hs to aid sleep when given in divided doses
• Increase fluids and fiber in diet if constipation occurs
• Rinse with water, take sips of fluid, sugarless gum, or hard candy for dry mouth
• Decrease stimulation in environment by dimming lights, avoiding loud noises
• Do not treat Parkinson-like reactions with levodopa; can cause agitation, worsening of the psychotic disorder
• This drug should not be discontinued abruptly following long-term use; withdraw gradually over a period of 2-3 wk

H

NURSING ALERT

Do not administer IV

A possible effect is neuroleptic malignant syndrome; symptoms include fever, fast or irregular heartbeat, fast breathing, increased CPK, sweating, weakness, muscle stiffness, seizures, loss of bladder control; if these occur, obtain medical intervention immediately; monitor VS, ECG, urine output and renal function; symptom management with medications, hydration, and cooling blankets

Evaluation

• Evaluate therapeutic response (ability to function in daily activities, to sleep throughout the night; emotional excitement, hallucinations, delusions, paranoia, thought patterns, and speech)
• Evaluate mental status (affect, impulsiveness, mood, orientation, LOC, sensorium, suicidal ideation, psychiatric symptoms)
• Monitor monthly bilirubin, CBC, AST, ALT, bilirubin liver functions, temp, UA
• Monitor and document orthostatic B/P and pulse monthly; report drops of 20 mm Hg to prescriber
• Monitor ECG, eyes, skin turgor
• Examine every 3 mo for abnormal movements, reflexes, gait, coordination; fine, involuntary wavelike movements of the tongue could indicate the beginning of tardive dyskinesia
• Monitor for dizziness, faintness, palpitations on rising
• Should not be discontinued abruptly following long-term use; gradual withdrawal over a period of 2 to 3 wk is advised

PATIENT AND FAMILY EDUCATION
Teach/instruct

• To take as directed at prescribed intervals for prescribed length of time

• That medication is most helpful when used as part of a comprehensive, multimodal treatment program
• Not to stop taking medication without prescriber approval
• That therapeutic effects may take up to 6 wk
• To increase fluids and fiber in diet if constipation or urinary retention occurs
• That a possible effect is neuroleptic malignant syndrome; symptoms include fever, fast or irregular heartbeat, fast breathing, sweating, weakness, muscle stiffness, seizures, loss of bladder control; if these occur, obtain medical help immediately
• To make sure medication is swallowed
• To take with food or milk if GI symptoms occur
• To rinse with water, take sips of fluid, sugarless gum, or hard candy for dry mouth

Warn/advise

• Not to discontinue medication quickly after long-term use; tapering should be supervised by prescriber
• To maintain meticulous oral hygiene, since oral candidiasis may occur
• To report any change or disturbance in vision, jaundice, tremors, or muscle twitching to prescriber right away
• To use caution in hot environments, baths or saunas; may impair regulation of body temp and increase the risk of heat stroke; in hot weather take extra precautions to stay cool
• To avoid strenuous exercise; fainting is possible
• To stay out of direct sunlight, especially between 10 AM and 3 PM, if possible; when outside, wear protective clothing, a hat, sunglasses; put on sun block that has a skin protection factor (SPF) of at least 15
• To avoid ingesting alcohol, other CNS depressants
• That drug may cause drowsi-

---

ness; be careful on bicycles, skates, skateboards, while driving, or with other activities requiring alertness
• To avoid OTC preparations (cough, hay fever, cold) unless approved by prescriber; serious drug interactions can occur
• To return for follow-up health care visits

STORAGE
• Store at room temp in tightly closed, light-resistant container

---

heparin calcium, heparin sodium

Brand Name(s): Calcilean✤, Calciparine, Hepalean✤, Hepalean-Lok✤, Heparin-Leo✤, Heparin-Lock Flush, Hep-Lock, Liquaemin

Classification: Anticoagulant

Pregnancy Category: C

AVAILABLE PREPARATION
Inj: 10 U/ml, 100 U/ml, 1000 U/ml, 2500 U/ml, 5000 U/ml, 7500 U/ml, 10,000 U/ml, 20,000 U/ml, 40,000 U/ml
Repository inj: 20,000 U/ml (120 U = 1 mg)

ROUTES AND DOSAGES
Infants and children: Initial 50 U/kg IV bolus; maintenance dosage 20-35 U/kg/hr as constant infusion /24 hr or 50-100 U/kg/dose q4h IV
Adults: Initial 5000-10,000 U IV bolus; maintenance dosage 20,000-40,000 U IV as constant infusion/24 hr or 5000-10,000 U q4-6h IV
Deep vein thrombosis prophylaxis: SC 5000 U/dose q8-12h until ambulatory
Heparin flush: Peripheral IV 1-2 ml of 10 U/ml sol q4h
Central lines: 2-3 ml of 100 U/ml sol q24h
IV administration
• Recommended concentration: Undiluted or dilute to desired concentration in NS, R, dextrose sol or lipids
• Maximum concentration: Undiluted
• IV push rate: Not established
• Intermittent infusion rate: 50-100 U/kg/dose IV
• Continuous infusion rate: 20-35 U/kg/hr for anticoagulation

MECHANISM AND INDICATIONS
Mechanism: Potentiates action of antithrombin, inactivating thrombin; prevents conversion of fibrinogen to fibrin
Indications: For prevention and treatment of deep vein thrombosis, pulmonary emboli, MI, open heart surgery, disseminated intravascular clotting, atrial fibrillation with embolization, and as an anticoagulant in transfusion and dialysis

PHARMACOKINETICS
Onset of action: SC 20-60 min
Peak: IV 5 min
Duration: IV 2-6 hr; SC 8-12 hr
Metabolism: Partially metabolized in reticulo-endothelial system
Excretion: Urine

CONTRAINDICATIONS AND PRECAUTIONS
• Contraindicated with hypersensitivity to heparin or any component, severe thrombocytopenia, subacute bacterial endocarditis, suspected intracranial hemorrhage, shock, severe hypotension, uncontrollable bleeding, hemophilia, ITP
• Use with caution with peptic ulcer disease, severe renal, hepatic, or biliary disease, menstruation, indwelling catheters, alcoholism, elderly, pregnancy, lactation

INTERACTIONS
Drug
• Increased action with other oral anticoagulants, salicylates, dextran, steroids, NSAIDs
• Decreased action with digitalis, tetracycline, antihistamine
Lab
• Increased T_3 uptake
• Decreased uric acid

SIDE EFFECTS

CNS: Fever, headache, chills
DERM: Urticaria, rash, pruritis
GI: Nausea, vomiting, diarrhea, anorexia, cramps
GU: Hematuria
HEME: Hemorrhage, thrombocytopenia
Local: Irritation, ulceration, SC necrosis (rare)

TOXICITY AND OVERDOSE

Clinical signs: Bleeding (nosebleeds, hematuria, easy bruising, petechiae, melena)
Treatment: Protamine sulfate (1 mg per 100 U heparin in previous 4 hr)

PATIENT CARE MANAGEMENT

Assessment
• Assess history of hypersensitivity to drug
• Assess blood studies (Hct, platelets, stool occult blood) q 3 mo
• Assess PT/INR
• Assess for bleeding (nosebleeds, bruising, petechiae, melena)

Interventions
• Administer at same time qd
• Do not administer IM
• Administer SC in abdomen; do not aspirate syringe; apply gentle pressure after removing syringe for 1 min

> **NURSING ALERT**
> Do not administer IM
> Use preservative-free heparin in neonates

Evaluation
• Evaluate therapeutic response (decreased deep vein thrombosis, other clot formation)
• Evaluate for bleeding (bruising, bleeding, gums, tarry stools, petechiae)
• Evaluate need for dosage change

PATIENT AND FAMILY EDUCATION

Teach/instruct
• To carry medical alert identification

• To use soft-bristle toothbrush, electric razor, avoid contact sports
• To report any signs of bleeding

Warn/advise
• Not to use aspirin

Encourage
• To comply with medication schedule, monitoring of blood studies

STORAGE

• Store at room temp

---

hepatitis B, immune globulin, human (HBIG)

Brand Name(s): H-BIG, Hep-B-Gammagee, HyperHep✿

Classification: Hepatitis B prophylaxis agent

Pregnancy Category: C

AVAILABLE PREPARATIONS

Inj: 0.5 ml single dose syringe; 1 ml, 5 ml multidose vials

ROUTES AND DOSAGES

Neonates born to HBs Ag-positive women: IM 0.5 ml within 12 hr of birth; repeat doses at 3 and 6 mo if hepatitis B vaccine is refused
Children and adults: IM 0.06 ml/kg within 7 days after exposure; repeat 28 days after exposure

MECHANISM AND INDICATIONS

Mechanism for postexposure prophylaxis of hepatitis B: Provides passive immunity to hepatitis B
Indications: Used for prophylaxis of neonates born to HBs Ag-positive women and for postexposure prophylaxis for children and adults following parenteral exposure, direct mucous membrane contact, or oral ingestion involving HBs Ag-positive materials

---

✿ Available in Canada.

PHARMACOKINETICS
Peak: 3-11 days (appears in serum within 1-6 days; persists 2-6 mo)
Half-life: 21 days

CONTRAINDICATIONS AND PRECAUTIONS
• Contraindicated with known hypersensitivity to thimerosal
• Use cautiously with history of systemic allergic reactions to human immune globulin preparations; pregnancy

INTERACTIONS
Drug
• Interference with response to live vaccines possible (e.g., MMR); administer live vaccines 2 wk before or 3 mo after HBIG

SIDE EFFECTS
DERM: Rash, pruritus
Local: Pain, redness at injection site
Other: Nausea, faintness, urticaria, angioedema, anaphylaxis

PATIENT CARE MANAGEMENT
Assessment
• Obtain history of hepatitis B exposure
• Assess history of hypersensitivity to thimerosal
Interventions
• Administer IM in lateral thigh, deltoid muscle, or upper outer quadrant of gluteal area, depending on pt's age
• Do not administer IV
• Emergency resuscitative equipment should be readily available for possible anaphylaxis
• Administer hepatitis B vaccine simultaneously but at different site as ordered

---
NURSING ALERT
Do not administer IV

Evaluation
• Monitor for allergic reaction (dyspnea, skin eruptions, pruritus)
• Reevaluate infants treated with HBIG at 12-15 mo to determine immune status

PATIENT AND FAMILY EDUCATION
Warn/advise
• To notify care provider of hypersensitivity, side effects
• That HBIG only provides temporary protection against hepatitis
• That a mild analgesic (acetaminophen) may alleviate discomfort, fever

STORAGE
• Store in refrigerator; do not freeze

---

homatropine hydrobromide
Brand Name(s): AK-Homatropine, Isopto Homatropine❦
Classification: Cycloplegic, mydriatic
Pregnancy Category: C

AVAILABLE PREPARATIONS
Ophthal sol: 2%, 5%

ROUTES AND DOSAGES
Mydriasis and Cycloplegia for Refraction
Children: Instill 1 gtt 2% sol immediately before procedure, repeat q 10 min prn
Adults: Instill 1-2 gtt 2% sol or 1 gtt 5% sol before procedure, repeat q 5-10 min prn
Uveitis
Children: Instill 1 gtt of 2% sol bid-tid
Adults: Instill 1-2 gtt 2% or 5% sol bid-tid up to q3-4h prn

MECHANISM AND INDICATIONS
Cycloplegic and mydriatic mechanism: Blocks response of iris sphincter muscle and the accommodative muscle of the ciliary body to cholinergic stimulation, resulting in dilation and loss of accommodation
Indications: Used in refraction, diagnostic ophthalmic procedures, and treatment of uveitis

---

❦ Available in Canada.

PHARMACOKINETICS
Peak: Cycloplegia 30-90 min; mydriasis 10-30 min
Duration: Cycloplegia 10-48 hr; mydriasis 6-96 hr

CONTRAINDICATIONS AND PRECAUTIONS
• Contraindicated with hypersensitivity to homatropine or any components, narrow-angle glaucoma, acute hemorrhage
• Use cautiously in infants and children (because of increased risk of cardiovascular and CNS effects); with hypertension, cardiac distress, increased intraocular pressure, pregnancy; in children with Down syndrome, spastic paralysis, or brain damage

INTERACTIONS
Drug
• Interference with antiglaucoma effects possible with use of ilocarpine, carbachol, cholinesterase

SIDE EFFECTS
CNS: Hallucinations, amnesia, ataxia, headache, drowsiness
CV: Tachycardia, hypotension, vasodilation
DERM: Allergic reactions, flushing, dryness, rash
EENT: Follicular conjunctivitis, blurred vision, increased intraocular pressure, stinging, exudate
GI: Decreased GI motility, abdominal distention in infants
GU: Bladder distention, urinary retention
Other: Fever, respiratory depression, coma

TOXICITY AND OVERDOSE
Clinical signs: Dry flushed skin, dry mouth, dilated pupils, hallucinations, delirium, tachycardia, decreased bowel sounds
Treatment: Induced emesis, activated charcoal, supportive care; for severe toxicity, physostigmine, propranolol

PATIENT CARE MANAGEMENT
Assessment
• Assess history of hypersensitivity to homatropine, any components

Interventions
• See Chapter 2 regarding instillation; wash hands before and after application; cleanse crusts, discharge from eye before application; after instillation, apply gentle pressure to lacrimal sac for 1 min to minimize systemic absorption; wipe excess medications from eye; do not flush medication from eye

> **NURSING ALERT**
> Discontinue if signs of systemic toxicity develop

Evaluation
• Monitor for signs of CNS disturbances (psychotic reactions, behavioral changes)
• Monitor blurred vision, photosensitivity lasting more than 72 hr; notify care provider

PATIENT AND FAMILY EDUCATION
Teach/instruct
• To use as directed at prescribed intervals for prescribed length of time
Warn/advise
• To notify care provider of hypersensitivity, side effects
• Not to let child rub or blink eyes
• To wait 5 min before using other ophthal preparations
• To wear dark glasses to reduce photophobia
• Not to engage in hazardous activities until effects have subsided
• To report any change in vision, difficult breathing, flushing

STORAGE
• Store at room temp, tightly sealed; do not freeze

♣ Available in Canada.

hyaluronidase

Brand Name(s): Wydase✤

Classification: Adjunctive agent to increase absorption of injected drugs; extravasation treatment (enzyme)

Pregnancy Category: C

AVAILABLE PREPARATIONS
Inj: Powder 150 U, 1500 U; sol 150 U/ml, add 150 U to sol

ROUTES AND DOSAGES
Adjunct to Increase Drug Absorption
Children and adults: Add 150 U to vehicle containing drug
Adjunct to Increase Absorption of Fuids (given by hypodermoclysis)
Neonate: Do not exceed 2 ml/min
Child <3 yrs: Do not exceed 200 ml/clysis
Children ≥3 yr and adults: Add 150 U to each liter of clysis sol; rate and volume not to exceed maintenance
Management of IV Extravasation
Reconstitute 150 U vial with 1 ml NS, then take 0.1 ml of this solution and dilute with 0.9 ml NS, to give 15 U/ml; using 25- or 26-gauge needle, inject 0.2 ml SC or ID into edge of extravasation site × 5, changing needles between injections

MECHANISM AND INDICATIONS
Mechanism: Modifies permeability of connective tissue through hydrolysis of hyaluronic acid
Indications: For use in increasing dispersion and absorption of other drugs; to increase rate of absorption of fluids given by hypodermoclysis; treatment of IV extravasations

PHARMACOKINETICS
Onset of action: SC or ID, immediate
Duration: 24-48 hr

CONTRAINDICATIONS AND PRECAUTIONS
• Contraindicated with hypersensitivity, CHF, hypoproteinemia; not for injection into injected, inflamed, or cancerous areas

INTERACTIONS
Drug
• Decreased effect with salicylates, cortisone, ACTH, estrogens, antihistamines
• Increased analgesia, increased absorption of anesthesia, decreased duration of action when used with local anesthetics

SIDE EFFECTS
CNS: Dizziness, chills
CV: Tachycardia, hypotension
GI: Nausea, vomiting
Local: Urticaria, irritation
Other: Overhydration with hypodermoclysis

TOXICITY AND OVERDOSE
Clinical signs: Overdose not reported

PATIENT CARE MANAGEMENT
Assessment
• Assess history of hypersensitivity to hyaluronidase
• Assess site before administration
Interventions
• Administer skin test for sensitivity before use
• Administer drug within first few min to 1 hr after extravasation occurs
Evaluation
• Evaluate therapeutic response (absence of pain, swelling after hypodermoclysis)
• Evaluate for overhydration in children <3 yr

PATIENT AND FAMILY EDUCATION
Teach/instruct
• About rationale for use
• To report unusual side effects

STORAGE
• Store at room temp

hydralazine hydrochloride

Brand Name(s): Apo-Hydralazine✚, Apresoline✚, Alazine, Hydralazine HCl, Novo-Hylazin✚, Nu-Hydral✚

Classification: Antihypertensive, vasodilator

Pregnancy Category: C

AVAILABLE PREPARATIONS
Inj: 20 mg/ml
Tabs: 10 mg, 25 mg, 50 mg, 100 mg

ROUTES AND DOSAGES
Children: IM/IV 0.1-0.2 mg/kg/dose (not to exceed 20 mg) q4-6hr prn; not to exceed 20 mg/24 hr or 1.7-3.5 mg/kg/24 hr divided q4-6h; PO 0.75-3.0 mg/kg/24 hr divided bid-qid, increase over 3-4 wk to maximum of 7.5 mg/kg/24 hr or 200 mg/24 hr
Adult: IM/IV 10-40 mg q4-6h prn; PO 10 mg qid, increase by 10-25 mg/dose q 2-5 days to maximum of 300 mg/24 hr

IV administration
- Recommended concentration: 20 mg/ml
- Maximum concentration: 20 mg/ml
- IV push rate: 0.2 mg/kg/min

MECHANISM AND INDICATIONS
Mechanism: Direct relaxation of arteriolar smooth muscle causes decreased B/P and reflex increase in cardiac function
Indications: For use in essential hypertension

PHARMACOKINETICS
Onset of action: PO 20-30 min, IM 5-10 min, IV 5-20 min
Peak: PO, IM 1 hr; IV 10-80 min
Duration: PO, IM 2-4 hr; IV 2-6 hr
Half-life: 2-8 hr
Metabolism: Liver
Excretion: 14% excreted unchanged in liver

CONTRAINDICATIONS AND PRECAUTIONS
- Contraindicated with hypersensitivity, CAD, mitral valvular heart disease, rheumatic heart disease
- Use cautiously with CVA, advanced renal disease, pregnancy, lactation

INTERACTIONS
Drug
- Increased tachycardia and angina with sympathomimetics
- Increased effects of β blockers
- Decreased B/P with MAOIs
- Increased diuretic effects with other diuretics

Lab
- Positive ANA titer possible
- Positive LE prep possible
- Blood dyscrasias (leukopenia, agranulocytosis, purpura, decreased Hgb and RBC count)

INCOMPATIBILITIES
- Aminophylline, ampicillin disodium edetate, chlorothiazide, ethacrynic acid, hydrocortisone, mephentermine, nitroglycerin, phenobarbital, verapamil, $D_{10}LR$

SIDE EFFECTS
CNS: Headache, tremors, dizziness, peripheral neuritis, malaise, depression
CV: Palpitations, flushing, tachycardia, edema, angina
DERM: Rash, pruritis
EENT: Nasal congestion
GI: Anorexia, nausea, vomiting, diarrhea
GU: Impotence, urinary retention, Na and water retention
HEME: Leukopenia, agranulocytosis, anemia
Other: Positive ANA, positive LE prep

TOXICITY AND OVERDOSE
Clinical signs: Hypotension, tachycardia, arrhythmias, facial flushing, shock
Treatment: Induce emesis, gastric lavage, activated charcoal; symptomatic and supportive care

PATIENT CARE MANAGEMENT
Assessment
- Assess history of hypersensitivity to hydralazine hydrochloride

---

✚ Available in Canada.

- Assess B/P q 5 min × 2 hr, then q1h × 2, then q4h
- Assess wt, I&O daily
- Assess electrolytes, blood studies (include ANA and LE prep)
- Assess VS (especially pulse)

Interventions
- Administer PO with food
- Administer IV push undiluted through stopcock with infusion pump; do not exceed rate of 0.2 mg/kg/min
- Administer to pt in recumbent position; keep pt recumbent 1 hr
- Monitor B/P closely

NURSING ALERT
Hydralazine has limited use in children; use only if benefit outweighs risk

Evaluation
- Evaluate therapeutic response (decreased B/P)
- Evaluate hydration status
- Evaluate for edema
- Evaluate for signs of wt gain, edema with long-term use

PATIENT AND FAMILY EDUCATION
Teach/instruct
- To take as directed at prescribed intervals for prescribed length of time
- About disease process and importance of complying with medication regime
- About side effects; to report unusual ones to care provider
Warn/advise
- To take medication with meals
- To avoid OTC preparations unless ordered by care provider

STORAGE
- Store at room temp in light-resistant container

---

hydrocortisone, hydrocortisone acetate, hydrocortisone butyrate, hydrocortisone cypionate, hydrocortisone sodium phosphate, hydrocortisone succinate, hydrocortisone valerate

Brand Names(s): hydrocortisone: AquaCort✤, Cortate✤, Cortef, Corter✤, Cortenema✤, Cortoderm✤, Emo-Cort Hycort✤, Hydrocortone, Prevex HCSarna-HC✤, Texacort✤; hydrocortisone acetate: Biosone, Cortacet✤, Corrtamed✤, Corticreme✤, Cortifoam✤, Cortiment✤, Cortisone Acetate-ICN✤, Cortone Suspension✤, Cortone Tablets✤, Hyderm✤, Rectocort✤; hydrocortisone butyrate: Locoid Cream, Ointment, Topical Solution; hydrocortisone cypionate: Cortef; hydrocortisone sodium phosphate: Hydrocortone Phosphate; hydrocortisone sodium succinate: A-Hydro-Cort✤, Lifocort, Solu-Cortef✤; hydrocortisone valerate: Westcort Cream 0.2%, Westcort Ointment 0.2%

Classification: Adrenocorticoid replacement

Pregnancy Category: C

AVAILABLE PREPARATIONS
Tabs: 5 mg, 10 mg, 20 mg (hydrocortisone)
Oral susp: 10 mg/5 ml (hydrocortisone cypionate)
Inj: 25 mg/ml, 50 mg/ml susp (hydrocortisone acetate); 50 mg/ml sol (hydrocortisone sodium phosphate); 100 mg/vial, 250 mg/vial, 500 mg/vial, 1000 mg/vial (sodium succinate)
Enema: 100 mg/60 ml (hydrocortisone)
Cream (top): 0.25%, 0.5%, 1%,

✤ Available in Canada.

2.5% (hydrocortisone); 0.2% (hydrocortisone valerate)

Ointment (top): 0.5%, (hydrocortisone); 0.5%, 1% (hydrocortisone acetate); 0.1% (hydrocortisone butyrate); 0.2% (hydrocortisone valerate)

ROUTES AND DOSAGES
Acute Adrenal Insufficiency
Infants and children <6 yr: IM/IV 1-2 mg/kg/dose bolus, then 25-150 mg/24 hr divided tid

Children >6 yr: IM/IV 1-2 mg/kg/dose bolus, then 150-250 mg/24 hr divided tid

Adults: IM/IV/SC 15-240 mg q12h

Physiologic Replacement
Children: PO 0.5-0.75 mg/kg/24 hr or 20-25 mg/m^2/24 hr divided q8h; IM 0.25-0.35 mg/kg/24 hr or 12-15 mg/m^2/24 hr qd

Antiinflammatory or Immunosuppressive
Infants and children: PO 2.5-10 mg/kg/24 hr or 75-300 mg/m^2/24 hr divided q6-8h; IM/IV 1-5 mg/kg/24 hr or 30-150 mg/m^2/24 hr divided q12-24h

Adults: IM/IV/SC 15-240 mg q12h

Congenital Adrenal Hyperplasia
PO, initial 30-36 mg/m^2/24 hr divided ⅓ dose q AM and ⅔ dose q PM, or ¼ q AM and midday and ½ q PM; maintenance 20-25 mg/m^2/24 hr in divided doses

Status Asthmaticus
Children: Loading IV 1-2 mg/kg/dose q6h for 24 hr; maintenance 0.5-1 mg/kg/dose q6h

Adults: IV 100-500 mg/dose q6h

Shock
Children: IM/IV initial 50 mg/kg (hydrocortisone succinate), then repeat q4h and/or q24h prn

Adults: IM/IV 500 mg-2 g q2-6h (hydrocortisone succinate)

Inflammation
Children and adults: Rectal, 1 application qd-bid for 2-3 weeks; top, apply bid-qid

IV administration
• Recommended concentration: Hydrocortisone sodium phosphate 50 mg/ml for IV push or dilute in D$_5$W or NS for IV infusion; hydrocortisone sodium succinate 50 or 125 mg/ml for IV push or dilute to 0.1-1 mg/ml in D$_5$NS, D$_5$W, or NS for IV infusion

• Maximum concentration: 50 mg/ml for hydrocortisone sodium phosphate, 125 mg/ml for hydrocortisone sodium succinate

• IV push rate: Over 30 sec (100 mg) to 10 min (≥500 mg)

• Intermittent infusion rate: Over 20-30 min

• Continuous infusion rate: Varies based on indication from bolus to 2 mg/kg over 8 hr

MECHANISM AND INDICATIONS
Mechanism: Replacement adrenocorticoid has actions similar to endogenous adrenocorticoids with both glucocorticoid and mineralocorticoid effects; antiinflammatory acts through synthesis of enzymes that decrease inflammation

Indications: Adrenal insufficiency, severe inflammation

PHARMACOKINETICS
Onset: 1-2 hr PO; 20 min IM/IV
Peak: 1-2 hr
Half-life: 30 min
Metabolism: Liver
Excretion: Urine

CONTRAINDICATIONS AND PRECAUTIONS
• Contraindicated with hypersensitivity, systemic fungal infections

• Use cautiously with pregnancy, lactation, latent amebiasis, GI ulceration, renal disease, hypertension, osteoporosis, diabetes, seizures, myasthenia gravis, CHF, tuberculosis, glaucoma, cataracts, psychosis, AIDS, liver disease

INTERACTIONS
Drug
• Decreased effect of hydrocortisone with barbiturates, phenytoin, rifampin, cholestyramine, colestipol, ephedrine, theophylline, antacids

• Decreased effects of anticoagulants, anticonvulsants, oral hypoglycemics, toxoids, vaccines

• Increased effect of hydrocortisone with salicylates, estrogen

• Increased risk of GI ulceration with other GI irritants

- Increased hypokalemia when used with amphotericin B and diuretics

Lab
- Suppressed reaction to allergy skin tests
- False negative on nitrobluetetrazolium tests for bacterial infection
- Altered thyroid function tests
- Increased cholesterol, glucose, urinary Ca
- Decreased K$^+$, Ca, T$_4$, T$_3$

INCOMPATIBILITIES

- Hydrocortisone phosphate with amobarbital, calcium gluconate, cephalothin, chloramphenicol, erythromycin, diazepam, heparin, kanamycin, metaraminol, methicillin, pentobarbital, phenobarbital, phenytoin, phytonadione, prochlorperazine, promazine, tetracycline, vancomycin, vitamin B complex with C, warfarin
- Hydrocortisone succinate with aminophylline, amobarbital, ampicillin, bleomycin, chlorpromazine, colistimethate, dimenhydrinate, diphenhydramine, doxorubicin, ephedrine, heparin, hyaluronidase, hydralazine, hydroxyzine, kanamycin, lidocaine, meperidine, nafcillin, netilmicin, pentobarbital, phenobarbital, prochlorperazine, promazine, promethazine, secobarbital, tetracycline, tolazoline, vancomycin, diazepam, phenytoin

SIDE EFFECTS

CNS: Euphoria, depression, flushing, sweating, headache, mood changes, insomnia, psychotic behavior, pseudotumor cerebri, nervousness
CV: Hypertension, CHF, edema
DERM: Acne, delayed healing, striae, ecchymosis, petechiae
EENT: Thrush, cataracts, glaucoma, blurred vision
ENDO: Suppression of hypothalamic–pituitary–adrenal axis (dependent on dosage, frequency, time, duration of therapy); highly variable from pt to pt; abrupt withdrawal can lead to nausea, fatigue, hypotension, hypoglyce-

mia, and other symptoms associated with adrenal insufficiency; this can be fatal
GI: Peptic ulcer, diarrhea, nausea, increased appetite, abdominal distention
HEME: Thrombocytopenia
MS: Fractures, osteoporosis, muscle weakness
Other: Pancreatitis, immunosuppression, hirsutism, cushingoid appearance, Na retention, hypokalemia, growth suppression in children, glucosuria

TOXICITY AND OVERDOSE

Clinical signs: Generally no severe symptoms noted even with massive doses; side effects as above; increased risk for suppression of endogenous secretion of adrenocorticoids
Treatment: Decrease drug gradually if possible

PATIENT CARE MANAGEMENT

Assessment
- Assess history of hypersensitivity to hydrocortisone
- Assess baseline wt, B/P, bone age, K$^+$, BG with long term therapy

Interventions
- Administer PO with food or milk to decrease GI distress
- Administer IM deeply; rotate injection sites; avoid deltoid; avoid SC administration in children
- Dosage may need to be increased for increased physiologic stress (trauma, surgery, febrile illness)

> **NURSING ALERT**
> Abrupt withdrawal of chronic doses can lead to potentially fatal adrenal crisis; long-term therapy should only be decreased by tapering dosage

Evaluation
- Evaluate therapeutic response (decreased inflammation)
- Monitor wt gain, linear growth, B/P, mental status
- Monitor hypokalemia (paresthesias, fatigue, nausea, vomiting, depression, polyuria, arrhythmias, weakness)

• Monitor symptoms of infection (fever, increased WBC) which may be masked by medication

PATIENT AND FAMILY EDUCATION
Teach/instruct
• To take as directed at prescribed intervals for prescribed length of time
• About implications of decreased immune response in relation to vaccinations and childhood illness exposures, especially chicken pox; to report febrile illness, other stress immediately
• About rationale for therapy
• That adrenal crisis can be life threatening; parents may be taught to administer IM in event that PO is not tolerated (acute illness in adrenal insufficiency)
Warn/advise
• To notify care provider of hypersensitivity, side effects (especially long term)
• Not to discontinue suddenly
• To inform all care providers of medication use
• To carry medical alert ID
• To restrict Na intake, increase K+ intake

STORAGE
• Store at room temp, unless otherwise noted on package insert

---

hydromorphone hydrochloride

Brand Name(s): Dilaudid✽, Dihydromorphone, Dilaudid-HP✽, Dilaudid-HP-Plus✽, Dilaudid-XP✽, Dilaudid Sterile Powder✽, Hydromorph Contin✽, PNS-Hydromorphone✽

Classification: Narcotic analgesic, agonist, opiate

Controlled Substance Schedule II

Pregnancy Category: C

AVAILABLE PREPARATIONS
Tabs: 1 mg, 2 mg, 3 mg, 4 mg
Rectal supp: 3 mg

Inj: 1 mg/ml, 2 mg/ml, 3 mg/ml, 4 mg/ml

ROUTES AND DOSAGES
Children >12 yr: PO: 2 mg q3-6h prn, may be increased to 4 mg q4-6h or 0.06 mg/kg q3-6h; rectal 3 mg q4-8h prn; IM/SC 1-2 mg q4-6h prn, may be increased to 3-4 mg q4-6h; IV 0.5-1 mg q3h prn; IV infusion 2-9 mg/hr; alternate parenteral dosing 0.015 mg/kg q3-4h
IV administration
• Recommended concentration: Dilute in at least 5 ml of SW, NS
• IV push rate: Very slow; each 2 mg over 2-5 min, administer through Y-tube or 3-way stopcock
• Continuous infusion: Dilute each 0.1-1 mg in 1 ml of NS to provide 0.1-1 mg/ml; deliver by narcotic syringe infusor; may be diluted in D_5W, D_5NS, ½NS, or NS for larger amounts and delivery through an infusion pump
• Continuous infusion rate (via controlled infusion device): 2-9 mg/hr

MECHANISM AND INDICATIONS
Mechanism: Binds to the opiate receptor in CNS; alters perception of and response to painful stimuli, while producing generalized CNS depression
Indications: Used to treat moderate or severe pain

PHARMACOKINETICS
Onset: PO, PR, SC, IM, 15-30 min; IV 10-15 min
Peak: PO, PR, SC, IM, 30-90 min; IV 15-30 min
Distribution: Widely distributed
Duration: PO, PR, SC, IM, 4-5 hr; IV 2-3 hr
Half-life: 2-4 hr
Metabolism: Liver
Excretion: Urine

CONTRAINDICATIONS AND PRECAUTIONS
• Contraindicated with hypersensitivity; avoid chronic use during pregnancy, lactation, with narcotic addiction
• Use cautiously with head trauma, increased ICP; severe re-

✽ Available in Canada.

nal, hepatic, or pulmonary disease; hypothyroidism, adrenal insufficiency, alcoholism, undiagnosed abdominal pain, severe heart disease, respiratory depression; use extreme caution in pts receiving MAOIs

INTERACTIONS
Drug
• Increased risk of coma, respiratory depression, hypotension with use of MAOIs
• Additive CNS depression with alcohol, antidepressants, antipsychotics, skeletal muscle relaxants, antihistamines, sedative or hypnotics.
• Withdrawal in narcotic-dependent pts with use of partial antagonists (buprenorphine, butorphanol, nalbuphine, pentazocine)
Lab
• Increased amylase and lipase

INCOMPATIBILITIES
• Alkalies, bromides, iodides, pentobarbital, prochlorperazine, NaHCO$_3$, thiopental

SIDE EFFECTS
CNS: Sedation, confusion, headache, euphoria, floating feeling, unusual dreams, hallucinations, dysphoria, dizziness
CV: Hypotension, bradycardia, palpitations
DERM: Sweating, flushing, rash, urticaria, bruising, flushing, pruritus
EENT: Miosis, diplopia, blurred vision
GI: Nausea, vomiting, constipation, anorexia, cramps
GU: Urinary retention, increased urinary output, dysuria
RESP: Respiratory depression
Other: Tolerance, physical and psychological addiction

TOXICITY AND OVERDOSE
Clinical signs: Respiratory depression, respiratory rate <8-10/min
Treatment: Supportive care; naloxone (dose may need to be repeated or naloxone infusion administered)

PATIENT CARE MANAGEMENT
Assessment
• Assess history of hypersensitivity to hydromorphone and related drugs
• Assess baseline VS, bowel and urinary function
• Assess pain (type, location, intensity)
Interventions
• Administer before pain becomes too severe; regularly scheduled administration may be more effective than prn administration
• May administer with non-narcotic analgesics to produce additive analgesic effects and permit lower narcotic dosages
• Discontinue gradually after long-term use to prevent withdrawal symptoms
• Administer antiemetic if nausea or vomiting occur
• Determine dosage interval based on pt response
• Institute safety measures (supervise ambulation, raise side rails, call light within reach)

> **NURSING ALERT**
> Use of controlled IV infusion should be reserved for critically ill oncology patients with pain uncontrollable by other methods or agents
>
> Rapid administration may lead to increased respiratory depression, hypotension, circulatory collapse; provide naloxone for IV administration

Evaluation
• Evaluate therapeutic response (decrease in severity of pain without significant alteration in LOC or respiratory status)
• Monitor VS, pain control 30-60 min after administration, CNS changes, respiratory dysfunction
• Evaluate side effects, hypersensitivity

• Evaluate for increased need for higher dosages with prolonged use

PATIENT AND FAMILY EDUCATION
Teach/instruct
• To take as directed at prescribed intervals for prescribed length of time
• About best time to request medication if ordered prn
• About use of PCA pump
Warn/advise
• That tolerance or dependence may occur with long term use
• That drug may cause drowsiness, dizziness, orthostatic hypotension; make position changes slowly, seek assistance with ambulation
• To avoid any activity that requires alertness
• To avoid concurrent use of alcohol, other CNS depressants
• To notify care provider of side effects, hypersensitivity
Encourage
• That coughing, deep breathing, and movement help to prevent respiratory complications

STORAGE
• Store at room temp
• Protect from light

---

hydroxychloroquine sulfate
Brand Name(s): Plaquenil Sulfate✦
Classification: Antimalarial
Pregnancy Category: C

AVAILABLE PREPARATIONS
Tabs: 200 mg (155 mg base)

ROUTES AND DOSAGES
Suppression or Chemoprophylaxis of Malaria
Children: PO 5 mg/kg once/wk, beginning 1-2 wk before exposure and continuing 6-8 wk after leaving endemic area; maximum 310 mg/kg/24 hr (regardless of wt)
Adults: PO 400 mg once/wk (on same day of each wk), beginning

1-2 wk before exposure and continuing 6-8 wk after leaving endemic area
Acute Malaria
Children: PO 10 mg/kg initial dose, followed by 5 mg/kg in 6 hr on 1st day; 5 mg/kg as single dose on 2nd and 3rd day
Adults: PO 800 mg initial dose, followed by 400 mg in 6 hr on 1st day; 400 mg as single dose on 2nd and 3rd day
Juvenile Rheumatoid Arthritis or Systemic Lupus Erythematosus
Children: 3-5 mg/kg/24 hr qd or divided bid; maximum 400 mg/24 hr or 7 mg/kg/24 hr
Rheumatoid Arthritis
Adults: 400-600 mg/24 hr qd with meals; increase until optimum response is achieved; maintenance 200-400 mg/24 hr qd
Lupus Erythematosus
Adults: 400 mg qd-bid until optimum response is achieved; maintenance 200-400 mg/24 hr

MECHANISM AND INDICATIONS
Mechanism: Inhibits replication of parasite by altering properties of DNA
Indications: Used in suppression and treatment of malaria caused by *Plasmodium malariae, P. ovale, P. falciparum, P. vivax;* also used to treat rheumatoid arthritis and systemic lupus erythematosus

PHARMACOKINETICS
Peak: 1-2 hr
Distribution: Widely distributed; concentrates in lungs, liver, erythrocytes, eyes, skin, kidneys
Half-life: 70-120 hr
Metabolism: Liver
Excretion: Urine, feces

CONTRAINDICATIONS AND PRECAUTIONS
• Contraindicated with prolonged therapy in children with known hypersensitivity to drug, retinal or visual field changes, porphyria
• Use cautiously with hepatic disease, with other hepatotoxic drugs; with G-6-PD deficiency,

blood dyscrasias, severe GI disease, neurologic disease, alcoholism, pregnancy, psoriasis, eczema

INTERACTIONS
Drug
• Decreased absorption with use of products containing Mg, kaolin, aluminum compounds

SIDE EFFECTS
CNS: Irritability, headache, nightmares, ataxia, convulsions, tinnitus, nystagmus, lassitude, fatigue, confusion, vertigo, hypoactive deep tendon reflexes
CV: Hypotension, heart block, asystole with syncope
DERM: Alopecia, eruptions, eczema, exfoliation, pruritus, flushing, pigmentation changes
EENT: Blurred vision, difficult focus, corneal changes, retinal changes, optic atrophy, labyrinthitis
GI: Nausea, vomiting, anorexia, diarrhea, cramps
HEME: Agranulocytosis, thrombocytopenia, anemia, leukopenia

TOXICITY AND OVERDOSE
Clinical signs: Visual or hearing alterations, headache
Treatment: Supportive care

PATIENT CARE MANAGEMENT
Assessment
• Assess history of hypersensitivity to hydroxychloroquine
• Assess history of travel or exposure
• Obtain blood samples to test for and identify organism
• Assess baseline ophthalmic test for long term therapy
Interventions
• Administer drug on same day of each wk for prophylaxis
• Give with meals to reduce gastric distress; tabs may be crushed, mixed with small amount of food or fluid

Evaluation
• Evaluate therapeutic response (decreased symptoms of malaria)
• Observe for side effects and monitor closely; obtain CBCs, ALT, AST, bilirubin, ophthalmologic, and audiometric tests during long term therapy
• Evaluate side effects, hypersensitivity (pruritus, rash, urticaria)
• Evaluate CBC for blood dyscrasias (malaise, fever, bruising, bleeding)
• Evaluate for ototoxicity (tinnitus, change in hearing, vertigo)
• Evaluate AST, ALT, bilirubin each week
• Evaluate for decreased reflexes in knee or ankle
• Evaluate ECG during therapy (depression of T-waves, increased QRS duration)

PATIENT AND FAMILY EDUCATION
Teach/instruct
• To take as directed at prescribed intervals for prescribed length of time
• To use sunglasses in bright sunlight to avoid photophobia
Warn/advise
• To notify care provider of hypersensitivity, side effects
• To exercise mosquito precautions while in infested area
• That urine may turn rust or brown
• To report hearing, visual problems, fever, fatigue, bleeding, bruising
Encourage
• To comply with prescribed regime

STORAGE
• Store at room temp in tight container
• Injection should be kept in cool environment

NURSING ALERT
Fatalities have occurred in children with just 3-4 tabs; keep out of reach

---

hydroxyurea

Brand Name(s): Hydrea ♣

Classification: Antineoplastic, selective DNA antimetabolite; cell cycle phase specific (S phase)

Pregnancy Category: D

AVAILABLE PREPARATIONS
Caps: 500 mg

ROUTES AND DOSAGES
• Dosage may vary in response to diagnosis, extent of disease, concurrent or previous therapy, protocol guidelines, physiologic parameters; consult current literature, protocol recommendations

CML

Doses titrated to peripheral blood counts; recommended PO dosage 10-30 mg/kg qd; majority of pts demonstrate control of symptoms and peripheral blasts with dosages of 1-3 g/24 hr

MECHANISM AND INDICATIONS
Mechanism: Exact mechanism unknown; drug diffuses passively into cells, blocking conversion of ribonucleotides to deoxyribonucleotides, causing immediate cessation of DNA synthesis; may also directly damage DNA by inhibiting incorporation of thymidine into DNA structure; may inhibit cellular repair of DNA; specific for S phase of cell cycle, causes cells to arrest in G-1 to S phase

Indications: Management of myeloproliferative disorders (including acute blast and chronic phases of CML, thrombocytopenia, polycythemia vera, hypereosinophilia); theoretically, might be useful as radiosensitizer because it synchronizes cells in radiosensitive G-1 phase; may be useful in sickle cell disease, since it causes increased production of hemoglobin F, associated with decreased incidence of hemolysis

PHARMACOKINETICS
Peak: 1-2 hr in serum; 3 hr in CSF

Distribution: Uptake rapid by cells; crosses blood–brain barrier

Half-life: 2-5.5 hr

Metabolism: 50% degraded in liver; also broken down by urease in intestinal bacteria

Excretion: 70%-80% unchanged in urine; CO_2 in expired air

CONTRAINDICATIONS AND PRECAUTIONS
• Contraindicated with hypersensitivity, active infections (especially chicken pox and herpes zoster), marked bone marrow suppression, pregnancy, lactation
• Use cautiously in pts who have previously received myelosuppressive chemotherapy or radiation therapy; with renal dysfunction

INTERACTIONS
Drug
• Reduced efficacy of ferrous iron
• Enhanced activity of iron chelating agents
• Administration with 5-FU blocks conversion of 5-FU to active metabolite; if leucovorin also administered, cytotoxicity of 5-FU is enhanced
• Enhanced cytotoxicity of cytarabine
• Enhanced efficacy of drugs that damage DNA possible, as hydroxyurea blocks cellular repair efforts

Lab
• Interference with triglyceride measurement by glycerol oxidase method
• Increased serum concentration of creatinine, BUN, uric acid

SIDE EFFECTS
CNS: Headache, vertigo, disorientation, seizures

DERM: Maculopapular rash, facial erythema; radiation recall phenomena; long term use may cause thinning of skin and erythema; alopecia (rare)

GI: Nausea, vomiting, diarrhea or constipation, stomatitis (rare)

GU: Dysuria, impairment of tubular dysfunction resulting in azotemia with increased BUN, creatinine, hyperuricemia, renal dysfunction

HEME: Bone marrow suppression

♣ Available in Canada.

with leukopenic nadir at 10 days; platelets, RBCs not generally significantly affected

TOXICITY AND OVERDOSE
Clinical signs: Prolonged myelosuppression
Treatment: Supportive measures (including blood transfusions, hydration, nutritional supplementation, broad-spectrum antibiotic therapy if febrile, electrolyte replacement)

PATIENT CARE MANAGEMENT
Assessment
• Assess history of hypersensitivity to hydroxyurea
• Assess history of previous treatment
• Assess efficacy of previous antiemetic therapy
• Assess baseline CBC, differential, platelet count
• Assess baseline renal function, (BUN, creatinine), liver function (alk phos LDH, AST, ALT, bilirubin), and serum uric acid function
Interventions
• Premedicate with antiemetic therapy if needed
• Contents of cap may be dissolved in liquid, taken immediately
• Provide supportive measures to maintain hemostasis, fluid, electrolyte, nutritional balance status
Evaluation
• Evaluate therapeutic response (CBC recovery)
• Evaluate CBC, differential, platelet count weekly
• Evaluate renal function, (BUN, creatinine), liver function (AST, ALT, LDH, alk phos, bilirubin), and serum uric acid function regularly

PATIENT AND FAMILY EDUCATION
Teach/instruct
• To have patient well hydrated before and after chemotherapy
• About importance of follow-up visits to monitor blood counts, serum chemistry values
• To take accurate temp; rectal temp contraindicated
• To notify care provider of signs of bleeding (bruising, epistaxis, bleeding gums), infection (fever, sore throat, fatigue)
Warn/advise
• About impact of body changes that may occur (hair loss, hyperpigmentation, nail ridging), how to minimize changes (wigs, caps, scarves, long sleeves)
• To avoid OTC preparations containing aspirin
• To report any alterations in behavior, sensation, perception; help to develop a plan of care to manage side effects, stress of illness or treatment
• That good oral hygiene with very soft toothbrush is imperative
• That dental work be delayed until blood counts return to baseline, with permission of caretaker
• To avoid contact with known viral, bacterial illnesses
• That close household contacts of child not be immunized with live polio virus; use inactivated form
• That children on chemotherapy not receive immunizations until immune system recovers sufficiently to mount necessary antibody response
• To report exposure to chicken pox in susceptible child immediately
• To report reactivation of herpes zoster virus (shingles) immediately
• If appropriate, ways to preserve reproductive patterns, sexuality (sperm banking, contraceptives)
Encourage
• Provision of nutritious food intake; consider nutrition consultation
• To use top anesthetics to control discomfort of mucositis; avoid spicy foods, commercial mouthwashes

STORAGE
• Store caps at room temp
• Protect from moisture

H

hydroxyzine hydrochloride, hydroxyzine pamoate

Brand Name(s): E-Vista, Hydroxacen, Multipax✿, Novo-Hydroxyzin✿, Quiess, Rezine, Vistazine; hydroxyzine hydrochloride: Anxanil, Apo-Hydroxide✿, Atarax✿; hydroxyzine pamoate: Hy-Pam, Vistaril

Classification: Antihistamine, antianxiety agent, antiemetic

Pregnancy Category: C

AVAILABLE PREPARATIONS
• Not available in generic form
Syrup: 10 mg/5 ml (Atarax) contains alcohol
Susp: 25 mg/5 ml (Vistaril)
Tabs: 10 mg, 25 mg, 50 mg, 100 mg (Anxanil, Atarax)
Caps: 25 mg, 50 mg, 100 mg (Hy-Pam, Vistaril)
Inj: Hydroxyzine hydrochloride 25 mg/ml, 50 mg/ml

DOSAGES AND ROUTES
Antihistamine, Antiemetic, Antipruritic
Children: PO 2 mg/kg/24 hr divided q6-8h; IM 0.5-1 mg/kg/dose q4-6h
Antiemetic
Adults: IM 25-100 mg/dose q4-6h prn
Anxiety
Adults: PO 25-100 mg qid, maximum 600 mg/24 hr
Preoperative Sedation
Adults: PO 50-100 mg; IM 25-100 mg
Pruritis
Adults: PO 25 mg tid-qid

MECHANISM AND INDICATIONS
Mechanism: Depresses subcortical levels of CNS, including limbic system and reticular formation; competes with histamine for H_1 receptor sites on effector cells in the GI tract, blood vessels, and respiratory tract

Indications: For use as a preoperative sedative, antihistamine, antiemetic, antipruritic; in the treatment of anxiety

PHARMACOKINETICS
Onset of action: PO 15-30 min
Duration: PO 4-6 hr
Half-life: PO 3 hr

CONTRAINDICATIONS AND PRECAUTIONS
• Contraindicated with hypersensitivity to this or any component of this medication; lactation, early pregnancy
• Use cautiously with kidney disease, liver disease; in elderly, debilitated pts, children with uncontrollable seizures

INTERACTIONS
Drug
• Increased CNS depressant effects with alcohol, analgesics, barbiturates, narcotics, antidepressants, antipsychotics
• Additive anticholinergic effects with anticholinergics
• Decreased effects of epinephrine
Lab
• Falsely elevated 17-OHCS
Nutrition
• Do not drink alcohol

SIDE EFFECTS
CNS: Dizziness, drowsiness, ataxia, confusion, depression, fatigue, headache, seizures, tremor, weakness
CV: Hypotension
GI: Dry mouth
Local: Pain at injection site
Other: Difficulty breathing, chest tightness, involuntary movements, wheezing

TOXICITY AND OVERDOSE
Clinical signs: Oversedation
Treatment: If orally ingested, monitor VS; lavage; administer IV norepinephrine for hypotension

PATIENT CARE MANAGEMENT
Assessment
• Assess history of hypersensitivity to drug
• Obtain baseline CBC, AST, ALT, bilirubin, creatinine
• Obtain baseline assessment of

✿ Available in Canada.

symptom treated (allergy, anxiety, itching, vomiting)

Interventions

- Usually administered PO prn
- Administer at hs for best sedative and anti-itching effects
- Shake susp well before pouring
- Do not crush coated tab; if necessary, consult prescriber for another form
- Administer IM to children by Z-track injection in midlateral muscles of the thigh
- Has been administered slowly by IV to oncology pts via central venous lines without problems
- Do not drink alcohol
- Take with food or milk if GI symptoms occur
- Rinse with water, take sips of fluid, sugarless gum, or hard candy for dry mouth

---

NURSING ALERT

Extravasation can result in sterile abscess, marked tissue induration

SC, intraarterial, and IV administration are not recommended since thrombosis and gangrene can occur

---

Evaluation

- Evaluate therapeutic response (symptoms of allergy, anxiety, itching, vomiting)
- Evaluate mental status (mood, sensorium, affect, impulsiveness, suicidal ideation, thoughts)
- Monitor orthostatic B/P; if systolic B/P drops 20 mm Hg, hold drug, notify prescriber

PATIENT AND FAMILY EDUCATION

Teach/instruct

- To take as directed at prescribed intervals for prescribed length of time
- To discontinue drug at first appearance of wheezing, breathing difficulty, or chest tightness; to contact prescriber immediately
- To keep this and all medications out of reach of children

Warn/advise

- To make sure medication is swallowed
- To consult pharmacist for expiration date of hydroxyzine (because it is taken on an as-needed basis)
- To avoid ingesting alcohol, other CNS depressants
- To avoid OTC cold, cough, antihistamine medications unless approved by prescriber
- May cause drowsiness; be careful on bicycles, skates, skateboards, while driving, or with other activities requiring alertness

STORAGE

- Store at room temp
- Protect from light

---

ibuprofen

Brand Name(s): Aches-N-Pain, Actiprofen✤, Advil✤, Apo-Ibuprofen✤, Cap-Profen, Children's Advil, Exedrin IS, Genpril, Haltran, Ibuprin, IBU-Tab, Ifen, Menadol, Medipren, Midol 200, Motrin✤, Motrin-IB✤, Novo-Profen✤, Nuprin, Nu-Ibuprofen✤, Pamprin-IB, PediaProfen, Rufen, Saleto-200, 400, 600, 800, Tab-Profen, Trendar, Uni-Pro

Classification: Non-narcotic analgesic, non-steroidal antiinflammatory agent, antipyretic, antirheumatic

Pregnancy Category: B (1st and 2nd trimester), D (3rd trimester)

AVAILABLE PREPARATIONS

Susp: 100 mg/5 ml
Tabs: 200 mg, 300 mg, 400 mg, 600 mg, 800 mg
Tabs (film coated): 200 mg, 300 mg, 400 mg, 600 mg, 800 mg

ROUTES AND DOSAGES
Juvenile Rheumatoid Arthritis
• Dosages established by clinicians, not by manufacturers
Children ≤20 kg: PO: 400 mg/24 hr maximum divided q6-8h
Children 20-30 kg: PO: 600 mg/24 hr maximum divided q6-8h
Children 30-40 kg: PO: 800 mg/24 hr maximum divided q6-8h
Menstrual Pain
Adolescents and adults: PO 200-400 mg q4-6h prn; maximum 1.2 g/24 hr
Fever
Children and adults: PO 5-10 mg/kg q6-8h; maximum 40 mg/kg/24 hr

MECHANISM AND INDICATIONS
Mechanism: Interferes with action of prostaglandins; has an effect on the hypothalmus; and acts to block peripheral nerve transfer
Indications: Used for management of inflammatory disorders (including rheumatoid arthritis); treatment of mild or moderate pain or dysmenorrhea; treatment of fever

PHARMACOKINETICS
Onset: Analgesia 30 min; antiinflammatory 1-2 wk
Peak: Analgesia 1-2 hr; antiinflammatory 1-2 wk
Duration: Analgesia 4-6 hr; antiinflammatory unknown
Half-life: 2-4 hr
Metabolism: Liver
Excretion: Urine
Distribution: Highly protein bound with distribution in body unknown

CONTRAINDICATIONS AND PRECAUTIONS
• Contraindicated with known hypersensitivity (cross sensitivity may exist with other NSAIDs, including aspirin), active GI bleeding or ulcer disease, severe renal or hepatic disease, asthma; use for children should be supervised by a health care provider
• Use cautiously in 1st and 2nd trimester of pregnancy; with bleeding disorders, GI disorders, cardiac disorders; in children

INTERACTIONS
Drug
• Additive adverse GI side effects with aspirin and other NSAIDs
• Increased risk of adverse renal reactions with concurrent chronic use of acetaminophen
• Decreased effectiveness of antihypertensive therapy possible
• Increased hypoglycemic effect of insulin or oral hypoglycemic agents possible
• Increased risk of bleeding with oral anticoagulant, cefamandole, cefoperazone, moxalactam, or plicamycin
• Increased serum lithium and increased risk of toxicity possible
• Increased risk of toxicity from methotrexate, verapamil, nifedipine
• Increased risk of ibuprofen toxicity with probenecid
• Increased risk of GI side effects with other drugs having similar effects such as corticosteroids, K^+, aspirin
• Potentiation of anticoagulant effects with drugs (e.g., aspirin, heparin, and coumarin)
• Increased risk of hematologic side effects with other drugs with same effect or with radiation
• Decreased serum level of ibuprofen possible when administered with aspirin
• Increased action of phenytoin and sulfonamides possible
Lab
• Prolonged bleeding time for 1-2 days; no effect on pro-time
• Increased ALT, AST, alk phos, LDH, transaminase, BUN, creatinine, K^+, urine glucose, urine protein
• Decreased BG, Hgb, Hct, CrCl possible
• Decreased urine output, uric acid possible
Nutrition
• Absorption is slowed, but not decreased, by food

SIDE EFFECTS
CNS: Headache, drowsiness, psy-

chic disturbances, dizziness, weakness, insomnia, confusion, fatigue, tremors, anxiety, depression
CV: Palpitations, tachycardia, peripheral edema, arrhythmias, hypertension
DERM: Urticaria, pruritus, sweating, rashes, purpura, alopecia, Stevens-Johnson syndrome
EENT: Dry mouth, blurred vision, tinnitus, amblyopia, cataracts, hearing loss
GI: Nausea, dyspepsia, vomiting, constipation, GI bleeding, discomfort, anorexia, diarrhea, jaundice, cholestatic hepatitis, flatulence, cramps, peptic ulcer
GU: Renal failure, hematuria, cystitis, polyuria, nephrotoxicity, oliguria, azotemia
HEME: Blood dyscrasias, prolonged bleeding time, neutropenia, agranulocytosis, aplastic anemia, thrombocytopenia, anemia
RESP: Bronchospasm, dyspnea, and anaphylaxis as allergic response

TOXICITY AND OVERDOSE
Clinical signs: Blurred vision, tinnitus, dizziness, nystagmus, apnea, cyanosis
Treatment: Supportive care, induce vomiting or gastric lavage, administer alkali solution and induce diuresis; may also use activated charcoal

PATIENT CARE MANAGEMENT
Assessment
• Assess history of hypersensitivity to ibuprofen, aspirin, other NSAIDs
• Assess pain (type, location, intensity), range of motion (if used for treatment of arthritis)
• Assess temp; note signs associated with fever (diaphoresis, tachycardia, malaise) if used for treatment of fever
• Assess cardiac status, renal function (BUN, creatinine, I&O), liver function (ALT, AST, bilirubin), CBC, differential, platelet count before anticipated long term treatment
• Perform audiometric, ophthalmic examination before long term treatment
• Assess history of peptic ulcer
Interventions
• May crush tab, mix with fluids or food; 800 mg tabs can be dissolved in water
• Administer with full glass of water; may administer with food, milk, or antacids to decrease GI irritation
• Administer 30 min ac or 2 hr after meals for rapid initial effect

> **NURSING ALERT**
> Pts who have asthma, aspirin-induced allergy, and nasal polyps are at increased risk for developing hypersensitivity reactions

Evaluation
• Evaluate therapeutic response (decreased pain, stiffness in joints; decreased swelling in joints; ability to move more easily; reduction in fever or menstrual cramping)
• Evaluate hepatic and renal labs with known dysfunction and bleeding time in pts with coagulation disorder
• Evaluate side effects, hypersensitivity

PATIENT AND FAMILY EDUCATION
Teach/instruct
• To take as directed at prescribed intervals for prescribed length of time
• Take with full glass of water; may administer with food, milk, antacids to decrease GI irritation
• Administer as soon as possible after onset of menses when used for the treatment of dysmenorrhea
• Partial arthritic relief usually occurs within 7 days, but maximum effectiveness may require 1-2 wks of continuous therapy
• Do not administer for >10 days for pain or >3 days for fever without consulting health care provider
• Consult health care provider if symptoms persist or worsen
• Antiinflammatory response may

not be seen for 1-2 wk, may take up to one mo

Warn/advise
- To avoid activities that require alertness until response is known
- To avoid concurrent use of alcohol, aspirin, acetaminophen, other OTC medications without consultation with health care provider
- To notify care provider of hypersensitivity, side effects
- To avoid sun, sunlamps

STORAGE
- Store at room temp
- Store in tightly closed, light-resisant container

---

idoxuridine (IDU)

Brand Name(s): Herplex✚, Herplex-D✚, Herplex Liquifilm, Stoxil Ophthalmic

Classification: Antiviral (pyrimidine nucleoside)

Pregnancy Category: C

AVAILABLE PREPARATIONS
Ophthal oint: 0.5%
Ophthal sol: 0.1%

ROUTES AND DOSAGES
Children and adults: Ophthal oint, instill 1 cm strip into conjunctival sac 5 times/24 hr q4h while awake, for 7 days; if no response after 7 days discontinue; do not use longer than 21 days; ophthal sol, instill 1 gtt into conjunctival sac q1h during the day and q2h during the night for 7 days; if no response after 7 days discontinue; do not use longer than 21 days

MECHANISM AND INDICATIONS
Antiviral mechanism: Blocks viral reproduction by interfering with DNA synthesis
Indications: Used for herpes simplex keratitis, CMV, varicella-zoster (alone or with corticosteroids)

PHARMACOKINETICS
Excretion: Urine

CONTRAINDICATIONS AND PRECAUTIONS
- Contraindicated with known hypersensitivity to idoxuridine or any component
- Use cautiously with known antibiotic hypersensitivity, corneal ulceration, corticosteroid applications, pregnancy

INTERACTIONS
Drug
- Precipitation of inactive ingredients or preservatives with use of boric acid preparations; do not use concomitantly

SIDE EFFECTS
EENT: Slow corneal wound healing, temporary visual haze, overgrowth of nonsusceptible organisms, irritation, pain, burning, or inflammation of eye, photophobia, mild edema of eyelid or cornea

TOXICITY AND OVERDOSE
Clinical signs: Toxicity of ingestion unknown; irritation with dermal exposure
Treatment: If ingested, induce emesis or perform gastric lavage; wash area with soap and water for dermal exposure

PATIENT CARE MANAGEMENT
Assessment
- Assess history of hypersensitivity to idoxuridine
- Obtain C&S; may begin therapy before obtaining results
- Assess eye for redness, swelling, discharge

Interventions
- See Chapter 2 regarding ophthal instillation; wash hands before, after application; cleanse crusts or discharge from eye before application; after instillation, apply gentle pressure to lacrimal sac for 1 min to minimize systemic absorption; wipe excess medication from eye; do not flush medication from eye

Evaluation
- Evaluate therapeutic response (decreased redness, inflammation, tearing, photophobia)
- Monitor for signs of allergic re-

---

action (itching, excessive tearing, redness, swelling)

PATIENT AND FAMILY EDUCATION
Teach/instruct
• To take as directed at prescribed intervals for prescribed length of time
Warn/advise
• To notify care provider of hypersensitivity, side effects, superinfection
• Not to share towels, wash cloths, bed linens, eye make-up with family member being treated
• To use sunglasses if photosensitivity occurs
• To keep hands away from eyes

STORAGE
• Store in refrigerator

---

ifosfamide
Brand Name(s): Ifex✤
Classification: Alkylating Agent
Pregnancy Category: D

AVAILABLE PREPARATIONS
Inj: 1 g, 2 g, 3 g vials

ROUTES AND DOSAGES
• Drug may vary in response to diagnosis, extent of disease, concurrent or previous therapy, protocol guidelines, physiologic parameters; consult current literature, protocol recommendations
Children: IV 1800 mg/m^2/24 hr for 3-5 days q3-4 wk, or 5000 mg/m^2 as single 24-hr infusion, or 3 g/m^2/24 hr for 2 days
Adults: IV 2000 mg/m^2/24 hr for 5 days, or 2400 mg/m^2/24 hr for 3 days q3-4 wk, or 5000 mg/m^2 as single 24 hr infusion
• Continuous infusion may be administered IV for 5 days; mesna begun simultaneously and repeated at specified intervals per protocol after ifosfamide
• Ifosfamide and mesna are compatible and may be mixed in same IV sol

IV administration
• Recommended concentration: 1 g reconstituted with 20 ml diluent, for 50 mg/ml; use SW or bacteriostatic water for inj; may be further diluted with SW, D$_5$W, ½NS, NS, D$_5$NS, or LR
• IV bolus/push rate: 50 mg/kg/24 hr; over 30 minutes, slowly

MECHANISM AND INDICATIONS
Mechanism: Activated by microsomes in the liver, is an analogue of cytoxan and is cell cycle phase non-specific; works by destroying DNA throughout the cell cycle by binding to protein and DNA, cross-links of cellular DNA, and interference of RNA transcription; causes an imbalance of growth that leads to cell death
Indications: Used to treat testicular cancer; also promising in treating recurrent lymphoma and soft tissue sarcomas; effective in tumors resistant to cytoxan

PHARMACOKINETICS
• In humans, exhibits dose-dependent pharmacokinetics
Peak: Serum, immediately after IV infusion/bolus push; CSF levels 38%-49% of plasma levels
Half-life: At doses of 3.8-5.0 g/m^2, plasma decay biphasic; half-life of elimination 16 hr, 50%-60% excreted in urine as parent drug; at doses 1.6-2.4 g/m^2, plasma decay monoexponential, half-life of elimination 6.9 hr, 12%-20% excreted unmetabolized in urine
Metabolism: Activated by microsomes in the liver
Excretion: 50% in urine, almost completely unchanged

CONTRAINDICATIONS AND PRECAUTIONS
• Contraindicated with pts in whom previous use has proven ineffective; with hypersensitivity to drug, with severely depressed bone marrow function, with active infections (especially chicken pox or herpes zoster), pregnancy, lactation
• Use cautiously with renal or hepatic impairment

✤ Available in Canada.

INTERACTIONS
Drug
- Increased risk of bleeding with aspirin or anticoagulants
- Increased ifosfamide effect with allopurinol
- Increased ifosfamide toxicity with barbiturates, chloral hydrate, phenytoin
- Increased hematologic toxicity with myelosuppressive agents
- Decreased ifosfamide effectiveness with corticosteroids

INCOMPATIBILITIES
- IV form incompatible with $NaHCO_3$ in sol

SIDE EFFECTS
CNS: Lethargy, confusion, somnolence, depressive psychosis, hallucinations, coma, dizziness, disorientation, cranial nerve dysfunction
CV: Supraventricular arrhythmias
DERM: Alopecia
GI: Nausea, vomiting, anorexia, diarrhea, sometimes constipation, elevated liver enzymes (especially alk phos, serum transaminase, BUN, creatinine)
GU: Dysuria, urinary frequency, hematuria, hemorrhagic cystitis (dose limiting), nephrotoxicity (elevated BUN, creatinine, decreased CrCl)
HEME: Leukopenia, thrombocytopenia, myelosuppression

TOXICITY AND OVERDOSE
Clinical signs: Hemorrhagic cystitis (dose-limiting) can occur in up to 50% of pts
Treatment: Mesna, extensive hydration

PATIENT CARE MANAGEMENT
Assessment
- Assess history of hypersensitivity to ifosfamide and related drugs (e.g., cyclophosphamide)
- Assess baseline VS, renal function (BUN, creatinine), cardiac and liver (ALT, AST, bilirubin, alk phos) function
- Assess baseline CBC, differential, platelet count, serum electrolytes
- Assess hydration status (SG) and assess for hematuria, dysuria, urinary frequency
- Assess neurologic and mental status before drug administration and on follow-up visits
- Assess urinary elimination pattern before each course of chemotherapy with ifosfamide
- Assess success of previous antiemetic therapy
- Assess history of previous treatment with special attention to other therapies that may predispose to renal or hepatic dysfunction

Interventions
- Premedicate with antiemetics and continue periodically through chemotherapy
- Maintain IV infusion rate and bolus rate over at least 30 min to decrease risk of cystitis
- Encourage small, frequent feedings of foods pt likes
- Administer IV fluids until pt is able to resume normal PO fluid intake
- Provide supportive measures to maintain hemostasis, fluid and electrolyte balance, and nutritional support

> **NURSING ALERT**
> Monitor closely for hemorrhagic cystitis
>
> Should only be administered with aggressive hydration and in combination with mesna, a protective, prophylactic agent for hemorrhagic cystitis

Evaluation
- Evaluate therapeutic response (decreased tumor size, spread of malignancy)
- Evaluate serum electrolytes, BUN, creatinine, bilirubin, alk phos, LDH, ALT, AST
- Evaluate CBC, differential, and platelet count at given intervals after chemotherapy
- Evaluate for signs and symp-

toms of infection (fever, fatigue, sore throat), bleeding (easy bruising, nose bleeds, bleeding gums)
• Evaluate I&O carefully, check wt daily; have pt empty bladder at least q2h
• Evaluate side effects, response to antiemetic regimen

PATIENT/FAMILY EDUCATION
Teach/instruct
• To have pt well-hydrated before and after chemotherapy
• About importance of follow-up to monitor blood counts, serum chemistry values, drug blood levels
• To take accurate temp; rectal temp contraindicated
• To notify care provider of signs of bleeding (bruising, epistaxis, bleeding gums), infection (fever, sore throat, fatigue)
Warn/advise
• About impact of body changes that might occur (hair loss, hyperpigmentation, nail ridging), how to minimize changes (wigs, caps, scarves, long sleeves)
• To avoid OTC products containing aspirin
• To report any alterations in behavior, sensation, perception; help to develop a plan of care to manage side effects, stress of illness or treatment
• To monitor bowel function and call if abdominal pain, constipation noted
• To immediately report any pain, discoloration at injection site (parenteral forms)
• That good oral hygiene with very soft toothbrush is imperative
• That dental work be delayed until blood counts return to baseline, with permission of the care provider
• To avoid contact with known viral, bacterial illnesses
• That household contacts of child not be immunized with live polio virus; inactivated form should be used
• That child not receive immunizations until immune system recovers sufficiently to mount needed antibody response
• To report exposure to chicken pox in susceptible child immediately
• To report reactivation of herpes zoster virus (shingles) immediately
• If appropriate, ways to preserve reproductive patterns, sexuality (sperm banking, contraceptives)
Encourage
• Provision of nutritious food intake; consider nutritional consultation
• To comply with bowel management program
• To use top anesthetics to control discomfort of mucositis; avoid spicy foods, commercial mouthwashes
• To maintain adequate fluid intake and void frequently to reduce risk of cystitis

STORAGE
• Store dry powder at room temp
• Reconstituted sol remains stable for 1 wk at room temp or 3 wks refrigerated; if reconstituted with SW, must be used within 6 hr

---

imipenem-cilastatin
Brand Name(s): Primaxin
Classification: Antibiotic (miscellaneous)
Pregnancy Category: C

AVAILABLE PREPARATIONS
Inj: 250 mg, 500 mg

ROUTES AND DOSAGES
• Dosages based on imipenem component
Premature neonates ≤7 days: IV 20 mg/kg/dose q12h for bacterial infections other than CNS infections
Full term neonates ≤7 days: IV 30 mg/kg/dose q12h
Full term neonates >7 days: IV 30 mg/kg/dose q8h
Children: IV 40-60 mg/kg/24 hr divided q6h; maximum 4 g/24 hr
Adults: IV 250 mg-1 g q6-8h maxi-

mum 50 mg/kg/24 hr or 4 g/24 hr, whichever is less

IV administration
• Recommended concentration: 2.5-7 mg/ml in D_5NS, $D_5\frac{1}{4}NS$, $D_5\frac{1}{2}NS$, D_5W, $D_{10}W$, or NS
• Maximum concentration: 7 mg/ml
• IV push rate: Not recommended
• Intermittent infusion rate: Over 20-60 min
• Continuous infusion: Not recommended

MECHANISM AND INDICATIONS

Antibiotic mechanism: Bactericidal; imipenem inhibits bacterial cell wall synthesis; cilastatin inhibits imipenem's enzymatic breakdown in kidneys
Indications: Effective against many gram-negative, gram-positive, and anaerobic bacteria including *Staphylococcus* and *Streptococcus* species, *E. coli, Klebsiella, Proteus, Enterobacter* species, *Pseudomonas aeruginosa,* and *Bacteroides;* used to treat septicemia, endocarditis, serious lower respiratory tract, urinary tract, skin, soft tissue, bone, joint, gynecologic, intra-abdominal infections

PHARMACOKINETICS

Peak: 20 min
Distribution: Widely distributed; low concentrations penetrate CSF
Half-life: 1 hr
Metabolism: Kidneys
Excretion: Urine

CONTRAINDICATIONS AND PRECAUTIONS

• Contraindicated with known hypersensitivity to imipenem or cilastatin
• Use cautiously with known hypersensitivity to penicillins or cephalosporins, history of seizures or impaired renal function, pregnancy, lactation

INTERACTIONS

Drug
• Increased serum concentration with use of probenecid
• Decreased bactericidal effects when given with chloramphenicol; give chloramphenicol a few hr after imipenem-cilastatin

Lab
• Increased liver function tests, BUN, alk phos, bilirubin, creatinine
• False positive Coombs' test

INCOMPATIBILITIES

• Aminoglycosides, all sol except those recommended for dilution by manufacturer; $NaHCO_3$; do not mix with any other bacteriostatic agent in syringe or sol

SIDE EFFECTS

CNS: Seizures, dizziness, encephalopathy, confusion
CV: Hypotension
GI: Nausea, vomiting, diarrhea, pseudomembranous colitis
Local: Thrombophlebitis, pain at injection site
Other: Hypersensitivity, bacterial or fungal superinfection

TOXICITY AND OVERDOSE

Clinical signs: CNS symptoms (myoclonic activity, confusion, seizures)
Treatment: Anticonvulsants; supportive care; hemodialysis

PATIENT CARE MANAGEMENT

Assessment
• Assess history of hypersensitivity to imipenem, cilastatin, penicillins, cephalosporins
• Obtain C&S; may begin therapy before obtaining results
• Assess renal function (BUN, creatinine, I&O), hepatic function (ALT, AST, bilirubin), hematologic function, (CBC, differential, platelet count) bowel pattern

Interventions
• Sol may range from colorless to yellow without affecting drug potency
• Do not premix IV with other medications; infuse separately
• Use large vein with small-bore needle to reduce local reaction; rotate site q48-72h
• Maintain age-appropriate fluid intake

♣ Available in Canada.

NURSING ALERT
Discontinue drug if signs of hypersensitivity, seizures, pseudomembranous colitis develop

Evaluation
• Evaluate therapeutic response (decreased symptoms of infection)
• Evaluate renal function (BUN, creatinine, I&O), hepatic function (ALT, AST, bilirubin), hematologic function (CBC, differential, platelet count), particularly in long-term therapy
• Monitor bowel pattern; diarrhea may be symptomatic of pseudomembranous colitis
• Continue anticonvulsants, monitor pts with known seizure disorders
• Observe for allergic reaction (rash, urticaria, pruritus)
• Observe for signs of superinfection (perineal itching, diaper rash, fever, malaise, redness, pain, swelling, drainage, rash, diarrhea, sore throat, change in cough or sputum)
• Evaluate IV site for vein irritation

PATIENT AND FAMILY EDUCATION
Teach/instruct
• To take as directed at prescribed intervals for prescribed length of time
Warn/advise
• To notify care provider of hypersensitivity, side effects, superinfection

STORAGE
• Store powder at room temp
• Reconstituted sol stable at room temp for 10 hr, refrigerated for 48 hr

imipramine hydrochloride, imipramine pamoate
Brand Name(s): Apo-Imipramine✿, Janimine, Tofranil✿ (imipramine hydrochloride); Tofranil-PM (imipramine pamoate)

Classification: Tricyclic antidepressant

Pregnancy Category: D

AVAILABLE PREPARATIONS
Tabs: 10 mg, 25 mg, 50 mg (imipramine hydrochloride)
Caps: 75 mg, 100 mg, 125 mg, 150 mg (imipramine pamoate)
Inj: 12.5 mg/ml (imipramine hydrochloride)

DOSAGES AND ROUTES
• Not approved for children <12 yr for depression and <6 yr for enuresis
• Children 6-12 yr may be more susceptible than adults to heart toxicity from this and related drugs.
• Tofranil-PM caps should not be used with children because of the increased potential for overdose caused by their high potency
Enuresis
Children ≥6 yr: PO initial 10-25 mg at hs; if response is inadequate after 1 wk, increase by 25 mg/24 hr; maximum 2.5 mg/kg/24 hr or 50 mg at hs if 6-12 yr or 75 mg at bedtime if >12 yr; usual dose 25-75 mg at hs (depending on the size of the child); Tofranil-PM caps should not be used to treat enuresis
Depression and Anxiety Disorders
Children ≥12 yr and adults: PO initial 1 mg/kg/24 hr; dose increases of 25% are made q4-5 days as tolerated to 3 mg/kg/24 hr in 2 divided doses; maximum 5 mg/kg/24 hr qd or divided qid; monitor carefully, especially with doses >3.5 mg/kg/24 hr; usual dose 25-75 mg/24 hr divided bid

Attention Deficit Disorder
PO 1-3 mg/kg/24 hr divided bid
Adjunct in Treatment of Severe, Chronic, or Neuropathic Pain
Children 6-12 yr: PO initial 0.2-0.4 mg/kg at hs; dose increases of 50% q 2-3 days; maximum 1-3 mg/kg/dose at hs
Older adolescents: PO initial 25-50 mg/24 hr; increase gradually; usual dose 30-40 mg/24 hr; maximum 200 mg/24 hr qd or divided bid
Adults: PO initial 25 mg/24 hr divided tid-qid; increase q wk by 10-25 mg/24 hr; usual dose 50-150 mg/24 hr; maximum 300 mg/24 hr; IM route rarely used; may be used for depression when patient is NPO, PO as soon as possible

MECHANISM AND INDICATIONS
Mechanism: Inhibits reuptake of serotonin and/or norepinephrine by presynaptic neuronal membrane, thus increasing their concentration
Indications: For use in treating enuresis in children ≥6 yr; in children ≥12 yr, effective in treating depression, anxiety, ADD, ADHD, panic disorder, anxiety-based school refusal, separation anxiety disorder, primary nocturnal enuresis, night terrors, sleepwalking; occasionally prescribed (unlabeled uses) to control chronic pain and neuropathic pain, and to treat binge eating and purging in bulimia

PHARMACOKINETICS
Onset of action: PO 4-6 wk; therapeutic antidepressant effects usually occur after 2-4 wk of continual use, optimal response may not occur until ≥3 mo of use
Peak: PO 1-2 hr; IM 30 min
Half life: 6-20 hr
Metabolism: Liver
Excretion: Urine, small amount in feces
Therapeutic level: Steady-state plasma levels of imipramine plus desipramine 150-300 ng/ml

CONTRAINDICATIONS AND PRECAUTIONS
• Contraindicated with hypersensitivity to this or any component of this medication, tricyclic antidepressants, or maprotiline; arrhythmia, lactation, recent heart attack, prostatic hypertrophy, undiagnosed syncope, have taken MAOIs within past 14 days
• Use cautiously with allergy to aspirin; angina, asthma, conduction disturbances, CHF, DM, known electrolyte abnormality with binging and purging, electroshock therapy, narrow-angle glaucoma, heart disease, family history of sudden cardiac death or cardiomyopathy, history of alcoholism, hyperthyroidism or receiving thyroid replacement, increased intraocular pressure, kidney disease, liver disease, paranoia, pregnancy, prostatism, schizophrenia, seizures, severe depression, suicidal tendencies, plan to have surgery under general anesthesia in the near future, Tourette syndrome, spasms of ureter or urethra, urinary retention

INTERACTIONS
Drug
• Increased sedation with alcohol, antihistamines, antipsychotics, barbiturates, benzodiazepines, chloral hydrate, CNS depressants, glutethimide, sedatives
• Increased hypotension with alpha methyldopa, β-adrenergic blockers, clonidine, diuretics
• Additive cardiotoxicity with quinidine, thioridazine, mesoridazine
• Additive anticholinergic toxicity with antihistamines, antiparkinsonians, GI antispasmodics and antidiarrheals, OTC sleeping medications, thioridazine
• Increased effects of adrenergic agents, anticholinergic agents, CNS depressants, decongestants, dicumarol, local anesthetics, stimulants, warfarin
• Decreased effects of antihypertensives, clonidine, ephedrine, guanadrel, guanethidine

♣ Available in Canada.

• Increased imipramine levels with phenothiazines
• Increased imipramine effects with cimetidine, estrogens, fluoxetine, methylphenidate, oral contraceptives, phenothiazines, ranitidine
• Decreased imipramine levels with barbiturates, cigarette smoking
• Decreased imipramine effects with barbiturates, carbamazepine, chloral hydrate, lithium, marijuana smoking, reserpine
• Within 14 days of use of MAOIs, hyperpyrexia, tachycardia, hypertension, seizures and death may occur
• Delirium with ethchlorvynol
• Increased drowsiness, mouth dryness, and tachycardia with marijuana smoking
• Severe high B/P or fever with amphetamine, cocaine, epinephrine, phenylpropanolamine
• Increased risk of heart rhythm disorders with thyroid preparations
• Anticonvulsant medications may need dosage adjustment because of changes in seizure patterns
• Increased gastric emptying time; may slow absorption and cause inactivation of some drugs

Lab
• Increased ALT, AST, alk phos, bilirubin, eosinophils, transaminase
• Decreased 5-HIAA, VMA, urinary catecholamines, platelets, WBCs
• Fluctuations in BG
• Liver toxicity may be mistaken for viral hepatitis

Nutrition
• Enhanced elimination of imipramine with ≥1 g of vitamin C
• Reduced elimination and prolonged effect of imipramine with antacids containing $NaHCO_3$
• Janimine contains the dye tartrazine (FD&C yellow #5), which can cause allergic reactions
• Inj contains sulfites, which can cause allergic reactions
• Do not drink alcohol

SIDE EFFECTS
• Imipramine has less sedation and anticholinergic effects than amitriptyline
• Imipramine is less likely to increase HR than other tricyclic antidepressants

CNS: Dizziness, drowsiness, abnormal dreaming, agitation, anxiety, confusion, delirium, delusions, disorientation, emotional instability, excitement, fainting, fatigue, hallucinations, headache, insomnia, irritability, lethargy, lightheadedness, mania, nervousness, nightmares, paresthesia, psychosis, psychomotor agitation, sedation, seizures, stimulation, tremors, unsteadiness, weakness

CV: ECG changes, hypotension, tachycardia, arrhythmias, CHF, heart block, thrombosis, hypertension, palpitations, ventricular flutter and fibrillation

DERM: Hives, itching, petechiae, photosensitivity, rash, sweating

EENT: Swelling of face or tongue, increased intraocular pressure, dry mouth, mydriasis, altered taste, tinnitus, irritation of tongue or mouth, blurred vision

GI: Diarrhea, dry mouth, abdominal complaints, increased appetite, constipation, cramps, epigastric distress, hepatitis, indigestion, jaundice, nausea, stuffy nose, paralytic ileus, stomatitis, vomiting, wt gain

GU: Urinary retention, impaired ejaculation, impaired erection, decreased or increased libido, galactorrhea, gynecomastia, impotence, kidney damage, inhibited orgasm, swelling of testicles

HEME: Agranulocytosis, abnormally low WBC and platelet counts, eosinophilia, leukopenia, thrombocytopenia

Other: Anaphylactoid reaction, fluctuations in BG, neuroleptic malignant syndrome

TOXICITY AND OVERDOSE
Clinical signs: Cardiotoxic effects of tricyclic antidepressants more frequent in children and adoles-

cents than in adults, especially at levels >300 ng/mol; plasma levels of desipramine or desipramine plus imipramine, potentially toxic >300 ng/mol; toxic >1000 ng/ml; early indication of toxicity or overdosage, agitation, arrhythmia, confusion, tachycardia; symptoms of overdose, hypothermia early, fever later; arrhythmia, confusion, drowsiness, hallucinations, hypotension, seizures, stupor, tremors, urinary retention

Treatment: Maintain normal temperature; monitor ECG, induce emesis, administer activated charcoal, lavage; administer anticonvulsant, correct acidosis with $NaHCO_3$, treat arrhythmias or seizures with physostigmine

PATIENT CARE MANAGEMENT

Assessment

- Assess history of hypersensitivity to drug or yellow dye
- Obtain baseline AST, ALT, bilirubin, ECG, cardiac examination, CBC, differential, leukocytes, orthostatic B/P and pulse, serum electrolytes
- Assess family history for sudden cardiac death and pt's history for cardiac disease, arrhythmias, syncope, seizure disorder or congenital hearing loss (associated with long QT syndrome)
- Obtain baseline BUN for pts with eating disorders
- Rule out functional disorder before starting a trial of therapy with imipramine for pts with enuresis

Interventions

- Cap may be opened, tab may be crushed for administration
- May be given without regard to meals
- Give with food or milk if GI symptoms occur
- Administer the dose at hs when prescribed qd
- If oversedation occurs during the day, pt may take entire dose at hs
- Administer medication in the AM if difficult to awaken or sluggish during the day
- Administer 1 hr before hs for enuresis; if ≥50 mg is administered, ½ may be administered in the late afternoon and half at hs, especially if child wets bed early in the night
- May need to limit food intake to avoid excessive wt gain
- Increase fluids and fiber in diet if constipation occurs
- Rinse with water, take sips of fluid, sugarless gum, or hard candy for dry mouth
- If used for ADD or ADHD, imipramine must be administered on weekends and holidays during the school year to maintain effectiveness
- Discontinue imipramine gradually over 3-4 wk; abrupt withdrawal after prolonged use may cause nausea, vomiting, diarrhea, headache, malaise, disturbed sleep, and vivid dreaming
- When imipramine is discontinued, it may be necessary to adjust dosages of other drugs taken concurrently

> **NURSING ALERT**
> Do not discontinue long-term, high-dosage therapy abruptly
>
> Tofranil-PM caps should not be used in children because of increased potential for overdose caused by their high potency

Evaluation

- Evaluate therapeutic response (ability to function in daily activities, to sleep throughout the night; if taken for depression, evaluate for symptoms of depression; if taken for attention deficit, obtain parent and teacher reports about attention and behavioral performance; if taken for enuresis, evaluate for bedwetting)
- Evaluate mental status (affect, mood, sensorium, impulsiveness, suicidal ideation, panic, psychiatric symptoms)
- With each dose increase above 3 mg/kg/24 hr, monitor and document ECG and orthostatic B/P and pulse

---

♣ Available in Canada.

• Monitor blood drug levels as appropriate
• Observe for deterioration of thinking or behavior
• At steady state monitor q 3-4 mo: Height, wt, AST, ALT, bilirubin, ECG, cardiac examination, CBC, differential, leukocytes, orthostatic B/P and pulse, intraocular pressure, serum electrolytes
• Monitor cardiac enzymes if receiving long-term therapy
• Examine ECG for flattening T-wave, bundle branch block, AV block, arrhythmias
• Evaluate cardiovascular parameters: HR >130/min, systolic B/P >130 mm Hg, diastolic B/P >85 mm Hg, PR interval >0.20 sec, QRS interval >0.12 sec, or no more than 30% over baseline, QT corrected >0.45 sec; notify care provider
• Assess for urinary retention and constipation; constipation is more likely to occur in children than adults
• If drug is successful for enuresis, it is usually used for about 3 mo; if enuresis occurs after drug is discontinued, imipramine may be restarted (but is not always successful)
• Taper down over 2 wk when discontinuing medication; withdrawal symptoms if drug is stopped suddenly are headache, nausea, vomiting, muscle pain, weakness, psychomotor activation
• Evaluate for early signs of toxicity (agitation, arrhythmia, confusion, tachycardia)

PATIENT AND FAMILY EDUCATION
Teach/instruct
• To take as directed at prescribed intervals for prescribed length of time
• That this medication is most helpful when used as part of a comprehensive multimodal treatment program
• To not stop taking this medication without prescriber approval
• That therapeutic effects may take 3-4 wk

• To increase fluids, fiber in diet if constipation occurs
• That a possible side effect is neuroleptic malignant syndrome; symptoms include fever, fast or irregular heartbeat, fast breathing, sweating, weakness, muscle stiffness, seizures, loss of bladder control; if these occur, obtain medical help immediately
• To make sure medication is swallowed
• To administer with food or milk if GI symptoms occur
• To rinse with water, take sips of fluid, sugarless gum, or hard candy for dry mouth
• Not to use OTC drugs without consulting prescriber
Warn/advise
• To know the expiration date of medication (it may be taken on a trial basis for enuresis)
• To return for follow-up visits as recommended
• To report excess fatigue, mood changes, wt change, and unusual symptoms
• To avoid ingesting alcohol, other CNS depressants
• That there may be increased suicide potential at beginning of therapy if given for depression
• That medication may cause drowsiness; be careful on bicycles, skates, skateboards, while driving, or with other activities requiring alertness; change position slowly when rising
• To stay out of direct sunlight, especially between 10 AM and 3 PM, if possible; when outside, wear protective clothing, hat, sunglasses; put on sun block that has skin protection factor (SPF) of at least 15

• That imipramine can inhibit sweating and impair the body's adaptation to hot environments, increasing the risk of heat stroke; avoid saunas, hot baths
• Not to discontinue medication quickly after long-term use; sudden discontinuation may cause headache, nausea, vomiting, muscle pain, weakness
• To keep this and all medications out of reach of children; as few as 10 pills can cause lethal cardiac arrhythmias in children

STORAGE
• Store at room temp in a tightly closed container; do not freeze parenteral sol
• Slight discoloration of sol does not preclude use, but do not use a marked red or yellow sol
• Expiration dates are 3-5 yr after manufacture

---

immune globulin intravenous

Brand Name(s): Gamimune N♣, Gammagard, Gammar-IV, IGIV, Iveegam, Sandoglobulin, Venoglobulin-I-1, Venoglobulin-S, Veno-S

Classification: Human serum immune globulin

Pregnancy Category: C

AVAILABLE PREPARATIONS
Inj: Multiple preparations available; differ according to immune globulin component, concentration, method of preparation, use of additives, pH, rate to be administered, cost, storage; most pharmacies stock only a few of the many preparations; familiarity with institutional product is prudent

ROUTES AND DOSAGES
• Dosage may vary in response to diagnosis, extent of disease, concurrent or previous therapy, response to therapy, institutional guidelines, product used, physiologic parameters; consult current literature, package insert

Immunodeficiency
Children and adults: IV 100-400 mg/kg/dose q 2-4 wk
ITP
IV initial, 400-1000 mg/kg/24 hr for 2-5 consecutive days; maintenance, 400-1000 mg/kg/dose q 3-6 wk based on clinical response and platelet count
Kawasaki Disease
400 mg/kg/24 hr for 4 days, or 2 g/kg as a single dose
Bone Marrow Transplant
400-500 mg/kg/dose q wk
Severe Systemic Viral and Bacterial Infections
Neonates: 500 mg/kg/24 hr for 2-6 days then q wk
Children: 500-1000 mg/kg/wk
IV administration
• Infusion rate: Varies with product and pt tolerance; initial infusion at slower rate but generally can be increased if no adverse reactions

MECHANISM AND INDICATIONS
Mechanism: Serum containing immune globulin; serum obtained from human serum or plasma, purified via cold liquid ethanol fractionation and standardized
Indications: Treat primary immune deficiencies; to prevent or modify potential CMV infection following bone marrow transplantation; autoimmune hemolytic disorders (such as ITP, hemolytic anemia, immune neutropenia); to reduce incidence of coronary artery aneurysms in Kawasaki Disease; to help prevent infections in lymphoproliferative disorders (such as CLL and multiple myeloma); help decrease number of infections in HIV patients; augment immune system of children on immunosuppressive chemotherapy, decreasing number of infections or viral illnesses

PHARMACOKINETICS
Peak: Immediately following infusion; levels decrease by about 50% by 3rd day, return to baseline by 21-28 days

Half-life: 22-25 days
Metabolism: Exact mechanism not fully described; great individual variability

CONTRAINDICATIONS AND PRECAUTIONS
• Contraindicated with known allergy to γ globulin or trimerosal; specific deficiency of IgA with antibodies to IgA if preparation contains IgA (Sandoglobulin, Gamimune-N)
• Use cautiously with pregnancy, lactation, pts with history of systemic allergic reactions

INTERACTIONS
Drugs
• Interference with antibody response, live virus vaccines

INCOMPATIBILITIES
• Incompatible in syringe or sol with any other drug

SIDE EFFECTS
CNS: Headache (especially in dosages >400 mg/kg/24 hr)
CV: Hypotension, chest tightness
GI: Nausea
Other: Full range allergic reactions including chills, flushing, fever, dizziness, diaphoresis, angioedema, anaphylaxis

TOXICITY AND OVERDOSE
Clinical signs: Precipitous drop in B/P, headache, chills generally signifies infusion too rapid
Treatment: Slow or stop infusion; supportive measures including analgesics, antihistamines, hydration, availability of epinephrine, vasopressors, O_2, corticosteroids

PATIENT CARE MANAGEMENT
Assessment
• Assess history of hypersensitivity to immune globulin infusion
• Assess history of systemic allergic response
• Assess reactions to immunizations
• Assess information regarding sensitivity to thimerosal
• Assess baseline VS (including B/P)
• Assess baseline IgG, IgA/IgM levels

• Assess baseline CBC, differential, platelet count, reticulocytes
• Assess hepatitis screen before initiation

Interventions
• Acquire knowledge about specific product being administered with regard to initial and maximum rate of infusion
• Premedicate with acetaminophen, diphenhydramine prn
• Monitor VS, B/P throughout infusion

Evaluation
• Evaluate therapeutic response (IgG, IgA, IgM levels if treating primary immunodeficiency, increased platelet count if treating ITP)
• Evaluate tolerance to particular product rate of infusion
• Evaluate for possibility of home administration
• Evaluate yearly hepatitis screen for pts on long-term therapy

PATIENT AND FAMILY EDUCATION
Teach/instruct
• To report headache, dizziness, fever, allergic reaction immediately
Warn/advise
• That chance of acquiring viral illness as result of receiving IV IgG is minute

STORAGE
• Varies with individual preparations

---

indomethacin sodium trihydrate

Brand Name(s): Indameth, Indocin, Indocin IV, Insocin SR, Indo-Lemmon

Classification: Non-narcotic analgesic, non-steroidal antiinflammatory

Pregnancy Category: B in first and second trimester, D in third trimester

---

AVAILABLE PREPARATIONS
Susp: 25 mg/5 ml

Tab: 25 mg, 50 mg
Cap (ext rel): 75 mg
Rectal supp: 50 mg
Inj: 1 mg

ROUTES AND DOSAGES
Juvenile Rheumatoid Arthritis
Children 2-14 yr: PO/PR 1-2 mg/kg/24 hr divided bid-qid; maximum 4 mg/kg/24 hr

Closure of Patent Ductus Arteriosus
Infant <2 days: IV 0.2 mg/kg, then 0.1 mg/kg × 2 doses after 12, 24 hr
Infant 2-7 days: IV 0.2 mg/kg then 0.2 mg/kg × 2 doses after 12, 24 hr
Infant >7 days: IV 0.2 mg/kg, then 0.25 mg/kg × 2 doses after 12, 24 hr

IV administration
• Recommended concentration: 0.5 or 1 mg/ml in preservative free SW or NS
• Maximum concentration: 1 mg/ml
• IV push rate: Over 20-35 min

MECHANISM AND INDICATIONS
Mechanism: Inhibits the synthesis of prostaglandins by decreasing enzyme needed for biosynthesis, has an effect on the hypothalamus and acts to block peripheral nerve transfer
Indications: Used to treat inflammatory disorders (including rheumatoid arthritis) and as an alternative to surgery in the management of patent ductus arteriosus closure (PDA) in premature neonates

PHARMACOKINETICS
Onset: PO/ (analgesic) 30 min; PO (antiinflammatory) up to 7 days
Peak: PO (analgesic) 0.5-2 hr; PO (antiinflammatory) 1-2 wk
Distribution: Widely distributed, highly bound to plasma proteins; crosses blood–brain barrier
Half-life: 2.6-11 hr (12-21 hr in neonate)
Duration: 4-6 hr
Metabolism: Liver
Excretion: Mainly in urine
Therapeutic level: 0.5-3 mcg/ml may be needed for antiinflamma-

tory action; 0.25 mcg/ml appears to be needed for closure of PDA

CONTRAINDICATIONS AND PRECAUTIONS
• Contraindicated with hypersensitivity to drug or to ingredients (suspensions may contain alcohol, parabens, or propylene glycol); cross-sensitivity may exist with other NSAIDs, active GI bleeding, ulcer disease, asthma, severe renal or hepatic disease
• Use cautiously with coagulation disorder, cardiac, renal, or hepatic dysfunction, hypertension, CHF, mental depression, systemic lupus erythematosus, pregnancy, lactation (animal studies suggest the possibility of premature closure of the ductus arteriosus in the fetus and prolonged pregnancy because of uterine prostaglandin inhibition; therefore use in the second half of pregnancy is not recommended), history of rectal lesions or bleeding (PR)

INTERACTIONS
Drug
• Decreased effectiveness with aspirin, phenobarbital
• Decreased effectiveness of antihypertensives or diuretics possible
• Additive adverse GI side effects with aspirin, other NSAIDs, corticosteroids, K^+
• Increased risk of bleeding with aspirin, oral anticoagulants, NSAIDs, cefamandole, cefoperazone, cefotetan, moxalactam, plicamycin
• Increased blood levels and possible increased toxicity with probenecid
• Increased risk of methotrexate, verapamil, or nifedipine toxicity possible
• Increased risk of developing hypoglycemia with insulin
• Increased risk of hematologic side effects with other drugs with the same effect or with radiation
• Increased serum lithium and digoxin levels possible
• Increased hyperkalemia with other drugs having the same effect such as K^+-sparing diuretics

- Increased levels of aminoglycoside in premature infants
- Decreased action of triamterene

Lab
- Prolonged bleeding time for 1 day; no effect on pro-time or whole blood clotting time
- Increased AST, ALT, alk phos, LDH, transaminase, BUN, creatinine, K^+, urine glucose, urine protein
- Decreased BG, plasma renin activity
- Decreased CrCl, serum Na, urine chloride, urine output, uric acid, K^+ and Na concentrations, urine osmolality possible

INCOMPATIBILITIES
- Do not use with antacids

SIDE EFFECTS
CNS: Headache, drowsiness, psychic disturbances (mood changes, depression) dizziness, fatigue, confusion, fever, potential intracranial hemorrhage with neonates receiving IV form, tremors, anxiety, insomnia
CV: Peripheral edema, arrhythmias, fluid retention, CHF, hypertension, palpitation
DERM: Rashes, urticaria, alopecia, Stevens-Johnson syndrome, purpura, pruritus, sweating
EENT: Blurred vision, tinnitus, amblyopia, cataracts, hearing loss
GI: Nausea, anorexia, dyspepsia, vomiting, constipation, GI bleeding, heartburn, pain, diarrhea, flatulence, cramps, peptic ulcer, dry mouth, gingivitis, jaundice, hepatitis, altered liver enzymes
GU: Nephrotoxicity, renal failure, hematuria, cystitis, polyuria, proteinuria, oliguria, dysuria
HEME: Inhibited platelet action, prolonged bleeding time, neutropenia, agranulocytosis, aplastic anemia, thrombocytopenia, anemia
RESP: Bronchospasm, dyspnea, anaphylaxis
Local: Phlebitis at IV site
Other: Allergic reactions, including anaphylaxis

TOXICITY AND OVERDOSE
Clinical signs: Blurred vision, tinnitus, nausea, vomiting, headache, dizziness, mental confusion, lethargy, paresthesias, numbness, convulsions
Treatment: Supportive care; empty stomach (induce vomiting or gastric lavage); activated charcoal

PATIENT CARE MANAGEMENT
Assessment
- Assess history of hypersensitivity to indocin, aspirin, other NSAIDs
- Assess history of asthma (at higher risk for allergy)
- Assess any visual disturbances and coagulation disorders
- Assess renal function (BUN, creatinine, I&O), liver function (ALT, AST, bilirubin)
- Perform audiometric, ophthalmic exam
- Assess limitation of movement, pain

Interventions
- Administer PO with food to decrease GI discomfort; however this may decrease drug absorption; may crush tab, administer with food; do not administer susp with antacid or liquid
- Supp should remain in rectum for 1 hr after administration
- Do not administer IV sol that is discolored or contains particulates; use immediately after reconstitution and discard unused portion

NURSING ALERT
Do not administer with antacids

May be a higher risk for allergic response with history of asthma

IV administration: Although indocin has been given IV push over 5-10 sec, rapid administration can cause a significant decrease in mesenteric artery and cerebral blood flow, which may contribute to development of necrotizing enterocolitis or cerebral ischemia

Evaluation
• Evaluate therapeutic response (decreased pain, stiffness, and swelling in joints; ability to move easily; evidence of closure of PDA)
• Evaluate liver function (ALT, AST, bilirubin), renal function (BUN, creatinine, I&O), audiometric, and ophthal exam
• Evaluate pain 1-2 hr after administration
• Evaluate side effects and hypersensitivities

PATIENT AND FAMILY EDUCATION
Teach/instruct
• To take as directed at prescribed intervals for prescribed length of time
• Not to take with antacids
• That pt may take with food (but this may interfere with drug absorption)
• That improvement may not be seen for about 2 wk to 1 mo
Warn/advise
• To avoid driving or other activities that require alertness until response to drug is known
• To avoid concurrent use of alcohol, aspirin, acetaminophen, other OTC medications without consulting health care provider
• To notify care provider of hypersensitivities or side effects
Encourage
• To inform physician or dentist of medication regimen before treatment or surgery

STORAGE
• Store at room temp
• Protect from light
• Do not freeze susp

---

influenza virus vaccine
Brand Name(s): Flu-Immune, FluViral S/F♣, Fluzone♣, Influenza Virus Vaccine Trivalent

Classification: Immunization

Pregnancy Category: C

AVAILABLE PREPARATIONS
Inj: 5 ml multidose vials

ROUTES AND DOSAGES
Children 6-35 mo: IM 1 or 2 0.25 ml doses yearly of subvirion, split, or purified-surface-antigen vaccine, at least 1 mo apart, with the 2nd dose before December if possible
Children 3-8 yr: IM 1 or 2 0.5 ml doses yearly of subvirion, split, or purified-surface-antigen vaccine at least 1 mo apart, with the 2nd dose before December if possible
Children 9-12 yr: IM 1 0.5 ml dose yearly of subvirion, split, or purified-surface-antigen vaccine
Children >12 yr and adults: IM 1 0.5 ml dose yearly of subvirion, split, purified-surface-antigen, or whole vaccine

MECHANISM AND INDICATIONS
Immunization mechanism: Induces antibody formation against influenza virus strains contained in the vaccine
Indications: Used for children >6 mo who have chronic illnesses (including chronic pulmonary or cardiovascular disorders, metabolic diseases (e.g., DM), renal dysfunction, hemoglobinopathies, immunosuppression, symptomatic HIV disease, children receiving long-term aspirin therapy); household members of high-risk patients should also be immunized

PHARMACOKINETICS
Onset of action: Adequate immune response within 2 wk after vaccination; response may be less in young children than in young adults

CONTRAINDICATIONS AND PRECAUTIONS
• Contraindicated in infants <6 mo, with a history of known hypersensitivity to eggs or any vaccine component (including thimerosal), previous hypersensitivity to an influenza vaccine; delay vaccination with unstable active neurological disorders, acute febrile illnesses
• Use cautiously with pregnancy

INTERACTIONS
Drug
• Increased serum levels of warfarin, theophylline possible
• Reduced antibody response with immunosuppressive therapy possible (including irradiation, corticosteroids, cytotoxic agents)

SIDE EFFECTSSITE
MS: Myalgia
Local: Pain, erythema at injection
Other: Fever, anaphylaxis

PATIENT CARE MANAGEMENT
Assessment
• Identify target population for immunization (children >6 mo with chronic illnesses)
• Assess history of hypersensitivity to eggs, any vaccine components, or previous influenza vaccines
Interventions
• Use subvirion, split, or purified-surface-antigen vaccine for children ≤ 12 yr to reduce incidence of febrile reactions
• Administer IM into deltoid muscle or lateral mid-thigh, depending on age, with appropriate precautions to avoid IV administration
• Vaccine is administered annually in autumn for protection against that year's influenza
• Emergency resuscitative equipment should be readily available for possible anaphylaxis
Evaluation
• Monitor pt for 20 min after administration for signs of anaphylaxis (urticaria, dyspnea, wheezing, drop in B/P)

PATIENT AND FAMILY EDUCATION
Warn/advise
• To notify care provider of hypersensitivity, side effects
• That mild analgesic (acetaminophen) may alleviate discomfort, fever
• That vaccination is required annually in autumn for protection against that year's influenza

STORAGE
• Store unopened and opened vials in refrigerator; do not freeze
• Discard previous year's vaccines

---

insulin
Brand Name(s): Humulin, Iletin I✤, Iletin II, Iletin II Pork✤, Novolin

Classification: Antidiabetic agent (pancreatic hormone)

Pregnancy Category: B

AVAILABLE PREPARATIONS 100 U/ml (except where indicated)
• Insulatard NPH, Insulatard NPH Human, Novolin N, Humulin N, Humulin R, Novolin R, Velosulin Human, Humulin 50/50, Humulin 70/30, Mixtard 70/30, Novolin 70/30, Humulin L, Humulin U, Novolin L, Iletin I, NPH Iletin II, NPH Purified Pork Isophane Insulin, Iletin I Regular, Regular Iletin II, Regular Iletin II (concentrated: 500 U/ml) Pork 500 U, Regular Purified Pork Insulin, Velosulin, Iletin I NPH, Iletin I Lente, Lente Iletin II, Lente Purified Pork, Semilente

ROUTES AND DOSAGES
Insulin Replacement in Diabetes
SC individualized based on BG; usual starting dose for newly diagnosed Type I diabetic is 0.5-0.6 U/kg/24 hr divided bid, divided between regular and NPH, generally ⅔ of total dose in the AM divided as ⅔ NPH and ⅓ regular; the PM dose is approximately ½ NPH and ½ regular
Diabetic Ketoacidosis
Use regular insulin only; IV 0.1 U/kg IV bolus, then 0.1 U/kg/hr by IV infusion until stabilized and acidosis is resolving
Hyperkalemia
0.05-0.1 U/kg/hr infused concomitantly with glucose; titrate dose to maintain desired BG concentration

---

✤ Available in Canada.

IV administration

- Recommended concentration: 0.2-1 U/ml in NS
- Maximum concentration: 100 U/ml
- IV push rate: Rapid
- Continuous infusion rate: 0.05-0.1 U/kg/hr

MECHANISM AND INDICATIONS

Mechanism: Increases glucose transport across cell membranes to reduce BG; also promotes glycogen synthesis, inhibits lipolysis, stimulates protein synthesis

Indications: Replacement of endogenous insulin in pts with Type I diabetes and pts with type II diabetes who are not adequately controlled with diet and oral medication

PHARMACOKINETICS

Onset: Regular ½ hr; semilente 1-3 hr; NPH 2-4 hr; lente 1-2½ hr; ultralente 4-8 hr

Peak: Regular 2-4 hr; semilente 2-8 hr; NPH 4-12 hr; lente 7-15 hr; ultralente 10-30 hr

Metabolism: Liver, muscle, kidneys

Excretion: Urine

CONTRAINDICATIONS AND PRECAUTIONS

- Contraindicated with hypersensitivity; do not use longer-acting insulin with diabetic ketoacidosis, circulatory collapse, or hyperkalemia
- Use cautiously with pregnancy

INTERACTIONS

Drug

- Increased risk of hypoglycemia with alcohol, β blockers, clofibrate, fenfluramine, MAOIs, salicylates, tetracycline, anabolic steroids, guanethidine
- Diminished insulin response with corticosteroids, thiazide diuretics, estrogens, thyroid hormone

Lab

- Increased VMA
- Decreased K^+, Ca, Mg, inorganic phosphate

INCOMPATIBILITIES

- Aminophylline, amobarbital, chlorothiazide, dobutamine, heparin, penicillin G, K^+, pentobarbital, phenobarbital, phenytoin, secobarbital, $NaHCO_3$, thiopental

SIDE EFFECTS

DERM: Urticaria, lipoatrophy, lipohypertrophy

METAB: Hypoglycemia, hyperglycemia (rebound or Somogyi)

Local: Stinging, warmth at injection site

Other: Anaphylaxis

TOXICITY AND OVERDOSE

Clinical signs: Hypoglycemic symptoms (including irritability, diaphoresis, tachycardia, confusion, lethargy, hunger, shakiness, headache, motor dysfunction, seizure, coma)

Treatment: Aimed at increasing BG; if able to swallow, administer oral glucose (juice, regular soda, hard candy) equivalent to 10-15 g glucose; if unresponsive administer bolus of IV glucose, glucagon, or epinephrine IV, IM, or SC

PATIENT CARE MANAGEMENT

Assessment

- Assess history of hypersensitivity to insulin (including its preservatives)
- Assess symptoms of hyper- or hypoglycemia, BG, urine ketones
- Assess pt's level of knowledge of insulin action and symptoms of hypoglycemia

Interventions

- Prime IV tubing first because insulin binds to plastic tubing
- Measure doses carefully
- Always put short-acting insulin in SC syringe before long-acting insulin
- Warm insulin to room temp before inj if stored in refrigerator
- Rotate or roll bottles to mix insulin; do not shake
- Administer insulin approximately ½ hr ac
- Rotate injection sites in a systematic manner to avoid overuse of one area

Evaluation

- Evaluate therapeutic response (BG generally between 80-180 or

as defined by care provider)
- Absence of symptoms of hypo- and hyperglycemia
- Improvement of electrolytes if pt was in diabetic ketoacidosis

PATIENT AND FAMILY EDUCATION
Teach/instruct
- To take as directed at prescribed intervals for prescribed length of time
- To ensure pt eats within ½ hr after regular insulin dose
- About signs, symptoms, and treatment of hypoglycemia, ketoacidosis
- To use glucagon for emergencies
- About modifying insulin dose related to diet and exercise

Warn/advise
- To notify care provider of hypersensitivity, side effects
- About range for BG and when to call for dosage adjustment
- To carry simple sugar at all times to treat hypoglycemia
- To wear medical alert identification
- To avoid OTC medications unless directed by care provider

STORAGE
- Vial currently in use can be stored at room temp if kept away from heat, direct sunlight, and freezing
- Extra supply of insulin should be stored in refrigerator
- Store concentrated insulin in a separate location to avoid accidental overdose

---

iodoquinol
Brand Name(s): Diodoquin ♣, Yodoxin
Classification: Amebicide
Pregnancy Category: C

AVAILABLE PREPARATIONS
Tabs: 210 mg, 650 mg

ROUTES AND DOSAGES
Children: PO 30-40 mg/kg/24 hr divided tid × 20 days; maximum 1.95 g/24 hr; do not repeat before 2-3 wk
Adults: PO 650 mg tid after meals × 20 days; maximum 2 g/24 hr

MECHANISM AND INDICATIONS
Mechanism: Contact amebicide effective in the lumen of the intestine
Indications: Used to treat acute and chronic amebiasis including *Entamoeba histolytica, Trichomonas vaginalis,* and *Balantidium coli*

PHARMACOKINETICS
Metabolism: Liver
Excretion: Feces, urine

CONTRAINDICATIONS AND PRECAUTIONS
- Contraindicated with known hypersensitivity to iodine or iodoquinol, hepatic or renal disease, preexisting optic neuropathy, severe thyroid disease
- Use cautiously with thyroid disease, neurological disorders, pregnancy

INTERACTIONS
Lab
- False positive PKU
- Increased protein-bound serum iodine concentrations possible, reflecting a decrease in iodine uptake

SIDE EFFECTS
CNS: Agitation, neuropathy, fever, headache, retrograde amnesia
DERM: Pruritus, rash, acne, alopecia, discolored skin
EENT: Optic neuritis, optic atrophy, visual impairment, sore throat
ENDO: Thyroid enlargement
GI: Nausea, vomiting, diarrhea, gastritis, anorexia, constipation, abdominal cramps, rectal irritation
HEME: Agranulocytosis (rare)

TOXICITY AND OVERDOSE
Clinical signs: Overdose may affect cardiovascular and respiratory functions

---

♣ Available in Canada.

Treatment: Discontinue drug and notify care provider; supportive care; emesis or gastric lavage if ingested within 4 hr; followed by activated charcoal

PATIENT CARE MANAGEMENT
Assessment
- Assess history of hypersensitivity to iodoquinol
- Inspect, record appearance and number of stools
- Obtain family history of home, sanitation, pets
- Obtain baseline ophthalmic exam

Interventions
- Administer PO with meals to avoid GI distress; tabs may be crushed, mixed with food or fluids
- Perform proper hygiene procedures; apply child's diapers securely to avoid leakage; dispose of diapers properly; practice good handwashing

NURSING ALERT
Discontinue medication if rash or ophthalmic symptoms develop

Evaluation
- Evaluate therapeutic response (decreased diarrhea)
- Stool cultures weekly, then 1-3 to 6-12 months after therapy is completed; stools should be free of parasites for 1 yr before patient is considered cured
- Monitor stools (number, pattern, character)
- Evaluate spread of infection to other household members
- Monitor for visual impairment
- Monitor for monilia overgrowth
- Monitor for skin eruptions

PATIENT AND FAMILY EDUCATION
Teach/instruct
- To take as directed at prescribed intervals for prescribed length of time
- To practice proper hygiene after bowel movements; good hand-

washing techniques; proper stool collection techniques

Warn/advise
- To notify care provider of hypersensitivity, side effects (fever, rash, chills)
- About importance of follow-up
- About importance of securing child's diaper and proper disposal of used diapers
- About transmission, prevention, proper food preparation and handling

Encourage
- To comply with medication regime and follow up care

STORAGE
- Store at room temp in light-resistant container

---

ipecac syrup
Brand Name(s): PMS-Ipecac ♣

Classification: Antidote (emetic)

Pregnancy Category: C

AVAILABLE PREPARATIONS
Syr: 70 mg/ml

ROUTES AND DOSAGES
Infants 6-12 mo: PO 5-10 ml followed by 10-20 ml/kg of water; repeat dose once if vomiting does not occur within 20 min
Children 1-12 yr: PO 15 ml followed by 10-20 ml/kg of water; repeat dose once if vomiting does not occur within 20 min
Adults: PO 30 ml followed by 200-300 ml of water; repeat dose once if vomiting does not occur within 20 min

MECHANISM AND INDICATIONS
Antidote mechanism: Irritates gastric mucosa, stimulates medullary chemoreceptor trigger zone to induce vomiting
Indications: Used to treat acute

♣ Available in Canada.

oral drug overdose and certain poisonings

PHARMACOKINETICS
Onset (of vomiting): Within 15-30 min after PO dose
Duration: 20-25 minutes; may last up to 60 min
Excretion: Urine

CONTRAINDICATIONS AND PRECAUTIONS
• Contraindicated in pts who are unconscious or semiconscious; with depressed or absent gag reflexes, seizures; with ingestions of strong bases or acids, volatile oils
• Use cautiously with cardiovascular disease, bulimia, pregnancy, lactation

INTERACTIONS
Drug
• Decreased effectiveness with use of activated charcoal; give charcoal after emesis has occurred
Nutrition
• Decreased effectiveness with use of milk, carbonated beverages

SIDE EFFECTS
CNS: Lethargy, tremors
CV: Cardiotoxicity, tachycardia, arrhythmias, atrial fibrillation
GI: Protracted vomiting, diarrhea
MS: Myopathy

TOXICITY AND OVERDOSE
Clinical signs: Usually associated with inadvertent substitution of ipecac fluid extract for ipecac syr; cardiac conduction disturbances, bradycardia, atrial fibrillation, tachycardia, hypotension, bloody diarrhea, protracted emesis, dyspnea, shock, seizures, coma
Treatment: Supportive care, gastric lavage or activated charcoal if vomiting does not occur; cardiac glycosides or pacemakers to counter cardiotoxicity

PATIENT CARE MANAGEMENT
Assessment
• Obtain complete history of ingestion and treatment initiated
• Assess LOC, contraindications to use of ipecac syr
• Assess VS
Interventions
• Use ipecac syr; do not use ipecac fluid extract, which is 14 times more potent and can cause death
• Provide appropriate amount of water before or after ipecac syr; do not use milk, carbonated beverages
• Gently bouncing child may increase emetic affects; keep pt active and moving about
• Repeat dose if no emesis within 20 min; do not administer activated charcoal concurrently
• Provide activated charcoal, gastric lavage, or other emergency equipment if ipecac syr is not effective in inducing emesis

> **NURSING ALERT**
> Use ipecac syr; do not use ipecac fluid extract (its potency may cause death)

Evaluation
• Evaluate therapeutic response (vomiting within 20-30 min of 1st or 2nd dose; no side effects of poison)
• Monitor VS, respiratory status; respiratory depression may occur
• Notify care provider if vomiting does not subside within 2-3 hr

PATIENT AND FAMILY EDUCATION
Teach/instruct
• About preventing poisonings, what to do in the event of ingestion
Advise/warn
• That family should have ipecac syr at home as well as the telephone number for poison control center

STORAGE
• Store at room temp

iron dextran

Brand Name(s): Dexatraron, Feostat, Hematran, Hydextran, InFed

Classification: Hematinic

Pregnancy Category: C

AVAILABLE PREPARATIONS

Inj: IM 50 mg/ml with phenol 0.5% (contains 50 mg elemental Fe/ml)
Inj: IV, IM: 50 mg/ml with NS (contains 50 mg elemental Fe/ml)

ROUTES AND DOSAGES

• Administer 0.5 ml test dose (0.25 ml in infants) before first infusion

Iron Deficiency Anemia

Children and adults: IM/IV: wt (kg) × 4.5 × (desired Hgb − pt's Hgb g%) = mg Fe needed; maximum dose: 5 mg/kg or 100 mg for infants and children and 100 mg for adults

IV administration

• Recommended concentration: Dilute in 50-100 ml NS
• Maximum concentration: 50 mg/ml
• IV push rate: <50 mg/min
• Intermittent infusion rate: Over >2 hr
• Continuous infusion rate: Daily iron requirement may be added to daily TPN solution

MECHANISM AND INDICATIONS

Mechanism: Iron is carried by transferrin to bone marrow and incorporated into hemoglobin
Indications: For use in iron deficiency anemia

PHARMACOKINETICS

Absorption: Gradually absorbed over wk/mo
Half-life: 6 hr or less
Excretion: Breast milk, urine, bile, feces

CONTRAINDICATIONS AND PRECAUTIONS

• Contraindicated with known hypersensitivity; anemias other than iron deficiency

• Use cautiously with juvenile rheumatoid arthritis, hepatic disease, significant allergies, asthma; pregnancy, lactation; do not give with oral iron

INTERACTIONS

Drug

• Increased toxicity with oral iron; do not use
• Decreased reticulocyte response with chloramphenicol

Lab

• Falsely elevated serum bilirubin
• Falsely decreased serum Ca
• Falsely positive Tc diphosphate bone scan, iron test

INCOMPATIBILITIES

• Do not mix with other drugs in syringe

SIDE EFFECTS

CNS: Headache transitory paresthesias, dizziness, malaise, syncope
CV: Hypotensive reaction, tachycardia, chest pain, shock
DERM: Rash, pruritis, urticaria, fever, sweating, chills, skin discoloration, pain at injection site, phlebitis, sterile abscess
GI: Nausea/vomiting, metallic taste
GU: Hematuria
MS: Arthralgia
Other: Anaphylactic reactions

TOXICITY AND OVERDOSE

Clinical signs: Iron toxicity, first phase nausea, vomiting, diarrhea, abdominal pain, hematemesis, melena
Treatment: Administer iron-chelating drug (deferoxamine)

PATIENT CARE MANAGEMENT

Assessment

• Assess history of hypersensitivity to iron dextran
• Assess blood studies before and during treatment (Hct, Hgb, reticulocyte count, bilirubin)

Interventions

• Discontinue oral iron
• Before administering drug, administer test dose
• Z-track method for IM, in upper outer quadrant of buttocks using 2″-3″ 19- or 20-G needle

---

✤ Available in Canada.

• Use IV dose only if pt has insufficient muscle mass to give IM

NURSING ALERT
Test dose of 0.25-0.5 ml should be administered before therapeutic dose; do not use with premature infants or neonates <4 mo

Evaluation
• Evaluate therapeutic response (increased serum iron levels)
• Monitor signs of allergic response
• Evaluate causes of iron deficiency

PATIENT AND FAMILY EDUCATION
Teach/instruct
• To report allergy symptoms which may occur 1-2 days after administration; call care provider
• About iron-rich diet

STORAGE
• Store at room temp

---

isoetharine hydrochloride

Brand Name(s): Bronkosol, Bronkometer

Classification: Bronchodilator (adrenergic)

Pregnancy Category: C

AVAILABLE PREPARATIONS
Aerosol: 340 mcg/dose, 20 metered doses/ml
Sol (for nebulization): 1% (10 mg/ml); also available as 0.062%, 0.08%, 0.11%, 0.125%, 0.14%, 0.167%, 0.17%, 0.2%, 0.25%, 0.5%

ROUTES AND DOSAGES
Children: (Safety/effectiveness not established. Dosage is accepted standard practice recommendations) via nebulizer, 0.01 ml/kg, minimum 0.1 ml, maximum 0.5 ml, q2-4h prn; metered dose inhaler, 1-2 INH q4-6h prn; nebulization 0.25-0.5 ml 1% sol (= 0.1-0.2 mg/kg/dose) diluted to 2 ml in NS (1:8-1:4 dilution) q4h prn

Adults: Aerosol 1-2 INH q3-4h prn; hand nebulizer, I PPB or O_2 aerosolization dosing, see package insert

MECHANISM AND INDICATIONS
Bronchodilation mechanism: Stimulates β_2 receptors selectively to relax bronchial smooth muscle, relieving bronchospasm, increasing vital capacity, and decreasing bronchial airway resistance; may also inhibit histamine release by stabilizing mast cells; acts on smooth muscles of the peripheral vasculature
Indications: Used to treat bronchial asthma, reversible bronchospasm that may occur in association with bronchitis, emphysema

PHARMACOKINETICS
Onset of action: 1-6 min
Peak: 15 min
Half-life: 1-4 hr duration of action
Metabolism: Liver, lungs, GI, other tissues
Excretion: Urine

CONTRAINDICATIONS AND PRECAUTIONS
• Contraindicated with hypersensitivity to drug or ingredients, including sulfites
• Use cautiously with hyperthyroidism, hypertension, acute coronary disease, angina, cardiac arrhythmia, limited cardiac reserve, in pts sensitive to sympathomimetic amines; safety for use in lactation has not been established

INTERACTIONS
Drug
• Increased risk of adverse reaction (because of direct cardiac stimulation) with epinephrine or other sympathomimetic amines; drug doses may be alternated
• Decreased bronchodilation, cardiac and vasodilation effects with β adrenergic blocking agents (propranolol)

SIDE EFFECTS
CNS: Headache, anxiety, tension, restlessness, insomnia, dizziness, excitement, irritability
CV: Tachycardia, hypertension,

♣ Available in Canada.

hypotension, angina, palpitations
GI: Nausea, vomiting
RESP: Cough, bronchial irritation, paradoxical bronchoconstriction, edema

TOXICITY AND OVERDOSE

Clinical signs: Tachycardia, palpitations, vomiting, nausea, headache, epinephrine-like side effects, B/P change, anxiety, restlessness, extreme tremor, insomnia, weakness, dizziness, excitation; paradoxical bronchospasm or cardiac arrest can occur with overuse
Treatment: Discontinue drug immediately; support vital functions and treat symptoms until pt stabilized; monitor VS closely; sedatives may be used to treat restlessness; use cardioselective β blockers cautiously to treat arrhythmias because they may induce asthma attack

PATIENT CARE MANAGEMENT
Assessment
• Assess hypersensitivity to isoetharine hydrochloride, sulfites, and related drugs
• Assess respiratory status, VS
Interventions
• Shake inhaler before use
• See Chapter 3 for inhaler instructions
• Wait 1-2 min between inhalations
• Keep spray away from eyes
• Do not administer with other sympathomimetic amines; alternate doses if needed
• See Chapter 3 for discussion of nebulizer use
• Maintain age-appropriate fluid intake
• Offer sips of fluids, rinse mouth to prevent irritation, dryness

> **NURSING ALERT**
> INH sol contains a sulfite; risk of anaphylaxis exists for sulfite-sensitive individuals
>
> Not for injection
>
> Discontinue drug if paradoxical bronchospasm occurs

Evaluation
• Evaluate therapeutic response (improved respiratory effort)
• Evaluate for signs of paradoxical bronchospasm, increased dyspnea, decreased effect of drug; side effects; hypersensitivity

PATIENT AND FAMILY EDUCATION
Teach/instruct
• To take as directed at prescribed intervals and for prescribed length of time
• To begin treatment at first sign of bronchospasm
• About correct inhaler or nebulizer techniques
• To allow 1-2 min between inhalations; to take no more than 2 inhalations at one time
• To increase fluid intake to liquefy secretions
• That rinsing of mouth after treatment will lessen dryness and irritation of mouth, throat
Warn/advise
• About risks of overuse (tolerance, paradoxical bronchospasm)
• Not to use more than prescribed amount or more frequently than prescribed
• To keep spray away from eyes
• To call provider if pt requires more than four aerosol treatments in 24 hr
• To report no effect from treatment, worsening or persistent symptoms, severe dyspnea, tachycardia, chest pain, palpitations, headache, nausea, dizziness
• That sputum may be pink to rust colored because of medication oxidation
• To avoid other adrenergic medications unless they are prescribed

STORAGE
• Store aerosol at room temp; do not puncture canister; do not place near heat or open flame
• Store sol at room temp; protect from light, store vial in pouch until used; do not use sol if it is pink or darker than slightly yellow, or if it contains a precipitate
• Keep out of reach of children

---

isoniazid (INH)

Brand Name(s): INH,
Isotamine✤, Laniazid,
Nydrazid, PMS-Isoniazid✤

Classification: Antitubercular (isonicotinic acid
hydrazine)

Pregnancy Category: C

AVAILABLE PREPARATIONS
Syr: 50 mg/5 ml
Tabs: 50 mg, 100 mg, 300 mg
Inj: 100 mg/ml

ROUTES AND DOSAGES
Infants and children: Treatment,
PO, IM 10-20 mg/kg/24 hr qd or
divided bid (maximum 300-500
mg/24 hr) or 20-40 mg/kg/dose
twice weekly (maximum 900 mg/
dose); prophylaxis, 10 mg/kg/24 hr
qd (maximum 300 mg/24 hr)
Adults: Treatment, PO, IM 5 mg/
kg/24 hr qd (usual 300 mg/24 hr) or
15 mg/kg/dose twice weekly (maximum 900 mg/dose); prophylaxis
300 mg qd

MECHANISM AND INDICATIONS
Antitubercular mechanism: Bacteriostatic or bactericidal; inhibits
bacterial cell wall synthesis by
interfering with lipid and DNA
synthesis
Indications: Effective against *Mycobacterium tuberculosis*, *M. bovis*, some strains of *M. kansasii*;
used with at least one other antitubercular agent to treat active
tuberculosis; used alone as prophylaxis for those closely exposed
to tuberculosis, for those with positive Mantoux skin test and chest
x-rays and bacteriologic studies
indicating nonprogressive tuberculosis, and for those who are
priorities per CDC guidelines

PHARMACOKINETICS
Peak: Oral 1-2 hr
Distribution: To all body tissues,
fluids including CSF
Half-life: Fast acetylators 0.5-1.5
hr; slow acetylators 2-5 hr

Metabolism: Liver
Excretion: Urine, feces, saliva

CONTRAINDICATIONS AND PRECAUTIONS
• Contraindicated with known hypersensitivity to isoniazid, with
acute liver disease or previous
history of hepatic damage during
isoniazid therapy
• Use cautiously with chronic hepatic or renal impairment, history
of seizures, alcoholism, pregnancy

INTERACTIONS
Drug
• Increased risk of hepatotoxicity,
seizures with daily use of alcohol
• Increased risk of CNS toxicity of
cycloserine
• Increased toxicity of phenytoin,
carbamazepine
• Increased coordination problems, psychotic episodes with use
of disulfiram
• Decreased absorption with use
of aluminum antacids
• Decreased effectiveness with
use of corticosteroids
• Increased metabolism to hepatotoxic metabolites with use of
rifampin
Lab
• Elevated liver function tests
Nutrition
• Flushing, palpitations, hypotension from tyramine-containing
foods (smoked fish, organ meats,
aged cheese, yeast vitamin supplements, broad bean pods)
• Headache, rash, flushing, palpitations, hypotension, diarrhea
from histamine-containing foods
(yeast extracts, sauerkraut, tuna)

SIDE EFFECTS
CNS: Paraesthesias of hands or
feet leading to peripheral neuropathy (particularly in slow acetylators, alcoholic, diabetic, or malnourished pts), seizures, psychosis
CV: Postural hypotension
EENT: Optic neuritis
ENDO/METAB: Hyperglycemia,
metabolic acidosis, pyridoxine deficiency
GI: Nausea, vomiting, epigastric
distress, constipation, jaundice,
hepatitis

✤ Available in Canada.

HEME: Agranulocytosis, hemolytic anemia, aplastic anemia, eosinophilia, leukopenia, neutropenia, thrombocytopenia, methemoglobinemia

Local: Pain induration, sterile abscesses at injection site

Other: Hypersensitivity (rash, fever, lymphadenopathy, vasculitis), rheumatic syndrome, systemic lupus erythematosus-like syndrome

TOXICITY AND OVERDOSE

Clinical signs: Initially GI upset, slurred speech, dizziness, visual hallucinations; CNS depression, respiratory distress, seizures with severe overdose

Treatment: Seizure control, gastric lavage, forced diuresis, hemodialysis or peritoneal dialysis; supportive care

PATIENT CARE MANAGEMENT

Assessment

• Assess history of hypersensitivity to isoniazid

• Obtain C&S; may begin therapy before obtaining results

• Assess renal function (BUN, creatinine, I&O), hepatic function (ALT, AST, bilirubin), hematologic function (CBC, differential, platelet count), ophthalmologic status

Interventions

• Administer PO 1 hr before or 2 hr after meals; may administer with food to reduce GI distress; tablet may be crushed, mixed with food or fluid

• Aluminum antacids should be administered 1 hr after medication

• If crystallization of IM sol occurs at low temp, warm to room temp to dissolve

• Injection is painful; administer deeply into large muscle mass, rotate injection sites

• Change from IM to PO form when tolerated

• Maintain age-appropriate fluid intake

• Treatment of active tuberculosis may continue from 9-24 mo; pro-

phylaxis may continue from 6-12 mo

• Pyridoxine may be prescribed to prevent peripheral neuropathy

> **NURSING ALERT**
> Discontinue if signs of hypersensitivity or hepatic impairment develop

Evaluation

• Evaluate therapeutic response (decreased TB symptoms, negative culture)

• Monitor hepatic function (ALT, AST, bilirubin), renal function (BUN, creatinine, I&O) hematologic function (CBC, differential, platelet count), ophthalmologic status

• Monitor for hepatic impairment (anorexia, jaundice, dark urine, malaise, fatigue, liver tenderness)

• Monitor DM control, if appropriate

• Monitor CNS toxicity (affect, behavioral changes)

• Monitor safety in case of postural hypotension

• Evaluate IM site for tissue damage

PATIENT AND FAMILY EDUCATION

Teach/instruct

• To take as directed at prescribed intervals for prescribed length of time

Warn/advise

• To notify care provider of hypersensitivity, side effects

• To comply with follow-up care

• To avoid use of alcohol, medications containing alcohol

STORAGE

• Store at room temp

• Protect from light, air

✢ Available in Canada.

isoproterenol, isoproterenol hydrochloride, isoproterenol sulfate

Brand Name(s): Aerolone, Isuprel, Vapo-Iso, Isuprel✦, Isuprel Mistometer, Norisodrine, Medihaler ISO

Classification: β-adrenergic agonist, sympathomimetic, bronchodilator

Pregnancy Category: C

AVAILABLE PREPARATIONS
Nebulizer inh: 0.25%, 0.5%, 1% (isoproterenol)
Aerosol inh: 120 mcg or 131 mcg/metered spray (isoproterenol hydrochloride); 80 mcg/metered spray (isoproterenol sulfate)
Tabs (SL): 10 mg, 15 mg
Inj: 200 mcg/ml

ROUTES AND DOSAGES
Bronchospasm in Mild Asthma
Children and adults: INH isoproterenol hydrochloride 6-12 inhalations of 0.25% nebulized sol dilute with NS to 2 ml, repeat q15 min prn; 3 treatment maximum; not to exceed 8 treatments/24 hr; aerosol 1-2 puffs up to 5×/24 hr

Acute Asthma Unresponsive to Inhalation Therapy
Children: IV infusion isoproterenol hydrochloride 0.05-2 mcg/kg/min
Adults: IV infusion isoproterenol hydrochloride 2-20 mg, repeat prn

Bradycardia (Atropine-Resistant)
Children: IV 0.1 mcg/kg/min IV; titrate to pt response; maximum rate 1 mcg/kg/min IV
Adults: IV 2-10 mcg/min IV; titrate to pt response

Shock
Children and adults: IV 0.05-1.5 mcg/kg/min continuous IV; titrate to pt response

IV administration
• Recommended concentration: 4-12 mcg/ml in dextrose sols, NS, LR
• Maximum concentration: 20 mcg/ml in D_5W or NS
• IV push rate: Not established for pediatric pts
• Intermittent infusion rate: Not recommended because of short half-life
• Continuous infusion rate: 0.02-1.6 mcg/kg/min

MECHANISM AND INDICATIONS
Mechanism: Relaxes bronchial smooth muscle, dilates trachea and main bronchi, increases cardiac contractility and HR
Indications: For use in asthma, COPD, emergency treatment for atropine-resistant bradycardia, shock

PHARMACOKINETICS
Absorption: Rapid
Half-life: 2.5-5 min
Metabolism: GI tract, liver, lungs
Excretion: Urine

CONTRAINDICATIONS AND PRECAUTIONS
• Contraindicated with hypersensitivity, preexisting cardiac arrhythmias, angina
• Use cautiously with cardiac disorders, renal disease, diabetes, hyperthyroidism; receiving cyclopropane or halothane anesthetics; pregnancy, lactation

INTERACTIONS
Drug
• Increased effects with epinephrine, other sympathomimetics
• Decreased effects with propranolol, other β blockers

INCOMPATIBILITIES
• Aminophylline, barbiturates, carbenicillin, lidocaine, $NaHCO_3$ in solution or syringe

SIDE EFFECTS
CNS: Nervousness, anxiety, headache, irritability, dizziness, insomnia, tremors

---

CV: Tachycardia, arrhythmias, chest pain, palpitations, changes in B/P
EENT: Parotid swelling, tinnitus
GI: Nausea, vomiting, diarrhea, dry mouth
METAB: Hyperglycemia
RESP: Bronchial irritation
Other: Sweating, flushing of face, skin

TOXICITY AND OVERDOSE
Clinical signs: Exaggeration of side effects, especially arrhythmias; nausea, vomiting, low B/P
Treatment: Supportive care, use sedatives, β blockers prn, with caution

PATIENT CARE MANAGEMENT
Assessment
• Assess history of hypersensitivity to drug
• Assess baseline, VS, B/P, breath sounds before treatment and frequently throughout
• Assess I&O
Interventions
• See Chapter 3 regarding use of nebulizer, inhaler
• Monitor ECG with IV dose
Evaluation
• Therapeutic response (increased B/P, decreased respiratory distress)
• Evaluate for adverse reactions (especially cardiac)

PATIENT AND FAMILY EDUCATION
Teach/instruct
• To take as directed at prescribed intervals for prescribed length of time
• About use of nebulizer, inhaler
Warn/advise
• To call care provider if symptoms worsen, or if pt requiring more than 3 treatments/24 hr
• About adverse reactions; report to care provider
• To rinse mouth after treatments; saliva and sputum may be pink-tinged after inhalation

STORAGE
• Store at room temp
• Keep away from heat, light

---

isotretinoin
Brand Name(s): Accutane, Acutane Roche✤, Isotrex✤
Classification: Anti-acne agent
Pregnancy Category: X

AVAILABLE PREPARATIONS
Caps: 10 mg, 20 mg, 40 mg

ROUTES AND DOSAGES
Adolescents and adults: PO 0.5 to 1 mg/kg/24 hr divided bid for 15-20 wk; maximum dosage for severe acne 2 mg/kg/24 hr divided bid

MECHANISM AND INDICATIONS
Mechanism: Decreases size and activity of sebaceous glands; also has antiinflammatory and keratinizing effects
Indications: Used to treat severe cystic acne unresponsive to standard therapy

PHARMACOKINETICS
Onset of action: Rapid
Half-life: 10-20 hr
Peak: 3 hr
Metabolism: Liver, possibly intestines
Excretion: Urine, biliary pathways

CONTRAINDICATIONS AND PRECAUTIONS
• *Contraindicated in pregnancy; begin therapy after negative pregnancy test and after confirmation that adequate birth control measures are being used;* with known hypersensitivity to isotretinoin, vitamin A
• Use cautiously with hepatic disease, photosensitivity, lactation

INTERACTIONS
Drug
• Additive toxic effects possible with vitamin supplement containing vitamin A
• Increased potential for pseudotumor cerebri with tetracycline, minocycline
Lab
• Increased plasma triglyceride

✤ Available in Canada.

levels, especially with alcohol consumption
• Increased liver function tests (AST, ALT, alk phos)
• Increased sedimentation rate
• Decreased RBC/WBC counts

SIDE EFFECTS
CNS: Depression, headache, lethargy, pseudotumor cerebri
DERM: Dry skin, peeling palms and toes, pruritis, urticaria, photosensitivity, skin rash, hirsutism, petechiae, hypo- or hyperpigmentation
EENT: Eye irritation, conjunctivitis, corneal deposits, contact lens intolerance, photophobia, dry nose, dry mouth, epistaxis
ENDO: Hyperglycemia
GI: Nausea, vomiting, anorexia, cheilitis, weight loss, abdominal pain
HEME: Thrombocytopenia, elevated platelet count, increased sedimentation rate

TOXICITY AND OVERDOSE
Clinical signs: Rare; would be extensions of side effects
Treatment: Discontinue drug

PATIENT CARE MANAGEMENT
Assessment
• *Assess for pregnancy with pregnancy test, have patient sign consent explaining teratogenic effects and confirming appropriate birth control measures*
• Assess history of hypersensitivity to drug
• Assess triglyceride levels, AST, ALT, sedimentation rate before, during, and after treatment
Interventions
• Advise patient to take PO with meals to increase absorption and decrease GI upset

> **NURSING ALERT**
> May be teratogenic to fetus; begin therapy only after negative pregnancy test; confirm appropriate birth control method before use

Evaluation
• Evaluate clinical response (decrease in size and quantity of lesions)
• Evaluate side effects; discontinue drug if symptoms of pseudotumor cerebri, visual disturbances, or inflammatory bowel disease develop

PATIENT AND FAMILY EDUCATION
Teach/instruct
• To take as directed at prescribed intervals for prescribed length of time
Warn/advise
• That an initial increase in acne may occur early in treatment
• To avoid sunlight, wear sunscreen when outside
• Not to become pregnant during or until 30 days after completing therapy
• Not to consume alcohol during treatment
• Not to use vitamin supplements containing vitamin A during treatment

STORAGE
• Store in light-resistant container at room temp

---

kanamycin sulfate

Brand Name(s): Kantrex, Klebcil

Classification: Antibiotic (aminoglycoside)

Pregnancy Category: D

AVAILABLE PREPARATIONS
Caps: 500 mg
Inj: 37.5 mg/ml, 250 mg/ml, 333 mg/ml

ROUTES AND DOSAGES
PO, IM, IV
Neonates <7 days, ≤2000 g: 7.5 mg/kg/dose q12h
Neonates <7 days, >2000 g: 10 mg/kg/dose q12h
Neonates 1-4 wk, ≤2000 g: 10 mg/kg/dose q12h

K

Neonates 1-4 wk, >2000 g: 10 mg/kg/dose q8h

Infants >4 wk/children: 15-30 mg/kg/24 hr divided q8-12h (maximum 1.5 g/24 hr)

Adults: 15 mg/kg/24 hr divided q8-12h (maximum 1.5 g/24 hr)

MECHANISM AND INDICATIONS

Antibiotic mechanism: Bactericidal; inhibits bacterial protein synthesis by binding directly to the 30S ribosomal subunit

Indications: Effective against many aerobic gram-negative and some aerobic gram-positive organisms including *E. coli, Enterobacter, Acinetobacter, Proteus, Neisseria gonorrhoeae, Haemophilus influenzae, Shigella, Klebsiella pneumoniae, Serratia marcescens, Staphylococcus;* used to treat severe systemic infections of CNS, respiratory, GI, urinary tracts, bone, skin and soft tissue; also used as preoperative agent for bowel surgery

IV administration

• Recommended concentration: 2.5-5 mg/ml in D_5NS, D_5W, $D_{10}W$, LR, or NS

• Maximum concentration: 5-6 mg/ml

• IV push rate: Not recommended

• Intermittent infusion: Over 30 min using constant-rate volumetric infusion device

• Continuous infusion: Not recommended

PHARMACOKINETICS

Peak: IM 1 hr; IV end of infusion

Half-life: Neonates 6-18 hr; children/adults 2-4 hr

Metabolism: Not metabolized

Excretion: Urine, bile

Therapeutic levels: Peak 15-30 mcg/ml; trough 5 mcg/ml

CONTRAINDICATIONS AND PRECAUTIONS

• Contraindicated with known hypersensitivity to kanamycin or any other aminoglycoside, intestinal obstruction (oral form), or renal failure

• Use cautiously in neonates and infants (because of renal immaturity); with impaired renal function, dehydration, 8th cranial nerve impairment, myasthenia gravis, parkinsonism, hypocalcemia, pregnancy, lactation

INTERACTIONS

Drug

• Increased risk of nephrotoxicity, ototoxicity, neurotoxicity with methoxyflurane, polymyxin B, vancomycin, amphotericin B, cisplatin, cephalosporins, other aminoglycosides

• Increased risk of ototoxicity with ethacrynic acid, furosemide, bumetanide, urea, mannitol

• Masked symptoms of ototoxicity with dimenhydrinate and other antiemetic or antivertigo drugs

• Synergistic antimicrobial activity against certain organisms with penicillins

• Increased risk of neuromuscular blockade with general anesthetics or neuromuscular blocking agents such as succinylcholine, tubocurarine

• Increased respiratory depression with opioids and analgesics

• Inactivated when administered with parenteral penicillin, carbenicillin, ticarcillin

• Inhibited vitamin K-producing bacteria in GI tract, thus potentiating action of oral anticoagulants (oral kanamycin)

Lab

• Increased LDH, BUN, non-protein nitrogen, serum creatinine levels

• Increased urinary excretion of casts

• Decreased serum Na

INCOMPATIBILITIES

• Amphotericin B, ampicillin, carbenicillin, cefoxitin, cephalothin, cephapirin, chlorpheniramine, colistimethate, heparin, hydrocortisone, methohexital, lincomycin, penicillins

SIDE EFFECTS

CNS: Headache, lethargy, neuromuscular blockade with respiratory depression

EENT: Ototoxicity (tinnitus, vertigo, hearing loss)

GI: Nausea, vomiting, diarrhea
GU: Nephrotoxicity (cells or casts in urine, oliguria, proteinuria, decreased CrCl, increased BUN, serum creatinine, and nonprotein nitrogen levels)
Other: Hypersensitivity reactions (eosinophilia, fever, rash, urticaria, pruritus), bacterial or fungal superinfections

TOXICITY AND OVERDOSE

Clinical signs: Ototoxicity, nephrotoxicity, neuromuscular toxicity
Treatment: Supportive care, hemodialysis or peritoneal dialysis; neuromuscular blockade reversed with Ca salts or anticholinesterases; if ingested within 4 hr, empty the stomach by induced emesis or gastric lavage, followed by activated charcoal

PATIENT CARE MANAGEMENT

Assessment

• Assess history of hypersensitivity to kanamycin or other aminoglycosides
• Obtain C&S; may begin therapy before obtaining results
• Assess renal function (BUN, creatinine, I&O), baseline wt, and hearing tests before beginning therapy

Interventions

• Sol should be colorless or clear to very pale yellow; do not use if dark yellow, cloudy, or containing precipitates
• Administer kanamycin at least 1 hr before or after other antibiotics (penicillins, cephalosporins)
• May administer PO without regard to meals; caps may be taken apart, mixed with food or fluid
• IM injection is painful; administer deeply into large muscle mass, rotate injection sites; do not inject more than 2 g of drug per injection site
• Do not premix IV with other medications; infuse separately, flush line with D_5W or NS
• Use large vein with small-bore needle to reduce local reaction; rotate site q48-72h

• Maintain age-appropriate fluid intake; keep pt well hydrated to reduce risk of renal toxicity
• Supervise ambulation, other safety measures with vestibular dysfunction
• Obtain drug levels after the 3rd dose; sooner in neonates or pts with rapidly changing renal function; peak levels drawn after end of 30-min IV infusion, 1 hr after IM injection; trough levels drawn within 30 min before next dose

> **NURSING ALERT**
> Discontinue if signs of ototoxicity, nephrotoxicity, hypersensitivity develop
> Do not administer IV push

Evaluation

• Evaluate therapeutic response (decreased symptoms of infection)
• Evaluate renal function (BUN, creatinine, I&O), daily wt, hearing evaluations
• Monitor signs of respiratory depression with IV infusion
• Observe for signs of superinfection (perineal itching, diaper rash, fever, malaise, redness, pain, swelling, drainage, rash, diarrhea, sore throat, change in cough or sputum)
• Evaluate IM site for tissue damage, IV site for vein irritation

PATIENT AND FAMILY EDUCATION

Teach/instruct

• To take as directed at prescribed intervals for prescribed length of time

Warn/advise

• To notify care provider of hypersensitivity, side effects, superinfection

STORAGE

• Store at room temp

K

ketoconazole

Brand Name(s): Nizoral, Nizoral Cream ✙

Classification: Antifungal

Pregnancy Category: C

AVAILABLE PREPARATIONS
Susp: 100 mg/5 ml
Tabs: 200 mg
Top cream: 2% (contains sodium sulfite)

ROUTES AND DOSAGES
Children ≥2 yr: PO 5-10 mg/kg/24 hr qd or divided bid; maximum 800 mg/24 hr; top, apply to affected area qd-bid
Adults: PO 200-400 mg/qd; maximum 1 g/24 hr; top, apply to affected area qd-bid

MECHANISM AND INDICATIONS
Mechanism: Alters permeability of cell wall; inhibits fungal biosynthesis of triglycerides and phospholipid; fungal enzymes that result in a buildup of toxic concentrations of hydrogen peroxide also inhibited
Indications: Used to treat fungal infections including candidiasis, oral thrush, blastomycosis, mucocandidiasis, paracoccidiomycosis, top form used to treat tinea corporis, tinea versicolor, tinea cruris, cutaneous candidiasis

PHARMACOKINETICS
Peak: 1-2 hr
Distribution: Minimal CNS penetration
Half-life: Biphasic, initial 2 hr, terminal 8 hr
Metabolism: Liver
Excretion: Feces, urine

CONTRAINDICATIONS AND PRECAUTIONS
• Contraindicated with lactation; in children <2 yr; with hypersensitivity to drug or any component; with CNS fungal infections; with concomitant use of terfenadine or astemizole
• Use cautiously with impaired hepatic functions, alcoholism, pregnancy

INTERACTIONS
Drug
• Increased action with cyclosporine, theophylline
• Severe hypoglycemia with oral hypoglycemics
• Disulfram reaction with alcohol
• Decreased absorption of antacids, H_2 blockers, anticholinergics, rifampin, isoniazid
• Increased anticoagulant affect with Coumarin anticoagulants
• Life-threatening arrhythmias with terfenadine and astemizole
• Hepatotoxicity with other hepatotoxic drugs
• Decreased levels of both drugs with use of phenytoin

SIDE EFFECTS
CNS: Lethargy, headache, vertigo
DERM: Pruritis, rash
ENDO/METAB: Adrenocortical insufficiency, gynecomastia
GI: Nausea, vomiting, abdominal discomfort, GI bleeding, hepatotoxicity
GU: Oligospermia
Local: Irritation, stinging

TOXICITY AND OVERDOSE
Clinical signs: Vertigo, tinnitus, headache, nausea, vomiting, diarrhea, signs of adrenal crisis
Treatment: Induced emesis, lavage; supportive measures

PATIENT CARE MANAGEMENT
Assessment
• Assess history of hypersensitivity to ketoconazole
• Obtain baseline hepatic function (ALT, AST, bilirubin)
• Review possible concomitant use of terfenadine, astemizole
Interventions
• Administer PO 2 hr before antacids or H_2 receptors
• Dissolve tab in 4 ml aqueous sol of 0.2% HCl; take through straw to avoid damaging tooth enamel
• Administer with food prn to decrease GI distress; tab may

✙ Available in Canada.

be crushed, administered with small amounts of food or fluids
• Avoid top use near eyes, mucous membranes

> **NURSING ALERT**
> Contraindicated for use with astemizole and terfenadine

Evaluation
• Evaluate therapeutic response (decreased fever, malaise, rash, negative culture)
• Monitor liver function tests q mo

PATIENT AND FAMILY EDUCATION
Teach/instruct
• To take as directed at prescribed intervals for prescribed length of time
Warn/advise
• To notify care provider of hypersensitivity, side effects
• That long-term therapy may be needed
• That therapy is to be monitored closely by care provider
• To avoid exposure to sunlight because of potential photosensitivity
• To take no other drugs, including OTCs, without consulting care provider
• To avoid hazardous activities with dizziness
Encourage
• To comply with prescribed regimen

STORAGE
• Store at room temp in tight containers

> **ketorolac**
> **Brand Name(s):** Toradol
> **Classification:** Nonsteroidal antiinflammatory
> **Pregnancy Category:** C

AVAILABLE PREPARATIONS
Tab: 10 mg

Inj: 15 mg, 30 mg, 60 mg (prefilled syringes)
Ophthal: 0.5% sol

ROUTES AND DOSAGES
Adolescents >16 yr and adults: PO 10 mg q4-6h, maximum 40 mg/24 hr; IM 30-60 mg loading dose, then 15-30 mg q6h; ophthal 1 gtt (0.25 mg) qid
• Do not use PO/IM >5 days

MECHANISM AND INDICATIONS
Mechanism: Inhibits prostaglandin synthesis by decreasing an enzyme needed for biosynthesis
Indications: Used to treat mild-to-moderate pain (short-term management only, up to 5 days); ophthal ketorolac is used for allergic conjunctivitis

PHARMACOKINETICS
Onset: 15-30 min
Peak: 50 min
Distribution: Highly plasma protein bound
Half-life: 6 hr
Duration: Dependent on dosage and route
Metabolism: Liver
Excretion: Urine

CONTRAINDICATIONS AND PRECAUTIONS
• Contraindicated with hypersensitivity, asthma, severe renal or hepatic disease, peptic ulcer
• Use cautiously in children; with pregnancy, lactation, bleeding disorders, hypertension, GI disorders, cardiac disorders, hypersensitivity to other antiinflammatory agents; in pts using high dosage salicylates

INTERACTIONS
Drug
• Increased action with phenytoin and sulfonamides
• Increased risk of bleeding with anticoagulants (heparin and dicumarol)
Lab
• Prolonged bleeding time possible

K

- Diminished clearance of drug in pts with reduced CrCl
- Increased liver enzymes (particularly ALT) possible

SIDE EFFECTS

CNS: Dizziness, drowsiness, tremors, somnolence, headaches, paresthesias
CV: Hypertension, flushing, syncope, pallor, fluid retention, edema
DERM: Purpura, rash, pruritus, sweating
EENT: Tinnitus, hearing loss, blurred vision
GI: Nausea, anorexia, vomiting, diarrhea, constipation, abdominal pain, dyspepsia, flatulence, cramps, dry mouth, peptic ulcer, bleeding, ulceration and perforation
GU: Nephrotoxicity, dysuria, hematuria, oliguria, azotemia, proteinuria, nephrotic syndrome
HEME: Blood dyscrasias
Local: Pain with IM injection; minor burning and stinging with ophthal sol

TOXICITY AND OVERDOSE

Clinical signs: Blurred vision, tinnitus may indicate toxicity
Treatment: Absence of experience with acute overdosage precludes characterization of sequelae and assessment of antidotal efficacy at this time

PATIENT CARE MANAGEMENT
Assessment

- Assess history of hypersensitivity to ketorolac or related drugs
- Assess baseline VS, renal function (BUN, creatinine, I&O), liver function (ALT, AST, bilirubin), Hgb, bleeding times
- Assess hepatic, GI, or cardiac dysfunction

Interventions

- Loading dose (IM) should only be administered once unless therapy has been interrupted for >15-40 hr
- Encourage around-the-clock management to ensure adequate pain relief

- Administer when pain is not too severe to enhance effectiveness (if ordered prn)
- Institute safety measures (supervise ambulation, raise side rails, call light within reach) until effects of medication are known

Evaluation

- Evaluate therapeutic response (decreased pain, stiffness, swelling in joints, ability to move easily; decreased menstrual pain and cramping)
- Monitor VS, pain control 30-60 min after administration; renal, liver, and blood studies
- Monitor for bruising or bleeding; test for occult blood in urine
- Evaluate side effects, hypersensitivity

PATIENT AND FAMILY EDUCATION
Teach/instruct

- To take as directed at prescribed intervals for prescribed length of time
- About best time to request medication if ordered prn

Warn/advise

- To notify care provider of side effects, hypersensitivity
- To avoid driving or other activities requiring alertness if dizziness or drowsiness occurs
- To avoid alcohol, aspirin products

STORAGE

- Store at room temp

---

lactulose

Brand Name(s): Acilac✤, Cephulac✤, Cholac, Chronulac, Comalose-R✤, Constilac, Constulose, Duphalac, Enulose, Gen-Lac✤, Gerelac, Lacutlax✤, PMS-Lactulose✤, Portalac

Classification: Hyperosmotic laxative; antihyperammonemic

Pregnancy Category: B

AVAILABLE PREPARATIONS
Sol: 10 g/15 ml

ROUTES AND DOSAGES
Hyperammonemic
Infants: PO 2.5 ml (1.7 g)-10 ml (6.7 g)/24 hr divided tid-qid
Older children and adolescents: PO 40 ml (27 g)-90 ml (60 g)/24 hr divided tid-qid; goal 2-4 soft stools/24 hr
Adult: PO initial 30 ml (20 g)-45 ml (30g) qh to induce rapid laxation, then adjust dosage to maintain goal; maintenance 30 ml (20 g)-45 ml (30 g) divided tid-qid; goal 2-4 soft stools/24 hr
Retention Enema
Adult: 300 ml diluted in 700 ml water or NS; retain for 30-60 min; may administer q4-6h prn
Chronic Constipation
Infants and children: PO 7.5 ml (5 g) qd
Adult: PO 10 ml (6.7 g)-20 ml (13.4 g)/24 hr; maximum 60 ml/24 hr

MECHANISM AND INDICATIONS
Mechanism: Produces osmotic effect in colon resulting from biodegradation by colonic bacterial flora into lactic, formic, and acetic acids; fluid accumulation produces distention, promotes increased peristalsis and bowel evacuation; bacterial degradation of lactulose in the colon acidifies colonic contents, results in retention of ammonia in the colon as ammonium ion, which is expelled with feces
Indications: For the prevention and treatment of portal-systemic encephalopathy including the stages of hepatic pre-coma and coma; also used in the treatment of chronic constipation

PHARMACOKINETICS
Absorption: Minimal
Onset: 24-48 hr
Metabolism: Colonic bacteria
Excretion: Primarily feces, urine

CONTRAINDICATIONS AND PRECAUTIONS
• Contraindicated with a low galactose diet
• Use cautiously with pregnancy, lactation; pts with symptoms of appendicitis; undiagnosed rectal bleeding; diabetes (contains up to 1.2 g lactose, up to 2.2 g galactose per 15 ml); pts undergoing colonoscopy (lactulose causes accumulation of hydrogen ion in bowel; a cleansing enema is required before procedure)

INTERACTIONS
Drug
• Interference with K^+ sparing diuretics or K^+ supplements with chronic use
• Concurrent use of other softeners or laxatives may give a false impression of adequate dosage when using lactulose as treatment for elevated ammonia levels
• Decreased colonic bacteria necessary to metabolize lactulose possible with neomycin and other antiinfective agents
Lab
• Decreased serum K^+ levels possible
• Increased blood Na, BG, and CO_2 levels
Nutrition
• Contains up to 1.2 g lactose and up to 2.2 g galactose; use with caution in patients with diabetes or who are on a low galactose diet

SIDE EFFECTS
GI: Cramping, diarrhea, flatulence, belching
Other: Increased thirst

TOXICITY AND OVERDOSE
Clinical signs: Diarrhea, abdominal cramping; infants, hyponatremia, dehydration
Treatment: Discontinue medication; supportive measures

PATIENT CARE MANAGEMENT
Assessment
• Assess history of hypersensitivity to lactulose
• Assess symptoms of appendicitis, rectal bleeding, hydration, LOC, and neurologic status
Interventions
• Pt should drink 8 oz glass of liquid with each dose
• PO contraindicated with de-

L

creased LOC because of risk of aspiration
• A low protein diet is recommended for pts undergoing therapy for elevated ammonia levels

Evaluation
• Evaluate therapeutic response (decreased constipation, decreased blood ammonia level)
• Evaluate for hypersensitivity, side effects
• Evaluate I&O, fluid and electrolyte status
• For pts undergoing therapy for hyperammonemia monitor ammonia levels, LOC, and neurologic parameters

PATIENT AND FAMILY EDUCATION
Teach/instruct
• To take as directed at prescribed intervals for prescribed length of time
• To drink 8 oz glass of fluid with each dose

Warn/advise
• To notify care provider if diarrhea occurs
• About signs of dehydration and electrolyte imbalance
• That a cleansing enema must be administered before the procedure if pt is to undergo colonoscopy, sigmoidoscopy, polypectomy during therapy

STORAGE
• Store at room temp

---

lamivudine (3TC)
Brand Name(s): Epivir
Classification: Antiviral
Pregnancy Category: C

AVAILABLE PREPARATIONS
Sol: 10 mg/ml
Tabs: 150 mg

ROUTES AND DOSAGES
Children 3 mo-12 yr: PO 4 mg/kg bid administered with zidovudine
Adults <50 kg: PO 2 mg/kg bid administered with zidovudine

Adults >50 kg: PO 150 mg bid administered with zidovudine

MECHANISM AND INDICATIONS
Mechanism: Potent and selective inhibitor of HIV-1 and HIV-2 replication; shows activity against zidovudine-resistant strains of HIV
Indications: Indicated for use in the treatment of children and adults with HIV infection in combination with zidovudine; based on clinical or immunological evidence of disease progression

PHARMACOKINETICS
Onset of action: Rapid
Half-life: Children: 2 hrs; adults: 3.7 hrs
Metabolism: Unknown
Elimination: Urine

CONTRAINDICATIONS AND PRECAUTIONS
• Contraindicated with hypersensitivity to drug or its components, lactation
• Use cautiously with pregnancy; in children (limited clinical data available); with hepatic and renal dysfunction; with pancreatitis; in patients with granulocyte count <1000 or Hgb <9.5

INTERACTIONS
Drug
• Increased levels of zidovudine with lamivudine
• Increased levels of lamivudine with trimethoprim-sulfamethoxazole
Lab
• Increased AST, ALT, alk phos, bilirubin
• Increased serum amylase
• Decreased absolute neutrophil count, Hgb, platelets

INCOMPATIBILITIES
• None reported

SIDE EFFECTS
CNS: Neuropathy, headache, insomnia, dizziness, depression
DERM: Rash
EENT: Taste change, hearing loss, photophobia
GI: Diarrhea, nausea, vomiting,

✦ Available in Canada.

abdominal pain, anorexia, dyspepsia, pancreatitis
HEME: Anemia, neutropenia, thrombocytopenia
RESP: Cough, nasal congestion
Other: Chills, fever, pain, malaise, myalgia, arthralgia

TOXICITY AND OVERDOSE
Not reported

PATIENT CARE MANAGEMENT
Assessment
• Assess history of hypersensitivity to drug
• Assess for previous history of pancreatitis (especially in pediatric pts)
• Assess baseline T-cell studies, CBC, differential
• Assess baseline liver function (AST, ALT, bilirubin, alk phos), renal function (BUN, creatinine)
• Assess baseline serum amylase (especially in pediatric pts)
• Assess baseline wt
Interventions
• May administer PO with or without food
• Administer bid with zidovudine

NURSING ALERT
Lamivudine may cause pancreatitis (especially in children)

Evaluation
• Evaluate therapeutic response (improved T-cell counts)
• Evaluate for side effects, hypersensitivity
• Evaluate for signs and symptoms of pancreatitis (abdominal pain, bloating, belching, increased serum amylase [esp. in pediatric pts])
• Monitor liver function (AST, ALT, bilirubin, alk phos), renal function (BUN, creatinine)
• Monitor baseline T-cell studies, CBC, differential
• Monitor serum amylase (especially in pediatric pts)
• Monitor wt

PATIENT/FAMILY EDUCATION
Teach/instruct
• To take as directed at prescribed intervals for prescribed length of time
• That GI complaints and insomnia usually resolve after 3-4 wks of treatment
• About side effects; to notify care provider
• That opportunistic infections and HIV-related complications can still occur while taking medication
• That patient remains contagious while taking this medication and should practice safe sex
Advise/warn
• To notify care provider of numbness, burning, tingling, pain or weakness in feet or hands
• That drug may cause dizziness
Encourage
• Intake of nutritious meals; consider nutrition consultation
• To verbalize fears, concerns; consider social work consultation

STORAGE
• Store at room temp in tightly closed container

---

leucovorin calcium
Brand Name(s): Folinic Acid, Citrovorum factor
Classification: Water-soluble vitamin in the folate group (an active metabolite of folic acid)
Pregnancy Category: C

AVAILABLE PREPARATIONS
Tabs: 5 mg, 10 mg, 15 mg, 25 mg
Inj: 3 mg/ml ampule
Powder for inj: 50 mg/vial, 100 mg/vial, 350 mg/vial

ROUTES AND DOSAGES
• Drug may vary in response to diagnosis, extent of disease, concurrent or previous therapy, protocol guidelines, physiologic parameters; consult current literature, protocol recommendations

---

Children and adults: PO/IM/IV 10 mg/m^2 q6h (per protocol) until methotrexate is cleared; dosage and duration of rescue dependent on serum methotrexate levels

IV/IM administration
• Recommendend concentration: Reconstitute 50 mg vial and 100 mg vial with 5 ml, 10 ml, respectively, with SW or bacteriostatic water (concentration 10 mg/ml); reconstitute 350 mg vial with 17 ml of SW or bacteriostatic water (concentration 20 mg/ml); can be further diluted with any common IV sol
• Infusion rate: Administer slow IVP over 5 min or IM beginning 24 hr after MTX infusion; infusion rate should not exceed 16 ml/min (160 mg leucovorin) because of Ca concentration of sol

MECHANISM AND INDICATIONS

Mechanism: Acts as an antidote for methotrexate and other folic acid antagonists by circumventing the biochemical block of the enzyme inhibitors (dihydrofolate reductase) to permit RNA and DNA synthesis
Indications: Used to treat accidental folic acid antagonist (methotrexate) overdose or delayed excretion of methotrexate; folinic acid rescue to prevent or decrease toxicity of massive methotrexate doses used to treat neoplasms such as osteosarcoma

PHARMACOKINETICS

Onset of action: IV 5 min; IM 10-20 min; PO 20-30 min
Peak: IV 10 min; IM 1 hr; PO 2-3 hr
Distribution: Distributed to all body tissues; the liver contains about ½ of the total body folate stores
Half-life: 3-6 hr
Metabolism: Primarily in liver; *in vivo* studies is show that leucovorin calcium is rapidly converted to tetrahydrofolic acid and derivatives which are the major transport and storage form of folate
Excretion: 50% of a single dose

excreted in 6 hr in urine (80%-90% of dose) and feces (8% of dose)

CONTRAINDICATIONS AND PRECAUTIONS

• Contraindicated with known hypersensitivity to drug or folic acid (possible cross-sensitivity)
• Use cautiously with pernicious anemia and other megaloblastic anemias secondary to lack of vitamin B$_{12}$, (a hemolytic remission may occur while neurologic manifestations remain progressive); use cautiously with pregnancy, lactation

INTERACTIONS
Drugs
• Increased toxicity of fluorouracil (severe enterocolitis, diarrhea, dehydration, death)
• Increased risk of epileptic effects with phenobarbital, phenytoin

INCOMPATIBILITIES
• Folic acid; foscarnet

SIDE EFFECTS
GI: Nausea, vomiting
DERM: Rash, pruritus, erythema, facial flushing, urticaria
RESP: Bronchospasm

TOXICITY AND OVERDOSE
Clinical signs: Allergic sensitization including anaphylactoid reactions and urticaria
Treatment: Supportive care

PATIENT CARE MANAGEMENT
Assessment
• Assess history of hypersensitivity to leucovorin
• Assess for concomitant use of antiepileptic medications (phenobarbital, phenytoin)
• For any complaints of nausea or vomiting; administer parenterally if present
• Assess success of previous antiemetic regimen
• Assess baseline VS and methotrexate level
• Assess for any 3rd space fluid accumulation (edema, decreased breath sounds, chest x-ray to assess pleural effusion), renal insufficiency, or inadequate hydration; higher dosages of leucovorin or

prolonged administration may be indicated

Interventions

- Administer oral leucovorin with antacids or milk
- Be sure doses are administered *on time* in order to rescue normal cells from methotrexate toxicity
- Encourage small, frequent feedings of foods pt likes
- Administer diphenhydramine as ordered for allergic reaction
- Administer IV fluids until pt able to resume normal PO intake

---

NURSING ALERT

Be sure to administer drug on time as ordered, do not hold doses; if pt cannot take PO, obtain IV order

Be sure leucovorin administration is 0-72 hours after completion of methotrexate infusion

Do not confuse leucovorin (folinic acid) with folic acid

Evaluation

- Evaluate therapeutic response (increased wt, orientation, absence of fatigue)
- Evaluate serum methotrexate levels
- Evaluate for signs or symptoms of allergic reaction (urticaria, chest tightness, wheezing)
- Evaluate for signs of infection (fever, fatigue, sore throat), bleeding (easy bruising, bleeding gums, nosebleeds)
- Evaluate for possible increased seizure activity if on antiepileptic medications
- Evaluate I&O, check wt daily
- Evaluate for side effects and response to antiemetic regimen

PATIENT AND FAMILY EDUCATION

Teach/instruct

- To take drug as directed at prescribed intervals for prescribed length of time to maximize its effectiveness and avoid fatal methotrexate toxicity
- To notify care provider of inability to take drug PO so IV doses can be administered
- To report any symptoms of itching, facial flushing, rash, or erythema; diphenhydramine may be taken to help relieve these side effects
- To have pt well-hydrated before and after chemotherapy
- About importance of follow-up to monitor blood counts, serum chemistry values, drug blood values
- To take accurate temp; rectal temp contraindicated
- To notify care provider of signs of bleeding (bruising, epistaxis, bleeding gums); infection (fever, sore throat, fatigue)

Warn/advise

- Regarding impact of body changes that may occur (hair loss, hyperpigmentation, nail ridging); how to minimize changes (wigs, caps, scarves, long sleeves)
- To avoid OTC products containing aspirin
- To report any alterations in behavior, sensation, perception; help to develop a plan of care to manage side effects, stress of illness or treatment
- To monitor bowel function and call if abdominal pain, constipation noted
- To immediately report any pain, discoloration at injection site (parenteral forms)
- That good oral hygiene with very soft toothbrush is imperative
- That dental work be delayed until blood counts return to baseline and with permission of care provider
- To avoid contact with known viral or bacterial illnesses
- That household contacts of child not be immunized with live polio virus; inactivated form should be used
- That child not receive immunizations until immune system recovers sufficiently to mount needed antibody response
- To report exposure to chicken pox in susceptible child immediately

L

- To report reactivation of herpes zoster virus (shingles) immediately
- If appropriate, ways to preserve reproductive patterns, sexuality (sperm banking, contraceptives)

Encourage
- Provision of nutritious food intake; consider nutritional consultation
- To comply with bowel management program
- To use top anesthetics to control discomfort of mucositis; avoid spicy foods, commercial mouthwashes

STORAGE
- Store at room temp protected from light
- Powder reconstituted with bacteriostatic water stable at room temp for 7 days; sols further diluted stable 24 hr

---

leuprolide acetate

Brand Name(s): Lupron ✤, Lupron Depot ✤, Lupron Depot-Ped ✤

Classification: Gonadotropin-releasing hormone agonist

Pregnancy Category: X

AVAILABLE PREPARATIONS
Inj: 5 mg/ml
Susp(Depot): 3.75 mg/ml

ROUTES AND DOSAGES
Children: IM (Depot preparation) 0.3 mg/kg/dose q 4 wks (minimum 7.5 mg); if desired effect is not achieved or if accelerated sexual maturity occurs, titrate upward in increments of 3.75 mg q 4 wk
SC: 50 mcg/kg/24 hr, titrate to pt response

MECHANISM AND INDICATIONS
Mechanism: Reduces testosterone to prepubertal levels in males, reduces estradiol levels to prepubertal levels in females enabling normal physical and psychological growth and development
Indications: For use in the treatment of children with central precocious puberty

PHARMACOKINETICS
- Limited information available
Half-life: 3 hr

CONTRAINDICATIONS AND PRECAUTIONS
- Contraindicated with women who are or may become pregnant; lactation
- Use cautiously with all children; if accelerated sexual maturity occurs after dosing, adjust dosage upward (see Routes and Dosages)

INTERACTIONS
Drug
- None reported
Lab
- Suppressed gonadal–pituitary hormones

INCOMPATIBILITIES
- None reported

SIDE EFFECTS
CNS: Nervousness, personality disorder, somnolence, emotional lability
CV: Syncope, vasodilation
DERM: Alopecia, local irritation or abscess at injection site, skin striae
ENDO/METAB: Accelerated sexual maturity (if dosage inadequate)
GI: Gingivitis, nausea, vomiting, dysphagia
GU: Incontinence, gynecomastia
RESP: Epistaxis

TOXICITY AND OVERDOSE
Clinical signs: Not reported in human studies

PATIENT CARE MANAGEMENT
Assessment
- Assess history of hypersensitivity to drug
- Assess for appropriateness of treatment, clinical diagnosis of central precious puberty (onset of secondary sexual characteristics earlier than 8 yr in females and 9 yr in males)
- Assess baseline evaluation studies to confirm diagnosis of central precocious puberty height, wt; sex

---

✤ Available in Canada.

steroid levels; adrenal steroid levels (to rule out congenital adrenal hyperplasia), β human chorionic gonadotropin level (to rule out chorionic gonadotropin-secreting tumor): pelvic/adrenal/testicular ultrasound (to rule out steroid-secreting tumor), computerized tomography (CT) of head (to rule out brain tumor), bone age advanced 1 yr beyond chronological age)
• Assess response to gonadotropin-releasing hormone test; a pubertal response confirms diagnosis

Interventions
• Withdraw 1 ml of diluent that comes pre-packaged with leuprolide acetate using a syringe with a 22 G needle, inject diluent into vial of powder, shake well to disperse particles, susp will appear milky, withdraw contents and inject at time of reconstitution, discard remaining susp
• Rotate IM injection sites
• Medication to be administered by care provider
• Consider discontinuation of drug before age 11 for females and age 12 for males

Evaluation
• Evaluate therapeutic response (reproductive organs will return to prepubertal state; linear growth will occur; menses, if present, will cease)
• Monitor gonadotropin-releasing hormone stimulation test, sex steroid levels 1-2 mo after start of therapy
• Measure bone age q 6-12 mo
• Monitor for signs of advancement of puberty; adjust dosage upward

PATIENT/FAMILY EDUCATION
Teach/instruct
• About need for therapy
• About potential side effects; notify care provider
• That during first 2 mo of therapy, females may experience menses or spotting; notify care provider if bleeding occurs beyond 2nd mo

Warn/advise
• To notify care provider of hypersensitivity
• To report signs of irritation at injection site
• To report signs of accelerated sexual maturity
• To expect to see linear growth

Encourage
• Family and child to discuss their questions and concerns related to diagnosis and treatment of central precocious puberty

STORAGE
• Store at room temp
• Discard reconstituted vials

---

levothyroxine sodium (T$_4$, L-thyroxine sodium)

Brand Name(s): Eltroxin✦, Levothyroid, Levothyroxine Sodium, Levoxine, PMS-Levothyroxine Sodium✦, Synthroid✦

Classification: Thyroid hormone (synthetic T$_4$)

Pregnancy Category: A

AVAILABLE PREPARATIONS
Inj: 200 mcg/vial, 500 mcg/vial
Tabs: 0.025 mg, 0.05 mg, 0.075 mg, 0.088 mg, 0.1 mg, 0.112 mg, 0.125 mg, 0.137 mg, 0.15 mg, 0.175 mg, 0.2 mg, 0.3 mg

ROUTES AND DOSAGES
Infants 0-6 mo: PO 25-50 mcg (8-10 mcg/kg) qd
Infants 6-12 mo: PO 50-75 mcg (6-8 mcg/kg) qd
Children 1-5 yr: PO 75-100 mcg (5-6 mcg/kg) qd
Children 6-12 yr: PO 100-150 mcg (4-5 mcg/kg) qd
Children >12 yr and adults: PO 100-200 mcg qd
• Dosage should be adjusted to keep TSH and T$_4$ within normal range
• Initial IV dose is ½ PO dose, with further adjustments based on lab results; for use when oral route

is unavailable for a prolonged period of time

MECHANISM AND INDICATIONS

Mechanism: Increases metabolic rates of tissues and regulates growth; essential for normal neurologic development in the first 2-3 yr of life

Indication: Replacement of endogenous thyroid hormone; standard hormonal content and predictable effects make this the usual drug of choice

PHARMACOKINETICS

Onset of action: Variable absorption from GI tract, 99% bound to serum proteins

Peak: 1-3 wk after initiation of oral therapy

Half-life: 6-7 days

Metabolism: Liver, kidneys, intestines, peripheral tissues

Excretion: Feces

CONTRAINDICATIONS AND PRECAUTIONS

• Contraindicated with thyrotoxicosis, acute MI, adrenal insufficiency (uncorrected)

• Use cautiously with cardiovascular disease, DM, adrenal insufficiency, pregnancy, lactation

INTERACTIONS

Drug

• Decreased effect of digoxin

• Increased effect of tricyclic antidepressants, sympathomimetics, anticoagulants

• Increased doses of insulin or oral antihyperglycemics may be required

• Decreased absorption of levothyroxine with cholestyramine

• Increased dose of levothyroxine may be required with estrogen or oral contraceptives

Lab

• Altered iodine (I¹³¹) uptake tests

Nutrition

• Soybean formulas can cause excessive fecal loss of levothyroxine

Incompatibilities

• Incompatible in syringe with all other drugs

SIDE EFFECTS

CNS: Insomnia, tremor, anxiety

CV: Tachycardia, palpitations, arrhythmias, hypertension, widened pulse pressure, angina

DERM: Partial loss of hair during initial therapy (temporary), sweating, allergic rash

GI: Change in appetite, nausea, diarrhea

GU: Menstrual irregularity

Other: Heat intolerance, fever

TOXICITY AND OVERDOSE

Clinical signs: Signs of hyperthyroidism (weight loss, anxiety, tachycardia, arrhythmias, insomnia, diarrhea, heat intolerance)

Treatment: Reduce GI absorption by gastric lavage or induced emesis; respiratory support; propranolol to control effects of increased sympathetic activity; gradually discontinue levothyroxine; reinstitute at lower dosage

PATIENT CARE MANAGEMENT

Assessment

• Assess history of hypersensitivity to levothyroxine, related drugs

• Assess pulse, B/P, I&O, T₃, T₄, TSH, height, wt, dry skin, constipation, cold intolerance

Interventions

• PO may be crushed, mixed with food or fluid; do not administer with soy formulas

• Administer qd at consistent time; administer in AM to reduce sleeplessness

• Stop medication 4 wk before radioactive iodine uptake test

• Do not premix with IV fluids or any medications

Evaluation

• Evaluate therapeutic response (absence of depression, increased wt loss, diuresis, absence of constipation, peripheral edema, cold intolerance, pale, cool dry skin, brittle nails, alopecia, coarse hair, menorrhagia, night blindness, paresthesias, syncope, stupor, coma, rosy cheeks)

• Monitor pulse, B/P

• Monitor growth (including head circumference in infants), bone

age, development, intellectual functioning, thyroid function tests
• Monitor for signs of overdose (nervousness, excitability, irritability, tachycardia, palpitations, angina pectoris, hypertension, nausea, diarrhea, wt loss, heat intolerance)

PATIENT AND FAMILY EDUCATION
Teach/instruct
• To take as directed at prescribed intervals for prescribed length of time
Warn/advise
• To notify care provider of hypersensitivity, side effects
• To notify care provider of symptoms of hypothyroidism or hyperthyroidism
• That temporary hair loss will occur in children
• Not to switch brands unless directed by care provider
• To avoid use of OTC or any medications (particularly those containing iodine) unless directed by care provider
• To avoid iodine food, iodized salt, soy beans, tofu, turnips, some seafood and breads
• To comply with follow-up care

STORAGE
• Store at room temp
• Protect from heat, humidity, light

lidocaine, lidocaine hydrochloride

Brand Name(s): Alphacaine, Anestacon, Dalcaine, Dilocaine, L-Caine, Lidocaine Parenteral✤, Lidodan Ointment✤, Lidodan Viscous✤, Lidoject, LidoPen Autoinjector, Nervocaine, Nulicaine, PMS-Lidocaine Viscous✤, Xylocaine, Xylocaine Dental Ointment (5%)✤, Xylocaine Endotracheal✤, Xylocain Jelly (2%)✤, Xylocaine Ointment (5%)✤, Xylocaine Oral Aerosol✤, Xylocaine Sterile Solution (4%)✤, Xylocaine Topical (4%)✤, Xylocaine Topical (5%)✤, Xylocaine Viscous✤, Xylocaine Viscous (2%)✤, Xylocord✤

Classification: Ventricular antiarrhythmic, local anesthetic

Pregnancy Category: B

AVAILABLE PREPARATIONS
Inj: 10, 20, 40, 100, 200 mg/ml vials
2, 4, 8, mg/ml with 5% dextrose
0.5%, 1%, 1.5%, 2%, 4% vials (local anesthetic)
1.5%, 5% with 7.5% dextrose (local anesthetic)
0.5%, 1%, 1.5%, 2% with epinephrine (local anesthetic)
Top oint: 2.5%, 5%
Top jelly: 2%
Top sol: 2%, 4%, 10%
Liquid, viscous: 2%

ROUTES AND DOSAGES
Local Anesthesia: ID, maximum 7 mg/kg/dose with epinephrine q2h, maximum 4.5 mg/kg/dose without epinephrine q2h, total maximum 500 mg; IV regional, maximum 3 mg/kg; epidural/caudal, use only preservative-free sol, administer test dose of 2-5 ml 5 min before the dose
Top: Apply to affected area 2.5%-5% preparation, maximum 3 mg/

L

kg/dose q2h; total maximum dose 200 mg

Antiarrhythmic

Children: ET, IV, single bolus 1 mg/kg/dose slowly; may repeat in 10-15 min × 2; maximum 3.0-4.5 mg/kg/hr; continuous infusion 20-50 mcg/kg/min IV

Adult: ET/IV, single bolus 1-1.5 mg/kg, may repeat in 5-10 min to total of 3 mg/kg, continuous infusion 2-4 mg/min

IV administration

• Recommended concentration: 0.2-2 mg/ml preferably in D_5W for IV infusion; 120 mg in 100 ml D_5W at 1 and 2.5 ml/kg/hr provides 20 and 50 mcg/kg/min, respectively

• Maximum concentration: 1-2 mg/ml for IV infusion; 20 mg/ml for IV push

• IV push rate: 0.35-0.7 mg/kg/min or 50 mg/min, whichever is less

• Intermittent infusion rate: Not recommended because of short half-life

• Continuous infusion rate: 10-50 mcg/kg/min

MECHANISM AND INDICATIONS

Antiarrhythmic mechanism: Suppresses automaticity, shortens effective refractory period and action potential of His-Purkinje fibers, suppresses ventricular depolarization during diastole

Local anesthetic mechanism: Blocks initiation and conduction of nerve impulses

Indications: Indicated for use in ventricular arrhythmias, including VT, and for use as a regional infiltrative anesthetic or topical anesthetic (sore throats, sunburn, pruritis, cold sores, oral pain)

PHARMACOKINETICS

Onset: IV, top: immediate; regional: 4-17 min

Peak: 2-5 min

Half-life: Biphasic, first: 7-30 min; second, infants 2-3 hr; adults 1.5-2 hrs

Metabolism: Liver

Excretion: Urine

CONTRAINDICATIONS AND PRECAUTIONS

• Contraindicated with known hypersensitivity, Stokes-Adams syndrome, or severe degrees of SA, AV, or intraventricular heart block; with inflammation or infection at puncture region or topical site

• Use cautiously with hepatic or renal disease (decrease dosage), heart failure, marked hypoxia, severe respiratory depression, hypovolemia or shock, incomplete heart block, bradycardia, AF, pregnancy, lactation

INTERACTIONS

Drug

• Lidocaine toxicity with cimetidine, β blockers

• Increased neuromuscular effects of succinylcholine

• Increased effects, toxicity with phenytoin, procainamide, propranolol, quinidine

• Hypertension possible with MAOIs, tricyclic antidepressants, phenothiazines

Lab

• Increased CPK levels with injections

SIDE EFFECTS

CNS: Lethargy, confusion, anxiety, agitation, paresthesias, slurred speech, muscle twitching, seizures, hallucinations, euphoria

CV: Bradycardia, hypotension, heart block, arrhythmias, myocardial depression

EENT: Blurred vision, diplopia, tinnitus, ototoxicity

GI: Nausea, vomiting

RESP: Status asthmaticus, respiratory depression, arrest

Local: Sensitization, rash, soreness at injection site, erythema, burning, stinging

TOXICITY AND OVERDOSE

Clinical signs: Seizures, respiratory depression, hypotension

Treatment: Discontinue drug, supportive measures, treat respiratory depression (airway, O_2), seizures, use vasopressors for hypotension

---

♣ Available in Canada.

PATIENT CARE MANAGEMENT
Assessment
- Assess history of hypersensitivity to lidocaine
- Assess ECG continuously with IV administration
- Assess VS, B/P continuously with IV administration
- Assess I&O
- Assess serum electrolytes
- Assess gag reflex if used orally before administration of any other fluids

Interventions
- Administer test dose before IV use
- Use cardiac monitor with all IV infusions
- Administer IV through infusion pump, not to exceed 4 mg/min
- ID for regional anesthesia, use lidocaine with epinephrine cautiously in areas of limited blood supply (ears, nose, fingers, toes, penis)
- Apply top to mouth with cotton swab or swish and gargle; sol is not to be swallowed (use only in child old enough to follow these directions)

Evaluation
- Evaluate therapeutic response (decreased arrhythmias, absence of pain in affected areas)
- Evaluate for hypersensitivity
- Evaluate ECG, serum lidocaine concentrations (therapeutic level 2-5 mcg/ml)
- Evaluate HR, respiratory rate
- Monitor for CNS effects; discontinue drug
- Monitor locally for sensitization

PATIENT AND FAMILY EDUCATION
Teach/instruct
- To take as directed at prescribed intervals for prescribed length of time
- About need for frequent monitoring
- Not to use drug on abraded skin
- That viscous liquid can decrease gag reflex; caution against ingesting food, candy, or chewing gum until gag reflex returns

- To report side effects to care provider

Encourage
- Provide support during treatment

STORAGE
- Store at room temp, avoid freezing and exposure to light
- Discard partially used vials containing no preservatives

---

lindane
Brand Name(s): G-well, Kwell, Kwellada♣, Lindane Lotion♣, Lindane Shampoo♣, PMS-Lindane, Scabene♣

Classification: Scabicide

Pregnancy Category: B

AVAILABLE PREPARATIONS
Top: Cream 1%, lotion 1%, shampoo 1%

ROUTES AND DOSAGES
Scabies
Children and adults: Top, apply a thin layer of lotion or cream and massage on skin from neck to toes (head to toes on infants); remove with soap and water after 8-12 hr; may reapply in 1 wk if needed

Pediculosis
Children and adults: Top, apply 15-30 ml of shampoo and lather for 5 min; rinse hair thoroughly and comb with fine tooth comb to remove nits; may repeat in 7 days if lice or nits still present; avoid contact with eyes, mucous membranes

MECHANISM AND INDICATIONS
Mechanism: Stimulates nervous system of arthropods resulting in seizures, death of arthropods
Indications: Used to treat scabies (*Sarcoptes scabiei*), head lice (*Pediculus capitis*), and crab lice (*Pediculus pubis*)

PHARMACOKINETICS
Peak: 6 hr after application
Distribution: Stored in body fat
Half-life: 17-22 hr in children

♣ Available in Canada.

Metabolism: Liver
Excretion: Urine, feces

CONTRAINDICATIONS AND PRECAUTIONS

• Contraindicated with known hypersensitivity to lindane or any component; in premature infants or neonates; with acutely inflamed, raw, or weeping skin; with known seizure disorders

• Use cautiously with infants, small children, pregnancy, lactation; consider alternative therapy for treatment of scabies in infants or small children (e.g., crotamiton or permethrin)

SIDE EFFECTS

CNS: Vertigo, restlessness, headache, ataxia, seizures
CV: Cardiac arrhythmias, pulmonary edema
DERM: Eczema eruptions, contact dermatitis, pruritus
GI: Nausea, vomiting, diarrhea, liver damage
GU: Kidney damage
HEME: Aplastic anemia

TOXICITY AND OVERDOSE

Clinical signs: Local irritation; inhaled vapors may be toxic resulting in cardiac arrhythmias, seizures, nausea, headaches
Treatment: Wash area thoroughly, discontinue treatment, and notify care provider

PATIENT CARE MANAGEMENT

Assessment

• Assess history of hypersensitivity to lindane

• Carefully inspect and note extent and amount of infestation

Interventions

• Take proper isolation precautions if the child is hospitalized during infestation.

• Administer top corticosteroids, antihistamines, top antibiotics as ordered

---

NURSING ALERT
Not for use in premature infants or neonates; use cautiously in infants and small children

---

Evaluation

• Evaluate therapeutic response (decreased nits, crusts, itching, papules)

• Evaluate skin for healing

• Evaluate for side effects (skin irritation)

• Evaluate all family members for infestation, treat with product if evident

PATIENT AND FAMILY EDUCATION

Teach/instruct

• To use as directed at prescribed intervals for prescribed length of time

• Family that this is a contagious condition, why it is necessary to treat

Warn/advise

• To notify care provider of hypersensitivity, side effects

• That all personal clothing and bedding must be washed in hot water or dry cleaned, and all personal articles such as hair care items need to be cleaned, in a sol of the drug

• That a fine tooth nit comb should be used to remove dead lice or nits from hair

• That pubic lice may be transmitted sexually; all sexual partners must be treated simultaneously

• To flush with water immediately if in contact with eyes

• To notify schools or day care facilities

• To consult care provider with infestation of eyebrows or lashes

• That itching may continue for 4-6 wk

• To reapply drug if accidentally washed off

• That oils may enhance absorption; if oil-based shampoos or creams are used, wash with shampoo or soap, then rinse and dry before applying product

Encourage

• Children should be instructed not to borrow clothes, brushes, combs

STORAGE

• Store at room temp in light-resistant container

✦ Available in Canada.

liothyronine sodium

Brand Name(s): Cytomel✦

Classification: Thyroid hormone (synthetic T_3)

Pregnancy Category: A

AVAILABLE PREPARATIONS
Tabs: 5 mcg, 25 mcg, 50 mcg

ROUTES AND DOSAGES
Children ≤3 yr: PO 5 mcg qd, increased by 5 mcg q 3-4 days until desired response occurs
Children >3 yr and adults: PO 50-100 mcg qd

MECHANISM AND INDICATIONS
Mechanism: Increases metabolic rates of tissues and regulates growth; essential for normal neurologic development in the first 2-3 yr of life
Indication: Replacement of endogenous thyroid hormone

PHARMACOKINETICS
Onset: Few hr
Peak: 24-72 hr
Distribution: Not firmly bound to serum proteins, readily available; may be preferred when rapid effect is desired or when GI absorption or peripheral conversion of T_4 to T_3 is impaired
Half-life: 2 ½ days

CONTRAINDICATIONS AND PRECAUTIONS
• Contraindicated with thyrotoxicosis, acute MI, adrenal insufficiency (uncorrected)
• Use cautiously with cardiovascular disease, DM, adrenal insufficiency, pregnancy, lactation

INTERACTIONS
Drug
• Decreased effect of digoxin
• Increased effect of tricyclics, sympathomimetics, anticoagulants
• May require higher doses of insulin/oral antihyperglycemics
• Decreased absorption of liothyronine with cholestyramine
• Increased dosage of liothyronine

may be necessary with estrogen or oral contraceptives
Lab
• Altered iodine (I^{131}) uptake tests

SIDE EFFECTS
CNS: Insomnia, tremor, anxiety
CV: Tachycardia, palpitations, arrhythmias, hypertension, widened pulse pressure, angina
DERM: Partial loss of hair during initial therapy (temporary), sweating, allergic rash
GI: Change in appetite, nausea, diarrhea
GU: Menstrual irregularity
Other: Heat intolerance, fever

TOXICITY AND OVERDOSE
Clinical signs: Signs of hyperthyroidism (wt loss, anxiety, tachycardia, arrhythmias, insomnia, diarrhea, heat intolerance)
Treatment: Reduce GI absorption by gastric lavage or induced emesis; respiratory support; propranolol to control effects of increased sympathetic activity; gradually discontinue liothyronine; reinstitute at lower dosage

PATIENT CARE MANAGEMENT
Assessment
• Assess history of hypersensitivity to liothyronine, related drugs
• Assess pulse, B/P, I&O, T_3, T_4, T_5H, height, wt, dry skin, constipation, cold intolerance
Interventions
• PO may be crushed, mixed with food or fluid; do not give with soy formulas
• Administer qd at consistent time; administer in AM to reduce sleeplessness
• Stop medication 4 wk before radioactive iodine uptake test
Evaluation
• Evaluate therapeutic response (absence of depression, increased wt loss, diuresis, absence of constipation, peripheral edema, cold intolerance, pale, cool dry skin, brittle nails, alopecia, coarse hair, menorrhagia, night blindness, paresthesias, syncope, stupor, coma, rosy cheeks)
• Monitor pulse, B/P

✦ Available in Canada.

- Monitor growth (including head circumference in infants), bone age, development, thyroid function tests
- Monitor for signs of overdose (nervousness, excitability, irritability, tachycardia, palpitations, angina pectoris, hypertension, nausea, diarrhea, wt loss, heat intolerance)

PATIENT AND FAMILY EDUCATION
Teach/instruct
- To take as directed at prescribed intervals for prescribed length of time
Warn/advise
- To notify care provider of hypersensitivity, side effects
- To notify care provider of symptoms of hypo- or hyperthyroidism
- That temporary hair loss will occur in children
- Not to switch brands unless directed by care provider
- To avoid use of OTC or any medications (particularly those containing iodine) unless directed by care provider
- To avoid iodine food, iodized salt, soy beans, tofu, turnips, some seafood and breads
- To comply with follow-up care

STORAGE
- Store at room temp
- Protect from heat, humidity, light

---

lithium
Brand Name(s): Cibalith-S, Eskalith, Lithane, Lithobid, Lithonate, Lithotabs✤
Classification: Antimanic
Pregnancy Category: D

AVAILABLE PREPARATIONS
Syr: lithium citrate 300 mg (8 mEq)/5 ml
Tabs: lithium carbonate 300 mg (8.12 mEq),
Caps: lithium carbonate 150 mg (4.06 mEq), 300 mg (8.12 mEq), 600 mg (16.24 mEq)

Tabs sus rel: lithium carbonate 300 mg (8.12 mEq)
Tabs ext rel: lithium carbonate 450 mg (12.18 mEq)

DOSAGES AND ROUTES
- Safety and effectiveness for use by children <12 yr not established. Dosage represents accepted standard practice recommendations.
Children: PO 15-60 mg/kg/24 hr divided tid-qid, or 2 doses with sus rel preparations; oral doses of lithium up to 1800 mg/24 hr are frequently necessary to maintain therapeutic blood levels of 1-1.5 mEq/L; dose should not exceed usual adult dosage
Adults: PO 1st day 300 mg taken tid 6 hr apart; 2nd day and thereafter, increase dose to 1200 mg/24 hr and later to 1800 mg/24 hr if needed and tolerated; may give in 3-4 divided doses; usual maintenance dose 600-1200 mg/24 hr taken in 3 divided doses; usual maximum maintenance dose 2400 mg/24 hr; total daily dosage should not exceed 3600 mg

MECHANISM AND INDICATIONS
Mechanism: It is not known if neurobiologic effects of lithium are related to its therapeutic benefits; lithium may alter Na and K+ ion transport across cell membrane in nerve and muscle cells; may also influence reuptake of tryptophan, serotonin, and norepinephrine in the brain
Indications: Treatment of choice for management of bipolar mood disorder and treatment of acute manic episodes; also helps to manage the depression phase of bipolar disorder; can augment the use of fluoxetine, sertraline, and paroxetine in treatment-resistant depression and obsessive compulsive disorder; useful in treating behaviorally disturbed children whose parents are known lithium responders; may be helpful in pts with ADHD who have a severe problem with temper, stress intolerance, impulsivity, and emotional lability, in these cases, the mood

---

✤ Available in Canada.

disorder is stabilized with lithium, then the psychostimulant is introduced; useful in treating pts with severely aggressive symptoms and emotionally unstable behavior disorders; unlabeled uses, prevention of cluster headaches, stimulation of production of WBCs

PHARMACOKINETICS

Onset of action: PO rapid; continual use on a regular schedule for 1-3 wk is usually necessary to determine effectiveness in correcting acute mania; several mo of continuous treatment may be required to correct depression

Peak: Non-sus rel preparations 0.5-2 hr; sus rel preparations 4-4.5 hr

Half-life: In healthy adults 16-32 hr; can increase to more than 36 hr in elderly or in pts with renal impairment

Metabolism: Not metabolized, excreted unchanged in urine

Excretion: Urine; small amounts in sweat and feces; not facilitated by diuretics; thiazides increase lithium concentration by 30%-50%; dialyzable, 50%-100%

Therapeutic levels: Reference range, acute mania, 0.6-1.5 mEq/L; protection against future episodes in most pts with bipolar disorder, 0.8-1 mEq/L; higher rate of relapse is described in pts who are maintained below 0.4 mEq/L (SI 0.4 mmol/L); occasionally, to achieve therapeutic effects, blood levels must be increased to 1.8 mEq/L in adolescents and 2 mEq/L in preadolescents

CONTRAINDICATIONS AND PRECAUTIONS

• Contraindicated with hypersensitivity to this or any component of lithium; brain trauma, lactation, severe cardiac disease, uncontrolled diabetes, uncorrected hypothyroidism, liver disease, schizophrenia; in pts unable to comply with the need for regular monitoring of lithium blood levels or at risk for pregnancy or dehydration and electrolyte imbalance, such as with binging and purging

• Use cautiously with children <12 yr long-term diarrhea, taking any diuretic or steroid drug, organic brain disease, DM, systemic infection, kidney disease, psoriasis, on a salt-restricted diet, low Na blood level, history of schizophrenic-like thought disorder, seizure disorder, long-term sweating, thyroid disease, urinary retention, vomiting; in pts who plan to have surgery under general anesthesia in the near future

INTERACTIONS

Drug

• Increased effects with bumetanide, ethacrynic acid, fluoxetine, furosemide, NSAIDs such as indomethacin, piroxicam, thiazide diuretics

• Decreased effects with acetazolamide, $NaHCO_3$, theophylline and related drugs, urea, urinary alkalinizers

• Increased hypothyroid effects with calcium iodide, potassium iodide, iodinated glycerol

• Increased the effects of chlorpromazine or other phenothiazines, tricyclic antidepressants possible

• Increased apathy, lethargy, drowsiness or sluggishness, accentuated lithium-induced tremor, and possibly increased risk of precipitating psychotic behavior possible with marijuana smoking

• Brain damage possible with haloperidol

• Hypothermia possible with diazepam

• Unpredictable effects possible with verapamil both lithium toxicity and decreased lithium blood levels have been reported

• Usually well tolerated with methyldopa, but in some susceptible individuals it may cause a severe neurotoxic reaction

• Increased renal clearance with $NaHCO_3$, acetazolamide, mannitol, aminophylline

• Interaction with carbamazepine, sympathomimetics

Lab

• Increased alk phos, cholesterol,

parathyroid hormone, platelet counts, TSH, WBC counts
• Decrease: blood thyroid hormone (T_3 and T_4) levels, blood uric acid

Nutrition
• May be taken with milk
• Avoid excessive salt intake and salt restriction
• Drink at least 8-12 glasses of liquids each 24 hr; avoid dehydration
• Avoid OTC preparations that contain iodides, such as some cough medicines and vitamin-mineral supplements; they may have an antithyroid effect when taken with lithium
• Do not drink alcohol
• Those with a sensitivity to tartrazine should not take Lithane tabs; they contain the dye tartrazine (yellow dye #5)

SIDE EFFECTS
CNS: Dizziness, drowsiness, headache, blackout spells, coma, confusion, dullness, fatigue, lethargy, malaise, memory loss, restlessness, sedation, seizures, spasmodic movements of extremities, stupor, tremor, twitching, unsteadiness, vertigo, weakness
CV: Decrease in B/P, arrhythmias, sinus node dysfunction
DERM: Acne, dry hair and skin, hair loss, hyperkeratosis, itching, worsening of psoriasis, rash
EENT: Blind spot, blurred vision, metallic taste, tinnitus, slurred speech, narrowing of visual field
ENDO/METAB: Goiter, nephrogenic diabetes insipidus (thirst, polyuria, polydipsia), hyponatremia, lithium-induced hypothyroidism, chronic kidney disease
GI: Appetite loss, diarrhea, dry mouth, nausea, abdominal pain, GI distress, loss of rectal control, vomiting, wt loss or gain
GU: Albuminuria, loss of bladder control, edema, inhibited erection, galactorrhea, glycosuria, gynecomastia, decreased libido, male infertility, polydipsia, polyuria, proteinuria
HEME: Leukocytosis

Other: Ankle swelling, unknown effects on developing bone, muscle hyperirritability, wt gain may occur in the first few mo of use

TOXICITY AND OVERDOSE
Clinical signs: Lithium has a low therapeutic index, levels required for therapeutic effects are close to levels that produce toxic symptoms; lithium blood levels >2.5 mEq/L carry a greater risk of toxicity than lower levels; toxic, >2 mEq/L (SI >2 mmol/L); toxicity may be caused by overdose or alteration in Na balance due to dehydration, changes in dietary habits, wt reduction diet, use of diuretics or NSAIDs, renal disease, or other causes of decreased renal blood flow; sweat contains lithium, so heavy perspiration does not cause elevated lithium levels; early signs of toxicity, altered consciousness, diarrhea, drowsiness, lack of coordination, muscle twitching, sluggishness, tremor, unsteadiness, or vomiting; these may occur at lithium levels 1.5-2 mEq/L; moderate to severe symptoms of lithium toxicity, blurred vision, coma, confusion, dizziness, giddiness, kidney failure, muscle spasms, nausea, ringing in the ears, seizures, slurred speech, staggering gait, stupor, coarse tremor, large output of urine, vertigo, vomiting, weakness, death; these may occur with blood levels >2 mEq/L.
Treatment: Lithium should be discontinued at the first signs of toxicity; for mild toxicity, lithium should be withheld until levels return to pt's usual therapeutic range; sudden discontinuation does not cause withdrawal symptoms; if it is not clear why the lithium level increased, do a urinalysis and 24 hr CrCl; for moderate to severe toxicity, if levels are <3.0 mEq/L and signs of intoxication are mild, if urine output is adequate, IV administration of NS is effective in reducing lithium levels, do not use diuretics; correct fluid and electrolyte abnormali-

ties; check lithium levels several times a day to make sure they are decreasing; lithium poisoning (levels >4.0 mEq/L) is a medical emergency, obtain a toxic screen, protect airway; if lithium was taken <4 hr before treatment, induce vomiting or gastric lavage, start dialysis

PATIENT CARE MANAGEMENT
Assessment
• Assess history of hypersensitivity to drug
• Obtain baseline medical history, physical examination, pulse, B/P, height, wt
• Obtain baseline BUN, creatinine, CBC, TSH, T_4 and T_3, serum electrolytes
• Obtain baseline urine for albuminuria, glycosuria, uric acid; if pt has kidney disease, obtain a 24 hr CrCl

Interventions
• Do not crush or chew slow or ext rel tabs; swallow whole; caps may be opened and regular tabs crushed for administration
• Give with food or milk if GI symptoms occur
• Avoid changes in Na content of diet
• Avoid dehydration; during initial treatment, give with 2-3 L of fluids/day; maintenance 1-2 L/day
• If a dose is missed, it should be given as soon as possible; if several hr have passed or if it is nearing time for the next dose, do not double dose in order to catch up (unless advised to do so by care provider)

NURSING ALERT
Lithium has a very narrow margin of safe use; blood level of lithium needed to be effective is very close to the level that can cause toxic effects

Evaluation
• Evaluate therapeutic response (ability to function in daily activities, to sleep throughout the night; aggression, depression, emotional lability, excitement, mania, obsessive compulsive disorder)
• Evaluate mental status (affect, mood, sensorium, impulsiveness, suicidal ideation, psychiatric symptoms)
• Assess for early signs of toxicity (altered consciousness, diarrhea, drowsiness, lack of coordination, muscle twitching, sluggishness, tremor, unsteadiness, vomiting)
• Regular evaluations of blood lithium levels are absolutely essential for safe and effective use of lithium; draw samples 8-12 hr after the last dose
• Monitor serum lithium every 3-4 days during initial therapy; after a change in dose, monitor within 5-7 days
• When steady state is reached, monitor serum lithium levels monthly; should not exceed 2 mEq/L during acute treatment phase; every 2 mo check for albuminuria, glycosuria, uric acid; CBC with differential; monitor renal, hepatic, thyroid, skin turgor, cardiovascular function; every 3-4 mo determine serum creatinine, TSH, thyroid gland size; monitor LOC, gait, motor reflexes, hand tremors, wt; evaluate Na intake (decreased Na intake with decreased fluid intake may lead to lithium retention, and increased Na and fluids may decrease lithium retention)
• If on long-term therapy, assess for hypothyroidism, goiter, reduced sugar tolerance, diabetes insipidus-like syndrome, serious kidney damage
• Lithium should be discontinued if symptoms of brain toxicity appear or if an uncorrectable diabetes insipidus-like syndrome develops
• Painful discoloration and coolness of the hands and feet may resemble Raynaud syndrome
• Avoid premature discontinuation; maximum response may take up to a yr of continuous treatment in some individuals; discontinua-

L

---

tion may result in recurrence of either mania or depression
• Stopping lithium is indicated if nausea and GI discomfort are severe and persistent

PATIENT AND FAMILY EDUCATION
Teach/instruct
• To take as directed at prescribed intervals for prescribed length of time
• That medication is most helpful when used as part of a comprehensive multimodal treatment program
• Not to stop taking medication without prescriber approval
• That therapeutic effects may take 1-3 wk to correct mania and up to several mo to correct depression
• About the need for adequate salt and fluid intake
• That lithium has a very narrow margin of safe use; to call prescriber with early signs of toxicity

Warn/advise
• About importance of regular follow-up care to determine lithium levels
• To guard against dehydration; be especially aware of hot weather, vigorous exercise, excessive sweating, sauna and steam rooms, hot baths and tubs
• To be aware that any illness that causes fever, sweating, vomiting, or diarrhea can result in changes in hydration; when ill, closely monitor for signs of toxicity
• That mild nausea and general discomfort may also appear during the first few days of treatment; these side effects are an inconvenience rather than a disabling condition, and usually become less over time, or if dosage is lowered or stopped
• That fine hand tremor, increased urination, and mild thirst may occur when starting therapy and may persist throughout treatment
• That medication may cause drowsiness; be careful on bicycles, skates, skateboards, while driv-

ing, or with other activities requiring alertness
• About the need for contraception if sexually active; lithium contraindicated in pregnancy

STORAGE
• Store at room temp in light-resistant containers

---

lomustine, CCNU
Brand Name(s): CeeNU✤
Classification: Antineoplastic, alkylating agent, nitrosourea, cell cycle phase nonspecific
Pregnancy Category: D

AVAILABLE PREPARATIONS
Caps: 10 mg, 40 mg, 100 mg

ROUTES AND DOSAGES
• Dosage may vary in response to diagnosis, extent of disease, concurrent or previous therapy, protocol guidelines, physiological parameters; consult current literature, protocol recommendations

Single Agent
Children: PO 75-150 mg/m^2 repeated q 6 wk
Adults: PO 100-130 mg/m^2/dose, repeated q 6-8 wk

Combination Therapy
PO 30-75 mg/m^2/dose

MECHANISM AND INDICATIONS
Mechanism: Decomposition results in metabolites that alkylate DNA molecule causing interference in DNA, RNA, and protein synthesis; crosses blood–brain barrier more effectively than carmustine
Indications: Brain tumors, lymphomas, malignant melanoma, ALL, Hodgkin's disease

PHARMACOKINETICS
Half-life: Prolonged plasma half-life of drug metabolites (16-48 hr) secondary to enterohepatic circulation, extensive protein binding, lipid solubility

---

✤ Available in Canada.

Distribution: Decomposes spontaneously with rapid distribution through plasma into cell; also distributes rapidly into CSF

Metabolism: Rapid spontaneous decomposition, also metabolized in liver

Excretion: 50% of metabolites excreted in urine within 24 hr, small amount in feces and through lungs as expired CO_2

CONTRAINDICATIONS AND PRECAUTIONS

• Contraindicated with known hypersensitivity to drug; in individuals with active infections (especially chicken pox or herpes zoster); with history of pulmonary function impairment; with pregnancy, lactation

• Use cautiously with compromised renal or hepatic function (drug may accumulate), those previously treated with bleomycin or chest radiation

INTERACTIONS
Drug

• Increased marrow suppression possible with cimetidine or theophylline derivatives

• Decreased antitumor activity of drug possible with phenobarbital

Lab

• Transient elevation of BUN, alk phos, AST, bilirubin possible

SIDE EFFECTS

CNS: Encephalopathy, dizziness, ataxia, optic neuritis, lethargy, seizures, sudden onset cortical blindness

DERM: Reversible alopecia

GI: Variable nausea, vomiting usually occurring 2-5 hr after dose, stomatitis, hepatotoxicity, anorexia

GU: Nephrotoxicity if therapy continues >15 mo or cumulative dose exceeds 1000 mg/m^2; nephrotoxicity insidious and progressive, must be suspected if renal size or glomerular filtration rate decreases; progressive azotemia

HEME: Cumulative myelosuppression with nadir of neutrophils and platelets at 4-5 wk with 1-2 wk recovery, myelodysplastic syndrome, ANLL

RESP: Pulmonary fibrosis possible if cumulative doses exceed 600-1040 mg/m^2; symptoms include nonproductive cough, dyspnea, tachypnea, basilar crepitant rales, normal chest x-ray or interstitial infiltrates; can progress to restrictive disease, causing ventilatory defects including resting hypoxemia, decreased CO_2 diffusing capacity

TOXICITY AND OVERDOSE

Clinical signs: Prolonged myelosuppression, pulmonary fibrosis, neurologic deterioration

Treatment: Supportive measures including blood transfusions, hydration, nutritional supplementation, broad-spectrum antibiotic coverage in event of fever, electrolyte replacement

PATIENT CARE MANAGEMENT
Assessment

• Assess history of hypersensitivity to nitrosourea

• Assess history of previous chemotherapy or radiation therapy, especially that might predispose pt to pulmonary fibrosis, hepatic or renal dysfunction

• Assess previous success with antiemetic therapy

• Assess baseline VS, oximetry, pulmonary function tests, chest radiograph

• Assess baseline CBC, differential, platelet count

• Assess baseline renal function (BUN, creatinine), liver function (AST, ALT, bilirubin, alk phos)

Interventions

• Ensure correct dosage of medication is administered on an empty stomach

• Administer antiemetic therapy before chemotherapy

• Monitor I&O, wt

• Provide supportive measures to maintain hemostasis, fluid, electrolyte, nutritional balance

NURSING ALERT
Drug causes delayed and
cumulative myelosuppression

Drug should be taken on an
empty stomach

Evaluation

- Evaluate therapeutic response evidenced by radiologic or clinical regression of tumor
- Evaluate CBC, differential, platelet count at least weekly
- Evaluate respiratory status frequently (including respiratory rate, oximetry, chest auscultation, and periodic chest x-rays)
- Evaluate renal function (BUN, creatinine, I&O), liver function (AST, ALT, bilirubin, alk phos) at regular intervals

PATIENT AND FAMILY EDUCATION

Teach/instruct

- To have pt well hydrated before and after chemotherapy
- About importance of follow-up to monitor blood counts, serum chemistry values (especially important because of delayed nadir)
- To take accurate temp; rectal temp contraindicated
- To notify care provider of signs of bleeding (bruising, epistaxis, bleeding gums), infection (fever, sore throat, fatigue)

Warn/advise

- About impact of body changes that may occur (hair loss, hyperpigmentation, nail ridging), how to minimize changes (wigs, caps, scarves, long sleeves)
- To avoid OTC preparations containing aspirin
- To report any alterations in behavior, sensation, perception; help to develop a plan of care to manage side effects, stress of illness or treatment
- That good oral hygiene with very soft toothbrush is imperative
- That dental work be delayed until blood counts returns to baseline, with permission of caretaker
- To avoid contact with known viral and bacterial illnesses
- That close household contacts of child not be immunized with live polio virus; use inactivated form
- That children on chemotherapy not receive immunizations until immune system recovers sufficiently to mount necessary antibody response
- To report exposure to chicken pox in susceptible child immediately
- To report reactivation of herpes zoster virus (shingles) immediately
- If appropriate, ways to preserve reproductive patterns, sexuality (sperm banking, contraceptives)

Encourage

- Provision of nutritious food intake; consider nutritional consultation
- To use top anesthetics to control discomfort of mucositis; to avoid spicy foods, commercial mouthwashes

STORAGE

- Stable at room temp in closed container for 2 yr

loracarbef
Brand Name(s): Lorabid
Classification: Antibiotic (carbacephem)
Pregnancy Category: B

AVAILABLE PREPARATIONS

Oral susp: 100 mg/5 ml, 200 mg/5 ml
Caps: 200 mg

ROUTES AND DOSAGES

Infants >6 mo and children: For acute otitis media, 30 mg/kg/24 hr divided q12h; for pharyngitis, tonsillitis or impetigo, 15 mg/kg/24 hr divided q12h
Adults: 200-400 mg q12h

MECHANISM AND INDICATIONS

Antibiotic mechanism: Bactericidal; inhibits bacterial cell-wall synthesis

---

❧ Available in Canada.

Indications: Effective against gram-negative and gram-positive organisms including *Haemophilus influenzae, E. coli, Proteus mirabilis, Klebsiella, Streptococcus pneumoniae, Str. pyogenes,* and *Staphylococcus aureus;* used to treat otitis media, upper and lower respiratory tract, urinary tract, and skin infections

PHARMACOKINETICS
Peak: 1 hr
Distribution: Distributes into middle ear fluid
Half-life: 1 hr
Metabolism: Not metabolized
Excretion: Urine

CONTRAINDICATIONS AND PRECAUTIONS
• Contraindicated with known hypersensitivity to loracarbef or cephalosporins
• Use cautiously with renal impairment, history of colitis, pregnancy, lactation

INTERACTIONS
Drug
• Increased serum concentrations with use of probenecid
• Decreased effectiveness with use of tetracyclines, erythromycins, chloramphenicol
• Increased nephrotoxicity possible with use of aminoglycosides, loop diuretics, ethacrynic acid, vancomycin
Lab
• False elevations of urine creatinine using Jaffe's reaction
• False positive Coombs' test
Nutrition
• Decreased absorption if given with food

SIDE EFFECTS
CNS: Dizziness, headache, fatigue, paresthesia, confusion
GI: Diarrhea, nausea, vomiting, anorexia, glossitis, abdominal pain, loose stools, flatulence, pseudomembranous colitis, jaundice, elevated liver function tests, bilirubin
GU: Vaginitis, pruritus, nephrotoxicity, renal failure, pyuria, dysuria, reversible interstitial nephritis
HEME: Leukopenia, thrombocytopenia, agranulocytosis, anemia, neutropenia, lymphocytosis, eosinophilia, pancytopenia, hemolytic anemia, leukocytosis, granulocytopenia
Other: Hypersensitivity, dyspnea, fever, bacterial or fungal superinfection

TOXICITY AND OVERDOSE
Clinical signs: Nausea, vomiting, epigastric distress, diarrhea
Treatment: Supportive care

PATIENT CARE MANAGEMENT
Assessment
• Assess history of hypersensitivity to loracarbef or cephalosporins
• Obtain C&S; may begin therapy before obtaining results
• Assess renal function (BUN, creatinine, I&O), hepatic function (ALT, AST, bilirubin), hematologic function (CBC, differential, platelet count), electrolytes (K$^+$, Na, Cl), particularly for long-term therapy; assess bowel pattern
Interventions
• Administer at least 1 hr before giving bacteriostatic antibiotics (tetracyclines, erythromycins, chloramphenicol)
• Administer PO 1 hr ac or 2 hr after meals
• Shake susp well before administering; caps may be taken apart, mixed with food or fluid
• Maintain age-appropriate fluid intake
• For group A β-hemolytic streptococcal infection, provide 10-day course to prevent risk of acute rheumatic fever or glomerulonephritis

> **NURSING ALERT**
> Discontinue drug if signs of toxicity, hypersensitivity, pseudomembranous colitis develop

---

✤ Available in Canada.

Evaluation
• Evaluate therapeutic response (decreased symptoms of infection)
• Monitor renal function (BUN, creatinine, I&O)
• Monitor bowel pattern; diarrhea may be symptomatic of pseudomembranous colitis
• Observe for signs of allergic reaction (rash, flushing, urticaria, pruritus)
• Monitor signs of bleeding (ecchymosis, bleeding gums, hematuria, daily stool guaiac)
• Observe for signs of superinfection (perineal itching, diaper rash, fever, malaise, redness, pain, swelling, drainage, rash, diarrhea, sore throat, change in cough or sputum)

PATIENT AND FAMILY EDUCATION
Teach/instruct
• To take as directed at prescribed intervals for prescribed length of time
Warn/advise
• To notify care provider of hypersensitivity, side effects, superinfection
• To avoid use of alcohol or medications containing alcohol
• To add live-culture yogurt or buttermilk to diet to prevent intestinal superinfection

STORAGE
• Store caps at room temp in tightly closed container
• Reconstituted susp stable for 14 days room temp; label date and time of reconstitution

---

lorazepam

Brand Name(s): Apo-Lorazepam✤, Ativan✤, Novo-Lorazem✤, Nu-Loraz✤

Classification: Tranquilizer, anticonvulsant, benzodiazepine

Controlled Substance Schedule IV

Pregnancy Category: C

AVAILABLE PREPARATIONS
Tabs: 0.5 mg, 1 mg, 2 mg
Oral sol: 2 mg/calibrated dropper
Inj: 2 mg/ml, 4 mg/ml

ROUTES AND DOSAGES
Anxiety or Sedation
Infants and children: PO 0.02-0.09 mg/kg/dose q4-8h; IV 0.02-0.09 mg/kg/dose q4-8h
Adults: PO 1-10 mg/24 hr divided bid-tid

Insomnia
Adults: PO 2-4 mg hs

Antiemetic
Children 2-15 yr: IV 0.05 mg/kg/dose q6-8h prn, maximum 2 mg/dose
Adults: PO 0.5-2 mg q4-6h prn; IV 0.5-2 mg q4-6h prn

Preoperative Medications
Children: IV 0.04-0.08 mg/kg/dose q6h prn
Adults: IM 0.05 mg/kg/dose given 2 hr before surgery (maximum 4 mg/dose)

Status Epilepticus
Neonates: IV 0.05-0.1 mg/kg/dose
Infants and children: IV 0.1 mg/kg; may repeat with 0.05 mg/kg in 10-15 min if seizures continue (Note: a single dose 0.25 mg/kg may be used; then 0.05 mg/kg in 10-15 min); maximum 4 mg/dose
Adults: IV 4 mg/dose, may repeat in 10-15 min; maximum 8 mg in 12 hr period

IV administration
• Recommended concentration: Dilute to 1 mg/ml in D_5W, NS, or SW
• Maximum concentration: 4 mg/ml

✤ Available in Canada.

• IV push rate: 2 mg/min or 0.05 mg/kg over 2-5 min

MECHANISM AND INDICATIONS

Mechanism: Depresses all levels of the CNS including the cortex, thalamus, and limbic systems, probably through the potentiation of neural inhibition, mediated by γ-aminobutyric acid (GABA).

Indications: Used to treat status epilepticus, chronic seizures, and insomnia; also used for preoperative sedation, antiemetic, and anxiolytic

PHARMACOKINETICS

Onset of action: IM 20-30 min
Peak: 1-2 hr
Distribution: Widely throughout body
Half-life: 10-16 hr
Metabolism: Liver
Excretion: Urine, feces (minimally)

CONTRAINDICATIONS AND PRECAUTIONS

• Contraindicated with known hypersensitivity to lorazepam or other benzodiazepines, preexisting CNS depression, narrow-angle glaucoma, severe uncontrolled pain, severe hypotension, pregnancy, and in comatose pts

• Use cautiously with impaired hepatic or renal function, organic brain syndrome, myasthenia gravis, Parkinson's disease, and in neonates (injectable sol may contain benzyl alcohol which has been associated with fatal gasping syndrome); injectable form may produce arteriospasm if inadvertently injected intraarterially, possibly resulting in gangrene and potentially leading to amputation

INTERACTIONS

Drug

• Additive effect with other CNS depressants (alcohol, narcotics, tranquilizers, anxiolytics, barbiturates)

• Decreased effectiveness of oral contraceptives, valproic acid

Lab

• Elevated liver function tests possible

INCOMPATIBILITIES

All medications in sol or syringe except cimetidine and ranitidine

SIDE EFFECTS

CNS: Related to CNS depression; drowsiness, sedation, behavioral changes (particularly in persons with brain damage, mental retardation, or mental illness), aggression, irritability, hyperactivity, confusion, depression, dizziness, tremor, vertigo, headache, insomnia, choreiform movements

CV: Palpitation, thrombophlebitis

DERM: Skin rash, hirsutism or hair loss

EENT: Hypersalivation, diplopia, nystagmus, abnormal eye movements, rhinorrhea, difficulty swallowing

GI: Dry mouth, thirst, sore gums, nausea, changes in appetite, anorexia, gastritis, constipation

GU: Dysuria, enuresis, urinary retention, nocturia

HEME: Anemia, leukopenia, thrombocytopenia, eosinophilia

RESP: Increased bronchial secretions, dyspnea, chest congestion

Other: Metabolic hypercalcemia, hepatomegaly, liver enzyme changes

TOXICITY AND OVERDOSE

Clinical signs: Ataxia, confusion, coma, decreased reflexes, hypotension

Treatment: Supportive care; vasopressors to treat hypotension; flumazenil used to reverse CNS depression

PATIENT CARE MANAGEMENT

Assessment

• Assess history of hypersensitivity to lorazepam, other benzodiazepines

• Review potential drug interactions if using for concurrent chronic therapy

• Assess hematologic function (CBC, differential, platelets), liver function (AST, ALT, bilirubin) before beginning therapy

---

✤ Available in Canada.

Interventions
- Administer PO with food or milk to reduce GI symptoms; tab may be crushed, mixed with food or fluid
- Do not use IM sol if discolored or if precipitate is present
- Administer deep into large muscle mass
- Administer slowly with frequent aspiration to prevent intraarterial injection and peripheral extravasation
- Provide emergency equipment in the event of hypotension
- Institute safety precautions (assist with ambulation, raise side rails) because of drowsiness or dizziness

---

NURSING ALERT

Do not inject intraarterially; may produce arteriospasm, resulting in gangrene

Injectable sol may contain benzyl alcohol, which has been associated with fatal gasping syndrome in neonates

---

Evaluation
- Evaluate therapeutic response (decreased anxiety or insomnia, seizure control)
- If used IV for status epilepticus, monitor VS q 15 min, CBC, differential, platelets, ALT, AST, bilirubin
- If used for chronic therapy, monitor hematologic function (CBC, differential, platelets), liver function (ALT, AST, bilirubin)
- Monitor for side effects (hypersensitivity, signs of physical dependency, mental status, increased depression, suicidal tendencies)

PATIENT AND FAMILY EDUCATION
Teach/instruct
- To take as directed at prescribed intervals for prescribed length of time
- To take with food or milk to decrease GI symptoms
- To notify care provider of hypersensitivity, side effects

Warn/advise
- Not to use for everyday stress longer than 4 mo unless directed by care provider
- About potential for physical dependency
- To avoid OTC preparations unless directed by care provider
- To avoid alcohol
- Not to discontinue suddenly after long-term use
- To avoid tasks requiring mental alertness (bikes, skates, skateboarding) until stabilized because of sedative effect of drug

Encourage
- To keep a seizure calendar to monitor effectiveness
- To comply with follow-up care, periodic laboratory testing

STORAGE
- Store tabs at room temp
- Store vials in refrigerator protected from light
- Vials stable at room temperature for 2 wks
- Reconstituted parenteral sol stable at room temp for 4 hr

---

lypressin
Brand Name(s): Diapid

Classification: Pituitary hormone (antidiuretic hormone)

Pregnancy Category: B

AVAILABLE PREPARATIONS
Nasal spray: 0.185 mg/ml

ROUTES AND DOSAGES
Children and adults: Intranasal 1-2 sprays in one or both nostrils

---

qid; an extra dose can be given hs to prevent nocturia

MECHANISM AND INDICATIONS

Mechanism: Acts at renal tubule to promote reabsorption of water and increase urine osmolality
Indications: Neurogenic (central) diabetes insipidus

PHARMACOKINETICS

Onset of action: Rapid
Peak: ½-2 hr
Half-life: 15 min
Metabolism: Liver, kidneys
Excretion: Urine

CONTRAINDICATIONS AND PRECAUTIONS

• Contraindicated with hypersensitivity to lypressin and other antidiuretic hormones
• Use cautiously with CAD, pts at risk from increased B/P, pregnancy

INTERACTIONS

Drug
• Increased effect with carbamazepine, chlorpropamide, clofibrate
• Decreased effect with demeclocycline, lithium, norepinephrine, heparin, alcohol

SIDE EFFECTS

CNS: Headache, dizziness, seizures, coma
EENT: Nasal irritation, congestion, rhinorrhea, conjunctivitis, pruritus of nasal passages
GI: Heartburn, nausea, abdominal cramps
GU: Possible fluid retention from overdose
Other: Chest tightness

TOXICITY AND OVERDOSE

Clinical signs: Anuria, drowsiness, headache, confusion, wt gain (water intoxication), decreased serum Na
Treatment: Water restriction, withdrawal of medication until polyuria occurs; severe cases may require osmotic diuresis alone or with furosemide

PATIENT CARE MANAGEMENT

Assessment
• Assess history of hypersensitivity to lypressin
• Assess I&O, wt, edema, nasal irritation, signs of water intoxication

Interventions
• Do not use outdated medication
• Have child blow nose gently before administering; position pt seated upright; administer onto nasal mucosa by squeezing bottle quickly and firmly into each nostril; advise pt not to inhale medication
• Provide appropriate fluid intake, especially in young children and those with impaired thirst mechanism

Evaluation
• Evaluate therapeutic response (appropriate I&O, absence of polyuria or anuria)
• Monitor wt (appropriate for age; same scale at same time of day); urine osmolality (appropriate for age); serum and urine electrolytes
• Monitor signs of water intoxication (behavioral changes, lethargy, disorientation, neuromuscular irritability)
• Evaluate nasal irritation, rhinorrhea (nasal inflammation will impair absorption)

PATIENT AND FAMILY EDUCATION

Teach/instruct
• To take as directed at prescribed intervals for prescribed length of time

Warn/advise
• To notify care provider of hypersensitivity, side effects (water intoxication)
• To notify care provider of cold or allergy symptoms
• To carry medication at all times because of short half-life
• Carry medical alert identification

STORAGE

• Store at room temp

♣ Available in Canada.

mafenide acetate

Brand Name(s): Sulfamylon

Classification: Topical antibacterial

Pregnancy Category: C

AVAILABLE PREPARATIONS
Cream: 8.5%

ROUTES AND DOSAGES
Children and adults: Top, apply $1/16$″ to cleansed, debrided wound or burn areas qd-bid; reapply as needed to keep wound or burn area covered

MECHANISM AND INDICATIONS
Mechanism: Interferes with bacterial cell wall metabolism
Indications: Bacteriostatic against many gram-positive and gram-negative organisms and several strains of anaerobes; used primarily to treat 2nd- and 3rd-degree burns

PHARMACOKINETICS
Onset of action: Absorbed and distributed rapidly
Elimination: Urine

CONTRAINDICATIONS AND PRECAUTIONS
• Contraindicated with known hypersensitivity to drug or other sulfa derivatives
• Use cautiously with renal failure, impaired pulmonary function, inhalation burns, pregnancy, lactation

INTERACTIONS
Drug
• None reported
Lab
• None reported

SIDE EFFECTS
DERM: Rash, erythema, blisters, urticaria, bleeding, excoriation of new skin, stinging, burning
HEME: Bone marrow suppression, eosinophilia, fatal hemolytic anemia
METAB: Metabolic acidosis, porphyria, hyperchloremia

RESP: Hyperventilation, tachypnea

TOXICITY AND OVERDOSE
Clinical signs: Diarrhea (if ingested), increased dermatologic side effects if over-applied
Treatment: Discontinue drug and clean skin thoroughly

PATIENT CARE MANAGEMENT
Assessment
• Assess history of hypersensitivity to this drug, sulfa drugs
• Assess baseline wound appearance.
• Assess baseline VS and wt
• Assess mental status, renal (BUN, creatinine) and respiratory function
Interventions
• Apply aseptically to clean, debrided wounds using sterile gloves
• Keep burned areas covered with cream at all times
• Premedicate for painful dressing changes prn
Evaluation
• Evaluate therapeutic response (wound healing, granulation tissue)
• Monitor for superinfection
• Monitor acid–base balance
• Monitor for fluid loss

PATIENT AND FAMILY EDUCATION
Teach/instruct
• To take as directed at prescribed intervals for prescribed length of time
• For home treatment, about appropriate burn care and drug application
• About signs of super-infection; to notify care provider
Warn/advise
• That treatment may continue until pt is ready for skin grafting
• About changes in respiratory activity
• About side effects; to notify care provider

STORAGE
• Store in tight, light-resistant containers
• Avoid excess heat

♣ Available in Canada.

magnesium sulfate

Brand Name(s): Magonate (OTC), mg-plus (OTC), Slow-Mag (OTC), Epsom salts

Classification: Saline laxative, anticonvulsant, electrolyte, mineral

Pregnancy Category: B

AVAILABLE PREPARATIONS

Granule: Approximately 40 mEq mg/5 g
Oral sol: 50%
Inj: 100 mg/ml, 125 mg/ml, 250 mg/ml, 500 mg/ml

ROUTES AND DOSAGES

Laxative
Children: PO 0.25 g/kg/24 hr
Adults: PO 10-30 g/24 hr

Parenteral Nutrition Solution
Children and adults: IV maintenance 31-62 mg/kg/24 hr (0.25-0.5 mEq/kg/24 hr) up to 2 g/24 hr (16-24 mEq/24 hr)

Hypomagnesemia
Neonates: IV 25-50 mg/kg/dose (0.2-0.4 mEq/kg/dose) q8-12h for 2 or 3 doses
Infants and children: IV 25-50 mg/kg/dose q4-6h for 3 or 4 doses

Seizures and Hypertension
Children: IM/IV 20-100 mg/kg/dose q4-6h prn; 200 mg/kg/dose with severe symptoms

IV administration
• Recommended concentration: ≤30 mg/ml in D$_5$W or NS
• Maximum concentration: 200 mg/ml
• I.V. push rate: Over ≥10 min, not to exceed 150 mg/min with ECG monitoring
• Intermittent infusion: Administer over 3-4 hr

MECHANISM AND INDICATIONS

Mechanism: Acts as a Ca channel blocker; effects transport of Na and K$^+$ across cell membranes by activating Na-K$^+$ ATPase
Indications: Activation of ATPase facilitates maintenance of resting potential, and may reduce arrhythmias; acts on the lipoprotein lipase to reduce serum cholesterol; used as an anticonvulsant in preeclampsia and eclampsia; to treat seizures in nephritis, during hypertension, and in encephalopathy; to prevent Mg deficiency in total parenteral nutrition; as a saline laxative

PHARMACOKINETICS

Onset of action: PO 3-6 hr; IV immediate; IM 60 min
Distribution: Widely throughout the body
Duration: IV 30 min; IM 3-4 hr
Excretion: Urine (unchanged)

CONTRAINDICATIONS AND PRECAUTIONS

• Contraindicated with known heart block, myocardial damage, respiratory depression, renal failure; avoid in pregnant women in last 2 hr of labor because of potential effects of hypotonia and respiratory depression in the newborn
• Use cautiously with digoxin and renal insufficiency, lactation

INTERACTIONS

Drug
• Increased CNS depression possible with alcohol, narcotics, anxiolytics, barbiturates, antidepressants, hypnotics, antipsychotics, or general anesthetics; decreased dosage may be necessary
• Increased, prolonged neuromuscular blocking action with succinylcholine, tubocurarine

SIDE EFFECTS

CNS: Hypotonia, depressed reflexes, flaccid paralysis, hypothermia, CNS depression
CV: Flushing sweating, hypotension, cardiac depression, bradycardia, increased PR interval, increase QRS duration
GI: Bitter taste, diarrhea, GI discomfort, electrolyte disturbance with prolonged use of laxative form
RESP: Respiratory arrest with high levels
Other: Hypocalcemia, pain at infusion site

TOXICITY AND OVERDOSE

Clinical signs: Sharp drop in B/P and respiratory paralysis; ECG changes increased PR and QRS interval; heart block and asystole; serum level >4, deep tendon reflexes may be depressed; ≥10, deep tendon reflexes may disappear, respiratory paralysis may occur, complete heart block may occur; >12 may be fatal

Treatment: Supportive care; requires artificial ventilation and IV Ca salt to reverse the respiratory depression and heart block; usual dosage is 5-10 mEq of Ca (10-20 ml of 10% calcium gluconate solution); in extreme cases peritoneal or hemodialysis may be required

PATIENT CARE MANAGEMENT
Assessment

• Take baseline VS; may also take baseline ECG and renal (BUN, creatinine, I&O) function studies
• If used in preeclampsia and eclampsia within 24 hr of delivery, watch newborn for signs of Mg toxicity, including neuromuscular and respiratory depression

Interventions

• Administer PO with orange or lemon juice to disguise taste; give early in day to allow for elimination to take place; encourage extra fluid intake
• Should be administered only by experienced clinicians who are familiar with the drug's actions and complications
• Monitor VS continuously during infusion; respiratory rate must be within norm for age group before next dose is administered
• Have emergency resuscitation drugs (calcium gluconate) available for IV administration
• Institute seizure precautions
• Monitor patellar reflex often and withhold next dose if diminished or absent
• Monitor I&O carefully; urinary output must be normal for age group or next dose is held
• Monitor contractions for intensity, monitor fetal HR reactivity; these may decrease if using the drug during labor
• Monitor Mg levels during IV administration
• Use infusion pump if available; rapid drip causes feeling of heat
• Monitor ECG for cardiac arrhythmias, hypotension, respiratory and CNS depression during IV administration

---

NURSING ALERT

Administer IV dose slowly; respiratory depression can occur

Have calcium gluconate available to treat overdose/ toxicity

Evaluation

• Evaluate therapeutic response (control of seizures, relief of constipation, restoration of normal electrolyte balance)
• Monitor Mg levels and clinical status to avoid overdose

PATIENT AND FAMILY EDUCATION
Teach/instruct

• About signs and symptoms of hypermagnesemia (flushing, sweating, confusion, CNS depression); notify care provider
• To take oral medication with orange or lemon juice to disguise taste
• To take early in day to allow time for elimination
• Encourage to take extra fluids during day
• To monitor number and amount of bowel movements if taken PO for constipation

STORAGE

• Store at room temp
• Avoid freezing

---

mannitol

Brand Name(s): Mannitol✤, Osmitrol✤, Resectisol

Classification: Osmotic diuretic

Pregnancy Category: C

AVAILABLE PREPARATIONS
Inj: 5%, 10%, 15%, 20%, 25%

ROUTES AND DOSAGES
Oliguria or Inadequate Renal Function
Children and adults: Test dose: IV 200 mg/kg (15% or 20% sol) (maximum 12.5 g) over 3-5 min to produce urine flow of 1 ml/kg/hr (discontinue if no urinary response within 2 hr); initial 0.5-1 g/kg/dose × 1 then maintenance

To Decrease Intraocular or Intraranial Pressure
Children and adults: IV 250 mg/kg (15%-25% sol) over 30-60 min (may give furosemide 1 mg/kg IV concurrently or 5 min before mannitol), may increase dose to 1 g/kg/dose prn

To Promote Diuresis in Drug Intoxication
0.25-0.5 g/kg/dose q4-6h 5%-10% sol continuous IV to maintain 100-500 ml urine output and positive fluid balance

IV administration
• Recommended concentration: 15%, 20%, 25%
• Maximum concentration: 25%
• IV push rate: Over 3-5 min for oliguria test dose
• Intermittent infusion rate: Over 20-30 min for cerebral edema or elevated ICP

MECHANISM AND INDICATIONS
Mechanism: Increases osmolality of plasma to increase water loss from tissues, including brain and CSF; enhances excretion of water and toxic substances from kidneys
Indications: For use in treatment of edema in acute renal failure, cerebral edema, pulmonary edema; to decrease intraocular ede-ma; to prevent renal damage from toxic overdoses of salicylates, barbiturates, lithium

PHARMACOKINETICS
Half-life: 1.1-1.6 hr
Distribution: Remains confined to extracellular space
Metabolism: Minimal amounts metabolized by liver
Excretion: Urine

CONTRAINDICATIONS AND PRECAUTIONS
• Contraindicated with anuric pts who do not respond to test dose; with severe pulmonary congestion, edema; with severe dehydration
• Use cautiously with cardiac, renal, or pulmonary dysfunction; hypovolemia, hyperkalemia, pregnancy

INTERACTIONS
Drug
• Increased renal excretion of lithium
• Increased diuretic effects with other diuretics
Lab
• Altered electrolyte balance

INCOMPATIBILITIES
• Incompatible with whole blood, potassium chloride, sodium chloride

SIDE EFFECTS
CNS: Headache confusion, rebound increased intracranial pressure 8-12 hr after diuresis, blurred vision, dizziness, seizures
CV: Tachycardia, chest pain, circulatory overload, CHF, orthostatic hypotension
GI: Nausea, vomiting, thirst
GU: Increased urination, urinary retention
METAB: Fluid and electrolyte imbalance, cellular dehydration, water intoxication
RESP: Dyspnea, wheeze, cough

TOXICITY AND OVERDOSE
Clinical signs: Polyuria, hypotension, dehydration, cardiovascular collapse
Treatment: Discontinue drug, supportive measures, hemodialysis

M

✤ Available in Canada.

PATIENT CARE MANAGEMENT
Assessment
- Assess weight qd
- Assess electrolytes (Na, K+)
- Assess fluid status
- Assess respiratory status
- Assess B/P lying, standing, sitting

Interventions
- Administer IV with filter, infusion pump
- Inject IV bolus slowly
- Avoid extravasation, check IV site frequently
- Do not administer with whole blood
- Measure VS, B/P, CVP, I&O q1h

Evaluation
- Evaluate hydration status, fluid and electrolyte balance
- Evaluate for signs of rebound increase in intracranial and intraocular pressure approximately 12 hr after infusion ends

PATIENT AND FAMILY EDUCATION
Teach/instruct
- That pt may experience thirst, dry mouth but may only drink fluids as ordered
- To change position slowly to prevent dizziness, orthostatic hypotension
- To report chest, back or leg pain, shortness of breath immediately

STORAGE
- Store at room temp

---

mebendazole
Brand Name(s): Vermox✤
Classification: Anthelmintic
Pregnancy Category: C

AVAILABLE PREPARATIONS
Tabs (chewable): 100 mg

ROUTES AND DOSAGES
Pinworms
Children >2 yr and adults: PO 100 mg once; repeat in 2 wk if needed

Hookworms, Roundworms, and Whipworms
Children >2 yr and adults: PO 100 mg bid × 3 days; may repeat in 3-4 wk if needed

MECHANISM AND INDICATIONS
Mechanism: Inhibits glucose and other nutrient uptake in intestine-dwelling helminths
Indications: Used to treat pinworms, hookworms, roundworms, whipworms

PHARMACOKINETICS
Peak: 2-4 hr
Half-life: 1-11.5 hr
Metabolism: Liver
Excretion: Feces, urine

CONTRAINDICATIONS AND PRECAUTIONS
- Contraindicated with known hypersensitivity to mebendazole or any component
- Use cautiously with pregnancy, lactation, children <2 yr

INTERACTIONS
Drug
- Increased metabolism possible with use of carbamazepine, phenytoin

SIDE EFFECTS
CNS: Vertigo, fever, headache
DERM: Rash, pruritus
EENT: Tinnitus
GI: Diarrhea, abdominal pain, nausea, vomiting, abnormalities in liver function tests
HEME: Neutropenia, anemia, leukopenia

TOXICITY AND OVERDOSE
Clinical signs: GI disturbance, altered mental state
Treatment: If ingested within 4 hr, induced emesis or gastric lavage, followed by activated charcoal; supportive care

PATIENT CARE MANAGEMENT
Assessment
- Assess history of hypersensitivity to mebendazole
- Obtain pinworm test at night when child is sleeping; worms migrate to perianal area to deposit

---

✤ Available in Canada.

eggs; use scotch tape with sticky side, expose buttocks and press tape to anal area; wash hands well
• If necessary, collect stool specimens in a clean, dry container to be examined

Interventions
• May be given without regard to meals, although if given after meals it may decrease GI symptoms; tab may be crushed, mixed with food or fluids
• Use effective hygiene techniques (including handwashing)

Evaluation
• Evaluate therapeutic response (expulsion of worms and 3 negative stool cultures after treatment)
• Evaluate for spread of infection to other household members
• Evaluate for side effects, hypersensitivity (rash, abdominal pain, diarrhea)

PATIENT AND FAMILY EDUCATION

Teach/instruct
• To take as directed at prescribed intervals for prescribed length of time
• About proper hygiene procedures, especially good handwashing techniques
• About how to prevent reinfection; change undergarments and bed linens, wash clothes and linens in hot water (do not shake bed linens into the air), frequent cleansing of perianal area
• To clean toilet every day with disinfectant
• To wash all fruits and vegetables before eating

Warn/advise
• To notify care provider of hypersensitivity
• That all family members to be evaluated and treated
• That ova are easily transmitted by hands, food, contaminated articles
• To keep fingernails clean, short
• That infected person should sleep alone with tight fitting underwear

Encourage
• To comply with treatment regime

STORAGE
• Store at room temp in tight container

---

mechlorethamine hydrochloride

Brand Name(s):
Mustargen✤

Classification: Antineoplastic, alkylating agent; cell cycle phase nonspecific

Pregnancy Category: D

AVAILABLE PREPARATIONS
Inj: 10 mg powder

ROUTES AND DOSAGES
• Dosages may vary in response to diagnosis, extent of disease, concurrent or previous therapy, protocol guidelines, physiological parameters; consult current literature, protocol recommendations

Hodgkin's Disease
IV 6 mg/m^2/dose administered on days 1 and 8 of 28 day cycle (classic MOPP therapy)

Other Lymphomas
IV dosage range 0.4 mg/kg/dose or 12-16 mg/m^2/dose with about 6 wk between doses

IV administration
• Recommended concentration: 1 mg/ml
• IV push rate: 1-3 min; must be given 15-20 min after reconstituted

MECHANISM AND INDICATIONS
Mechanism: Analogue of mustard gas, a bifunctional alkylating agent that causes abnormal DNA base pairing, interfering with DNA replication; also causes cross-linking and depuration of DNA resulting in single strand breaks in helix; inhibits glycolysis, cell respiration, protein synthesis
Indications: Most frequently used in treatment of Hodgkin's disease; frequently in non-Hodgkin's lymphoma, diffuse lymphocytic lymphoma; occasionally used in adults for multiple myeloma, CLL

M

✤ Available in Canada.

PHARMACOKINETICS
• Pharmacokinetic studies have not been performed; as drug enters body fluid, it is chemically transformed and active drug is no longer present; cellular uptake of highly reactive drug derivative is almost immediate
Excretion: >50% inactive metabolites in urine within 24 hr

CONTRAINDICATIONS AND PRECAUTIONS
• Contraindicated with history of hypersensitivity to drug, with evidence of chronic or suppurative inflammation; children with active infections (especially chicken pox and herpes zoster [shingles]); pregnancy, lactation
• Use cautiously in peripheral IV (drug is powerful vesicant)

INTERACTIONS
Drug
• Increased alkylating action with glutathione-depleting agents
• Increased neurotoxicity in pts who have received procarbazine or cyclophosphamide
• Decreased local effects with sodium thiosulfate
Lab
• Increased blood and urine concentrations of uric acid possible
• Decreased serum cholinesterase
Incompatibilities
• None reported

SIDE EFFECTS
CNS: Drowsiness, headache, seizures, progressive muscular paralysis, fever, coma, temporary aphasia
CV: Thrombosis, thrombophlebitis; often subsequent use of same vein is impossible
DERM: Reversible alopecia, severe vesicant, pruritus, hyperpigmentation
EENT: Tinnitus, deafness
GI: Nausea, vomiting in about 90% of pts within 3 hr (lasts about 8 hr), anorexia, metallic taste, diarrhea, stomatitis
GU: Amenorrhea, impaired spermatogenesis
HEME: Myelosuppressive (primary effect on leukocytes and platelets); nadir in 8-14 days, may last for 10-20 days; lymphopenia within 24 hr; mild anemia
Other: Severe allergic reaction, anaphylaxis rare; second malignancies (ANLL and non–Hodgkin's Lymphoma)

TOXICITY AND OVERDOSE
Clinical signs: Prolonged myelosuppression, signs of neurologic deterioration
Treatment: Supportive measures including blood transfusions, hydration, nutritional supplementation, broad spectrum antibiotic coverage if febrile, electrolyte replacement

PATIENT CARE MANAGEMENT
Assessment
• Assess history of previous hypersensitivity reaction to drug
• Assess history of previous chemotherapy, radiation therapy
• Assess previous history that may predispose to greater risk of cardiac, hepatic, renal dysfunction
• Assess baseline CBC, differential, platelet count
• Assess baseline renal function (BUN, creatinine), liver function (bilirubin, alk phos, LDH, AST, ALT)
• Assess success of previous antiemetic regimens
• Assess integrity of oral mucosa
• Assess baseline VS
Interventions
• Administer antiemetic therapy before chemotherapy
• Ensure absolute patency of IV
• Do not place IV over joint; if extravasation occurs, joint may become immobilized
• In event of extravasation, inject site with thiosulfate and apply ice for 6-12 hr
• Active agent as administered; gown, gloves should be worn by care provider administering drug (it is a potent vesicant, irritant)
• Monitor I&O; administer IV fluids until child is able to resume normal oral intake
• Provide supportive therapy to maintain hemostasis, fluid, electrolyte, nutritional balance

---

♣ Available in Canada.

NURSING ALERT

Drug is a powerful vesicant; if there is any consideration of infiltration, area should be injected with sodium thiosulfate and ice should be applied

Drug is in active form when diluted for administration; use every precaution to avoid exposure to skin or mucous membrane

Drug must be administered within 15-20 min after reconstitution

Evaluation
• Evaluate therapeutic response through radiologic or clinical demonstration of tumor regression
• Evaluate CBC, differential, platelet counts at least weekly
• Evaluate renal function (BUN, creatinine), liver function (alk phos, LDH, AST, ALT, bilirubin) before each cycle

PATIENT AND FAMILY EDUCATION
Teach/instruct
• To have pt well hydrated before and after chemotherapy
• The importance of follow-up to monitor blood counts, chemistry values
• To take accurate temp; rectal temp contraindicated
• To notify care provider of signs of bleeding (bruising, epistaxis, bleeding gums), infection (fever, sore throat, fatigue)
Warn/advise
• About impact of body changes that may occur (hair loss, hyperpigmentation, nail ridging), how to minimize changes (wigs, caps, long sleeves)
• To avoid OTC products containing aspirin
• To report any alterations in behavior, sensation, perception; help to develop a plan of care to manage side effects, stress, illness or treatment
• To immediately report any signs

of pain or inflammation at injection site
• That good oral hygiene with very soft toothbrush is imperative
• That dental work may be delayed until blood counts return to baseline, with permission of care provider
• To avoid contact with known viral and bacterial illnesses
• That close household contacts of child not receive live polio vaccine; inactivated form should be used
• That children on chemotherapy not receive immunizations until immune system recovers sufficiently to mount appropriate antibody response
• To report exposure to chicken pox in susceptible child immediately
• To report reactivation of herpes zoster (shingles) immediately
• If appropriate, ways to preserve reproductive patterns, sexuality (sperm banking, contraceptives)
Encourage
• Provision of nutritious food intake; consider nutritional consultation
• To use top anesthetics to control discomfort of mucositis; to avoid spicy foods, commercial mouthwashes

STORAGE
• Store at room temp
• Administer within 15-20 min after reconstitution

M

---

medrysone
Brand Name(s): HMS Liquifilm✚

Classification: Ophthalmic antiinflammatory agent (corticosteroid)

Pregnancy Category: C

AVAILABLE PREPARATIONS
Ophthal sol: 1%

ROUTES AND DOSAGES
Children: Safety and effectiveness not established
Adults: Ophthalmic, instill 1 gtt

into conjunctival sac bid-qid up to q4h

MECHANISM AND INDICATIONS

Antiinflammatory mechanism: Inhibits inflammatory response by suppression of migration of leukocytes and reversal of increased capillary permeability
Indications: Used to treat allergic conjunctivitis, vernal conjunctivitis, episcleritis, and ophthalmic epinephrine sensitivity reaction

PHARMACOKINETICS

Metabolism: Liver
Excretion: Urine, feces

CONTRAINDICATIONS AND PRECAUTIONS

• Contraindicated with known hypersensitivity to medrysone; with ocular fungal, viral, tubercular, or acute untreated purulent bacterial infections
• Use cautiously in children <2 yr because of increased risk of systemic effects; in pts with corneal abrasions, glaucoma, cataracts, DM, pregnancy

SIDE EFFECTS

EENT: Transient stinging, burning, corneal thinning, increased intraocular pressure, glaucoma, damage to optic nerve, defects in visual acuity, cataracts
Other: Adrenal suppression with excessive dosages or long-term use

PATIENT CARE MANAGEMENT

Assessment

• Assess history of hypersensitivity to medrysone
• Assess eye inflammation

Interventions

• Shake sol well before instillation; wash hands before, after application; cleanse crusts or discharge from eye before application; after instillation, apply gentle pressure to lacrimal sac for 1 min to minimize systemic absorption; wipe excess medication from eye; do not flush medication from eye

• Gradually taper drug to prevent disease exacerbation if used for long-term therapy

> **NURSING ALERT**
> Discontinue drug if signs of local irritation, infection, systemic absorption, hypersensitivity, or visual changes develop

Evaluation

• Evaluate therapeutic response (decreased inflammation); discontinue if no improvement after several days of treatment
• Monitor for symptoms of adrenal suppression
• Monitor for signs of skin irritation or ulceration, hypersensitivity, or infection
• Monitor tonometry measurements q 2-3 wk on chronic therapy

PATIENT AND FAMILY EDUCATION

Teach/instruct

• To use as directed at prescribed intervals for prescribed length of time

Warn/advise

• To notify care provider of hypersensitivity, side effects
• To notify care provider if there is no improvement after 1 wk of treatment, if condition worsens, or if eye pain, itching, or swelling develop
• To wear dark glasses to reduce photophobia
• To taper medication after long-term therapy
• Not to use ophthal preparations unless prescribed by care provider
• Not to use this medication for any new eye inflammation

STORAGE

• Store at room temp in tightly closed container, protected from light
• Do not freeze

✤ Available in Canada.

melphalan, L-phenylalanine mustard

Brand Name(s): Alkeran, l-PAM

Classification: Alkylating agent

Pregnancy Category: D

AVAILABLE PREPARATIONS

Tabs: 2 mg
Inj: 50 mg, 100 mg ampules (experimental)

ROUTES AND DOSAGES

• Drug may vary in response to diagnosis, extent of disease, concurrent or previous therapy, protocol guidelines, physiologic parameters; consult current literature, protocol recommendations
Children and adults: PO 6 mg/24 hr, maintenance 2 mg/24 hr; adjust dosage as required, on basis of blood counts; after 2-3 weeks of treatment, drug is discontinued for up to 4 weeks, following counts weekly, restarting drug once counts recovered; or PO 0.15 mg/kg × 7 days or 0.25 mg/kg/24 hr × 4 days, repeated at 4-6 week intervals; IV 16 mg/m²/dose at 2 week intervals for 4 doses, then repeat monthly as per protocol
• Melphalan usually administered with prednisone

IV administration

• Recommended concentration: Reconstitute 50 mg vial with 10 ml diluent for 5 mg/ml; can further dilute with NS to final maximum concentration 0.45 mg/ml for peripheral administration or 2 mg/ml for central administration; give immediately after reconstitution
• IV infusion rate: Slow, over 30-45 min; do not exceed 10 mg/min

MECHANISM AND INDICATIONS

Mechanism: A derivative of nitrogen mustard; cell cycle phase nonspecific; prevents cell replication by causing breaks and cross-linkages in DNA strands, interferes with RNA transcription causing an imbalance of growth that leads to miscoding, breakage, and eventually cell death
Indications: Used to treat multiple myeloma, ovarian cancer, rhabdomyosarcoma, neuroblastoma

PHARMACOKINETICS

Half-life: 90 min
Distribution: Rapidly distributed throughout total body water; into CSF in low concentration following IV administration
Absorption: Variable from the GI tract
Metabolism: Spontaneous hydrolysis in plasma
Excretion: 20%-50% in feces over 6 days; 50% in urine within 24 hr

CONTRAINDICATIONS AND PRECAUTIONS

• Contraindicated with known hypersensitivity; with disease known to be resistant to the drug; hypersensitivity to chlorambucil (may have cross-sensitivity to melphalan), severely depressed bone marrow function, active infection (especially chicken pox or herpes zoster), anemia or CLL, pregnancy, lactation

INTERACTIONS

Drug

• Increased risk of bleeding with anticoagulants or aspirin
• Decreased effectiveness of anti-gout agents
• Additive toxicity possible with other bone marrow suppressants
• Decreased effectiveness of killed-virus vaccines, increased risk of toxicity from live-virus vaccines

SIDE EFFECTS

DERM: Alopecia, rash, pruritus, dermatitis
GI: Nausea, vomiting, wt loss
GU: Infertility, amenorrhea
HEME: Thrombocytopenia, leukopenia, agranulocytosis, bleeding
RESP: Pneumonitis, pulmonary fibrosis, persistent cough
Other: Anaphylaxis, fever

M

TOXICITY AND OVERDOSE

Clinical signs: Immediate effects of overdose are vomiting, diarrhea, ulcerations of mouth, hemorrhage of GI tract; ANLL and myeloproliferative syndromes occur as secondary cancers

Treatment: Monitor blood counts closely and offer supportive care (antibiotics, transfusions)

PATIENT CARE MANAGEMENT

Assessment

• Assess history of hypersensitivity to melphalan

• Assess baseline CBC, platelet count, renal function (BUN, serum uric acid, urine CrCl), liver function (ALT, AST, LDH, bilirubin) before chemotherapy

• Assess baseline VS

• Assess for any signs or symptoms of infection (fever, fatigue, sore throat), bleeding (easy bruising, bleeding gums, nose bleeds)

• Assess oral mucosa and skin integrity

• Assess baseline pulmonary status, lung sounds

• Assess success of previous antiemetic therapy

Interventions

• Premedicate with antiemetics 1 hour before administration of oral dose, continue prn

• Administer total daily dose in one dose on an empty stomach

• Encourage small, frequent feedings of foods pt likes

• Provide supportive measures to maintain hemostasis, fluid and electrolyte balance, nutritional support

> **NURSING ALERT**
> Administer antiemetics 1 hr before melphalan to decrease nausea and vomiting
>
> Administer oral melphalan on empty stomach for better absorption

Evaluation

• Evaluate therapeutic response (decreased tumor size, spread of malignancy)

• Evaluate CBC, platelet count, renal function (BUN, serum uric acid, urine CrCl), liver function (ALT, AST, LDH, bilirubin) at given intervals after chemotherapy

• Evaluate for signs or symptoms of infection (fever, fatigue, sore throat), bleeding (epistaxis, bruising, bleeding gums), changes in skin integrity (rashes, alopecia, urticaria); develop a plan to manage symptom distress

• Evaluate for side effects, response to antiemetic regimen

• Evaluate lung sounds (pulmonary status) and oral mucosa

PATIENT AND FAMILY EDUCATION

Teach/instruct

• To have pt well-hydrated before and after chemotherapy

• About importance of follow-up to monitor blood counts, serum chemistry values, drug blood levels

• To take accurate temp; rectal temp contraindicated

• To notify care provider of signs of bleeding (bruising, epistaxis, bleeding gums), infection (fever, sore throat, fatigue)

Warn/advise

• About impact of body changes that may occur (hair loss, hyperpigmentation, nail ridging), how to minimize changes (wigs, caps, scarves, long sleeves)

• To avoid OTC products containing aspirin

• To report any alterations in behavior, sensation, perception; help to develop a plan of care to manage side effects, stress of illness or treatment

• To monitor bowel function, call if abdominal pain, constipation noted

• To immediately report any pain, discoloration at injection site (parenteral forms)

• That good oral hygiene with very soft toothbrush is imperative

- That dental work be delayed until blood counts return to baseline, with permission of care provider
- To avoid contact with known viral or bacterial illnesses
- That household contacts of child not be immunized with live polio virus; inactivated form should be used
- That child not receive immunizations until immune system recovers sufficiently to mount needed antibody response
- To report exposure to chicken pox in susceptible child immediately
- To report reactivation of herpes zoster virus (shingles) immediately
- If appropriate, ways to preserve reproductive patterns, sexuality (sperm banking, contraceptives)
- To report cough or dyspnea

Encourage
- Provision of nutritious food intake; consider nutritional consultation
- To comply with bowel management program
- To use top anesthetics to control discomfort of mucositis; avoid spicy foods, commercial mouthwashes

STORAGE
- Store at room temp
- Protect from light
- Use reconstituted parenteral form within 1 hr

---

meperidine

Brand Name(s): Demerol♣, Mepergan♣, Meperidine♣, Pethidine

Classification: Narcotic analgesic, opiate agonist

Controlled Substance Schedule II

Pregnancy Category: B, D (in labor)

AVAILABLE PREPARATIONS
Oral sol: 50 mg/5 ml
Tabs: 50 mg, 100 mg
Inj: 25 mg, 50 mg, 75 mg, 100 mg vials
IV inf: 10 mg/ml injection

ROUTES AND DOSAGES
Children: PO not recommended, SC/IM/IV 0.5-2 mg/kg/dose q3-4h prn; maximum 100 mg/dose or 1.5 mg/kg/hr
Adults: PO/SC/IM/IV 50-150 mg/dose q3-4h prn

IV administration
- Recommended concentration: 0.6-10 mg/ml with SW or NS
- Maximum concentration: Not established; recommend sol be diluted for IV administration
- IV push rate: Not recommended
- Intermittent infusion rate: Very slow; do not exceed 25 mg over 1 min
- Continuous infusion rate: 0.3-1.5 mg/kg/hr in D-LR, D-R, D-S, D_5W, $D_{10}W$, LR, NS, or ½NS

MECHANISM AND INDICATIONS
Mechanism: Depresses pain impulse transmission at the spinal cord level by interacting with opioid receptors
Indications: Used to treat moderate-to-severe pain

PHARMACOKINETICS
Onset of action: PO 15 min; IM 10-15 min; SC 10-15 min; IV immediate
Peak: PO 60 min; IM 30-50 min; SC 40-60 min; IV 5-7 min
Half-life: 2.4-4 hr
Duration: 2-4 hr
Metabolism: Liver
Excretion: Urine
Distribution: Widely distributed

CONTRAINDICATIONS AND PRECAUTIONS
- Contraindicated with hypersensitivity to drug, respiratory depression, comatose, elevated CSF pressure, pregnancy, lactation; preparations with metabisulfite contraindicated with sulfite hypersensitivity
- Use cautiously with asthma, hepatic or renal dysfunction, atrial

M

♣ Available in Canada.

flutter, tachycardia, colitis, hypothyroidism, neonates, pts who have taken MAOIs in last 14 days, undiagnosed abdominal pain

INTERACTIONS
Drug
• Increased risk of coma, respiratory depression, hypotension (may even result in unpredictable fatal reaction) with MAOIs
• Additive CNS depression with alcohol, antihistamines, sedatives or hypnotics
• Withdrawal in narcotic-dependent patients with partial antagonists (buprenorphine, butorphanol, nalbuphine, pentazocine)
• Antagonized action possible with phenothiazines
• Decreased effects of diuretics in CHF
• Increased effects of neuromuscular-blocking agents possible
Lab
• Increased serum amylase and lipase (delay drawing blood for these tests for 24 hr after administration)
• Decreased serum and urine 17-KS, 17-OHCS

INCOMPATIBILITIES
• Incompatible with aminophylline, amobarbital, furosemide, heparin, hydrocortisone, methicillin, methylprednisolone, morphine, pentobarbital, phenobarbital, secobarbital, phenytoin, NaHCO₃, thiopental

SIDE EFFECTS
CNS: Sedation, confusion, headache, euphoria, floating feeling, unusual dreams, hallucinations, dysphoria, insomnia, coma, increased ICP (normeperidine is a toxic metabolite of meperidine excreted through kidneys; it is a cerebral irritant, and accumulation can cause effects ranging from dysphoria and irritable mood to seizure, even in young, otherwise healthy persons)
CV: Circulatory depression potentially life threatening, orthostatic hypotension, palpitation, bradycardia, tachycardia (more common than with other opiates)

DERM: Rash, erythema, urticaria, pruritus, facial flushing indicates hypersensitivity reaction, sweating, bruising
EENT: Miosis, diplopia, blurred vision, tinnitus, depressed corneal reflex
GI: Nausea, vomiting, constipation, anorexia, cramps, biliary spasm, increased serum amylase and lipase
GU: Urinary retention, oliguria
RESP: Respiratory depression
Other: Tolerance, physical and psychological dependence

TOXICITY AND OVERDOSE
Clinical signs: Respiratory and circulatory depression
Treatment: Supportive care; naloxone (dose may need to be repeated or naloxone infusion administered); vasopressors

PATIENT CARE MANAGEMENT
Assessment
• Assess history of hypersensitivity to meperidine or related drugs
• Assess rationale for use (should be used for very brief courses in pts who have demonstrated allergy or intolerance to morphine or hydromorphone)
• Assess baseline VS, renal status
• Assess pain (type, location, intensity)
Interventions
• Administer PO with food or milk to minimize GI irritation; syr should be diluted in half glass of water
• Rapid IV administration may lead to increased respiratory depression, hypotension, circulatory collapse; have naloxone readily available
• IV infusion may be administered with PCA pump (first choice drugs are morphine and hydromorphone)
• Determine dosing interval by pt response
• Administer when pain is not too severe to enhance drug's effectiveness
• Concurrent administration with nonnarcotic analgesics may have

additive analgesic effects, permitting lower narcotic doses
• Institute safety measures (supervise ambulation, raise side rails, call light within reach)

NURSING ALERT
Rapid IV administration may cause increased respiratory depression, hypotension, circulatory collapse; have naloxone available

Evaluation
• Evaluate therapeutic response (decreased pain without significant alteration in LOC or respiratory status)
• Monitor VS, pain control (for 30-60 min after administration), CNS changes
• Evaluate for side effects, hypersensitivity

PATIENT AND FAMILY EDUCATION
Teach/instruct
• To take as directed at prescribed intervals for prescribed length of time
• About best time to request medication (if ordered prn)
• About how to use PCA pump if appropriate
Warn/advise
• To notify care provider of hypersensitivity, side effects
• That tolerance and dependence may occur with long-term use
• That drug may cause drowsiness, dizziness, orthostatic hypotension; to make position changes slowly and seek assistance with ambulation
• Avoid alcohol, OTC medications
Encourage
• To drink adequate amounts of fluids
• That coughing, deep breathing, and movement help to avoid respiratory complications

STORAGE
• Store at room temp
• Protect from light
• Avoid freezing sol

---

mephobarbital
Brand Name(s): Mebaral, Mentaban, Mephoral
Classification: Anticonvulsant, nonspecific CNS depressant (barbiturate)
Controlled Substance Schedule IV
Pregnancy Category: D

AVAILABLE PREPARATIONS
Tabs: 32 mg, 50 mg, 100 mg, 200 mg

ROUTES AND DOSAGES
Children: PO 4-10 mg/kg/24 hr divided q6-8h; initially smaller doses may be administered and increased over 4-5 days prn
Adults: PO 200-600 mg/24 hr in divided doses

MECHANISM AND INDICATIONS
Mechanism: Acts to increase seizure threshold in motor cortex by depressing monosynaptic and polysynaptic transmission in CNS; the physiological inhibition is mediated by γ-aminobutyric acid (GABA) (however, the effect may not be entirely mediated by GABA)
Indication: Used to treat generalized tonic-clonic, absence, myoclonic, mixed-type seizures, and as a sedative to relieve anxiety and tension

PHARMACOKINETICS
Onset of action: 30-60 min
Duration: 6-8 hr
Half-life: 34 hr
Absorption: After oral dose, 50% from GI tract
Metabolism: Liver, metabolized to phenobarbital
Excretion: Urine
Therapeutic levels: Phenobarbital 15-40 mcg/ml

CONTRAINDICATIONS AND PRECAUTIONS
• Contraindicated with known sensitivity to barbiturates; pregnancy (because of respiratory de-

pression and neonatal coagulation defects); with porphyria or marked hepatic impairment (may exacerbate porphyria); respiratory distress or status asthmaticus (may cause respiratory depression)

• Use cautiously with alcohol, CNS depressants, MAOIs, narcotic analgesics, anticoagulants, lactation; abrupt withdrawal could precipitate seizures

INTERACTIONS
Drug
• Excessive depression possible with alcohol and other CNS depressants
• Increased hepatic metabolism of oral anticoagulants
• Decreased barbiturate levels, efficacy possible with rifampin
Lab
• Elevated liver function tests; alk phos, ammonia
• Decreased bilirubin, Ca

SIDE EFFECTS
CNS: Dizziness, headache, confusion, paradoxical excitation, exacerbation of existing pain, drowsiness, nightmares, hallucinations
CV: Hypotension, bradycardia
DERM: Urticaria, rash, blisters, purpura, erythema multiforme, Stevens-Johnson syndrome
GI: Nausea, vomiting, epigastric pain, constipation
HEME: Megaloblastic anemia, agranulocytosis, thrombocytopenia
Other: Psychological and physical dependence

TOXICITY AND OVERDOSE
Clinical signs: CNS and respiratory depression, areflexia, oliguria, tachycardia, hypotension, hypothermia, coma; shock may occur in a massive overdose
Treatment: Supportive symptomatic care; in pts with intact gag reflex, induce vomiting with ipecac, follow with repeated doses of activated charcoal (repeated doses reduce half-life), usual dose is 30-60 g q4-6h for 3-4 days unless patient does not have a BM thus causing the charcoal to be retained

in GI tract; alkalinization with IV NaHCO₃ also helps to promote elimination; hemodialysis may be required; monitor VS, fluid, electrolyte balance

PATIENT CARE MANAGEMENT
Assessment
• Assess for history of hypersensitivity to barbiturates; respiratory depression, hepatic impairment
• Assess baseline laboratory studies including CBC, differential and liver function (ALT, AST, bilirubin, alk phos)
• Assess seizure type; determine appropriate anticonvulsant for this type of seizure
Interventions
• Initiate at modest dosage
• Increase dosage and level up as needed to control seizures (to the point of intolerable side effects)
• If drug is only partially effective, another anticonvulsant may be initiated in same way
• If drug is not effective, gradually withdraw and another anticonvulsant may be initiated
• If break-through seizures occur at times when serum levels are at trough or peak, frequency of dosing may be increased to provide more even coverage
Evaluation
• Evaluate therapeutic response (seizure control, decreased anxiety); initially done more frequently until seizures are controlled, then q 3-6 mo or in case of seizure breakthrough or side effects
• Monitor anticonvulsant levels periodically

PATIENT AND FAMILY EDUCATION
Teach/instruct
• To take as directed; not to change dosage independently or withdraw suddenly
• About process for initiating anticonvulsant drugs, need for frequent visits (especially initially)
• About rationale for measuring serum levels, how these should be obtained (peak/trough)

✤ Available in Canada.

- That unpleasant side effects may decrease as pt becomes more used to drug
- That drug initially may be more sedating until pt becomes used to it; avoid hazardous tasks (bike, skates, skateboards) that require mental alertness until drug side effects have stabilized

Warn/advise

- To avoid use of other drugs with CNS depressant effects (such as antihistamines, analgesics, alcohol) because these may increase sedative effect
- That drug may decrease effectiveness of oral contraceptives; it may be necessary to use a different birth control method
- To make other health care providers aware of their medications in order to avoid drug interactions
- To inform care provider if pregnancy should occur while taking drug
- To report serious side effects immediately (any signs of unusual bleeding, bruising, skin eruptions, fever, chills, sore throat, mouth ulcers, edema, disturbances in mood, alertness, coordination)

Encourage

- To keep a record of any seizures (seizure calendar)

STORAGE

- Store in a light-resistant container

6-mercaptopurine

Brand Name(s): Puri-nethol♣

Classification: Antineoplastic, purine antimetabolite; cell cycle phase specific (S phase); immunosuppressant

Pregnancy Category: D

AVAILABLE PREPARATIONS
Tabs: 50 mg

ROUTES AND DOSAGES

- Dosage may vary in response to diagnosis, extent of disease, concurrent or previous therapy, protocol guidelines, physiological parameters; consult current literature, protocol recommendations
- PO, induction 2.5-5 mg/kg/24 hr or 75-100 mg/m²/24 hr; maintenance 1.5-2.5 mg/kg/24 hr or 40-50 mg/m²/24 hr qd

ALL Induction (POMP)
PO 500-700 mg/m²/24 hr for 5 days with dosage escalations on subsequent cycles

ALL Remission Maintenance
PO 50 mg/m²/24 hr qd for several consecutive days; usually administered in conjunction with methotrexate

Regional Enteritis and Ulcerative Colitis
PO 1.5-2.5 mg/kg/24 hr

MECHANISM AND INDICATIONS
Mechanism: Exact mechanism unknown; readily enters cell and is converted to active form; thought to act as false metabolite (is chemically similar to purine base hypoxanthine); inhibits enzymes required for DNA, RNA synthesis
Indications: Used in combination chemotherapy for induction, maintenance for ALL, non-Hodgkin's lymphoma, diffuse histiocytic and undifferentiated lymphoma; immunosuppressant for autoimmune diseases such as regional enteritis, ulcerative colitis; may also be useful in chronic granulocytic leukemia, CML (maintenance and blast crises)

PHARMACOKINETICS
Peak: PO 1-2 hr after ingestion, absorption influenced by food in stomach
Distribution: Widely into total body water; enormous individual variability in absorption across GI tract

M

Half-life: PO triphasic, terminal half-life 10 hr
Metabolism: Liver
Excretion: Urine

CONTRAINDICATIONS AND PRECAUTIONS

• Contraindicated with history of hypersensitivity to drug; when previous use has proven ineffective; pts with active infections (especially chicken pox and herpes zoster); previous treatment with 6-thioguanine, if that therapy was not effective (generally complete cross-resistance), pregnancy, lactation

• Use cautiously with impaired hepatic function, generalized edema

INTERACTIONS
Drug

• Reduced metabolism of 6-MP by xanthine oxidase; if concomitant use, dose reduction of 6-MP required (long half-life of allopurinol metabolites must be noted in conjunction with this interaction)

• Decreased cellular uptake of methotrexate possible

• Interferes with anticoagulant effect of warfarin

• Reduced toxicity to normal cells possible with adenosine

• Increased hepatotoxicity possible with doxorubicin

• Increased bioavailability of oral 6-MP with oral methotrexate

Lab

• False increase in BG, uric acid levels when sequential multiple analyzer is used

• Increased concentration of uric acid in blood, urine

SIDE EFFECTS

CNS: None reported with PO administration

GI: Mucositis, hepatotoxicity (increased alk phos, AST, ALT, bilirubin, jaundice); hepatitis, often evidenced by abdominal pain with increased tenderness in right hypochondrium

GU: Hematuria, crystalluria, (may be accompanied by flank pain or alterations in serum creatinine)

HEME: Mild myelosuppression (most effect on leukocytes and platelets, nadir day 15-16 after 5 day course)

Other: Fever

TOXICITY AND OVERDOSE

Clinical signs: Prolonged myelosuppression, hepatic necrosis

Treatment: Supportive measures including blood transfusions, hydration, nutritional supplementation, broad-spectrum antibiotic therapy if febrile, electrolyte replacement

PATIENT CARE MANAGEMENT
Assessment

• Assess history of hypersensitivity to drug

• Assess history of previous treatment with attention to other therapies that might predispose to hepatic dysfunction

• Assess success of previous antiemetic therapy

• Assess baseline CBC, differential, platelet count

• Assess baseline renal function (BUN, creatinine, uric acid), and liver function (bilirubin, alk phos, LDH, AST, ALT)

• Assess baseline VS

Interventions

• Administer antiemetic therapy before chemotherapy; repeat during infusion

• Administer PO at hs; avoid taking with milk

• Monitor I&O; administer IV fluids until child is able to resume normal fluid intake

• Provide supportive measures to maintain hemostasis, fluid, electrolyte, nutritional status

---

✤ Available in Canada.

NURSING ALERT

Initial drug metabolism occurs almost exclusively in liver; liver function must be monitored closely

Concomitant use of allopurinol and 6-MP requires a significant dosage reduction in 6-MP

Evaluation

- Evaluate therapeutic response to treatment through hematologic recovery
- Evaluate CBC, differential, platelet count at least once per week
- Evaluate renal function (BUN, creatinine, uric acid), liver function (bilirubin, alk phos, LDH, AST, ALT) at regular intervals

PATIENT AND FAMILY EDUCATION
Teach/instruct

- To take as directed at prescribed intervals for prescribed length of time
- To take tab hs; avoid taking with milk
- To have patient well hydrated before and after chemotherapy
- About the importance of follow-up to monitor blood counts, serum chemistry values
- To take accurate temp; rectal temp contraindicated
- To notify care provider of signs of bleeding (bruising, epistaxis, bleeding gums), infection (fever, sore throat, fatigue)

Warn/advise

- About impact of body changes that may occur (hair loss, hyperpigmentation, nail ridging), how to minimize changes (wigs, caps, scarves, long sleeves)
- To avoid OTC preparations containing aspirin
- To report any alterations in behavior, sensation, perception; help to develop a plan of care to manage side effects, stress of illness or treatment

- That good oral hygiene with very soft toothbrush is imperative
- That dental work be delayed until blood counts return to baseline, with permission of caretaker
- To avoid contact with known viral, bacterial illnesses
- That close household contacts of child not be immunized with live polio virus; use inactivated form
- That children on chemotherapy not receive immunizations until immune system recovers sufficiently to mount necessary antibody response
- To report exposure to chicken pox in susceptible child immediately
- To report reactivation of herpes zoster virus (shingles) immediately
- If appropriate, ways to preserve reproductive patterns, sexuality (sperm banking, contraceptives)

Encourage

- Provision of nutritious food intake; consider nutritional consultation
- To use top anesthetics or systemic analgesics to control discomfort of mucositis; avoid spicy foods, commercial mouthwashes

STORAGE

- Store tabs at room temp
- Protect from light

---

mesna

Brand Name(s): Mesnex, Uromitexam✦

Classification: Sulfydryl

Pregnancy Category: B

AVAILABLE PREPARATION
Inj: 100 mg/ml

ROUTES AND DOSAGES

- Drug may vary in response to diagnosis, extent of disease, concurrent or previous therapy, protocol guidelines, physiologic param-

---

eters; consult current literature, protocol recommendations

Children and adults: IV, fractionated dosing schedule of IV bolus infusions which equal the total dose of ifosfamide; can be given 15 min before ifosfamide, then just after with 2-3 more doses at given hours; PO 2 × IV dose, with carbonated beverage or juice

IV administration

• Recommended concentration: 20 mg/ml; dilute with NS, D_5W, D_5NS, or LR to desired concentration

• Maximum concentration: Each 100 mg (1 ml) must be diluted in a minimum of 4 ml D_5W, NS, D_5NS, or LR

• Infusion rate: Administer by slow IV push or IV infusion over 15-30 min

MECHANISM AND INDICATIONS

Mechanism: Reacts with urotoxic ifosfamide metabolites; is rapidly metabolized by the metabolite dimesna; in the kidney, dimesna is reduced to mesna which binds to the ifosfamide metabolites acrolein and 4-hydroxy-ifosfamide, resulting in their detoxification

Indications: Used whenever ifosfamide is being administered (usually 15 min before ifosfamide, immediately after ifosfamide infusion, then 3 more times with vigorous hydration); used to reduce the risk of hemorrhagic cystitis when ifosfamide or high doses of cyclophosphamide are used in treating lymphomas, brain tumors, Ewing's sarcoma, and relapsed osteosarcoma

PHARMACOKINETICS

Onset of action: Immediate

Peak: Immediately following infusion

Half-life: 0.36-1.7 hr (mesna and dimesna); terminal 7 hr

Metabolism: Rapidly oxidized to its only metabolite, dimesna and remains in the intravascular compartment

Excretion: Urine (majority in 4 hr)

CONTRAINDICATIONS AND PRECAUTIONS

• Contraindicated with known hypersensitivity to the drug or thiol-containing compounds, pregnancy, lactation

INTERACTIONS

Lab

• False positive: Urine ketones

INCOMPATIBILITIES

• Do not mix with cisplatin

SIDE EFFECTS

GI: Nausea, vomiting, soft stool, diarrhea, dysgeusia, bad taste in mouth

Other: Headache, fatigue, hypotension

• Because mesna is given with other drugs (ifosfamide or cyclophosphamide), it is difficult to determine which side effects are solely attributable to mesna

TOXICITY AND OVERDOSE

Clinical signs: Allergic reactions, diarrhea, fatigue, headache, hematuria, hypotension, limb pain, nausea

Treatment: Supportive care

PATIENT CARE MANAGEMENT

Assessment

• Assess history of hypersensitivity to mesna

• Assess baseline VS, renal function (BUN, creatinine, urine output)

• Assess hydration status (SG); for ketones and glucose in urine; for dysuria, urinary frequency

• Assess success of antiemetic regimen

• Assess history of previous treatment with special attention to other therapies that may predispose to renal or urinary dysfunction

Interventions

• Measure I&O and check urine every void for SG, heme, ketones, glucose

• Administer IV fluids with inadequate PO

• Provide supportive measures to maintain hemostasis, fluid or electrolyte balance, and nutritional support

Evaluation
- Evaluate therapeutic response (absence of hemorrhagic cystitis)
- Evaluate I&O carefully, renal function (BUN, creatinine)
- Evaluate side effects, response to antiemetic regimen

PATIENT AND FAMILY EDUCATION

Teach/instruct
- To take all doses of mesna and to drink plenty of fluids before and after chemotherapy
- To report any pain on urination or blood in urine immediately
- About the importance of follow-up to monitor blood counts, serum chemistries, drug blood levels

Warn/advise
- To report any alterations in behavior, sensation, perception; help to develop a plan of care to manage side effects, stress of illness or treatment
- If appropriate, ways to preserve reproductive patterns, sexuality (sperm banking, contraceptives)

Encourage
- To drink plenty of fluids and void frequently

STORAGE
- Reconstituted sol stable for 24 hr at room temp; recommended that sol be refrigerated and used within 6 hr

---

metaraminol bitartrate
Brand Name(s): Aramine ❦
Classification: Vasopressor
Pregnancy Category: C

AVAILABLE PREPARATIONS
Inj: 10 mg/ml

ROUTES AND DOSAGES

Hypotension
Children: SC/IM 0.1 mg/kg/dose or 3 mg/m²/dose
Adults: SC/IM 2-10 mg/dose

Hypotension in Severe Shock
Children: IV 0.01 mg/kg/dose or 0.03 mg/m²/dose; may follow by IV infusion prn of 5 mcg/kg/min titrated to maintain desired B/P, diluted 1 mg/25 ml NS or D_5W
Adults: IV 0.5-5 mg/dose; may follow with IV infusion prn of 1-4 mcg/kg/min titrated and diluted 100 mg/500 ml NS or D_5W to maintain desired B/P

IV administration
- Recommended concentration: 1 mg/25 ml NS or D_5W
- Maximum concentration: May administer undiluted
- IV push rate: ≤1 min
- Continuous infusion rate: Titrate to maintain desired B/P

MECHANISM AND INDICATIONS
Vasopressor mechanism: Stimulates α-adrenergic receptors, resulting in increased peripheral vascular resistance; also produces a positive inotropic effect on the heart
Indications: Used to treat hypotension caused by hemorrhage, reactions to medications, surgical complications, and shock caused by trauma

PHARMACOKINETICS
Onset of action: IM within 10 min; IV 1-2 min
Metabolism: Not metabolized; effects of drug terminated by absorption into tissues and by urinary excretion
Excretion: Urine

CONTRAINDICATIONS AND PRECAUTIONS
- Contraindicated with allergy to sulfites; anesthesia using cyclopropane or halothane; with profound hypoxia or hypercapnia
- Use cautiously with hypertension, hyperthyroidism, diabetes, heart disease, cirrhosis, peripheral vascular disease, acidosis, pregnancy, lactation

INTERACTIONS

Drug
- Increased vasopressor response with atropine

- Increased risk of arrhythmias with digoxin
- Increased vasopressor effects with MAOIs or tricyclic antidepressants
- Decreased vasopressor effects with α-adrenergic blocking agents
- Decreased vasopressor effects with β blockers

Lab
- None reported

INCOMPATIBILITIES
- Do not mix with other medications

SIDE EFFECTS
CNS: Anxiety, restlessness, headache, dizziness, tremor, faintness
CV: Arrhythmias, peripheral and visceral vasoconstriction, hypotension, hypertension, palpitations, tachycardia, bradycardia
ENDO: Hyperglycemia
GI: Nausea, vomiting
Other: Pallor, sweating, fever, respiratory distress

TOXICITY AND OVERDOSAGE
Clinical signs: Severe hypertension, cerebral hemorrhage, seizures, arrhythmia, acute pulmonary edema, cardiac arrest
Treatment: Discontinue drug; supportive measures include sympatholytic agents, antiarrhythmic agents

PATIENT CARE MANAGEMENT
Assessment
- Assess history of hypersensitivity to drug, sulfites
- Assess blood volume depletion, correct before administering drug
- Assess VS

Interventions
- Inject IV into largest veins possible, avoid extravasation; if extravasation occurs, treat infiltrate site promptly with phentolamine
- Wait at least 10 min before giving subsequent doses
- Monitor VS and heart rhythm during and after drug administration until pt is stable
- Emergency drugs and equipment must be readily available

- Measure I&O
- Be available to support pt or family

Evaluation
- Evaluate therapeutic response (increased B/P)
- Evaluate for excessive vasopressor response
- Evaluate for evidence of tolerance to drug
- Monitor electrolyte balance, fluid balance

PATIENT AND FAMILY EDUCATION
Warn/advise
- That patient will be closely monitored while receiving drug

STORAGE
- Store at room temp in light-resistant container; avoid temp below −20° C

---

methadone hydrochloride

Brand Name(s): Dolophine, Methadone

Classification: Narcotic analgesic, opiate agonist

Controlled Substance Schedule II

Pregnancy Category: B

AVAILABLE PREPARATIONS
Oral sol: 5 mg/5 ml, 10 mg/5 ml
Tabs: 5 mg, 10 mg; 40 mg dispersible
Inj: 10 mg/ml

ROUTES AND DOSAGES
Children and adults: PO 0.05-0.2 mg/kg/dose q6-8h; SC/IM: 0.1 mg/kg/dose q6-8h

MECHANISM AND INDICATIONS
Mechanism: Depresses pain impulse transmission at spinal cord level by interacting with opioid receptors; alters perception of and response to painful stimuli while producing generalized CNS depression
Indications: Used to treat severe pain, narcotic withdrawal

✦ Available in Canada.

PHARMACOKINETICS
Onset of action: PO 30-60 min; IM/SC: 10-20 min
Peak: PO 90-120 min; IM/SC: 60-120 min
Distribution: Widely distributed, 90% bound to plasma protein
Half-life: 1-1.5 days
Duration: PO 4-12 hrs; IM/SC: 4-6 hr; cumulative: 22-48 hr
Metabolism: Liver
Excretion: Urine

CONTRAINDICATIONS AND PRECAUTIONS
• Contraindicated with known hypersensitivity to drug, pregnancy, lactation
• Use cautiously with head trauma, increased ICP; severe renal, hepatic, or pulmonary disease; hypothyroidism, adrenal insufficiency, undiagnosed abdominal pain; with pts receiving MAOIs

INTERACTIONS
Drug
• Additive CNS depression with alcohol, narcotics, sedatives or hypnotics, antipsychotics, skeletal muscle relaxants, rifampin, phenytoin
• Unpredictable, potentially fatal reactions possible with MAOIs
• Withdrawal in narcotic-dependent pts with use of partial antagonists (buprenorphine, butorphanol, nalbuphine, pentazocine)
Lab
• Increased amylase and lipase levels

SIDE EFFECTS
CNS: Sedation, confusion, headache, euphoria, floating feeling, unusual dreams, hallucination, dysphoria, dizziness
CV: Hypotension, bradycardia, palpitations
DERM: Sweating, flushing, rash, urticaria, bruising, pruritus
EENT: Miosis, diplopia, blurred vision, tinnitus
GI: Nausea, vomiting, constipation, anorexia, cramps, biliary tract spasm
GU: Urinary retention, increased urinary output, dysuria
RESP: Respiratory depression
Other: Tolerance, physical/psychological dependence

TOXICITY AND OVERDOSE
Clinical signs: Respiratory depression
Treatment: Supportive care; naloxone; vasopressors

PATIENT CARE MANAGEMENT
Assessment
• Assess history of hypersensitivity to methadone, related drugs
• Assess pain (type, location, intensity)
• Assess baseline VS
• Assess GI and renal function (BUN, creatinine, I&O)
Interventions
• Administer PO with food or milk to minimize GI irritation; for pts in chronic severe pain, oral sol containing 5-10 mg/5 ml is recommended on a fixed-dosage schedule
• IM is preferred parenteral route for repeated doses; SC administration may cause local irritation; rotate injection sites
• Determine dosage interval based on pt response
• Administer when pain is not too severe to enhance effectiveness
• Around-the-clock dosing may be more effective than prn administration
• Concurrent administration with non-narcotic analgesics may have additive analgesic effects and permit lower narcotic dosages
• Institute safety measures (support ambulation, raise siderails, call light within reach)

> **NURSING ALERT**
> Cumulative effects of this medication may necessitate periodic dosage adjustments
>
> To prevent withdrawal symptoms, medication should be discontinued gradually after long-term use

Evaluation
• Evaluate therapeutic response (decrease in pain without significant side effects)
• Monitor VS, pain control 30-60 min after administration, CNS changes
• Evaluate side effects, hypersensitivity

PATIENT AND FAMILY EDUCATION
Teach/instruct
• To take as directed at prescribed intervals for prescribed length of time
• About best way to request medication if ordered prn
Warn/advise
• That drug may cause drowsiness or dizziness; orthostatic hypotension; make position changes slowly; seek assistance with ambulation
• To avoid concurrent use of alcohol, other CNS depressants
• To notify care provider of hypersensitivity, side effects
• Tolerance or dependence may occur with long term use
• Withdrawal symptoms may occur (nausea, vomiting, cramps, fever, faintness, anorexia) with discontinuation of drug
Encourage
• To cough, breath deeply, and move to avoid respiratory complications

STORAGE
• Store at room temp
• Protect from light

---

methenamine hippurate, methenamine mandelate

Brand Name(s): Hiprex, Urex (methenamine hippurate); Mandameth, Mandelamine (methenamine mandelate)

Classification: Urinary tract antiseptic (formaldehyde pro-drug)

Pregnancy Category: C

AVAILABLE PREPARATIONS
Oral susp: 250 mg/5 ml, 500 mg/5 ml
Granules: 1 g
Tabs: 500 mg, 1 g
Tabs (enteric-coated): 250 mg, 500 mg, 1 g
Tabs (film-coated): 500 mg, 1 g

ROUTES AND DOSAGES
Children 6-12 yr: PO Methenamine hippurate 25-50 mg/kg/24 hr divided q12h; methenamine mandelate 50-75 mg/kg/24 hr divided q6h
Adults: PO Methenamine hippurate 1 g bid; methenamine mandelate 1 g qid after meals and at hs

MECHANISM AND INDICATIONS
Antibacterial mechanism: Hydrolyzed in acidic urine to ammonia and formaldehyde (which are bactericidal)
Indications: Effective against UTIs caused by *E. coli, Klebsiella, Enterobacter, Proteus mirabilis, P. morganii, Serratia, Citrobacter*

PHARMACOKINETICS
Peak: 2 hr
Half-life: 3-6 hr
Metabolism: Liver
Excretion: Urine

CONTRAINDICATIONS AND PRECAUTIONS
• Contraindicated with known hypersensitivity to methenamine hippurate or methenamine mandelate; with severe renal or he-

---

patic impairment, severe dehydration
• Use cautiously with history of renal disease; with pregnancy, lactation

INTERACTIONS
Drug
• Decreased effectiveness with use of urine alkalinizing agents ($NaHCO_3$ acetazolamide)
• Insoluble precipitate in urine with use of sulfonamides
Lab
• False elevation in catecholamine and 17-OHCS
• False decrease in 5-hydroxyindoleacetic acid and estriol
• Abnormal liver function tests

SIDE EFFECTS
DERM: Rashes
GI: Nausea, vomiting, diarrhea
GU: Urinary tract irritation, dysuria, urinary frequency, hematuria, albuminuria

PATIENT CARE MANAGEMENT
Assessment
• Assess history of hypersensitivity to methenamine hippurate or methenamine mandelate
• Obtain C&S; may begin therapy before obtaining results
• Assess I&O, urine pH (<5.5 for maximum effect), hepatic function (ALT, AST, bilirubin)
Interventions
• Administer PO after meals to reduce GI distress
• Shake susp well before administering; tab may be crushed, mixed with food or fluid; enteric- and film-coated tabs should be swallowed whole
• Maintain urine pH <5.5; large doses of ascorbic acid (6-12 g/24 hr) may be necessary
• Maintain adequate hydration with high fluid intake to prevent crystalluria
Evaluation
• Evaluate therapeutic response (decreased urinary pain, frequency, urgency, negative culture)
• Monitor I&O, urine pH, hematuria, hepatic function (ALT, AST, bilirubin)

• Monitor for allergic reaction (fever, flushing, rash, urticaria, pruritus)

PATIENT AND FAMILY EDUCATION
Teach/instruct
• To take as directed at prescribed intervals for prescribed length of time
Warn/advise
• To notify care provider of hypersensitivity, side effects
• To maintain high fluid intake
• Not to take antacids, alkalinizing agents, $NaHCO_3$
• To eat foods that acidify urine (meats, eggs, fish, gelatin products, prunes, plums, cranberries); to avoid alkaline foods (vegetables, milk, peanuts)

STORAGE
• Store at room temp

---

methicillin sodium
Brand Name(s): Staphcillin
Classification: Antibiotic (penicillinase-resistant penicillin)
Pregnancy Category: B

AVAILABLE PREPARATIONS
Inj: 1 g, 4 g, 6 g, 10 g
ROUTES AND DOSAGES
Meningitis
Neonates 0-4 wk, <1200 g: IM/IV 50 mg/kg/dose q12h
Neonates ≤7 days, <2000 g: IM/IV 50 mg/kg/dose q12h
Neonates >7 days, <2000 g: IM/IV 50 mg/kg/dose q8h
Neonates <7 days, >2000 g: IM/IV 50 mg/kg q8h
Neonates >7 days, >2000 g: IM/IV 50 mg/kg/dose q6h
Infants >1 mo-children <40 kg: IM/IV 100-400 mg/kg/24 hr divided q4-6h
Adults: IM/IV 4-12 g/24 hr divided q4-6h; maximum 12 g/24 hr
Other Infections
Neonates 0-4 wk, <1200 g: IM/IV 25 mg/kg/dose q12h
Neonates ≤7 days, <2000 g: IM/IV 25 mg/kg/dose q12h

Neonates >7 days, <2000 g: IM/IV 25 mg/kg/dose q8h
Neonates <7 days, >2000 g: IM/IV 25 mg/kg q8h
Neonates >7 days, >2000 g: IM/IV 25 mg/kg/dose q6h
Infants >1 mo-children <40 kg: IM/IV 100-400 mg/kg/24 hr divided q4-6h
Adults: IM/IV 4-12 g/24 hr divided q4-6h; maximum 12 g/24 hr
IV administration
• Recommended concentration: 2-20 mg/ml in D_5NS, $D_5\frac{1}{2}NS$, D_5W, LR, NS, or SW
• Maximum concentration: 20 mg/ml
• IV push rate: 200 mg/ml in older children, adults
• Intermittent infusion rate: Over 15-30 min

MECHANISM AND INDICATIONS
Antibiotic mechanism: Bactericidal; inhibits bacterial cell wall synthesis by adhering to bacterial penicillin-binding proteins
Indications: Effective against gram-positive cocci, including *Staphylococcus aureus, Streptococcus pyogenes, Str. viridans, Str. faecalis, Str. bovis,* and *Str. pneumoniae,* and infections caused by penicillinase-producing *Staphylococcus;* used to treat meningitis, respiratory tract, skin, soft tissue, bone, joint infections

PHARMACOKINETICS
Peak: IM 0.5 hr; IV end of infusion
Distribution: Into body tissue, fluids, CNS (only with inflamed meninges)
Half-life: Neonates 0.9-3.9 hr; children 0.8-1.6 hr
Metabolism: Liver
Excretion: Urine, bile
Therapeutic level: 0.81-6.3 mcg/ml

CONTRAINDICATIONS AND PRECAUTIONS
• Contraindicated with known hypersensitivity to methicillin, penicillins, cephalosporins
• Use cautiously in neonates; with impaired renal function; with history of colitis or other GI disorders; with pregnancy

INTERACTIONS
Drug
• Synergistic antimicrobial activity against certain organisms with aminoglycosides
• Increased serum concentrations with probenecid
• Decreased effectiveness with tetracyclines, erythromycins, chloramphenicol
Lab
• False positive serum uric acid
• False positive Coombs' test
• False positive urine protein

INCOMPATIBILITIES
• Aminophylline, ascorbic acid, cephalothin, chloramphenicol, chlorpromazine, codeine, hydrocortisone sodium succinate, levorphanol, lincomycin, metaraminol, methadone, methohexital, morphine, promethazine, sodium bicarbonate, vancomycin

SIDE EFFECTS
CNS: Neuropathy; seizures with high dosages
GI: Glossitis, stomatitis, pseudomembranous colitis, intrahepatic cholestasis, diarrhea
GU: Interstitial nephritis
HEME: Eosinophilia, hemolytic anemia, transient neutropenia, thrombocytopenia, agranulocytosis
Local: Vein irritation, thrombophlebitis
Other: Hypersensitivity reactions (chills, fever, edema, rash, urticaria, anaphylaxis), bacterial or fungal superinfection

TOXICITY AND OVERDOSE
Clinical signs: Neuromuscular irritability, seizures
Treatment: Supportive care; gastric lavage; minimally removed by hemodialysis

PATIENT CARE MANAGEMENT
Assessment
• Assess history of hypersensitivity to methicillin, penicillin, cephalosporins
• Obtain C&S; may begin therapy before obtaining results
• Assess renal function (BUN, cre-

atinine, I&O), hepatic function (ALT, AST, bilirubin), hematologic function (CBC, differential, platelet count), particularly for long-term therapy

Interventions
• Administer penicillins at least 1 hr before bacteriostatic antibiotics (tetracyclines, erythromycins, chloramphenicol)
• Discard reconstituted sol that has darkened to deep orange and developed hydrogen sulfide odor at room temp
• IM injection is painful; administer slowly and deeply into large muscle mass, rotate injection sites
• Do not mix IV with any other drug and only with sol per package insert; infuse separately
• Use large vein with small-bore needle to reduce local reaction; rotate site q48-72h
• Maintain age-appropriate fluid intake

NURSING ALERT
Discontinue if signs of hypersensitivity, interstitial nephritis, pseudomembranous colitis develop

Do not infuse rapidly; seizures may develop

Evaluation
• Evaluate therapeutic response (decreased symptoms of infection)
• Monitor for signs of superinfection (perineal itching, diaper rash, fever, malaise, redness, pain, swelling, drainage, rash, diarrhea, sore throat, change in cough or sputum)
• Observe for sign of allergic reactions (wheezing, tightness in chest, urticaria), especially within 15-30 min of first dose
• Monitor renal function (BUN, creatinine, I&O), hepatic function (ALT, AST, bilirubin), electrolyte levels, particularly K^+ and Na
• Monitor for signs of bleeding (ecchymosis, bleeding gums, hematuria, daily stool guaiac); monitor pro-times and platelet counts

• Evaluate IM site for tissue damage, IV site for vein irritation

PATIENT AND FAMILY EDUCATION
Teach/instruct
• To take as directed at prescribed intervals for prescribed length of time
Warn/advise
• To notify care provider of hypersensitivity, side effects, superinfection

STORAGE
• Store powder at room temp
• Reconstituted IM sol stable refrigerated 4 days, room temp 3 days
• IV sol stable at room temp 4 hr at dilution 2 mg/ml, 8 hr at dilution 10-30 mg/ml; label date, time, dilution

---

methimazole
Brand Name(s): Tapazole✤
Classification: Antithyroid agent
Pregnancy Category: D

M

AVAILABLE PREPARATIONS
Tabs: 5 mg, 10 mg

ROUTES AND DOSAGES
Children: PO initial dose 0.4 mg/kg/24 hr divided q8h; maintenance 0.2 mg/kg/24 hr divided q8h; maximum 30 mg/24 hr
Adults: PO initial dose 15-60 mg/24 hr divided q8h; maintenance 5-30 mg/24 hr divided q8h

MECHANISM AND INDICATIONS
Antithyroid mechanism: Inhibits synthesis of thyroid hormone and iodothyronine; does not affect stored T_4 and T_3
Indications: Used to treat hyperthyroidism

PHARMACOKINETICS
Onset of action: 30-40 min
Peak: 1 hr
Half-life: 5-13 hr
Metabolism: Liver
Excretion: Urine, bile

✤ Available in Canada.

CONTRAINDICATIONS AND PRECAUTIONS
• Contraindicated with hypersensitivity to drug, pregnancy (3rd trimester), lactation
• Use cautiously in pts at risk for agranulocytosis; with hepatic disease, pregnancy (1st and 2nd trimesters), doses >40 mg/24 hr

INTERACTIONS
Drug
• Increased effects of anticoagulants
• Increased risk of agranulocytosis with bone marrow depressants
• Increased risk of hepatic toxicity with hepatotoxic agents
Lab
• Hypoprothrombinemia and bleeding possible
• Altered pancreas, thyroid function tests

SIDE EFFECTS
CNS: Headache, paresthesias, drowsiness, vertigo
DERM: Rash, urticaria, pruritus, lupus-like syndrome, hyperpigmentation
GI: Diarrhea, nausea, vomiting, hepatitis, jaundice
GU: Nephritis
Other: Agranulocytosis, leukopenia, granulocytopenia, thrombocytopenia

TOXICITY AND OVERDOSE
Clinical signs: Nausea, vomiting, epigastric distress, fever, headache, joint pain, pruritus, edema
Treatment: Supportive treatment

PATIENT CARE MANAGEMENT
Assessment
• Assess history of hypersensitivity to methimazole, related drugs
• Assess T_3, T_4, TSH, CBC, pulse, BP, wt, temp, symptoms of hyperthyroidism
Interventions
• Tabs may be crushed, mixed with food or fluids
• Administer with meals to decrease GI distress
• Administer at consistent times to maintain adequate drug serum levels
• Discontinue 4 wk before radioactive iodine uptake test

NURSING ALERT
Can cause agranulocytosis; pt's complaints of fever, sore throat, mouth sores should be evaluated immediately

---

Evaluation
• Evaluate therapeutic response (wt gain; decreased pulse, B/P, T_4)
• Monitor for signs of bone marrow suppression (sore throat, fever, fatigue)
• Monitor for signs of overdose (peripheral edema, heat intolerance, diaphoresis, palpitations, arrhythmias, severe tachycardia, increased temp, CNS irritability)
• Monitor for signs of hypersensitivity (rash, enlarged cervical lymph nodes)
• Monitor for signs of hypoprothrombinemia (bleeding, petechiae, ecchymosis)
• Monitor CBC, pulse, B/P

PATIENT AND FAMILY EDUCATION
Teach/instruct
• To take as directed at prescribed intervals for prescribed length of time
Warn/advise
• To notify care provider of hypersensitivity, side effects (especially rash, sore throat, fever, mouth sores)
• To notify care provider of symptoms of hypo- or hyperthyroidism
• That response may take several mo of therapy
• To avoid use of OTC drugs or any medications (particularly those containing iodine) unless directed by care provider
• To avoid iodine food, iodized salt, soy beans, tofu, turnips, some seafood and breads
• Not to discontinue medication abruptly; thyroid crisis may occur

STORAGE
• Store at room temp
• Protect from heat, humidity, light

♣ Available in Canada.

methocarbamol

Brand Name(s): Delaxin, Marbaxin, Robaxin❦, Robaxin Injectable❦, Robaxin-750❦, Robaxisal, Robomol

Classification: Skeletal muscle relaxant

Pregnancy Category: C

AVAILABLE PREPARATIONS
Tabs: 500 mg, 750 mg
Inj: 100 mg/ml

ROUTES AND DOSAGES
Tetanus
Children: IV 15 mg/kg/dose; may repeat q6h prn; maximum 1.8 g/m^2/24 hr for 3 days only
Adults: 1-2 g by direct IV, followed by additional 1-2 g; repeat with 1-2 g q6h until NG tube or oral treatment possible
Muscle Spasm
Adults: PO 1.5 g qid; IM/IV 1 g q8h; maximum 3 g/24 hr for 3 consecutive days
IV administration
• Recommended concentration: May give undiluted
• IV push rate: Not to exceed 300 mg/min
• Intermittent infusion rate: May dilute as desired in D$_5$W or NS

MECHANISM AND INDICATIONS
Mechanism: CNS depressant, also has skeletal muscle relaxant effects
Indications: For use in treatment of acute muscle spasm; tetanus management

PHARMACOKINETICS
Onset of action: PO <30 min; IV immediate
Peak: 1-2 hr
Half-life: 0.9-1.8 hr
Metabolism: Liver
Excretion: Urine

CONTRAINDICATIONS AND PRECAUTIONS
• Contraindicated with known hypersensitivity to drug
• Use cautiously with renal disease, liver disease, seizures, myasthenia gravis, pregnancy, lactation

INTERACTIONS
Drug
• Increased CNS depression with alcohol, narcotics, anxiolytics, tricyclic antidepressants, psychotics
Lab
• False increase for VMA, urinary 5 HIAA

INCOMPATIBILITIES
• Incompatible with other drugs in sol or syringe

SIDE EFFECTS
CNS: Drowsiness, lightheadedness, syncope, vertigo, seizures
CV: Hypotension, bradycardia
DERM: Phlebitis, pain at injection site, sloughing with IV extravasation
EENT: Diplopia, nystagmus, blurred vision, conjunctivitis, nasal congestion
GI: Nausea, vomiting, anorexia, metallic taste
GU: Discoloration of urine (black, blue, brown, green)
HEME: Hemolysis
Other: Hypersensitivity reactions

TOXICITY AND OVERDOSE
Clinical signs: Extreme drowsiness, cardiac arrhythmias, nausea, vomiting
Treatment: Induce emesis, gastric lavage, maintain airway, have emergency equipment and medications available

PATIENT CARE MANAGEMENT
Assessment
• Assess history of hypersensitivity to drug
• Assess CBC, differential, liver function (AST, ALT, bilirubin)
• Assess baseline VS, B/P
Interventions
• Do not administer SC
• Keep pt supine 10-15 min after IV administration; assist with ambulation
• Obtain VS, B/P frequently during IV administration

M

> **NURSING ALERT**
> Do not use in children <12 yr
> except for management of
> tetanus

Evaluation
- Evaluate therapeutic response (decreased spasticity, pain)
- Evaluate for extravasation; discontinue immediately, inform care provider
- Evaluate side effects (especially levels of CNS depression)

PATIENT AND FAMILY EDUCATION
Teach/instruct
- To take as directed at prescribed intervals for prescribed length of time
- That drug may discolor urine
- That drug may cause dizziness and drowsiness; to use caution in hazardous activities; to rise slowly from lying position
- Not to take drug with alcohol, other CNS or OTC drugs

STORAGE
- Store at room temp

---

methotrexate

Brand Name(s): Amethopterin, Folex, Mexate

Classification: Antimetabolite (folic acid antagonist)

Pregnancy Category: D

AVAILABLE PREPARATIONS
Tabs: 2.5 mg (scored)
Inj (sodium): 2.5 mg/ml, 25 mg/ml
Inj (sodium, preservative free): 25 mg
Inj (powder, sodium): 20 mg, 25 mg, 50 mg, 100 mg, 250 mg

ROUTES AND DOSAGES
- Drug may vary in response to diagnosis, extent of disease, concurrent or previous therapy, protocol guidelines, physiologic parameters; consult current literature, protocol recommendations

Juvenile Rheumatoid Arthritis
Children: PO/IM 5-15 mg/m^2/wk as single dose or in 3 divided doses 12 hr apart

Rheumatoid Arthritis
Adults: PO 7.5 mg once weekly or 2.5 mg q12h for 3 doses/wk; maximum 20 mg/wk

Acute Lymphoblastic Leukemia
Children and adolescents: PO/IM/IV induction 3.3 mg/m^2 24 hr for 4-6 wk or until remission occurs; maintenance 20-30 mg/m^2 (2.5 mg/kg) q wk or 2 ×/wk

Burkitt's Lymphoma
Children and adolescents: PO 10-25 mg/24 hr for 4-8 days with 1 wk rest intervals; may also give IV or IM

Osteosarcoma
Children and adolescents: IV 12 g/m^2 (maximum 20 g) administered over 4 hr repeated weekly × 2 with leucovorin rescue

Meningeal Leukemia
Intrathecally 10-15 mg/m^2 (maximum 12-15 mg); may be administered every 2-5 days until the CSF has cleared; remove CSF volume approximately equivalent to volume of methotrexate to be instilled, inject over 30-60 sec and only if easy flow of blood-free spinal fluid

IV administration
- Recommended concentration: Reconstitute each 5 mg with 2 ml preservative-free D$_5$W or NS
- Maximum concentration: 25 mg/ml; may further dilute with D$_5$W or NS before use as high dosage methotrexate

MECHANISM AND INDICATIONS
Mechanism: Blocks the enzyme dihydrofolate reductase (DHFR) which inhibits conversion of folic acid to tetrahydrofolic acid resulting in inhibition of the key precursors of DNA, RNA, and cellular proteins; may synchronize malignant cells in the S-phase; at high plasma levels, passive entry of the drug into the tumor cells can potentially overcome drug resistance
Indications: Used in treatment of ALL, osteogenic sarcoma, Bur-

---

kitt's lymphoma; juvenile rheumatoid arthritis

PHARMACOKINETICS

Onset of action: 3-12 hr
Peak: IV immediately after injection; IM within 0.5-1 hr; PO 1-4 hr
Distribution: Widely distributed into body tissues, with highest concentration in kidneys, gall bladder, spleen, liver, skin
Half-life: Plasma 2 hr; terminal 8-15 hr
Absorption: Completely absorbed from GI tract
Metabolism: Liver
Excretion: Urine; small amounts feces, bile

CONTRAINDICATIONS AND PRECAUTIONS

• Contraindicated with known hypersensitivity to drug, pregnancy, lactation
• Use cautiously and at modified dosage with impaired hepatic or renal function, bone marrow suppression, aplasia, leukopenia, thrombocytopenia, anemia, infection, peptic ulcer, ulcerative colitis; in very young, elderly, or debilitated pts

INTERACTIONS

Drug

• Increased risk of toxicity with salicylates, sulfonamides, phenytoin, some antibacterials (tetracycline, chloramphenicol), alcohol, PABA, NSAIDs, probenecid
• Decreased serum phenytoin levels possible
• Antagonized methotrexate effect with folic acid derivatives
• Decreased immune response to routine immunizations
• Decreased effectiveness of methotrexate with use of folic acid preparations (including vitamins)

INCOMPATIBILITIES

• Incompatible with bleomycin, fluorouracil, idarubicin, metoclopramide, prednisolone, ranitidine

SIDE EFFECTS

CNS: Arachnoiditis within hours of intrathecal administration; subacute neurotoxicity, necrotizing demyelinating leukoencephalopathy (a few years later), headache, drowsiness, dizziness, confusion, blurred vision
DERM: Urticaria, pruritus, hyperpigmentation, melena, erythematous rashes, folliculitis, vasculitis, dermatitis, photosensitivity
EENT: Pharyngitis, gingivitis, mucositis, tinnitus
GI: Stomatitis, nausea, vomiting, diarrhea, anorexia, ulcerations and bleeding of mucous membranes, acute hepatic toxicity (elevated transaminase levels), chronic hepatic toxicity (cirrhosis, hepatic fibrosis, atrophy)
GU: Nephropathy, tubular necrosis, infertility, spontaneous abortion
HEME: WBC and platelet count nadirs, anemia, leukopenia, thrombocytopenia (all are dose related), myelosuppression
RESP: Pulmonary fibrosis, pulmonary interstitial infiltrates, pneumonitis, cough, dyspnea, chest pain, hypoxemia
Other: Alopecia, hyperuricemia, osteoporosis (in children with long-term use), chills, fever, undue fatigue, malaise, myalgias

TOXICITY AND OVERDOSE

Clinical signs: Urinary pH <7; with high dosages, urine should be alkalinized (pH >7) before, during, and after drug administration because methotrexate is a weak acid that can crystallize in the kidneys with an acid pH
Treatment: Adequate pre- and post-hydration must also be administered during high-dose therapy, with leucovorin rescue administered on time to prevent excessive toxicity and facilitate maximum therapeutic response to methotrexate

PATIENT CARE MANAGEMENT

Assessment

• Assess history of hypersensitivity to methotrexate
• Assess baseline VS, CBC, differential, platelet count, renal function (BUN, creatinine, I&O), hepatic function (ALT, AST, LDH,

M

bilirubin, alk phos), pulmonary function
• Assess hydration status, fluid and electrolyte balance
• Assess neurologic status
• Assess success of previous antiemetic therapy
• Assess history of previous treatment with special attention to other therapies that may predispose to renal, pulmonary, or hepatic dysfunction

Interventions
• Premedicate with antiemetics and continue periodically through chemotherapy
• Offer small, frequent feedings of foods pt likes
• Administer IV fluids until pt able to resume normal PO intake
• Administer leucovorin calcium within 12 hr to prevent tissue damage
• Provide measures to maintain hemostasis, fluid and electrolyte balance, nutritional support

> **NURSING ALERT**
>
> Teach and encourage diligent mouth care to decrease risk of superinfection in mouth
>
> Leucovorin rescue is necessary with high dosage of methotrexate and should be administered as ordered; do not skip or hold doses; if unable to take PO, obtain IV order immediately
>
> Warn pts to stay out of direct sunlight; use highly protective sunblock when exposed

Evaluate
• Evaluate therapeutic response (decreased tumor size, spread of malignancy)
• Monitor CBC, differential, platelet count, renal function (BUN, creatinine, I&O), hepatic function (ALT, AST, LDH, bilirubin, alk phos)
• Evaluate CNS effects of drug (dizziness, blurred vision, malaise)
• Evaluate pt for back and flank pain; if necessary, slow down infusion; if pain occurs, give analgesics

(don't use ASA, NSAIDs as they displace methotrexate from serum albumin)
• Evaluate for symptoms of increased CSF pressure (seizures, paresis, headache, nausea, vomiting, fever, brain atrophy)
• Evaluate for signs of infection or bleeding
• Evaluate I&O carefully, check wt daily
• Evaluate side effects, response to antiemetic regimen

PATIENT AND FAMILY EDUCATION
Teach/instruct
• To have pt well-hydrated before and after chemotherapy
• About importance of follow-up to monitor blood counts, serum chemistry values, drug blood values
• To take accurate temp; rectal temp contraindicated
• To notify care provider of signs of bleeding (bruising, epistaxis, bleeding gums), infection (fever, sore throat, fatigue)
• To take leucovorin as ordered on schedule; not to stop taking drug until instructed by care provider
• To report any cough or dyspnea
Warn/advise
• About impact of body changes that may occur (hair loss, hyperpigmentation, nail ridging), how to minimize changes (wigs, caps, scarves, long sleeves)
• To avoid OTC products containing aspirin
• To avoid sun if possible; wear sunscreen, long sleeves or pants
• To report any alterations in behavior, sensation, perception; help to develop a plan of care to manage side effects, stress of illness or treatment
• To immediately report any CNS effects or symptoms of increased CSF pressure (headache, dizziness, nausea or vomiting, blurred vision, malaise) to care provider
• To monitor bowel function and call care provider if abdominal pain or constipation are noted
• To immediately report any pain,

discoloration at injection site (parenteral forms)
- That good oral hygiene with very soft toothbrush is imperative
- That dental work be delayed until blood counts return to baseline, with permission of care provider
- To avoid contact with known viral, bacterial illnesses
- That household contacts of child not be immunized with live polio virus; inactivated form should be used
- That child not receive immunizations until immune system recovers sufficiently to mount needed antibody response
- To report exposure to chicken pox in susceptible child immediately
- To report reactivation of herpes zoster virus (shingles) immediately
- If appropriate, ways to preserve reproductive patterns, sexuality (sperm banking, contraceptives)

Encourage
- Provision of nutritional food intake; consider nutritional consultation
- To comply with bowel management program
- To maintain adequate fluid intake, to void frequently
- To use top anesthetics to control discomfort of mucositis; avoid spicy foods, commercial mouthwashes

STORAGE
- Store at room temp
- Protect from light, moisture
- If prepared without preservative, use sol immediately; may be stable for up to 14 days with preservative

methyldopa

Brand Name(s): Aldomet♣, Amodopa tabs, Apo-Methyldopa♣, Novo-Medopa♣, Nu-Medopa♣

Classification: Antihypertensive

Pregnancy Category: B

AVAILABLE PREPARATIONS
Tabs: 125 mg, 250 mg, 500 mg
PO susp: 250 mg/5 ml
Inj: 250 mg/5 ml

ROUTES AND DOSAGES
Management of Hypertension
Children: PO 10 mg/kg/24 hr divided q6-12h; increase prn q2h; maximum 65 mg/kg/24 hr or 3 g/24 hr, whichever is less
Adults: PO 250-750 mg q8-12h
Hypertensive Crisis
Children: IV initial 2-4 mg/kg/dose; if no effect in 4-6 hr, double the dose; maintenance 20-40 mg/kg/24 hr divided q6-8h
Adults: IV initial 2-4 mg/kg/dose; if no effect in 4-6 hr, double the dose; maintenance 250-1000 mg q6h

IV administration
- Recommended concentration: Dilute dose in 50-100 ml D_5W or use 10 mg/ml
- Maximum concentration: 10 mg/ml
- IV push rate: Not recommended
- Intermittent infusion rate: Over 30-60 min

MECHANISM AND INDICATIONS
Mechanism: Stimulates inhibitory α-adrenergic receptors, acting as false transmitter, resulting in decreased arterial pressure
Indications: For use in hypertension

PHARMACOKINETICS
Onset: PO peak 2-4 hr, duration 12-24 hr; IV peak 2 hr, duration 10-16 hr
Metabolism: Liver, intestines
Excretion: Urine

CONTRAINDICATIONS AND PRECAUTIONS

• Contraindicated with hypersensitivity to drug, hepatic disease, blood dyscrasias
• Use cautiously with diuretics and other antihypertensives, renal failure, lactation

INTERACTIONS
Drug
• Increased hypoglycemia with tolbutamide
• Increased action of anesthetics
• Increased antihypertensive effect with other antihypertensives, fenfluramine, verapamil
• Decreased effect of phenothiazines or tricyclic antidepressants
• Dementia and sedation possible with haloperidol
Lab
• False elevation of urine catecholamine
• Altered uric acid, serum creatinine, AST levels

INCOMPATIBILITIES
• Incompatible with amphotericin B, methohexital, tetracycline

SIDE EFFECTS
CNS: Headache, sedation, weakness, dizziness, decreased mental acuity, involuntary choreoathetoid movements, nightmares, depression, psychic disturbances
CV: Bradycardia, orthostatic hypotension, aggravated angina, edema, wt gain, myocarditis
EENT: Dry mouth, nasal stuffiness
GI: Diarrhea, pancreatitis, GI upset, hepatic necrosis (rare)
HEME: Hemolytic anemia, reversible granulocytopenia, thrombocytopenia, leukopenia
Other: Gynecomastia, rash, drug induced fever, impotence

TOXICITY AND OVERDOSE
Clinical signs: Sedation, hypotension, impaired AV conduction, coma
Treatment: Induce emesis, gastric lavage, administer activated charcoal, treat symptomatically and supportively

PATIENT CARE MANAGEMENT
Assessment
• Assess history of hypersensitivity to drug
• Assess CBC and differential, platelet count, renal function (protein, BUN, creatinine), liver function (AST, ALT, bilirubin), VS, B/P before, during, after treatment
Interventions
• Infuse IV dose slowly with infusion pump over 30-60 min, concentration ≤10 mg/ml
• Check B/P q 30 min (minimum) during IV infusion
• Monitor I&O, daily wt
Evaluation
• Evaluate therapeutic response (decreased B/P)
• Evaluate for signs of tolerance which may develop after 2-3 wk

PATIENT AND FAMILY EDUCATION
Teach/instruct
• To take as directed at prescribed intervals for prescribed length of time
• About adverse effects, to report immediately to care provider
• To avoid sudden position changes
Warn/advise
• To take drug at hs to reduce sedating effects
• To avoid hazardous activities

STORAGE
• Store in tight containers

---

methylphenidate hydrochloride

Brand Name(s): Methidate, PMS-Methylphenidate♣, Ritalin♣, Ritalin-SR♣

Classification: Central nervous system stimulant

Controlled Substance Schedule II

Pregnancy Category: C

AVAILABLE PREPARATIONS
Tabs: 5 mg, 10 mg, 20 mg
Tabs: Sus rel 20 mg

DOSAGES AND ROUTES
Attention Deficit Disorder
• Medication is prescribed for some children <6 yr; safety and effectiveness not established

Children 6-12 yr: PO initial 0.3 mg/kg/dose 2.5-5 mg/dose given on school days before breakfast and lunch; increase by 0.1 mg/kg/dose or by 5-10 mg/24 hr at weekly intervals, checking for clinical effects; a 3rd dose may be added at 4 PM; administration on weekends and during vacations is determined by need; usual dose 0.5-1 mg/kg/24 hr (5-20 mg/dose), maximum dose 2 mg/kg/24 hr or 60 mg/24 hr

Children >12 yr: PO usual dosage range 5-20 mg bid-tid

Narcolepsy
Children >12 yr: PO 10 mg bid-tid, 30-45 min ac; may increase to 40-60 mg/24 hr

MECHANISM AND INDICATIONS
Mechanism: Blocks reuptake mechanism of dopaminergic neurons, increases release of norepinephrine, exact action unknown; may prevent flooding of sensory impulses into the cortex so they enter in a more integrated manner; resulting stimulation of the brain improves alertness and concentration, increases attention span and learning ability

Indications: Used as drug of first choice for treating attention deficit disorder (ADD) and attention deficit disorder with hyperactivity (ADHD) in children and adolescents; also effective in control of narcolepsy, to treat children with behavior problems such as severe distractibility, short attention span, impulsive behavior, mild-to-moderate depression, extreme mood changes that are not stress-induced

PHARMACOKINETICS
Onset of action: ½-1 hr; for narcolepsy, ADD, ADHD continual use on a regular schedule for 3-4 wk is usually necessary to determine this drug's effectiveness

Half-life: 2-4 hr
Duration: 3-6 hr; 8 hr for sus rel tabs; sus rel not as effective in some children, its duration of action may not be as long as equivalent of 10 mg of methylphenidate in the AM and at noon
Absorption: Slow and incomplete from GI tract
Metabolism: Liver
Excretion: Urine, feces

CONTRAINDICATIONS AND PRECAUTIONS
• Contraindicated with hypersensitivity to methylphenidate or any component; lactation; Tourette syndrome or family history of Tourette syndrome; glaucoma; motor tics; members of family with known and untreated substance abuse disorders; in pts experiencing agitation; with moderate-to-severe anxiety; nervous tension, emotional depression
• Use cautiously with angina, cardiac disease, EEG abnormalities, history of alcoholism or drug dependence, hypertension, psychosis, seizures, severe depression, taking or have taken in past 14 days any MAOIs

INTERACTIONS
Drug
• Increased effects of tricyclic antidepressants, coumarin, ephedrine, imipramine, primidone, phenobarbital, phenybutazine, phenytoin, pseudoephedrine, warfarin
• Decreased effects of bretylium, guanethidine
• Significant change in seizure pattern possible with anticonvulsants; dosage adjustments may be necessary for proper control
• MAOIs may potentiate effects of methylphenidate; do not use within 14 days of MAOIs or vasopressors
• Interaction with isocarboxazid, pargyline, phenelzine, phenylbutazone, selegiline, tranylcypromine

Lab
• Increased prothrombin time
• Decreased RBC, WBC, or platelet counts

Nutrition
• Excessive rise in B/P possible with tyramine; avoid foods high in tyramine (aged cheeses, sausages, cured fish and meats, liver; beverages prepared from meat or meat extracts)
• Increased irritability and stimulation possible with coffee, tea, cola, chocolate
• Avoid drinking alcohol

SIDE EFFECTS
CNS: Hyperactivity, insomnia, restlessness, talkativeness, akathisia, depression, dizziness, drowsiness, dyskinesia, dysphoria, headache, irritability, lethargy, mania, motor tics, nervousness, psychosis, seizures, tearfulness, Tourette syndrome, unusual movements, zombie-like appearance
CV: Palpitations, tachycardia, arrhythmias, chest pain, hypertension, hypotension
DERM: Bruising, erythema multiforme, hives, peeling skin, rash, red skin, scalp hair loss, purpura
EENT: Bleeding gums, blurred vision
GI: Abdominal discomfort, anorexia, dry mouth, nausea, weight loss
GU: Uremia
HEME: Anemia, eosinophilia, leukopenia, thrombocytopenia
Other: Erythema, fever, interdose rebound of ADHD symptoms, joint pain, potential for serious psychological dependence, possible slowing of growth in childhood (growth rebound occurs during drug holidays), paradoxical reactions with aggravation of initial symptoms for which the drug was prescribed

TOXICITY AND OVERDOSE
Clinical signs: Agitation, coma, confusion, delirium, dry mouth, fever, hallucinations, headache, hypertension, hyperthermia, irritability, muscle twitching, paranoia, toxic psychosis, seizures, sweating, tachycardia, tremors, violence, vomiting
Treatment: Protect airway if unconscious or seizing; administer fluids; administer short-acting barbiturate before lavage; treat severe hypertension or tachyarrhythmias with propranolol, high fever with cooling blanket, seizure with IV benzodiazepines with repeated dosing if necessary; use adrenergic blocking agents judiciously; delirium or psychosis usually respond to an antipsychotic agent; hemodialysis or peritoneal dialysis

PATIENT CARE MANAGEMENT
Assessment
• Assess history of hypersensitivity to drug
• Obtain history of previous drug reactions and risk factors for developing motor tics or Tourette syndrome
• Obtain baseline height, wt, pulse, B/P, CBC, platelet counts, UA
• Assess height and wt and plot on growth grid
• If child has diabetes, obtain BG and urine glucose; insulin changes may be necessary with decreased appetite

Interventions
• Regular tab may be crushed; sus rel tab should not be crushed or chewed
• Regular tab usually prescribed bid, 30-45 min before breakfast and lunch; if 3rd dose needed, administer before 4 PM to avoid insomnia
• Sus rel tab is given qd, in early AM
• Administer dose(s) at same time every day
• If appetite is lost, may be given with or after breakfast and lunch
• For dry mouth rinse with water, take sips of fluid, sugarless gum, hard candy
• There should be drug holidays (periodic discontinuation of methylphenidate) when school is not in session, to assess pt's requirements and to decrease tolerance

and limit suppression of growth and wt
- If drug has been used for months or years, do not discontinue abruptly; supervise carefully during withdrawal to prevent severe depression and erratic behavior
- When medicine is stopped, there may be a withdrawal depression, with tearfulness or crying for no apparent reason

Evaluation
- Evaluate therapeutic response (ability to function in daily activities to sleep throughout the night and be awake throughout the day; concentration, hyperactivity; obtain parent and teacher reports about attention and behavioral performance)
- Discontinue drug if methylphenidate does not manage ADD within 1 mo
- Evaluate mental status (affect, aggressiveness, mood, sensorium, impulsiveness)
- Monitor pulse, B/P, height, wt, CBC, and platelet counts every 3 to 4 mos and at times of dosage increases
- Evaluate growth periodically
- Observe for signs of bleeding, bruising, abnormal movements at each visit
- If discontinuing drug, monitor for withdrawal symptoms (depression, headache, lethargy, muscle pain, nausea, increased sleeping, vomiting, weakness)

PATIENT AND FAMILY EDUCATION
Teach/instruct
- To take as directed at prescribed intervals for prescribed length of time
- That medication is most helpful when it is used as part of a comprehensive multimodal treatment program
- To not stop taking this medication without prescriber approval; must be tapered off under supervision of prescriber over several wk to minimize withdrawal symptoms

- That therapeutic effects may take 3-4 wk
- To increase fluids and fiber in diet if constipation occurs
- That methylphenidate does not appear to predispose pt to future substance abuse
- To make sure medication is swallowed

Warn/advise
- That pt may feel more tired at the end of the day and should get needed rest
- That consumption of caffeine, such as coffee, tea, cola, chocolate, may increase stimulation and irritability
- To avoid OTC medications unless approved by prescriber
- To avoid ingesting alcohol, other CNS depressants
- That medication may cause drowsiness; be careful on bicycles, skates, skateboards, while driving, with other activities requiring alertness
- To report any signs of bleeding, fever, sore throat, bruising
- To report changes in behavior, ability to concentrate
- About need for periodic drug-free holidays

STORAGE
- Store at room temp in a tightly covered, light-resistant container

M

---

methylprednisolone, methylprednisolone acetate, methylprednisolone sodium succinate

Brand Name(s): Depo-Medrol✤, Medrol, Solu-medrol✤

Classification: Glucocorticoid

Pregnancy Category: C

AVAILABLE PREPARATIONS
Tabs (methylprednisolone): 2 mg, 4 mg, 8 mg, 16 mg, 24 mg, 32 mg

---

Inj (methylprednisolone acetate): 20 mg/ml, 40 mg/ml, 80 mg/ml
Inj (methylprednisolone sodium succinate): 40 mg/vial, 125 mg/ vial, 500 mg/vial, 1 g/vial, 2 g/vial

ROUTES AND DOSAGES

• Depends on condition being treated and pt response; IM or IV therapy generally reserved for pts unable to take PO or for emergency situations
• Drug may vary in response to diagnosis, extent of disease, concurrent or previous therapy, protocol guidelines, physiologic parameters; consult current literature, protocol recommendations

Antiinflammatory/Immuno-suppressive
PO/IV/IM 0.16-0.8 mg/kg/24 hr divided q6-12h

Status Asthmaticus
Children: IV loading 1-2 mg/kg/ dose once; maintenance 0.5-1 mg/ kg/dose q6h
Adults: IM/IV 10-250 mg/dose q4-6h

IV administration

• Recommended concentration: 2.5 mg/ml in D_5NS, D_5W, or NS for IV infusion; 40, 62.5, 63.5, or 125 mg/ml for IV push (available commercially)
• Maximum concentration: 125 mg/ml for IV push
• IV push rate: Over 1-5 min for lower doses
• Intermittent infusion: Over 20-60 min

MECHANISM AND INDICATIONS

Mechanism: Decreases inflammation mainly by stabilizing leukocyte lysosomal membranes; suppresses immune response, stimulates bone marrow, influences protein, fat, and carbohydrate metabolism
Indications: Used for antiinflammatory or immunosuppressant effects in the treatment of hematologic, allergic, neoplastic, inflammatory, or autoimmune conditions

PHARMACOKINETICS

Onset of action: PO/IV rapid; IM slow

Peak: PO 1-2 hr; IM 4-8 days
Duration: PO 30-36 hr; IM 1-4 wk
Metabolism: Liver
Excretion: Inactive metabolites in urine; small amounts of unmetabolized drug in urine, bile

CONTRAINDICATIONS AND PRECAUTIONS

• Contraindicated with allergy to any component of the formulation, (certain injectable forms contain sulfites which can cause an allergic reaction in sensitive pts), with systemic fungal infections, acute or active infection, chicken pox, or herpes zoster
• Use cautiously with GI ulceration or renal disease, hypertension, osteoporosis, varicella, DM, seizures, CHF, emotional instability, psychotic tendencies, pregnancy

INTERACTIONS
Drug

• Increased risk of GI bleeding or distress with aspirin, indomethacin, other NSAIDs
• Decreased action of dexamethasone possible with barbiturates, phenytoin, rifampin
• Decreased effects of oral anticoagulants possible
• Enhanced K^+-wasting effects of methylprednisolone with K^+-depleting drugs such as thiazide diuretics
• Decreased response of skin-test antigens
• Decreased antibody response, increased risk of neurologic complications with toxoids and vaccines

SIDE EFFECTS

• Most reactions are dosage and duration dependent
CNS: Euphoria, insomnia, psychotic behavior, pseudotumor cerebri
CV: CHF, hypertension, edema
DERM: Delayed wound healing, acne, various skin eruptions
EENT: Cataracts, glaucoma
ENDO/METAB: Hypokalemia, hyperglycemia, glucose intolerance, growth suppression

---

✤ Available in Canada.

GI: Peptic ulcer, GI irritation, increased appetite, pancreatitis
Other: Muscle weakness, osteoporosis, hirsutism, susceptibility to infection; acute adrenal insufficiency may follow increased stress (infection, surgery, trauma) or abrupt withdrawal after long-term therapy; after abrupt withdrawal, there may be rebound inflammation, fatigue, weakness, arthralgia, fever, dizziness, lethargy, depression, fainting, orthostatic hypotension, dyspnea, anorexia, hypoglycemia; after prolonged use, sudden withdrawal may be fatal

TOXICITY AND OVERDOSE
Clinical signs: Acute ingestion is rarely a clinical problem
Treatment: Decrease drug gradually if possible

PATIENT CARE MANAGEMENT
Assessment
• Assess history of hypersensitivity to drug or related drugs
• Assess baseline VS (especially B/P), serum electrolytes (K+, Ca, BG), cardiac function, renal function (BUN, creatinine, urine CrCl), liver function (ALT, AST, LDH, bilirubin, alk phos)
• Assess baseline wt, I&O, hydration status (SG)
• Assess baseline neurologic and mental status before starting therapy
• Assess baseline growth and development status
• Assess history of previous treatment with special attention to other therapies that may predispose to renal, cardiac, or hepatic dysfunction
Interventions
• Administer PO with food to decrease GI upset
• Administer IM deeply in large muscle mass; rotate injection sites
• Monitor wt, VS (especially B/P), I&O

• Provide supportive measures to maintain, fluid and electrolyte balance, nutritional support
• Administer K+ supplements as indicated
• Provide low Na, high protein, high K+ diet

> **NURSING ALERT**
> Administer with food to decrease chances of GI irritation
>
> Provide low-Na diet high in K+ and protein
>
> Do not stop drug abruptly if pt has been on long-term therapy; must be titrated over time
>
> Do not confuse Solu-Medrol with Solu-Cortef hydrocortisone sodium succinate
>
> Avoid SC injection; atrophy and abscesses may develop

Evaluation
• Evaluate therapeutic response (decreased inflammation)
• Monitor VS (especially B/P), serum electrolytes (K+, BG, Ca)
• Monitor I&O, check wt regularly
• Evaluate for signs of depression or psychotic episodes, especially with high-dose therapy
• Evaluate BG in pts with history of diabetes
• Evaluate growth and development in children on prolonged therapy
• Evaluate for signs or symptoms of infection (fever, fatigue, sore throat)

PATIENT/FAMILY EDUCATION
Teach/instruct
• About importance of follow-up to monitor serum chemistry values
• To notify care provider of signs of infection (fever, sore throat, fatigue), delayed healing
• About the possibility of weakening bones (osteoporosis) and need for proper exercise, diet, limitations for pts on prolonged therapy

M

- Not to stop drug abruptly or without care provider's consent because of possible side effects
- To take medication in the AM with food for best results, less GI upset
- About cushingoid symptoms, to report sudden wt gain or swelling for pt and family of pt on long-term therapy

Warn/advise
- To avoid OTC products containing aspirin NSAIDs
- To report any alterations in behavior; help to develop a plan of care to manage side effects, stress of illness or treatment
- To immediately report any pain, discoloration at injection site (parenteral forms)
- To avoid contact with known viral, bacterial illnesses
- That household contacts of child not be immunized with live polio virus; inactivated form should be used
- That child not receive immunizations until immune system recovers sufficiently to mount needed antibody response
- To report exposure to chicken pox in susceptible child immediately
- To report reactivation of herpes zoster virus (shingles) immediately
- About signs and symptoms of adrenal insufficiency (fatigue, muscle weakness, joint pain, fever, anorexia, nausea, dyspnea, dizziness, fainting)
- That pts with diabetes may need more insulin while taking steroids; monitor BG carefully
- That pts on long-term therapy have periodic ophthal examinations
- To limit the amount of salt or salty foods when on steroids; Use low Na, high K+, high protein diet
- About impact of body changes that may occur (weight gain, Cushingoid syndrome), how to minimize them (loose clothing, decrease salt intake)

Encourage
- Pts experiencing excessive wt gain to decrease salt intake; to eat a high protein, high K+ diet; nutritional consultation may be needed
- To wear medical alert identification indicating steroid use

STORAGE
- Store at room temp in tight containers
- Protect from light

---

methysergide maleate
Brand Name(s): Sansert✤
Classification: Serotonin antagonist; ergot derivative
Pregnancy Category: X

AVAILABLE PREPARATIONS
Tabs: 2 mg

ROUTES AND DOSAGES
Adults: PO 4-8 mg/24 hr with meals; given for 3 wks; if no improvement drug is unlikely to be helpful; may only be taken over a 6-mo period, then a drug-free interval of 3-4 wk must follow before the next 6-mo course

MECHANISM AND INDICATIONS
Mechanism: Inhibits vasoconstrictor and pressor effects of 5-HT, blocks amine action on extravascular and smooth muscles, other cells; as an ergot derivative, it has some vasoconstrictor and oxytocic activity; it is not clear why methysergide is effective in migraine other vascular headaches; exact mechanism unknown
Indications: Useful for the prophylactic treatment of migraine and other vascular headaches; not helpful when given during the acute attack; has also been used to treat diarrhea and malabsorption in pts with carcinoid, and in postgastrectomy dumping syndrome (both of these conditions have a 5-HT-mediated component)

✤ Available in Canada.

PHARMACOKINETICS
Onset of action: 1-2 days
Peak: Unknown
Half-life: 10 hr
Metabolism: Liver
Excretion: Urine, as metabolites and unchanged drug

CONTRAINDICATIONS AND PRECAUTIONS
• Contraindicated with hypersensitivity to ergot and tartrazine (some preparations contain tartrazine); with peripheral vascular disease, severe arteriosclerosis, pulmonary disease, severe hypertension, phlebitis, serious infections, pregnancy, lactation
• Use with caution with impairment of hepatic and renal function; pts who receive long-term therapy may develop retroperitoneal fibrosis, pleuropulmonary fibrosis, fibrotic thickening of cardiac valves; fibrosis has rarely occurred when therapy is interrupted for 3-4 wks q 6 mo

INTERACTIONS
Drug
• Increased vasoconstriction with β blockers
• Decreased effectiveness of narcotic analgesics

SIDE EFFECTS
CNS: Tremors, anxiety, overstimulation, insomnia, dizziness, mild euphoria, confusion, visual disturbances, paresthesias, drowsiness, lethargy, mental depression; rebound headaches may occur if methysergide is discontinued abruptly; drug should be discontinued gradually over 2-3 wk
CV: Retroperitoneal fibrosis, valvular thickening, palpitations, tachycardia, postural hypertension, angina, vascular insufficiency, thrombophlebitis, ECG changes, cardiac fibrosis

DERM: Flushing, rash, alopecia
GI: Nausea, vomiting, diarrhea, heartburn, abdominal pain, wt loss or gain; these symptoms may be decreased if taken with meals
MS: Arthralgia, myalgia
RESP: Pleuropulmonary fibrosis

TOXICITY AND OVERDOSE
Clinical signs: Hyperactivity, spasms in limbs, increased vasoconstriction beginning with cold extremities and weakness, impaired mental function, impaired circulation
Treatment: Discontinue medication; supportive care with symptomatic treatment

PATIENT CARE MANAGEMENT
Assessment
• Assess history of hypersensitivity to ergot, tartrazine
• Assess for presence of preexisting conditions that would contraindicate use (peripheral vascular disease, severe arteriosclerosis, pulmonary disease, severe hypertension, phlebitis, serious infections, pregnancy)
• Assess wt, VS (particularly B/P)
• Assess for any evidence of peripheral edema
• Assess characteristics of migraine including frequency, intensity, duration, precipitating foods or activities
Interventions
• Initially dosage needs to be titrated to pt's response; start with lower dosage and increase at weekly intervals up to 8 mg/24 hr
• Administer with meals to reduce GI symptoms

M

494 • metoclopramide

Signs and symptoms of toxicity
include hyperactivity, spasms
in limbs, increased vasoconstriction beginning with cold
extremities and weakness,
impaired mental function,
impaired circulation; stop
administration of drug; supportive care with symptomatic
treatment

It takes about 1-2 days for the
protective effects to develop,
and about as long for it to pass
off when treatment is ended;
rebound headaches not uncommon when treatment is stopped

Pts who receive long-term
therapy may develop retroperitoneal fibrosis, pleuropulmonary fibrosis, fibrotic thickening
of the cardiac valves; fibrosis
rarely occurs when therapy is
interrupted for 3-4 wk q 6 mo

Evaluation
• Evaluate therapeutic response
(decrease in frequency, intensity,
duration of headache)
• Evaluate periodically the effectiveness of treatment and monitor
for potential adverse effects

**PATIENT AND FAMILY
EDUCATION**
Teach/instruct
• To take as prescribed, do not
change dosage or discontinue
without prescriber instruction
• To take the drug with or right
after a meal in order to decrease
adverse GI symptoms
Warn/advise
• About potential side effects, to
report to care provider (particularly dyspnea, paresthesias, urinary problems; any pain in the
abdomen, chest, back, or legs)
• To avoid use of OTC medications
to prevent potential serious drug
interactions
• That it will take some time to
titrate dosage, and to determine
effectiveness; not likely to see immediate response

• That drug will need to be
stopped for 3-4 wks q 6 mo
• That drug may cause drowsiness
• About potential for orthostatic
hypotension; to make position
changes from lying to standing
slowly
• To report suspected pregnancy
immediately
Encourage
• To keep a record of headaches
(frequency, duration, intensity) to
determine effectiveness of treatment

STORAGE
• Store at room temp in light-
resistant container

---

metoclopramide
Apo-Metoclop♣, Clopra,
Maxeran♣, Maxolon,
Reclomide, Reglan♣

Classification: Antiemetic,
gastrointestinal stimulant

Pregnancy Category: B

AVAILABLE PREPARATIONS
Tabs: 5 mg, 10 mg
Syr: 5 mg/5 ml
Sol: (conc) 10 mg/ml
Inj: 5 mg/ml

ROUTES AND DOSAGES
• Oral preparation appears
equally effective as comparable IV
dose
**Prevention of Chemotherapy-
Associated Nausea and Vomiting**
PO/IV 1-3 mg/kg/dose beginning
30 min before chemotherapy, repeated q2h; or 2 mg/kg/dose 30
min before chemotherapy, repeating same dose q2h × 2, then
q3h × 3; or 3 mg/kg/dose 30 min
before chemotherapy, repeated 90
min following chemotherapy; or 1
mg/kg/dose for maximum of 4
doses; or continuous infusion beginning with loading dose of 1-2
mg/kg followed by infusion of 0.3-
0.5 mg/kg/hr

♣ Available in Canada.

Facilitate Small Bowel Intubation and Radiologic Examination

Children <6 yr: IV 0.1 mg/kg
Children 6-14 yr: IV 2.5-5 mg
Children >14 yr and adults: IV 10 mg over 1-2 min

Treatment of Gastroesophageal Reflux

Children 1-6 yr: PO/IM/IV 0.1-0.2 mg/kg/dose qid 30 min ac and hs
Children >12 yr and adults: PO/IM/IV 2.5-10 mg qid 30 min ac and hs

IV administration

• Recommended concentration: 0.4-3.2 mg/ml in D$_5$½NS, D$_5$W, LR, NS, or R
• Maximum concentration: 5 mg/ml
• IV push rate: Over 1-2 min in adults; if dose <10 mg
• Intermittent infusion rate: Over 15 min in children; if dose >10 mg
• Continuous infusion rate: 0.5-1.2 mg/kg/hr during emetogenic chemotherapy

MECHANISM AND INDICATIONS

Mechanism: Dopamine antagonist, functions by blocking chemoreceptor trigger zone through antagonizing peripheral and central dopamine receptors; stimulates tone and strength of gastric contractions, increases peristaltic activity of duodenum and jejunum, facilitating gastric emptying; relaxes lower esophageal and pyloric sphincter, duodenal bulb
Indications: Prevention of chemotherapy-associated nausea and vomiting; management of GERD; aid to small bowel intubation and radiologic studies

PHARMACOKINETICS

Onset of action: IV 1-3 min; PO 30-60 min; IM 10-15 min
Distribution: To most body tissues and fluids (including brain)
Duration: 1-2 hr
Half-life: 4-6 hr
Metabolism: Not extensively metabolized; small amount in liver
Excretion: 85% unchanged in urine, small amount in feces

CONTRAINDICATIONS AND PRECAUTIONS

• Contraindicated with history of hypersensitivity to drug or to sulfonamides; in situations where increase in gastric motility contraindicated (intestinal obstruction, perforation); with epilepsy; with other drugs that may cause EPS; with pheochromocytoma (may precipitate a hypertensive crisis)
• Use cautiously in children (increased incidence of EPS and CNS effects); in pts taking MAOIs; with pregnancy, lactation

INTERACTIONS

Drug

• Concurrent administration of diphenhydramine or lorazepam should prevent EPS
• Enhanced antiemetic effects with addition of dexamethasone or diphenhydramine
• Action negated with anticholinergic drugs, narcotic analgesics
• Increased effect with alcohol, cyclosporine, succinylcholine
• Increased effect of MAOIs
• Altered rate of absorption of other PO medications (inhibits absorption of digoxin and cimetidine)
• Increased incidence of EPS with antipsychotic drugs
• Increased incidence of CNS depression with antihypertensives, other CNS depressants

Lab

• Increased serum aldosterone, prolactin possible

INCOMPATIBILITIES

• IV form incompatible with ampicillin, calcium gluconate, cephalothin, chloramphenicol, cisplatin, erythromycin, methotrexate, penicillin G potassium, NaHCO$_3$

SIDE EFFECTS

CNS: Sedation, drowsiness, restlessness, vertigo, dysphoria, EPS, dystonic reaction, akathisia, hallucinations, headache, insomnia, tardive dyskinesia
CV: Transient hypertension or hypotension, arrhythmias, may cause methemoglobinemia in pre-

M

mature and full-term neonates at dosages >0.5 mg/kg/24 hr

DERM: Rash

EENT: Periorbital edema, oculogyric crisis

ENDO: Prolactin secretion, loss of libido

GI: Diarrhea, dry mouth, constipation

TOXICITY AND OVERDOSE

Clinical signs: Disorientation, excessive drowsiness, EPS, dystonic reactions

Treatment: Supportive care, including administration of diphenhydramine or benzatropine; symptoms should disappear within 24 hr

PATIENT CARE MANAGEMENT

Assessment

• Assess history of hypersensitivity to drug

• Assess baseline VS

• Assess history of previous antiemetic therapy

• Assess history of previous adverse response to drug

Interventions

• Administer before metoclopramide

• Continue to monitor VS

Evaluation

• Evaluate therapeutic effect (decreased nausea and vomiting, decreased GERD symptoms)

• Evaluate for signs of EPS up to 24 hr after antiemetic therapy ends

PATIENT AND FAMILY EDUCATION

Teach/instruct

• To take as directed at prescribed intervals for prescribed length of time

• That drug may produce drowsiness, dizziness; any activity (e.g., driving) that requires intense concentration should be delayed 24 hr after drug administration

• To report any involuntary movements of face, limbs, eyes immediately

• To take medication as ordered

Encourage

• To report perceived effectiveness of drug

STORAGE

• Store at room temp in light-resistant container

• IV sol stable for 48 hrs if protected from light

---

metocurine iodide

Brand Name(s): Metubine Iodide

Classification: Neuromuscular blocking agent; methyl analog of tubocurarine

Pregnancy Category: C

AVAILABLE PREPARATIONS

Inj: 2 mg/ml

ROUTES AND DOSAGES

Adult: IV 2-4 mg if giving cyclopropane as anesthetic; 1.5-3 mg if giving ether; 4-7 mg if giving nitrous oxide

IV administration

• Infusion rate: Slow push over 1-2 min by qualified careprovider; anticholinesterase available to reverse neuromuscular blockade

MECHANISM AND INDICATIONS

Mechanism: A competitive neuromuscular blocking agent that acts to interrupt transmission of nerve impulses at skeletal neuromuscular junction; combines with cholinergic receptor sites at the endplates in skeletal muscle and competitively blocks transmitter action of acetylcholine; this inhibits contractile activity in skeletal muscle resulting in muscle paralysis; effect is reversible with cholinesterase inhibitors (e.g., edrophonium, neostigmine, and physostigmine); acts primarily on the skeletal neuromuscular junction, is virtually devoid of CNS effects because of its inability to penetrate blood–brain barrier

Indications: Adjuvant in surgical anesthesia; advantage is the ability to obtain necessary degree of

---

muscular relaxation without using dangerously high concentrations of anesthetic; used to facilitate endotracheal intubation, skeletal muscle relaxation during mechanical ventilation, surgery, or general anesthesia, and in the reduction of fractures/dislocations

PHARMACOKINETICS
Onset of action: 30-60 sec
Peak: 3-5 min
Duration: 35-90 min
Half-life: 3½ hr; distributed slowly, this explains slow decline in plasma concentration after a single dose even in cases of renal failure
Metabolism: Liver
Excretion: Urine, small amount in bile; about ½-⅔ unchanged

CONTRAINDICATIONS AND PRECAUTIONS
• Contraindicated with hypersensitivity to iodides (Note: Neuromuscular blocking agents should be administered only by anesthesiologists and other clinicians with extensive training, with facilities for respiratory and cardiovascular resuscitation readily available)
• Use cautiously with pregnancy, lactation; cardiac, hepatic, renal, respiratory disease; neuromuscular disease (myasthenia gravis), electrolyte imbalance; dehydration; when histamine release is hazardous (asthma)

INTERACTIONS
Drug
• Increased neuromuscular blockade with aminoglycosides, clindamycin, lincomycin, quinidine, local anesthetics, polymyxin antibiotics, lithium, narcotic analgesics, thiazides, enflurane, isoflurane
• Arrhythmias possible with theophylline

INCOMPATIBILITIES
• All barbiturates in sol or syringe

SIDE EFFECTS
CV: Bradycardia, tachycardia, increased or decreased B/P
DERM: Rash, flushing, pruritus, urticaria

EENT: Increased secretions
RESP: Prolonged apnea, bronchospasm, cyanosis, respiratory depression
Other: Histamine-like wheals when injected SC or intraarterially; bronchospasm, hypotension, excessive bronchial and salivary secretion

TOXICITY AND OVERDOSE
Clinical signs: Prolonged apnea, bronchospasm, cyanosis, respiratory depression
Treatment: Supportive symptomatic care; mechanical ventilation may be required; anticholinesterase (edrophonium, neostigmine, atropine) to reverse neuromuscular blockade

PATIENT CARE MANAGEMENT
Assessment
• Assess history of hypersensitivity to iodine
• Assess for preexisting conditions requiring caution (pregnancy; cardiac, hepatic, or renal disease; lactation; electrolyte imbalances; neuromuscular, respiratory diseases)
• Assess electrolytes (Na, K⁺) before procedure; electrolyte imbalances (K^+, Mg) may increase action of drug
Interventions
• Monitor therapeutic response (paralysis of jaw, eyelid, head, neck, rest of the body)
• Monitor for allergic reactions (rash, fever, respiratory distress, pruritus); drug should be discontinued
• Monitor VS (pulse, respirations, airway, B/P) until fully recovered; characteristics of respirations (rate, depth, pattern), strength of hand grip
• Monitor I&O for urinary frequency, hesitancy, retention

M

NURSING ALERT

Like its parent compound, d-tubocurarine, metocurine iodide may produce typical histamine-like wheals when injected SC or intraarterially; also bronchospasm, hypotension, excessive bronchial and salivary secretion; this could be problematic when histamine release is a hazard (asthma)

Neuromuscular blocking agents should be administered only by anesthesiologists and other clinicians with extensive training, with facilities for respiratory and cardiovascular resuscitation readily available

Evaluation
- Evaluate effectiveness of neuromuscular blockade (degree of paralysis); use nerve stimulator
- Monitor for recovery (decreased paralysis of face, diaphragm, arm, rest of the body)

PATIENT AND FAMILY EDUCATION
Teach/instruct
- Provide reassurance if communication is difficult during recovery
- That often postoperative stiffness occurs; this is normal and will subside

STORAGE
- Store in light-resistant container in cool area

---

metolazone
Brand Name(s): Diulo, Mykrox, Zaroxolyn♣
Classification: Diuretic
Pregnancy Category: D

AVAILABLE PREPARATIONS
Tabs: 0.5 mg, 2.5 mg, 5 mg, 10 mg
Oral susp: 1 mg/ml (not commercially available)

ROUTES AND DOSAGES
Children: PO 0.2-0.4 mg/kg/24 hr divided qd or bid
Edema
Adults: PO 5-20 mg/24 hr qd
Hypertension
Adults: PO 2.5-5mg/24 hr qd

MECHANISM AND INDICATIONS
Diuretic mechanism: Inhibits Na reabsorption in distal tubules, promoting more excretion of water, Na, Cl, K+, Mg
Indications: Edema, hypertension, CHF

PHARMACOKINETICS
Onset of action: 1 hr
Peak: 2 hr
Half-life: 8 hr
Metabolism: None (remains unchanged)
Excretion: Urine

CONTRAINDICATIONS AND PRECAUTIONS
- Contraindicated with hypersensitivity to thiazides or sulfonamides, anuria, lactation
- Use cautiously with hypokalemia, renal disease, hepatic disease, gout, COPD, lupus, diabetes

INTERACTIONS
Drug
- Synergism possible with furosemide
- Increased toxicity of lithium and non-depolarizing skeletal muscle relaxants
- Decreased effects of oral hypoglycemic agents, methenamine
- Decreased absorption of thiazides, cholestyramine, colestipol
- Decreased hypotensive response with indomethacin, salicylates
- Hyperglycemia, hyperuricemia, hypotension with diazoxide

Lab
- Increased Ca, amylase, parathyroid test, creatinine, BUN
- Decreased PBI

SIDE EFFECTS
CNS: Syncope, neuropathy, dizziness, parasthesias, depression, impotence, drowsiness, fatigue, weakness, insomnia, headache

---

♣ Available in Canada.

CV: Orthostatic hypotension, volume depletion, chest pain, palpitations, irregular pulse
DERM: Rash, urticaria, purpura, photosensitivity
EENT: Blurred vision
GI: Hepatitis, jaundice, nausea, vomiting, pancreatitis, anorexia, GI distress, diarrhea, constipation, cramping, abdominal bloating
GU: Polyuria, frequency, uremia, glycosuria
Other: Fever, chills, aplastic anemia, leukopenia, agranulocytosis, thrombocytopenia, hypokalemia, hypomagnesemia, hyponatremia, hypochloremia

TOXICITY AND OVERDOSE
Clinical signs: Orthostatic hypotension, dizziness, drowsiness, syncope, electrolyte imbalances, lethargy, coma
Treatment: Gastric lavage, supportive measures to maintain hydration, electrolytes, respirations, CV status, renal status

PATIENT CARE MANAGEMENT
Assessment
• Assess hypersensitivity to drug, thiazides, sulfonamides
• Assess baseline wt, VS, B/P, hydration status
• Assess baseline electrolytes (K⁺, Na, PO_4, Ca)
Interventions
• Administer PO in AM to avoid nocturia
• May administer with food if nausea occurs
Evaluation
• Evaluate therapeutic response (decreased edema, decreased B/P, improved cardiovascular status)
• Evaluate for hypersensitivity, side effects
• Monitor VS, daily wt
• Evaluate labs (electrolytes)
• Monitor for signs of metabolic alkalosis, electrolyte imbalances

PATIENT AND FAMILY EDUCATION
Teach/instruct
• To take as directed at prescribed

intervals for prescribed length of time
• About need for medication
• To take medication early in day, to take with food if nausea occurs
• To monitor wt daily
Warn/advise
• Notify care provider of hypersensitivity, side effects
• To identify and report signs of electrolyte imbalance (e.g., weakness, fatigue, muscle cramps, paresthesias, confusion, nausea, vomiting, diarrhea, headache, dizziness, palpitations)
Encourage
• To increase intake of K⁺-rich foods (e.g., bananas, citrus fruits, tomatoes, dates, raisins, potatoes, apricots)
• To restrict salt and high-Na foods
• To notify care provider with sudden increases or decreases in wt
STORAGE
• Store at room temp in tight, light-resistant container

---

metoprolol tartrate
Brand Name(s): Apo-Metoprolol✦, Apo-Metoprolol (Type L)✦, Betaloc✦, Betaloc Durules✦, Lopresor✦, Lopressor, Novo-Metoprol✦, Nu-Metop✦, PMS-Metoprolol-B✦

Classification: β-blocker, antihypertensive

Pregnancy category: C

AVAILABLE PREPARATIONS
Tabs: 50 mg, 100 mg
Inj: 1 mg/ml
ROUTES AND DOSAGES
Hypertension
Adults: PO 50 mg bid or 100 mg qd; may give 200-450 mg in divided doses
Myocardial Infarction
IV early treatment, 5 mg q2 min × 3, then 50 mg PO 15 min after last dose; 50 mg PO q6h × 48 hr; PO late treatment, 100 mg bid × 3 mo

IV administration
- Recommended concentration: 1 mg/ml
- IV push rate: Over 1 min

MECHANISM AND INDICATIONS

β-blocker, antihypertensive mechanisms: Decreases B/P through β-blocking effects without reflex tachycardia or significant reduction in HR, reduces elevated plasma renins; decreases rate of SA node conduction at high dosages by blocking β_2-adrenergic receptors in bronchial and smooth muscle

Indications: Angina, mild-to-moderate hypertension, decreased mortality during acute MI

PHARMACOKINETICS

Onset of action: PO 1 hr; IV 5 min
Peak: PO 2-4 hr; IV 20 min
Half-life: 3-4 hr
Metabolism: Liver
Excretion: Urine

CONTRAINDICATIONS AND PRECAUTIONS

- Contraindicated with hypersensitivity to β-blockers, sinus bradycardia, 2nd- or 3rd-degree heart block, cardiogenic shock, CHF, bronchial asthma
- Use cautiously with pts undergoing major surgery, diabetes, CAD, COPD, bronchospasm; thyroid, renal, hepatic disease; during pregnancy, lactation

INTERACTIONS

Drug
- Increased hypotension and bradycardia with reserpine, hydralazine, methyldopa, prazosin, anticholinergics
- Increased hypoglycemic effects with insulin
- Decreased antihypertensive effects with indomethacin, sympathomimetics
- Decreased bronchodilation effects of theophylline

Lab
- Increased BUN, creatinine, liver function tests

INCOMPATABILITIES

- Incompatible with any drug in syringe or soluset

SIDE EFFECTS

CNS: Confusion, fatigue, memory loss, insomnia, dizziness, hallucinations, depression, anxiety, headaches, nightmares
CV: Bradycardia, hypotension, palpitations, CHF, arrhythmias, heart block, cardiac arrest
DERM: Alopecia, dry skin, rash, purpura, pruritus, urticaria
EENT: Dry mouth, burning eyes, sore throat
GI: Nausea, vomiting, constipation, cramps, colitis, diarrhea, flatulence, hiccups
GU: Impotence
RESP: Dyspnea, bronchospasm, wheezing
Other: Agranulocytosis, eosinophilia, thrombocytopenia

TOXICITY AND OVERDOSE

Clinical signs: Bradycardia, hypotension, bronchospasm, cardiac failure
Treatment: Gastric lavage for recent ingestion; supportive measures as necessary, including IV atropine for bradycardia, IV theophylline for bronchospasm, vasopressors for hypotension; may need hemodialysis

PATIENT CARE MANAGEMENT

Assessment
- Assess history of hypersensitivity to drug, β-blockers
- Assess baseline VS, B/P, wt, hydration, ECG
- Assess baseline electrolytes, renal function (BUN, creatinine), liver function (ALT, AST, bilirubin)

Interventions
- Tabs may be crushed or swallowed whole

Evaluation
- Evaluate therapeutic response (decreased B/P)
- Evaluate side effects, hypersensitivity
- Monitor daily wt, VS, B/P, hydration status
- Evaluate electrolytes, renal

✤ Available in Canada.

function (BUN, creatinine), liver function (ALT, AST, creatinine)

PATIENT AND FAMILY EDUCATION
Teach/instruct
• To take as directed at prescribed intervals for prescribed amount of time
• About need for medication
• To take medication with meals
Warn/advise
• To notify care provider of hypersensitivity, side effects
• Not to discontinue medication abruptly
• To avoid OTC preparations unless directed by care provider

STORAGE
• Store at room temp in tightly sealed container

---

metronidazole
Flagyl, MetroGel, Metro IV, Protostat

Classification: Amebicide, antibiotic, anaerobic

Pregnancy Category: B

AVAILABLE PREPARATIONS
Tabs: 250 mg, 500 mg
Inj: 5 mg/ml, powder for injection 500 mg
Top: Gel 0.75%

ROUTES AND DOSAGES
Anaerobic Infections
Neonates 0-4 wk, <1200 g: PO/IV 7.5 mg/kg q48h
Neonates ≤7 days, 1200-2000 g: PO/IV 7.5 mg/kg/24 hr qd
Neonates ≤7 days, >2000 g: PO/IV 15 mg/kg/24 hr divided q12h
Neonates >7 days, 1200-2000 g: PO/IV 15 mg/kg/24 hr divided q12h
Neonates >7 days, >2000 g: PO/IV 30 mg/kg/24 hr divided q12h
Infants and children: PO/IV 30 mg/kg/24 hr divided q6h
Adults: PO/IV 30 mg/kg/24 hr divided q6h; maximum 4 g/24 hr

Amebiasis
Infants and children: PO 35-50 mg/kg/24 hr divided q8h
Adults: PO/IV 500-750 mg q8h
Other Parasitic Infections
Infants and children: PO 15-30 mg/kg/24 hr divided q8h
Adults: 250 mg q8h or 2 g qd
Antibiotic-Associated Pseudomembranous Colitis
Infants and children: PO 20 mg/kg/24 hr divided q6h; maximum 4 g/24 hr
Adults: PO/IV 250-500 mg tid-qid × 10-14 days
Acne Rosacea
Top, apply thin film to affected areas bid

IV administration
• Recommended concentration: 5-8 mg/ml in D_5W, LR, or NS
• Maximum concentration: 8 mg/ml
• IV push rate: Not recommended
• Intermittent infusion rate: Over 60 min

MECHANISM AND INDICATIONS
Mechanism: Interacts with DNA to cause a loss of structure and strand breakage, thus inhibiting protein synthesis and causing cell death in organisms
Indications: Used to treat anaerobic bacterial and protozoal infections in amebiasis, trichomoniasis; skin, CNS, intraabdominal, systemic anaerobic infections; antibiotic-associated pseudomembranous colitis; top used to treat acne rosacea

PHARMACOKINETICS
Peak: 1-2 hr
Distribution: Widely into body tissues, fluids, and erythrocytes
Half-life: Neonates 25-75 hr; adults 6-8 hr
Metabolism: 30%-60% in liver
Excretion: Urine, feces

CONTRAINDICATIONS AND PRECAUTIONS
• Contraindicated with known hypersensitivity to metronidazole or any component, severe renal or hepatic disease, CNS disorders,

blood dyscrasias, pregnancy (1st trimester), lactation
• Use cautiously with coexisting candidiasis, alcoholism, pregnancy (2nd and 3rd trimesters)

INTERACTIONS
Drug
• Increased hypoprothrombinemia with oral anticoagulants
• Disulfiram reaction possible with alcohol
• Acute psychosis possible with disulfiram
• Increased metabolism of metronidazole with phenobarbital
Lab
• False decrease in ALT, AST

INCOMPATIBILITIES
• Any drug in syringe or sol; interacts with aluminum to form a precipitate

SIDE EFFECTS
CNS: Vertigo, confusion, seizures, headache, peripheral neuropathy, fever
DERM: Rash, urticaria, pruritus, flushing
GI: Anorexia, nausea, dry mouth, diarrhea, furry tongue, metallic taste
GU: Dark or reddish urine, burning, dysuria, cystitis, polyuria, pelvic pressure
HEME: Leukopenia
Local: Thrombophlebitis with IV infusion
Other: Disulfiram-type reaction with alcohol; bacterial or fungal superinfection (especially candidiasis)

TOXICITY AND OVERDOSE
Clinical signs: Nausea, vomiting, ataxia, neurologic symptoms (seizures)
Treatment: Induced emesis and gastric lavage followed by activated charcoal, cathartic; supportive care; diazepam or phenytoin for seizure control

PATIENT CARE MANAGEMENT
Assessment
• Assess history of hypersensitivity to metronidazole

• Inspect and record appearance of stool, obtain cultures
• Obtain family history of home, sanitation condition, pets
• Assess baseline hematologic function (CBC, differential, platelet count)
• Obtain baseline ophthalmic exam
Interventions
• Administer PO with meals to reduce GI distress; tabs may be crushed, mixed with food or fluid
• Do not mix IV with other drugs; infuse separately
• Avoid aluminum-containing equipment during IV preparation and administration (syringe needles, hubs)
• Rotate IV site q48-72h
• For top application; cleanse affected area; apply thin film
• Maintain age-appropriate fluid intake
• Perform proper hygiene procedures (good handwashing, ensure tight-fitting diapers to prevent leakage, proper disposal of feces)

> **NURSING ALERT**
> Avoid use of aluminum equipment during IV preparation and administration
>
> Do not administer IV push

Evaluation
• Evaluate therapeutic response (decreased symptoms of infection)
• Monitor stool pattern and stool cultures weekly during therapy, 1, 3, 6 mo after therapy is discontinued
• Monitor ophthalmic exams during therapy
• Monitor for neurotoxicity (peripheral neuropathy, seizures, dizziness, incoordination)
• Monitor for allergic reaction (fever, rash, itching, chills)
• Monitor for superinfection (fever, monilial growth, fatigue, malaise)
• Monitor renal function (BUN, creatinine, I&O), hematologic

function (CBC, differential, platelet count)
• Evaluate IV site for vein irritation, extravasation, thrombophlebitis
• Evaluate spread of infection to other household members

PATIENT AND FAMILY EDUCATION
Teach/instruct
• To take as directed at prescribed intervals for prescribed length of time
Warn/advise
• To notify care provider of hypersensitivity, side effects, superinfection
• About measures to prevent disease transmission (hand washing before meals, after defecation with liquid soap, proper food preparation and handling, proper disposal of feces and stool culture collection)
• To comply with follow-up care

STORAGE
• Store at room temp in light-resistant container

---

mezlocillin sodium
Brand Name(s): Mezlin
Classification: Antibiotic (extended-spectrum penicillin)
Pregnancy Category: B

AVAILABLE PREPARATIONS
Inj: 1 g, 2 g, 3 g, 4 g

ROUTES AND DOSAGES
Neonates ≤7 days: IM/IV 150 mg/kg/24 hr divided q12h
Neonates >7 days, <2000 g: IM/IV 225 mg/kg/24 hr divided q8h
Neonates >7 days, >2000 g: IM/IV 300 mg/kg/24 hr divided q6h
Infants and children: IM/IV 200-300 mg/kg/24 hr divided q4-6h; maximum 24 g/24 hr
Adults: IM/IV 1-4 g q4-6h; maximum 24 g/24 hr

IV administration
• Recommended concentration: 100 mg/ml in D_5W, NS, or SW for IV push; 10-20 mg/ml in $D_5\frac{1}{4}NS$, $D_5\frac{1}{2}NS$, D_5W, $D_{10}W$, LR, NS, R, or SW for IV infusion
• Maximum concentration: 100 mg/ml for IV push
• IV push rate: Over 3-5 min
• Intermittent infusion rate: Over 10-30 min

MECHANISM AND INDICATIONS
Antibiotic mechanism: Bactericidal; inhibits bacterial cell wall synthesis by adhering to bacterial penicillin-binding proteins
Indications: Effective against gram-positive and gram-negative organisms including *Staphylococcus aureus, Streptococcus viridans, Str. pneumoniae, Str. faecalis, Neisseria gonorrhoeae, Clostridium perfringens, C. tetani, Bacteroides, E. coli, Haemophilus influenzae, Klebsiella, Proteus mirabilis, P. vulgaris, Morganella morganii, Enterobacter, Serratia, Pseudomonas aeruginosa, Shigella, Citrobacter.* Used to treat septicemia, meningitis; respiratory tract, GU tract, intraabdominal, skin, and soft tissue infections

PHARMACOKINETICS
Peak: Neonates IM, IV 30 min; children 2-7 yr IV 5 min
Distribution: Widely distributed; highest concentration in urine, bile; penetrates CNS with inflamed meninges
Half-life: Neonates 2.4-4.47 hr; children 0.83-0.97 hr
Metabolism: Liver
Excretion: Urine, bile

CONTRAINDICATIONS AND PRECAUTIONS
• Contraindicated with known hypersensitivity to mezlocillin, penicillins, or cephalosporins
• Use cautiously with impaired renal function, history of bleeding problems, hypokalemia, pregnancy

INTERACTIONS
Drug
• Synergistic antimicrobial activity against certain organisms with aminoglycosides, clavulanic acid
• Increased serum concentrations with probenecid
• Increased serum concentrations of methotrexate
• Decreased effectiveness with erythromycins, tetracyclines, chloramphenicol

Lab
• False-positive urine protein with all tests except those using bromophenol blue (Albustix, Albutest, Multi Stix)
• Increased liver function tests
• False positive Coombs' test

INCOMPATIBILITIES
• Aminoglycosides, amphotericin B, chloramphenicol, ciprofloxacin, meperidine, polymyxin B, promethazine, verapamil

SIDE EFFECTS
CNS: Neuromuscular irritability, seizures
ENDO / METAB: Hypokalemia
GI: Nausea, diarrhea, vomiting, pseudomembranous colitis
GU: Acute interstitial nephritis
HEME: Bleeding with high dosages, neutropenia, eosinophilia, leukopenia, thrombocytopenia
Local: Pain at injection site; phlebitis, vein irritation with IV injection
Other: Hypersensitivity reactions (edema, fever, chills, rash, pruritus, urticaria, anaphylaxis), bacterial or fungal superinfections

TOXICITY AND OVERDOSE
Clinical signs: Neuromuscular hypersensitivity; seizures may result from high CNS concentrations
Treatment: Supportive care; hemodialysis

PATIENT CARE MANAGEMENT
Assessment
• Assess history of hypersensitivity to mezlocillin, penicillins, or cephalosporins
• Obtain C&S; may begin therapy before obtaining results

• Assess renal function (BUN, creatinine, I&O), hepatic function (ALT, AST, bilirubin), hematologic function (CBC, differential, platelet count); K^+ levels (with long-term therapy)

Interventions
• Administer penicillins at least 1 hr before bacteriostatic antibiotics (tetracyclines, erythromycins, chloramphenicol)
• Darkening of powder or unconstituted sol with storage does not affect potency of drug
• If precipitate forms in refrigerated reconstituted sol, redissolve by raising temp to 37° C in warm water bath for 20 min, then shake vigorously
• IM injection painful; administer slowly and deeply into large muscle mass, rotate injection sites
• Do not premix IV with other drugs (particularly aminoglycosides); infuse separately
• Use large vein with small-bore needle to reduce local reaction; rotate site q48-72h
• Maintain age-appropriate fluid intake

NURSING ALERT
Discontinue drug if signs of hypersensitivity, bleeding complications, pseudomembranous colitis develop

Do not infuse rapidly; seizures may result

Evaluation
• Evaluate therapeutic response (decreased symptoms of infection)
• Monitor signs of superinfection (perineal itching, diaper rash, fever, malaise, redness, pain, swelling, drainage, rash, diarrhea, sore throat, change in cough or sputum)
• Observe for signs of allergic reaction (wheezing, tightness in chest, urticaria), especially within 20-30 min of first dose
• Monitor bowel pattern; diarrhea may be symptomatic of pseudomembranous colitis

---

- Monitor renal function (BUN, creatinine, I&O), hepatic function (ALT, AST, bilirubin), electrolyte levels (particularly K^+ and Na)
- Monitor for signs of bleeding (ecchymosis, bleeding gums, hematuria, daily stool guaiac)
- Monitor pro-times and platelet counts
- Evaluate IM site for tissue damage and IV site for vein irritation

PATIENT AND FAMILY TEACHING
Teach/instruct
- To take as directed at prescribed intervals for prescribed length of time
Warn/advise
- To notify care provider of hypersensitivity, side effects, superinfection

STORAGE
- Store powder at room temp
- Reconstituted sol stable at room temp 24-72 hr depending on sol used for admixture

---

miconazole, miconazole nitrate

Brand Name(s): Miconazole: Monistat IV; miconazole nitrate: Micatin✤, Monistat 3, Monistat 3 Dual-Pak Package✤, Monistat 3 Vaginal Ovules✤, Monistat 7, Monistat 7 Cream✤, Monistat 7 Vaginal Suppositories✤, Monistat 7 Dual-Pak Package✤, Monistat-Derm, Monistat-Derm Cream✤

Classification: Antifungal
Pregnancy Category: C

AVAILABLE PREPARATIONS
Inj: 10 mg/ml
Top: Cream, lotion, powder 2%
Vag: Cream 2%; supp 100 mg, 200 mg

ROUTES AND DOSAGES
Neonates: IV 5-15 mg/kg/24 hr divided q8-24h (Safety and effectiveness not established. Dosage represents accepted standard practice recommendations.)
Infants >1 yr and children: IV 15-40 mg/kg/24 hr divided q8h; maximum 15 mg/kg/dose
Adults: IV Initial 200 mg; maintenance 1.2-3.6 g/24 hr divided q8h or IT 20 mg q1-2 days (use undiluted miconazole injection)
Infants, children, and adults: Top, apply to affected area bid; vag, insert one application of cream or 100 mg suppository q hs × 7 days or 200 mg suppository q hs × 7 days

IV administration
- Recommended concentration: 1-6 mg/ml in $D_5\frac{1}{4}NS$, D_5W, or NS
- Maximum concentration: 6 mg/ml
- IV push rate: Not recommended
- Intermittent infusion rate: Over 30-60 min; over 1-2 hr for larger doses given to adolescents or adults

MECHANISM AND INDICATIONS
Mechanism: Damages fungal cell wall membrane, causing increased permeability that leads to leaking of cell nutrients
Indications: Top/vag forms used to treat skin mucous membrane fungal infections and *Candida albicans;* IV form used to treat severe systemic fungal infections and fungal meningitis

PHARMACOKINETICS
Distribution: Distributes into body tissues, fluids, joints; poor penetration into CSF, urine, saliva, sputum
Half-life: Multiphasic, initial 40 min, secondary 126 min, terminal 24 hr
Metabolism: Liver
Excretion: Urine

CONTRAINDICATIONS AND PRECAUTIONS
- Contraindicated with known hypersensitivity to miconazole, polyoxyl 35 castor oil, or any component
- Use IV form cautiously with hepatic or renal insufficiency, children <2 yr, pregnancy, lactation

✤ Available in Canada.

INCOMPATIBILITIES
Drug
• Decreased antifungal effectiveness of both drugs with amphotericin B
• Increased risk of severe hypoglycemia with sulfonylureas
• Increased PT with warfarin
Lab
• False positive urine protein possible with tests other than bromphenol blue reagent test

SIDE EFFECTS
CNS: Arachnoiditis and 12th cranial nerve palsy (IT form), headache, fever, vertigo
CV: Tachycardia, arrhythmias
DERM: Maceration, hives, rash, pruritus
ENDO / METAB: Hyperlipidemia, hyponatremia
GI: Nausea, vomiting, diarrhea
GU: Pelvic cramps
HEME: Transient anemia, thrombocytopenia, thrombocytosis
Local: Irritation, burning, itching, phlebitis
Other: Anaphylactoid reactions

TOXICITY AND OVERDOSE
Clinical signs: GI complaints and altered mental status
Treatment: If ingested within 4 hr, induce emesis or gastric lavage, followed by activated charcoal and osmotic cathartic; supportive care

PATIENT CARE MANAGEMENT
Assessment
• Assess history of hypersensitivity to miconazole, polyoxyl 35 castor oil, any components
• Obtain culture to identify organism
• Assess baseline hematologic function (CBC, differential, platelet count), lipids (cholesterol, triglycerides), electrolytes (Ca, Na)
Interventions
• Do not administer IV at mealtime to avoid gastric distress
• Initial test dose of 200 mg should administered under direct medical supervision to determine possible hypersensitivity; ensure that emergency equipment is available
• Administer antihistamine to reduce pruritus, antiemetic to reduce nausea or vomiting as ordered; decreasing IV rate may reduce nausea or vomiting
• Do not mix with other drugs; administer separately
• To reduce vein irritation, use central venous catheter or change IV site q48h
• Fungal meningitis requires IT therapy in addition to IV
• Cleanse and dry affected area well before top application as ordered; massage area until cream disappears; use of lotion for intertriginous areas reduces maceration
• Insert vaginal application high into vagina
• Maintain age-appropriate fluid intake

> **NURSING ALERT**
> Initial IV test dose should be administered under direct medical supervision to determine possible hypersensitivity

Evaluation
• Evaluate therapeutic response (decreased fever, malaise, rash, size/number of lesions, negative C&S)
• Monitor hematologic function (CBC, differential, platelet count), electrolytes (Ca, Na), lipids (cholesterol, triglycerides)
• Monitor for cardiac arrhythmias during IV infusion
• Monitor pruritus (may continue several wk after therapy is complete)
• Evaluate IV site for vein irritation, phlebitis
• Evaluate response to top therapy; improvement usually evident in 1-2 wk; continue for at least 1 mo; reevaluate diagnosis if without improvement in 4 wk

---

✤ Available in Canada.

PATIENT AND FAMILY EDUCATION
Teach/instruct
• To take as directed at prescribed intervals for prescribed length of time
Warn/advise
• To notify care provider of hypersensitivity, side effects
• That pruritic rash may persist for several wk after therapy is discontinued
• To avoid use of OTC creams, lotions, ointments unless directed by care provider (top forms)
• To avoid use of occlusive dressings (top forms)
• About proper hygiene (top forms); to change socks, avoid tight fitting shoes if feet are infected
• About how to prevent vaginal reinfection; to abstain from sexual intercourse during therapy (vag forms)
• To notify care provider if no improvement within 4 wk or recurrence of symptoms within 2 wk

STORAGE
• Store top, vag forms at room temp
• Reconstituted IV sol stable at room temp for 24 hr

---

midazolam hydrochloride
Brand Name(s): Versed

Classification: Anticonvulsant, benzodiazepine, sedative

Controlled Substance Schedule IV

Pregnancy Category: D

AVAILABLE PREPARATIONS
Inj: 1 mg/ml, 5 mg/ml

DOSAGES AND ROUTES
Children: IM 0.07-0.08 mg/kg 30-60 min before surgery; intranasal 0.2-0.4 mg/kg administered by a 1 ml needleless syringe to the nares over 15 sec; IV 0.035 mg/kg/ dose, repeat over several min as required to achieve desired sedative effect, up to a total dose of 0.1-0.2 mg/kg

Adolescents >12 yr: IV 0.5 mg q 3-4 min until effect is achieved

IV administration
• Recommended concentration: Dilute with D_5W or NS to concentration of 0.25 mg/ml
• IV push rate: Conscious sedation, over 2-3 min; anesthesia induction, over 30 sec

MECHANISM AND INDICATIONS
Mechanism: Increased action of γ-aminobutyric acid (GABA), a major inhibitory neurotransmitter in the brain, depressing all levels of the CNS (including limbic system and reticular formation)
Indications: For use in conscious sedation for procedures, preoperative sedation, general anesthesia induction

PHARMACOKINETICS
Onset of action: IM within 15 min; IV within 1-5 min
Peak: IM 30-60 min; intranasal 10 min
Duration: IM averages 2 hr, up to 6 hr; intranasal 60 min
Absorption: Intranasal rapid
Half-life: 1-4 hr; increased with cirrhosis, CHF, obesity, in the elderly
Metabolism: Liver
Excretion: Urine, small amount in feces; crosses blood–brain barrier

CONTRAINDICATIONS AND PRECAUTIONS
• Contraindicated with hypersensitivity to this medication, any component, other benzodiazepines; alcohol intoxication, CNS depression, coma, narrow-angle glaucoma, uncontrolled pain, shock, pregnancy
• Use cautiously with chills, CHF, COPD, kidney or liver impairment, pulmonary disease, debilitated or elderly pts

M

INTERACTIONS
Drug
- Increased sedation and respiratory depression with alcohol, barbiturates, CNS depressants
- Increased hypnotic effect with analgesics, droperidol, fentanyl, narcotic agonists
- Decreased sedative effects with theophylline
- Increased serum concentrations with cimetidine

INCOMPATIBILITIES
- Incompatible mixed in a syringe with dimenhydrinate, pentobarbital, perphenazine, prochlorperazine, ranitidine

SIDE EFFECTS
CNS: Amnesia, retrograde amnesia, anxiety, ataxia, chills, confusion, dizziness, drowsiness, euphoria, excitement, headache, insomnia, paresthesia, sedation, slurred speech, tremors, weakness
CV: Bigeminy, bradycardia, cardiac arrest, hypotension, nodal rhythm, PVCs, tachycardia
DERM: Hives, itching, pain, rash
EENT: Loss of balance, blocked ears, nystagmus, blurred vision, double vision
GI: Nausea, vomiting, hiccups, increased salivation, acidic taste
Local: Pain or swelling at injection site
RESP: Apnea, bronchospasm, coughing, dyspnea, laryngospasm, respiratory depression
Other: Physical and psychological dependence with prolonged use

TOXICITY AND OVERDOSE
Clinical signs: Respiratory depression or arrest
Treatment: Monitor VS; administer O_2, vasopressors, physostigmine; resuscitate as needed

PATIENT CARE MANAGEMENT
Assessment
- Assess history of hypersensitivity to drug
- Obtain medical history, assess for risk factors
- Assess respiratory rate, HR, B/P

Interventions
- Have resuscitation equipment nearby before administering midazolam
- Administer IM injection deep into large muscle mass
- Compatible mixed in a syringe with atropine, chlorpromazine, diphenhydramine, droperidol, fentanyl, glycopyrrolate, hydroxyzine, meperidine, metoclopramide, morphine, promazine, promethazine, or trimethobenzamide

---

NURSING ALERT
Midazolam may cause respiratory depression or arrest; hypoxic encephalopathy and deaths have occurred; have resuscitation equipment readily available; monitor HR, respiratory rate, O_2 saturation during administration

---

Evaluation
- Evaluate therapeutic response (induction of sedation, general anesthesia)
- Monitor VS, heart rhythm
- Evaluate for anterograde amnesia
- Monitor injection site for redness, pain, and swelling

PATIENT AND FAMILY EDUCATION
Teach/instruct
- That amnesia may occur and events may not be remembered
Warn/advise
- To avoid hazardous activities until awake, oriented, and at normal strength

STORAGE
- Store at room temp

---

milrinone lactate
Brand Name(s): Primacor
Classification: Inotropic, vasodilator
Pregnancy Category: C

♣ Available in Canada.

AVAILABLE PREPARATIONS
Inj: 1 mg/ml

ROUTES AND DOSAGES
Adult: IV 50 mcg/kg bolus, maintenance infusion of 0.375-0.75 mcg/kg/min; maximum total dose 1.13 mg/kg/24 hr

IV administration
- Recommended concentration: 1 mg/ml
- IV push rate: Over 10 min
- Continuous infusion rate: 0.375-0.75 mcg/kg/min

MECHANISM AND INDICATIONS
Inotropic, vasodilator mechanisms: Reduces preload and afterload by direct relaxation of vascular smooth muscle
Indications: Management of CHF that has not responded to other treatment; may be used in conjunction with digitalis

PHARMACOKINETICS
Onset of action: 2-5 min
Peak: 10 min
Half-life: 4-6 hr
Metabolism: Liver
Excretion: Urine

CONTRAINDICATIONS AND PRECAUTIONS
- Contraindicated with hypersensitivity, severe pulmonic valve and aortic disease, acute MI
- Use cautiously with renal or hepatic disease, elderly pts, atrial flutter, fibrillation, pregnancy, lactation

INTERACTIONS
Drug
- Increased hypotension with antihypertensives

INCOMPATIBILITIES
None

SIDE EFFECTS
CNS: Headache, tremors
CV: Arrhythmias, hypotension, angina
GI: Nausea, vomiting, anorexia, abdominal pain, jaundice, hepatic failure
Other: Hypokalemia, thrombocytopenia

TOXICITY AND OVERDOSE
Clinical signs: Severe hypotension
Treatment: Supportive measures as necessary

PATIENT CARE MANAGEMENT
Assessment
- Assess history of hypersensitivity to drug
- Assess baseline VS, B/P, wt, hydration status
- Assess baseline electrolytes, renal function (BUN, creatinine), hematologic function (CBC, platelets)

Interventions
- Use large vein with small bore needle; rotate site q48-72h

Evaluation
- Evaluate therapeutic response (increased cardiac output, decreased shortness of breath, fatigue, edema)
- Evaluate for side effects, hypersensitivity
- Evaluate VS, B/P frequently
- Evaluate electrolytes, renal function (BUN, creatinine), hematologic functions (CBC, platelets)

PATIENT AND FAMILY EDUCATION
Teach/instruct
- About need for medication
Warn/advise
- To notify care provider of hypersensitivity, side effects
Provide
- Emotional support as indicated

STORAGE
- Store at room temp

M

---

minocycline hydrochloride
Brand Name(s): Dynacin, Minocin✦

Classification: Antibiotic (tetracycline)

Pregnancy Category: D

AVAILABLE PREPARATIONS
Oral susp: 50 mg/5 ml
Caps: 50 mg, 100 mg

Tabs: 50 mg, 100 mg
Inj: 100 mg

ROUTES AND DOSAGES
• Not recommended for children <8 yr
Children >8 yr: PO/IV initial 4 mg/kg/dose, then 4 mg/kg/24 hr divided q12h
Adults: PO/IV initial 200 mg, then 100 mg q12h or 50 mg q6h (maximum 400 mg/24 hr)

Chlamydia Trachomatis
Adult: PO 100 mg bid for 7 days

IV administration
• Recommended concentration: 100-200 mcg/ml in D_5W, NS
• Maximum concentration: 200 mcg/ml
• Intermittent infusion rate: Over 6 hr

MECHANISM AND INDICATIONS
Antibiotic mechanism: Bacteriostatic; inhibits bacterial protein synthesis by binding reversibly to ribosomal units
Indications: Active against many gram-positive and gram-negative organisms, *Mycoplasma, Rickettsia, Chlamydia,* and spirochetes; may be more active against staphylococci than other tetracyclines; used to treat syphilis, *Chlamydia trachomatis,* gonorrhea, lymphogranuloma venereum, rickettsial infection, mycoplasma pneumonia, inflammatory acne, and for *Neisseria meningitidis* prophylaxis

PHARMACOKINETICS
Peak: 2-3 hr
Distribution: Accumulates in adipose tissue
Half-life: 11-26 hr
Metabolism: Liver
Excretion: Urine, feces

CONTRAINDICATIONS
• Contraindicated with pregnancy, lactation, children <8 yr (because of risk of permanent discoloration of teeth, enamel defects, and retardation of bone growth); pts with known hypersensitivity to tetracyclines

• Use cautiously with impaired renal or hepatic function

INTERACTIONS
Drug
• Decreased bactericidal effects of penicillins
• Increased effects of oral anticoagulants
• Decreased absorption with antacids containing aluminum, Ca, Mg; laxatives continuing Mg, oral iron, zinc, $NaHCO_3$
• Increased effects of digoxin
• Increased risk of nephrotoxicity from methoxyflurane
Lab
• False positive for urine catecholamines
Nutrition
• Decreased oral absorption if given with food or dairy products

INCOMPATIBILITIES
• Do not mix with other drugs

SIDE EFFECTS
CNS: Light-headedness; dizziness from vestibular toxicity
CV: Pericarditis
DERM: Maculopapular and erythematous rashes, photosensitivity, increased pigmentation, urticaria, discolored nails and teeth
GI: Anorexia, epigastric distress, nausea, vomiting, diarrhea, dysphagia, glossitis, enterocolitis, inflammatory anogenital lesions
GU: Reversible nephrotoxicity from outdated minocycline, increased BUN level
HEME: Neutropenia, eosinophilia
Local: Thrombophlebitis with IV injection
Other: Hypersensitivity, bacterial or fungal superinfection

TOXICITY AND OVERDOSE
Clinical signs: GI disturbance
Treatment: Antacids; if ingested within 4 hr, empty stomach by gastric lavage; supportive care

PATIENT CARE MANAGEMENT
Assessment
• Assess history of hypersensitivity to tetracyclines
• Obtain C&S; may begin therapy before obtaining results

♣ Available in Canada.

- Assess renal function (BUN, creatinine, I&O), hepatic function (ALT, AST, bilirubin), hematologic function (CBC, differential, platelet count) particularly for long-term therapy, bowel pattern

Interventions

- Check expiration dates; nephrotoxicity may result from outdated minocycline
- If pt is receiving concurrent penicillins, administer penicillins at least 1 hr before minocycline
- Administer PO 1 hr ac or 2 hr after meals; administer with water to prevent esophageal irritation
- Do not administer within 1 hr of hs to prevent eosphageal reflux
- Do not give with milk, dairy products, $NaHCO_3$, oral iron, zinc, antacids
- Shake suspension well before administering
- Tabs may be crushed, caps taken apart and mixed with food or fluid
- Do not mix IV with other medications, sols containing Ca; infuse separately
- Use large vein with small-bore needle to reduce local reaction; rotate site q48-72h
- Maintain age-appropriate fluid intake

> **NURSING ALERT**
> Discontinue drug if signs of toxicity, hypersensitivity, renal dysfunction, superinfection, erythema to sun (ultraviolet) exposure, or pseudomembranous colitis develop
>
> Do not administer IV push

Evaluation

- Evaluate therapeutic response (decreased symptoms of infection)
- Monitor signs of superinfection (perineal itching, diaper rash, fever, malaise, redness, pain, swelling, drainage, rash, diarrhea, sore throat, change in cough or sputum)
- Observe for signs of allergic reaction (rash, pruritus, angioedema)

- Monitor bowel patterns; diarrhea may be symptomatic of pseudomembranous colitis
- Monitor renal function (BUN, creatinine, I&O), hepatic function (ALT, AST, bilirubin), hematologic function (CBC, differential, platelet count)
- Evaluate IV site for vein irritation; replace IV route with oral therapy as soon as possible to prevent thrombophlebitis

PATIENT AND FAMILY TEACHING

Teach/instruct

- To take as directed at prescribed intervals for prescribed length of time

Warn/advise

- To notify care provider of hypersensitivity, side effects, superinfection
- Not to use outdated medication
- To avoid sun (ultraviolet light) exposure

STORAGE

- Store tabs, caps at room temp in airtight, light-resistant containers
- Reconstituted oral susp stable at room temp for 14 days; label date and time of reconstitution
- Reconstituted parenteral forms stable for 24 hr at room temp

M

---

mitomycin

Brand Name(s): Mutamycin ❧

Classification: Antineoplastic, antibiotic; cell cycle phase nonspecific (although maximum effect occurs in late G_1 and early S phase)

Pregnancy Category: D

AVAILABLE PREPARATIONS

Inj: 5 mg, 20 mg, 40 mg powder

ROUTES AND DOSAGES

- Dosage may vary in response to diagnosis, extent of disease, concurrent or previous therapy, protocol guidelines, physiologic pa-

---

❧ Available in Canada.

rameters; consult current literature, protocol recommendations

Single Agent

IV 10-20 mg/m^2/dose × 1, repeat q6-8 wk or 2 mg/m^2/dose × 1 for 5 days, rest for 2 days, and repeat for 5 more days; cycle q6-8 wk

IV administration

• Recommended concentration: 20-40 mcg/ml for IV infusion; 0.5/ml for IV push

• IV push rate: Slow, over 5-10 min

• Intermittent infusion rate: Variable; through central line

MECHANISM AND INDICATIONS

Mechanism: Alkylating agent that causes cross-linking between complementary DNA base pairs and subsequent breakage of DNA strands, halting DNA and RNA synthesis; also generates O_2 free radical formation, causing breakage of DNA strands

Indications: Generally used in treatment of adult malignancies such as squamous cell carcinoma of anus, pleural mesothelioma, recurrent colorectal or breast cancer, recurrent or metastatic cancer of stomach, pancreas, esophagus, lung; has potential for pediatric use in recurrent sarcomas and resistant leukemias

PHARMACOKINETICS

Distribution: Rapid with uptake in muscles, eyes, lungs, intestines, stomach; does not cross blood–brain barrier

Half-life: 1 hr

Metabolism: Primarily in liver, also deactivated in kidneys, spleen, brain, heart

Excretion: Urine, bile

CONTRAINDICATIONS AND PRECAUTIONS

• Contraindicated in children with previous hypersensitivity, with active infections (especially chicken pox and herpes zoster), pregnancy, lactation

• Use cautiously in children with evidence of impaired renal or hepatic function, any evidence of coagulation disorder

INTERACTIONS

Drug

• Increased cardiotoxicity of doxorubicin possible

Lab

• Increased serum creatinine, BUN possible

INCOMPATIBILITIES

• Blenoxane

• Decreased stability in D_5W because of lower pH of sol; dilute in NS, LR

SIDE EFFECTS

CNS: Malaise, lethargy, weakness lasting for several days to weeks, paraesthesias

CV: Venous irritation, phlebosclerosis, hemolytic anemia, progressive renal failure with cardiopulmonary decompensation (fatal about 3-4 wk after diagnosis)

GI: Moderate nausea, vomiting (may be delayed), stomatitis, diarrhea, prolonged anorexia

GU: Glomerular damage resulting in renal failure (hemolytic uremic syndrome) exacerbated by blood transfusions (incidence increases to 28% in pts having received cumulative dose >70 mg/m^2)

HEME: Delayed cumulative myelosuppression (complicates dosing schedule), particularly affecting leukocytes, platelets (nadirs occur 4-5 wks after administration; recovery often takes 2-3 wk)

RESP: Interstitial pneumonia, pulmonary fibrosis (cumulative doses >50-60 mg/m^2); acute bronchospasm in adults approximately 4-12 hrs after receiving mitomycin with Vinca

Other: Reversible alopecia, fever; thrombocytopenia, consumptive coagulopathy, renal failure; syndrome mimics hemolytic uremic syndrome but now recognized as separate entity consisting of microangiopathic hemolytic anemia, consumptive microangiopathy; clinical findings include intravascular hemolysis, activation of fibrinolytic system, consumption of clotting factors, renal failure, hypertension (fatal about 3-4 wk after diagnosis)

✤ Available in Canada.

TOXICITY AND OVERDOSE

Clinical signs: Prolonged myelosuppression, evidence of pulmonary fibrosis, evidence of renal failure related to microangiopathic hemolytic anemia, consumptive microangiopathy

Treatment: Supportive measures including blood transfusion (may exacerbate hemolytic uremic syndrome), hydration, nutritional supplementation, broad spectrum antibiotic coverage if febrile, electrolyte replacement

PATIENT CARE MANAGEMENT

Assessment

- Assess history of hypersensitivity to mitomycin
- Assess history of previous chemotherapy, radiation therapy, with attention to any that might predispose to greater risk of pulmonary, cardiac, or renal complications
- Assess baseline ECG, echocardiogram, pulmonary function tests
- Assess baseline VS, oximetry
- Assess success of previous antiemetic therapy
- Assess baseline CBC, differential, platelet count
- Assess baseline renal function (BUN, creatinine), liver studies function (alk phos, LDH, AST, ALT, bilirubin)
- Assess baseline UA

Interventions

- Administer antiemetic therapy before chemotherapy
- Ensure absolute patency of IV before administration
- Do not place IV over joint; if extravasation occurs, joint may become immobilized
- Monitor I&O; provide IV fluids until child able to resume normal PO intake
- Provide supportive measures to maintain hemostasis, fluid, electrolyte, nutritional balance

> **NURSING ALERT**
>
> Drug is severe vesicant; ensure patency of IV line just before administration of drug; if infiltration occurs, area may be treated by top application of DMSO q6h for 14 days
>
> Drug can cause progressive and ultimately fatal syndrome of hemolytic anemia, consumptive angiopathy, hypertension, and progressive renal failure; assess UA, bleeding tendencies, and B/P frequently

Evaluation

- Evaluate therapeutic response (radiologic or clinical demonstration of tumor regression)
- Evaluate CBC, differential, platelet count at least weekly
- Evaluate renal function (BUN, creatinine), liver function (alk phos, LDH, AST, ALT, bilirubin) before each cycle
- Evaluate UA routinely with special attention to bleeding
- Evaluate cardiac status through periodic ECG, echocardiogram
- Evaluate pulmonary function tests regularly

PATIENT AND FAMILY EDUCATION

Teach/instruct

- To have patient well hydrated before and after chemotherapy
- About importance of follow-up to monitor blood counts, serum chemistry values, UA
- To take accurate temp; rectal temp contraindicated
- To notify care provider of signs of bleeding (bruising, epistaxis, bleeding gums), infection (fever, sore throat, fatigue)

Warn/advise

- About impact of body changes that may occur (hair loss, hyperpigmentation, nail ridging), how to minimize changes (wigs, caps, scarves, long sleeves)
- To avoid OTC preparations containing aspirin
- To report any alterations in behavior, sensation, perception; help

M

to develop a plan of care to manage side effects, stress of illness or treatment

- That urine may be discolored (green) for 48 hr
- To report any signs of hematuria
- That good oral hygiene with very soft toothbrush is imperative
- That dental work be delayed until blood counts returns to baseline, with permission of caretaker
- To avoid contact with known viral and bacterial illnesses
- That close household contacts of child not be immunized with live polio virus; use inactivated form
- That children receiving chemotherapy not receive immunizations until immune system recovers sufficiently to mount necessary antibody response
- To report chicken pox exposure in susceptible child immediately
- To report herpes zoster virus (shingles) reactivation immediately
- If appropriate, ways to preserve reproductive patterns, sexuality (sperm banking, contraceptives)

Encourage
- Provision of nutritious food intake; consider nutritional consultation
- To use top anesthetics to control discomfort of mucositis; avoidance of spicy foods, commercial mouthwashes

STORAGE
- Intact vial stable at room temp for lot life
- Reconstituted sol stable 7 days at room temp 14 days under refrigeration; protect from light
- Diluted in IV sol, stable in D_5W about 3 hr, NS for 12-24 hr, LR 24-43 hr

---

mitoxantrone
Brand Name(s): Novantrone

Classification: Antineoplastic, synthetic androstenedione; cell cycle phase non-specific

Pregnancy Category: D

AVAILABLE PREPARATIONS
Inj: 2 mg/ml

ROUTE AND DOSAGES
- Dosage may vary in response to diagnosis, extent of disease, concurrent or previous therapy, protocol guidelines, physiological parameters; consult current literature, protocol recommendations

ANLL Induction Therapy
Children ≤2 yr: IV 0.4 mg/kg/dose for 3-5 days
Children >2 yr and adults: IV 12 mg/m^2/24 hr for 3 days or 10-12 mg/m^2/24 hr for 5 days

Single Agent for Advanced Solid Tumors
Children: IV 18-20 mg/m^2/dose q 3-4 wks
Adults: 12-14 mg/m^2/dose q 3-4 wk
- Cumulative cardiotoxic dose is about 160 mg/m^2 if pt has had no previous anthracycline therapy; cumulative dose should not exceed 120 mg/m^2 if pt previously treated with anthracycline or chest radiation

IV administration
- IV push rate: Bolus injection diluted in 10-20 ml D_5W or NS over 1-2 min
- Intermittent infusion rate: Over 15-30 min
- Continuous infusion rate: 24 hrs/day for 5 days; 14-day continuous infusions reported

MECHANISM AND INDICATIONS
Mechanism: Exact mechanism of cytotoxicity unknown; intercalates with DNA, inhibits activity of DNA topoisomerase II causing single- and double-stranded breaks in helix; binds to intracellular proteins which may impair cell division; cytotoxic to both proliferating and non-proliferating cells, but rapidly dividing cells are more sensitive to effects
Indications: Predominantly used in ANLL, but also may have potential for use in ALL, CML (blast phase), lymphoma, ovarian cancer, some solid tumors

---

✤ Available in Canada.

PHARMACOKINETICS
Distribution: Rapid uptake from plasma into liver, pancreas, thyroid, spleen, heart, bone marrow
Half-life: Terminal half-life prolonged, median 12 days because of slow release of drug from formed blood elements
Metabolism: Liver
Excretion: Urine, bile

CONTRAINDICATIONS AND PRECAUTIONS
• Contraindicated with previous hypersensitivity to drug; children with active infections (especially chicken pox and herpes zoster); pts who have received cumulative lifetime dose, pregnancy, lactation
• Use cautiously with peripheral IV; hepatic dysfunction, generalized edema (adjust dosage)

INTERACTIONS
Drug
• Synergistic effect against leukemia cells with high-dosage cytarabine
• Very active in relapsed myeloid leukemias with etoposide
Lab
• Increased in AST, ALT, alk phos, bilirubin possible

INCOMPATIBILITIES
• Forms precipitate with heparin

SIDE EFFECTS
CV: Less cardiotoxic than anthracyclines but remains a concern; cumulative lifetime dose should not exceed 160 mg/m^2; phlebitis, venous discoloration
DERM: Reversible alopecia (infrequent); can be a selective loss of white hair in CML pts
GI: Nausea, vomiting, stomatitis; reversible hepatic dysfunction
GU: Green urine, hyperuricemia
HEME: Myelosuppression (most commonly affecting leukocytes, nadir at 10-14 days, recovery by 21 days)
Other: Allergic reaction (hypotension, urticaria, dyspnea, rashes)

TOXICITY AND OVERDOSE
Clinical signs: Prolonged myelosuppression, signs of cardiac toxicity
Treatment: Supportive measures including blood transfusions, hydration, nutritional supplementation, broad spectrum antibiotic coverage if febrile, electrolyte replacement

PATIENT CARE MANAGEMENT
Assessment
• Assess history of hypersensitivity to mitoxantrone
• Assess history of previous chemotherapy and radiation therapy, especially any that may predispose to greater risk of cardiac or hepatic dysfunction
• Assess cumulative anthracycline therapy
• Obtain baseline ECG, echocardiogram
• Assess baseline VS, oximetry
• Assess CBC, differential, platelet count
• Assess renal function (BUN, creatinine), liver function (bilirubin, alk phos, LDH, AST, ALT) function
• Assess success of previous antiemetic therapy
Interventions
• Administer antiemetic therapy before chemotherapy
• Ensure absolute potency of IV before administration
• Monitor I&O; provide IV hydration until child is able to resume PO fluid intake
• Provide supportive measures to maintain hemostasis, fluid, electrolyte, nutritional balance

> **NURSING ALERT**
> Drug has presumed cardiotoxic effects; cumulative lifetime dose should not exceed 160 mg/m^2; 120 mg/m^2 if previous anthracycline or chest radiation received; resting HR, ECG and echocardiograms should be monitored regularly

M

Evaluation
• Evaluate therapeutic response (demonstration of tumor regression)
• Evaluate CBC, differential, platelet count at least weekly
• Evaluate cardiac status through periodic ECG, echocardiogram
• Evaluate renal function (BUN, creatinine), liver function (AST, ALT, LDH, alk phos, bilirubin)

PATIENT AND FAMILY EDUCATION
Teach/instruct
• To have pt well-hydrated before and after chemotherapy
• About importance of follow-up to monitor blood counts, serum chemistry values
• To take accurate temp, rectal temp contraindicated
• To notify care provider of signs of bleeding (bruising, epistaxis, bleeding gums), infection (fever, sore throat, fatigue)

Warn/advise
• About impact of body changes that may occur (hair loss, hyperpigmentation, nail ridging), how to minimize changes (wigs, caps, scarves, long sleeves)
• To avoid OTC products containing aspirin
• To report any alterations in behavior, sensation, perception; help to develop a plan of care to manage side effects, stress of illness or treatment
• That urine may be discolored for up to 48 hr
• To call immediately if bleeding or bruising noted
• To call immediately if pain, swelling, erythema at injection site
• That good oral hygiene with very soft toothbrush is imperative
• That dental care be delayed until blood counts return to baseline and with provider approval
• To avoid contact with known bacterial and viral illnesses
• That close household contacts of child not be immunized with live polio virus; inactivated form should be used
• That children on chemotherapy not be immunized until the immune system recovers sufficiently to mount appropriate antibody response
• That exposure to chicken pox in susceptible child be reported immediately
• That reactivation of herpes zoster virus (shingles) be reported immediately
• If appropriate, ways to preserve reproductive patterns, and sexuality (sperm banking, contraceptives)

Encourage
• Provision of nutritious food intake; consider nutritional consultation
• To use top anesthetics to control pain of mucositis; avoid spicy foods, commercial mouthwashes

STORAGE
• Sol has no preservative but is chemically stable for yrs at room temp, under refrigeration, or frozen
• Sol itself has bacteriostatic qualities and, if entered aseptically, a multidose vial can be kept for 7 days at room temp, 14 days under refrigeration

---

morphine
Brand Name(s): Astramorph, Duramorph, Infumorph 200, Infumorph 500, Morphine HP✚, M.O.S.-Sulfate✚, MS, MS-Contin✚, MS-IR✚, MS-04, OMS Concentrate, Oramorph-SR✚, RMS, Roxanol, Roxanol SR, Statex✚

Classification: Narcotic analgesic, opiate agonist

Controlled Substance Schedule II

Pregnancy Category: B

AVAILABLE PREPARATIONS
Tabs: 15 mg, 30 mg

Tabs, soluble: 10 mg, 15 mg, 30 mg
Tabs, ext rel: 30 mg
Tabs, controlled rel: 15 mg, 30 mg, 60 mg, 100 mg
Oral sol: 2 mg/ml, 4 mg/ml, 20 mg/ml
Rectal supp: 5 mg, 10 mg, 20 mg, 30 mg
Inj: 0.5 mg/ml, 1 mg/ml, 2 mg/ml, 4 mg/ml, 5 mg/ml, 8 mg/ml, 10 mg/ml, 15 mg/ml
IV infusion device: 1 mg/ml or 5 mg/ml

ROUTES AND DOSAGES
Infants and children: PO 0.3 mg/kg/dose q3-4h prn starting dose; sus rel 0.3-0.6 mg/kg/dose q12h prn; IM/IV/SC 0.1-0.2 mg/kg/dose q2-4h prn starting dose (maximum 15 mg/dose); continuous infusion for postoperative pain 0.01-0.04 mg/kg/hr; for sickle cell or cancer pain 0.025-2 mg/kg/hr (begin with lowest dose)
Adults: PO 10-30 mg q4h prn; sus rel 15-30 mg q8-12h prn; IM/IV/SC 2.5-15 mg/dose q2-6h prn; continuous infusion 0.8-10 mg/hr

IV administration
• Recommended concentration: 0.1-1 mg/ml in D_5W for continuous infusion by controlled infusion device; 1 mg/kg in 100 ml D_5W infused at 2 ml/hr delivers 0.02 mg/kg/hr; 1 or 5 mg/ml for multiple slow injections
• Maximum concentration: 1 mg/ml for continuous infusion; 5 mg/ml for IV push
• IV push rate: Over 4-5 min

MECHANISM AND INDICATIONS
Mechanism: Depresses pain impulse transmission at the spinal cord level by interacting with opioid receptors; alters perception of and response to painful stimuli while producing generalized CNS depression
Indications: Used to treat moderate-to-severe pain

PHARMACOKINETICS
Onset: PO, PR variable, IM 10-30 min; SC 20 min; IV immediate
Peak: PO variable; PR 20-60 min; IM 30-60 min; SC 50-90 min; IV 20 min
Distribution: Widely distributed
Half-life: 2.5-3 hr
Duration: PO variable (ext rel 8-12 hr); PR 4-5 hr; IM 4-5 hr; SC 4-5 hr; IV 2-5 hr
Metabolism: Liver
Excretion: Urine

CONTRAINDICATIONS AND PRECAUTIONS
• Contraindicated with hypersensitivity, respiratory depression, comatose, elevated ICP, hemorrhage, bronchial asthma, premature infants, neonates
• Use cautiously with asthma; hepatic, renal or pulmonary disease; atrial flutter, tachycardia, colitis, hypothyroidism, undiagnosed abdominal pain, pregnancy, lactation

INTERACTIONS
Drug
• Increased risk of coma, respiratory depression, hypotension (may even result in unpredictable fatal reaction) with use of MAOIs
• Additive CNS depression with alcohol, antihistamines, sedatives or hypnotics
• Precipitation of withdrawal possible in narcotic-dependent pts with use of partial antagonists (buprenorphine, butorphanol, nalbuphine, pentazocine)
• Antagonized action possible with phenothiazines
• Decreased effects of diuretics in CHF
• Increased effects of neuromuscular-blocking agents possible
Lab
• Increased serum amylase and lipase (delay drawing blood for these tests for 24 hr after administration
• Decreased serum and urine 17-KS, 17-OHCS

INCOMPATIBILITIES
• Aminophylline, amobarbital, heparin, meperidine, methicillin, pentobarbital, phenobarbital, phenytoin, $NaHCO_3$, thiopental

M

SIDE EFFECTS

CNS: Dizziness, sedation, confusion, headache, euphoria, floating feeling, unusual dreams, hallucinations, dysphoria, insomnia, coma, restlessness, insomnia

CV: Palpitation, bradycardia, tachycardia (more common than with other opiates), orthostatic hypotension, circulatory depression is potentially life threatening

DERM: Rash, erythema, urticaria, pruritus, facial flushing indicates hypersensitivity reaction, sweating, bruising

EENT: Miosis, diplopia, blurred vision, tinnitus

GI: Nausea, vomiting, constipation, anorexia, cramps, biliary tract pressure, biliary spasm, increased serum amylase and lipase

GU: Urinary retention, oliguria

RESP: Respiratory depression

Other: Tolerance, physical and psychological dependence

TOXICITY AND OVERDOSE

Clinical signs: Respiratory and circulatory depression

Treatment: Supportive care; naloxone (dose may need to be repeated or naloxone infusion administered), vasopressors

PATIENT CARE MANAGEMENT

Assessment

• Assess history to hypersensitivity to morphine

• Assess baseline VS, renal function (BUN, creatinine)

• Assess pain (type, location, intensity) before and 30-60 minutes after administration

Interventions

• Administer PO with food or milk to reduce GI irritation; tabs may be crushed, mixed with food or fluid; controlled or ext rel tabs must be swallowed whole; dilute oral sol in at least 30 ml fluid

• Rapid IV administration may lead to increased respiratory depression, hypotension, circulatory collapse; ensure naloxone is readily available

• If using continuous and interval dosing (PCA), ensure that the continuous dose is not greater than 20% of the total dose ordered

• Determine dosing interval by patient response; administer when pain is not too severe to enhance its effectiveness; administer concurrently with non-narcotic analgesics may have additive analgesic effects and permit lower narcotic dosages

• Institute safety measures (support ambulation, raise side rails, call light within reach)

> **NURSING ALERT**
> Rapid administration may cause increased respiratory depression, hypotension, circulatory collapse; provide naloxone for IV use

Evaluation

• Evaluate therapeutic response (decreased pain without significant alteration in LOC or respiratory status)

• Monitor VS, pain control 30-60 min after administration, CNS changes

PATIENT AND FAMILY EDUCATION

Teach/instruct

• To take as directed at prescribed intervals for prescribed length of time (if on home care management)

• About best time to request medication (if ordered prn)

• About use of PCA pump, if appropriate

Warn/advise

• That tolerance or dependence may occur with long-term use

• That medication may cause drowsiness, dizziness, orthostatic hypotension; to make position changes slowly; to seek assistance with ambulation

• To avoid alcohol, OTC medications

Encourage

• To maintain adequate fluid intake, coughing, and deep breathing exercises to avoid respiratory stasis

---

✦ Available in Canada.

STORAGE
- Store at room temp
- Protect from light, moisture
- Avoid freezing sol

mupirocin
Brand Name(s): Bactroban ♣
Classification: Topical antibacterial
Pregnancy Category: B

AVAILABLE PREPARATIONS
Top: Oint: 2%

ROUTES AND DOSAGES
Children and adults: Top, apply small amount to affected area tid

MECHANISM AND INDICATIONS
Antibacterial mechanism: Inhibits bacterial protein synthesis
Indications: Used for superficial skin infections (impetigo, folliculitis, infected eczema) caused by *Staphylococcus aureus,* group A β hemolytic streptococcus, *Str. pyogenes*

PHARMACOKINETICS
Absorption: Minimal or no measurable systemic absorption
Excretion: Urine

CONTRAINDICATIONS AND PRECAUTIONS
- Contraindicated with known hypersensitivity to mupirocin or polyethylene glycol
- Use cautiously with prolonged use; may result in overgrowth of non-susceptible organisms (including fungi); should not be used on mucosal surfaces or on skin areas where absorption of large amounts is possible

INTERACTIONS
Drug
- None
Lab
- None

SIDE EFFECTS
DERM: Minor local burning, itching, stinging, or pain; contact dermatitis; increased exudate

TOXICITY AND OVERDOSE
- None reported

PATIENT CARE MANAGEMENT
Assessment
- Assess history of hypersensitivity to drug
- Assess affected area for infected, crusted lesions
Interventions
- Wash hands well before and after applying drug
- Apply drug to clean, dry lesions tid
- May cover lesions with gauze if needed
Evaluation
- Evaluate therapeutic response (lesions diminished in size, number)

PATIENT AND FAMILY EDUCATION
Teach/instruct
- To take as directed at prescribed intervals for prescribed length of time
- To wash hands well before and after contact with lesions
- To trim fingernails to reduce spread and irritation resulting from scratching
- To notify care provider if irritation, inflammation, or increased exudate occurs
- To notify provider if no improvement noted within 3-5 days

STORAGE
- Store in tight containers

nafcillin sodium
Brand Name(s): Nafcil, Nallpen, Unipen ♣
Classification: Antibiotic (penicillinase-resistant penicillin)
Pregnancy Category: B

AVAILABLE PREPARATIONS
Oral susp: 250 mg/5 ml

Caps: 250 mg
Tabs: 500 mg
Inj: 500 mg, 1 g, 1.5 g, 2 g, 4 g

ROUTES AND DOSAGES
PO
Neonates: 30-40 mg/kg/24 hr divided q6-8h
Infants and children: 50-100 mg/kg/24 hr divided q6h
Adults: 250-1000 mg q4-6h
IM/IV
Neonates ≤7 days, < 2000 g: 50 mg/kg/24 hr divided q12h
Neonates > 7 days, < 2000 g: 75 mg/kg/24 hr divided q8h
Neonates ≤7 days, > 2000 g: 50-75 mg/kg/24 hr divided q8h
Neonates > 7 days, > 2000 g: 75-100 mg/kg/24 hr divided q6h
Infants and children: IM 100-200 mg/kg/24 hr divided q12h; IV 100-200 mg/kg/24 hr divided q6h
Adults: 500-2000 mg q4-6h; maximum 12 g/24 hr
IV administration
• Recommended concentration: 2-40 mg/ml in D_5W, NS, R, or SW for IV infusion; dilute dose in 15-30 ml NS or SW for IV push
• Maximum concentration: 40 mg/ml for IV infusion
• IV push rate: Over 5-10 min
• Intermittent infusion rate: Over 15-60 min

MECHANISM
AND INDICATIONS
Antibiotic mechanism: Bactericidal; inhibits bacterial cell wall synthesis by adhering to bacterial penicillin-binding proteins
Indications: Effective against gram-positive cocci including *Staphylococcus aureus, Streptococcus viridans, Str. pneumoniae,* and infections caused by penicillinase-producing *Staphylococcus;* used to treat meningitis, respiratory tract, skin, soft tissue, bone, and joint infections

PHARMACOKINETICS
Peak: PO/IM 0.5-2.0 hr; IV, end of infusion
Distribution: Penetrates CNS with inflamed meninges

Half-life: Neonates 1.2-5.5 hr; children 0.75-1.9 hr
Metabolism: Liver
Excretion: Urine, bile

CONTRAINDICATIONS
AND PRECAUTIONS
• Contraindicated with known hypersensitivity to nafcillin, penicillins, or cephalosporins
• Use cautiously with neonates, impaired renal or hepatic function, history of colitis or other GI disorders, pregnancy

INTERACTIONS
Drug
• Synergistic antimicrobial effect against certain organisms with aminoglycosides.
• Increased serum concentrations with probenecid
• Decreased antimicrobial effectiveness with tetracyclines, erythromycins, chloramphenicol
• Increased risk of bleeding with anticoagulants.
Lab
• False positive urine protein
Nutrition
• Decreased absorption if given with meals, acidic fruit juices, citrus fruits, or acidic beverages (e.g., cola drinks)

INCOMPATIBILITIES
• Aminoglycosides, aminophylline, ascorbic acid, bleomycin, hydrocortisone sodium succinate, labetalol, meperidine, methyl-prednisolone, promazine, verapamil, sol with pH <5.0 or >8.0

SIDE EFFECTS
GI: Nausea, vomiting, diarrhea, pseudomembranous colitis
GU: Hematuria, acute interstitial nephritis
HEME: Transient leukopenia, neutropenia, granulocytopenia, thrombocytopenia with high dosages
Local: Vein, irritation, thrombophlebitis
Other: Hypersensitivity reactions (chills, fever, rash, pruritus, urticaria, anaphylaxis), bacterial or fungal superinfection

---

✤ Available in Canada.

TOXICITY AND OVERDOSE

Clinical signs: Neuromuscular irritability, seizures

Treatment: Supportive care; if ingested with 4 hrs, empty stomach by induced emesis or gastric lavage, followed by activated charcoal

PATIENT CARE MANAGEMENT

Assessment

• Assess history of hypersensitivity to nafcillin, penicillins, or cephalosporins

• Obtain C&S; may begin therapy before obtaining results

• Assess renal function (BUN, creatinine, I&O), hepatic function (ALT, AST, bilirubin), hematologic function (CBC, differential, platelet count), particularly for long-term therapy

Interventions

• Administer penicillins at least 1 hr before bacteriostatic antibiotics (tetracyclines, erythromycins, chloramphenicol)

• Administer PO 1 hr ac or 2 hr after meals; administer with water; avoid acidic beverages; shake suspension well before administering; caps may be taken apart, tabs crushed and mixed with food or fluid

• Caps and tabs buffered with calcium carbonate may interact with other medications

• Do not reconstitute IM with bacteriostatic water containing benzoyl alcohol for neonates

• Injection is painful; administer slowly and deeply into large muscle mass and rotate injection sites

• Do not mix IV with any other drug

• Use large vein with small-bore needle; rotate site q48-72h

• Infuse only through patent tubing; extravasation can cause severe skin damage; hyaluronidase can be used to treat extravasation

• Maintain age-appropriate fluid intake

> **NURSING ALERT**
>
> Discontinue drug if signs of hypersensitivity, interstial nephritis, pseudomembranous colitis develop
>
> Do not infuse rapidly; seizures may develop
>
> Extravasation can cause severe skin damage

Evaluation

• Evaluate therapeutic response (decreased symptoms of infection)

• Monitor signs of superinfection (perineal itching, diaper rash, fever, malaise, redness, pain, swelling, drainage, rash, diarrhea, sore throat, change in cough or sputum)

• Observe for signs of allergic reaction (wheezing, tightness in chest, urticaria), especially within 20-30 min of first dose

• Monitor renal function (BUN, creatinine, I&O) and hepatic function (ALT, AST, bilirubin), electrolyte levels, particularly K^+ and Na

• Monitor for signs of bleeding (ecchymosis, bleeding gums, hematuria, daily stool guaiac); monitor pro-times and platelet counts

• Evaluate IM site for tissue damage, IV site for vein irritation, extravasation

PATIENT AND FAMILY EDUCATION

Teach/instruct

• To take as directed at prescribed intervals for prescribed length of time

Warn/advise

• To notify care provider of hypersensitivity, side effects, superinfection

STORAGE

• Store powder, caps, tabs at room temp, tabs protected from light

• Reconstituted susp stable refrigerated 7 days; label date and time of reconstitution

• IM sol stable refrigerated for 7 days, room temp 3 days; IV sol at concentrations 2-40 mg/ml stable in specific concentration at room temp 24 hr, refrigerated 96 hr

---

nalbuphine

Brand Name: Nubain, Nalbuphine HCI

Classification: Narcotic analgesic, opiate agonist/ antagonist and partial agonist

Controlled Substance Schedule II

Pregnancy Category: B

AVAILABLE PREPARATIONS
Inj: 10 mg/ml, 20 mg/ml

ROUTES AND DOSAGES
Children and adults: SC/IM/IV 0.1 mg/kg q 3-6h prn; maximum single dose 20 mg, maximum dose 160 mg/24 hr (Safety and effectiveness in children not established. Dosage represents accepted standard practice recommendations.)

IV administration
• Recommended concentration: Undiluted
• IV push rate: May give each 10 mg over 3-5 min

MECHANISM AND INDICATIONS
Mechanism: Depresses pain impulse transmission at the spinal cord level by interacting with opioid receptors; alters perception of and response to painful stimuli while producing generalized CNS depression
Indications: Used to treat moderate-to-severe pain

PHARMACOKINETICS
Onset of action: IM/SC < 15 min; IV 2-3 min
Peak: IM 60 min; SC unknown; IV 30 min
Distribution: Widely distributed
Half-life: 5 hr
Duration: IM/SC/IV 3-6 hr
Metabolism: Liver
Excretion: Urine

CONTRAINDICATIONS AND PRECAUTIONS
• Contraindicated with hypersensitivity to the drug or bisulfites
• Use cautiously with hepatic, renal, or pulmonary disease; increased ICP; respiratory depression; hypothyroidism; adrenal insufficiency; undiagnosed abdominal pain; pregnancy (has been used during labor but may cause respiratory depression in the newborn); lactation

INTERACTIONS
Drug
• Increased risk of coma, respiratory depression, hypotension (may even result in unpredictable fatal reaction) with MAOIs
• Additive CNS depression with alcohol, antihistamines, sedatives/ hypnotics
• Withdrawal in narcotic-dependent patients (who have not been detoxified) with narcotic analgesic agonist
• Increased effects of neuromuscular-blocking agents
Lab
• Increase serum amylase, lipase; delay drawing blood for these tests for 24 hr after drug administration

INCOMPATIBILITIES
• Pentobarbital, diazepam, nafcillin

SIDE EFFECTS
CNS: Sedation, confusion, headache, euphoria, floating feeling, unusual dreams, hallucinations, dysphoria (with high dosages), dizziness, vertigo
CV: Orthostatic hypotension, palpitation, bradycardia
DERM: Rash, urticaria, pruritus, flushing, sweating, bruising, clammy feeling
EENT: Miosis (with high dosages), diplopia, blurred vision, tinnitus
GI: Nausea, vomiting, constipation, anorexia, cramps, ileus, dry mouth
GU: Urinary urgency and retention, dysuria, increased urinary output
RESP: Respiratory depression

✤ Available in Canada.

Other: Tolerance, physical and psychological dependence

TOXICITY AND OVERDOSE

Clinical signs: Respiratory depression
Treatment: Supportive care, naloxone (dose may need to be repeated or naloxone infusion administered), vasopressors

PATIENT CARE MANAGEMENT

Assessment

• Assess history of hypersensitivity to nalbuphine or related drugs
• Assess baseline VS, pain (type, location, intensity)
• Assess renal function (BUN, creatinine, I&O), GI complications, CNS changes

Interventions

• Administer IM deep into well-developed muscle; rotate injection sites
• Determine dosing interval based on response; administer when pain is not too severe to enhance its effectiveness; concurrent administration with non-narcotic analgesics may have additive analgesic effects and permit lower narcotic dosages
• Institute safety measures (supervise ambulation, raise side rails, call light within reach)

Evaluation

• Evaluate therapeutic response (decrease in pain without significant alteration in LOC or respiratory status)
• Evaluate renal function (BUN, creatinine), CNS, VS
• Evaluate pain 15-30 min after administration
• Evaluate side effects, hypersensitivity
• Monitor for withdrawal reactions in narcotic-dependent individuals

PATIENT AND FAMILY EDUCATION

Teach/instruct

• About best time to request medication (if ordered prn)
• That frequent mouth rinses, good oral hygiene, sugarless gum, or candy may decrease dry mouth

Warn/advise

• That drug may cause drowsiness, dizziness, orthostatic hypotension; make position changes slowly, seek assistance with ambulation
• That tolerance or dependence may occur with long-term use
• To avoid OTC medications, alcohol, other CNS depressants
• To notify care provider of hypersensitivity, side effects

Encourage

• To maintain adequate fluid intake, coughing, deep breathing exercises to avoid respiratory complications

STORAGE

• Store at room temp in tightly covered, light-resistant container

---

nalidixic acid

Brand Name(s): NegGram✚

Classification: Urinary tract antiseptic (quinolone antibiotic)

Pregnancy Category: B

AVAILABLE PREPARATIONS

Oral susp: 250 mg/5 ml
Tabs: 250 mg, 500 mg, 1 g

ROUTES AND DOSAGES

Children >3 mo: PO 55 mg/kg/24 hr divided q6h; suppressive therapy 33 mg/kg/24 hr divided q6h
Adults: PO 1 g qid for 14 days; suppressive therapy 500 mg qid

MECHANISM AND INDICATIONS

Antimicrobial mechanism: Inhibits microbial synthesis of DNA
Indications: Used to treat UTIs caused by *E. coli, Klebsiella, Enterobacter, Proteus mirabilis, P. vulgaris, P. morganii*

PHARMACOKINETICS

Peak: 1-2 hr
Distribution: Significant antibacterial concentrations only in urinary tract
Half-life: 6-7 hr

N

Metabolism: Liver
Excretion: Urine, feces

CONTRAINDICATIONS AND PRECAUTIONS

• Contraindicated with infants <3 mo, with known hypersensitivity to nalidixic acid, seizure disorders, G-6-PD deficiency, or liver failure
• Use cautiously with renal or hepatic impairment, pregnancy

INTERACTIONS
Drug
• Increased effects of oral anticoagulants
• Decreased absorption with antacids
• Additive effects with other photosensitizing drugs
Lab
• Falsely elevated urinary VMA
• False elevation of urine 17-KS and 17-OHCS

SIDE EFFECTS

CNS: Drowsiness, weakness, headache, dizziness, vertigo, convulsions in epileptic patients, confusion, hallucinations
DERM: Pruritus, photosensitivity, urticaria, rash
EENT: Sensitivity to light, change in color perception, diplopia, blurred vision
GI: Abdominal pain, nausea, vomiting, diarrhea
HEME: Eosinophilia, thrombocytopenia, leukopenia, hemolytic anemia
Other: Angioedema, fever, chills, increased intracranial pressure, bulging fontanelles in infants and children

TOXICITY AND OVERDOSE

Clinical signs: Toxic psychosis, seizures, increased intracranial pressure, metabolic acidosis, lethargy, nausea, vomiting
Treatment: Gastric lavage after recent ingestion; supportive care, increased fluid administration

PATIENT CARE MANAGEMENT
Assessment
• Assess history of hypersensitivity to nalidixic acid

• Obtain C&S; may begin therapy before obtaining results
• Assess I&O, urine pH (<5.5 for maximum effect), hematologic function (CBC, differential, platelet count), renal function (BUN, creatinine), hepatic function (ALT, AST, bilirubin)

Interventions
• Administer PO with food or milk to reduce GI distress
• Shake susp well before administering; tab may be crushed, mixed with food or fluid
• Provide diet limited in alkaline foods (milk, dairy products, peanuts, vegetables); avoid alkaline antacids, NaHCO$_3$
• Maintain urine pH <5.5
• Maintain age-appropriate fluid intake

> **NURSING ALERT**
> Discontinue drug if signs of hypersensitivity, seizures, toxic psychosis, increased intracranial pressure, photosensitivity develop

Evaluation
• Evaluate therapeutic response (decreased dysuria, frequency, urgency, negative culture)
• Monitor I&O, urine pH, hematologic function (CBC, differential, platelet count), renal function (BUN, creatinine), hepatic function (ALT, AST, bilirubin), particularly with long-term therapy
• Monitor for CNS symptoms (insomnia, vertigo, headache, drowsiness, seizures)
• Monitor for allergic reaction (fever, flushing, rash, urticaria, pruritus)

PATIENT AND FAMILY EDUCATION
Teach/instruct
• To take as directed at prescribed intervals for prescribed length of time
Warn/advise
• To notify care provider of hypersensitivity, side effects
• To avoid alkaline foods or medi-

---

cations (e.g., milk, dairy products, peanuts, vegetables, alkaline antacids, $NaHCO_3$)
• To avoid sunlight or use sunscreen to prevent burning; photosensitivity may continue up to 3 mo after the end of therapy

STORAGE
• Store tabs at room temp

---

naloxone
Brand Name: Narcan
Classification: Narcotic antagonist
Pregnancy Category: B

AVAILABLE PREPARATIONS
Inj: 0.02 mg/ml, 0.4 mg/ml, 1 mg/ml vials

ROUTES AND DOSAGES
Narcotic-Induced Respiratory or CNS Depression
Children <5 yr, <20 kg: IV/IM/SC 0.1 mg/kg q2-3 min as needed until opiate effects are reversed
Children >5 yr, ≥20 kg, and adults: IV/IM/SC 0.1 mg/kg (minimum individual dose 2 mg); subsequent doses of 0.1 mg/kg q2-3 min prn; when repeated dose is required, may use continuous infusion (0.04-0.16 mg/kg/hr) following titration of intermittent doses
Postoperative Respiratory Depression
Children and adults: IV/IM/SC 0.01-0.02 mg/kg q2-3 min until response obtained, with additional doses q1-2 h prn
IV administration
• Recommended concentration: 4 mcg/ml in D_5W or NS for continuous infusion, 0.4 or 1 mg/ml for IV push
• Maximum concentration: 1 mg/ml for IV push
• IV push rate: Rapid (seconds)
• Continuous infusion: 0.024-0.16 mg/kg/hr

MECHANISM AND INDICATIONS
Mechanism: Competitively blocks the effects of narcotics (e.g., CNS and respiratory depression, without producing any agonist [narcotic like] effects)
Indications: Used to treat respiratory depression induced by narcotics, pentazocine, propoxyhene

PHARMACOKINETICS
Onset of action: IV 1-2 min, IM/SC: 2-5 min
Peak: Unknown
Distribution: Rapidly distributed to tissues
Half-life: 30-100 min
Duration: IV 45 min, IM/SC 45-60 min
Metabolism: Liver
Excretion: Urine

CONTRAINDICATIONS AND PRECAUTIONS
• Contraindicated with known hypersensitivity to drug, in treatment of respiratory depression not caused by narcotics
• Use cautiously with cardiovascular disease, narcotic-dependent pts (may precipitate severe withdrawal), pregnancy (may cause withdrawal in mother and fetus if mother is narcotic-dependent), lactation, neonates of narcotic-dependent mothers

INTERACTIONS
Drug
• Withdrawal in narcotic-dependent patients
• Antagonized postoperative analgesia
Lab
• Interference with urine VMA, 5-HIAA, urine glucose

INCOMPATIBILITIES
• Alkaline drugs, bisulfites, sulfites

SIDE EFFECTS
CNS: Seizures (rare), drowsiness, nervousness
CV: Hypotension, hypertension (increased systolic when given in high dosages), tachycardia (these effects seen most often with CV

N

disease or with use of cardiac drugs), arrhythmias, ventricular tachycardia
GI: Nausea, vomiting (rare), hepatotoxicity
HEME: Prolonged PTT
RESP: Hyperpnea, pulmonary edema

TOXICITY AND OVERDOSE
• No clinical experience with overdose in humans

PATIENT CARE MANAGEMENT
Assessment
• Assess amount of opiate received (if possible)
• Assess VS, LOC
• Assess cardiac status, respiratory dysfunction
Interventions
• Have resuscitative equipment and drugs readily available
• Repeat doses as necessary (effects of some narcotics may last longer than effects of naloxone)

> **NURSING ALERT**
> May also be given via ET tube if no available access
>
> If no response is seen after 2 or 3 doses, respiratory depression probably is not caused by narcotics

Evaluation
• Evaluate therapeutic response (adequate ventilation and alertness without significant pain)
• Evaluate side effects, hypersensitivity
• Evaluate level of pain following administration if used to treat postoperative respiratory depression, because naloxone also reverses analgesic effects of narcotics
• Monitor for signs and symptoms of narcotic withdrawal (severity depends on dosage of naloxone, narcotic involved, degree of physical dependence)
• Evaluate ABGs

PATIENT AND FAMILY EDUCATION
Teach/instruct
• About purpose and effects of naloxone (as medication becomes effective)
• About possible change in narcotic administration because of respiratory effects of medication

STORAGE
• Store at room temp in light-resistant container

---

naltrexone hydrochloride
Brand Name(s): ReVia✤, Trexan
Classification: Narcotic antagonist
Pregnancy Category: C

AVAILABLE PREPARATIONS
Tabs: 50 mg

ROUTES AND DOSAGES
• Naltrexone has been tested only in adults, and there is limited information about use in pts <18 yr; (Although routinely used in pediatrics, safety and effectiveness have not been established. Dosage represents accepted standard practice recommendation for this age group and route.)
Self-Injurious Behavior, Social Withdrawal, Hyperactivity, Stereotypy
Children: PO 0.5-1.5 mg/kg qd
Narcotic Addiction
Adults: PO 25 mg qd; may administer 25 mg 1 hr later if there are no withdrawal symptoms; maintenance 50 mg/24 hr

MECHANISM AND INDICATIONS
Mechanism: Competes with narcotics at narcotic receptor sites
Indications: For use in treating self-injurious behavior, social withdrawal, hyperactivity, and stereotypy in some cases of autistic disorder and mentally retarded indi-

---

✤ Available in Canada.

viduals; also used to treat narcotic addiction

PHARMACOKINETICS
Onset of action: PO 15-30 min
Peak: 1-2 hr
Duration: Dose-dependent
Half-life: 4 hr
Metabolism: Liver
Excretion: Urine

CONTRAINDICATIONS AND PRECAUTIONS
• Contraindicated with hypersensitivity to naltrexone or any component, hepatitis, hepatic failure, narcotic dependence
• Use cautiously with pregnancy, lactation

INTERACTIONS
Drug
• Decreased effects of narcotics
Lab
• Increased PT

SIDE EFFECTS
CNS: Drowsiness, stimulation, anxiety, confusion, mental depression, dizziness, flushing, hallucinations, headache, irritability, mood changes, nervousness, restlessness, sedation, seizures, trouble sleeping
CV: Increased B/P, hypertension, pulmonary edema, tachycardia
DERM: Rash, bruising, hives, itching
EENT: Cough, earache; aching, burning, swollen eyes; hearing loss, hoarseness, runny or stuffy nose, nosebleeds, sinus problems, sneezing, sore throat, tinnitus, blurred vision
GI: Diarrhea, heartburn, nausea, vomiting, abdominal cramping or pain, anorexia, constipation, hepatitis, increased thirst, wt gain
GU: Male sexual problems, discomfort while urinating, frequent urination
HEME: Agranulocytosis, hemolytic anemia, leukopenia, neutropenia, thrombocytopenia
RESP: SOB, wheezing
Other: Chills, fever, swollen glands, joint or muscle pain, swelling, unusual tiredness, withdrawal symptoms

PATIENT CARE MANAGEMENT
Assessment
• Assess history of hypersensitivity to drug
• Assess ability to function in daily activities, to sleep throughout the night; self-injurious behavior, social withdrawal hyperactivity, stereotypy, narcotic addiction
• Assess mental status (mood, sensorium, affect, impulsiveness, suicidal ideation, thoughts)
• If used for narcotic addiction, obtain baseline ABGs including PO_2 and PCO_2
Interventions
• Rinse with water, take sips of fluid, sugarless gum, or hard candy for dry mouth
Evaluation
• Evaluate therapeutic response (ability to function in daily activities; to sleep throughout the night; discontinuation of self-injurious behavior, social withdrawal, hyperactivity, stereotypy, narcotic addiction)
• Evaluate mental status (mood, sensorium, affect, impulsiveness, suicidal ideation, thoughts)
• Evaluate for early signs of withdrawal in narcotic-dependent individuals
• Monitor pulse, B/P
• Monitor character, rate, and rhythm of respirations

PATIENT AND FAMILY EDUCATION
Teach/instruct
• To take as directed at prescribed intervals for prescribed length of time
• That this medication is most helpful when used as part of a comprehensive multimodal treatment program
• Not to discontinue medication without prescriber approval
• To tell all care providers that patient is using naltrexone
• That naltrexone also blocks the useful effects of narcotics; always use a non-narcotic medicine to treat pain, diarrhea, or cough

N

Warn/advise

• Not to try to overcome effects of naltrexone by taking very large amounts of narcotics; this could cause coma or death

• That drug may cause drowsiness; to be careful on bicycles, skates, skateboards, while driving, with other activities requiring alertness

• To carry medical alert identification stating that pt is taking naltrexone

STORAGE

• Store in tight container

• Protect from heat, direct light

---

naproxen/naproxen sodium

Brand Name(s): Anaprox✤, Anaprox DS✤, Apo-Napro-Na✤, Apo-Napro-Na-D5✤, Apo-Naproxen✤, Naprosyn✤, Naxen✤, Novo-Naprox✤, Novo-Naprox Sodium✤, Novo-Naprox Sodium-DS✤, Nu-Naprox✤, PMS-Naproxen✤, SynFlex✤, SynFlex DS✤

Classification: Nonsteroidal antiinflammatory agent, antipyretic, antirheumatic

Pregnancy Category: B

AVAILABLE PREPARATIONS
Susp: 125 mg/5 ml
Tabs: 250, 275, 375, 500 mg
Tabs, film coated: 275, 550 mg
Naproxen sodium: 220 mg = 200 mg base; 550 mg = 500 mg base; 275 mg = 250 mg base

ROUTES AND DOSAGES
Juvenile Rheumatoid Arthritis/Inflammatory Diseases
Children: PO naproxen, 10-15 mg/kg/24 hr divided bid (maximum 1000 mg/24 hr)
Analgesia
Children >2 yr: PO naproxen, 5-7 mg/kg/dose q8-12h prn
Analgesia and Dysmenorrhea
Adults: PO naproxen, initially 500 mg, followed by 250 mg q6-8h prn (maximum 1250 mg/24 hr); naproxen sodium, initially 550 mg, followed by 275 mg q6-8h prn (maximum 1375 mg/24 hr)

MECHANISM AND INDICATIONS
Mechanism: Interferes with action of prostaglandins; has effect on hypothalamus; acts to block peripheral nerve transfer; inhibits prostaglandin synthesis by decreasing an enzyme needed for biotransfer
Indications: Used in the management of inflammatory disorders, including rheumatoid arthritis; mild or moderate pain, dysmenorrhea, fever

PHARMACOKINETICS
Onset of action: Analgesia 60 min, antiinflammatory 14 days
Peak: Analgesia 2-4 hr, antiinflammatory 4 wk
Distribution: Highly protein bound
Duration: Analgesia up to 7 hr
Half-life: 10-20 hr
Metabolism: Liver
Excretion: Urine

CONTRAINDICATIONS AND PRECAUTIONS
• Contraindicated with known hypersensitivity, (cross sensitivity may exist with other NSAIDs, including aspirin), active GI bleeding, ulcer disease, severe renal or hepatic disease, asthma; children <2 yr

• Use cautiously during 1st and 2nd trimester of pregnancy; with bleeding, GI and cardiac disorders; with hypertension, asthma, CHF, mental depression, systemic lupus erythematosus; with children 2-14 yr (use should be supervised by health care provider)

INTERACTIONS
Drug
• Decreased naproxen levels with aspirin

• Decreased effectiveness of antihypertensive therapy possible

• Increased hypoglycemic effect of insulin or oral hypoglycemic agents possible

---

✤ Available in Canada.

• Increased risk of bleeding with oral anticoagulant, cefamandole, cefoperazone, cefotetan, moxalactam, plicamycin
• Increased hyperkalemia with other drugs having the same effect (K⁺-sparing diuretics)
• Increased serum lithium level, increased toxicity possible
• Increased risk of methotrexate toxicity
• Increased blood drug levels with probenecid, increased risk of toxicity
• Increased risk of GI side effects with other drugs having similar effects (corticosteroids, K⁺, aspirin)
• Increased anticoagulant effects with aspirin, heparin, coumarin
• Increased risk of hematologic side effects with other drugs with same effect or with radiation
• Increased risk of photosensitivity with other photosensitizing agents
• Increased risk of adverse renal effects with gold compounds or chronic use of acetaminophen

Lab
• Prolonged bleeding time for about 1-4 days; no effect on pro-time or whole clotting time
• Increased ALT, AST, alk phos, LDH, transaminase, BUN, creatinine, K⁺, urine glucose, urine protein
• False increase in 17-KS delay for 72 hrs after last naproxen dose
• Decreased BG, plasma renin activity
• Decreased urine output and uric acid possible

Nutrition
• Food slows but does not reduce extent of absorption

INCOMPATIBILITIES
• Do not mix susp with antacids or other liquid before administration

SIDE EFFECTS
CNS: Headache, drowsiness, weakness, insomnia, confusion, fatigue, tremors, fever, anxiety, mood changes, depression
CV: Palpitations, tachycardia, peripheral edema, arrhythmias, hypertension, fluid retention, CHF, anaphylaxis
DERM: Urticaria, pruritus, sweating, rashes, purpura, alopecia, Stevens-Johnson syndrome
EENT: Blurred vision, tinnitus, amblyopia, cataracts, hearing loss
GI: Nausea, dyspepsia, vomiting, constipation, GI bleeding, discomfort, anorexia, diarrhea, jaundice, cholestatic hepatitis, flatulence, cramps, peptic ulcer, GI ulceration, perforation
GU: Renal failure, hematuria, cystitis, polyuria, nephrotoxicity, oliguria, azotemia
HEME: Blood dyscrasias, prolonged bleeding time, neutropenia, agranulocytosis, aplastic anemia, thrombocytopenia, anemia
RESP: Bronchospasm, dyspnea, anaphylaxis as allergic response

TOXICITY AND OVERDOSE
Clinical signs: Blurred vision, tinnitus (toxicity); drowsiness, heartburn, indigestion, nausea or vomiting (overdose)
Treatment: Supportive care; empty stomach; use activated charcoal

PATIENT CARE MANAGEMENT
Assessment
• Assess history of hypersensitivity to naproxen, aspirin, other NSAIDs
• Assess pain (type, location, intensity), range of motion (if taken for arthritis)
• Assess cardiac function, renal function (BUN, creatinine, I&O), liver function (ALT, AST, bilirubin), CBC, differential, platelet count before anticipated long-term treatment
• Perform audiometric, ophthal examination before long term treatment
• Assess history of peptic ulcer and any GI irritation
Interventions
• Do not mix susp with antacid or other liquid before administration
• Give with full glass of water; may administer with food, milk, or antacids to decrease GI irritation

• For rapid initial effect, administer 30 min ac or 2 hr after meals

---

NURSING ALERT

Not recommended to be given with other NSAIDs

Pts who have asthma, aspirin-induced allergy, and nasal polyps are at increased risk for developing hypersensitivity reactions

---

Evaluation
• Evaluate therapeutic response (decreased pain, stiffness in joints; decreased swelling in joints; ability to move more easily; reduction in menstrual cramping)
• Evaluate hepatic and renal labs in pts with known dysfunction, bleeding time with coagulation disorder
• Evaluate for side effects, hypersensitivity reactions

PATIENT AND FAMILY EDUCATION
Teach/instruct
• To take as directed at prescribed intervals for prescribed length of time
• To administer as soon as possible after the onset of menses for dysmenorrhea
• That film-coated tabs cannot be accurately divided; it is recommended that children use susp or regular tabs instead
• To take with full glass of water; may take with food, milk, or antacids to decrease GI irritation (except for susp)
• That antiinflammatory response may not be seen for 2 wk

Warn/advise
• To notify care provider of hypersensitivity, side effects
• That partial arthritic relief usually occurs within 2 wks, but maximum effectiveness may require 2-4 wk of continuous therapy
• To avoid activities that require alertness until response to medication is known
• To avoid concurrent use of alcohol, aspirin, acetaminophen, steroids, other OTC medications without consultation with health care provider
• To avoid sun and sunlamps, wear protective clothing when in sun to prevent photosensitivity reactions

STORAGE
• Store at room temp
• Protect from light
• Do not freeze susp

---

nedocromil sodium

Brand Name(s): Tilade

Classification: Antiinflammatory

Pregnancy Category: B

AVAILABLE PREPARATIONS
Aerosol inhaler: 3.5 mg/metered spray

ROUTES AND DOSAGES
Asthma, Symptomatic and Maintenance Therapy
Children >12 yr and adults: Aerosol inhaler, 2 inhalations qid; if good clinical response, reduce to 2 inhalations tid (in pts whose only medication needed is occasional inhaled oral β-agonists and who have no serious exacerbations with respiratory infections), then after several weeks of good control decrease to 2 inhalations bid

MECHANISM AND INDICATIONS
Antiinflammatory mechanism: Inhibits activity of and release of mediators (histamine, leukotrienes, prostaglandins) from a variety of inflammatory cell types associated with asthma (e.g., eosinophils, neutrophils, macrophages, mast cells, monocytes, platelets); inhibits bronchoconstrictor response to inhaled antigen; has no intrinsic bronchodilator, antihistamine, or glucocorticoid activity
Indications: For maintenance therapy in mild to moderate bronchial asthma; not indicated for the

---

reversal of acute bronchospasm or status asthmaticus

PHARMACOKINETICS
Onset of action: Approximately 2 wk until beneficial effect is seen
Peak: 5-90 min
Half-life: 1.5 hr
Metabolism: Not metabolized, excreted unchanged
Excretion: Urine, feces

CONTRAINDICATIONS AND PRECAUTIONS
• Contraindicated with hypersensitivity to nedocromil sodium or other ingredients; not for reversal of acute bronchospasm, status asthmaticus
• Use cautiously if inhaled or systemic steroid therapy is reduced at all (because nedocromil has not been shown to be a substitute for total dose of steroids); with lactation; in children <12 yr

INTERACTIONS
Lab
• Elevated ALT possible

SIDE EFFECTS
CNS: Headache
CV: Sensation of warmth
DERM: Rash
GI: Bad taste, nausea, abdominal pain, dyspepsia
RESP: Bronchospasm, cough
Other: Arthritis, tremor

TOXICITY AND OVERDOSE
Clinical signs: No experience to date; unlikely to require more than observation and discontinuation of drug if necessary

PATIENT CARE MANAGEMENT
Assessment
• Assess history of hypersensitivity to nedocromil sodium and related drugs
• Assess baseline respiratory status
• Assess medication history, other asthma medications taken
Interventions
• Shake inhaler well before administration; see Chapter 3 for discussion of inhaler use
• Use only with mouthpiece dispensed

NURSING ALERT
Nedocromil sodium is not indicated for reversal of acute bronchospasm, or status asthmaticus

Evaluation
• Evaluate therapeutic response (improved respiratory status; decreased need for bronchodilators; decreased severity of asthma symptoms)
• Evaluate whether or not systemic or inhaled steroids have been reduced; monitor closely
• Evaluate for hypersensitivity, adverse effects

PATIENT AND FAMILY EDUCATION
Teach/instruct
• To take as directed at prescribed intervals for prescribed length of time
• About correct use and care of inhaler
• To rinse mouth or gargle after use to decrease aftertaste and dryness
• If also using a prescribed inhaled bronchodilator, to use 5-15 min before using nedocromil for increased drug penetration into bronchial tree
Warn/advise
• That drug is not a bronchodilator, will not reverse acute asthma
• To continue drug during acute exacerbations (if tolerated)
• That this is a preventive medication; may take two wk for full effect
• That drug must be used regularly (even if pt is symptom-free)
• To continue other treatments until full benefit achieved, then consult provider
• To report cough, bronchospasm to provider

STORAGE
• Store at room temp
• Do not freeze, puncture, incinerate, or place near heat
• Keep out of reach of children

neomycin, polymyxin B, and hydrocortisone

Brand Name(s): AK Spore HC, Cortatrigen, Cortisporin cream, Cortisporin ophthalmic susp♣, Cortisporin otic sol or susp, Ocutricin HC, Otomycin TPN, Diospor HC♣

Classification: Antibiotic (otic, ophthal, top); corticosteroid (otic, ophthal, top)

Pregnancy Category: C

AVAILABLE PREPARATIONS
Oint, ophthal oint: Neomycin sulfate 5 mg, bacitracin 400 U, polymyxin B 5000 U, hydrocortisone 10 mg/g
Otic sol, otic susp, ophthal susp: Neomycin sulfate 5 mg, polymyxin B 10,000 U, hydrocortisone 10 mg/ml

ROUTES AND DOSAGES
Children: Otic sol/susp, 3 gtt in affected ear tid-qid; top oint, apply thin layer to affected area bid-qid; ophthal susp, 1-2 gtt in affected eye q3-4h; ophthal oint, ½″ ribbon to inside of lower lid q3-4h
Adults: Otic sol/susp, 4 gtt in affected ear tid-qid; top oint, apply thin layer to affected area bid-qid; ophthal susp, 1-2 gtt in affected eye q3-4h; ophthal oint, ½″ ribbon to inside of lower lid q3-4h

MECHANISM AND INDICATIONS
Mechanism: Suppression of inflammatory response, antiinfective action
Indications: For use in corticosteroid-responsive dermatoses with secondary infection

PHARMACOKINETICS
Absorption: Minimal
Distribution: Top
Metabolism: Liver
Excretion: Urine, feces

CONTRAINDICATIONS AND PRECAUTIONS
• Contraindicated with known hypersensitivity to hydrocortisone, polymyxin B, bacitracin, neomycin; with herpes simplex, vaccinia, varicella; perforated tympanic membrane
• Use cautiously with chronic otitis media when perforated tympanic membrane is possible; avoid prolonged use

INTERACTIONS
• None known

INCOMPATIBILITIES
• None known

SIDE EFFECTS
DERM: Contact dermatitis
EENT: Otic toxicity; burning, swelling, pruritus, stinging
Local: Sensitization to neomycin, secondary infections

TOXICITY AND OVERDOSE
• Not reported

PATIENT CARE MANAGEMENT
Assessment
• Assess history of hypersensitivity to drug (especially neomycin)
• Assess for appropriateness of treatment
• Assess for signs of perforated tympanic membrane; do not administer
Interventions
• Instill otic drops into affected ear with pt lying on side; keep pt still for 5 min for maximum penetration
• Treat for 10 days maximum
Evaluation
• Evaluate therapeutic response (decreased infection and inflammation)
• Evaluate for signs of hypersensitivity; discontinue immediately

PATIENT AND FAMILY EDUCATION
Teach/instruct
• To take as directed at prescribed intervals for prescribed length of time
Warn/advise
• To notify care provider if no improvement noted in 3-5 days
• That stinging may occur with administration, may cause tempo-

---

♣ Available in Canada.

rary blurred vision with ophthal administration
• Not to allow tip of tube or bottle to come into contact with affected area(s)

STORAGE
• Store at room temp

---

neomycin sulfate

Brand Name(s): Drotic, Micifradin✤, Micifradin Sulfate, Myciguent✤, Neomycin Sulfate, Otocort

Classification: Antibiotic (aminoglycoside)

Pregnancy Category: C

AVAILABLE PREPARATIONS
Oral sol: 125 mg/5 ml
Tabs: 500 mg
Otic sol (with hydrocortisone): 0.25%, 0.5%
Top cream: 0.5%
Top oint: 0.5%

ROUTES AND DOSAGES
Premature infants and neonates: PO 50 mg/kg/24 hr divided q6h
Infants and children: PO 50-100 mg/kg/24 hr divided q6h
Adults: PO 500-2000 mg q6-8h

Hepatic Encephalopathy
Children: PO, acute, 2.5-7.0 g/m²/24 hr divided q6h for 5-7 days (maximum 12 g/24 hr); chronic 2.5 g/m²/24 hr divided qid
Adults: PO 4-12 g/24 hr divided q4-6h

Preoperative Intestinal Antisepsis
Neonates ≥8 days: PO 50 mg/kg/24 hr divided q6h
Children: PO 90 mg/kg/24 hr divided q4h for 3 days; 1st dose to be preceded by saline cathartic
Adults: PO 1 g q1h for 4 doses, then 1 g q4h for the balance of 24 hr; 1st dose to be preceded by saline cathartic

Otitis Externa
Children and adults: Otic, instill 2-5 gtt into auditory canal tid-qid

Skin Infections, Burns, Skin Grafts
Children and adults: Top, apply to affected area bid-tid

MECHANISM AND INDICATIONS
Antibiotic mechanism: Bactericidal; inhibits bacterial protein synthesis by binding directly to the 30S ribosomal subunit
Indications: Effective against many aerobic gram-negative and some aerobic gram-positive organisms including *Pseudomonas aeruginosa, E. coli, Enterobacter, Klebsiella pneumoniae, Proteus vulgaris;* used to treat severe systemic infections of CNS, respiratory, GI, urinary tracts, eye, bone, skin, and soft tissue; also used for hepatic coma and preoperatively to sterilize bowel; otic used for otitis externa; top used for skin infections, minor burns, skin grafts

PHARMACOKINETICS
Peak: PO 1-4 hr
Half-life: 2-3 hr
Metabolism: Slight hepatic metabolism
Excretion: Urine, feces

CONTRAINDICATIONS AND PRECAUTIONS
• Contraindicated with known hypersensitivity to neomycin or any other aminoglycoside; intestinal obstruction (oral form); renal failure; otic form contraindicated with perforated tympanic membrane; top form contraindicated with ulcerations, large areas of involvement, extensive burns
• Use cautiously with neonates and infants (because of renal immaturity), impaired renal function, intestinal mucosal ulcerations, large skin wounds, dehydration, 8th cranial nerve impairment, myasthenia gravis, parkinsonism, hypocalcemia, pregnancy, lactation

INTERACTIONS
Drug
• Increased risk of nephrotoxicity, ototoxicity, neurotoxicity with

N

✤ Available in Canada.

methoxyflurane, polymyxin B, vancomycin, amphotericin B, cisplatin, cephalosporins, other aminoglycosides
• Increased risk of ototoxicity with ethacrynic acid, furosemide, bumetanide, urea, mannitol
• Masked symptoms of ototoxicity with dimenhydrinate, other antiemetic or antivertigo drugs
• Synergistic antimicrobial activity against certain organisms with penicillins
• Increased risk of neuromuscular blockade with general anesthetics or neuromuscular blocking agents (succinylcholine, tubocurarine)
• Increased effects of oral anticoagulants
• Decreased effects of digoxin, methotrexate

Lab
• Increased LDH, BUN, nonprotein nitrogen, serum creatinine levels
• Increased urinary excretion of casts
• Decreased serum Na

SIDE EFFECTS

CNS: Headache, lethargy, neuromuscular blockade with respiratory depression
DERM: Rash, urticaria, contact dermatitis
EENT: Ototoxicity (tinnitus, vertigo, hearing loss); itching, irritation of ear (otic)
GI: Nausea, vomiting, diarrhea, pseudomembranous colitis
GU: Nephrotoxicity (cells or casts in urine, oliguria, proteinuria, decreased creatinine clearance, increased BUN, serum creatinine, non-protein nitrogen levels)
Other: Hypersensitivity reactions (eosinophilia, fever, rash, urticaria, pruritus), bacterial or fungal superinfection

TOXICITY AND OVERDOSE

Clinical signs: Ototoxicity, nephrotoxicity, neuromuscular toxicity
Treatment: Supportive care, hemodialysis or peritoneal dialysis; neuromuscular blockade reversed with Ca salts or anticholinesterases; if ingested within 4 hr, empty stomach by induced emesis or gastric lavage, followed by activated charcoal

PATIENT CARE MANAGEMENT

Assessment
• Assess history of hypersensitivity to neomycin or other aminoglycosides.
• Obtain C&S; may begin therapy before obtaining results
• Assess ear and skin for redness, drainage, swelling
• Assess renal function (BUN, creatinine, I&O), baseline wt, hearing tests before beginning therapy

Interventions
• Administer neomycin at least 1 hr before or after other antibiotics (penicillins, cephalosporins)
• May administer PO without regard to meals; tabs may be crushed, mixed with food or fluid
• For preoperative intestinal antisepsis, provide low-residue diet and cathartic immediately before administering oral neomycin; follow-up enemas may be necessary to completely empty bowel
• Maintain age appropriate fluid intake; keep pt well hydrated to reduce risk of renal toxicity
• Supervise ambulation, other safety measures with vestibular dysfunction
• Before otic instillation, remove impacted cerumen by irrigation; clean stopper with alcohol; warm sol slightly before instilling; direct drops toward auditory canal, not the tympanic membrane; after instillation, gently massage anterior ear to aid entry of drops; use cotton pledgets as needed; help child to avoid playing with ears or pledgets
• Wash hands before and after top application; before application, cleanse area with soap and water, dry well; apply quantity sufficient to completely cover lesions

NURSING ALERT
Discontinue drug if signs of ototoxicity, nephrotoxicity, hypersensitivity, pseudomembranous colitis, intestinal obstruction, ulcerations develop

Evaluation

• Evaluate therapeutic response (decreased symptoms of infection)
• Evaluate renal function (BUN, creatinine, I&O), daily wt and hearing evaluations
• Observe for signs of superinfection (perineal itching, diaper rash, fever, malaise, redness, pain, swelling, drainage, rash, diarrhea, sore throat, change in cough or sputum)

PATIENT AND FAMILY EDUCATION
Teach/instruct

• To take as directed at prescribed intervals for prescribed length of time
Warn/advise

• To notify care provider of hypersensitivity, side effects, superinfection
• To avoid use of OTC creams, ointments, lotions unless directed by care provider if using top forms

STORAGE

• Store at room temp
• Reconstituted oral sol stable for 7 days refrigerated

neostigmine bromide

Brand Name(s): Prostigmin

Classification: Muscle stimulant; cholinesterase inhibitor

Pregnancy Category: C

AVAILABLE PREPARATIONS
Tabs: 15 mg
Inj: 0.25 mg/ml, 0.5 mg/ml, 1 mg/ml

ROUTES AND DOSAGES
Myasthenia Gravis (Diagnosis)
Children: IM 0.025-0.04 mg/kg as a single dose
Adults: IM 0.022 mg/kg as a single dose
Myasthenia Gravis (Treatment)
Children: PO 0.333 mg/kg or 10 mg/m^2 6 ×/24 hr; IM/IV/SC 0.01-0.04 mg/kg q2-4h
Adults: PO 15 mg q3-4h; IM/IV/SC 0.5-2.5 mg q1-3h
Reversal of Nondepolarizing Neuromuscular Blockade After Surgery in Conjunction with Atropine or Glycopyrrolate
Infants: IV 0.025-0.1 mg/kg/dose
Children: IV 0.025-0.08 mg/kg/dose
Adults: IV 0.5-2.5 mg; total dose not to exceed 5 mg
Bladder Atony
Adults: IM/SC prevention, 0.25 mg q4-6h for 2-3 days; treatment: 0.5-1 mg q3h for 5 doses after bladder has emptied
IV administration
• Recommended concentration: Undiluted
• IV infusion rate: Slow, over several min

MECHANISM AND INDICATIONS
Mechanism: Acts by blocking the destruction of acetylcholine by acetylcholinesterase, thereby promoting transmission of nerve impulses across myoneural junction
Indications: Used in treatment of myasthenia gravis; to prevent and treat postoperative bladder distention and urinary retention; to reverse the effects of nondepolarizing neuromuscular blocking agents after surgery

PHARMACOKINETICS
Onset of action: PO 2-4 hr after dose; SC/IM 10-30 min; IV 1-20 min
Half-life: 50-80 min (increased in renal dysfunction)
Metabolism: 15%-25% binding to

plasma proteins; hydrolyzed by cholinesterases and metabolized by microsomal enzymes in the liver

Excretion: Urine

CONTRAINDICATIONS AND PRECAUTIONS

• Contraindicated with known hypersensitivity to neostigmine bromide, cholinergics, or bromides; with obstructions of urinary or intestinal tract; bradycardia, hypotension

• Use cautiously with bronchial asthma, epilepsy, peritonitis, vagotonia, hyperthyroidism, cardiac arrhythmia, peptic ulcer disease, recent coronary occlusion, pregnancy, lactation

INTERACTIONS
Drug

• Reverse cholinergic effect on muscle with procainamide, quinidine

• Decreased cholinergic effects with corticosteroids, if corticosteroids are stopped cholinergic effects of neostigmine may increase and affect muscle strength

• Prolonged respiratory depression with succinylcholine

• Additive toxicity with other cholinergic drugs

• Decreased B/P with ganglionic blockers; usually preceded by abdominal symptoms.

• Antagonized effects of neostigmine with Mg

SIDE EFFECTS

CNS: Dizziness, headache, muscle weakness, confusion, nervousness, sweating, convulsions

CV: Arrhythmias, bradycardia, hypotension

DERM: Rash (from bromide)

EENT: Miosis, increased tearing, accommodation spasms; diplopia, conjunctival hyperemia

GI: Nausea, vomiting, diarrhea, abdominal cramping, excessive salivation

RESP: Bronchospasm, bronchoconstriction, respiratory depression

Other: Muscle cramping

TOXICITY AND OVERDOSE

Clinical signs: Headache, nausea, vomiting, diarrhea, blurred vision, miosis, excessive tearing, bronchospasm, increased bronchial secretions, hypotension, incoordination, excessive sweating, muscle weakness, cramps, fasiculations, paralysis, bradycardia or tachycardia, excessive salivation, restlessness or agitation

Treatment: Discontinue drug immediately; supportive symptomatic care especially support for respiration; atropine may be given to block muscarinic effect, but will not reverse paralytic effects on skeletal muscle; care must be taken not to overdose with atropine because it could cause development of a bronchial plug

PATIENT CARE MANAGEMENT
Assessment

• Assess history of hypersensitivity to neostigmine bromide, cholinergics, bromides

• Assess for pre-existing conditions (asthma, peptic ulcer disease, epilepsy, obstructions of urinary or intestinal tract, bradycardia, hypotension, cardiac arrhythmias, recent coronary occlusion)

• Assess pt needs carefully; dosage must be individualized according to severity of the disease and pt's response

• Assess baseline VS

• Be aware of all other medications to avoid potential interactions

Interventions

• Administer PO dose with food or milk to decrease GI irritation

• Observe closely for cholinergic reaction, particularly with parenteral preparations

• Atropine should be readily available to treat hypersensitivity reactions

• Monitor VS

• All other cholinergic drugs should be discontinued during neostigmine therapy to avoid risk of additive toxicity

---

✤ Available in Canada.

• Prolonged use may result in decreased response; may restore response by reducing dosage or stopping for a few days
• May administer concurrently with atropine to relieve or eliminate adverse reaction; however, atropine may mask some of the symptoms of neostigmine overdose

---

NURSING ALERT
Multiple interactions with other medications

Use with corticosteroids may also decrease cholinergic effects; if corticosteroids are stopped cholinergic effects of neostigmine may increase and affect muscle strength

Use with succinylcholine may prolong respiratory depression by inhibiting plasma esterase, causing delayed succinylcholine hydrolysis

Use with other cholinergic drugs may cause additive toxicity

Use with ganglionic blockers may decrease B/P critically; usually preceded by abdominal symptoms

If muscle weakness is severe, try to differentiate whether it is result of drug toxicity or exacerbation of myasthenia gravis; one method is to administer a test dose of edrophonium IV; if weakness is drug-induced it will aggravate weakness, if disease-related it will be temporarily relieved

May administer concurrently with atropine to relieve or eliminate adverse reaction; however atropine may mask some of the symptoms of neostigmine overdose

---

Evaluation
• Evaluate therapeutic response; may develop resistance, evaluate regularly for effectiveness
• Evaluate for potential side effects

• If muscle weakness is severe, try to differentiate whether it is result of drug toxicity or exacerbation of myasthenia gravis; administer a test dose of edrophonium IV; if weakness is drug-induced it will aggravate weakness, if disease-related it will be temporarily relieved

PATIENT AND FAMILY EDUCATION
Teach/instruct
• Emphasize need to take exactly as prescribed; take a missed dose as soon as possible; however, if it is almost time for next dose eliminate the missed dose and return to usual schedule; do not double the dose
• Encourage to take with food or milk to decrease adverse GI effects
Warn/advise
• To discontinue drug if hypersensitivity, skin rash, difficulty breathing should occur
• To carry medical alert identification specifying myasthenia gravis and drugs taken
Encourage
• To keep a record of changes in muscle strength, particularly noting times of greatest weakness in order to individualize dosage to pt need

STORAGE
• Avoid direct heat
• Protect from light

---

netilmicin sulfate
Brand Name(s): Netromycin
Classification: Antibiotic (aminoglycoside)
Pregnancy Category: D

AVAILABLE PREPARATIONS
Inj: 10 mg/ml, 25 mg/ml, 100 mg/ml

ROUTES AND DOSAGES
Neonates <6 wk: IM/IV 2-3.25 mg/kg/dose q12h
Children 6 wk-12 yr: IM/IV 1.8-2.7

mg/kg/dose q8h or 2.7-4 mg/kg/dose q12h
Children >12 yr and adults: 3-6.5 mg/kg/24 hr divided q8-12h
IV administration
• Recommended concentration: 2-3 mg/ml in D_5W, NS
• Maximum concentration: 3 mg/ml
• IV push rate: Not recommended
• Intermittent infusion rate: Over 30-120 min
• Continuous infusion rate: Not recommended

MECHANISM AND INDICATIONS

Antibiotic mechanism: Bactericidal; inhibits bacterial protein synthesis by binding directly to the 30S ribosomal subunit
Indications: Effective against many aerobic gram-negative and some aerobic gram-positive organisms including *Pseudomonas aeruginosa, E. coli, Enterobacter, Citrobacter, Staphylococcus, Klebsiella pneumoniae, Proteus mirabilis, Serratia, Shigella, Salmonella, Acinetobacter, Neisseria;* used to treat severe systemic infections of CNS, respiratory, GI, urinary tracts, bone, skin, soft tissue

PHARMACOKINETICS

Peak: IM/IV 1-2 hr
Distribution: Does not cross blood–brain barrier; accumulates in renal cortex
Half-life: Neonates 8 hr; infants 4.5 hr; children 1.5-2 hr; adults 2-3 hr
Metabolism: Not metabolized
Excretion: Urine, bile
Therapeutic levels: Peak 6-10 mcg/ml; trough 0.5-2 mcg/ml

CONTRAINDICATIONS AND PRECAUTIONS

• Contraindicated with known hypersensitivity to netilmicin, any other aminoglycoside, bisulfites; renal failure
• Use cautiously with neonates and infants (because of renal immaturity); with impaired renal function, dehydration, 8th cranial nerve impairment, myasthenia gravis, parkinsonism, hypocalcemia, pregnancy, lactation

INTERACTIONS

Drug
• Increased risk of nephrotoxicity, ototoxicity, neurotoxicity with methoxyflurane, polymyxin B, vancomycin, capreomycin, cisplatin, cephalosporins, amphotericin B, other aminoglycosides
• Increased risk of ototoxicity with ethacrynic acid, furosemide, bumetanide, urea, mannitol
• Masked symptoms of ototoxicity with dimenhydrinate, other antiemetic or antivertigo drugs
• Synergistic antimicrobial activity against certain organisms with penicillins
• Increased risk of neuromuscular blockade with general anesthetics, neuromuscular blocking agents (e.g., succinylcholine, tubocurarine)

Lab
• Increased LDH, BUN, nonprotein nitrogen, serum creatinine levels
• Increased urinary excretion of casts
• Decreased serum Na

INCOMPATIBILITIES

• Amphotericin B, carbenicillin, cefamandole, cephalothin, dopamine, erythromycin, furosemide, heparin, ticarcillin

SIDE EFFECTS

CNS: Headache, lethargy, neuromuscular blockade with respiratory depression
EENT: Ototoxicity (tinnitus, vertigo, hearing loss)
GI: Diarrhea, pseudomembranous colitis
GU: Nephrotoxicity (cells or casts in the urine, obliguria, proteinuria, decreased CrCl, increased BUN, non-protein nitrogen, serum creatinine)
Other: Hypersensitivity reactions (eosinophilia, fever, rash, urticaria, pruritus), bacterial or fungal superinfection

TOXICITY AND OVERDOSE
Clinical signs: Ototoxicity, nephrotoxicity, neuromuscular toxicity
Treatment: Supportive care, hemodialysis or peritoneal dialysis; neuromuscular blockade reversed with Ca salts or anticholinesterases

PATIENT CARE MANAGEMENT
Assessment
• Assess history of hypersensitivity to netilmicin, other aminoglycosides
• Obtain C&S; may begin therapy before obtaining results
• Assess renal function (BUN, creatinine, I&O), baseline wt, hearing tests before beginning therapy
Interventions
• Administer netilmicin at least 1 hr before or after other antibiotics (penicillins, cephalosporins)
• Sol should be colorless or clear to very pale yellow; do not use if dark yellow, cloudy, or containing precipitates
• Administer IM deep into large muscle mass, rotate injection sites; do not inject more than 2 g per injection site
• Do not premix IV with other medications; infuse separately, flush line with D₅W or NS
• Use large vein with small-bore needle to reduce local reaction; rotate site q48-72h
• Maintain age-appropriate fluid intake; keep pt well hydrated to reduce risk of renal toxicity
• Supervise ambulation, other safety measures with vestibular dysfunction
• Obtain drug levels after the 3rd dose (sooner in neonates or pts with rapidly changing renal function); peak levels drawn 30 min after end of 30 min IV infusion, 1 hr after IM injection; trough levels drawn within 30 min before next dose

> **NURSING ALERT**
> Discontinue drug if signs of ototoxicity, nephrotoxicity, hypersensitivity, pseudomembranous colitis develop
>
> Do not administer IV push

Evaluation
• Evaluate therapeutic response (decreased symptoms of infection)
• Evaluate renal function (BUN, creatinine, I&O), daily wt, hearing evaluations
• Monitor signs of respiratory depression with IV infusion
• Observe for signs of superinfection (perineal itching, diaper rash, fever, malaise, redness, pain, swelling, drainage, rash, diarrhea, sore throat, change in cough or sputum)
• Evaluate IM site for tissue damage, IV site for vein irritation

PATIENT AND FAMILY EDUCATION
Teach/instruct
• To take as directed at prescribed intervals for prescribed length of time
Warn/advise
• To notify care provider of hypersensitivity, side effects, superinfection

STORAGE
• Store powder at room temp
• Reconstituted sol stable for 72 hr

---

niacin (vitamin B₃)
Brand Name(s): Niac, Niacels, Nicobid, Nicotinex, Slo-Niacin

Classification: Water-soluble vitamin, antilipemic, peripheral vasodilator

Pregnancy Category: A (C if dosage exceeds RDA)

AVAILABLE PREPARATIONS
Tabs: 20 mg, 25 mg, 50 mg, 100 mg (niacin)

Caps, timed rel: 125 mg, 300 mg, 400 mg
Elixir: 50 mg/5 ml
Niacinamide
Tabs: 50 mg, 100 mg, 500 mg (niacinamide)
Inj: 100 mg/ml

ROUTES AND DOSAGES
Dietary Supplement
• See Appendix F, Table of Recommended Daily Dietary Allowances
Pellagra
• Dosage depends on severity of niacin deficiency
Children: PO 50-100 mg/dose tid (maximum 300 mg/24 hr); IV/SC/IM 100-300 mg/24 hr
Adults: PO 50-100 mg tid-qid (maximum 500 mg/24 hr); SC/IM 50-100 mg 2-5 times/24 hr; IV 25-50 mg bid
Adjunct in Hyperlipidemia
Adults: 1.5-3 g/24 hr divided tid after meals; may be increased to 6 g/24 hr
Peripheral Vascular Disease
Adults: 250-800 mg/24 hr divided tid

IV administration
• IV indicated when oral administration not acceptable (nausea, vomiting, preoperative or postoperative condition, malabsorption syndromes)
• Recommended concentration: 2 mg/ml
• IV push rate: 2 mg/min

MECHANISM AND INDICATIONS
Mechanism: Acts as a coenzyme in fat metabolism, tissue respiration, and energy production; nicotinic acid and nicotinamide function identically as vitamins, but have different pharmacological effects; nicotinic acid lowers blood cholesterol and triglyceride levels, acts as a vasodilator of peripheral vessels; nicotinamide does not affect blood lipid levels; niacin deficiency is called pellagra and is characterized by dermatitis, diarrhea, dementia
Indications: Treatment and prevention of niacin deficiency (pellagra); niacin requirements may also be increased during periods of increased caloric intake; nicotinic acid is used in the treatment of high blood cholesterol levels which have not responded well to diet changes or wt loss

PHARMACOKINETICS
Peak: 45 min
Half-life: 45 min
Metabolism: Liver
Excretion: Urine

CONTRAINDICATIONS AND PRECAUTIONS
• Contraindicated with bleeding, liver disease, hypotension, active peptic ulcer, drug hypersensitivity
• Use cautiously with diabetes, gallbladder disease, glaucoma, gout, history of jaundice or peptic ulcer, schizophrenia, pregnancy; some products may contain tartrazine and should not be given to those sensitive to yellow dye #5

INTERACTIONS
Drug
• Increased risk of side effects possible with other OTC or prescription drugs with niacin
• Increased vasodilation reaction and hypotension with β-blockers
• Decreased niacin levels with isoniazid
• Altered requirements for pts with diabetes taking insulin
Lab
• Altered glucose tolerance tests
• Increased uric acid levels
• Altered liver function tests and PT
• Hypoalbuminemia possible

INCOMPATIBILITIES
• Alkali, erythromycin, kanamycin

SIDE EFFECTS
CNS: Headaches, restlessness, dizziness
CV: Hypotension, tachycardia
DERM: Rash, hives, itching, dry skin, tingling or yellowing of skin, flushing of chest, face, or neck
EENT: Visual dimming
GI: Nausea, vomiting, diarrhea, stomach pain, flatulence, heartburn, increased GI motility
GU: Glycosuria, hyperuricemia

✦ Available in Canada.

Other: Sensation of warmth

TOXICITY AND OVERDOSE
Clinical signs: Overdose seldom occurs as niacin is water soluble and is not stored in the body; megadosing could cause problems in pts with renal dysfunction
Treatment: Discontinue use

PATIENT CARE MANAGEMENT
Assessment
• Assess history of hypersensitivity to vitamin B$_3$
• Obtain dietary history to assess intake; niacin deficiency rarely occurs alone, is often associated with other micronutrient deficiencies
• Determine vitamin deficiency by obtaining baseline blood levels for suspected deficient vitamins
• Assess hepatic function (ALT, AST, bilirubin) and BG levels
Interventions
• PO preferred route; administer with meals if GI symptoms occur

---

NURSING ALERT
Avoid megadosing

If problems with side effects, administer 30 mg aspirin, 30 min before each dose of niacin or nicotinic acid

---

Evaluation
• Evaluate therapeutic response (normal serum levels, decreased deficiency symptoms)
• Observe for hypersensitivity, side effects
• Monitor liver function tests (AST, ALT, bilirubin); discontinue drug if abnormal
• Monitor BG; monitor diabetics for decreased glucose tolerance
• Monitor pts with gallbladder or liver disease for bleeding

PATIENT AND FAMILY EDUCATION
Teach/instruct
• To take as directed at prescribed intervals for prescribed length of time

• About a balanced diet to meet all micronutrient requirements; see Appendix F, Table of Recommended Daily Dietary Allowances
Warn/advise
• To notify care providers of hypersensitivity, side effects
• That pt may experience skin flushing, sensation of warmth in neck, face, ears; tingling, headache, itching within first few hours of taking drug; these effects are temporary and should decrease with continued therapy; if not, take 30 mg of aspirin 30 min before each dose
• Avoid sudden changes in posture if dizzy
Encourage
• Encourage a balanced diet to assure adequate vitamin intake; common sources of niacin are chicken, beef, liver, eggs, milk products, peas, beans, peanuts, enriched cereals, wheat germ

STORAGE
• Store at room temp in tightly sealed container
• Protect sol from freezing

N

---

niclosamide
Brand Name(s): Niclocide
Classification: Anthelmintic
Pregnancy Category: B

AVAILABLE PREPARATIONS
Tabs (chewable): 500 mg

ROUTES AND DOSAGES
Beef/Pork/Fish Tapeworm
Children 11-34 kg: PO 1 g (2 tabs) once
Children >34 kg: PO 1.5 g (3 tabs) once
Adults: PO 2 g (4 tabs) once
Dwarf Tapeworm
Children 11-34 kg: PO 1 g (2 tabs) for 1 day, then 500 mg (1 tab) qd × 6 days
Children >34 kg: PO 1.5 g (3 tabs) for 1 day, then 1 g (2 tabs) qd × 6 days
Adults: PO 2 g (4 tabs) qd × 7 days

MECHANISM AND INDICATIONS

Mechanism: Inhibits synthesis of ATP in mitochondria
Indications: Used to treat intestinal dwarf (beef, pork, fish) tapeworm infections

PHARMACOKINETICS

Excretion: Feces

CONTRAINDICATIONS AND PRECAUTIONS

• Contraindicated with known hypersensitivity to niclosamide
• Use cautiously in pregnancy, lactation, children <2 yr

SIDE EFFECTS

CNS: Drowsiness, vertigo, fever, headache, restlessness
DERM: Rash, pruritus
EENT: Bad taste, oral irritation
GI: Abdominal pain, bloating, nausea, vomiting, diarrhea, transient rise in AST

TOXICITY AND OVERDOSE

Clinical signs: Abdominal pain, nausea, vomiting
Treatment: Fast acting laxative and enema; do not induce vomiting

PATIENT CARE MANAGEMENT

Assessment

• Assess history of hypersensitivity to niclosamide
• Diagnose through stool culture

Interventions

• Tab to be chewed or crushed; mix with small amount of water to form paste, do not swallow whole; give after breakfast, follow with fluid
• For dwarf tapeworm, treat all family members
• A mild laxative is indicated for constipated children to cleanse bowel before starting drug
• Use effective handwashing techniques

Evaluation

• Evaluate therapeutic response (expulsion of worm); pt should have 3 negative stool cultures after completion of treatment
• Persistent tapeworm segments or ova excreted on or after the 7th day of therapy indicate failure; repeat course of treatment
• Evaluate spread of infection to other household members and treat as needed
• Evaluate for side effects, hypersensitivity (rash, abdominal pain, diarrhea)

PATIENT AND FAMILY EDUCATION

Teach/instruct

• To take as directed at prescribed intervals for prescribed length of time
• About proper hygiene procedures (especially good handwashing techniques)
• About how to prevent reinfection (change undergarments and bed linens; wash clothes and linens in hot water; do not shake bed linens into the air; frequent cleansing of perianal area)
• To clean toilet every day with disinfectant
• To wash all fruits and vegetables before eating
• To drink fruit juice; aids in worm expulsion by eliminating accumulation in intestinal mucosa

Warn/advise

• To notify care provider of hypersensitivity
• That all family members need to be evaluated and treated

Encourage

• To comply with treatment regime

STORAGE

• Store at room temp in tight container

---

nifedipine
Adalat♣, Adalat PA 10♣,
Adalat PA 20♣, Adalat XL♣,
Apo-Nifed, Gen-Nifedipine♣,
Nifedipine, Novo-Nifedin♣,
Nu-Nifed♣, Procardia,
Procardia XL♣

Classification: Antianginal,
antihypertensive, calcium
channel blocker

Pregnancy Category: C

AVAILABLE PREPARATIONS
Caps: 10 mg, 20 mg
Tabs, sus rel: 30 mg, 60 mg, 90 mg

ROUTES AND DOSAGES
Children: For hypertension, PO
0.25-0.5 mg/kg q6-8h, for cardiomyopathy, PO 0.5-0.9 mg/kg/24 hr
divided q6-8h
Adult: PO 10 mg tid, may increase
to 10-30 mg tid or qid (maximum
30 mg/dose, 180 mg/24 hr); sus rel
30-60 mg qd, may increase q7-14
days to maximum of 120 mg qd

MECHANISM
AND INDICATIONS
Antianginal mechanism: Inhibits
Ca ions across cell membrane during cardiac depolarization; relaxes
coronary vascular smooth muscle;
dilates coronary arteries; decreases myocardial O_2 consumption by reducing afterload; increases myocardial O_2 delivery by
inhibiting coronary artery spasm
*Antihypertensive/cardiomyopathy
mechanisms:* Dilates systemic arteries, resulting in decreased total
peripheral resistance, decreased
systemic B/P; slightly increases
HR, decreases afterload and increases cardiac index
Indications: Vasospastic angina,
chronic stable angina, essential
hypertension, cardiomyopathy

PHARMACOKINETICS
Onset of action: 20 min
Peak: 30 min-2 hr; sus rel 6 hr,
then steady state
Half-life: 2-5 hr
Metabolism: Liver

Excretion: Urine, feces (98% metabolites)

CONTRAINDICATIONS
AND PRECAUTIONS
• Contraindicated with known hypersensitivity
• Use cautiously with CHF, aortic
stenosis (especially if on other β-
blockers), sick sinus syndrome,
2nd- or 3rd-degree heart block,
hypotension, hepatic injury, renal
disease, pregnancy, lactation

INTERACTIONS
Drug
• Increased angina, CHF, hy-
potension, arrhythmias possible
with other β blockers
• Increased effects of theophyl-
line, digitalis, fentanyl, coumadin
• Increased nifedipine level with
cimetidine
• Decreased effects with quinidine
Lab
• Increased alk phos, CPK, LDH,
AST, ALT, BUN, creatinine
• Decreased platelets
• Positive direct Coombs' with or
without hemolytic anemia

INCOMPATIBILITIES
• None

SIDE EFFECTS
CNS: Dizziness, drowsiness, headache, fatigue, light-headedness,
flushing, weakness, syncope, anxiety, depression, insomnia, paresthesia, tinnitus, blurred vision,
nervousness, photosensitivity
CV: Arrhythmia, peripheral
edema, CHF, hypotension, palpitations, MI, tachycardia, pulmonary
edema, worsening angina
EENT: Nasal congestion
GI: Nausea, vomiting, heartburn,
diarrhea, constipation, dry mouth
GU: Nocturia, polyuria; sexual difficulties
RESP: Dyspnea, cough
Other: Rash, pruritis, fever, chills,
muscle cramps, hair loss

TOXICITY AND OVERDOSE
Clinical signs: Peripheral vasodi-
lation, hypotension
Treatment: Defibrillation, atropine

for AV block, vasopressors for hypotension, basic support measures

PATIENT CARE MANAGEMENT
Assessment
• Assess history of hypersensitivity to drug
• Assess baseline VS, ECG
Interventions
• Administer PO ac, hs; titrate dose over 7-14 days, more rapidly if pt is hospitalized and closely monitored
• When discontinuing, dosage should be reduced slowly with close monitoring
• Pt should swallow caps whole without breaking, crushing, or chewing
• For rapid antihypertensive effect, may administer SL by puncturing cap and placing in buccal mucosa, or chewing
Evaluation
• Evaluate therapeutic response (decreased B/P, decreased angina)
• Evaluate for side effects, hypersensitivity
• Regularly monitor HR, rhythm, B/P

PATIENT AND FAMILY EDUCATION
Teach/instruct
• Take as directed at prescribed intervals for prescribed length of time
• To swallow caps whole without breaking, crushing, or chewing
Warn/advise
• Notify care provider of hypersensitivity, side effects
• That hypotensive effects or worsening of angina with initial dosage or titration may occur; reassure that condition is temporary, encourage compliance
• To avoid hazardous activities until stabilized on drug and dizziness disappears
• To limit caffeine, avoid alcohol
• To avoid taking OTC preparations unless directed by care provider
• That medication should not be discontinued abruptly; should be gradually reduced

• That missed doses should be taken as soon as possible unless very close to time for next dose; do not double the dose
• To notify provider for irregular heartbeat, SOB, swelling of hands and feet, pronounced dizziness, constipation, nausea, hypotension
Encourage
• To comply with medical regimen including diet, exercise, stress reduction, medications
Provide
• Emotional support as indicated
STORAGE
• Store at room temp in tightly sealed, light-resistant container

---

nitrofurantoin, nitrofurantoin macrocrystals
Brand Name(s): Apo-Nitrofurantoin✤, Furadantin, Furalan, Furan, Furanite, Macrodantin✤

Classification: Urinary tract antiseptic (nitrofuran)

Pregnancy Category: B

AVAILABLE PREPARATIONS
Oral susp: 25 mg/5 ml
Tabs: 50 mg, 100 mg
Caps: 50 mg, 100 mg
Caps (macrocrystal): 25 mg, 50 mg, 100 mg
Caps (macrocrystal / monohydrate): 100 mg

ROUTES AND DOSAGES
Infants >1 mo and children: PO 5-7 mg/kg/24 hr divided q6h (maximum 400 mg/24 hr); prophylaxis, 1-2.5 mg/kg/24 hr divided q12-24h (maximum 400 mg/24 hr)
Adults: PO 50-100 mg q6h; prophylaxis 50-100 mg hs

MECHANISM AND INDICATIONS
Antibiotic mechanism: Bacteriostatic in low concentrations; possibly bactericidal in high concen-

---

✤ Available in Canada.

trations; may inhibit bacterial enzymes

Indications: Used to treat UTIs caused by many gram-positive and gram-negative urinary pathogens including *E. coli, Staphylococcus aureus,* enterococci, *Klebsiella, Proteus, Enterobacter*

PHARMACOKINETICS
Peak: Microcrystals 30 min
Half-life: 20-60 min
Metabolism: Liver
Excretion: Urine, bile

CONTRAINDICATIONS AND PRECAUTIONS
• Contraindicated in infants <1 mo, with known hypersensitivity to nitrofurantoin, severe renal impairment, pregnancy at term
• Use cautiously with G-6-PD deficiency, anemia, asthma, vitamin B deficiency, diabetes, electrolyte abnormalities, pregnancy, lactation

INTERACTIONS
Drug
• Increased serum concentrations, increased toxicity with probenecid, sulfinpyrazone
• Decreased absorption with magnesium antacids
• Antagonistic antibacterial effect of nalidixic acid
• Increased absorption with anticholinergic drugs
Lab
• Anemia, abnormal liver function tests
Nutrition
• Increased absorption when given with food

SIDE EFFECTS
CNS: Peripheral neuropathy, headache, dizziness, drowsiness, ascending polyneuropathy with high doses or renal impairment
DERM: Maculopapular, erythematous, or eczematous eruption, pruritus, urticaria, exfoliative dermatitis, Stevens-Johnson syndrome
GI: Anorexia, nausea, vomiting, abdominal pain, diarrhea, hepatitis

HEME: Hemolysis in patients with G-6-PD deficiency, agranulocytosis, thrombocytopenia
Other: Asthma exacerbation, anaphylaxis, hypersensitivity, transient alopecia, drug fever, urinary tract bacterial superinfection, pulmonary sensitivity (chest pain, cough, fever, chills, dyspnea)

TOXICITY AND OVERDOSE
Clinical signs: Vomiting
Treatment: Induced emesis; supportive care, increased fluid administration

PATIENT CARE MANAGEMENT
Assessment
• Assess history of hypersensitivity to nitrofurantoin
• Obtain C&S; may begin therapy before obtaining results
• Assess I&O, urine pH (<5.5 for maximum effect), hematologic function (CBC, differential, platelet count), renal function (BUN, creatinine), hepatic function (ALT, AST, bilirubin)
Interventions
• Administer PO with food to increase absorption
• Shake susp well before administering; cap may be taken apart, tabs crushed and mixed with food or fluid
• To prevent discoloration of teeth from oral susp, crushed tablet, or opened capsules, provide fluids with administration of dose and oral hygiene afterward
• Administer oral preparations 1 hr apart from Mg antacids; avoid administering with nalidixic acid
• Maintain age-appropriate fluid intake

> **NURSING ALERT**
> Discontinue drug if signs of hypersensitivity, hemolysis, peripheral neuropathy, pulmonary reaction develop

Evaluation
• Evaluate therapeutic response (decreased dysuria, frequency, urgency, negative culture)

• Monitor I&O, urine pH, hematologic function (CBC, differential, platelet count), renal function (BUN, creatinine), hepatic function (ALT, AST, bilirubin), particularly with long-term therapy

• Monitor for CNS symptoms (insomnia, vertigo, headache, drowsiness, seizures), signs of peripheral neuropathy (paresthesia, dysesthesia of lower extremities, muscle weakness, tingling), signs of pulmonary reaction (cough, dyspnea, chest tightness, wheezing)

• Monitor for allergic reaction (fever, flushing, rash, urticaria, pruritus)

PATIENT AND FAMILY EDUCATION
Teach/instruct
• To take as directed at prescribed intervals for prescribed length of time
Warn/advise
• To notify care provider of hypersensitivity, side effects
• That urine may turn brown or rust-yellow
STORAGE
• Store at room temp in airtight, light-resistant containers
• Contact with any metal other than stainless steel will cause decomposition

---

nitroglycerin
Brand Name(s): Deponit, Minitran✤, Nitro-bid, Nitro-bid IV, Nitro-bid Plateau Caps, Nitrocine, Nitrocine Timecaps, Nitrodisc, Nitro-dur✤, Nitrogard, Nitrogard-SR✤, Nitroglycerin, Nitroglycerine in 5% Dextrose Injection✤, Nitroglycerin Transdermal, Nitroglyn✤, Nitrol✤, Nitrolingual, Nitrolingual Spray✤, Nitrong-SR✤, Nitrostat✤, Transderm-Nitro✤, Tridil✤

Classification: Coronary vasodilator

Pregnancy Category: C

AVAILABLE PREPARATIONS
Buccal tabs: 1 mg, 2 mg, 3 mg
Aerosol: 0.4 mg/metered spray
Caps: 2.5 mg, 6.5 mg, 9 mg
Ext rel tabs: 2.6 mg, 6.5 mg, 9 mg
SL tabs: 0.15 mg, 0.3 mg, 0.4 mg, 0.6 mg
Inj: 0.5 mg/ml, 0.8 mg/ml, 5 mg/ml, 10 mg/ml
Oint: 2%
Transdermal: 2.5 mg/24 hr, 5 mg/24 hr, 7.5 mg/24 hr, 10 mg/24 hr, 15 mg/24 hr

ROUTES AND DOSAGES
Sublingual
Adult: 0.2-0.6 mg q 5 min × 3 doses
IV
Children: 0.25-0.5 mcg/kg/min; maximum dosage 5 mcg/kg/min
Adult: 5 mcg/min; increase by 5 mcg/min to maximum dosage of 20 mcg/min
Top
1-2″ q8h; increase to 4″ q4h prn
Transdermal
1 pad (2.5-15 mg/24 hr) qd to hair-free site
IV administration
• Recommended concentration: 50-100 mcg/ml in D₅W or NS
• Maximum concentration: 400 mcg/ml
• Continuous infusion rate: 0.5-20 mcg/kg/min

✤ Available in Canada.

MECHANISM AND INDICATIONS

Vasodilator mechanism: Dilates blood vessels, decreasing preload and afterload, thereby decreasing left ventricular end diastolic pressure and systemic vascular resistance

Indications: Angina, CHF, hypertension

PHARMACOKINETICS

Onset of action: IV 1-2 min, SL 1-3 min, spray 2 min, tabs 3 min, oint 20-60 min, sus rel 40 min, transdermal 40-60 min

Peak: Variable

Half-life: 1-4 min

Metabolism: Liver

Excretion: Urine

CONTRAINDICATIONS AND PRECAUTIONS

• Contraindicated with known hypersensitivity to medication, severe anemia, increased intracranial pressure, cerebral hemorrhage, severe hypotension, pericarditis, pericardial tamponade

• Use cautiously with glaucoma, hypotension, MI

INTERACTIONS

Drug

• Increased effects with β blockers, diuretics, antihypertensives, anticoagulants, alcohol

Lab

• Decreased serum cholesterol levels

INCOMPATIBILITIES

• Any medication in sol or syringe

SIDE EFFECTS

CNS: Headache, flushing, dizziness, weakness

CV: Hypotension, tachycardia, syncope, palpitations

DERM: Rash, pallor, sweating, cutaneous vasodilation

EENT: Dry mouth, sublingual burning

GI: Nausea, vomiting

Other: Methemoglobinemia

TOXICITY AND OVERDOSE

Clinical signs: Hypotension, throbbing headache, palpitations, visual disturbances, flushing, sweating, nausea, vomiting, colic, bloody diarrhea, respiratory difficulties, bradycardia, heart block, increased intracranial pressure, confusion, fever, paralysis, hypoxia, cyanosis, metabolic acidosis, coma, convulsions, cardiac collapse

Treatment: Gastric lavage, activated charcoal; monitor ABGs and methemoglobin level; supportive measures as necessary

PATIENT CARE MANAGEMENT

Assessment

• Assess history of hypersensitivity to drug

• Assess baseline VS, B/P

Interventions

• Do not administer PO, SL, top to children

• IV infusions should be prepared in glass bottle, administered with nonpolyvinyl chloride tubing

• May administer acetaminophen if headache occurs

Evaluation

• Evaluate therapeutic response (decrease or prevention of angina)

• Monitor VS, B/P regularly

PATIENT AND FAMILY EDUCATION

Teach/instruct

• To take as directed at prescribed intervals for prescribed length of time

• About need for medication

• To place buccal tab between lip and gum or between cheek and gum; swallow sus rel tabs whole; dissolve SL tabs under tongue and do not swallow; spray aerosol under tongue and do not inhale

Warn/advise

• To notify care provider of hypersensitivity, side effects

• That medication may cause headache; treat with acetaminophen

• To avoid hazardous activities until treatment is well-established

Provide

• Emotional support as indicated

STORAGE

• Store at room temp in tightly sealed light-resistant container

---

♣ Available in Canada.

nitroprusside sodium

Brand Name(s): Nitropress, Sodium Nitroprusside

Classification: Peripheral vasodilator, antihypertensive

Pregnancy Category: C

AVAILABLE PREPARATIONS
Inj: 50 mg/5 ml vial

ROUTES AND DOSAGES
Children and adults: IV 0.3-0.5 mcg/kg/min; titrate to desired effect; usual dose 3-4 mcg/kg/min; maximum 10 mcg/kg/min

IV administration
• Recommended concentration: 100 mcg/ml
• Maximum concentration: 200 mcg/ml
• Continuous infusion rate: 0.5-12 mcg/kg/min

MECHANISM AND INDICATIONS
Vasodilator, antihypertensive mechanisms: Reduces preload and afterload by directly relaxing arteriolar and venous smooth muscle
Indications: Hypertension

PHARMACOKINETICS
Onset of action: 1-2 min
Peak: 2 min
Half-life: Variable
Metabolism: Liver
Excretion: Urine

CONTRAINDICATIONS AND PRECAUTIONS
• Contraindicated with known hypersensitivity to drug, with compensatory hypertension
• Use cautiously with renal, hepatic insufficiency, hypothyroidism, pregnancy, lactation

INTERACTIONS
Drug
• Increased hypotension with other antihypertensives, general anesthetics, ganglionic blockers
• Hypertension with epinephrine
Lab
• Increased creatinine

INCOMPATIBILITIES
• Any medication in sol or syringe

SIDE EFFECTS
CNS: Agitation, dizziness, diminished reflexes, headache, loss of consciousness, twitching, restlessness
CV: Palpitations, hypotension
DERM: Rash, sweating, flushing
EENT: Blurred vision, tinnitus
GI: Nausea, vomiting, abdominal pain
GU: Impotence, renal insufficiency
Other: Acidosis

TOXICITY AND OVERDOSE
Clinical signs: Severe response to any of above side effects and tolerance to medication's antihypertensive effects
Treatment: Discontinue medication immediately; administer amylnitrite inhalations q min for 15-30 sec until 3% sodium nitrite sol can be obtained; administer sodium nitrite IV at 2.5-5 ml/min to total dose of 10-15 ml; administer sodium thiosulfate 12.5 g in 50 ml D_5W IV over 10 min; repeat infusion at half-dose if necessary; supportive measures as necessary

PATIENT CARE MANAGEMENT
Assessment
• Assess history of hypersensitivity to drug
• Assess baseline wt, VS, B/P, ECG, hydration status
• Assess baseline electrolytes, liver function tests (ALT, AST, bilirubin), renal function (BUN, creatinine)
Interventions
• Wrap IV tubing with foil to protect medication from light
Evaluation
• Evaluate therapeutic response (stabilization, decreased B/P)
• Evaluate for hypersensitivity, side effects
• Evaluate electrolytes, liver function tests (ALT, AST, bilirubin), renal function (BUN, creatinine)
• Monitor VS, B/P, ECG continually
• Monitor serum thiocyanate levels q72h because of risk of cyanide toxicity

---

✤ Available in Canada.

PATIENT AND FAMILY EDUCATION

Teach/instruct
- About need for medication
- That VS and B/P will need to be monitored frequently

Warn/advise
- To notify care provider of hypersensitivity, side effects

STORAGE
- Store at room temp
- Protect from light

---

norepinephrine bitartrate
Brand Name(s): Levophed✤
Classification: Vasopressor
Pregnancy Category: D

AVAILABLE PREPARATIONS
Inj: 1 mg/ml

ROUTES AND DOSAGES
Children: IV 0.05-0.1 mcg/kg/min, then titrate to maintain desired B/P; 1 mcg/kg/min for cardiac life support
Adult: IV 8-12 mcg/min, then titrate to maintain desired B/P; maintenance 2-4 mcg/min

IV administration
- Recommended concentration: 4 mcg/ml
- Maximum concentration: Not established
- IV push rate: Not recommended
- Intermittent infusion: Not recommended

MECHANISM AND INDICATIONS
Vasopressor mechanism: Stimulates α- and β-adrenergic receptors, causing vasoconstriction, increased contractility and HR, thereby increasing B/P, improving coronary blood flow, and increasing cardiac output
Indications: Severe hypotension

PHARMACOKINETICS
Onset of action: 1-2 min
Peak: 2 min
Half-life: 1 min

Metabolism: Liver
Excretion: Urine (metabolites)

CONTRAINDICATIONS AND PRECAUTIONS
- Contraindicated with known hypersensitivity to medication, arrhythmias, ventricular fibrillation, pheochromocytoma, severe peripheral vascular disease, hypoxia, hypovolemia, pregnancy
- Use cautiously with known sensitivity to sulfites, hypertension, hyperthyroidism, lactation

INTERACTIONS
Drug
- Increased arrhythmias with general anesthetics
- Increased pressor effects with tricyclic antidepressants, MAOIs, antihistamines, guanethidine, β blockers, atropine, methyldopa
- Decreased action of norepinephrine with α blockers

INCOMPATIBILITIES
- NaHCO$_3$

SIDE EFFECTS
CNS: Headache, insomnia, dizziness, weakness, restlessness, tremors, convulsions
CV: Hypertension, angina, palpitations, tachycardia, bradycardia, arrhythmias
GI: Nausea, vomiting
GU: Decreased urine output
RESP: Dyspnea, apnea, pallor
Local: Necrosis and tissue sloughing with extravasation, gangrene
Other: Thyroid swelling, photophobia, sweating, cerebral hemorrhage, metabolic acidosis, hyperglycemia, hyperthermia

TOXICITY AND OVERDOSE
Clinical signs: Severe hypertension, photophobia, pharyngeal pain, intense sweating, vomiting, cerebral hemorrhage, convulsions, arrhythmias
Treatment: Supportive measures as necessary; administer atropine for bradycardia, phentolamine for extravasation, propranolol for arrhythmias

N

✤ Available in Canada.

PATIENT CARE MANAGEMENT

Assessment
• Assess history of hypersensitivity to drug, sulfites
• Assess baseline VS, B/P, ECG, hydration status

Interventions
• Correct hypovolemia before administration
• Administer into large vein; if extravasation occurs, infiltrate site with 10-15 ml NS and 10 mg phentolamine using a fine-gauge needle
• Do not use discolored sol
• Protect sol from light

Evaluation
• Evaluate therapeutic response (stabilization, increased B/P)
• Evaluate for side effects, hypersensitivity
• Monitor IV site carefully
• Monitor VS, B/P, ECG, hydration throughout infusion

PATIENT AND FAMILY EDUCATION

Teach/instruct
• About need for medication
• That VS will need to be monitored frequently

Warn/advise
• To notify care provider of hypersensitivity, side effects

Provide
• Emotional support as indicated

STORAGE
• Store at room temp
• Protect from light

---

nortriptyline hydrochloride

Brand Name(s): Aventyl✤, Aventyl HCL, Pamelor

Classification: Tricyclic antidepressant

Pregnancy Category: D

AVAILABLE PREPARATIONS
Sol: 10 mg/5 ml
Caps: 10 mg, 25 mg, 75 mg

DOSAGES AND ROUTES
• Safety and effectiveness for use by children <6 yr not established

Depression
Children 6-12 yr: PO, daily dosage for major depressive disorder ranges from 1-3 mg/kg/24 hr divided bid-qid; maximum 2 mg/kg/24 hr; plasma levels should not exceed 150 ng/ml
Adults: PO, initial 25 mg tid-qid; may increase as needed and tolerated, by 10-25 mg/24 hr at 1 wk intervals, up to 150 mg/24 hr; usual maintenance 50-100 mg/24 hr; maximum 150 mg/24 hr

Nocturnal Enuresis
Children 6-7 yr: PO 10 mg 30 min before hs
Children 8-11 yr: PO 10-20 mg 30 min before hs
Children >11 yr and adolescents: PO 25-35 mg 30 min before hs

MECHANISM AND INDICATIONS
Mechanism: Blocks reuptake of norepinephrine and serotonin into CNS neurons, increasing action of norepinephrine and serotonin
Indications: For use in treating depression, ADHD, panic disorder, anxiety-based school refusal, separation anxiety disorder, bulimia, primary nocturnal enuresis, night terrors, sleepwalking; also used to manage chronic, severe pain

PHARMACOKINETICS
Onset of action: 4-19 days
Half-life: 18-28 hr
Metabolism: Liver
Excretion: Urine
Therapeutic level: Children, 60-100 ng/ml; adults, 50-150 ng/ml

CONTRAINDICATIONS AND PRECAUTION
• Contraindicated with hypersensitivity to this medication or any component, cardiac disease, arrhythmia, narrow angle glaucoma, MAOIs taken within past 14 days, recent MI, prostatic hypertrophy, undiagnosed syncope
• Use cautiously with family history of sudden cardiac death or cardiomyopathy; severe depression, diabetes, known electrolyte

---

✤ Available in Canada.

abnormality with binging and purging, electroshock therapy, history of glaucoma, hyperthyroidism, increased intraocular pressure, seizures, suicidal, surgery under general anesthesia planned for the near future, urinary retention

• Use cautiously with pregnancy, lactation

INTERACTIONS
Drug
• Risk of hyperpyretic crisis, convulsions, hypertensive episode within 14 days of MAOIs
• Increased sedation with alcohol, antihistamines, antipsychotics, barbiturates, benzodiazepines, chloral hydrate, glutethimide, sedatives
• Increased hypotension with methyldopa, β-adrenergic blockers, clonidine, diuretics
• Additive cardiotoxicity with quinidine, thioridazine, mesoridazine
• Additive anticholinergic toxicity with antihistamines, antiparkinsonians, thioridazine, OTC sleeping medications, GI antispasmodics, antidiarrheals
• Increased effects of alcohol, barbiturates, benzodiazepines, CNS depressants and stimulants, dicoumarol, epinephrine, warfarin
• Decreased effects of clonidine, ephedrine, guanethidine
• Increased tachycardia possible with marijuana
• Increased effects with cimetidine, oral contraceptives, methylphenidate, phenothiazines, quinidine
• Decreased effects with barbiturates, cigarette smoking
• Confusion, disorientation, hallucinations with disulfiram
• Impaired heart rhythm and function with thyroid preparations
Lab
• Increased ALT, AST, alk phos, serum bilirubin, BG
• Decreased VMA, 5-HIAA, WBC, platelet counts
• Falsely elevated urinary catecholamines

• Fluctuation in BG levels
• Liver toxicity may be mistaken for viral hepatitis
Nutrition
• Oral sol contains 4% alcohol

SIDE EFFECTS
CNS: Dizziness, drowsiness, anxiety, confusion, delusions, disorientation, fainting, hallucinations, headache, insomnia, light-headedness, nightmares, seizures, stimulation, tremors, unsteady gait, weakness
CV: Tachycardia, orthostatic hypotension, arrhythmia, ECG changes, hypertension, palpitations
DERM: Hives, itching, photosensitivity, rash, sweating
EENT: Blurred vision, mydriasis, taste changes, tinnitus
GI: Constipation, dry mouth, increased appetite, cramps, epigastric distress, hepatitis, paralytic ileus, indigestion, jaundice, nausea, stomatitis, vomiting
GU: Urinary retention, galactorrhea, gynecomastia, increased or decreased libido, male impotence, inhibited female orgasm, swelling of testicles, acute renal failure
HEME: Agranulocytosis, bone marrow depression, eosinophilia, thrombocytopenia
Other: Fluctuation of BG levels, fever, leukopenia, peripheral neuritis

TOXICITY AND OVERDOSE
Clinical signs: Agitation, coma, confusion, dilated pupils, drowsiness, hallucinations, hypotension, hypothermia, palpitations, seizures, deep sleep, stupor, tachycardia, tremors, urinary retention
Treatment: Monitor VS, ECG; induce emesis, lavage; administer activated charcoal; anticonvulsant; correct acidosis with $NaHCO_3$ to increase protein binding and decrease free fraction; correction of acidosis may decrease cardiovascular toxicities; avoid disopyramide, procainamide, quinidine; lidocaine, phenytoin or propranolol may be necessary; reserve physostigmine for

---

✦ Available in Canada.

refractory life-threatening anticholinergic toxicities; for life-threatening arrhythmias or seizures in children, administer slow IV physostigmine 0.01-0.03 mg/kg/dose, up to 0.5 mg/dose over 2-3 min, repeat in 5 min, maximum total dose 2 mg; in adolescents and adults, 2 mg/dose physostigmine, may repeat 1-2 mg in 20 min and give 1-4 mg slow IV over 5-10 min if signs and symptoms recur

PATIENT CARE MANAGEMENT
Assessment
• Assess history of hypersensitivity to drug
• Obtain general physical examination (including thorough cardiac examination)
• Examine family history for sudden cardiac death and pt's history for cardiac disease, arrhythmias, syncope, seizure disorder or congenital hearing loss (associated with prolonged QT syndrome)
• Assess ability to function in daily activities and sleep throughout the night
• Assess mental status (mood, sensorium, affect, impulsiveness, suicidal ideation, thoughts)
• Obtain baseline orthostatic B/P, pulse
• Obtain baseline CBC, leukocytes, differential, AST, ALT, bilirubin, serum electrolytes, ECG, wt
• In pts with eating disorders, obtain BUN

Interventions
• PO may be given without regard to meals; may be given with milk; may mix concentrate with a small amount of fruit juice, water, or milk; caps may be opened
• If sedation occurs with day administration, entire dose may be administered hs
• Rinse with water, take sips of fluid, sugarless gum, or hard candy for dry mouth
• Increase fluids and fiber in diet if constipation occurs
• Do not drink alcohol
• If GI symptoms occur, give with food or milk

• If electroshock therapy is to be administered, hold nortriptyline

> **NURSING ALERT**
> Do not administer at the same time as or within 14 days of MAOIs; may cause a hypertensive crisis, high fever, seizures

Evaluation
• Evaluate therapeutic response (improved depression, ability to function in daily activities, to sleep throughout the night); if prescribed for attention deficit, assess activity level, impulsivity, distractibility, attending, obtain parent and teacher reports about attention and behavioral; if taken for depression, evaluate for symptoms of depression
• Evaluate mental status (mood, sensorium, affect, impulsiveness, suicidal ideation, thoughts)
• Careful cardiac monitoring with dosage increases; monitor ECG for flattening of T wave, bundle branch block, AV block, arrhythmias
• Monitor for constipation, urinary retention
• Monitor wt; nortriptyline may increase appetite
• Monitor blood levels as needed
• Monitor orthostatic B/P, pulse; if systolic B/P drops 20 mm Hg, hold drug, notify prescriber
• Monitor cardiac enzymes with long-term therapy
• Evaluate need for nortriptyline at least every 6 mo
• Do not discontinue abruptly; if it is not tapered, symptoms include headache, nausea, vomiting, muscle pain, weakness

PATIENT AND FAMILY EDUCATION
Teach/instruct
• To take as directed at prescribed intervals for prescribed length of time
• That sometimes this medicine must be taken for 2-3 wk before improvement is noticed

- That medication is most helpful when used as part of a comprehensive multimodal treatment program
- About the importance of returning for follow-up visits
- Not to discontinue medication without prescriber approval

Warn/advise

- To avoid ingesting alcohol, other CNS depressants.
- That medication may cause drowsiness; be careful on bicycles, skates, skateboards, while driving, with other activities requiring alertness
- To stay out of direct sunlight (especially between 10 AM and 3 PM) if possible; if pt must be outside, to wear protective clothing, a hat, sunglasses; pt should put on sunblock that has a skin protection factor (SPF) of at least 15
- To use caution when exposed to heat; drug may impair body's adaptation to hot environments, increasing risk of heat stroke; avoid saunas, hot tubs, hot baths
- Not to discontinue medication quickly after long-term use

STORAGE

- Store at room temp in a tightly covered, light-resistant container

---

nystatin

Brand Name(s):
Mycostatin✤, Nadostine✤, Nilstat✤, Nyaderm✤, Nystat-Rx, Nystex, PMS-Nystatin✤

Classification: Antifungal

Pregnancy Category: B

AVAILABLE PREPARATIONS

Oral susp: 100,000 U/ml
Troche: 200,000 U
Tabs: 500,000 U
Top powder, oint, cream: 100,000 U/g
Vag supp: 100,000 U

ROUTES AND DOSAGES
Oral Candidiasis
Neonates: PO 50,000 U (0.5 ml) to each side of mouth qid after meals (total 100,000 U/dose)
Infants: PO 100,000 U (1 ml) to each side of mouth qid after meals (total 200,000 U/dose)
Children and adults: PO 400,000-600,000 U (4-6 ml) qid after meals; troche 200,000-400,000 U (1-2 troches) 4-5 ×/day after meals; continue oral therapy for 48 hr after symptoms have resolved

Intestinal Infection
Adults: PO 500,000-1,000,000 U q8h

Cutaneous Candidal Infection
Children and adults: Top, apply to affected area tid-qid

Vaginal Candidiasis
Children and adults: Insert 1 vag supp qhs × 2 wk

MECHANISM AND INDICATIONS

Mechanism: Binds sterols in fungal cell membrane, causing increased permeability, leading to leaking of cell nutrients
Indications: Used to treat oral, intestinal, and vaginal fungal infections caused by *Candida* species

PHARMACOKINETICS

Onset: Symptomatic relief 24-72 hr
Excretion: Feces

CONTRAINDICATIONS AND PRECAUTIONS

- Contraindicated with known hypersensitivity to nystatin or any component
- Use cautiously with pregnancy, lactation

SIDE EFFECTS

DERM: Contact dermatitis, Stevens-Johnson syndrome
GI: Nausea, vomiting, diarrhea
Local: Irritation

TOXICITY AND OVERDOSE

Clinical signs: Local irritation
Treatment: Supportive care; toxicity negligible

PATIENT CARE MANAGEMENT
Assessment

- Assess history of hypersensitivity to nystatin, any components

N

• Assess mouth for characteristic white patches

Interventions

• Administer PO after meals, after mouth has been cleaned of food residue; shake susp well, swab inside of entire mouth area in infants and young children; have older children swish susp and hold in mouth several minutes before swallowing; troches should be allowed to dissolve in mouth for 30 min; do not chew, crush, or swallow whole; wait 30 min after administration to give additional fluids or foods

• Apply top lotion or cream sparingly to affected area using gloves or swabs; use cream in intertriginous areas; use powder in moist intertriginous areas; apply powder carefully so infant or child does not inhale particles; do not use occlusive dressings

• Insert vaginal applicator high into vagina

Evaluation

• Evaluate therapeutic response (decrease in size or number of lesions, decreased itching, negative *Candida* culture)

• Monitor for allergic reaction (burning, stinging, swelling, redness)

• Evaluate for predisposing factors (antibiotic therapy, pregnancy, DM, sexual partner infection)

PATIENT AND FAMILY EDUCATION

Teach/instruct

• To take as directed at prescribed intervals for prescribed length of time

Warn/advise

• To notify care provider of hypersensitivity, side effects

• About proper hygiene (oral forms); wash all pacifiers, bottle nipples in hot soapy water after each use; remove dentures before each rinse and at night

• That relief from itching may occur after 24-72 hr of therapy

• To avoid contact with eyes (top forms)

• To avoid use of occlusive dressings (top forms)

• About proper hygiene (top forms), change socks, avoid tight fitting shoes if feet are infected

• About how to prevent vag reinfection; to abstain from sexual intercourse during therapy

STORAGE

• Store all forms except vag supp at room temp

• Protect from light, air, heat, moisture

• Store vag supp in refrigerator; avoid freezing

---

omeprazole

Brand Name(s): Losec✤, Prilosec

Classification: Gastric acid pump inhibitor; antiulcer agent

Pregnancy Category: C

AVAILABLE PREPARATIONS

Delayed release caps: 20 mg

ROUTES AND DOSAGES

Infants and children: PO, has been administered at 0.7 mg/kg/24 hr; may administer 0.7 mg/kg/dose q12h (0.7 = 3.3 mg/kg/hr) (Safety and effectiveness not established. Dosage represents accepted standard practice recommendations.)

Gastroesophageal Reflux

Adults: PO 20 mg qd; 40 mg qd for 4-8 wk has reportedly been used for esophagitis associated with GERD refractory to usual therapy

Hypersecretory Conditions

Adults: PO 60 mg qd; doses up to 120 mg tid have been administered

Duodenal Ulcer

Adults: PO 20 mg qd; 40 mg qd has reportedly been used for disease refractory to usual therapy for 4-6 wk

---

Gastric Ulcer
Adults: PO 20 mg qd; can be increased to 40 mg qd for gastric ulcer refractory to other treatment regimens; if healing has not occurred within 4 wk, an additional 4 wk of treatment is recommended

MECHANISM AND INDICATIONS
Mechanism: Gastric acid pump inhibitor; inhibits H^+/K^+ ATPase system at the secretory surface of gastric parietal cell which results in inhibition of transport of hydrogen ions into gastric lumen
Indications: Used in therapy for duodenal ulcer, severe erosive esophagitis, poorly responsive GERD, long-term therapy of pathologic hypersecretory conditions

PHARMACOKINETICS
Onset of action: Within 1 hr
Half-life: 0.5-1 hr (with normal hepatic function)
Peak concentration: 0.5-3.5 hr
Peak effect: Within 2 hr
Duration: Up to 72 hr (96 hr required for full restoration of acid production)
Metabolism: Liver
Excretion: Urine, feces

CONTRAINDICATIONS AND PRECAUTIONS
• Contraindicated with sensitivity to omeprazole
• Use cautiously in pregnancy, lactation, hepatic insufficiency

INTERACTIONS
Drug
• Altered bioavailability of drug, dose forms (e.g., enteric-coated) with pH dependent absorption
• Prevention of degradation of acid-labile drugs possible
• Impaired elimination of drugs requiring hepatic metabolism
• Reduced absorption of ampicillin (esters), iron salts, ketoconazole
• Increased blood concentration of anticoagulants, diazepam, phenytoin
• Increased leukopenic or thrombocytopenic effects of bone marrow depressants

Lab
• Increased alk phos, ALT, AST
• Increased serum gastrin levels during first 2 wk of therapy, then normalized levels after discontinuation of omeprazole

SIDE EFFECTS
CNS: Dizziness, headache, drowsiness, fatigue
DERM: Skin rash, itching
GI: Constipation, diarrhea, nausea, vomiting, flatulence, abdominal pain
GU: Urinary tract infection, hematuria, proteinuria
HEME: Anemia, eosinopenia, leukocytosis, neutropenia, pancytopenia, thrombocytopenia

TOXICITY AND OVERDOSE
Clinical signs: No reported experience to date with overdose of omeprazole
Treatment: Supportive measures

PATIENT CARE MANAGEMENT
Assessment
• Assess history of hypersensitivity to omeprazole
• Obtain baseline assessment of GI symptoms, hepatic function (ALT, AST, bilirubin), CBC
Interventions
• Suggested dosage schedule is ac, preferably the first AM meal
• Caps must be taken whole, not chewed, crushed, or opened
Evaluation
• Evaluate therapeutic response (absence of epigastric pain, swelling, fullness)
• Evaluate for hypersensitivity, side effects
• Evaluate CBC and hepatic function (ALT, AST, bilirubin)

PATIENT AND FAMILY EDUCATION
Teach/instruct
• To take as directed at prescribed intervals for prescribed length of time
• To continue taking even after symptoms subside
Warn/advise
• To notify care provider if side effects occur

♣ Available in Canada.

- To avoid smoking, caffeine, alcohol, which might exacerbate symptoms
- To avoid OTC drugs unless directed by care provider

STORAGE
- Store at room temp in a tightly closed container, protect from light

---

ondansetron

Brand Name(s): Zofran

Classification: Antiemetic, selective 5HT$_3$ receptor antagonist

Pregnancy Category: B

AVAILABLE PREPARATIONS
Inj: 2 mg/ml
Tabs: 4 mg, 8 mg

ROUTES AND DOSAGES
- Most dosage studies have been done using IV preparation; oral form less well-absorbed across GI tract; for moderately emetogenic chemotherapy, oral tab dosages have been established based on recommended IV dosing; in therapy with higher degree of emetogenic potential, oral dosages may need to be increased

Children 4-11 yr: PO 4 mg 30 min before chemotherapy; repeat 4 and 8 hr after initial dose; IV (children >3 yr) 0.15 mg/kg 30 min before chemotherapy; repeat 4 and 8 hr after initial dose

Children >11 yr and adults: PO 8 mg 30 min before chemotherapy; repeat 4 and 8 hr after initial dose; IV 0.15 mg/kg 30 min before chemotherapy; repeat 4 and 8 hr after initial dose

IV administration
- Intermittent infusion: Dilute in 50 ml of NS, D$_5$W, D$_5$½NS, D$_5$NS; infuse over 15 min

MECHANISM AND INDICATIONS
Mechanism: Binds to 5-HT$_3$ serotonin receptors on vagal nerve terminals and in chemoreceptor trigger zone in CNS; in response to chemotherapy, mucosal cells secrete serotonin which affects 5-HT$_3$ receptors, evoking vagal discharge, causing vomiting
Indications: Prevention of chemotherapy-associated nausea and vomiting; may also aid in treatment of postoperative nausea and vomiting

PHARMACOKINETICS
Onset of action: IV immediate, PO 1-2 hr
Peak action: 1-1.5 hr
Half-life: Children >15, adults 3-4 hr; shorter in children <15 yr
Metabolism: Liver
Excretion: Urine, feces

CONTRAINDICATIONS AND PRECAUTIONS
- Contraindicated with hypersensitivity to drug
- Use cautiously with impaired liver function, pregnancy, lactation

INTERACTIONS
Drug
- Does not inhibit cytochrome P-450 drug metabolism enzyme system of liver
Lab
- Transient increase in AST, ALT, bilirubin; may cause hypokalemia

INCOMPATIBILITIES
- Acyclovir, aminophylline, amphotericin-B, ampicillin, ampicillin with sulbactam, cefoperazone, fluorouracil, furosemide, ganciclovir, lorazepam, methylprednisolone, mezlocillin, piperacillin; precipitates in alkaline sol

SIDE EFFECTS
CNS: Faintness, dizziness, headache, EPS, grand mal seizure (rare)
CV: Orthostatic hypotension, tachycardia, chest pain, ECG changes
EENT: Transient blurred vision
GI: Abdominal pain or discomfort, constipation with multiple day regimens, dry mouth

TOXICITY AND OVERDOSE
- Have not been reported

PATIENT CARE MANAGEMENT

Assessment
- Assess hypersensitivity history to drug
- Assess baseline VS
- Assess effectiveness of previous antiemetic therapy

Interventions
- Administer 30 min before initiating chemotherapy
- Repeat dosages at appropriate intervals

Evaluation
- Therapeutic response (control of nausea, vomiting)

PATIENT AND FAMILY EDUCATION

Teach/instruct
- To take medication as directed
- To report any adverse effect (especially involuntary movements of eyes, face, limbs)

Encourage
- To report perceived effectiveness of agent

STORAGE
- Store tabs at room temp
- Inj sol stable at room temp in ambient lighting for 48 hr in NS, D_5W, D_5NS, $D_5\frac{1}{2}NS$

---

oxacillin sodium

Brand Name(s): Bactocill

Classification: Antibiotic (penicillinase-resistant penicillin)

Pregnancy Category: B

AVAILABLE PREPARATIONS
Oral susp: 250 mg/5 ml
Caps: 250 mg, 500 mg
Inj: 250 mg, 500 mg, 1 g, 2 g, 4 g, 10 g

ROUTES AND DOSAGES
Neonates ≤7 days, <2000 g: IM/IV 25 mg/kg q12h
Neonates >7 days, wt <2000 g: IM/IV 25 mg/kg q8h
Neonates ≤7 days, wt >2000 g: IM/IV 25 mg/kg q8h
Neonates >7 days, wt >2000 g: IM/IV 25 mg/kg q6h
Children >1 mo, <40 kg: PO 50-100 mg/kg/24 hr divided q6h; IM/IV 100-200 mg/kg/24 hr divided q6h; maximum 12 g/24 h
Children >40 kg and adults: PO 500-1000 mg q4-6h; IM/IV 250-2000 mg q4-6h (maximum 20 g/24 hr)

IV administration
- Recommended concentration: 0.5-4.0 mg/ml in compatible IV sol for infusion; 50-100 mg/ml in NS or SW for IV push
- Maximum concentration: 100 mg/ml for IV push
- IV push rate: Over 10 min
- Intermittent infusion: Over 15-30 min

MECHANISM AND INDICATIONS
Antibiotic mechanism: Bactericidal; inhibits bacterial cell wall synthesis by adhering to bacterial penicillin-binding proteins
Indications: Effective against gram-positive cocci (including, *Staphylococcus aureus, S. epidermidis, Streptococcus pneumoniae*), and infections caused by penicillinase-producing *Staphylococcus;* used to treat meningitis, respiratory tract, skin, soft tissue, bone, joint infections

PHARMACOKINETICS
Peak: PO, IM 0.5 hr; IV end of infusion
Distribution: Penetrates CNS with inflamed meninges
Half-life: Neonates 1.5 hr; children 0.5-1.0 hr
Metabolism: Liver
Excretion: Urine, bile

CONTRAINDICATIONS AND PRECAUTIONS
- Contraindicated with known hypersensitivity to oxacillin, penicillins, cephalosporins
- Use cautiously in neonates, with impaired renal or hepatic function, history of colitis or other GI disorders, pregnancy

O

INTERACTIONS
Drug
• Synergistic antimicrobial activity against certain organisms with aminoglycosides
• Increased serum concentrations with probenecid
• Decreased effectiveness with erythromycins, tetracyclines, chloramphenicol
Lab
• False positive urine protein
• Increased liver function tests
Nutrition
• Decreased absorption if given with meals, acidic fruit juices, citrus fruits, or acidic beverages (e.g., cola drinks)

INCOMPATIBILITIES
• Amikacin, levarterenol, metaraminol, tetracycline, verapamil

SIDE EFFECTS
CNS: Neuropathy, neuromuscular irritability, seizures
GI: Oral lesions, diarrhea, pseudomembranous colitis, intrahepatic cholestasis, hepatitis, elevated lever enzymes
GU: Interstitial nephritis, transient hematuria, proteinuria
HEME: Granulocytopenia, thrombocytopenia, eosinophilia, hemolytic, anemia, transient neutropenia
Local: Thrombophlebitis
Other: Hypersensitivity reactions (fever, chills, rash, urticaria, anaphylaxis), bacterial or fungal superinfection

TOXICITY AND OVERDOSE
Clinical signs: Neuromuscular hypersensitivity, seizures
Treatment: Supportive care; if ingested within 4 hr, empty stomach by induced emesis or gastric lavage, followed with activated charcoal

PATIENT CARE MANAGEMENT
Assessment
• Assess history of hypersensitivity to oxacillin, penicillins, or cephalosporins
• Obtain C&S; may begin therapy before obtaining results
• Assess renal function (BUN, creatinine, I&O), hepatic function (ALT, AST, bilirubin), hematologic function (CBC, differential, platelet count), particularly for long-term therapy
Interventions
• Administer penicillins at least 1 hr before bacteriostatic antibiotics (tetracyclines, erythromycins, chloramphenicol)
• Administer PO 1 hr ac or 2 hr after meals; administer with water; avoid acidic beverages
• Refrigerate susp; shake well before administering
• Caps may be taken apart, mixed with food or fluid
• Reconstitute IM with SW or NS for injection per package insert
• Injection is painful; administer deeply into large muscle mass and rotate injection sites
• Do not mix IV with any other drugs, particularly aminoglycosides; infuse separately
• Use large vein with small-bore needle to reduce local reaction; rotate site q48-72h
• Maintain age-appropriate fluid intake

> **NURSING ALERT**
> Discontinue drug if signs of hypersensitivity, interstitial nephritis, or pseudomembranous colitis develop
>
> Do not infuse rapidly; seizures may result

Evaluation
• Evaluate therapeutic response (decreased symptoms of infection)
• Monitor signs of superinfection (perineal itching, diaper rash, fever, malaise, redness, pain, swelling, drainage, rash, diarrhea, sore throat, change in cough or sputum)
• Observe for signs of allergic reaction (wheezing, tightness in chest, urticaria), especially within 20-30 min of first dose
• Monitor renal function (BUN, creatinine, I&O), hepatic function (ALT, AST, bilirubin), electrolyte

levels (particularly K^+ and Na)
• Monitor for signs of bleeding (ecchymosis, bleeding gums, hematuria, daily stool guaiac); monitor pro-times and platelet counts
• Evaluate IM site for tissue damage, IV site for vein irritation

PATIENT AND FAMILY EDUCATION
Teach/instruct
• To take as directed at prescribed intervals for prescribed length of time
Warn/advise
• To notify care provider of hypersensitivity, side effects, superinfection

STORAGE
• Store powder, caps at room temperature
• Reconstituted susp stable refrigerated 7 days, room temp 3 days; label date, time of reconstitution
• Diluted parenteral sol stable for minimum of 6 hr; see package insert

---

oxandrolone

Brand Name(s): Oxandrin, Oxandrolone

Classification: Anabolic steroid

Controlled Substance Schedule III

Pregnancy Category: X

AVAILABLE PREPARATIONS
Tabs: 2.5 mg

ROUTES AND DOSAGES
Turner's Syndrome
PO 0.05-0.125 mcg/kg/24 hr qd (Safety and effectiveness not established. Dosage represents accepted standard practice recommendations.)
Reversal of Catabolism
PO 0.25 mg/kg/24 hr qd for 2-4 wk; continuous therapy should not exceed 3 mo

MECHANISM AND INDICATIONS
Anabolic mechanism: Promotes tissue development, growth; increases K^+, Ca, PO_4, Cl, and N levels
Indications: To reverse corticosteroid-induced catabolism, promote tissue development in debilitated pts, osteoporosis, Turner's syndrome

PHARMACOKINETICS
Metabolism: Liver
Excretion: Urine

CONTRAINDICATIONS AND PRECAUTIONS
• Contraindicated with severe renal and cardiac disease, hepatic disease, undiagnosed genital bleeding, pregnancy, lactation, hypersensitivity to drug
• Use cautiously with diabetes, CAD, hypercalcemia

INTERACTIONS
Drug
• Potentiates warfarin-type anticoagulants
• Increased fluid and electrolyte retention possible with corticosteroids
Lab
• Altered glucose tolerance, thyroid function tests, metyrapone test
• Increased sulfobromophthalein retention
• Increased serum Na, K^+, Ca, PO_4, cholesterol

SIDE EFFECTS
Androgenic: Females: deepening of voice, clitoral enlargement, premature epiphyseal closure; prepubertal males: premature epiphyseal closure, priapism, phallic enlargement; post-pubertal males: testicular atrophy, oligospermia, impotence, gynecomastia, epididymitis
CNS: Headache, anxiety, dizziness, fatigue, paresthesias, depression
CV: Edema, hypertension
DERM: Acne, oiliness, hirsutism, flushing, sweating
GI: Nausea, vomiting, diarrhea, gastroenteritis, constipation, wt gain, cholestatic jaundice, change in appetite

---

♣ Available in Canada.

GU: Bladder irritability, hematuria

Other: Hypersensitivity, hypercalcemia

PATIENT CARE MANAGEMENT
Assessment
• Assess history of hypersensitivity to oxandrolone
• Assess growth rate, bone age, pubertal status (Tanner stage), wt, K^+, Na, Cl, Ca, ALT, AST, bilirubin, hypoglycemia for pts with diabetes

Interventions
• Administer with food if GI upset occurs
• Restrict salt in diet if edema occurs

Evaluation
• Evaluate therapeutic response (monitor pubertal status, bone age for appropriate progression; increased growth velocity may occur as puberty progresses)
• Evaluate for signs of virilization in females (increased libido, deepening of voice, breast tissue, enlarged clitoris, menstrual irregularities) and gynecomastia, impotence, testicular atrophy in males
• Monitor for signs of hypoglycemia in diabetics
• Monitor edema, hypertension, cardiac symptoms, jaundice
• Monitor bone age q 6 mo (bone age advancement should not exceed increase in linear growth)
• Monitor priapism (may need to decrease dosage)
• Monitor K^+, Na, Cl, Ca, ALT, AST, bilirubin
• Monitor signs of hypercalcemia (lethargy, polyuria, polydipsia, nausea, vomiting, constipation)

PATIENT AND FAMILY EDUCATION
Teach/instruct
• To take as directed at prescribed intervals for prescribed length of time
• About anticipated changes in body image with adolescents

Warn/advise
• To notify care provider of hypersensitivity, side effects (GI distress, diarrhea, jaundice, priapism, menstrual irregularities)
• Not to discontinue medication suddenly
• That excess hair growth in females and acne are reversible when medication is discontinued
• That sexually active pts need to practice contraception when taking this medication
• About the dangers of steroid use to improve athletic performance

STORAGE
• Store at room temp

---

oxymethalone
Brand Name(s): Anadrol, Anapolon 50✤

Classification: Anabolic steroid, antianemic

Controlled Substance Schedule III

Pregnancy Category: X

AVAILABLE PREPARATIONS
Tabs: 50 mg

ROUTES AND DOSAGES
Erythropoietic Effect
Children and adults: PO 1-5 mg/kg/24 hr to maximum of 100 mg qd

MECHANISM AND INDICATIONS
Mechanism: Stimulates kidney's production of erythropoietin, increasing red blood mass and volume; stimulates receptors to promote growth and development of male sex organs, maintains secondary sex characteristics in androgen-deficient males

Indications: For use with pts who have anemia caused by myelotoxic drugs, deficient RBC production, aplastic anemia, or myelofibrosis; also used to offset protein breakdown associated with prolonged corticosteroid use, to treat wt loss caused by severe illness

PHARMACOKINETICS
Half-life: 9 hr
Metabolism: Liver
Excretion: Urine

✤ Available in Canada.

CONTRAINDICATIONS AND PRECAUTIONS

• Contraindicated with severe renal or cardiac disease (may compound fluid and electrolyte retention), hypersensitivity to anabolic steroids, hepatic dysfunction, infants, pregnancy, lactation
• Use cautiously with epilepsy, hyperlipidemia, liver disease, migraine, history of artery disease caused by hypercholesteremic drug manifestations; may also cause enhancement of physical appearance

INTERACTIONS
Drug
• Prolonged blood clotting times with oral anticoagulants
• May need to adjust levels with insulin
• May need to decrease levels of oral hypoglycemic agents
• Increased possibility of fluid overload with adrenalcorticosteroids
Lab
• Altered glucose tests, electrolytes, serum creatinine
• Decreased thyroid function tests, HDL
• Increased liver function, blood coagulation tests; LDL

SIDE EFFECTS
Androgenic: Females: virilization; prepubertal males: gonadal changes, premature epiphyseal closure; post-pubertal: impotence, testicular atrophy
CNS: Stimulation, sleeplessness, depression, behavior disturbances
CV: Edema
DERM: Acne, flushing, sweating, hirsutism
ENDO: Breast enlargement
GI: Nausea, vomiting, diarrhea, wt gain, appetite changes
GU: Bladder irritation, menstrual irregularities
Other: Fluid and Na retention, iron deficiency anemia, hepatotoxicity, hypercalcemia, liver cell tumor, blood lipid changes with risk of arteriosclerosis, premature epiphyseal closure

TOXICITY AND OVERDOSE
Clinical signs: Hepatotoxic effects (hepatocellular carcinoma), cholestasis, jaundice, hepatitis, abnormal healing
Treatment: Discontinue medication

PATIENT CARE MANAGEMENT
Assessment
• Assess history of hypersensitivity to oxymetholone
• Assess growth rate, bone age, pubertal status (Tanner stage) wt, K^+, Na, Cl, Ca, AST, ALT, bilirubin
• Assess hypoglycemia for pts with DM
Interventions
• Administer with food if GI upset occurs
• Restrict salt in diet if edema occurs

> **NURSING ALERT**
> Drug should be discontinued if hypercalcemia, edema, drug reaction, or noticeable signs of sexual changes occur

Evaluation
• Evaluate therapeutic response (normal hematologic values
• Evaluate signs of virilization in females (increased libido, deepening of voice, breast tissue, enlarged clitoris, menstrual irregularities) and gynecomastia, impotence, testicular atrophy in males
• Monitor for signs of hypoglycemia in diabetic pts
• Monitor for edema, hypertension, cardiac symptoms, jaundice
• Monitor bone age q 6 mo (bone age advancement should not exceed increase in linear growth)
• Monitor priapism (may need to decrease dosage)
• Monitor K^+, Na, Cl, Ca, ALT, AST, bilirubin
• Monitor for signs of hypercalcemia (lethargy, polyuria, polydip-

sia, nausea, vomiting, constipation)

PATIENT AND FAMILY EDUCATION
Teach/instruct
• To take as directed at prescribed intervals for prescribed length of time
• About anticipated changes in body image with adolescents
Warn/advise
• To notify care provider of hypersensitivity, side effects (GI distress, diarrhea, jaundice, priapism, menstrual irregularities)
• Not to discontinue medication suddenly
• That excess hair growth in females and acne are reversible when medication is discontinued
• That sexually active pts need to practice contraception when taking this medication
• About the dangers of steroid use to improve athletic performance

STORAGE
• Store at room temp in air tight, light-resistant container

---

oxymorphone
Brand Name(s):
Numorphan, Numorphan H.P.

Classification: Narcotic analgesic, opiate agonist

Controlled Substance Schedule II

Pregnancy Category: B

AVAILABLE PREPARATIONS
Rectal supp: 5 mg
Inj: 1.5 mg/ml

ROUTES AND DOSAGES
Children >50 kg and adults: PR 5 mg q4-6h prn; SC/IM 1-1.5 mg q4-6h prn; IV 0.5 mg q4-6h prn
IV administration
• Recommended concentration: May be diluted in 5 ml of SW or NS
• IV push: Over 2-5 min through Y-tube or 3-way stopcock

MECHANISM AND INDICATIONS
Mechanism: Inhibits ascending pain pathways in CNS; increases pain threshold; alters pain experience
Indications: Used to treat moderate-to-severe pain

PHARMACOKINETICS
Onset of action: IM/SC 10-15 min; IV 5-10 min; PR 15-30 min
Peak: IM/SC/IV 60-90 min
Duration: IM/SC 2-6 hr; IV/PR 3-6 hr
Metabolism: Liver
Excretion: Urine

CONTRAINDICATIONS AND PRECAUTIONS
• Contraindicated with hypersensitivity to the drug
• Use cautiously with hepatic and renal disease, increased ICP, respiratory depression, pregnancy, lactation, severe cardiac disease

INTERACTIONS
Drug
• Increased effects with other CNS depressants (alcohol, narcotics, sedative or hypnotics, antipsychotics, skeletal muscle relaxants)
Lab
• Increased serum amylase

INCOMPATIBILITIES
• Unknown

SIDE EFFECTS
CNS: Drowsiness, sedation, confusion, headache, euphoria, dizziness, vertigo
CV: Palpitation, bradycardia, changes in B/P
DERM: Rash, urticaria, pruritus, flushing, sweating, bruising
EENT: Miosis, diplopia, blurred vision, tinnitus
GI: Nausea, vomiting, constipation, anorexia, cramps
GU: Urinary retention, dysuria, increased urinary output
RESP: Respiratory depression
Other: Tolerance, physical and psychological dependence

TOXICITY AND OVERDOSE
Clinical signs: Respiratory depression

Treatment: Supportive care, naloxone (dose may need to be repeated or naloxone infusion administered), vasopressors

PATIENT CARE MANAGEMENT
Assessment
• Assess history of hypersensitivity to oxymorphone or related drugs
• Assess baseline VS, pain (type, location, intensity)
• Assess renal status (BUN, creatinine, I&O), respiratory function, CNS changes
Interventions
• Determine dosing interval by pt response; administer when pain is not too severe to enhance its effectiveness; coadministration with non-narcotic analgesics may have additive analgesic effects and permit lower narcotic dosages
• Institute safety measures (supervise ambulation, raise side rails, call light within reach)

NURSING ALERT

Only for use in children and adults >50 kg

When administering IV, naloxone and emergency equipment need to be readily available

---

Evaluation
• Evaluate therapeutic response (decrease in pain without significant alteration in LOC or respiratory status)
• Evaluate VS, renal status (BUN, creatinine), CNS changes
• Evaluate pain 15-30 min after administration
• Evaluate for side effects, hypersensitivity

PATIENT AND FAMILY EDUCATION
Teach/instruct
• About best time to request medication (if ordered prn)
Warn/advise
• That medication may cause drowsiness, dizziness, hypotension; to make position changes slowly, seek assistance with ambulation
• That tolerance or dependence may occur with long-term use
• To avoid other OTC medications, alcohol, other CNS depressants
• To notify care provider of hypersensitivity, side effects
Encourage
• To maintain adequate fluid intake; to practice coughing, perform deep breathing exercises to avoid respiratory complications

STORAGE
• Store at room temp in tightly covered, light-resistant container

---

oxytetracycline hydrochloride
Brand Name(s): Terramycin
Classification: Antibiotic (tetracycline)
Pregnancy Category: D

AVAILABLE PREPARATIONS
Caps: 250 mg
Tabs: 250 mg
Inj: 50 mg/ml 125 mg/ml
ROUTES AND DOSAGES
• Not recommended for children <8 yr
Children >8 yr: PO 25-50 mg/kg/24 hr divided q6h (maximum 2 g/24 hr); IM 15-25 mg/kg/24 hr divided q8-12h
Adults: PO 250-500 mg q6h; IM 100 mg q8-12h

MECHANISM AND INDICATIONS
Antibiotic mechanism: Bacteriostatic; inhibits bacterial protein synthesis by binding reversibly to ribosomal units
Indications: Effective against gram-positive and gram-negative organisms, *Mycoplasma, Rickettsia, Chlamydia,* and spirochetes; used to treat syphilis, *C. trachomatis,* lymphogranuloma venereum, mycoplasma pneumonia, early stages of Lyme disease, rickettsial infections

---

♣ Available in Canada.

PHARMACOKINETICS
Peak: 2-4 hr
Distribution: Concentrates in hepatic system
Half-life: 6-12 hr
Metabolism: Liver
Excretion: Urine, feces

CONTRAINDICATIONS AND PRECAUTIONS
• Contraindicated with pregnancy, lactation, children <8 yr (risk of permanent discoloration of teeth, enamel defects, retardation of bone growth), with known hypersensitivity to any tetracycline
• Use cautiously with impaired renal or hepatic function

INTERACTIONS
Drug
• Decreased bactericidal effects of penicillins
• Increased effects of oral anticoagulants
• Decreased absorption with antacids containing aluminum, Ca, Mg, laxatives containing Mg, oral iron, zinc, $NaHCO_3$
• Increased effects of digoxin
• Increased risk of nephrotoxicity from methoxyflurane
Lab
• False positive urine catecholamines
Nutrition
• Decreased oral absorption if given with food or dairy products

SIDE EFFECTS
CNS: Dizziness, headache, increased intracranial pressure
CV: Pericarditis
DERM: Maculopapular and erythematous rashes, urticaria, photosensitivity, increased pigmentation, discolored nails and teeth
GI: Anorexia, nausea, vomiting, diarrhea, glossitis, dysphagia, enterocolitis, inflammatory anogenital lesions
GU: Reversible nephrotoxicity with outdated oxytetracycline
HEME: Neutropenia, eosinophilia
METAB: Elevated BUN
Other: Hypersensitivity, bacterial or fungal superinfection

TOXICITY AND OVERDOSE
Clinical signs: GI disturbance
Treatment: Antacids; if ingested within 4 hr, empty stomach by gastric lavage; supportive care

PATIENT CARE MANAGEMENT
Assessment
• Assess history of hypersensitivity to tetracyclines
• Obtain C&S; may begin therapy before obtaining results
• Assess renal function (BUN, creatinine, I&O), hepatic function (ALT, AST, bilirubin), hematologic function (CBC, differential, platelet count) (particularly for long-term therapy), bowel pattern
Interventions
• Check expiration dates; nephrotoxicity may result from outdated oxytetracycline
• If pt is receiving penicillins concurrently, administer penicillins at least 1 hr before tetracycline
• Administer PO 1 hr ac or 2 hr after meals; administer with water to prevent esophageal irritation; do not administer within 1 hr of hs to prevent esophageal reflux; do not administer with milk or dairy products, $NaHCO_3$, oral iron, zinc, antacids
• Tabs may be crushed, capsules taken apart and mixed with food or fluid
• Administer IM deeply into large muscle mass, rotate injection sites
• Maintain age-appropriate fluid intake

> **NURSING ALERT**
> Discontinue drug if signs of toxicity, hypersensitivity, renal dysfunction, superinfection, erythema to sun or ultraviolet light exposure, or pseudomembranous colitis develop

Evaluation
• Evaluate therapeutic response (decreased symptoms of infection)
• Monitor for signs of superinfection (perineal itching, diaper rash, fever, malaise, redness, pain, swelling, drainage, rash, diarrhea, sore

throat, change in cough or sputum)

• Observe for signs of allergic reaction (rash, pruritus, angioedema)

• Monitor bowel pattern; diarrhea may be symptomatic of pseudomembranous colitis

• Monitor renal function (BUN, creatinine, I&O), hepatic function (ALT, AST, bilirubin), hematologic function (CBC, differential, platelet count)

• Evaluate IM site for tissue damage

PATIENT AND FAMILY EDUCATION
Teach/instruct
• To take as directed at prescribed intervals for prescribed length of time
Warn/advise
• To notify care provider of hypersensitivity, side effects, superinfection

• Not to use outdated medications

• To avoid sun or ultraviolet light exposure

STORAGE
• Store at room temp in airtight, light-resistant containers

---

paclitaxel
Brand Name(s): Taxol✦
Classification: Antineoplastic; spindle inhibitor
Pregnancy Category: D

AVAILABLE PREPARATIONS
Inj: 30 mg/5 ml ampule

ROUTES AND DOSAGES
• Drug may vary in response to diagnosis, extent of disease, concurrent or previous therapy, protocol guidelines, physiologic parameters; consult current literature, protocol recommendations
Children and adults: IV 135-250 mg/m^2 as a 24 hr continuous infusion q 3 wk

IV administration
• Recommended concentration: Dilute with NS, D$_5$W, D$_5$NS, or D$_5$LR to a final paclitaxel concentration of 0.03-1.2 mg/ml

• Paclitaxel is extremely hydrophobic; therefore, it must be mixed in a sol with Cremophor and dehydrated alcohol

• Sol may appear hazy; use in-line filtration for administration

• Do not use polyvinyl chloride infusion bags or administration sets; use only glass bottles, polypropylene, polyolefin bags or administration sets

MECHANISM AND INDICATIONS
Mechanism: Prevents depolymerization of cellular microtubules, inhibiting normal reorganization of the microtubule network necessary for mitosis and other vital cellular functions
Indications: Used to treat metastatic ovarian cancer after failure of first-line or subsequent therapy; 2nd line therapy in Ewing's osteosarcoma, and testicular cancer

PHARMACOKINETICS
Half-life: Terminal 5.5-17.5 hr
Metabolism: Liver
Excretion: Bile; minimal amount of unchanged drug in urine

CONTRAINDICATIONS AND PRECAUTIONS
• Contraindicated with known hypersensitivity to the drug or to polyoxyethylated castor oil (Cremophor, a vehicle used in sol), with baseline neutrophil counts <1500/mm^3, platelet count <100,000/mm^3; severely depressed bone marrow function, active infections (especially chicken pox or herpes zoster), pregnancy, lactation

• Use cautiously in pts who have received previous radiation therapy (may display more frequent or more severe myelosuppression), previous cardiotoxic drugs which may have affected cardiac function or output; with hepatic impairment

INTERACTIONS
Drug
• Inhibited paclitaxel metabolism possible with ketoconazole
• Additive myelosuppressive effects possible with cisplatin

INCOMPATIBILITIES
• Do not mix with other medications in syringe or sol

SIDE EFFECTS
CNS: Peripheral neuropathy (tingling, numbness), mild paresthesias
CV: Bradycardia, hypotension, abnormal ECG, chest pain, arrhythmias
DERM: Alopecia, radiation recall dermatitis
GI: Nausea, vomiting, diarrhea, mucositis, elevated liver enzymes (ALT, AST, bilirubin, alk phos)
HEME: Neutropenia, leukopenia, thrombocytopenia, anemia, bleeding
Other: Myalgias, arthralgia, phlebitis, cellulitis at injection site, hypersensitivity reaction (anaphylaxis)

TOXICITY AND OVERDOSE
Clinical signs: Allergic reactions have been reported with too-rapid an infusion; hypotension, significant neurotoxicity, generalized erythema, acute dyspnea, myalgias, nausea, vomiting, and myelosuppression have also been reported
Treatment: Slow infusion rate; pretreat with dexamethasone; supportive care

PATIENT CARE MANAGEMENT
Assessment
• Assess history of hypersensitivity to paclitaxel
• Assess baseline VS, CBC, serum electrolytes, liver function (ALT, AST, LDH, bilirubin, alk phos), baseline cardiac function before each course
• Assess success of previous antiemetic therapy
• Assess history of previous treatment with special attention to other therapies that may predispose pt to cardiac or hepatic dysfunction

Interventions
• Premedicate with corticosteroids (dexamethasone) and antihistamines to decrease incidence and severity of hypersensitivity reaction; premedicate with antiemetics and continue periodically throughout chemotherapy
• If pt has significant cardiac conduction abnormalities, continuous cardiac monitoring should be performed with each paclitaxel infusion
• Encourage small, frequent meals of foods pt likes
• Provide supportive measures to maintain hemostasis, fluid and electrolyte balance, and nutritional support

NURSING ALERT
Take precautions to avoid extravasation

Preparation and administration of parenteral form of drug are associated with carcinogenic, mutagenic, and teratogenic risks for health care personnel; safe handling, preparation, and administration of this drug are imperative

Health care providers must use in-line filtration when administering paclitaxel

Evaluation
• Therapeutic response (decreased tumor size; spread of malignancy)
• Evaluate CBC, platelet count, serum electrolytes, liver function (ALT, AST, LDH, bilirubin, alk phos) at given intervals after chemotherapy
• Evaluate for signs of infection (fever, fatigue, sore throat), bleeding (easy bruising, nosebleeds, bleeding gums)
• Evaluate for side effects and response to antiemetic regimen

PATIENT AND FAMILY EDUCATION
Teach/instruct
• To report immediately signs of peripheral neuropathy (tingling or burning sensations, numbness in extremities)
• About importance of follow-up to monitor blood counts, serum chemistry values, drug blood values
• To take accurate temp; rectal temp contraindicated
• To notify care provider of signs of bleeding (bruising, epistaxis, bleeding gums), infection (fever, sore throat, fatigue)
Warn/advise
• About impact of body changes that may occur (hair loss, hyperpigmentation, nail ridging), how to minimize changes (wigs, caps, scarves, long sleeves)
• To avoid OTC products containing aspirin
• To report any alterations in behavior, sensation, perception; help to develop a plan of care to manage side effects, stress of illness or treatment
• To manage bowel function, call care provider if abdominal pain or constipation are noted
• To immediately report any pain, discoloration at injection site (parenteral forms)
• That good oral hygiene with very soft toothbrush is imperative
• That dental work be delayed until blood counts return to baseline, with permission of the care provider
• To avoid contact with known viral or bacterial illnesses
• That household contacts of child not be immunized with live polio virus; inactivated form should be used
• That child not receive immunizations until immune system recovers sufficiently to mount needed antibody response
• To report exposure to chicken pox in susceptible child immediately

• To report reactivation of herpes zoster virus (shingles) immediately
• If appropriate, ways to preserve reproductive patterns, sexuality (sperm banking, contraceptives)
Encourage
• Provision of nutritious food intake; consider nutritional consultation
• To comply with bowel management program
• To use top anesthetics to control discomfort of mucositis; avoid spicy foods, commercial mouthwashes

STORAGE
• Diluted sol stable 27 hr at room temp
• Store in glass bottles

---

pancreatin
Brand Name(s): Creon, Dizymes, Donnazyme, Hi-Vegi-Lip, Pancreatin 5X USP Tablets, Pancreatin 8X USP Tablets

Classification: Digestant (pancreatic enzyme)

Pregnancy Category: C

AVAILABLE PREPARATIONS
Caps, sus rel: 8000 USP U lipase activity, 30,000 USP U amylase activity, 13,000 USP U protease activity (Creon)
Tabs, enteric coated: 6750 USP U lipase, 43,750 USP U amylase, 41,250 USP U protease (Dizymes); 2000 USP U lipase, 60,000 USP U amylase, 60,000 USP U protease (Hi-Vegi-Lip)
Tabs: 1000 USP U lipase, 12,500 USP U amylase, 12,500 USP U protease (Donnazyme); 12,000 USP U lipase, 60,000 USP U amylase, 60,000 USP U protease (Pancreatin 5X USP); 22,500 USP U lipase, 180,000 USP U amylase, 180,000 USP U protease (Pancreatin 8X USP)

ROUTES AND DOSAGES

• Dosage depends on condition being treated and digestive requirements as related to diet; considerable variation exists

Infants 6 mo-1 yr: PO 2000 USP U lipase with meals/feedings

Children 1-6 yr: PO 4000-8000 USP U lipase with meals, 4000 USP U lipase with snacks

Children 7-12 yr: PO 4000-12,000 USP U lipase with meals and snacks

Adults: PO 4000-16,000 USP U lipase with meals and snacks

MECHANISM AND INDICATIONS

Mechanism: Enzyme concentrate from hog pancreas; contains lipase, amylase, and protease enzymes; enhances the digestion of proteins, starches, and fats; activity increased in neutral or slightly alkaline environments

Indications: Used to supplement or replace naturally occurring pancreatic enzymes; used in pancreatic deficiency diseases (such as cystic fibrosis of the pancreas, chronic pancreatitis, pancreatectomy, pancreatic duct obstruction)

PHARMACOKINETICS

Absorption: Not absorbed; acts locally in GI tract

Excretion: Feces

CONTRAINDICATIONS AND PRECAUTIONS

• Use with extreme caution with known hypersensitivity to hog protein, pancreatin, acute pancreatitis

• Use cautiously with pregnancy, lactation

INTERACTIONS

Drug

• Decreased effectiveness possible with Ca- and Mg-containing antacids

• Decreased response to oral iron possible

• Enhanced absorption possible with antacids and H_2-blockers

Lab

• Hyperuricosuria, hyperuricemia with extremely high dosages

SIDE EFFECTS

• Most commonly seen in association with high dosages

GI: Diarrhea, nausea, cramping; irritation of oral mucosa when tabs are held in the mouth

Other: Allergic sneezing, rash, lacrimation

TOXICITY AND OVERDOSE

Clinical signs: Transient GI upset (diarrhea, cramping, nausea), hyperuricosuria, hyperuricemia

Treatment: Supportive care

PATIENT CARE MANAGEMENT

Assessment

• Assess history of hypersensitivity to pancreatin, hog protein

• Assess baseline GI function (particularly bowel pattern, nutritional status)

Interventions

• Administer ac or with meals; caps may be opened, contents mixed with food; enteric coated tabs should not be crushed or chewed

• Avoid administration with Ca- or Mg-containing antacids

• Administer oral iron preparations separately

Evaluation

• Evaluate therapeutic response (improved digestion of food and absorption of nutrients)

• Evaluate GI function, wt, nutritional parameters

• Evaluate for hyperuricosuria, hyperuricemia (blood in urine, joint pain, swelling of lower legs, feet)

PATIENT AND FAMILY EDUCATION

Teach/instruct

• To take as directed at prescribed intervals for prescribed length of time

• To take with adequate fluids to prevent oral mucosal irritation; oral mucosa of infants should be inspected and remaining enzyme should be wiped away

• About proper administration techniques for prescribed preparation

---

✤ Available in Canada.

- Reinforce nutritional education with pt

Warn/advise
- To report hypersensitivity, side effects to care provider
- To avoid inhalation of cap contents
- That pancreatic enzyme dosage forms are not interchangeable

STORAGE
- Store in tight container at room temp

---

pancrelipase

Brand Name(s): Cotazym, Cotazym-S, Digess 8000✤, Ilozyme, Ku-Zyme HP, Pancrease✤, Pancrease MT✤, Pancrease MT 4, Pancrease MT 10, Pancrease MT 16, Protilase, Ultrase MT 12, Ultrase MT 20, Ultrase MT 24, Viokase✤, Zymase

Classification: Digestant (pancreatic enzyme)

Pregnancy Category: C

AVAILABLE PREPARATIONS
Cap: 8000 USP U lipase activity, 30,000 USP U amylase activity, 30,000 USP U protease activity (Cotazym, Ku-Zyme HP); 5000 USP U lipase, 20,000 USP U amylase, 20,000 USP U protease (Cotazym-S); 10,000 USP U lipase, 30,000 USP U amylase, 30,000 USP U protease (Pancrease MNT-10); 16,000 USP U lipase, 48,000 USP U amylase, 48,000 USP U protease (Pancrease MT 16); 12,000 USP U lipase, 24,000 USP U amylase, 24,000 USP U protease (Zymase)
Cap, ext rel: 4000 USP U lipase, 12,000 USP U amylase, 12,000 USP U protease (Pancrease MT 4); 4000 USP U lipase, 20,000 USP U amylase, 25,000 USP U protease (Pancrease, Protilase)
Tab: 11,000 USP U lipase, 30,000 USP U amylase, 30,000 USP U protease (Ilozyme); 8000 USP U lipase, 30,000 USP U amylase, 30,000 USP U protease (Viokase)
Powder: 16,800 USP U lipase, 70,000 USP U protease, 70,000 USP amylase/0.7 g (Viokase Powder)

ROUTES AND DOSAGES
- Dosage depends upon pt's degree of maldigestion and malabsorption, fat content of diet, enzymatic activity of preparation

Pancreatic Insufficiency
- Dosage for children <6 mo not established
Children 6 mo-1 yr: 2000 U with each meal/feeding
Children 1-6 yr: 4000-8000 U with each meal; 4000 U with snacks
Children 7-12 yr: 4000-12,000 U with each meal and snacks
Children >12 yr and adults: 4000-16,000 U with each meal and snacks

Pancreatectomy or Obstruction of Pancreatic Ducts
Adults: 8000-16,000 U q2h

MECHANISM AND INDICATIONS
Mechanism: Enzyme concentrate from hog pancreas; contains lipase, amylase, and protease enzymes
Indications: Used to supplement or replace naturally occurring pancreatic enzymes; used in pancreatic deficiency diseases (such as cystic fibrosis of the pancreas, chronic pancreatitis, pancreatectomy, pancreatic duct obstruction); treatment of steatorrhea associated with the post-gastrectomy syndrome and bowel resection, and for decreasing malabsorption in these pts

PHARMACOKINETICS
Enhances the digestion of proteins, starches, and fats; the activity of pancrelipase is greater in neutral or faintly alkaline environments; the lipolytic activity of pancrelipase is 12 times that of pancreatin; both the proteolytic and amylolytic activities of pancrelipase are 4 times those of pancreatin

---

✤ Available in Canada.

CONTRAINDICATIONS AND PRECAUTIONS
• Contraindicated with acute pancreatitis
• Use cautiously, if at all, with hypersensitivity to hog protein, pancrelipase, and pancreatin
• Use cautiously with pregnancy, lactation, acute exacerbations of chronic pancreatitis

INTERACTIONS
Drug
• Decreased effectiveness possible with Ca- and Mg-containing antacids
• Enhanced absorption possible with antacids and H_2 blockers
• Decreased absorption of oral iron possible

Lab
• Increased uric acid possible in blood and urine

SIDE EFFECTS
• Side effects are most commonly associated with high dosages
GI: Diarrhea, nausea, abdominal cramping, intestinal obstruction (uncommon); irritation of the oral mucosa when tabs are held in the mouth
Other: Allergic (skin rash, hives); sensitization (shortness of breath, stuffy nose, wheezing, tightness in chest induced by repeated inadvertent inhalation of powder form or powder from opened capsules); hyperuricemia, hyperuricosuria (blood in urine, joint pain, swelling of feet or lower legs)

TOXICITY AND OVERDOSE
Clinical signs: Diarrhea, intestinal upset
Treatment: Supportive care

PATIENT CARE MANAGEMENT
Assessment
• Assess history of hypersensitivity to pancrelipase, pancreatin, hog protein
• Assess baseline GI function (particularly bowel pattern, nutritional status)

Interventions
• Administer before or with meals; caps may be opened, contents sprinkled on or mixed with food; enteric coated caps should not be crushed or chewed
• Administer oral iron preparations separately
• Avoid administering with Ca- and Mg-containing antacids

Evaluation
• Evaluate therapeutic response (improved digestion of food and absorption of nutrients)
• Evaluate for hypersensitivity, side effects
• Evaluate GI function, wt, nutritional parameters
• Evaluate for hyperuricosuria, hyperuricemia (blood in urine, joint pain, swelling of lower legs)

PATIENT AND FAMILY EDUCATION
Teach/instruct
• To take as directed at prescribed intervals for prescribed length of time
• To take with adequate fluids to prevent oral mucosal irritation; oral mucosa of infants should be inspected and wiped clean of any remaining enzyme
• Reinforce nutritional education with pt
• About proper administration techniques for prescribed preparation

Warn/advise
• To report hypersensitivity, side effects to care provider
• To avoid inhalation of powder or cap contents
• That pancreatic enzyme dosage forms are not interchangeable

STORAGE
• Store Cotazym, Cotazym-S, Ilozyme, Ku-Zyme HP, Zymase in tight containers at room temp
• Open containers should be stored in a dry place (a desiccant may be useful)
• Store Pancrease, Pancrease MT delayed-release caps in a dry place in tightly closed containers at room temp

---

✤ Available in Canada.

- Open preparations should not be refrigerated
- Store Viokase in a dry place in a tightly closed container at ≤25° C

---

pancuronium bromide

Brand Name(s):
Pancuronium Bromide
Injection✤, Pavulol✤,
Pavulon

Classification: Neuromuscular blocking agent

Pregnancy Category: C

AVAILABLE PREPARATIONS
Inj: 1 mg/ml, 2 mg/ml

ROUTES AND DOSAGES
Neonates: IV, test dose of 0.02 mg/kg recommended by manufacturer to assess responsiveness (neonates particularly sensitive to non-depolarizing agents)
Infants and children: IV 0.08-0.15 mg/kg initially, then 0.02-0.2 mg/kg repeated prn or 0.1 mg/kg/hr as continuous infusion
Adults: IV 0.04-0.1 mg/kg then 0.01 mg/kg q½-1h

IV administration
- Recommended concentration: 1-2 mg/ml or dilute to 0.01-0.8 mg/ml in D$_5$NS, D$_5$W, LR, or NS
- Maximum concentration: 1-2 mg/ml
- IV push rate: Rapid (seconds)
- Continuous IV infusion: 0.1 mg/kg/hr

MECHANISM AND INDICATIONS
Mechanism: Interrupts the transmission of nerve impulse at the skeletal neuromuscular junction; antagonizes acetylcholine by competitively binding to cholinergic sites on motor endplates, resulting in muscle paralysis; reversible with edrophonium, neostigmine, and physostigmine
Indications: Used as an adjunct in surgical anesthesia to facilitate endotracheal intubation and skeletal muscle relaxation during mechanical ventilation or surgery

PHARMACOKINETICS
Onset of action: 30-45 sec
Peak effects: 2-3 min
Duration: 40-60 min (depending on dose)
Half-life: 110 min
Metabolism: Liver
Excretion: Urine (55%-70% unchanged)

CONTRAINDICATIONS AND PRECAUTIONS
- Contraindicated with known hypersensitivity to bromide ion; injectable sol may contain benzyl alcohol, doses of 99-234 mg/kg associated with fatal gasping syndrome in neonates (metabolic acidosis, hypotension, CNS depression, cardiovascular collapse)
- Use cautiously with pregnancy, renal and hepatic disease, lactation, children <2 yr, fluid and electrolyte imbalances, neuromuscular disease, dehydration, respiratory disease

INTERACTIONS
Drug
- Increased neuromuscular blockade with aminoglycosides, clindamycin, lincomycin, quinidine, local anesthetics, polymyxin antibiotics, lithium, narcotic analgesics, thiazides, enflurane, isoflurane, verapamil, magnesium sulfate, furosemide
- Arrhythmias possible with theophylline

INCOMPATIBILITIES
- Do not mix with barbiturates in sol or syringe

SIDE EFFECTS
CV: Bradycardia, tachycardia, increased or decreased B/P
DERM: Rash, flushing, pruritus, urticaria, sweating, salivation
EENT: Increased secretions
MS: Weakness
RESP: Prolonged apnea, broncho-

P

✤ Available in Canada.

spasm, cyanosis, respiratory depression

Other: Endogenous histamine release may occur with mivacurium (erythema, hypotension, bradycardia or tachycardia)

TOXICITY AND OVERDOSE

Clinical signs: Prolonged apnea, bronchospasm, cyanosis, respiratory depression

Treatment: Supportive, symptomatic care; mechanical ventilation may be required; anticholinesterase to reverse neuromuscular blockade (edrophonium or neostigmine, atropine)

PATIENT CARE MANAGEMENT

Assessment

• Assess history of hypersensitivity to bromide ion
• Assess for preexisting conditions requiring caution (pregnancy, lactation, renal or hepatic disease, fluid and electrolyte imbalance, neuromuscular disease, dehydration, respiratory disease)
• Assess electrolytes (Na, K^+) before procedure; electrolyte imbalances (K^+, Mg) may increase action of drug

Interventions

• Monitor VS (pulse, respirations, airway, B/P) until fully recovered; characteristics of respirations (rate, depth, pattern); strength of hand grip
• Monitor therapeutic response (paralysis of jaw, eyelid, head, neck, rest of the body)
• Monitor I&O for urinary frequency, hesitancy, retention
• Monitor for allergic reactions (rash, fever, respiratory distress, pruritus); *drug should be discontinued if noted*
• Instill artificial tears (q2h) and covering to eyes to protect the cornea

---

NURSING ALERT

Injectable sol may contain benzyl alcohol as a preservative; benzyl alcohol in doses of 99-234 mg/kg has been associated with a fatal gasping syndrome in neonates; clinical signs include metabolic acidosis, hypotension, CNS depression, cardiovascular collapse

Should be administered only by experienced clinicians familiar with the drug's actions and complications

Administer only in facilities where intubation, artificial respiration, O_2 therapy, and antagonists are immediately available

---

Evaluation

• Monitor effectiveness of neuromuscular blockade (degree of paralysis) using nerve stimulator
• Monitor for recovery (including decreased paralysis of face, diaphragm, arm, rest of the body)

PATIENT AND FAMILY EDUCATION

Warn/advise

• That postoperative stiffness often occurs; is normal, and will subside

Provide

• Reassurance to pt if communication is difficult during recovery

STORAGE

• Refrigerate; stable ≤6 mo at room temp
• Do not store in plastic containers or syringes
• Use only fresh sol

---

paraldehyde
Brand Name(s): Paral

Classification: Anticonvulsant; cyclic ether

Controlled Substance Schedule IV

Pregnancy Category: C

AVAILABLE PREPARATIONS
Oral, rectal liquid: 1 g/ml
Inj: 1 g/ml

ROUTES AND DOSAGES
Seizures
Children: PR, dilute with cottonseed or olive oil as retention enema or with 200 ml NS for enema, 0.3 ml/kg q4-6h or 1 ml/yr of age, not to exceed 5 ml, may repeat in 1 hr prn; IM 0.15 ml/kg; IV 5 ml/90 ml NS, begin infusion at 5 ml/hr, titrate to pt response
Adults: IM 5-10 ml (divide 10 ml into two injections); IV 0.2-0.4 ml/kg in NS
Sedation
Children: PO/PR/IM 0.15 ml/kg
Adults: PO/PR 4-10 ml; IM 5 ml; IV 3-5 ml (used only in emergency)
Tetanus
Adults: IM 5-10 ml prn; IV 4-5 ml or 12 ml by gastric tube q4h diluted with water
Alcohol Withdrawal
Adults: PO/PR 5-10 ml, not to exceed 60 ml; IM 5 ml q4-6h × 24 hr, then q6h on following days, not to exceed 30 ml
IV administration
• Recommended concentration: Dilute 1 ml/20 ml of NS for injection
• Infusion rate: Administer ≤21 ml over 3-5 min

MECHANISM AND INDICATIONS
Mechanism: Exact mechanism of action unknown; acts as a CNS depressant; has a strong aromatic odor and a disagreeable taste, can be irritating to throat and stomach, may cause nerve injury when given IM
Indications: Used to treat status

epilepticus, tetanus-induced seizures, alcohol withdrawal; also used as a sedative/hypnotic

PHARMACOKINETICS
Onset of action: IV 10-15 min; PR slower
Peak: 1-2 hr
Duration: IV 6-8 hr; PR 4-6 hr
Half-life: 7.5 hr
Metabolism: Liver (70%-80%)
Excretion: Urine

CONTRAINDICATIONS AND PRECAUTIONS
• Contraindicated with known hypersensitivity, gastroenteritis with ulceration
• Use cautiously with pregnancy, asthma, hepatic and pulmonary disease

INTERACTIONS
Drug
• Increased blood levels of paraldehyde with alcohol, CNS depressants, general anesthetics, disulfiram
• Crystallization in kidneys with sulfonamides

INCOMPATIBILITIES
• Incompatible with chlorpromazine, prochlorperazine
• Incompatible in plastic; do not mix with any other drugs for administration

SIDE EFFECTS
CNS: Stimulation, drowsiness, dizziness, confusion, convulsion, headache, flushing, hallucinations, coma
CV: Pulmonary edema, pulmonary hemorrhage, circulatory collapse, respiratory depression
DERM: Rash, erythema, local irritation, pain, sloughing, fat necrosis
GI: Foul breath, irritation
GU: Nephrosis

TOXICITY AND OVERDOSE
Clinical signs: Rapid, labored respiratory movements; acidosis, bleeding, gastritis, muscular irritability, azotemia, oliguria, albuminuria, leukocytosis, fatty changes in liver and kidney with toxic hepatitis and nephrosis, pul-

P

monary hemorrhages, edema, dilatation of right ventricle
Treatment: Treat metabolic acidosis with $NaHCO_3$; hemodialysis may be needed to support renal function and treat acidosis

PATIENT CARE MANAGEMENT
Assessment
• Assess history of hypersensitivity, gastroenteritis with ulceration
• Assess for pregnancy, asthma, hepatic or pulmonary disease
• Assess baseline labs, including CBC, differential, platelets, liver function (ALT, AST, bilirubin, alk phos)
Interventions
• Administer PO with juice or milk to mask taste and smell, to decrease GI symptoms
• Use only glass containers or rubber tubing
• Administer IM injection deep in large muscle using Z-track method in order to prevent tissue sloughing; do not exceed 5 ml/site
• Monitor VS q 30 min after parenteral administration
• Monitor for signs and symptoms of respiratory dysfunction (respiratory depression, character, rate, rhythm); *if respirations <10/min or if the pupils are dilated, do not administer*
• Ensure that room is well ventilated to remove exhaled drug

NURSING ALERT

Monitor for signs and symptoms of respiratory dysfunction (respiratory depression, character, rate, rhythm); if respirations are <10/min or if the pupils are dilated, *do not administer*

Do not use plastic equipment for administration; use glass syringes or rubber tubing

---

Evaluation
• Evaluate therapeutic response (increased sedation, decreased seizures)

• Monitor mental status (mood, sensorium, affect, memory)
• Monitor Hct, Hgb, RBC, serum folate, vitamin D (if on long-term therapy)
• Monitor liver function (AST, ALT, bilirubin, creatinine)
• Monitor for signs of jaundice, hepatitis

PATIENT AND FAMILY EDUCATION
Teach/instruct
• That drug should be used as instructed; dosage should not be increased or decreased independently
• To give with juice or milk to help cover taste and smell and to decrease GI symptoms
• To administer only with glass containers or rubber tubing
Warn/advise
• To monitor for signs and symptoms of respiratory dysfunction (respiratory depression, character, rate, rhythm); *if respirations <10/min or if the pupils are dilated, do not administer*
• That paraldehyde is a CNS depressant; avoid activities that require alertness
• That dependency may result with long-term use
• That after long-term use, should be tapered over several wk

STORAGE
• Store in tightly closed containers; do not expose to light or air
• Use only fresh supply; do not use if brown, odor is vinegary, or if container has been open >24 hr

---

paroxetine
Brand Name(s): Paxil
Classification: Antidepressant
Pregnancy Category: B

AVAILABLE PREPARATIONS
Tabs: 20 mg, 30 mg

DOSAGES AND ROUTES
• Safety and effectiveness not established in children <12 yr

Adolescents and adults: PO initial 10-20 mg qd in AM: after 4 wk if no clinical improvement, dosage may be increased by 10 mg/24 hr each wk until desired response or maximum dose (50 mg/24 hr) is reached

MECHANISM AND INDICATIONS
Mechanism: Inhibits uptake of serotonin (but not norepinephrine uptake) in CNS neurons
Indications: For use in major depressive disorder in adults and adolescents (particularly when there may be a greater risk of drug overdose); to treat adults and adolescents with anorexia and obsessive compulsive disorder

PHARMACOKINETICS
Onset of action: Therapeutic effect may take 2-3 wk
Peak: 6-8 hr
Half-life: 1-7 days
Metabolism: Liver
Excretion: Feces, urine

CONTRAINDICATIONS AND PRECAUTIONS
• Contraindicated with hypersensitivity to this medication or any component; within 14 days of administration of MAOIs
• Use cautiously with kidney or liver disease; history of mania or seizures; children; lactation

INTERACTIONS
Drug
• Hypertensive crisis, high fever, seizures possible within 14 days of MAOIs
• Increased bleeding with warfarin
• Increased agitation with L-tryptophan
• Increased paroxetine levels with cimetidine
• Decreased paroxetine levels with phenobarbital, phenytoin
• Increased side effects with highly protein-bound drugs
• Increased digoxin levels possible
Lab
• Increased alk phos, serum bilirubin, BG
• Decreased VMA, 5-HIAA

• Falsely elevated urinary catecholamines
Nutrition
• Do not drink alcohol

SIDE EFFECTS
CNS: Agitation, anxiety, apathy, delusions, dizziness, abnormal dreams, drowsiness, euphoria, fatigue, hallucinations, headache, nervousness, insomnia, psychosis, sedation, tremor
CV: Vasodilation, orthostatic hypotension, palpitations
DERM: Rash, sweating
EENT: Cough, nasal congestion, dry mouth, sinus headache, sinusitis, visual changes, pharyngitis
GI: Anorexia, constipation, cramps, diarrhea, dry mouth, dyspepsia, flatulence, nausea, taste changes, vomiting
GU: Amenorrhea, cystitis, dysmenorrhea, decreased libido, impotence, urinary frequency, UTI
HEME: Leukopenia, anemia, lymphocytosis, leukocytosis
RESP: Dyspnea, respiratory infection
Other: Arthritis, fever, muscle pain, myasthenia, myopathy, weakness

PATIENT CARE MANAGEMENT
Assessment
• Assess history of hypersensitivity to drug
• Obtain baseline medical examination (including wt and orthostatic B/P)
• Assess baseline mental status (affect, mood, sensorium, impulsiveness, suicidal ideation)
• Obtain baseline CBC, differential, AST, ALT, bilirubin, creatinine
Interventions
• Administer PO qd in AM
• Tabs may be crushed if pt cannot swallow them whole
• If oversedation occurs during the day, take before hs
• Pt should not drink alcohol
• Take with food or milk if GI symptoms occur

P

• Increase fluids and fiber in diet if constipation occurs
• Rinse with water, take sips of fluid, sugarless gum, hard candy for dry mouth
• May cause headache, nausea, vomiting, muscle pain, weakness if withdrawn suddenly

> **NURSING ALERT**
> Do not take at the same time as or within 14 days of administration of MAOIs; may cause hypertensive crisis, high fever, seizures

Evaluation
• Evaluate therapeutic response (ability to function in daily activities, to sleep throughout night; symptoms of depression)
• Evaluate mental status (mood, sensorium, affect, impulsiveness, suicidal ideation, panic, thought organization)
• Evaluate for signs of urinary retention, constipation
• Monitor for orthostatic B/P changes; if systolic B/P drops 20 mm Hg, hold drug and notify care provider
• Monitor wt, CBC, differential

PATIENT AND FAMILY EDUCATION
Teach/instruct
• To take as directed at prescribed intervals for prescribed length of time
• To make sure PO medication is swallowed
• That this medicine must sometimes be taken for 2-3 wk before improvement is noticed
• That this medication is most helpful when used as part of a comprehensive multimodal treatment program
Warn/Advise
• To avoid ingesting alcohol, other CNS depressants
• That this medication may cause drowsiness; be careful on bicycles, skates, skateboards, while driving, with other activities requiring alertness

• Not to discontinue medication without prescriber approval

STORAGE
• Store at room temp

---

pemoline
Brand Name(s): Cylert✤
Classification: Central nervous system stimulant
Controlled Substance Schedule IV
Pregnancy Category: B

AVAILABLE PREPARATIONS
Tabs: 18.75 mg, 37.5 mg, 75 mg
Chewable tabs: 37.5 mg

DOSAGES AND ROUTES
Children >6 yr: PO initial, 37.5 mg qd in AM; increase by 18.75 mg/24 hr at weekly intervals; effective dose range 56.25-75 mg/24 hr; range 0.5-3 mg/kg/24 hr; maximum 112.5 mg/24 hr
• Do not use in children <6 yr
• Tolerance may develop over time and require dosage adjustment; seems to be more, rather than less, effective as children mature; as the child ages, dosage may be adjusted downward while still maintaining same level of effectiveness

MECHANISM AND INDICATIONS
Mechanism: Increases mental alertness by stimulating the brain; exact mechanism not fully understood, but may block reuptake mechanism of dopaminergic neurons
Indications: For use in treating children with behavior problems (such as hyperactivity, attention deficit disorder, severe distractibility, inability to concentrate, short attention span, impulsive behavior, and extreme mood changes that are not induced by stress) effective in treating narcolepsy

PHARMACOKINETICS
Onset of action: 2-4 wk
Peak: 2-4 hr

✤ Available in Canada.

Half-life: children 7-8 hr; adults 12 hr
Duration: 8 hr
Metabolism: Liver; wide variability (200%-300%), resulting in unpredictable reactions of children and adolescents
Excretion: Urine

CONTRAINDICATIONS AND PRECAUTIONS

• Contraindicated with hypersensitivity to this medication or any component, aplastic anemia, liver disease, psychosis, seizures, Tourette syndrome
• Use cautiously with history of drug dependence; kidney disease, children <6 yr, pregnancy, lactation

INTERACTIONS
Drug
• Additive CNS-stimulating effect with other CNS stimulants, ephedrine, pseudoephedrine, sympathomimetics
• Decreased seizure threshold; anticonvulsant dosage may need adjustment
• Altered insulin requirements possible in diabetics
Lab
• Increased ALT, AST, alk phos, LDH
Nutrition
• Increased stimulation and irritability possible with caffeine (coffee, tea, cola, chocolate)
• Avoid alcohol ingestion
• The 37.5 mg tab and the 37.5 mg chewable tab contain FD&C yellow dye #6

SIDE EFFECTS
CNS: Hyperactivity, insomnia, restlessness, anorexia, aggressiveness, depression, dizziness, drowsiness, Gilles de la Tourette syndrome, hallucinations, headache, irritability, movement disorders, nervousness, seizures, stimulation
CV: Tachycardia with overdose
DERM: Rash
GI: Abdominal pain, anorexia, diarrhea, hepatitis, jaundice, increased liver enzymes, liver damage, nausea, weight loss
HEME: Aplastic anemia
Other: Growth suppression in children, wt loss

TOXICITY AND OVERDOSE
Clinical signs: Agitation, confusion, delirium, false sense of well-being, hallucinations, headache, hypertension, hyperthermia, irritability, muscle trembling or twitching, nervousness, paranoia, dilated pupils, restlessness, seizures, tachycardia, toxic psychosis, violent behavior, vomiting
Treatment: Provide supportive care; if unconscious or seizing, protect airway; treat high fever with cooling blanket; treat seizure with IV benzodiazepines, with repeated dosing if necessary; treat severe hypertension or tachyarrhythmias with propranolol; delirium or psychosis usually respond to an antipsychotic agent; use adrenergic blocking agents judiciously

PATIENT CARE MANAGEMENT
Assessment
• Assess history of hypersensitivity to drug
• Assess risk factors for developing motor tics or Tourette syndrome
• Obtain baseline height, wt recorded on growth grids, pulse, B/P
• Obtain baseline ALT, AST, bilirubin, creatinine, alk phos
• Do not administer pemoline if liver enzymes are elevated
Interventions
• Chewable tab must be chewed before swallowing; do not swallow whole
• Administer medication in AM (as early in the day as possible to avoid insomnia at night) and at least 6 hr before hs
• This medication must be given on weekends (because two days off pemoline reduces serum levels and therapeutic benefit)
• Treatment of ADHD should include drug holidays (periodic stop-

ping of stimulant medication) to assess pt's requirements, to decrease tolerance, limit suppression of linear growth and wt

• Discontinuation requires several wk for drug to fully dissipate from bloodstream; because it has a build-up effect, it should be discontinued gradually

• Pemoline can usually be discontinued by adolescence

Evaluation

• Monitor ALT, AST, bilirubin, creatinine at least q 6 mo before treatment; elevated liver enzymes occur in 1%-3% of children receiving this medication; if this occurs, pemoline should be discontinued

• Monitor and record pulse, B/P, height, wt every 3-4 mo and at times of dosage increases; plot height and wt on growth grid; if growth rate is slowing, drug is usually discontinued for several mo

• Assess for abnormal movements at each visit

• Evaluate therapeutic response (ability to function in daily activities, to sleep throughout the night); obtain parent and teacher reports about attention and behavioral performance

• Evaluate mental status (mood, sensorium, affect, impulsiveness, aggressiveness, suicidal ideation, psychiatric symptoms

PATIENT AND FAMILY EDUCATION

Teach/instruct

• To take as directed at prescribed intervals for prescribed length of time

• That medication is most helpful when used as part of a comprehensive multimodal treatment program

• To not stop taking medication without prescriber approval

• That therapeutic effects may take 3-4 wk

• That missed doses should be taken as soon as possible, then go back to regular schedule; if very close to next dose, skip it and go back to regular schedule; do not double dose

• That insomnia and anorexia often decrease with continued therapy or lowering of dosage

Warn/advise

• That pemoline can produce dependence, has been abused by adults; use for children only as prescribed

• To minimize caffeine consumption (coffee, tea, cola, chocolate), avoid alcohol ingestion

• To avoid OTC preparations unless approved by prescriber

• To ensure medication is swallowed

• To avoid ingesting alcohol, other CNS depressants

• That medication may cause drowsiness; be careful on bicycles, skates, skateboards, while driving, with other activities requiring alertness

• To report to prescriber behavior changes, school performance, uncontrolled movement, yellowing of the skin, other unexpected occurrences

• To return for scheduled health care visits so behavior, growth, and liver function can be monitored

• Not to discontinue medication without prescriber approval; needs to be tapered off over several wk

STORAGE

• Store at room temp in a tightly sealed container, away from heat and direct light

---

penicillamine

Brand Name(s):
Cuprimine✤, Depen✤

Classification: Antidote (copper, lead poisoning), antirheumatic agent

Pregnancy Category: D

AVAILABLE PREPARATIONS
Caps: 125 mg, 250 mg

✤ Available in Canada.

Tabs: 250 mg

ROUTES AND DOSAGES
Rheumatoid Arthritis
Children: PO initial 3 mg/kg/24 hr (maximum 250 mg/24 hr) for 3 mo, then 6 mg/kg/24 hr (maximum 500 mg/24 hr) divided bid for 3 mo to a maximum 10 mg/kg/24 hr divided tid-qid
Adults: PO 125-250 mg/24 hr; may increase dose q1-3 mo to 1-1.5 g/24 hr; doses >500 mg/24 hr should be divided

Wilson's Disease
• Doses titrated to maintain urinary copper excretion >1 mg/24 hr
Infants and children: PO 20 mg/kg/24 hr divided bid-qid (maximum 1 g/24 hr)
Adults: PO 1 g/24 hr divided qid (maximum 2g/24 hr)

Cystinuria
• Doses titrated to maintain urinary cystine excretion at <100-200 mg/24 hr
Children: PO 30 mg/kg/24 hr divided qid (maximum 4 g/24 hr)
Adults: PO 2 g/24 hr divided q6h (range 1-4 g/24 hr)

Lead Poisoning
Children: PO 25-40 mg/kg/24 hr divided bid-tid (maximum 1.5 g/24 hr)
Adults: PO 1-1.5 g/24 hr divided q8-12h

MECHANISM AND INDICATIONS
Antidote mechanism: Chelates with lead, copper, mercury, iron, other heavy metals to form stable, soluble complexes which are excreted in urine; combines with cystine to form a more soluble compound and prevent the formation of cystine calculi
Antirheumatic mechanism: Depresses circulating IgM rheumatoid factor levels and *in vitro* depresses T cell (but not B cell) activity
Indications: Used to treat Wilson's disease, cystinuria, adjunct in treatment of rheumatoid arthritis, lead poisoning

PHARMACOKINETICS
Peak: 1-2 hr
Metabolism: Liver
Excretion: Urine, feces

CONTRAINDICATIONS AND PRECAUTIONS
• Contraindicated with hypersensitivity to penicillamine, possibly penicillin; rheumatoid arthritis with renal or hepatic insufficiency; with previous penicillamine-related aplastic anemia or agranulocytosis, during pregnancy in pts with cystinuria
• Use cautiously in pts who receive a second course of therapy (may have become more sensitized with greater risk of allergic reaction); in pts who develop proteinuria not associated with Goodpasture syndrome

INTERACTIONS
Drug
• Increased risk of adverse hematologic and renal effects with gold, antimalarials, immunosuppressants, oxyphenbutazone, phenylbutazone
Lab
• Positive ANA possible with or without clinical systemic lupus erythematosus-like syndrome
• Elevated liver function tests possible, not necessarily indicating significant hepatotoxicity
Nutrition
• Decreased absorption when given with meals

SIDE EFFECTS
CNS: Peripheral sensory and motor neuropathies, myasthenic syndrome
DERM: Rash, pruritus, pemphigus, increased friability of skin, hirsutism
EENT: Optic neuritis
GI: Oral lesions, nausea, vomiting, hypogeusia, hepatic dysfunction
HEME: Leukopenia, thrombocytopenia, eosinophilia, aplastic anemia
Other: Lymphadenopathy, pneumonitis, allergic reactions, systemic lupus erythematosus-like syndrome

P

✤ Available in Canada.

TOXICITY AND OVERDOSE
Clinical signs: No information available
Treatment: Supportive care; induced vomiting or gastric lavage followed by activated charcoal; hemodialysis

PATIENT CARE MANAGEMENT
Assessment
• Assess history of hypersensitivity to penicillamine, penicillin
• Assess hematologic function (CBC, differential, platelet count), renal function (BUN, creatinine, I&O), hepatic function (ALT, AST, bilirubin), heavy metal blood concentration

Interventions
• Administer PO 1 hr ac or 2 hr after meals, other medications; provide large amounts of water
• Tabs may be crushed, capsules taken apart and mixed with food or fluid
• Administer pyridoxine, sulfurated potash as ordered for pts with Wilson's disease

Evaluation
• Evaluate therapeutic response (decreased symptoms of Wilson's disease, cystinuria, rheumatoid arthritis, decreasing blood lead concentrations)
• Monitor hematologic function (CBC, differential, platelet count), renal function (BUN, creatinine, I&O), hepatic function (ALT, AST, bilirubin)
• Monitor allergic reaction (rash, joint pains, easy bruising)
• Monitor symptoms of fever, chills, sore throat, fatigue; notify care provider if these develop

PATIENT AND FAMILY EDUCATION
Teach/instruct
• To take as directed at prescribed intervals for prescribed length of time
• About sources of lead poisoning, ways to prevent further exposure or poisoning

Warn/advise
• To notify care provider of hypersensitivity, side effects

• That clinical improvement may not be noticeable for 3 mo with Wilson's disease, rheumatoid arthritis, cystinuria
• That exacerbations of rheumatoid arthritis may occur during penicillamine therapy
• To maintain a low copper diet (by excluding liver, broccoli, chocolate, nuts) with Wilson's disease; to take sulfurated potash as directed
• That compliance with follow-up care is critical

STORAGE
• Store at room temp in tight container

---

penicillin G benzathine

Brand Name(s): Bicillin, Bicillin Injectable Preparations (Benzathine Penicillin G Compound)♣, Bicillin L-A, Megacillin, Permapen

Classification: Antibiotic (natural penicillin)

Pregnancy Category: B

AVAILABLE PREPARATIONS
Tabs: 200,000 U
Inj: 300,000 U/ml, 600,000 U/ml

ROUTES AND DOSAGES
Neonates: IM 50,000 U/kg once
Children ≤12 yr: PO 25,000-90,000 U/kg/24 hr divided q6-8h
Children <27 kg: IM 300,000-600,000 U once
Children ≥27 kg: IM 900,000-1.2 million U once
Children >12 yr and adults: PO 400,000-600,000 U q4-6h
Adults: IM 600,000-2.4 million U once

Syphilis, Early
Infants and children: IM 50,000 U/kg once (maximum 2.4 million U/dose
Adults: IM 2.4 million U once

Syphilis, >1 yr Duration
Infants and children: IM 50,000

♣ Available in Canada.

U/kg q wk × 3 wk (maximum 2.4 million U/dose)
Adults: IM 2.4 million U q wk × 3 wk
Rheumatic Fever Prophylaxis
Infants and children: IM 25,000 U/kg q 3-4 wk; maximum 1.2 million U/dose
Adults: IM 1.2 million U q 3-4 wk or 600,000 U q 2 wk

MECHANISM AND INDICATIONS

Antibiotic mechanism: Bactericidal; inhibits bacterial cell wall synthesis by adhering to penicillin-binding proteins
Indications: Effective against gram-positive and gram-negative organisms including *Staphylococcus aureus, Streptococcus pyogenes, Str. viridans, Str. faecalis, Str. bovis, Str. pneumoniae, Neisseria gonorrhoeae, Bacillus anthracis, Clostridium perfringens, C. tetani, Corynebacterium diphtheriae, Listeria monocytogenes, E. coli, Proteus mirabilis, Salmonella, Shigella, Enterobacter, Streptobacillus moniliformis;* used to treat respiratory tract infections, otitis media, scarlet fever, skin and soft tissue infections, GI infections; for prophylaxis of rheumatic fever and syphilis

PHARMACOKINETICS

Peak: PO 6 hr; IM 13-24 hr
Half-life: 0.5-1.0 hr
Metabolism: Hydrolyzed to penicillin
Excretion: Urine

CONTRAINDICATIONS AND PRECAUTIONS

• Contraindicated with known hypersensitivity to any other penicillins or to cephalosporins
• Use cautiously with impaired renal function, pregnancy

INTERACTIONS
Drug
• Synergistic antimicrobial activity against some organisms with aminoglycosides
• Increased serum concentrations with probenecid
• Decreased effectiveness with tetracyclines, erythromycins, chloramphenicol
• Decreased effectiveness of oral contraceptives
• Increased serum concentrations of methotrexate
• Prolonged half-life with use of salicylates, NSAIDs
Lab
• False positive urine protein except with those tests using bromophenol blue—Albustix, Albutest, Multistix
• False positive Coombs' test
Nutrition
• Decreased absorption if given with meals, acidic fruit juices, citrus fruits, acidic beverages (such as colas)

SIDE EFFECTS

CNS: Neuropathy, seizures at high dosages
GI: Diarrhea, epigastric distress, vomiting, nausea, pseudomembranous colitis
GU: Acute interstitial nephritis
HEME: Hemolytic anemia, leukopenia, eosinophilia, thrombocytopenia
Local: Sterile abscess with injection
Other: Hypersensitivity (rash, urticaria, maculopapular eruptions, exfoliative dermatitis, chills, fever, edema, anaphylaxis), arthralgia, bacterial or fungal superinfections, serum sickness (erythema multiforme, rashes, urticaria, polyarthritis, fever)

TOXICITY AND OVERDOSE

Clinical signs: Neuromuscular irritability, seizures
Treatment: If ingested within 4 hr, empty stomach by induced emesis or gastric lavage, followed by activated charcoal; supportive care, hemodialysis

PATIENT CARE MANAGEMENT
Assessment
• Assess history of hypersensitivity to penicillins or cephalosporins
• Obtain C&S; may begin therapy before obtaining results
• Assess renal function (BUN, creatinine, I&O), hepatic function

(ALT, AST, bilirubin), hematologic function (CBC, differential, platelet count), particularly for long-term therapy, bowel pattern

Interventions

• Administer penicillins at least 1 hr before bacteriostatic antibiotics (tetracyclines, erythromycins, chloramphenicol)

• Administer PO 1 hr ac or 2 hr after meals; administer with water; avoid acidic beverages; tabs may be crushed, mixed with food or fluid

• Shake IM well before withdrawing

• Administer deeply into large muscle mass; aspirate to avoid intravascular injection; do not inject more than 2 g per injection site; rotate injection sites

• Injection is painful; if child complains of or shows symptoms of severe pain, use alternate site

• Maintain age-appropriate fluid intake

NURSING ALERT

Discontinue drug if signs of immediate hypersensitivity or pseudomembranous colitis develop

Do not administer IV; do not inject into peripheral nerves or blood vessels

Provide emergency equipment and medications for possible immediate hypersensitivity reaction

---

Evaluation

• Evaluate therapeutic response (decreased symptoms of infection)

• Monitor signs of superinfection (perineal itching, diaper rash, fever, malaise, redness, pain, swelling, drainage, rash, diarrhea, sore throat, change in cough or sputum

• Observe for signs of allergic reaction (wheezing, tightness in chest, urticaria); reaction may occur in 30 min to 10 days

• Monitor bowel pattern; diarrhea may be symptomatic of pseudomembranous colitis

• Monitor renal function (BUN, creatinine, I&O), hepatic function (ALT, AST, bilirubin), hematologic function (CBC, differential, platelet count)

• Monitor for signs of bleeding (ecchymosis, bleeding gums, hematuria, daily stool guaiac), especially with long-term therapy

• Evaluate IM site for tissue damage

PATIENT AND FAMILY EDUCATION

Teach/instruct

• To take as directed at prescribed intervals for prescribed length of time

Warn/advise

• To notify care provider of hypersensitivity, side effects, superinfection

STORAGE

• Store tabs at room temp in airtight container

• Store IM preparations in refrigerator

---

penicillin G potassium, penicillin G sodium

Brand Name(s): Acrocillin, Burcillin-G, Crystapen✤, Deltapen, Pentids, Pfizerpen

Classification: Antibiotic (natural penicillin)

Pregnancy Category: B

AVAILABLE PREPARATIONS

Oral susp: 200,000 U/5 ml, 400,000 U/5ml

Tabs: 200,000 U, 250,000 U, 400,000 U, 500,000 U, 800,000 U

Inj: 0.2 million U, 0.5 million U, 1 million U, 5 million U, 10 million U, 20 million U

ROUTES AND DOSAGES

Neonates <4 wk, <1200 g: IM/IV 50,000-100,000 U/kg/24 hr divided q12h

Neonates <7 days, <2000 g: IM/IV 50,000-100,000 U/kg/24 hr divided q12h

---

✤ Available in Canada.

Neonates ≥7 days, <2000 g: IM/IV 75,000-225,000 U/kg/24 hr divided q8h

Neonates <7 days, >2000 g: IM/IV 75,000-150,000 U/kg/24 hr divided q8h

Neonates ≥7 days, >2000 g: IM/IV 100,000-200,000 U/kg/24 hr divided q6h

Infants ≥1 mo and children <12 yr: PO 25,000-90,000 U/kg/24 hr divided q6-8h; IM/IV 25,000-400,000 U/kg/24 hr divided q4-6h (maximum 24 million U/24 hr)

Children ≥12 yr and adults: PO 200,000-800,000 U/kg/24 hr; IM/IV 2-24 million U/24 hr divided q4-6h

• Use higher dosage recommendation for treatment of meningitis

Congenital Syphilis

Neonates <7 days: IM/IV 100,000 U/kg/24 hr divided q12h; treat for 10-14 days

Neonates 7-28 days: IM/IV 150,000 U/kg/24 hr divided q8h; treat for 10-14 days

Infants >28 days: IM/IV 200,000 U/kg/24 hr divided q6h; treat for 10-14 days

IV administration

• Recommended concentration: 50,000-500,000 U/ml in D_5W, NS, or SW

• Maximum concentration: 1 million U/ml in D_5W, NS, or SW

• Intermittent infusion rate: Over 15-30 min

MECHANISM AND INDICATIONS

Antibiotic mechanism: Bactericidal; inhibits bacterial cell wall synthesis by adhering to penicillin-binding proteins

Indications: Effective against nonpenicillinase producing gram-positive and gram-negative organisms including *Staphylococcus aureus*, *Streptococcus pyogenes*, *Str. viridans*, *Str. faecalis*, *Str. bovis*, *Str. pneumoniae*, *Neisseria gonorrhoeae*, *N. meningitidis*, *Bacillus anthracis*, *Clostridium perfringens*, *C. tetani*, *Corynebacterium diphtheriae*, *Listeria monocytogenes*, *Bacteroides*, *Streptobacillus moniliformis*, spirochetes including *Treponema pallidum*, *Actinomyces;* used to treat empyema, gangrene, anthrax, gonorrhea, mastoiditis, septicemia, meningitis, osteomyelitis, pneumonia, tetanus, UTI, pericarditis, endocarditis; as prophylaxis against rheumatic fever

PHARMACOKINETICS

Peak: PO 30 min; IM 15-30 min; IV end of infusion

Distribution: Widely distributed throughout body; CSF with inflamed meninges

Half-life: Infants <6 days, 3.2-3.4 hr; infants 7-14 days, 0.9-2.2 hr; older infants/children, 0.5-0.7 hr

Metabolism: Partially metabolized by liver

Excretion: Urine, bile

CONTRAINDICATIONS AND PRECAUTIONS

• Contraindicated with known hypersensitivity to any other penicillin or to cephalosporins

• Use cautiously with impaired renal function, pregnancy; use during lactation may result in sensitization of infant

INTERACTIONS

Drug

• Synergistic antimicrobial activity against some organisms with aminoglycosides

• Increased serum concentrations with probenecid

• Decreased effectiveness with tetracyclines, erythromycins, chloramphenicol

• Decreased effectiveness of oral contraceptives

• Increased serum concentrations of methotrexate

• Prolonged half-life with salicylates, NSAIDs

• Hypokalemia possible with K^+-sparing diuretics

Lab

• False positive urine protein except with those tests using bromophenol blue—Albustix, Albutest, MultiStix

• False positive Coombs' test

Nutrition

• Decreased absorption if given with meals, acidic fruit juices, cit-

P

rus fruits, acidic beverages (e.g., colas)

INCOMPATIBILITIES
• Acid, alkaline media; aminoglycosides, aminophylline, amphotericin B, ascorbic acid, cephalothin, chlorpromazine, dextran, dopamine, heparin, hydroxyzine, lincomycin, metaraminol, metoclopramide, pentobarbital, phenytoin, prochlorperazine, promazine, promethazine, NaHCO₃, thiopental, trifluoperazine, vancomycin

SIDE EFFECTS
CNS: Neuropathy, seizures at high dosages
CV: CHF with high dosages of penicillin G sodium
GI: Diarrhea, epigastric distress, vomiting, pseudomembranous colitis
GU: Acute interstitial nephritis
HEME: Hemolytic anemia, leukopenia, eosinophilia, thrombocytopenia
METAB: Possible potassium poisoning (hyperreflexia, convulsions, coma)
Local: Pain, induration, sterile abscesses, tissue sloughing at injection site; phlebitis and thrombophlebitis with IV injection
Other: Hypersensitivity (rash, urticaria, maculopapular eruptions, exfoliative dermatitis, chills, fever, edema, anaphylaxis), arthralgia, bacterial or fungal superinfection, serum sickness (erythema multiforme, rashes, urticaria, polyarthritis, fever)

TOXICITY AND OVERDOSE
Clinical signs: Neuromuscular irritability, seizures
Treatment: If ingested within 4 hr, empty stomach by induced emesis or gastric lavage, followed by activated charcoal; supportive care; hemodialysis

PATIENT CARE MANAGEMENT
Assessment
• Assess history of hypersensitivity to penicillins or cephalosporins
• Obtain C&S; may begin therapy before obtaining results
• Assess renal function (BUN, creatinine, I&O), hepatic function (ALT, AST, bilirubin), hematologic function (CBC, differential, platelet count), particularly for long-term therapy; bowel pattern
Interventions
• Administer penicillins at least 1 hr before bacteriostatic antibiotics (tetracyclines, erythromycins, chloramphenicol)
• Administer PO 1 hr ac or 2 hr after meals; administer with water; avoid acidic beverages; shake suspension well before administering; tabs may be crushed, mixed with food or fluid
• When reconstituting IM direct stream of diluent against sides of vial while rotating vial; shake vigorously
• Injection is painful; administer deeply into large muscle mass, rotate injection sites
• Do not premix IV with other medications, particularly strong acidic or basic medications; inactivated by acids, alkalis, oxidizing agents, carbohydrate sols with alkaline pH
• Use large vein with small-bore needle to reduce local reaction; rotate site q48-72h
• Maintain age-appropriate fluid intake
• For group A β-hemolytic streptococcal infection, provide 10-day course of treatment to prevent risk of acute rheumatic fever or glomerulonephritis

NURSING ALERT

Discontinue drug if signs of immediate hypersensitivity, pseudomembranous colitis develop

Too-rapid IV administration or excessive dosage may cause electrolyte imbalance or seizures

Provide emergency equipment and medications for possible immediate hypersensitivity reaction

Evaluation
- Evaluate therapeutic response (decreased symptoms of infection)
- Monitor signs of superinfection (perineal itching, diaper rash, fever, malaise, redness, pain, swelling, drainage, rash, diarrhea, sore throat, change in cough or sputum)
- Observe for signs of allergic reaction (wheezing, tightness in chest, urticaria); reaction may occur in 30 min-10 days
- Monitor bowel patterns; diarrhea may be symptomatic of pseudomembranous colitis
- Monitor renal function (BUN, creatinine, I&O), hepatic function (ALT, AST, bilirubin), hematologic function (CBC, differential, platelet count); monitor electrolytes (K^+, Na), particularly if more than 10 million U administered IV
- Monitor for signs of bleeding (ecchymosis, bleeding gums, hematuria, daily stool guaiac), especially with long-term therapy
- Evaluate IM site for tissue damage, IV site for vein irritation and extravasation

PATIENT AND FAMILY EDUCATION
Teach/instruct
- To take as directed at prescribed intervals for prescribed length of time
Warn/advise
- To notify care provider of hypersensitivity, side effects, superinfection

STORAGE
- Store powder, tabs at room temp in airtight containers
- Reconstituted susp stable refrigerated 14 days, room temp 7 days; label date and time of reconstitution
- Parenteral sol stable refrigerated 7 days, room temp 24 hr

penicillin G procaine

Brand Name(s): Ayercillin♣, Crysticillin AS, Duracillin AS, Pfizerpen AS, Wycillin

Classification: Antibiotic (natural penicillin)

Pregnancy Category: B

AVAILABLE PREPARATION
Inj: 300,000 U/ml, 500,000 U/ml, 600,000 U/ml

ROUTES AND DOSAGES
Neonates: Avoid use in neonates because of greater risk of sterile abscesses and procaine toxicity; IM 50,000 U/kg/24 hr qd
Infants and children: IM 25,000-50,000 U/kg/24 hr qd (maximum 4.8 million U/24 hr)
Adults: IM 600,000-4.8 million U/24 hr qd or divided q12h
Congenital Syphilis
Neonates and children < 12 yr: IM 50,000 U/kg/24 hr qd for 10-14 days
Children ≥12 yr and adults: IM 600,000 U qd for 8 days
Syphilis, >1 yr Duration
Children ≥12 yr and adults: IM 600,000 U qd for 10-15 days
Gonorrhea
Infants and children: PO probenecid 25 mg/kg (maximum 1 g/dose) 30 min before IM procaine penicillin 100,000 U/kg once
Adults: PO probenecid 1 g 30 min before IM procaine penicillin 4.8 million U once

MECHANISM AND INDICATIONS
Antibiotic mechanism: Bactericidal; inhibits bacterial cell wall

P

---

synthesis by adhering to penicillin-binding proteins

Indications: Effective against gram-positive and gram-negative organisms including *Staphylococcus aureus, Streptococcus pyogenes, Str. viridans, Str. faecalis, Str. bovis, Str. pneumoniae, Neisseria gonorrhoeae, N. meningitidis, Bacillus anthracis, Clostridium perfringins, C. tetani, C. diphtheriae, Listeria monocytogenes, Bacteroides, Streptobacillus moniliformis,* spirochetes including *Treponema pallidum, Actinomyces;* used to treat empyema, gangrene, anthrax, gonorrhea, syphilis, mastoiditis, septicemia, meningitis, osteomyelitis, pneumonia, tetanus, UTIs; prophylaxis against rheumatic fever

PHARMACOKINETICS
Peak: 1-4 hr
Distribution: Poor penetration across blood–brain barrier despite inflamed meninges
Half-life: 0.5-1.0 hr
Metabolism: Hydrolyzed to penicillin
Excretion: Urine

CONTRAINDICATIONS AND PRECAUTIONS
• Contraindicated with known hypersensitivity to any other penicillin, cephalosporins, procaine, formaldehyde sulfoxylate (in Crysticillin)
• Use cautiously with neonates (increased risk of sterile abscesses and procaine toxicity); with impaired renal function; pregnancy

INTERACTIONS
Drug
• Synergistic antimicrobial activity against some organisms with aminoglycosides
• Increased serum concentrations with probenecid
• Decreased effectiveness with tetracyclines, erythromycins, chloramphenicol
• Decreased effectiveness of oral contraceptives
• Increased serum concentrations of methotrexate

• Prolonged half-life with use of salicylates, NSAIDs
Lab
• False positive urine protein except with those tests using bromophenol blue—Albustix, Albutest, MultiStix
• False positive Coombs' test

SIDE EFFECTS
CNS: Neuropathy, seizures at high dosage
GI: Diarrhea, epigastric distress, vomiting, nausea, pseudomembranous colitis
GU: Acute interstitial nephritis
HEME: Hemolytic anemia, leukopenia, eosinophilia, thrombocytopenia
Local: Pain, sterile abscess with injection
Other: Hypersensitivity (rash, urticaria, maculopapular eruptions, exfoliative dermatitis, chills, fever, edema, anaphylaxis), arthralgia, bacterial or fungal superinfection, serum sickness (erythema multiforme, rashes, urticaria, polyarthritis, fever)

TOXICITY AND OVERDOSE
Clinical signs: Neuromuscular irritability, seizures
Treatment: Supportive care; hemodialysis

PATIENT CARE MANAGEMENT
Assessment
• Assess history of hypersensitivity to penicillins, cephalosporins, procaine, formaldehyde sulfoxylate (if using Crysticillin)
• Obtain C&S; may begin therapy before obtaining results
• Assess renal function (BUN, creatinine, I&O), hepatic function (ALT, AST, bilirubin), hematologic function (CBC, differential, platelet count) (particularly for long-term therapy), bowel pattern
Interventions
• Administer penicillin at least 1 hr before bacteriostatic antibiotics (tetracyclines, erythromycins, chloramphenicol)
• Shake IM sol well before withdrawing

♣ Available in Canada.

• Administer deeply into large muscle mass; aspirate to avoid intravascular injection; do not inject more than 2 g per injection site; rotate injection sites
• Injection is painful; if child complains of or shows symptoms of severe pain, use alternate site
• Maintain age-appropriate fluid intake

NURSING ALERT

Discontinue drug if signs of immediate hypersensitivity, pseudomembranous colitis develop

Do not administer IV; do not inject into peripheral nerves or blood vessels

Provide emergency equipment and medications for possible immediate hypersensitivity reaction

---

Evaluation
• Evaluate therapeutic response (decreased symptoms of infection)
• Monitor signs of superinfection (perineal itching, diaper rash, fever, malaise, redness, pain, swelling, drainage, rash, diarrhea, sore throat, change in cough or sputum)
• Observe for signs of allergic reaction (wheezing, tightness in chest, urticaria); reaction may occur in 30 min-10 days
• Monitor for transient toxic reaction to procaine (erythema, wheal, flare, eruption), which may occur immediately and subside after 15-30 min
• Monitor bowel pattern; diarrhea may be symptomatic of pseudomembranous colitis
• Monitor renal function (BUN, creatinine, I&O), hepatic function (ALT, AST, bilirubin), hematologic function (CBC, differential, platelet count)
• Monitor for signs of bleeding (ecchymosis, bleeding gums, hematuria, daily stool guaiac), especially with long-term therapy

• Evaluate IM site for tissue damage

PATIENT AND FAMILY EDUCATION
Teach/instruct
• To take as directed at prescribed intervals for prescribed length of time
Warn/advise
• To notify care provider of hypersensitivity, side effects, superinfection

STORAGE
• Store in refrigerator

---

penicillin V, penicillin V potassium

Brand Name(s): Betapen-VK, Bopen V-K, Cocillin V-K, Nadopen-V♣, Lanacillin VK, Ledercillin VK, Penapar VK, Pen-Vee♣, Pen-Vee K, Pfizerpen VK, Robicillin-VK, Uticillin VK, V-Cellin K, Veetids

Classification: Antibiotic (natural penicillin)

Pregnancy Category: B

AVAILABLE PREPARATIONS
Oral susp: 125 mg/5 ml, 250 mg/5 ml
Tabs: 125 mg, 250 mg, 500 mg

ROUTES AND DOSAGES
Children >1 mo-12 yr: PO 15-62.5 mg/kg/24 hr divided q6-8h
Children >12 yr and adults: PO 250-500 mg q6h
Group A β-Hemolytic Streptococci
Children and adults: PO 125-250 mg tid
Rheumatic Fever/Pneumococcal Prophylaxis
Children < 5 yr: PO 125 mg bid
Children ≥5 yr and adults: PO 250 mg bid
Lyme Disease
Children < 9 yr: PO 25-50 mg/

---

kg/24 hr divided q8h for 10-30 days; maximum 1-2 g/24 hr

Endocarditis Prophylaxis for Dental Surgery (see Appendix H)

Children < 27 kg: PO 1 g 1 hr before procedure, then 500 mg 6 hr after procedure

Children ≥27 kg and adults: PO 2 g 30-60 min before procedure, then 1 g 6 hr after procedure

MECHANISM AND INDICATIONS

Antibiotic mechanism: Bactericidal; inhibits bacterial cell wall synthesis by adhering to penicillin-binding proteins

Indications: Effective against gram-positive and gram-negative organisms including *Staphylococcus aureus, Streptococcus pyogenes, Str. viridans, Str. faecalis, Str bovis, Str. pneumoniae, Neisseria gonorrhoeae, N. meningitidis, Bacillus anthracis, Clostridium perfringens, C. tetani, C. diphtheriae, Listeria monocytogenes, Streptobacillus moniliformis,* spirochetes including *Treponema pallidum, Actinomyces;* used to treat otitis media, upper respiratory infections, Lyme disease; used for prophylaxis in endocarditis, pneumococcal infections, rheumatic fever

PHARMACOKINETICS

Peak: 0.5-1.0 hr
Half-life: 1 hr
Metabolism: Liver
Excretion: Urine

CONTRAINDICATIONS AND PRECAUTIONS

• Contraindicated with known hypersensitivity to penicillins or cephalosporins; in neonates
• Use cautiously with impaired renal function, pregnancy

INTERACTIONS

Drug
• Synergistic antimicrobial activity against some organisms with aminoglycosides
• Increased serum concentrations with probenecid
• Decreased effectiveness with tetracyclines, erythromycins, chloramphenicol
• Decreased effectiveness of oral contraceptives
• Prolonged half-life with salicylates and NSAIDs
• Hypokalemia possible with K⁺-sparing diuretics

Lab
• False positive urine protein except with those tests using bromophenol blue—Albustix, Albutest, Multistix
• False positive Coombs' test

Nutrition
• Decreased absorption if administered with meals, acidic fruit juices, citrus fruit, acidic beverages (such as colas)

SIDE EFFECTS

CNS: Neuropathy; seizures at high dosages

GI: Diarrhea, epigastric distress, vomiting, nausea, pseudomembranous colitis

HEME: Hemolytic anemia, leukopenia, eosinophilia, thrombocytopenia

Other: Hypersensitivity (rash, urticaria, maculopapular eruptions, exfoliative dermatitis, chills, fever, edema, anaphylaxis); arthralgia, bacterial or fungal superinfection

TOXICITY AND OVERDOSE

Clinical signs: Neuromuscular hypersensitivity, seizures

Treatment: If ingested within 4 hr, empty stomach by induced emesis or gastric lavage, followed by activated charcoal; supportive care

PATIENT CARE MANAGEMENT

Assessment
• Assess history hypersensitivity to penicillin or cephalosporins
• Obtain C&S; may begin therapy before obtaining results
• Assess renal function (BUN, creatinine, I&O), hepatic function (ALT, AST, bilirubin), hematologic function (CBC, differential, platelet count), particularly for long-term therapy; bowel pattern

Interventions
• Administer penicillins at least 1

✦ Available in Canada.

hr before bacteriostatic antibiotics (tetracyclines, erythromycins, chloramphenicol)
• Administer PO 1 hr ac or 2 hr after meals; administer with water; avoid acidic beverages; shake susp well before administering; tabs may be crushed, mixed with food or fluid
• Maintain age-appropriate fluid intake
• For group A β-hemolytic streptococcal infection, provide 10-day course of treatment to prevent risk of acute rheumatic fever or glomerulonephritis

> **NURSING ALERT**
> Discontinue drug if signs of immediate hypersensitivity, pseudomembranous colitis develop
> Provide emergency equipment and medications for possible immediate hypersensitivity reaction

Evaluation
• Evaluate therapeutic response (decreased symptoms of infection)
• Monitor signs of superinfection (perineal itching, diaper rash, fever, malaise, redness, pain, swelling, drainage, rash, diarrhea, sore throat, change in cough or sputum)
• Observe for signs of allergic reaction (wheezing, tightness in chest, urticaria); reaction may occur in 30 min-10 days
• Monitor bowel pattern; diarrhea may be symptomatic of pseudomembranous colitis
• Monitor renal function (BUN, creatinine, I&O), hepatic function (ALT, AST, bilirubin), hematologic function (CBC, differential, platelet count)
• Monitor for signs of bleeding (ecchymosis, bleeding gums, hematuria, daily stool guaiac

PATIENT AND FAMILY EDUCATION
Teach/instruct
• To take as directed at prescribed

intervals for prescribed length of time
Warn/advise
• To notify care provider of hypersensitivity, side effects, superinfection

STORAGE
• Store powder, tabs at room temp
• Reconstituted susp stable refrigerated 14 days; label date and time of reconstitution

---

pentamidine isethionate

Brand Name(s): NebuPent, Pentacarinat✤, Pentam-300

Classification: Antibiotic, antiprotozoal

Pregnancy Category: C

AVAILABLE PREPARATIONS
Inj: 300 mg
Inhal: 300 mg

ROUTES AND DOSAGES
Prevention of *Pneumocystis carinii* Pneumonia
Children < 5 yr: IM/IV (IV preferred) 4 mg/kg q mo or biweekly; inhal 8 mg/kg/dose or 150 mg/dose q 3 wk or q mo using Respigard II Inhaler
Children ≥5 yr: IM/IV (IV preferred) 4 mg/kg q mo or biweekly; inhal 300 mg/dose in 6 ml water q 3 wk or q mo using Respigard II Inhaler
Adult: Inhal 300 mg q 4 wk using Respigard II Inhaler
Treatment of *Pneumocystis carinii* Pneumonia
Children: IM/IV (IV preferred) 4 mg/kg/24 hr qd for 10-14 days
Adults: IM/IV (IV preferred) 4 mg/kg/24 hr qd for 14 days
Trypanosomiasis
Children: 4 mg/kg/24 hr qd for 10 days
IV administration
• Recommended concentration: 1-2.5 mg/ml in D_5W or NS

- Maximum concentration: 6 mg/ml
- IV push rate: Not recommended
- Intermittent infusion rate: Over ≥60 min

MECHANISM AND INDICATIONS

Mechanism: Blocks parasite reproduction by interfering with RNA/DNA, phospholipid, and protein synthesis

Indications: Used to prevent *Pneumocystis carinii* pneumonia; to treat trypanosomiasis, visceral leishmaniasis

PHARMACOKINETICS

Peak: IM 30-60 min
Distribution: Binds extensively with body tissues
Half-life: Terminal 6.4-9.4 hr
Excretion: Urine (33%-66%)

CONTRAINDICATIONS AND PRECAUTIONS

- Contraindicated with known hypersensitivity to pentamidine isethionate, any component
- Use cautiously with DM, renal or hepatic dysfunction, hypertension, hypotension, pregnancy

INTERACTIONS

Drug
- Increased nephrotoxicity with aminoglycosides, amphotericin B, capreomycin, colistin, cisplatin, methoxyflurane, polymyxin B, vancomycin

INCOMPATIBILITIES

- Do not use with other drugs in syringe or sol

SIDE EFFECTS

CNS: Vertigo, fever, fatigue, confusion
CV: Hypotension, arrhythmia, tachycardia
DERM: Rash, itching, Stevens-Johnson Syndrome
ENDO/METAB: Hypoglycemia, hyperglycemia, hypocalcemia, hyperkalemia
GI: Nausea, vomiting, diarrhea, anorexia, metallic taste, pancreatitis, elevated liver enzymes
GU: Renal toxicity or failure, elevated BUN, creatinine
HEME: Leukopenia, thrombocytopenia, neutropenia, anemia
Local: Pain at injection site, abscess, thrombophlebitis
Other: Fever, anaphylaxis; with aerosolized solution, irritation of airway, cough, bronchospasm, conjunctivitis

TOXICITY AND OVERDOSE

Clinical signs: Hypoglycemia, hyperglycemia, renal toxicity
Treatment: Supportive care

PATIENT CARE MANAGEMENT

Assessment
- Assess history of hypersensitivity to pentamidine isethionate
- Assess baseline hematologic function (CBC, differential, platelet count), renal function (BUN, creatinine, I&O), hepatic function (ALT, AST, bilirubin), VS, ECG, electrolytes (BG, K^+, Ca)

Interventions
- IM injection is painful; administer deep into large muscle; IV route preferred
- Provide emergency equipment for resuscitation with IV administration
- Administer IV with patient lying down because of severe hypotension
- Do not use low-pressure aerosol (< 20 psi); flow rate should be 5-7 L/min (40-50 psi) air or O_2 source over 30-45 min until chamber is empty
- Health care personnel who administer aerosolized therapy, a cough-producing procedure, should be aware of the possibility of secondary exposure to tuberculosis from pts with undiagnosed pulmonary disease
- Maintain age-appropriate hydration
- Monitor B/P continuously during administration to monitor for hypotension; ECG

♣ Available in Canada.

NURSING ALERT

Health care personnel who administer aerosolized therapy (a cough-producing procedure) should be aware of possibility of secondary exposure to TB from pts with undiagnosed pulmonary disease

Pt should receive parenteral pentamidine while lying down because of severe hypotension; monitor B/P continuously during infusion

Evaluation
- Evaluate therapeutic response (decreased fever, improved respiratory effort)
- Monitor VS (B/P q2-4h after infusion until stable), ECG
- Monitor hematologic function (CBC, differential, platelet count), renal function (BUN, creatinine, I&O), hepatic function (ALT, AST, bilirubin), electrolytes status (glucose, K$^+$, Ca)
- Monitor respiratory status (rate, effort, wheezing, dyspnea)
- Monitor CNS status (dizziness, confusion, hallucinations)
- Evaluate IV site for vein irritation, induration, abscess

PATIENT AND FAMILY EDUCATION
Teach/instruct
- To take as directed at prescribed intervals for prescribed length of time

Warn/advise
- To notify care provider of hypersensitivity, side effects, superinfection

STORAGE
- Store powder in refrigerator, away from light
- Reconstituted sol stable 48 hr at room temp; discard unused portions

pentobarbital sodium

Brand Name(s): Nembutal, Nembutal Sodium✤, Nembutal Sodium Solution, Nova-Rectal✤, Pentobarbital Sodium, Pentogen

Classification: Sedative, hypnotic, barbiturate

Controlled Substance Schedule II (supp Schedule III)

Pregnancy Category: D

AVAILABLE PREPARATIONS
Elixir: 18.2 mg/5 ml
Caps: 50 mg, 100 mg
Inj: 50 mg/ml for parenteral use
Supp: 30 mg, 60 mg, 120 mg, 200 mg rectal

ROUTES AND DOSAGES
Sedation
Children: PO/PR/IM 2-6 mg/kg/24 hr divided tid; maximum 100 mg/dose
Adults: PO/PR/IM 20-40 mg bid-qid

Insomnia
Children 2 mo-1 yr: PR 30 mg; IM 2-6 mg/kg/dose up to maximum 100 mg/dose
Children 1-4 yr: PR 30-60 mg; IM 2-6 mg/kg/dose up to maximum 100 mg/dose
Children 5-12 yr: PR 60 mg; IM 2-6 mg/kg/dose up to maximum 100 mg/dose
Children 12-14 yr: PR 60-120 mg; IM 2-6 mg/kg/dose up to maximum 100 mg/dose
Adults: PO 100-200 mg hs; PR 120-200 mg; IM 150-200 mg

Preanesthetic Medication
Infants and children ≤5 yr: PR 5 mg/kg
Children >5 yr: IM 5 mg/kg
Adults: PO/IM 150-200 mg in two divided doses

Anticonvulsant
Children: IM/IV initially, 50 mg or 3-8 mg/kg; additional doses may be administered after 1 min
Children >5 yr: IM 5 mg/kg
Adults: IV 100 mg; additional

P

doses may be administered after 5 min; maximum dose 500 mg

Elevated Intracranial Pressure, Therapeutic Coma

Children and adults: IV loading dose 5-15 mg/kg infused over 60-120 min; then maintenance with 1.5-3.5 mg/kg/hr; adjust dosage with renal or hepatic dysfunction

IV administration

• Recommended concentration: 50 mg/ml for slow IV push, or dilute in SW, LR, NS for continuous infusion

• Maximum concentration: 50 mg/ml for slow IV push

• IV push rate: Over 10-30 min not to exceed 50 mg/min

• Intermittent infusion: Over 10-30 min not to exceed 50 mg/min

MECHANISM AND INDICATIONS

Mechanism: As a sedative/hypnotic, drug acts throughout the CNS as a non-selective depressant and decreases both presynaptic and postsynaptic membrane excitability by facilitating the action of γ-aminobutyric acid (GABA); as an anticonvulsant, drug suppresses the spread of seizure discharges by enhancing the effect of GABA

Indications: Used to treat insomnia (short-term use), status epilepticus, and severe seizures, and is used to induce coma with increased intracranial pressure, Reye syndrome, and post-drowning

PHARMACOKINETICS

Onset of action: PO/PR 15-60 min; IM 10-25 min; IV immediate
Peak: PO/PR 30-60 min
Duration: PO/PR 1-4 hr
Half-life: 35-50 hr
Metabolism: Liver
Excretion: Urine

CONTRAINDICATIONS AND PRECAUTIONS

• Contraindicated with known hypersensitivity to barbiturates, bronchopneumonia, status asthamaticus, severe respiratory distress, porphyria, depressed or suicidal pts; pts with tartrazine hypersensitivity should not use 100 mg Nembutal Sodium caps (contain Yellow Dye #5); avoid prolonged use of high dosages because of potential for physical or psychological dependence

• Use with caution with acute or chronic pain, pregnancy, cardiovascular disease, hypertension, hypotension, renal or hepatic dysfunction

INTERACTIONS

Drug

• Increased CNS and respiratory depressant effects of other sedative-hypnotics, antihistamines, narcotics, antidepressants, tranquilizers, alcohol

• Enhanced metabolism of anticoagulants; may need to increase anticoagulant dosage

• Enhanced hepatic metabolism of digitoxin (not digoxin), corticosteroids, oral contraceptives, other estrogens, theophylline, other xanthines, doxycycline

• Decreased absorption of griseofulvin from the GI tract, impaired effectiveness

• Decreased metabolism of pentobarbitol, possible increased toxicity with valproic acid, phenytoin, disulfiram, MAOIs

• Increased hepatic metabolism (decreased levels) of pentobarbital with rifampin

Lab

• False positive phentolamine test

• Impaired absorption of cyanocobalamin

• Decreased serum bilirubin concentrations in neonates, pts with epilepsy, congenital nonhemolytic unconjugated hyperbilirubinemia

• EEG patterns may show a low-voltage, fast activity; this change may persist for some time after discontinuation of therapy

INCOMPATIBILITIES

• All other medications in sol or syringe

SIDE EFFECTS

CNS: Drowsiness, lethargy, dizziness, CNS depression, increased dreams or nightmares, rebound

---

✤ Available in Canada.

insomnia, potential for seizures after acute withdrawal or decreased dosage; mental confusion; paradoxical excitement, confusion, agitation
CV: Hypotension (after rapid IV administration), bradycardia, circulatory collapse
DERM: Rash, urticaria, exfoliative dermatitis, Stevens-Johnson syndrome
GI: Nausea, vomiting, diarrhea, constipation
Local: Thrombophlebitis, pain, tissue necrosis with extravasation
RESP: Laryngospasm, bronchospasm, respiratory depression
Other: Angioedema, vitamin K deficiency and bleeding in newborns of mothers treated during pregnancy; hyperalgesia in low dosages or in pts with chronic pain

TOXICITY AND OVERDOSE
Clinical signs: Unsteady gait, slurred speech, sustained nystagmus, somnolence, confusion, respiratory depression, pulmonary edema, areflexia, coma; shock syndrome with tachycardia and hypotension may occur; jaundice, hypothermia followed by fever and oliguria; profound coma may be produced by concentrations >10 mcg/ml; concentrations >30 mcg/ml may be fatal
Treatment: Supportive and symptomatic; monitor VS, I&O, labs; maintain body temp, support ventilation and pulmonary function prn; use vasopressors and IV fluids to support cardiac function and circulation; if ingested recently and pt is conscious with intact gag reflex, induce emesis with ipecac; or perform gastric lavage with cuffed ET tube to prevent aspiration; follow with activated charcoal or saline cathartic; may be helpful to alkalinize urine to remove drug from the body; hemodialysis may be necessary in overdose

PATIENT CARE MANAGEMENT
Assessment
• Assess history of hypersensitivity to barbiturates, tartrazine
• Rule out preexisting respiratory disease, porphyria
• Assess for cautious use with pregnancy, depression, acute or chronic pain, cardiovascular disease, hypotension, hypertension, renal or hepatic dysfunction
• Assess current health status and medications to avoid potential interactions
• Obtain baseline hematologic function (CBC, differential, platelets), liver function (ALT, AST, bilirubin, alk phos)
Interventions
• Administer PO ½-1 hr before hs for sleeplessness on empty stomach; tab may be crushed, mixed with food or fluid
• Monitor VS q 30 min after parenteral administration
• Monitor for signs and symptoms of respiratory dysfunction (respiratory depression, character, rate, rhythm); if respirations are <10 min or if pupils are dilated, do not administer
• IM injections are administered deep in large muscle mass to prevent tissue sloughing or abscess; no more than 5 ml/site
• Administer injection within 30 min of mixing with SW
• Do not mix with other medications for injection; do not administer if sol contains precipitate
• Ensure that equipment is available for potential emergency when administering IV
• Provide emergency equipment in the event of respiratory depression (particularly when administered IV)

P

NURSING ALERT
Rapid administration of loading dose may cause hypotension because of peripheral vasodilatation; if hypotension occurs, decrease rate of infusion or treat with IV fluids and vasopressors

Administer IV only with resuscitative equipment available

IV should be administered only by qualified person (nurse anesthetist, anesthesiologist)

Administer alone; do not mix with other drugs; do not use if sol contains precipitate

Respiratory depression, apnea, laryngospasm, and hypotension may result from rapid administration

IM dose should be administered deep in large muscle mass to prevent tissue sloughing and abscesses; tissue necrosis may result from extravasation

Monitor for signs and symptoms of respiratory dysfunction (respiratory depression, character, rate, rhythm); if respirations are <10/min or if pupils are dilated, *do not administer*

Evaluation
• Evaluate therapeutic response (ability to sleep at night, decrease in early morning awakening if taking for insomnia); if taking for seizures monitor seizure frequency, intensity, duration
• Monitor mental status (mood, sensorium, affect, memory)
• Monitor blood studies if on long-term therapy, (Hct, Hgb, RBCs, serum folate, vitamin D)
• Monitor liver function with AST, ALT, bilirubin; if elevated, drug is usually discontinued
• Monitor PT/INR in pts taking anticoagulants
• Monitor for signs and symptoms of barbiturate toxicity (hypotension, pupillary constriction; cold, clammy skin; cyanosis of lips; insomnia; nausea, vomiting, hallucinations, delirium, weakness, coma); mild symptoms may occur in 8-12 hr without the drug
• Monitor for signs and symptoms of blood dyscrasias (fever, sore throat, bruising, rash, jaundice, epistaxis)
• Evaluate for signs and symptoms of physical dependency

PATIENT AND FAMILY EDUCATION
Teach/instruct
• To take as directed at prescribed intervals and for prescribed length of time
• That oral dose may be administered whole or crushed; usually administered on empty stomach ½-1 hr before hs for sleeplessness
Warn/advise
• That it may take 1-2 nights before benefit of treatment for insomnia is noticed
• That morning "hangover" is common effect
• About potential side effects, to report these to primary health care provider
• That drug is not indicated for long-term use
• About risks of physical and psychological dependency
• About depressive effects; to avoid activities that require alertness when taking drug
• Avoid other CNS depressants, alcohol, and be sure that all prescribers are aware that pt is taking this drug

STORAGE
• Store oral and injectable preparations at room temp
• Store rectal supp in refrigerator

permethrin

Brand Name(s): Elimite, Nix, Nix Cream Rinse✦, Nix Dermal Cream✦

Classification: Pediculicide

Pregnancy Category: B

AVAILABLE PREPARATIONS
Top: Cream 5%, cream rinse 1%

ROUTES AND DOSAGES
Head Lice
Children >2 mo and adults: Top, after hair has been washed with shampoo, rinsed with water, and towel dried, apply a sufficient volume to saturate hair and scalp; shake well before using, avoid contact with eyes; leave on for 10 min, rinse with water, remove remaining nits with fine-tooth comb; may repeat in 1 wk if nits or lice are present

Scabies
Children >2 mo and adults: Top, apply cream from head to toe, massage in well; leave on 8-14 hr before washing off with water; for infants also apply on hairline, neck, scalp, forehead; may reapply in 1 wk if live mites reappear

MECHANISM AND INDICATIONS
Mechanism: Disrupts Na ion influx through nerve cell membrane channels in parasites; this results in delayed repolarization, paralysis, death of the lice
Indications: Used to treat *Pediculus humanus capitis* (head lice) and its nits, *Sarcoptes scabiei* (scabies)

PHARMACOKINETICS
Metabolism: Liver
Excretion: Urine

CONTRAINDICATIONS AND PRECAUTIONS
• Contraindicated with known hypersensitivity to pyrethyroid, pyrethrin, or chrysanthemums; acute inflammation of scalp
• Use cautiously with lactation, pregnancy, head rash; for external use only

SIDE EFFECTS
DERM: Pruritus, erythema, rash, burning, stinging, tingling, numbness, edema

TOXICITY AND OVERDOSE
Clinical signs: Local irritation
Treatment: Wash thoroughly with soap and water, discontinue treatment, and notify care provider

PATIENT CARE MANAGEMENT
Assessment
• Assess history of hypersensitivity to permethrin
• Carefully inspect and note extent and amount of infestation
Interventions
• Take proper isolation precautions if the child is hospitalized during infestation
• Administer top corticosteroids, antihistamines, top antibiotics as ordered

> **NURSING ALERT**
> Formulation contains formaldehyde, which is a contact allergen

Evaluation
• Evaluate therapeutic response (decreased crusts, nits, itching, papules in skin folds)
• Evaluate for side effects (skin irritation)
• Evaluate all family members for infestation; treat if positive

PATIENT AND FAMILY EDUCATION
Teach/instruct
• Take as directed at prescribed intervals for prescribed length of time
• That family must understand this is a contagious condition, why it is necessary to treat
Warn/advise
• That all personal clothing and bedding must be washed in hot water or dry cleaned, all personal articles (e.g., hair care items) need to be cleaned in a sol of drug
• That a fine-tooth nit comb should be used to remove dead lice and nits from hair

P

✦ Available in Canada.

• That pubic lice may be transmitted sexually; all sexual partners must be treated simultaneously
• To flush with water immediately if drug comes in contact with eyes
• To notify care provider of hypersensitivity, side effects
• To notify schools and day care facilities
• To consult care provider with infestation of eyebrows or lashes
• That itching may continue for 4-6 wk
• To reapply drug if accidentally washed off

Encourage
• Children should be instructed not to borrow clothes, brushes, combs

STORAGE
• Store at room temp
• Do not re-use empty container

---

phenazopyridine

Brand Name(s): Azo-Standard, Baridium, Eridium, Geridium, Pyrazodine, Pyridiate, Pyridin, Pyridium, Urodine, Urogesic, Viridium

Classification: Non-narcotic analgesic; urinary anesthetic

Pregnancy Category: B

AVAILABLE PREPARATIONS
Tabs: 100 mg, 200 mg

ROUTES AND DOSAGES
Children: PO 12 mg/kg/24 hr divided tid (treatment should not exceed 2 days if used with an antibiotic for UTI)
Adults: PO 100-200 mg tid (treatment should not exceed 2 days if used with an antibiotic for UTI)

MECHANISM AND INDICATIONS
Mechanism: Acts locally on urinary tract mucosa to produce analgesic or local anesthetic effects; exact mechanism of action unknown

Indications: Used to treat urinary tract symptoms of pain, itching, burning, urgency, frequency; these symptoms may occur in association with infection or following urologic procedures

PHARMACOKINETICS
Onset: Unknown
Peak: 5-6 hr
Half-life: Unknown
Duration: 6-8 hr
Metabolism: Liver
Distribution: Unknown
Excretion: Urine

CONTRAINDICATIONS AND PRECAUTIONS
• Contraindicated with known sensitivity, glomerulonephritis, pregnancy, lactation, severe hepatitis, uremia renal failure
• Use cautiously with renal insufficiency, hepatitis

INTERACTIONS
Drug
• None significant
Lab
• Interference with bilirubin, urinary glucose tests, urinalysis, PSP excretion, urinary ketones, steroids, proteins (tests based on color reactions)
• False positive urine glucose possible

SIDE EFFECTS
CNS: Headache, vertigo
DERM: Rash, urticaria, skin pigmentation
GI: Nausea, hepatotoxicity, vomiting, GI bleeding, diarrhea, heartburn, anorexia
GU: Renal failure, orange-red urine
HEME: Thrombocytopenia, agranulocytosis, leukopenia, neutropenia, hemolytic anemia, methemoglobinemia

TOXICITY AND OVERDOSE
Clinical signs: Methemoglobinemia
Treatment: Supportive care; methylene blue 1-2 mg/kg IV or 100-200 mg vitamin C PO

PATIENT CARE MANAGEMENT

Assessment
• Assess history of hypersensitivity to phenazopyridine, related drugs
• Assess for urgency, frequency, pain on urination
• Assess renal function (BUN, creatinine, I&O), liver function (ALT, AST, bilirubin)

Interventions
• Administer with or following meals to decrease GI irritation
• Tabs may be crushed or taken whole

NURSING ALERT

May require discontinuation if jaundice of skin and sclera develop (this may indicate an accumulation of the drug caused by impaired renal function)

Evaluation
• Evaluate therapeutic response (decrease in pain and burning on urination)
• Evaluate labs, urine, stools, skin coloring
• Evaluate for side effects, hypersensitivity

PATIENT AND FAMILY EDUCATION

Teach/instruct
• To take as directed at prescribed intervals for prescribed length of time
• That drug causes reddish-orange discoloration of urine that may stain clothing or bedding; sanitary napkins may be worn to avoid stains
• To discontinue after pain is relieved, but to continue to take concurrent prescribed antibiotic until finished

Warn/advise
• To notify care provider of hypersensitivity, side effects

STORAGE
• Store at room temp

---

phenobarbital, phenobarbital sodium

Brand Name(s): Barbita, Luminal, Solfoton

Classification: Anticonvulsant, sedative/hypnotic, barbiturate

Controlled Substance Schedule IV

Pregnancy Category: D

AVAILABLE PREPARATIONS
Oral sol: 15 mg/5 ml, 20 mg/5 ml
Elixir: 20 mg/5 m
Caps: 16 mg
Tabs: 8 mg, 15 mg, 16 mg, 30 mg, 32 mg, 60 mg, 65 mg, 100 mg
Inj: 30 mg/ml, 60 mg/ml, 65 mg/ml, 130 mg/ml
Powder for inj: 120 mg/ampule
Caps: 100 mg phenytoin, with 16 mg, 32 mg phenobarbital

ROUTES AND DOSAGES

Anticonvulsant
Neonates: IV loading dose 15-20 mg/kg in a single or divided dose; maintenance PO/IV 4-5 mg/kg/24 hr divided qd-bid, assess serum concentration, increase to 5 mg/kg/24 hr if needed
Infants and children: IV loading dose 10-20 mg/kg in a single or divided dose; in some pts may give additional 5 mg/kg/dose q 15-30 min until seizure is controlled or a total dose of 40 mg/kg is given; maintenance PO/IV, infants <1 yr, 5-8 mg/kg/24 hr divided qd-bid; children 1-5 yr, 6-8 mg/kg/24 hr divided qd-bid, children 5-12 yr, 4-6 mg/kg/24 hr divided qd-bid
Children >12 yr and adults: IV loading dose 300-800 mg initial, followed by 120-240 mg/dose at 20 min intervals until seizure is controlled or a total dose of 1-2 g; maintenance PO/IV 1-3 mg/kg/24 hr in divided doses of 50-100 mg bid-tid

Sedation
Children: PO 2 mg/kg/dose tid
Adults: PO/IM 30-120 mg/24 hr divided bid-tid

P

Insomnia
Children: PO 3-6 mg/kg/dose hs
Adults: PO/IM 100-320 mg hs
Preoperative Sedation
Children: IM/IV 1-3 mg/kg/dose
60-90 min before surgery
Adults: IM/IV 100-200 mg 60-90
min before surgery
Hyperbilirubinemia
Neonates: PO/IM 5-10 mg/kg/24 hr
or up to 10 mg/kg/24 hr for the first
few days after birth divided bid-tid
Chronic Cholestasis
Children <12 yr: PO 2-12 mg/kg/24
hr divided bid-tid
Adults: PO 90-180 mg/24 hr di-
vided bid-tid
IV administration
• Recommended concentration:
30, 60, 65, or 130 mg/ml undiluted
or dilute in equal volume of D-LR,
D-R, D-S, D_5W, $D_{10}W$, LR, NS,
½NS, or R
• Maximum concentration: 130
mg/ml
• IV push rate: Over 3-5 min; in
infants/children do not exceed 2
mg/kg/min or 30 mg/min, adults 60
mg/min
• Intermittent infustion: <2 mg/
kg/min

**MECHANISM
AND INDICATIONS**
Mechanism: Suppresses spread of
seizure discharges by enhancing
the effect of γ-aminobutyric acid
(GABA); both the presynaptic
and postsynaptic discharges are
decreased, raising the seizure
threshold
Indications: Used to treat generalized tonic-clonic, partial, neonatal,
and febrile seizures; used to prevent and treat neonatal hyperbilirubinemia and to lower bilirubin
in chronic cholestasis; also used
for sedation

PHARMACOKINETICS
Onset of action: PO 1 hr, IV 5 min
Peak: PO 1-6 hr; IV 30 min
Distribution: Widely throughout
the body
Half-life: 5-7 days; neonates 45-
500 hr; infants 20-133 hr; children
37-73 hr; adults 53-140 hr; because of long half-life, 3-4 wk of

therapy needed to reach a true
steady state
Duration: PO 6-10 hr; IV 4-10 hr
Metabolism: Liver
Excretion: Urine
Therapeutic levels: 10-20 mcg/ml

**CONTRAINDICATIONS
AND PRECAUTIONS**
• Contraindicated with known
hypersensitivity to barbiturates,
sulfites (in some preparations);
bronchopneumonia, status asthmaticus, severe respiratory distress; severe pain, depressed or
suicidal pts, porphyria; in treating
seizures when LOC is important
(head trauma); lactation
• Use with caution with pregnancy, hypovolemic shock, CHF,
respiratory dysfunction or depression, hepatic or renal impairment,
history of barbiturate addiction,
chronic or acute pain, elderly pts
• Some preparations may contain
benzyl alcohol as a preservative;
administration of benzyl alcohol in
doses 99-234 mg/kg has been associated with a fatal gasping syndrome in neonates; clinical signs
include metabolic acidosis, hypotension, CNS depression, cardiovascular collapse

INTERACTIONS
Drug
• Decreased serum concentration
or decreased effectiveness of ethosuximide, warfarin, oral contraceptives, chloramphenicol, griseofulvin, doxycycline, β blockers,
theophylline, corticosteroids, tricyclic antidepressants, cyclosporine, quinidine, haloperidol, phenothiazines
• Inhibited metabolism, increased
serum levels of phenobarbital with
valproic acid, methyphenidate,
chloramphenicol, propoxyphene
• Increased CNS and respiratory
depression, especially when giving
loading dose of phenobarbital,
with benzodiazepines or other
CNS depressants
Lab
• Increased serum phosphatase
levels possible

Nutrition
• Decreased vitamin D and folate levels possible

INCOMPATIBILITIES
• Atropine, benzquinamide, brompheniramine, butorphanol, cefazolin, cephalothin, chlordiazepoxide, chlorpheniramine, chlorpromazine, cimetidine, clindamycin, codeine, dimenhydrinate, droperidol, erythromycin, glycopyrrolate, hydrocortisone, insulin, kanamycin, levarterenol, levorphanol, meperidine, methadone, midazolam, morphine, nalbuphine, opium, penicillins, pentazocine, phenytoin, prochlorperazine, promazine, promethazine, ranitidine, streptomycin, succinylcholine, tetracycline, triflupromazine, vancomycin, NaHCO$_3$, fructose sol

SIDE EFFECTS
CNS: Drowsiness, lethargy, dizziness, CNS depression, paradoxical excitement, confusion, agitation, hyperexcitability (especially in children), increased dreams or nightmares, rebound insomnia, potential for seizures after acute withdrawal or decreased dosage
CV: Hypotension (after rapid IV administration), bradycardia, circulatory collapse
DERM: Rash, urticaria, exfoliative dermatitis, Stevens-Johnson syndrome
EENT: Miosis
GI: Epigastric pain, nausea, vomiting, diarrhea, constipation
Local: Thrombophlebitis, pain, possible tissue necrosis at extravasation site
RESP: Laryngospasm, bronchospasm, respiratory depression
Other: Angioedema, vitamin K deficiency, bleeding in newborns of mothers treated during pregnancy; hyperalgesia in low dosages or with chronic pain

TOXICITY AND OVERDOSAGE
Clinical signs: Unsteady gait, slurred speech, sustained nystagmus, somnolence, confusion, respiratory depression, pulmonary edema, areflexia, coma; shock syndrome with tachycardia and hypotension may occur; jaundice, hypothermia followed by fever and oliguria; profound coma may be produced by concentrations >10 mcg/ml; concentrations >30 mcg/ml may be fatal
Treatment: Supportive, symptomatic care; monitor VS, I&O, labs; maintain body temp; support ventilation and pulmonary function prn; use vasopressors and IV fluids to support cardiac function and circulation; if ingestion was recent, induce emesis in pt who is conscious and has intact gag reflex with ipecac; if emesis is contraindicated, use gastric lavage, follow with charcoal or saline cathartic; it may be helpful to alkalinize urine to remove drug from the body; hemodialysis may be necessary in overdose

PATIENT CARE MANAGEMENT
Assessment
• Assess history of hypersensitivity to barbiturates, sulfites
• Assess preexisting physical condition and current medications to avoid potential interactions
• Assess baseline hematologic function (CBC, differential), liver function (ALT, AST, bilirubin, alk phos)
• Assess seizure type; determine the appropriate anticonvulsant for this type of seizure
Interventions
• Oral sol may be administered with water or juice to improve taste
• Do not crush or chew ext rel forms, must be swallowed whole
• Use reconstituted parenteral sol within 30 min (phenobarbital hydrolyzes in sol and on exposure to air)
• Do not use injectable sol if it contains precipitate
• Administer IM dose deep into large muscle mass to prevent injury to tissues
• Ensure that emergency resuscitation equipment is available when administering IV

P

- When administering full loading dose over a short period of time for status epilepticus in adults, full ventilatory support will be necessary
- Monitor VS frequently during IV administration
- Use large vein to avoid extravasation
- Initiate at modest dosage
- Increase dosage prn to control seizures, to the point of intolerable side effects
- If only partially effective, another anticonvulsant may be initiated in the same way
- If drug is not effective, gradually withdraw and initiate another anticonvulsant
- If break-through seizures occur when serum levels are at trough or peak, frequency of administration may be increased to provide more-even coverage
- Provide for pt safety with seizure precautions

NURSING ALERT

Some preparations may contain benzyl alcohol as a preservative; administration of benzyl alcohol in doses of 99-234 mg/kg has been associated with a fatal gasping syndrome in neonates; clinical signs include metabolic acidosis, hypotension, CNS depression, cardiovascular collapse

Evaluation

- Evaluate therapeutic response (seizure control); initially done more frequently until seizures are controlled, then q 3-6 mo, with seizure break throughs, or with side effects
- Evaluate LOC before and frequently during therapy to determine effectiveness of drug
- Evaluate neurologic status to assess possible alterations or deterioration
- Monitor seizure character, frequency, duration for changes
- Monitor PT/INR carefully in pts taking anticoagulants

- Evaluate children carefully; premature infants more susceptible to depressant effects of barbiturates because of immature hepatic metabolism; toddlers and older children may experience hyperactivity or excitement
- Monitor anticonvulsant levels periodically

PATIENT AND FAMILY EDUCATION
Teach/instruct

- To take as directed at prescribed intervals; do not alter dosage independently or withdraw drug suddenly
- That oral sol may be administered with water or juice to improve taste
- That ext rel form should not be crushed or chewed
- About process for initiating anticonvulsant drugs and need for frequent visits (especially initially)
- That full therapeutic effects are not seen for 2-3 wks unless a loading dose is used
- About rationale for measuring serum levels, how these should be obtained (peak/trough)

Warn/advise

- About potential side effects; to report serious side effects immediately (rashes, disturbances in mood, alertness, coordination)
- That unpleasant side effects may decrease as pt becomes more used to the drug
- That the drug initially may be more sedating until pt becomes used to it; avoid hazardous tasks (bike, skates, skateboard) that require mental alertness until stabilized
- About potential for physical and psychological dependence with prolonged use
- To avoid use of other CNS depressants (antihistamines, analgesics, alcohol, many OTC cold and flu preparations); may increase sedative effect
- To make other health care providers aware of medications to avoid potential drug interactions

---

✦ Available in Canada.

• To inform care provider if pregnancy occurs while taking the drug

Encourage

• To keep a record of any seizures (seizure calendar)

STORAGE

• Store at room temp
• Discard parenteral sol if a precipitate is visible

---

phentolamine mesylate

Brand Name(s): Regitine

Classification: α-adrenergic blocker, antihypertensive, cutaneous vasodilator

Pregnancy Category: C

AVAILABLE PREPARATIONS
Inj: 5 mg/ml

ROUTES AND DOSAGES
Diagnosis of Pheochromocytoma
Children: IM/IV 0.05-0.1 mg/kg/dose; maximum dose 5 mg
Adult: IM/IV 5 mg
Hypertension
Children: IM/IV 0.05-0.1 mg/kg dose 1-2 hr before pheochromocytomectomy
Adult: IM/IV 5 mg 1-2 hr before pheochromocytomectomy
Treatment of Extravasation
Children and adults: Inject 5-10 mg in 10 ml of NS into affected area
IV administration
• Recommended concentration: 5 mg/ml
• Maximum concentration: 5 mg/ml
• IV push rate: 5 mg/min

MECHANISM AND INDICATIONS
Antihypertensive mechanism: Blocks α-adrenergic receptors, dilating peripheral blood vessels and thereby lowering peripheral resistance, preload and afterload, and decreasing B/P
Cutaneous vasodilator mechanism: Blocks epinephrine- and norepinephrine-induced vasodilation
Indications: Hypertension, pheochromocytoma, treatment of dermal necrosis after norepinephrine, dopamine, or phenylephrine extravasation

PHARMACOKINETICS
Onset of action: Immediately
Peak: IV 2 min; IM 15-20 min
Half-life: 19 min
Metabolism: Liver
Excretion: Urine

CONTRAINDICATIONS AND PRECAUTIONS
• Contraindicated with known hypersensitivity to medication, MI, coronary insufficiency, angina
• Use cautiously with gastritis, peptic ulcer, pts receiving other antihypertensives

INTERACTIONS
Drug
• Increased effects of epinephrine, antihypertensives

INCOMPATIBILITIES
• Iron salts

SIDE EFFECTS
CNS: Dizziness, weakness, lethargy, flushing
CV: Hypotension, tachycardia, shock, arrhythmias, palpitations, angina, hypertension, MI
EENT: Dry mouth, nasal congestion
GI: Nausea, vomiting, diarrhea, abdominal pain, hyperperistalsis, increased secretions
Local: Tissue sloughing, necrosis at IV site
Other: Hypoglycemia

TOXICITY AND OVERDOSE
Clinical signs: Hypotension, dizziness, syncope, tachycardia, vomiting, lethargy, shock
Treatment: Supportive measures as necessary; use norepinephrine to increase B/P; do not use epinephrine

PATIENT CARE MANAGEMENT
Assessment
• Assess history of hypersensitivity to drug

♣ Available in Canada.

- Assess baseline VS, B/P, wt, hydration status
- Assess baseline electrolytes

Interventions
- Test for pheochromocytoma; have pt rest in supine position until B/P stabilized; inject dose rapidly IVP after effects of venipuncture on B/P have passed; record B/P immediately after injection, at 30 sec intervals for first 3 min, and 1 min intervals for 7 min; test is positive if B/P decreases at least 35 mm Hg systolic, 25 mm Hg diastolic
- Monitor closely for extravasation
- For treatment of dermal necrosis, use 25 or 27 G needle, inject medication at edge of extravasation site, wrap loosely with sterile dressing for 2 hr to absorb drainage; do not apply heat

Evaluation
- Evaluate therapeutic response (decreased B/P, diminished dermal necrosis)
- Evaluate for side effects, hypersensitivity
- Monitor VS, B/P
- Evaluate electrolytes

PATIENT AND FAMILY EDUCATION
Teach/instruct
- To take as directed at prescribed intervals for prescribed length of time
- About need for medication
- Not to take sedatives or narcotics for at least 24 hr before phentolamine test

Warn/advise
- To notify care provider of hypersensitivity, side effects
- To avoid hazardous activities until therapy is well established
- To avoid OTC preparations unless directed by care provider

Encourage
- Reassure pt that adverse effects should diminish after several doses

Provide
- Emotional support as indicated

STORAGE
- Store at room temp

---

phenylephrine hydrochloride

Brand Name(s): Dionephrine✽, Mydrine✽, Neo-Synephrine✽, Neo-Synephrine Parenteral✽, Navahistine Decongestant✽; *Nasal products:* Allerest, Neo-synephrine, Sinex; *Ophthalmic:* Ak-Dilate, Ak-Nefrin, Isopto Frin, Mydfrin, Neo-synephrine, Prefin Liquifilm

Classification: Adrenergic, vasoconstrictor

Pregnancy Category: C

AVAILABLE PREPARATIONS
Nasal drops: 0.125%, 0.16%, 0.2%, 0.25%
Nasal spray: 0.25%, 0.5%, 1%
Nasal gel: 0.5%
Ophthal sol: 0.12%, 2.5%, 10%
Inj: 10 mg/ml (1%)

ROUTES AND DOSAGES
Hypotension
Children: IM/SC 0.1 mg/kg/dose q1-2h prn, maximum dose 5 mg; IV 5-20 mcg/kg/dose q 10-15 min prn; infusion 0.1-0.5 mcg/kg/min, titrate to desired effect
Adults: IM/SC 2-5 mg q1-2h prn, maximum dose 5 mg; IV 0.1-0.5 mg/dose q 10-15 min prn; infusion 1-4 mcg/kg/min, titrate to desired effect

Supraventricular Tachycardia
Children: IV 5-10 mcg/kg/dose
Adults: IV 0.25-0.5 mg/dose; may double and repeat dose q 5 min until desired effect is achieved

Nasal Decongestant
Children <6 yr: Nasal sol, 2-3 gtt of 0.125% sol q4h prn
Children 6-12 yr: Nasal sol/spray, 2-3 gtt or 1-2 sprays of 0.25% sol q4h prn

---

✽ Available in Canada.

Children >12 yr and adults: Nasal sol/spray 2-3 gtt or 1-2 sprays of 0.25% or 0.5% sol q4h prn

Pupillary Dilation

Children and adults: Ophthal, 1 gtt 2.5% sol in each eye 15 min before exam

IV administration

• Recommended concentration: 1 mg/ml
• Maximum concentration: 1 mg/ml
• IV push rate: Over 1 min; do not exceed 5 mg
• Intermittent infusion rate: 5-20 mcg/kg q 10-15 min
• Continuous infusion rate: Children 0.1-0.5 mcg/kg/min; adults 1-4 mcg/kg/min

MECHANISM AND INDICATIONS

Vasoconstrictor mechanism: Selective α_1-receptor agonist that causes contraction of blood vessels
Indications: Hypotension, paroxysmal supraventricular tachycardia, shock, nasal congestion, pupillary dilation

PHARMACOKINETICS

Onset of action: IV immediate; IM/SC 15-20 min
Peak: Variable
Half-life: Variable
Metabolism: Liver
Excretion: Unknown

CONTRAINDICATIONS AND PRECAUTIONS

• Contraindicated with known hypersensitivity to medication, severe CAD, ventricular fibrillation, tachyarrhythmias, pheochromocytoma, glaucoma, peripheral or vascular thrombosis, severe hypertension
• Use cautiously with hyperthyroidism, bradycardia, partial heart block, diabetes, acute pancreatitis, hepatitis, pregnancy

INTERACTIONS

Drug

• Decreased action with α blockers
• Increased arrhythmias with general anesthetics, epinephrine, digoxin, levodopa, guanadrel, guanethidine

• Increased pressor effects with oxytocics, tricyclic antidepressants, MAOIs
• Increased effects of both phenylephrine and thyroid hormones when used together

Lab

• Decreased intraocular pressure
• False normal tonometry readings

INCOMPATIBILITIES

• Alkaline sol including $NaHCO_3$, iron salts, phenytoin

SIDE EFFECTS

CNS: Headache, anxiety, tremor, insomnia, dizziness, restlessness, nervousness, lightheadedness, weakness, paresthesias, seizures
CV: Palpitations, tachycardia, hypertension, ectopy, angina, bradycardia
DERM: Sweating, blanching, necrosis, tissue sloughing with extravasation, gangrene
EENT: Blurred vision; iris floaters; glaucoma; burning, stinging, or dryness of nasal mucosa; rebound myosis; rebound nasal congestion
GI: Nausea, vomiting
RESP: Respiratory distress

TOXICITY AND OVERDOSE

Clinical signs: Severe adverse reactions, palpitations, paresthesias, vomiting, arrhythmias, hypertension
Treatment: Supportive measures as necessary; atropine sulfate to block reflex bradycardia; phentolamine to treat hypertension; propranolol to treat arrhythmias; levodopa to reduce excessive mydriatic effects

PATIENT CARE MANAGEMENT

Assessment

• Assess history of hypersensitivity to drug
• Assess baseline VS, B/P, ECG, hydration status

Interventions

• Administer through large vein, monitor carefully for extravasation; administer 10-15 ml NS with 5-10 mg of phentolamine through

P

---

a fine needle if infiltration occurs
- Correct hypovolemia before administration
- Apply pressure to lacrimal sac during and for 1-2 min after ophthal instillation to prevent systemic absorption
- Do not touch applicator tip to any surface to prevent contamination
- Rinse tip of bottle or dropper of nasal preparations with hot water after use; dry with clean tissue
- Use lowest effective dosage to reduce risk of rebound congestion

Evaluation
- Evaluate therapeutic response (increased B/P with stabilization, decreased nasal congestion, pupil dilation)
- Evaluate for side effects, hypersensitivity
- Monitor VS, B/P, ECG continuously

PATIENT AND FAMILY EDUCATION
Teach/instruct
- To take as directed at prescribed intervals for prescribed length of time
- Not to use if sol is brown or contains precipitate
- To wash hands before ophthal application; use finger to apply pressure to lacrimal sac during and for 1-2 min after instillation
- To keep bottle and dropper of nasal preparations clean
- To blow nose gently to clear nasal passages before using nasal medication
- About correct method of nasal instillation
- To increase fluid intake to help keep secretions liquid

Warn/advise
- To notify care provider of hypersensitivity, side effects
- To discontinue medication if dizziness or chest pain occur
- To use sunglasses to protect eyes from sunlight, bright lights if using ophthal
- To avoid using OTC medications unless directed by care provider

STORAGE
- Store at room temp in tightly sealed, light-resistant container

---

phenytoin, phenytoin sodium, phenytoin sodium (extended), phenytoin sodium (prompt)

Brand Name(s): Dilantin✦, Dilantin Capsules, Dilantin Injection✦, Diphenylan, Diphenylan Sodium, Phenytoin Oral Suspension

Classification: Anticonvulsant, hydantoin derivative, antiarrhythmic

Pregnancy Category: D

AVAILABLE PREPARATIONS
Tabs, chewable: 50 mg (phenytoin)
Oral susp: 30 mg/5 ml, 125 mg/5 ml (phenytoin)
Caps: 30 mg, 100 mg (phenytoin sodium); 30 mg, 100 mg (phenytoin sodium extended); 30 mg, 100 mg (phenytoin sodium prompt)
Inj: 50 mg/ml (phenytoin sodium)

ROUTES AND DOSAGES
Status Epilepticus/ Anticonvulsant
- An IV loading dose may be administered to reach therapeutic serum levels more quickly or with status epilepticus; maintenance dose may then be administered
Neonates: IV loading dose 15-20 mg/kg in a single or divided dose; maintenance dose, initial 4-8 mg/kg/24 hr divided bid-tid
Children 6 mo-3 yr: IV loading dose 10-20 mg/kg in a single or divided dose; maintenance dose 8-10 mg/kg/24 hr divided qd-tid
Children 4-6 yr: IV loading dose 10-20 mg/kg in a single or divided dose; maintenance dose 7.5-9 mg/kg/24 hr divided qd-tid
Children 7-9 yr: IV loading dose 10-20 mg/kg in a single or divided dose; maintenance dose 7-8 mg/kg/24 hr divided qd-tid

---

✦ Available in Canada.

Children 10-16 yr: IV loading dose 10-20 mg in a single or divided dose; maintenance dose 6-7 mg/kg/24 hr divided qd-tid

Adults: IV loading dose 15-18 mg in a single or divided dose; maintenance dose 5-6 mg/kg/24 hr divided qd-tid

• IM administration only used temporarily in pts unable to take medication PO; usual PO dose should be reduced by ½ and administered IM; when pt is able to return to PO route, administer ½ of usual PO dose because of the possibility of slow release from IM sites

• PO loading doses may be administered initially to achieve therapeutic levels more quickly

Children and adults: PO loading dose 15-20 mg/kg/24 hr divided bid-tid 8-12 hr apart to decrease GI effects; maintenance dose 5 mg/kg/24 hr or 250 mg/m²/24 hr divided bid-tid (usual dose 5-8 mg/kg/24 hr or 200 mg/24 hr; maximum dose 300 mg/24 hr)

Seizure Patients Receiving Phenytoin Who Have Missed One or More Doses and Have Subtherapeutic Levels

Neonates: IV loading dose 10-25 mg/kg in NS infused slowly at a rate not to exceed 0.5 mg/kg/min

Children: IV 5-7 mg/kg not to exceed 50 mg/min; lower dose may be repeated in 30 min if necessary

Adults: 100-300 mg; not to exceed 50 mg/min

Arrhythmia

Children: IV loading dose 1.25 mg/kg q 5 min, may be repeated up to a total loading dose of 15 mg/kg; PO/IV maintenance dose 5-10 mg/kg/24 hr divided bid

Adults: IV loading dose 1.25 mg/kg q 5 min, may be repeated up to a total loading dose of 15 mg/kg; PO/IV maintenance dose 250 mg qid on day 1; 250 mg divided bid on days 2-3, then 300-400 mg/24 hr divided qd-qid

IV administration

• Recommended concentration: 50 mg/ml (commercially available) or may dilute with NS

• Maximum concentration: 50 mg/ml

• IV push rate/intermittent infusion: Neonates, infants, young children 0.5-3 mg/kg/min; older children, adults 50 mg/min

• Therapeutic reference range: 10-20 mcg/ml; toxicity is determined clinically; some pts may require serum levels outside suggested therapeutic range

MECHANISM AND INDICATIONS

Mechanism: Stabilizes central motor cortex and peripheral neuronal membranes; decreases flux on Na ions that normally flow during action potentials or during chemically induced depolarization; prolongs refractory period and suppresses ventricular pacemaker; shortens action potential in heart

Indications: Used to treat generalized tonic–clonic, simple partial, and complex partial seizures and to prevent seizures after head trauma; also used to control ventricular arrhythmias, particularly those induced by digitalis

PHARMACOKINETICS

Onset of action: Varies with different preparations and dosages

Peak: 3-12 hr

Distribution: Widely throughout the body

Half-life: 6-24 hr

Metabolism: Liver

Excretion: Urine

Therapeutic level: 7.5-20 mcg/ml

CONTRAINDICATIONS AND PRECAUTIONS

• Contraindicated with known hypersensitivity to phenytoin; some preparations contain sodium bisulfite and are contraindicated with known sulfite allergy; with heart block, sinus bradycardia; with pregnancy, lactation

• Use cautiously with hepatic or renal dysfunction (especially in uremic pts with decreased protein-binding); respiratory depression, CHF (especially IV); IM administration not recommended because it is painful and drug absorption is erratic

P

INTERACTIONS
Drug
• Increased phenytoin serum levels with acute alcohol intake, amiodarone, chloramphenicol, chlordiazepoxide, cimetidine diazepam, dicumarol, disulfiram, estrogens, H_2-antagonist, halothane, isoniazid, methylphenidate, phenothiazines, phenylbutazone, salicylates, succinimides, sulfonamides, tolbutamide, trazodone, trimethoprim

• Decreased phenytoin serum levels with chronic alcohol abuse, rifampin, cisplatin, vinblastine, bleomycin, folic acid, reserpine, sucralfate; ingestion times of phenytoin and antacids containing Ca should be staggered in pts with low serum phenytoin levels to prevent absorption difficulties

• Increased or decreased phenytoin serum levels with phenobarbital, sodium valproate, valproic acid, carbamazepine

• Decreased serum concentrations and effectiveness of other anticonvulsants (valproic acid, ethosuximide, primidone); warfarin, oral contraceptives, corticosteroids, cyclosporin, theophylline, chloramphenicol, rifampin, doxycycline, quinidine, mexiletine, disopyramide, dopamine, nondepolarizing skeletal muscle relaxants

• Competition for protein binding sites with sulfisoxazole, phenylbutazone, valproate, salicylates

• Increased phenytoin metabolism (decreased phenytoin serum levels) with carbamazepine; reduced serum levels of carbamazepine also possible

• Enhanced metabolism of corticosteroids, oral contraceptives

• Increased rate of clearance of theophylline, decreased plasma levels of phenytoin when given together

• Interaction with phenobarbital; increased biotransformation of phenytoin possible; decreased inactivation of phenytoin by competitive inhibition possible; reduced oral absorption of phenytoin, resulting in increased serum concentration possible

Lab
• Increased levels of BG, alk phos, γ-glutamyl transpeptidase (GGT) possible

• Decreased serum levels of PBI possible

• Decreased values for dexamethasone or metyrapone tests possible

Nutrition
• Decreased serum concentration of phenytoin, possible with continuous NG feeds

INCOMPATIBILITIES
• Any drug in sol or syringe

SIDE EFFECTS
CNS: Ataxia, slurred speech, confusion, dizziness, insomnia, nervousness, twitching, dyskinesias, headache, CNS depression, lethargy, drowsiness, irritability

CV: Hypotension, bradycardia, ventricular fibrillation, cardiovascular collapse, asystole (with rapid IV administration)

DERM: Photosensitivity, purpuric dermatitis, scarlatiniform or morbilliform rash; bullous exfoliative rash, Stevens-Johnson syndrome; lupus erythematous, hirsutism, coarsening of facial features

GI: Nausea, vomiting, gingival hyperplasia (especially in children), constipation

HEME: Thrombocytopenia, leukopenia, agranulocytosis, pancytopenia, macrocytosis, megaloblastic anemic, blood dyscrasias, lymphadenopathy

EENT: Nystagmus, blurred vision, diplopia

Local: With IV or IM administration, pain, venous irritation, thrombophlebitis, necrosis, inflammation at injection site, purple glove syndrome

Other: Periarteritis nodosa, lymphadenopathy, hyperglycemia, osteomalacia, hypertrichosis

TOXICITY AND OVERDOSAGE
Clinical signs: Drowsiness, nausea, vomiting, nystagmus, ataxia, dysarthria, tremor, slurred speech;

hypotension, respiratory depression, coma and death may follow
Treatment: Gastric lavage or emesis; supportive treatment including careful monitoring of VS, fluid and electrolyte balance; hemodialysis or peritoneal dialysis may be helpful

PATIENT CARE MANAGEMENT
Assessment
• Assess seizure type, determine appropriate anticonvulsant for this type of seizure
• Assess history hypersensitivity to phenytoin or sulfites
• Assess carefully for preexisting conditions, current medications in order to avoid potential interactions; drug interactions are frequent, particularly with drugs metabolized in the liver; check the serum levels to avoid either increased or decreased levels
• Assess baseline CBC, differential, liver function (ALT, AST, bilirubin, alk phos)
Interventions
• Initiate at modest dosage
• Increase dosage and level prn to control seizures, to the point of intolerable side effects
• If only partially effective, another anticonvulsant may be initiated in the same way
• If drug is not effective, gradually withdraw and initiate another anticonvulsant
• If break-through seizures occur when serum levels are at trough or peak, frequency may be increased to provide more-even coverage
• May be administered PO with food to reduce GI effects; shake sol well to assure adequate mixing
• IV solution should be clear to light yellow; do not use if sol contains precipitate
• IV doses should be mixed in NS, used within 1 hr; will precipitate in D_5; do not refrigerate sol, do not mix with other drugs; use in-line filter; after administration, flush IV tubing to clear with NS
• When administering IV, continuous monitoring of ECG, B/P, and respiratory status is essential
• If administering IV bolus, deliver slowly (50 mg/min); IV push or constant infusion administered too quickly may cause hypotension and circulatory collapse
• Use larger veins to administer IV to prevent discoloration associated with purple glove syndrome
Evaluation
• Evaluate therapeutic response (seizure control); initially done more frequently until seizures are controlled, then q 3-6 mo, if seizure breakthrough occurs, or with side effects
• Monitor anticonvulsant levels periodically

PATIENT AND FAMILY EDUCATION
Teach/instruct
• To take drug as prescribed, not to change dosage independently or withdraw drug suddenly
• About process for initiating anticonvulsant drugs, need for frequent visits (especially initially)
• About rationale for measuring serum levels, how these should be obtained (peak/trough)
• That PO dose may be taken with food if GI distress occurs
• That contents of oral sol settle; shake well before administering to avoid under- or overdosing
• That phenytoin may cause gingival hyperplasia; pts must be instructed in good mouth care (including regular brushing and flossing); schedule regular dental visits
• That oral or nasogastric feeding may interfere with absorption of oral susp; dose should be separated from feedings as much as possible; with tube feedings, the line should be flushed before and after dose
• That pink or reddish-brown discoloration of urine is harmless
Warn/advise
• About potential side effects; encourage to report serious side effects immediately (drowsiness, nausea, vomiting, nystagmus, ataxia, dysarthria, tremor, slurred

speech, hypotension, respiratory depression)
• That unpleasant side effects may decrease as pt becomes more used to the drug
• That drug may initially be more sedating; avoid hazardous tasks (bike, skates, skateboard) that require mental alertness until stabilized on drug
• To avoid alcohol, other CNS depressants, OTC drugs
• To make other health care providers aware of medications in order to avoid drug interactions
• To inform care provider if pregnancy should occur while taking drug

Encourage
• To keep a record of any seizures (seizure calendar)

STORAGE
• Store at room temp in tightly closed containers
• Avoid freezing oral and parenteral sol

---

physostigmine sulfate, physostigmine salicylate

Brand Name(s): Physostigmine sulfate: Eserine, Isopto; physostigmine salicylate: Antilirium

Classification: Antimuscarinic antidote, antiglaucoma agent (cholinesterase inhibitor)

Pregnancy Category: C

AVAILABLE PREPARATIONS
Inj (salicylate): 1 mg/ml
Oint, ophthal: 0.25%
Sol, ophthal: 0.25%;, 0.5%

ROUTES AND DOSAGES
Reversal of Anticholinergic Effects:
Children: IV 0.01-0.03 mg/kg/dose, may repeat after 15-20 min to maximum total dose of 2 mg; for maintenance, the lowest effective test dose should be repeated q30-60 min if life-threatening signs or symptoms recur
Adults: IM/IV/SC:0.5-2 mg to start, repeat q 20 mins until desired response occurs

Preanesthetic Reversals of Anticholinergic Effects of Atropine or Scopolamine
Children and adults: IM/IV administer twice the dose, based on weight, of the anticholinergic drug dosage

Glaucoma
Children and adults: Ophth 1-2 gtt of 0.25% or 0.5% solution q4-8h (up to qid), ointment can be instilled at night

IV administration
• Recommended concentration: Administer undiluted
• Maximum concentration: 1 mg/ml
• IV push rate: Over 5 min not to exceed 0.5 mg/min in children or 1 mg/min in adults (bradycardia and convulsions have occurred following more rapid injection); atropine sulfate should be available to reverse signs and symptoms of life-threatening physostigmine excess; it is preferable to wait for life-threatening symptoms to diminish if possible; dose 0.5 mg atropine/1 mg physostigmine

MECHANISM AND INDICATIONS
Mechanism: Blocks the destruction of acetylcholine by acetylcholinesterase, promoting the transmission of nerve impulses across the myoneural junction
Indications: Used to reverse the toxic effects of anticholinergic drugs; also used to treat wideangle glaucoma

PHARMACOKINETICS
Peak: IV 5 min, persists 45-60 min; PO 2 mins and persists 12-36 hr
Half-life: 1-2 hr
Absorption: Readily absorbed, freely crosses the blood–brain barrier, reversing both central and peripheral anticholinergic effects
Metabolism: Liver (cholinesterase hydrolyzes physostigmine relatively quickly)

✦ Available in Canada.

Excretion: Only small amount of physostigmine is excreted; exact mode of excretion unknown

CONTRAINDICATIONS AND PRECAUTIONS

• Contraindicated with known sensitivity to cholinesterase inhibitors and sulfite sensitivity (some preparations contain sulfites); with narrow angle glaucoma (may cause pupillary blockage and result in increased intraocular pressure); with obstructions of the urinary or intestinal tract (because of its stimulatory effect on smooth muscle); with bradycardia or hypotension (may exacerbate these conditions); with DM or CVS disorders

• Use cautiously with bronchial asthma (may precipitate bronchospasm); with epilepsy (may stimulate CNS); with peritonitis, vagotonia, hyperthyroidism, or cardiac arrhythmias (may exacerbate these conditions); with peptic ulcer disease (may increase gastric acid secretions); with recent coronary occlusion (may stimulate the cardiovascular system); with pregnancy

• Injectable solution may contain benzyl alcohol as a preservative; administration of benzyl alcohol in doses ranging from 99-234 mg/kg has been associated with a fatal gasping syndrome in neonates; clinical signs include metabolic acidosis, hypotension, CNS depression, cardiovascular collapse

INTERACTIONS
Drug

• Antagonized cholinergic effect on muscle with procainamide, quinidine

• Increased neuromuscular blockade with systemic administration of succinylcholine, bethanechol, methacholine

• Additive toxicity possible with other cholinergic drugs

• Retarded corneal healing possible with ophthal oints

Lab

• Elevated ALT, AST, amylase possible

INCOMPATIBILITIES

• Incompatible with most drugs in sol or syringe

SIDE EFFECTS

CNS: Headache, browache, convulsions, confusion, restlessness, muscle twitching, muscle weakness, ataxia, hallucinations, excitability

CV: Bradycardia, hypotension, cardiac irregularities

EENT: Blurred vision, conjunctivitis, miosis, ocular burning, tearing, spasms with accommodation, twitching of eyelid, myopia, retinal detachment, hemorrhage of vitreous, erythema of conjunctiva and ciliary body, opacities of the lens, obstruction of the nasolacrimal canals, paradoxical increased intraocular pressure, activation of latent iritis or uveitis, iris cysts (more often in children)

GI: Nausea, vomiting, increased salivation, increase in gastric and intestinal secretions, epigastric pain, diarrhea

GU: Urinary urgency, incontinence

RESP: Increase tracheobronchial secretions, bronchiolar constriction, bronchospasm

Other: Allergic reaction, sweating; drug should be discontinued if hypersensitivity, difficulty breathing, incoordination, restlessness, agitation or skin rash should occur

TOXICITY AND OVERDOSE

Clinical signs: Headache, nausea, vomiting, diarrhea, blurred vision, miosis, myopia, excessive tearing, bronchospasm, increased bronchial secretions, hypotension, incoordination, excessive sweating, muscle weakness, cramps, fasciculations, paralysis, bradycardia, tachycardia, excessive salivation, restlessness, agitation

Treatment: Supportive, symptomatic care; discontinue drug immediately; atropine may be given to block neostigmine's muscarinic effect, but it will not reverse paralytic effects on skeletal muscle; care must be taken not to overdose with atropine because it could

P

cause development of a bronchial plug

PATIENT CARE MANAGEMENT
Assessment
• Assess history of hypersensitivity to physostigmine or sulfites
• Assess pt needs carefully; dosage must be individualized according to severity of disease and response of pt
• Be aware of all other medications to avoid potential interactions
• Assess for preexisting conditions in order to avoid potential side effects
Interventions
• Observe sol for discoloration; do not use if darkened
• Observe closely for cholinergic reactions (especially with the parenteral forms)
• Ensure that atropine is available to reduce or reverse hypersensitivity reactions
• Administer concurrently with atropine as needed to relieve or eliminate adverse reaction
• See Chapter 2 regarding ophthal instillation; have pt lie down or tilt head back; after instillation, gently pinch nasal bridge for 1-2 min to reduce systemic absorption; after instilling ointment, close eyelids and roll eye; wait 5 min before instilling other eye preparations

---

NURSING ALERT

Injectable sol may contain benzyl alcohol as a preservative; administration of benzyl alcohol in doses of 99-234 mg/kg has been associated with a fatal gasping syndrome in neonates; clinical signs include metabolic acidosis, hypotension, CNS depression, cardiovascular collapse

Drug should be discontinued if hypersensitivity, difficulty breathing, incoordination, restlessness, agitation, skin rash occur

---

Evaluation
• Monitor regularly for drug effectiveness
• Monitor for potential side effects
PATIENT AND FAMILY EDUCATION
Teach/instruct
• About how to instill ophthal medications
Warn/advise
• About potential side effects; to report should any of these occur (particularly abdominal cramps, excessive salivation, diarrhea)
• That blurred vision may occur with initial doses
• Miosis causes difficulty in adapting to the dark; pt should use caution while driving at night or performing hazardous tasks (bike, skates, skateboard) in poor light

---

phytonadione (vitamin K)

Brand Name(s): Aqua-MEPHYTON, Konakion, Mephyton

Classification: Fat-soluble vitamin, blood coagulant

Pregnancy Category: C

AVAILABLE PREPARATIONS
Tabs: 5 mg
Inj: 2 mg/ml, 5 mg/ml, 10 mg/ml, 25 mg/ml, 37.5 mg/ml

ROUTES AND DOSAGES
Dietary Supplement
See Appendix F, Table of Recommended Daily Dietary Allowances
Hypoprothrombinemia
Caused by Malabsorption of Vitamin K
Infants and children: PO 2.5-5 mg/24 hr, IM/IV 1-2 mg as single dose
Adults: PO 2.5-25 mg/24 hr, IM/IV 10 mg as single dose
Hypoprothrombinemia
Caused by Oral Anticoagulants
Infants: IM/IV/SC 1-2 mg/dose q4-8h
Children and Adults: PO/SC/IM

2.5-10 mg, may repeat in 12-48 hr after PO dose or 6-8 hr after IM/SC dose per PT/INR

Prevention of Neonatal Hemorrhagic Disease
Neonates: SC/IM 0.5-1.0 mg immediately after birth; repeat in 6-8 hr if needed

IV administration
- IM/SC preferred; use IV only with severe hemorrhagic disease and physician present
- Recommended concentration: AquaMEPHYTON, dilute in 5-10 ml D_5NS, D_5W, NS
- IV push rate: Do not exceed 1 mg/min
- Intermittent infusion rate: Over 15-30 min

MECHANISM AND INDICATIONS
Mechanism: Vitamin K is a fat-soluble vitamin important in the hepatic formation of active prothrombin and other blood coagulation factors; phytonadione is the synthetic form, also fat-soluble, requires the presence of bile salts for absorption; AquaMEPHYTON is the injectable form of vitamin K
Indications: Treatment and prevention of hypoprothrombinemia or vitamin K deficiency

PHARMACOKINETICS
Peak: Inj 3-6 hr
Metabolism: Liver
Excretion: Feces

CONTRAINDICATIONS AND PRECAUTIONS
- Contraindicated during last few wk of pregnancy, with hypersensitivity to vitamin K or analogues
- Use cautiously with hepatic disease, neonates, pregnancy

INTERACTIONS
Drug
- Interference with action of vitamin K with antibiotics
- Antagonized action of warfarin, other oral anticoagulants
- Decreased absorption of fat-soluble form of vitamin K with mineral oil

Lab
- Falsely elevated urine steroid levels

INCOMPATIBILITIES
- Vitamin C, vitamin B_{12}, dextran, pentobarbital, phenobarbital, phenytoin, vancomycin

SIDE EFFECTS
CNS: Headache, dizziness, convulsive movements
CV: Rapid weak pulse, transient hypotension following IV administration, cardiac arrhythmias
DERM: Rash, pruritus, urticaria, sweating, flushing
GI: Nausea, vomiting
Local: Hematoma at injection site, swelling, pain
Other: Anaphylaxis

TOXICITY AND OVERDOSE
Clinical signs: Fatigue, weakness; hyperbilirubinemia, fatal kernicterus, hemolytic anemia in neonates
Treatment: Discontinue treatment; supportive care

PATIENT CARE MANAGEMENT
Assessment
- Assess history of hypersensitivity to vitamin K
- Obtain baseline blood clotting factors (PT/INR)
- Assess for other medication use to assure optimum absorption and use
- Assess bile acid production; pts with bile deficiency will require concomitant bile salts

Interventions
- Administer 2 hrs after or before mineral oil
- Mix SC/IM with NS, D_5W
- Do not administer IV without direct medical supervision
- May need adjustment of anticoagulant medication dosage

> **NURSING ALERT**
> IM/SC routes preferred over IV; use IV only with severe hemorrhagic disease with physician present

Evaluation
• Evaluate therapeutic response (decreased bleeding tendencies, normal blood clotting factors)
• Monitor PT/INR
• Monitor for signs of hypersensitivity (flushing, weakness, tachycardia, hypotension) when giving injectable form
• Monitor dietary intake; should not increase amounts of foods high in vitamin K when taking medications

PATIENT AND FAMILY EDUCATION
Teach/instruct
• To take as directed at prescribed intervals for prescribed length of time
• Review rationale for therapy, stress importance of compliance; any missed doses should be taken as soon as possible; report missed doses to health care provider
Warn/advise
• To notify care provider of hypersensitivity, side effects
• To inform other caregivers and dentist of medication use
• To avoid OTC medications (especially those containing aspirin, salicylates, or drugs that interact with the anticoagulant effect)
• To consult with care provider before taking other medications
Encourage
• Encourage balanced diet; foods containing vitamin K should remain constant; increase or decrease in foods high in vitamin K can affect therapy (common sources include leafy green vegetables, fish, pork or beef liver, green tea, tomatoes)

STORAGE
• Store at room temp in an airtight, light-resistant container
• Protect from moisture and heat

---

pimozide
Brand Name(s): Orap✦
Classification: Neuroleptic
Pregnancy Category: C

AVAILABLE PREPARATIONS
Tabs: 2 mg (not available as generic)

DOSAGES AND ROUTES
Tourette Syndrome
Children <12 yr: PO dose must be determined by prescriber; not recommended for use in any childhood condition other than Tourette syndrome; although Tourette syndrome often begins between the ages of 2 and 15 yr, pimozide is not recommended for use in patients <12
Adolescents and adults: PO initial 1-2 mg/24 hr divided bid; maximum dose 10 mg/24 hr

MECHANISM AND INDICATIONS
Mechanism: Acts in CNS to help control symptoms of Tourette syndrome
Indications: For use in treatment of symptoms of Tourette syndrome that have not responded to other treatments

CONTRAINDICATIONS AND PRECAUTIONS
• Contraindicated with hypersensitivity to this medication or any component, to other neuroleptics; coma, history of abnormal heart rhythm, diseases other than Tourette syndrome
• Use cautiously with history of breast cancer; cardiac, kidney, or liver disease; glaucoma, low K^+ level, enlarged prostate

INTERACTIONS
Drug
• Increased risk of arrhythmias with antipsychotics, disopyramide, maprotiline, procainamide, quinidine, tricyclic antidepressants
• Increased anticholinergic effects with anticholinergics
• Cause of tics may be masked by

✦ Available in Canada.

amphetamines, methylphenidate, pemoline
• Interacts with alcohol, amoxapine, antianxiety drugs, antiarrhythmic drugs, barbiturates, deserpidine, methyldopa, metoclopramide, metyrosine, narcotic pain relievers, phenothiazines, phenytoin, promethazine, Rauwolfia alkaloids, reserpine, sedatives, trimeprazine

Nutrition
• May contain sulfite preservatives which can cause allergic reactions in sensitive pts

SIDE EFFECTS
CNS: Akathisia, behavior changes, mental depression, dizziness, drowsiness, fainting, handwriting changes, headache, insomnia, lightheadedness, mood changes, abnormal movements, nervousness, neuroleptic malignant syndrome, parkinsonian symptoms, rigidity, seizures, shuffling walk, tardive dyskinesia, tiredness, tremor, weakness
CV: Arrhythmias, B/P changes, chest pain, orthostatic hypotension, palpitations, tachycardia
DERM: Discoloration, irritation, unusually pale skin, rash, sweating, yellow eyes or skin
EENT: Loss of balance, cataracts, eyes sensitive to light, spots before eyes, inability to move eyes, dry mouth, swallowing problems, swelling around eyes, taste changes, sore throat, blurred vision
GI: Appetite changes, belching, constipation, diarrhea, dry mouth, nausea, increased salivation, stomach upset, thirst, vomiting, wt changes
GU: Impotence, galactorrhea, gynecomastia, menstrual irregularities, loss of sex drive, urinary incontinence
Other: Dyspnea, fever, mask-like face, muscle tightness and cramps, muscle spasms, speech problems, swelling of the face

TOXICITY AND OVERDOSE
Clinical signs: Dizziness, drowsiness, dyspnea, severe uncontrolled movements, tiredness, tremors, weakness
Treatment: Withhold drug; supportive care

PATIENT CARE MANAGEMENT
Assessment
• Assess history of hypersensitivity to drug
• Obtain baseline medical history, physical exam
• Assess symptoms of Tourette syndrome; assess ability to function in daily activities, to sleep throughout the night
• Assess mental status (mood, sensorium, affect, impulsiveness, suicidal ideation, thoughts)

Interventions
• Pt should not drink alcohol
• Rinse mouth with water, take sips of fluid, sugarless gum, hard candy for dry mouth
• Increase fluids and fiber in diet if constipation occurs

> **NURSING ALERT**
> Neuroleptic malignant syndrome and tardive dyskinesia are possible side effects

Evaluation
• Evaluate therapeutic response (symptoms of Tourette syndrome, ability to function in daily activities, to sleep throughout the night)
• Evaluate mental status (mood, sensorium, affect, impulsiveness, suicidal ideation, thoughts)
• Monitor for symptoms of tardive dyskinesia; symptoms include rhythmic involuntary movements of the tongue, face, mouth, jaw, arms, or legs, and fine worm-like movements of the tongue
• Monitor for symptoms of neuroleptic malignant syndrome; symptoms include fever, fast or irregular heartbeat, fast breathing, sweating, weakness, muscle stiffness, seizures, loss of bladder control; if these occur, obtain medical intervention immediately; monitor VS, ECG, urine output, renal function; manage symptoms with

P

medications, hydration, cooling blankets
• Tic intensity and frequency may increase during periodic gradual withdrawals from medication; allow 1-2 drug-free wk to pass before concluding that tic increase is caused by disease rather than drug withdrawal

PATIENT AND FAMILY EDUCATION
Teach/instruct
• To take as directed at prescribed intervals for prescribed length of time
• To ensure that medication is swallowed
• That medication is most helpful when used as part of a comprehensive multimodal treatment program
• Not to discontinue medication without prescriber approval
• That some side effects continue after pimozide is discontinued including lip smacking or puckering, puffing of cheeks, rapid or worm-like movements of the tongue, uncontrolled chewing movements, uncontrolled movements of arms and legs
Warn/advise
• To avoid ingesting alcohol, other CNS depressants
• To tell physicians, dentists, other health care providers that you are taking pimozide before any surgery, dental treatment, or emergency treatment is done (in order to avoid medications that interact with pimozide)
• That this medication may cause drowsiness; be careful on bicycles, skates, skateboards, while driving, with other activities requiring alertness
• To immediately report signs of tardive dyskinesia (fine worm-like movement of tongue, rhythmical involuntary movements of tongue, face, mouth, or jaw; involuntary movements of arms and legs)
• To immediately report signs of neuroleptic malignant syndrome (fever, muscle rigidity, irregular pulse, B/P, heart rhythm, increased HR, sweating)

STORAGE
• Store away from heat, direct light
• Do not store in damp places; heat or moisture may cause the medicine to break down

---

piperacillin sodium
Brand Name(s): Pipracil✹
Classification: Antibiotic (extended-spectrum penicillin)
Pregnancy Category: B

AVAILABLE PREPARATIONS
Inj: 2 g, 3 g, 4 g, 40 g

ROUTES AND DOSAGES
Neonates: IM/IV 150-200 mg/kg/24 hr divided q12h (Safety and effectiveness not established. Dosage represents accepted standard practice recommendations.)
Infants and children <12 yr: IM/IV 200-300 mg/kg/24 hr divided q4-6h (maximum 24 g/24 hr) (Safety and effectiveness not established. Dosage represents accepted standard practice recommendations.)
Children with cystic fibrosis: IM/IV 300-600 mg/kg/24 hr divided q4-6h (Safety and effectiveness not established. Dosage represents accepted standard practice recommendations.)
Children >12 yr and adults: IV 2-4 g q4-6h or IM 2-3 g q6-12h (maximum 24 g/24 hr)
IV administration
• Recommended concentration: 200 mg/ml in D_5NS, D_5W, NS, SW for IV push; 10-20 mg/ml in D_5NS, D_5W, LR, NS for IV infusion
• Maximum concentration: 200-300 mg/ml for IV push
• IV push rate: Over 3-5 min
• Intermittent infusion rate: Over 30-60 min

✹ Available in Canada.

MECHANISM AND INDICATIONS

Antibiotic mechanism: Bactericidal; inhibits bacterial cell wall synthesis by adhering to bacterial penicillin-binding proteins.

Indications: Active against many gram-positive and gram-negative organisms including *Staphylococcus aureus, Streptococcus pyogenes, Str. viridans, Str. faecalis, Str. pneumoniae, Neisseria gonorrhoeae, N. meningitidis, Clostridium perfringens, C. tetani, Bacteroides, E. coli, Klebsiella, Proteus mirabilis, P. vulgaris, Morganella morganii, Enterobacter, Citrobacter, Pseudomonas aeruginosa, Serratia, Acinetobacter;* used to treat septicemia, serious lower respiratory, intraabdominal, urinary tract, gynecologic, skin, bone, joint, and gonococcal infections

PHARMACOKINETICS

Peak: IM 30-50 min; IV 20-30 min
Distribution: Widely distributed; highest concentrates in urine, bile; penetrates CNS with inflamed meninges
Half-life: 0.5-1.5 hr
Metabolism: Not significantly metabolized
Excretion: Urine, bile

CONTRAINDICATIONS AND PRECAUTIONS

• Contraindicated with known hypersensitivity to piperacillin, penicillins, cephalosporins
• Use cautiously with impaired renal function, history of bleeding problems, hypokalemia, pregnancy

INTERACTIONS
Drug

• Synergistic antimicrobial activity against certain organisms with aminoglycosides, clavulanic acid
• Increased serum concentrations with probenecid
• Increased serum concentrations of methotrexate
• Decreased effectiveness with tetracyclines, erythromycin, chloramphenicol
• Increased risk of bleeding with use of anticoagulants

Lab

• False positive urine protein
• False positive Coombs' test
• Increased liver function tests

INCOMPATIBILITIES

• Aminoglycosides, amphotericin B, chloramphenicol, lincomycin, polymyxin B, promethazine, tetracycline, vitamins B and C

SIDE EFFECTS

CNS: Neuromuscular irritability, headache, dizziness
ENDO/METAB: Hypokalemia
GI: Nausea, diarrhea, vomiting
GU: Acute interstitial nephritis
HEME: Bleeding with high dosages, neutropenia, eosinophilia, leukopenia, thrombocytopenia
Local: Pain at injection site; vein irritation, phlebitis with IV injection
Other: Hypersensitivity reaction (edema, fever, chills, rash, pruritus, urticaria, anaphylaxis), bacterial or fungal superinfection

TOXICITY AND OVERDOSE

Clinical signs: Neuromuscular hypersensitivity; seizures may result from high CNS concentration
Treatment: Supportive care; hemodialysis

PATIENT CARE MANAGEMENT
Assessment

• Assess history of hypersensitivity to piperacillin, penicillins, cephalosporins
• Obtain C&S; may begin therapy before obtaining results
• Assess renal function (BUN, creatinine, I&O), hepatic function (ALT, AST, bilirubin), hematologic function (CBC, differential, platelet count); K$^+$ levels if on long-term therapy

Interventions

• Administer penicillins at least 1 hr before bacteriostatic antibiotics (tetracyclines, erythromycins, chloramphenicol)
• IM injection is painful; administer deeply into large muscle mass, rotate injection site
• Do not premix IV with other

P

---

medications (particularly aminoglycosides); infuse separately
• Use large vein with small-bore needle to reduce local reaction; rotate site q48-72h
• Maintain age-appropriate fluid intake

NURSING ALERT
Discontinue drug if signs of hypersensitivity, bleeding complications, pseudomembranous colitis develop

Do not infuse rapidly; seizures may result

Evaluation
• Evaluate therapeutic response (decreased symptoms of infection)
• Monitor signs of superinfection (perineal itching, diaper rash, fever, malaise, redness, pain, swelling, drainage, rash, diarrhea, sore throat, change in cough or sputum)
• Observe for signs of allergic reaction (wheezing, tightness in chest, urticaria), especially within 20-30 min of first dose
• Monitor bowel pattern; diarrhea may be symptomatic of pseudomembranous colitis
• Monitor renal function (BUN, creatinine, I&O), hepatic function (ALT, AST, bilirubin), electrolyte levels (particularly K^+ and Na)
• Monitor for signs of bleeding (ecchymosis, bleeding gums, hematuria, daily stool guaiac); monitor PT/INR platelet counts
• Evaluate IM site for tissue damage, IV site for vein irritation

PATIENT AND FAMILY EDUCATION
Teach/instruct
• To take as directed at prescribed intervals for prescribed length of time
Warn/advise
• To notify care provider of hypersensitivity, side effects, superinfection

STORAGE
• Store powder at room temp
• Reconstituted sol stable at room temp 24 hr, refrigerated 7 days

---

piperacillin sodium/ tazobactam sodium
Brand Name(s): Zosyn
Classification: Antibiotic (extended-spectrum penicillin)
Pregnancy Category: B

AVAILABLE PREPARATIONS
Inj: 2.25 g (2 g piperacillin, 0.25 g tazobactam), 3.375 g (3 piperacillin, 0.375 g tazobactam), 4.5 g (4 g piperacillin, 0.5 g tazobactam)

ROUTES AND DOSAGES
Infants <6 mo: IV 150-300 mg piperacillin/kg/24hr divided q6-8h (Safety and effectiveness not established. Dosage represents accepted standard practice recommendations.)
Infants >6 mo and children: IV 300-400 mg piperacillin/kg/24 hr divided q6-8h (Safety and effectiveness not established. Dosage represents accepted standard practice recommendations.)
Adults: IV 3.375 g q6h
IV administration
• Because safety and effectiveness have not been established for infants or children, there are no specific pediatric IV administration guidelines
Adult IV administration
• Recommended concentration: Dilute with small amount compatible sol; do not use LR; may dilute further
• Intermittent infusion rate: Over 30 min

MECHANISM AND INDICATIONS
Mechanism: Piperacillin is bactericidal; inhibits bacterial cell wall synthesis by adhering to bacterial penicillin-binding proteins; tazo-

---

bactam improves piperacillin's bacterial activity against β-lactamase-producing strains resistant to penicillins and cephalosporins

Indications: Active against many gram-positive and gram-negative organisms (see piperacillin sodium) and is effective for resistant *Staphylococcus aureus,* resistant *E. coli, Bacteroides fragilis, B. ovatus, B. thetaiotaomicron,* and *B. vulgatus;* used to treat medium-to-severe infections of respiratory and GU tracts, skin, and bone caused by piperacillin-resistant β-lactamase-producing strains of bacteria

PHARMACOKINETICS
Peak: Completion of IV
Distribution: Widely distributed; highest concentrations in urine, bile
Half-life: 0.7-1.2 hr
Duration: 6 hr
Metabolism: Not significantly metabolized
Excretion: Urine, bile

CONTRAINDICATIONS AND PRECAUTIONS
• Contraindicated with known hypersensitivity to penicillins, cephalosporins, or β-lactamase inhibitors
• Use cautiously with pregnancy, lactation, children <age 12 yr, with CHF

INTERACTIONS
Drug
• Decreased effectiveness of piperacillin with use of tetracycline, erythromycins, aminoglycosides IV
• Increased piperacillin serum concentrations with use of probenecid
Lab
• False positive for urine glucose using copper-reduction method
• False positive for urine protein, Coombs' test
• Decreased Hct, Hgb, electrolytes
• Increased platelet count, esosinphilia, neutropenia, leukopenia, serum creatinine, PTT, AST, ALT, alk phosphatase, bilirubin, BUN, electrolytes

INCOMPATIBILITIES
• Aminoglycosides, amphotericin B, chloramphenicol, lincomycin, polymyxin B, promethazine, tetracycline, vitamin B with C, LR

SIDE EFFECTS
CNS: Lethargy, hallucinations, anxiety, depression, twitching, coma, convulsions
ENDO/METAB: Hypokalemia, hypernatremia
GI: Nausea, vomiting, diarrhea, elevated AST, ALT, abdominal pain, glossitis, pseudomembranous colitis
GU: Oliguria, proteinuria, hematuria, vaginitis, moniliasis, glomerulonephritis
HEMA: Anemia, increased bleeding time, bone marrow depression
Local: Vein irritation, phlebitis with IV injection
Other: Hypersensitivity reaction (edema, fever, chills, rash, pruritus, urticaria, anaphylaxis), bacterial or fungal superinfection

TOXICITY AND OVERDOSE
Clinical signs: Neuromuscular hypersensitivity; seizures may result from high CNS concentration
Treatment: Supportive care, hemodialysis

PATIENT CARE MANAGEMENT
Assessment
• Assess history of hypersensitivity to piperacillin, tazobactam, penicillins, cephalosporins, β-lactamase inhibitors.
• Obtain C&S; may begin therapy before obtaining results
• Assess renal function (BUN, creatinine, I&O), hepatic function (ALT, AST, bilirubin), hematologic function (CBC, differential, platelet count), K+ levels (if on long term therapy)
Interventions
• Administer penicillins at least 1 hr before bacteriostatic antibiotics (tetracycines, erythromycins, chloramphenicol)
• Do not premix IV with other

P

medications (particularly aminoglycosides); infuse separately
• Use large vein with small-bore needle to reduce local reaction; rotate sites q48-72h
• Maintain age-appropriate fluid intake

> **NURSING ALERT**
> Discontinue drug if signs of hypersensitivity, bleeding complications, pseudomembranous colitis develop
>
> Do not infuse rapidly; seizures may result

Evaluation
• Evaluate therapeutic response (decreased symptoms of infection)
• Monitor for signs of superinfection (perineal itching, diaper rash, fever, malaise, redness, pain, swelling, drainage, rash, diarrhea, sore throat, change in cough or sputum)
• Observe for signs of allergic reaction (wheezing, tightness in chest, urticaria), especially in first 20-30 min of first dose
• Monitor bowel pattern; diarrhea may be symptomatic of pseudomembranous colitis
• Monitor renal function (BUN, creatinine, I&O), hepatic function (ALT, AST, bilirubin), electrolyte levels (particularly K^+ and Na)
• Monitor for signs of bleeding (ecchymosis, bleeding gums, hematuria, daily stool guaiac); monitor pro-times and platelet counts
• Evaluate IV site for vein irritation

PATIENT AND FAMILY TEACHING
Teach/instruct
• To take as directed at prescribed intervals for prescribed length of time
Advise/warn
• To notify care provider of hypersensitivity, side effects, superinfection

STORAGE
• Store powder at room temp

• Use single-dose vials immediately after reconstitution
• Unused portion stable at room temp for 24 hr or refrigerated for 48 hr

---

piperazine
Brand Name(s): Piperazine
Classification: Anthelmintic
Pregnancy Category: B

AVAILABLE PREPARATIONS
Syr: 500 mg/5 ml
Tabs: 250 mg

ROUTES AND DOSAGES
Pinworm
Children and adults: PO 65 mg/kg/24 hr qd × 7 days (maximum 2.5 g/24 hr); may repeat in 1 wk if needed
Roundworm
Children: PO 75 mg/kg/24 hr qd × 2 days (maximum 3.5 g/24 hr); if infection is severe, repeat after 1 wk
Adults: PO 3.5 g qd × 2 days (maximum 3.5 g/24 hr); if infection is severe, repeat after 1 wk

MECHANISM AND INDICATIONS
Mechanism: Causes muscle paralysis of worm, leading to expulsion by normal peristalsis
Indications: Used to treat pinworm and roundworm; alternative to first-line agents mebendazole or pyrantel pamoate

PHARMACOKINETICS
Excretion: Urine

CONTRAINDICATIONS AND PRECAUTIONS
• Contraindicated with known hypersensitivity to piperazine or any components, seizure disorder, liver or kidney impairment
• Use cautiously with anemia, malnutrition, pregnancy, lactation; avoid prolonged use because of neurotoxicity

---

✦ Available in Canada.

INTERACTIONS
Drug
- Antagonistic action with pyrantel pamoate
- Increased EPS, seizures with use of phenothiazines

Lab
- Decreased serum uric acid possible

SIDE EFFECTS
CNS: Vertigo, weakness, seizures, tremors, headaches, fevers
DERM: Urticaria, erythema multiforme, photodermatitis
EENT: Visual disturbances
GI: Nausea, vomiting, diarrhea
HEME: Hemolytic anemia
RESP: Cough, bronchospasm, rhinorrhea

TOXICITY AND OVERDOSE
Clinical signs: Nausea, vomiting, confusion, weakness, ataxia, seizures, coma
Treatment: Gastric lavage followed by activated charcoal; monitor fluid and electrolytes; manage seizures with diazepam; supportive care

PATIENT CARE MANAGEMENT
Assessment
- Assess history of hypersensitivity to piperazine
- Obtain pinworm test during night or when child is sleeping, worms migrate to perianal area; use sticky side of scotch tape, expose buttocks, press tape to anal area

Interventions
- May be given with food, but more effective on an empty stomach; tab may be crushed
- Use laxatives only if pt is constipated
- Use effective hygiene techniques (especially handwashing)

> **NURSING ALERT**
> Observe closely for neurotoxicity effects

Evaluation
- Evaluate therapeutic response (expulsion of worms)

- Monitor stools; should have 3 negative cultures after treatment
- Evaluate spread of infection to other household contacts, treat as necessary
- Evaluate side effects, hypersensitivity (rash, itching, headache, seizures, fevers, vertigo, weakness), and adverse effects closely

PATIENT AND FAMILY EDUCATION
Teach/instruct
- To take as directed at prescribed intervals for prescribed length of time
- About proper hygiene procedures (especially good handwashing techniques)
- About how to prevent reinfection; to change undergarments and bed linens; to wash clothes and linens in hot water; not to shake bed linens into the air; to frequently cleanse perianal area
- To clean toilet every day with disinfectant
- To wash all fruits and vegetables before eating
- To drink fruit juice; aids in worm expulsion by eliminating accumulation in intestinal mucosa

Warn/advise
- To notify care provider of hypersensitivity, side effects
- That all family members need to be evaluated and treated
- That urine may turn orange or red
- To avoid hazardous activities because drowsiness may occur
- That seizures may recur in pts who are controlled on medications

Encourage
- To comply with treatment regime

STORAGE
- Store at room temp in tight container

P

plasma protein factor

Brand Name(s): Plasma-nate❀, Plasmatein, PPF Protenate, Plasma-Plex

Classification: Plasma volume expander (blood derivative)

Pregnancy Category: C

AVAILABLE PREPARATIONS
Inj: 5% in 50 ml, 250 ml, 500 ml vials

ROUTES AND DOSAGES
Shock
Children: IV 22-33 ml/kg at 5-10 ml/min
Adult: IV 250-500 ml at 10 ml/min
Hypoproteinemia
Adults: IV 1000-1500 ml qd, maximum infusion rate 8 ml/min
IV administration
• Recommended concentration: Do not dilute
• IV push rate: Not recommended
• Continuous infusion rate: Child 5-10 ml/min; adult 8-10 ml/min

MECHANISM AND INDICATIONS
Mechanism: Causes fluid shift from interstitial spaces into circulation, expanding blood volume
Indications: For use in shock and hypoproteinemia

PHARMACOKINETICS
Distribution: Intravascular space, extravascular sites (including skin, muscle, bone)
Metabolism: Liver (as protein/energy source)

CONTRAINDICATIONS AND PRECAUTIONS
• Contraindicated with severe anemia, heart failure, pts undergoing cardiopulmonary bypass, with increased blood volume
• Use cautiously with liver or renal failure, restricted salt intake, poor cardiac reserve

INTERACTIONS
Lab
• Increased plasma protein levels
• Falsely increased alk phos

INCOMPATIBILITIES
• Incompatible with sol containing alcohol, norepinephrine

SIDE EFFECTS
CNS: Headache, fever, chills, paraesthesias, flushing
CV: Hypotension, fluid overload, irregular pulse
DERM: Rash, urticaria, erythema
GI: Nausea, vomiting, increased salivation
RESP: Dyspnea, pulmonary edema
Other: Hypersensitivity (flushing, chills, dyspnea, chest tightness, cyanosis, shock)

TOXICITY AND OVERDOSE
Clinical signs: Circulatory overload, pulmonary edema, hypervolemia
Treatment: Decrease rate of infusion, discontinue drug

PATIENT CARE MANAGEMENT
Assessment
• Assess history of hypersensitivity to blood products
• Assess VS, B/P, CVP frequently
• Assess I&O
• Assess blood studies (Hct, electrolytes, serum protein)
Interventions
• Do not dilute IV, infuse through pump
• Do not use sol that is cloudy or contains sediment
• Discard unused portion
• Avoid rapid IV infusion; individualize rate
Evaluation
• Evaluate for signs of fluid overload
• Evaluate B/P, slow or stop infusion if hypotension occurs
• Monitor I&O, Hct, electrolyte levels
• Evaluate for signs of allergic reaction

PATIENT AND FAMILY EDUCATION
Teach/instruct
• About rationale for therapy; be available to provide support
• That drug is derived from hu-

❀ Available in Canada.

man blood; risk for blood-borne infections low

STORAGE
- Store at room temp
- Do not freeze

---

pneumococcal polysaccharide vaccine
Brand Name(s): Pneumo-vax✤

Classification: Immuniza-tion

Pregnancy Category: C

AVAILABLE PREPARATIONS
Inj: Single dose or 5-dose vials

ROUTES AND DOSAGES
Children >2 yr/adults: IM/SC 0.5 ml one time

MECHANISM AND INDICATIONS
Immunization mechanism: Induces antibody production against *Streptococcus pneumoniae,* thus preventing pneumococcal disease
Indications: Used to prevent pneumococcal disease in pts >2 yr with chronic illnesses

PHARMACOKINETICS
Onset of action: Adequate immune response 2-3 wk after administration

CONTRAINDICATIONS AND PRECAUTIONS
- Contraindicated with known hypersensitivity to any component of the vaccine including phenol; children <2 yr; Hodgkin's disease pts immunized <10 days before or during treatment, or who have received extensive chemotherapy or nodal irradiation; revaccination contraindicated except for adults at highest risk of fatal pneumococcal infection who were initially vaccinated with Pneumococcal Vaccine Polyvalent, MSD, (14-valent) without serious reaction ≥4 yr previously, children at highest risk for pneumococcal infection (with asplenia, sickle cell disease,

nephrotic syndrome) who would be ≤10 yr at revaccination
- Use cautiously with severely compromised cardiac or pulmonary function, pregnancy; delay vaccination with febrile respiratory illnesses

INTERACTIONS
Drug
- Decreased response with immunosuppressive therapy; delay vaccination until 10-14 days after completion of therapy

SIDE EFFECTS
Local: Pain, erythema at injection site
MS: Myalgia
Other: Fever, anaphylaxis

PATIENT CARE MANAGEMENT
Assessment
- Identify target population for immunization (children >2 yr with chronic illness associated with risk of pneumococcal disease)
- Assess history of hypersensitivity to any vaccine components
Interventions
- Administer IM/SC into deltoid muscle or lateral mid-thigh, depending on age, with appropriate precautions to avoid IV or ID administration
- Administer vaccine as one-time dose
- Ensure that emergency resuscitative equipment is readily available for possible anaphylaxis
- Continue penicillin prophylaxis against pneumococcal infection if pt requires such prophylaxis
Evaluation
- Monitor for 20 min after administration for signs of anaphylaxis (urticaria, dyspnea, wheezing, drop in B/P)

PATIENT AND FAMILY EDUCATION
Warn/advise
- To notify care provider of hypersensitivity, side effects
- That a mild analgesic (acetaminophen) may alleviate discomfort, fever
- That required penicillin prophy-

P

✤ Available in Canada.

laxis for pneumococcal infection should continue

STORAGE
• Store unopened and opened vials in refrigerator

---

podophyllum resin

Brand Name(s): Podofilm♣, Pod-Ben 25, Podophyllin

Classification: Keratolytic

Pregnancy Category: X

AVAILABLE PREPARATIONS
Top sol: 11.5%, 25%

ROUTES AND DOSAGES
• For application by care provider only; do not dispense to pt

Keratoses, Epitheliomatoses
Children and adults: Top, apply to lesion qd; let dry, remove dead tissue, reapply prn

Warts
Children and adults: Top, apply to wart for 30-60 min, then wash thoroughly, apply weekly prn

MECHANISM AND INDICATIONS
Mechanism: Arrests mitosis of cells, interferes with chromosomal activity
Indications: For use with venereal warts, keratoses, superficial epitheliomas

PHARMACOKINETICS
Absorption: Systemic absorption minimal if applied for short periods

CONTRAINDICATIONS AND PRECAUTIONS
• Contraindicated with known hypersensitivity to drug, pregnancy, lactation
• Use cautiously, applying only to affected area and protecting surrounding skin with petroleum

INTERACTIONS
Drug
• Increased tissue necrosis when used with other keratolytics

SIDE EFFECTS
CNS: Peripheral neuropathy
GI: Nausea, vomiting
HEME: Thrombocytopenia, leukopenia
Local: Irritation at site of application

TOXICITY AND OVERDOSE
Clinical signs: CNS toxicity (paresthesias, neuritis, lethargy, stupor, paralysis, coma, death)
Treatment: Remove drug; supportive care

PATIENT CARE MANAGEMENT
Assessment
• Assess history of hypersensitivity to drug
• Assess lesions to determine appropriate treatment
• Assess baseline and serial CBC with differential
Interventions
• Apply only to affected area; cover surrounding skin with petrolatum
• Do not apply to broken or inflamed skin
• Apply only for short periods of time
Evaluation
• Evaluate therapeutic response (decreased size and number of lesions)
• Monitor for allergic reactions
• Evaluate for thrombocytopenia, leukopenia
• Evaluate for signs, symptoms of CNS toxicity

PATIENT AND FAMILY EDUCATION
Warn/advise
• That discomfort at application site is expected after 24 hr, lasting 2-4 days
• To use soap and water to clean application area and to remove drug

STORAGE
• Store at room temp in light-resistant container

---

polythiazide
Brand Name(s): Renese
Classification: Diuretic, antihypertensive
Pregnancy Category: C

AVAILABLE PREPARATIONS
Tabs: 1 mg, 2 mg, 4 mg

ROUTES AND DOSAGES
Children: PO 0.02-0.08 mg/kg qd
Adult: PO 1-4 mg qd

MECHANISM AND INDICATIONS
Diuretic mechanism: Inhibits Na reabsorption in the cortical diluting nephron tubule, promoting urinary excretion of Na and water and relieving edema
Antihypertensive mechanism: Exact mechanism unclear but thought to be caused by direct arteriolar vasodilatation and decreased peripheral resistance
Indications: Edema, hypertension

PHARMACOKINETICS
Onset of action: 3 hr
Peak: 5 hr
Half-life: 27 hr
Metabolism: Liver
Excretion: Urine, feces

CONTRAINDICATIONS AND PRECAUTIONS
• Contraindicated with known hypersensitivity to medication or other sulfonamides, anuria
• Use cautiously with severe renal, hepatic disease; pts taking digoxin

INTERACTIONS
Drug
• Increased hypotensive effects of other antihypertensives
• Increased hyperglycemia, hypotension, hyperuricemia with diazoxide
• Increased levels of lithium, amphetamines, quinidine
• Decreased effects of methenamine mandelate
• Decreased absorption with cholestyramine, colestipol

Lab
• Increased BG, urate, cholesterol, triglycerides
• Interference with parathyroid tests

SIDE EFFECTS
CNS: Dizziness, vertigo, paresthesias, headache, weakness, restlessness
CV: Hypotension, dehydration, hypercholesterolemia, hypertriglyceridemia
DERM: Rash, dermatitis, photosensitivity, purpura
GI: Nausea, vomiting, anorexia, heartburn, cramps, diarrhea, constipation, pancreatitis, jaundice
HEME: Aplastic anemia
Other: Agranulocytosis, leukopenia, thrombocytopenia, hyperuricemia, gout, hyperglycemia, hyponatremia, hypochloremia, hypercalcemia, hypokalemia, metabolic alkalosis, pneumonitis, vasculitis, muscle spasm

TOXICITY AND OVERDOSE
Clinical signs: GI irritation, hypermotility, diuresis, lethargy, coma
Treatment: Induce emesis or gastric lavage for recent ingestion; supportive measures as necessary

PATIENT CARE MANAGEMENT
Assessment
• Assess history of hypersensitivity to drug, sulfonamides
• Assess baseline VS, B/P, wt, hydration status
• Assess baseline electrolytes, renal function (BUN, creatinine) serum uric acid
Interventions
• Administer PO in AM to prevent nocturia
• May administer with food if nausea occurs
Evaluation
• Evaluate therapeutic response (decreased B/P, decreased edema)
• Evaluate for side effects, hypersensitivity

P

• Evaluate electrolytes, renal function (BUN, creatinine), serum uric acid regularly
• Monitor wt, I&O regularly

PATIENT AND FAMILY EDUCATION
Teach/instruct
• About need for medication; to take for prescribed amount of time
• That medication should be administered in AM to prevent nocturia
• That urination will be more frequent
• To monitor wt regularly, to report increased wt or edema
Warn/advise
• To notify care provider of side effects, hypersensitivity
• To identify signs of electrolyte imbalance (weakness, fatigue, muscle cramps, paresthesias, confusion, nausea, vomiting, diarrhea, headache, palpitations, dizziness); to report them immediately
• About how to identify photosensitivity reactions
• To avoid hazardous activities until treatment is well established
• To immediately report SOB, chest pain, back or leg pain
Encourage
• To increase intake of K+-rich foods (including bananas, citrus fruits, potatoes, tomatoes, raisins, dates, apricots), to restrict salt intake and high-Na foods
• That regular medical follow-up will be necessary

STORAGE
• Store at room temp

---

potassium salts
Brand Name(s): Potassium acetate, potassium bicarbonate: Klor-con, EF, K-Lyte, quic-K; potassium chloride: Kaochlor, Kaon-a, Kato, Kay Ciel, K-Dur, K-tab, Potachlor, Rum-K, Slow K, Ten-K; potassium gluconate: Kaon, Kolyum

Classification: Potassium supplement (electrolyte)

Pregnancy Category: C

AVAILABLE PREPARATIONS
Inj: 2 mEq/ml, 4 mEq/ml (acetate); 1.5 mEq/ml, 2 mEq/ml, 3 mEq/ml (chloride)
Liquid: 10 mEq/15 ml, 15 mEq/15 ml, 20 mEq/15 ml, 30 mEq/15 ml, 40 mEq/15 ml, 45 mEq/15 ml (chloride)
Liquid, sugarfree: 20 mEq/15 ml (gluconate)
Tabs, effervescent: 20 mEq, 25 mEq, 50 mEq (chloride); 25 mEq, 50 mEq (bicarbonate)
Tabs, sus rel: 6.7 mEq, 8 mEq, 10 mEq (chloride)
Tabs: 2 mEq, 5 mEq (gluconate)
Powder: 15 mEq, 20 mEq, 25 mEq (chloride); 20 mEq/packet (gluconate)
Caps, controlled release: 8 mEq, 10 mEq (chloride)

ROUTES AND DOSAGES
• Doses listed as mEq of K+
Normal Daily Requirement
Neonates: PO/IV 2-6 mEq/kg/24 hr
Children: PO/IV 2-3 mEq/kg/24 hr
Adults: PO/IV 40-80 mEq/kg/24 hr
Prevention of Hypokalemia During Diuretic Therapy
Children: PO 1-2 mEq/kg/24 hr in 1-2 divided doses
Adults: PO 20-40 mEq/kg/24 hr in 1-2 divided doses
Treatment of Hypokalemia
Children: PO/IV 2-5 mEq/kg/24 hr
Adults: PO/IV 40-100 mEq/kg/24 hr
IV administration
• Recommended concentration: <40 mEq/L in DLR, D_5LR, D_5NS,

✦ Available in Canada.

$D_5W, D_{10}W, D_{20}W, LR, NS, \frac{1}{2}NS, R$
• Maximum concentration: <80 mEq for IV infusion; greater concentrations may be used as bolus; rate not to exceed 0.5-1 mEq/kg/hr
• IV push rate: Contraindicated
• Intermittent infusion rate: <0.5-1 mEq/kg/hr
• Continuous infusion rate: (Dilute before administration)
• Children, 0.5-1 mEq/kg/hr (maximum 1 mEq/kg/hr); adults, 10 mEq/hr (maximum 40 mEq) to infuse over 2-3 hr

MECHANISM AND INDICATIONS

Mechanism: K^+ is necessary for transmission of nerve impulses, cardiac contraction, maintenance of normal renal function, acid base balance, carbohydrate metabolism, gastric secretion
Indications: For use in treatment or prevention of hypokalemia

PHARMACOKINETICS

Absorption: PO rapid, IV immediate
Excretion: Urine

CONTRAINDICATIONS AND PRECAUTIONS

• Contraindicated with severe renal impairment, hyperkalemia, Addison's disease, acute dehydration, K^+-sparing diuretics
• Use cautiously with cardiac or renal disease, acidosis, pregnancy, lactation

INTERACTIONS

Drug
• Hyperkalemia with K^+-sparing diuretics, captopril, salt substitutes containing K^+
• Increased GI upset with NSAIDs, heparin
• Decreased K^+ effects with corticosteroids
Nutrition
• Foods high in K^+ can increase hyperkalemia; salt substitutes may be high in K^+

INCOMPATIBILITIES

• Amikacin, amphotericin B, dobutamine, fat emulsion, potassium G sodium

SIDE EFFECTS

CNS: Confusion, paresthesias of extremities, headache, lethargy, weakness
CV: Hypotension, cardiac arrhythmias, heart block, cardiac arrest, ECG changes (prolonged PR interval; wide QRS complexes; peaked, tented T waves; depressed ST segments)
DERM: Rash, pallor, cold extremities
GI: Nausea, vomiting, diarrhea, abdominal pain, ulceration of small bowel
GU: Oliguria
Local: Postinfusion phlebitis

TOXICITY AND OVERDOSE

Clinical signs: Increased serum K^+, (listed side effects are signs of hyperkalemia), K^+ levels of 8-11 mEq/L may cause death from arrhythmias and cardiac arrest
Treatment: Discontinue K^+ supplementation, gastric lavage if K^+ level >6.5 mEq/L; provide supportive therapy, continuous ECG monitoring, infuse $NaHCO_3$, D_{10} or D_{25} with insulin, dialysis and sodium polystyrene sulfonate resin may be necessary

PATIENT CARE MANAGEMENT

Assessment
• Assess ECG baseline and during treatment
• Assess serum K^+ levels (normal = 3.5-5.0)
• Assess I&O; notify care provider for decreased urinary output
• Assess VS, B/P baseline and during treatment
Interventions
• Administer IV diluted in large volume of parenteral sol; administer slowly by IV infusion; do not administer IM or SC
• Do not administer K^+ in the immediate post-op period until urine flow established
• Administer through large-bore needle in large vein when possible
• If rate of IV infusion exceeds 0.5 mEq K^+/kg/hr, pt should receive continuous ECG monitoring
• Administer PO ac or with meals;

P

may administer with small amounts of juice

Evaluation

• Evaluate therapeutic response (decreased muscle weakness, decreased thirst, normalizing ECG, normal cardiac rate and rhythm
• Evaluate serum K^+ levels

PATIENT AND FAMILY EDUCATION

Teach/instruct

• To take as directed at prescribed intervals for prescribed length of time
• To administer PO with or before meals; may administer with small amounts of juice
• Symptoms of hyperkalemia (lethargy, confusion, diarrhea, nausea, vomiting, fainting), report to health care provider
• Symptoms of hypokalemia (fatigue, weakness, polydipsia, polyuria), report to health care provider

Warn/advise

• About importance of keeping regular follow-up appointments
• About foods high in K^+ (citrus fruits, bananas, raisins, potatoes); excess intake of these foods may cause hyperkalemia
• To take caps, powders, tabs with ample fluid
• That K^+ sol should be administered with fruit juices

STORAGE

• Store at room temp in tightly covered, light-resistant containers

---

praziquantel
Brand Name(s): Biltricide
Classification: Anthelmintic
Pregnancy Category: B

AVAILABLE PREPARATIONS

Tabs: 600 mg

ROUTES AND DOSAGES

Schistosomiasis

Children >4 yr and adults: PO 20 mg/kg/dose bid-tid for 1 day at 4-6 hr intervals

Flukes

Children and adults: PO 75 mg/kg/24 hr divided q8h for 1-2 days

Cysticercosis

Children and adults: PO 50 mg/kg/24 hr divided q8h for 14 days (administer steroids before praziquantel for neurocysticercosis)

Tapeworms

Children and adults: PO 10-20 mg/kg as one dose

MECHANISM AND INDICATIONS

Mechanism: Causes contraction and paralysis of worm musculature, leading to dislodgement; worms carried to liver for phagocytosis

Indications: Used to treat schistosomiasis, liver flukes, lung flukes, intestinal flukes, tapeworms

PHARMACOKINETICS

Peak: 1-3 hr
Distribution: Crosses blood–brain barrier
Half-life: 48-90 min
Metabolism: Liver
Excretion: Urine

CONTRAINDICATIONS AND PRECAUTIONS

• Contraindicated with known hypersensitivity to praziquantel; lactation
• Use cautiously with severe hepatic disease, seizure disorders, children <4 yr, pregnancy

SIDE EFFECTS

CNS: Vertigo, drowsiness, malaise, fever, headaches, increased seizure activity
DERM: Rash, pruritus, urticaria
GI: Abdominal pain, nausea, vomiting, anorexia, diarrhea, increased liver enzymes

PATIENT CARE MANAGEMENT

Assessment

• Assess history of hypersensitivity to praziquantel
• Assess for parasites in stool cultures
• Diagnose lung fluke infestation using sputum tests
• Obtain dietary histories (inges-

---

tion of raw fish, improperly cooked meat, recent travel)
• Assess baseline liver function tests (AST, ALT, bilirubin)
Interventions
• Administer with meals, follow with water to minimize GI discomfort
• Tabs are very bitter, may cause vomiting or gagging if not completely swallowed; do not crush or chew; may score into 4 segments, mix with small amount of food or fluids
• Administer corticosteroid as ordered to reduce CNS effects
• Use effective hygiene techniques (especially handwashing)
• Administer laxatives before treatment to cleanse bowel
Evaluation
• Evaluate therapeutic response (expulsion of worms)
• Evaluate for CSF reaction (headache, high fever)
• Evaluate spread of infection to other household members; treat as necessary

PATIENT AND FAMILY EDUCATION
Teach/instruct
• To take as directed at prescribed intervals for prescribed length of time
• About proper hygiene procedures (especially good handwashing techniques)
• About how to prevent reinfection; to change undergarments and bed linens; to wash clothes and linens in hot water; not to shake bed linens into the air; to frequently cleanse perianal area
• To clean toilet every day with disinfectant
• To wash all fruits and vegetables before eating
• To refrain from breastfeeding on day of treatment and for 72 hr after
Warn/advise
• To notify care provider of hypersensitivity
• That all family members need to be checked and treated
• To avoid hazardous activities since drowsiness may occur

Encourage
• To comply with treatment regime
STORAGE
• Store at room temp in tight container

**prednisolone,
prednisolone acetate,
prednisolone sodium
phosphate,
prednisolone tebutate**

Brand Name(s): Blephamide, Delta-Cortef, Diopred♣, Inflamase Forte♣, Inflamase Mild♣, Optho-Tate♣, Pediapred♣, Pred Forte♣, Pred Mild♣, Prelone

Classification: Glucocorticoid

Pregnancy Category: C

AVAILABLE PREPARATIONS
Tabs: 5 mg (prednisolone)
Syr: 15 mg/5 ml (prednisolone)
Oral liquid: 5 mg/5 ml (prednisolone sodium phosphate)
Inj: 25, 50, 100 mg/ml (prednisolone acetate); 20 mg/ml (prednisolone sodium phosphate); 20 mg/ml (prednisolone tebutate)
Ophthal susp: 0.12%, 0.125%, 1% (prednisolone acetate)

ROUTES AND DOSAGES
Antiinflammatory or Immunosuppressive
Children and adolescents: PO/IV 0.1-2 mg/kg/24 hr divided qd-qid
Acute Asthma
Children and adolescents: PO 1-2 mg/kg/24 hr qd or divided bid × 3-5 days; IV 2-4 mg/kg/24 hr divided tid-qid
Nephrotic Syndrome
Children and adolescents: PO initial, 2 mg/kg/24 hr divided tid-qid until urine is protein-free for 5 days or for maximum 28 days (maximum 80 mg/24 hr); if proteinuria persists, 4 mg/kg/dose qod for additional 28 days (maximum

P

♣ Available in Canada.

120 mg/24 hr); maintenance 2 mg/kg/dose qod × 28 days, then taper over 4-6 wk

Conjunctivitis, Corneal Injury
Children and adolescents: Ophthal 1-2 gtt into conjunctival sac q1h during day, q2h at night until desired response, then 1 gtt q4h

IV administration
• Recommended concentration: May be administered without further dilution; may be added to NS or D_5W for IV infusion; may be administered by slow IV push
• IVP push rate: Slow (over at least 1 min); if tingling or burning slow infusion rate

MECHANISM AND INDICATIONS

Mechanism: Decreases inflammation mainly by stabilizing leukocyte lysosomal membranes; suppresses immune response, stimulates bone marrow, influences protein, fat, and carbohydrate metabolism

Indications: Used for antiinflammatory or immunosuppressant effects in treatment of severe inflammation, asthma, immunosuppression, neoplasms; in acute life-threatening infections with massive antibiotic therapy, supplemental therapy for severe allergic reactions, shock unresponsive to conventional therapy; ophthal used in palpebral and bulbar conjunctivitis, corneal injury

PHARMACOKINETICS

Onset of action: IV/IM/PO rapid
Peak: IV/IM 1 hr; PO 1-2 hr
Absorption: Rapid, primarily into lymph
Duration: PO 30-36 hr; IM up to 4 wk
Metabolism: Liver
Excretion: Urine

CONTRAINDICATIONS AND PRECAUTIONS

• Contraindicated with known hypersensitivity to this drug or sulfites; systemic fungal infections, acute or active infections, chicken pox, herpes zoster
• Use cautiously with GI ulceration, renal disease, hypertension, osteoporosis, varicella, DM, seizures, CHF, emotional instability, psychotic tendencies, tuberculosis, ocular herpes simplex, thromboembolytic tendencies, pregnancy

INTERACTIONS

Drug
• Increased GI bleeding or distress with aspirin, indomethacin, other NSAIDs
• Decreased action possible with barbiturates, phenytoin, rifampin
• Decreased effects of oral anticoagulants possible
• Potentiates cyclosporin
• Enhanced K^+-wasting effects of prednisolone with K^+-depleting drugs (thiazide diuretics, amphotericin-B, digitalis products)
• Decreased response of skin-test antigens
• Decreased antibody response, increased risk of neurologic complications with toxoids and vaccines

Lab
• Increased serum cholesterol, Na, BG levels possible
• Decreased serum Ca and K^+ levels possible

INCOMPATIBILITIES

• Calcium gluconate, calcium gluceptate, dimenhydrinate, methotrexate, polymixin B, prochlorperazine, promazine, promethazine

SIDE EFFECTS

• Most reactions are dosage- and duration-dependent
CNS: Euphoria, insomnia, psychotic behavior, pseudotumor cerebri
CV: CHF, hypertension, edema with fluid or electrolyte imbalance, increased intracranial pressure, euphoria
EENT: Cataracts, glaucoma
ENDO/METAB: Hypokalemia, hyperglycemia, glucose intolerance, growth suppression, cushingoid state
DERM: Delayed wound healing, acne, skin eruptions
GI: Peptic ulcer, GI irritation, increased appetite, pancreatitis

✦ Available in Canada.

GU: Menstrual irregularities, decrease in spermatozoa

Other: Muscle weakness, osteoporosis, hirsutism, susceptibility to infection, spontaneous fractures; acute adrenal insufficiency may follow increased stress (infection, surgery, trauma) or abrupt withdrawal after long therapy; after abrupt withdrawal, there may be rebound inflammation, fatigue, weakness, arthralgias, fever, dizziness, lethargy, depression, fainting, orthostatic hypotension, dyspnea, anorexia, hypoglycemia; may be fatal

TOXICITY AND OVERDOSE

Clinical signs: Acute ingestion is rarely a clinical problem

Treatment: Decrease drug gradually (if possible)

PATIENT CARE MANAGEMENT

Assessment

• Assess history of hypersensitivity to prednisolone, related drugs
• Assess baseline VS (especially B/P), serum electrolytes (K+, Ca, Na, BG), cardiac function, renal function (BUN, creatinine, urine CrCl), liver function (ALT, AST, LDH, bilirubin, alk phos)
• Assess baseline wt, I&O, hydration status (SG), dysuria, urinary frequency
• Assess neurologic and mental status before starting therapy
• Assess baseline growth and development status
• Assess history of previous treatment with special attention to other therapies that may predispose pt to renal, hepatic, or cardiac dysfunction

Interventions

• Administer PO with food to decrease GI irritation
• Administer IM deeply in large muscle mass; rotate injection sites
• Prednisolone sodium phosphate should only be administered IV; never use IV administration with acetate or tebutate
• Monitor I&O, wt, VS (especially B/P)
• Provide supportive measures to maintain fluid and electrolyte balance, nutritional support
• Administer K+ supplements as indicated
• Provide low-Na, high-protein, high-K+ diet
• See Chapter 2 regarding ophthal instillation; shake susp before instillation, wash hands before and after; cleanse crusts and discharge from eye, apply gentle pressure with finger to lacrimal sac for 1 min to minimize systemic absorption, wipe excess medication from eye; do not flush medication from eye; wait 5-10 min before instilling another eye preparation

---

NURSING ALERT

Do not confuse with prednisone

Administer with food to decrease GI irritation

Provide low-Na, high-K+, high-protein diet

Do not stop drug abruptly with long-term therapy; dosage must be tapered over time

Administer IV dose over at least 1 min

Do not administer acetate or tebutate IV

Evaluation

• Evaluate therapeutic response (decreased inflammation)
• Monitor VS (especially B/P), serum electrolytes (K+, BG, Ca)
• Monitor I&O, check wt regularly
• Monitor for any signs of depression or psychotic episodes (especially with high-dosage therapy)
• Monitor BG in pts with history of diabetes
• Monitor growth and development in children on prolonged therapy
• Monitor for signs or symptoms of infection (fever, fatigue, sore throat)

P

PATIENT AND FAMILY EDUCATION
Teach/instruct
- To take as directed at prescribed intervals for prescribed length of time
- About importance of follow-up to monitor, serum chemistry values
- To notify care provider of signs of infection (fever, sore throat, fatigue), signs of delayed healing
- About the possibility of weakening bones with prolonged therapy (osteoporosis) and the need for proper exercise, diet, limitations
- Not to stop drug abruptly or discontinue without consent of care provider because of possible side effects associated with abrupt withdrawal
- To take medication in AM with breakfast for best results and less GI upset
- About cushingoid symptoms with long-term therapy; to report sudden wt gain or swelling
Warn/advise
- To avoid OTC products containing aspirin, NSAIDs
- To report any alterations in behavior; help to develop a plan of care to manage side effects, stress of illness or treatment
- To avoid contact with known viral or bacterial illnesses
- That household contacts of child not be immunized with live polio virus; inactivated form should be used
- That child not receive immunizations until immune system recovers sufficiently to mount needed antibody response
- To report exposure to chicken pox in susceptible child immediately
- To report reactivation of herpes zoster virus (shingles) immediately
- To notify care provider of signs or symptoms of adrenal insufficiency (fatigue, muscle weakness, joint pain, fever, anorexia, nausea, dyspnea, dizziness, fainting)
- That pts with diabetes may need more insulin while on steroids; monitor BG carefully

- That pts on long-term therapy need to have periodic ophthal examinations
- To limit the amount of salt or salty foods while on steroids; use low-Na, high-K+, high-protein diet
- About impact of body changes that may occur (wt gain, cushingoid syndrome), how to minimize them (loose clothing, decrease salt intake)
Encourage
- That pts experiencing excessive wt gain need to decrease salt intake; to eat a high-protein, high-K+ diet; a nutritional consultation may be needed
- To wear medical alert identification as a steroid user

STORAGE
- Store all forms at room temp in tight containers
- Protect from light

---

prednisone
Brand Name(s): Apo-Prednisolone♣, Deltasone♣, Liquid Pred, Meticorten, Orasone, Ptenicen-M, Sterapred, Winpred♣

Classification: Glucocorticoid

Pregnancy Category: C

AVAILABLE PREPARATIONS
Tabs: 1 mg, 2.5 mg, 5 mg, 10 mg, 20 mg, 50 mg
Oral sol: 5 mg/5 ml
Oral sol (concentrate): 5 mg/ml
Syr: 5 mg/5 ml

ROUTES AND DOSAGES
Antiinflammatory or Immunosuppressive
Children and adolescents: PO 0.5-2 mg/kg/24 hr or 25-60 mg/m²/24 hr divided q6-12h
Asthma, Acute Exacerbation
Children and adolescents: PO 0.5-2 mg/kg/24 hr × 3-5 days (maximum 20-40 mg/24 hr)
Chronic Refractory Asthma
Children and adolescents: PO 5-10 mg qd or 10-40 mg qod

♣ Available in Canada.

Nephrotic Syndrome

Children and adolescents: PO initial, 2 mg/kg/24 hr divided tid-qid until urine is protein-free for 5 days or for maximum 28 days (maximum 80 mg/24 hr); if proteinuria persists, 4 mg/kg/dose qod for additional 28 days (maximum 120 mg/24 hr); maintenance, 2 mg/kg/dose qod × 28 days, then taper over 4-6 wk

Physiologic Replacement

Children and adolescents: PO 4-5 mg/m^2/dose divided bid

MECHANISM AND INDICATIONS

Mechanism: Decreases inflammation mainly by stabilizing leukocyte lysosomal membranes; suppresses immune response, stimulates bone marrow, influences protein, fat, carbohydrate metabolism

Indications: Used for antiinflammatory or immunosuppressant effects in treatment of severe inflammation, asthma, immunosuppression, neoplasms, adrenocortical insufficiency

PHARMACOKINETICS

Half-life: 3.4-3.8 hr; excretion half-life 3-5 hr

Absorption: Readily absorbed from the GI tract

Peak: 1-2 hr

Duration: 30-36 hr

Metabolism: Liver

Excretion: Urine

CONTRAINDICATIONS AND PRECAUTIONS

• Contraindicated with history of hypersensitivity to prednisone, systemic fungal infections, acute or active infections, chicken pox or herpes zoster

• Use cautiously with GI ulceration, non-specific ulcerative colitis, renal disease, hypertension, thromboembolytic disorders, impaired hepatic function, tuberculosis, hypoalbuminemia, ocular herpes simplex, osteoporosis, varicella, DM, seizures, CHF, emotional instability, psychotic tendencies, pregnancy

INTERACTIONS

Drug

• Increased risk of GI bleeding or distress with aspirin, indomethacin, other NSAIDs

• Decreased action possible with barbiturates, phenytoin, rifampin

• Decreased effects of oral anticoagulants possible

• Decreased seizure threshold possible in pts taking anticonvulsants (phenytoin)

• Enhanced K$^+$-wasting (hypokalemia) effects of prednisone with K$^+$-depleting drugs (thiazide diuretics, amphotericin-B)

• Decreased response of skin-test antigens

• Decreased antibody response, increased risk of neurologic complications with toxoids and vaccines

• Increased hyperglycemia with asparaginase

Lab

• Increased serum cholesterol, Na, BG possible

• Decreased serum Ca, K$^+$ possible

• Decreased plasma cortisol or adrenal function assessed by ACTH stimulation possible

SIDE EFFECTS

• Most reactions are dose- and duration-dependent

CNS: Euphoria, insomnia, psychotic behavior, pseudotumor cerebri

CV: CHF, hypertension, edema

DERM: Delayed wound healing, acne, skin eruptions, increased sweating, facial edema

EENT: Cataracts, glaucoma

ENDO/METAB: Hypokalemia, hyperglycemia, glucose intolerance, growth suppression, cushingoid state

GI: Peptic ulcer, GI irritation, increased appetite, pancreatitis

Other: Muscle weakness, osteoporosis, hirsutism, susceptibility to infection, vertebral compression fractures, aseptic necrosis of femoral and humeral heads, pathologic fractures of long bones, acute adrenal insufficiency may

P

♣ Available in Canada.

follow increased stress (infection, surgery, trauma) or abrupt withdrawal after long therapy; after abrupt withdrawal, there may be rebound inflammation, fatigue, weakness, arthralgia, fever, dizziness, lethargy, depression, fainting, orthostatic hypotension, dyspnea, anorexia, hypoglycemia; may be fatal

TOXICITY AND OVERDOSE
Clinical signs: Acute ingestion is rarely a clinical problem
Treatment: Decrease drug gradually (if possible)

PATIENT CARE MANAGEMENT
Assessment
• Assess history of hypersensitivity to prednisone, related drugs
• Assess baseline VS (especially B/P), serum electrolytes (K+, Ca, Na, BG), cardiac function, renal function (BUN, creatinine, urine CrCl), liver function (ALT, AST, LDH, bilirubin, alk phos)
• Assess baseline wt, hydration status (SG), I&O
• Assess neurologic and mental status before starting therapy
• Assess baseline growth and development
• Assess history of previous treatment with special attention to other therapies that may predispose pt to renal, cardiac, or neurologic dysfunction

Interventions
• Administer medication with food whenever possible to decrease GI upset
• Monitor wt, I&O, and VS (especially B/P)
• Provide supportive measures to maintain fluid and electrolyte balance, nutritional support
• Administer K+ supplements as indicated
• Provide low-Na, high-protein, high-K+ diet

NURSING ALERT

Do not confuse with prednisolone

Administer with food to decrease chances of GI irritation

Provide low-Na, high-K+, high-protein diet

Do not stop drug abruptly if pt has been on long-term therapy; must be tapered over time

Drug has a bitter taste; place in caps (especially for children)

Evaluation
• Evaluate therapeutic response (decreased inflammation)
• Monitor VS (especially B/P), serum electrolytes (K+, BG, Ca)
• Monitor I&O, check wt regularly
• Evaluate for any signs of depression or psychotic episodes (especially with high-dosage therapy)
• Evaluate BG in pts with a history of diabetes
• Assess growth and development in children on prolonged therapy
• Assess for signs or symptoms of infection (fever, fatigue, sore throat)

PATIENT AND FAMILY EDUCATION
Teach/instruct
• To take as directed at prescribed intervals and for prescribed length of time
• About importance of follow-up to monitor serum chemistry values
• To notify care provider of signs of infection (fever, sore throat, fatigue) or delayed healing
• About the possibility of weakening bones (osteoporosis) with prolonged therapy; need for proper exercise, diet, limitations
• Not to stop drug abruptly or discontinue without care provider's consent because of possible side effects associated with abrupt withdrawal
• To take medication in the AM with breakfast to achieve best results and to decrease GI distress
• About cushingoid symptoms with long-term therapy; to report

---

✤ Available in Canada.

sudden wt gain or swelling

Warn/advise
• To avoid OTC products containing aspirin, NSAIDs
• To report any alterations in behavior; help to develop a plan of care to manage side effects, stress of illness or treatment
• To avoid contact with known viral or bacterial illnesses
• That household contacts of child not be immunized with with live polio virus; inactivated form should be used
• That child not receive immunizations until immune system recovers sufficiently to mount needed antibody response
• To report exposure to chicken pox in susceptible child immediately
• To report reactivation of herpes zoster virus (shingles) immediately
• To notify care provider of signs or symptoms of adrenal insufficiency (fatigue, muscle weakness, joint pain, fever, anorexia, nausea, dyspnea, dizziness, fainting)
• That pts on long-term therapy have periodic ophthal examinations
• That pts with diabetes may need more insulin while taking steroids; monitor BG carefully
• To limit the amount of salt or salty foods when taking steroids; use low-Na, high-K+, high-protein diet
• About impact of body changes that may occur (wt gain, cushingoid syndrome), how to minimize them (loose clothing, decrease salt intake)

Encourage
• That pts experiencing excessive wt gain to decrease salt intake; to eat a high-protein, high-K+ diet; nutritional consultation may be needed
• To wear medical alert identification as a steroid user

STORAGE
• Store all forms at room temp in tight containers
• Protect from light

primidone
Brand Name(s): Apo-Primidone♣, Midone, Mysoline, Neurosyn, Sertan
Classification: Anticonvulsant, barbiturate analog
Pregnancy Category: D

AVAILABLE PREPARATIONS
Tabs: 50 mg, 250 mg
Susp: 250 mg/5 ml

ROUTES AND DOSAGES
Neonates: PO 12-20 mg/kg/24 hr divided bid-qid; begin with lower dosage and titrate upwards
Children <8 yr: PO initial, 50-125 mg/24 hr given hs, increase by 50-125 mg/24 hr q 3-7 days; usual dosage 10-25 mg/kg/24 hr divided tid-qid
Children >8 yr and adults: PO initial, 125-250 mg/24 hr administered hs; increase by 125-250 mg/24 hr q 3-7 days; usual dosage 750-1500 mg/24 hr divided tid-qid; maximum dose 2 g/24 hr

MECHANISM AND INDICATIONS
Mechanism: Metabolized to two active metabolites, phenylethylmalonamide (PEMA) and phenobarbital; acts as a CNS depressant; anticonvulsant action has been attributed primarily to phenobarbital which acts to suppress presynaptic and postsynaptic discharges resulting in a lowering of the seizure threshold; the other metabolites are also responsible for seizure control, but mechanism(s) is not clearly understood
Indications: Used to treat all types of seizures except absence seizures

PHARMACOKINETICS
Absorption: Rapid and complete; primidone, and PEMA bound to plasma in small amounts, phenobarbital 50% plasma-bound; presence of phenobarbital in serum may be delayed a few days upon initiation of therapy
Peak: 3 hr

Half-life: 5-15 hr (phenobarbital), 16 hr (PEMA)

Metabolism: Liver, to 2 main metabolites, phenylethylmalonamide (PEMA), phenobarbital

Excretion: Urine, 40% unchanged; remainder unconjugated PEMA and small amounts of phenobarbital

Therapeutic serum levels: Primidone 5-12 mcg/ml; phenobarbital 10-30 mcg/ml

CONTRAINDICATIONS AND PRECAUTIONS

• Contraindicated with known hypersensitivity to barbiturates; porphyria, pregnancy, severe respiratory disease, status asthmaticus

INTERACTIONS
Drug

• Excessive depression with alcohol, other CNS depressants including narcotic analgesics
• Increased primidone levels with isoniazid, phenytoin
• Decreased effects possible with adrenocorticosteroids, anticoagulants, antidepressants, carbamazepine, dacarbazine, quinidine, phenytoin
• Increased metabolism of theophylline

Lab

• False positive phentolamine test
• Decreased serum bilirubin possible

Nutrition

• Increased excretion of ascorbic acid possible
• Decreased absorption of vitamin B_{12}, decreased level of vitamin D

SIDE EFFECTS

CNS: Stimulation, drowsiness, dizziness, confusion, sedation, headache, flushing, hallucinations, coma, psychosis, ataxia, vertigo

DERM: Rash, edema, alopecia, lupus-like syndrome

EENT: Diplopia, nystagmus, edema of the eyelids

GI: Nausea, vomiting, anorexia

GU: Impotence, polyuria

HEME: Thrombocytopenia, leukopenia, neutropenia, eosinophilia, megaloblastic anemia, decreased serum folate level, lymphadenopathy

TOXICITY AND OVERDOSE

Clinical signs: Similar to symptoms of barbiturate intoxication (CNS and respiratory depression, oliguria, tachycardia, hypotension, hypothermia; coma, areflexia, shock may occur)

Treatment: Supportive care; monitor VS, I&O, electrolytes (Na, K+); support ventilation and pulmonary function prn; use vasopressors and IV fluids to support cardiac function and circulation; with recent ingestion, induce emesis in conscious pt with ipecac; if emesis is contraindicated, use gastric lavage followed by charcoal or saline cathartic; it may be helpful to alkalinize the urine and force diuresis; hemodialysis may be necessary

PATIENT CARE MANAGEMENT
Assessment

• Assess history of hypersensitivity to barbiturates
• Assess seizure type and determine appropriate anticonvulsant for this type of seizure
• Assess preexisting physical condition and current medications to avoid potential interactions
• Assess baseline laboratory studies, including CBC, differential and liver function (ALT, AST, bilirubin, alk phos)
• Drug interactions are frequent, particularly with drugs metabolized in liver; check serum levels to avoid either increased or decreased levels

Interventions

• Initiate drug at modest dosage
• Increase dosage/level prn to control seizures, to the point of intolerable side effects
• Initiate another drug concurrently if 1st drug is only partially effective
• If not effective, discontinue and initiate a new medication
• If break-through seizures are occurring at times of trough serum levels or toxicity at times of peak,

increase frequency of administration

- Shake PO susp well before administering each dose

Evaluation

- Evaluate therapeutic response (seizure control); initially done more frequently until seizures are controlled, then q 3-6 mo, or if seizure breakthrough or side effects occur
- Monitor anticonvulsant levels periodically
- Monitor PT/INR in pts taking anticoagulants
- Evaluate neurologic status (alterations or deterioration)
- Evaluate for signs and symptoms of toxicity

PATIENT AND FAMILY EDUCATION

Teach/instruct

- To take as prescribed, not to change dosage independently or withdraw drug suddenly
- That contents of oral sol settle; shake well before administration to avoid over- or under-dosing
- About process for initiating anticonvulsant drugs, need for frequent visits (especially initially)
- Rationale for measuring serum levels, how these should be obtained (peak/trough)

Warn/advise

- About potential side effects, encourage to report serious side effects immediately (drowsiness, hyperirritability, mental confusion, rash, fever)
- That unpleasant side effects may decrease as pt becomes more used to the drug
- That drug initially may be more sedating until pt becomes used to it; avoid hazardous tasks (bike, skates, skateboard) that require mental alertness until stabilized
- To make other health care providers aware of this medication in order to avoid drug interactions
- To inform care provider if pregnancy should occur while taking drug

Encourage

- To keep a record of any seizures (seizure calendar)

STORAGE

- Store in tightly closed containers at room temp, avoid freezing
- Expiration date is 5 yr from manufacture date

probenecid

Brand Name(s): Benemid✤, Benuryl✤, Probalan

Classification: Uricosuric agent (sulfonamide derivative)

Pregnancy Category: B

AVAILABLE PREPARATIONS

Tabs: 500 mg

ROUTES AND DOSAGES

Adjunct to penicillin/cephalosporin treatment

Children 2-14 yr or <50 kg: PO initial 25 mg/kg as single dose, maintenance 40 mg/kg/24 hr divided qid (maximum single dose 500 mg)

Children >14 yr or >50 kg and adults: PO 500 mg qid

Hyperuricemia

Adults: PO 250 mg bid for 1 wk; increase to 500 mg bid; increase q 4 wk if needed to maximum 2-3 g/24 hr

Single-Dose Penicillin Treatment of Gonorrhea

Adults: PO 1 g administered with oral penicillin or 1 g 30 min before IM penicillin

MECHANISM AND INDICATIONS

Uricosuric mechanism: Competitively inhibits reabsorption of uric acid at the proximal convoluted tubule, thus promoting its excretion and reducing serum uric acid levels; increase plasma levels of weak organic acids (penicillins, cephalosporins) by competitively inhibiting their renal tubular secretion

Indications: Used to treat gonorrhea, hyperuricemia in gout, gouty arthritis, as adjunct to penicillin or cephalosporin treatment

P

✤ Available in Canada.

PHARMACOKINETICS
Peak: 2-4 hr
Half-life: 4-17 hr
Metabolism: Liver
Excretion: Urine

CONTRAINDICATIONS AND PRECAUTIONS
• Contraindicated with known hypersensitivity to probenecid, children <2 yr; pts with severe hepatic or renal impairment, blood dyscrasias, acute gout, uric acid kidney stones
• Use cautiously with history of peptic ulcer, renal impairment, severe respiratory disease, pregnancy, lactation

INTERACTIONS
Drug
• Increased or prolonged effects of penicillins, cephalosporins, other β-lactam antibiotics
• Increased toxicity of dapsone, aminosalicylic acid, methotrexate, nitrofurantoin, sulfa drugs, indomethacin, rifampin, naproxen
• Increased activity of oral anticoagulants
• Decreased action of oral hypoglycemics
• Decreased action with alcohol, salicylates, nitrofurantoin, diazoxides, diuretics
Lab
• False-positive urine glucose possible

SIDE EFFECTS
CNS: Headache, dizziness
CV: Hypotension
EENT: Sore gums
GI: Anorexia, nausea, vomiting, gastric distress
GU: Urinary frequency, renal colic, hematuria, uric acid stones
HEME: Leukopenia, hemolytic or aplastic anemia
Other: Hair loss, increased gouty arthritis attacks, fever, sweating, flushing, hypersensitivity

TOXICITY AND OVERDOSE
Clinical signs: Nausea, vomiting, stupor, coma, tonic-clonic seizures
Treatment: Supportive care; induced emesis or gastric lavage

PATIENT CARE MANAGEMENT
Assessment
• Assess history of hypersensitivity to probenecid
• Assess renal function (BUN, creatinine, I&O), uric acid levels, respiratory status, electrolytes, CO_2
Interventions
• Administer PO with food, milk, or prescribed antacids to reduce GI distress; tab may be crushed, mixed with food or fluid
• Maintain adequate hydration with high fluid intake to prevent formation of uric acid stones; maintain alkaline urine
• Provide low-purine diet, avoiding organ meats, anchovies, sardines, meat gravy, dried beans, meat extracts

> **NURSING ALERT**
> Discontinue if signs of hypersensitivity, rash, leukopenia, hemolytic or aplastic anemia develop

Evaluation
• Evaluate therapeutic response (absence of pain, stiffness in joints)
• Monitor renal function (BUN, creatinine, I&O), uric acid, electrolytes, CO_2
• Monitor for CNS symptoms (confusion, twitching, hyporeflexia, headache, stimulation)

PATIENT AND FAMILY EDUCATION
Teach/instruct
• To take as directed at prescribed intervals for prescribed length of time
Warn/advise
• To notify care provider of hypersensitivity, side effects
• To avoid use of alcohol or medications containing alcohol, high-purine foods, OTC medications (including aspirin)
• To maintain high fluid intake
• Not to use for pain, inflammation; not to increase during gouty attack

---

STORAGE
• Store at room temp

> ### procainamide hydrochloride
> **Brand Name(s):** Apo-Procainamide ✤, Procan SR ✤, Promine, Pronestyl ✤, Pronestyl SR ✤, Rhythmin, Sub-quin
>
> **Classification:** Antiarrhythmic
>
> **Pregnancy Category:** C

AVAILABLE PREPARATIONS
Tabs: 250 mg, 375 mg, 500 mg
Tabs, sus rel: 250 mg, 500 mg, 750 mg, 1 g
Caps: 250 mg, 375 mg, 500 mg
Inj: 100 mg/ml, 500 mg/ml

ROUTES AND DOSAGES
Infants: IV load 1 mg/kg/dose infused over 5 min, maintenance 20-80 mcg/kg/min continuous IV
Children: PO 15-50 mg/kg/24 hr divided q3-6h, maximum dose 4 g/24 hr; IV load 2-6 mg/kg/dose infused over 5 min, maintenance 20-80 mcg/kg/min continuous IV, maximum 100 mg/dose or 2 g/24 hr; IM 20-30 mg/kg/24 hr divided q4-6h, maximum dose 4 g/24 hr
Adults: PO 250-500 mg/dose q3-6h, may increase to 1500 mg/dose; IV load 50-100 mg/dose, repeat q5 min prn to maximum dose of 1-1.5 g, maintenance 1-6 mg/min continuous IV; IM loading dose 1 g once, maintenance 250 mg/dose q3h

IV administration
• Recommended concentration: 20-30 mg/ml loading, 2-4mg/ml continuous infusion
• Maximum concentration: 2-4 mg/ml; dilute in IV fluid to infuse ≤50 mg/min
• IV push rate: Over 5 min, do not exceed 50 mg/min
• Intermittent infusion rate: Loading dose over 25-30 min

• Continuous infusion rate: 20-80 mcg/kg/min

MECHANISM AND INDICATIONS
Antiarrhythmic mechanism: Decreases myocardial excitability and conduction velocity in atria, bundle of His, and ventricle; prolongs PR and QT interval
Indications: PVCs, atrial arrhythmias, PAT, atrial fibrillation, ventricular tachycardia

PHARMACOKINETICS
Onset of action: 10-30 min
Peak: 1 hr
Half-life: 2½-4¾ hr
Metabolism: Liver
Excretion: Urine

CONTRAINDICATIONS AND PRECAUTIONS
• Contraindicated with known hypersensitivity, complete heart block, digitalis toxicity, myasthenia gravis, prolonged QT interval, Torsades de Pointes
• Use cautiously with 1st- or 2nd-degree block or bundle branch block, CHF, renal or hepatic disease, respiratory depression

INTERACTIONS
Drug
• Increased effects of procainamide with neuromuscular blockers, cimetidine
• Increased effects of anticholinergics, antihypertensives
• Decreased effects of procainamide with barbiturates
• Additive or antagonistic effects with other antiarrhythmics
Lab
• Invalidated bentiromide
• Interference with edrophonium test, ANA titer, Coombs' test
• Decreased leukocytes, platelets possible
• Increased bilirubin, lactic dehydrogenase, alk phos, ALT, AST

INCOMPATIBILITIES
• Phenytoin

SIDE EFFECTS
CNS: Confusion, dizziness, headache, depression, convulsions, hallucinations, psychosis, restlessness, irritability, weakness

P

✤ Available in Canada.

CV: Hypotension, bradycardia, heart block, cardiac collapse or arrest, ventricular fibrillation
DERM: Rash, edema, pruritus, swelling, urticaria
GI: Anorexia, nausea, vomiting, diarrhea, hepatomegaly, bitter taste
Other: Lupus, agranulocytosis, thrombocytopenia, neutropenia, hemolytic anemia, fever

TOXICITY AND OVERDOSE

Clinical signs: Severe hypotension, widening of QRS complex, junctional tachycardia, intraventricular conduction delay, ventricular fibrillation, nausea, vomiting, oliguria, lethargy, confusion
Treatment: Induce vomiting, gastric lavage, inactivated charcoal for recent ingestion; supportive measures (including cardiovascular and respiratory support); phenylephrine or norepinephrine for severe hypotension; hemodialysis if necessary

PATIENT CARE MANAGEMENT

Assessment
• Assess history of hypersensitivity to drug
• Assess baseline VS, B/P, ECG
• Assess baseline ANA titer, CBC
Interventions
• Do not crush sus rel tabs
• Monitor VS and B/P continuously when initiating IV therapy
Evaluation
• Evaluate therapeutic response (decrease in arrhythmias)
• Evaluate for side effects, hypersensitivity
• Monitor ECG regularly
• Evaluate labs (ANA titer, CBC regularly)
• Monitor procainamide levels; therapeutic procainamide levels are 3-10 mcg/ml

PATIENT AND FAMILY EDUCATION

Teach/instruct
• To take as directed at prescribed intervals for prescribed length of time

• About need for frequent monitoring, blood studies
Warn/advise
• To notify care provider of side effects, hypersensitivity
Provide
• Emotional support as indicated

STORAGE

• Store at room temp

---

procarbazine

Brand Name(s): Matulane✤
Classification: Antineoplastic, cell cycle phase specific (S and G2 phase)
Pregnancy Category: D

AVAILABLE PREPARATIONS

Caps: 50 mg

ROUTES AND DOSAGES

• Dosage may vary in response to diagnosis, extent of disease, concurrent or previous therapy, protocol guidelines, physiologic parameters; consult current literature, protocol recommendations
Single Agent
PO 50-200 mg/m^2/24 hr, generally for 14 days; calculate dose to nearest 50 mg; 50 mg/m^2/24 hr for 1 wk, then increase to 100 mg/m^2/24 hr until maximum disease response or evidence of leukopenia or thrombocytopenia occurs, dosage then maintained at 50 mg/m^2/24 hr until evidence of toxicity is noted; continual low-dosage regimens may increase risk of drug-induced malignancies
Combination Chemotherapy for Hodgkin's Disease
PO 100 mg/m^2/24 hr for 14 days repeated at varying intervals
Combination Chemotherapy for Brain Tumors
PO 75-100 mg/m^2/24 hr repeated q 4-6 wk

MECHANISM AND INDICATIONS

Mechanism: Exact mechanism unknown; multiple reactive intermediates formed after microsomal metabolism; intermediates induce chromosomal damage, demonstrate antimitotic effects by prolonging interphase, inhibit DNA, RNA, protein synthesis; effect on DNA similar to effect of ionizing radiation or bifunctional alkylating agents

Indications: Hodgkin's disease, non-Hodgkin's lymphoma, brain tumors, malignant melanoma, multiple myeloma; polycythemia vera, lupus erythematous, graph versus host disease

PHARMACOKINETICS

Peak: 1 hr (serum); 30-90 min (CSF)

Distribution: Rapid; distributes widely in liver, kidney, intestine, skin, CNS, CSF

Metabolism: Liver, kidney biotransformation

Excretion: 25%-75% in urine within 24 hr (metabolites); also expired from lungs as methane and CO_2

CONTRAINDICATIONS AND PRECAUTIONS

• Contraindicated with pregnancy, lactation, history of hypersensitivity to drug; active infection (especially chicken pox or herpes zoster); poor bone marrow reserve
• Use cautiously with impaired hepatic or renal function

INTERACTIONS

Drug

• Nausea, vomiting, headache, visual disturbances, respiratory difficulty, weakness, vertigo, confusion, diaphoresis, thirst, chest pain, decreased B/P possible with alcohol
• Hypertensive crises, tremors, excitation, cardiac palpitations, chest pain, fevers, seizures possible with concurrent use of antidepressants and MAOIs
• Additive CNS depression, respiratory depression possible with narcotic analgesics, antihistamines, phenothiazines, barbiturates, antihypertensives such as methyldopa
• Increased incidence of neurotoxicity with mechlorethamine
• Concurrent administration of antioxidants may prevent spermatotoxicity without compromising therapeutic efficacy

Nutrition

• Hypertensive crisis, fever, seizures possible with tyramine-rich foods (dark beer, cheese, wine, bananas, yogurt, Brewer's yeast, pickled herring, chicken liver)

SIDE EFFECTS

CNS: Paraesthesias, neuropathies, vertigo, ataxia, headache, frequent nightmares, depression, insomnia, nervousness, hallucinations, tremors, coma, convulsions

CV: May precipitate hypertensive crisis if administered concurrently with tricyclic antidepressants, MAOIs, narcotic analgesics, tyramine-rich foods

DERM: Reversible alopecia, pruritus, flushing, hyperpigmentation, photosensitivity, reactivation of herpetic lesions

EENT: Nystagmus, diplopia, papilledema, photophobia, retinal hemorrhages, altered hearing ability, inability to focus eyes

GI: Nausea, vomiting, diarrhea (with tolerance increasing over repeated daily dosing); anorexia, protracted diarrhea, stomatitis, dry mouth, hepatic dysfunction, jaundice, GI bleeding, dysphagia, abdominal pain, constipation

GU: Azoospermia, cessation of menses always occurs; hematuria, urinary frequency, nocturia

HEME: Prolonged myelosuppression affecting all cell lines, recovery in 4-6 wk; hemolysis in patients with G-6-PD deficiency

RESP: Rare hypersensitivity reaction characterized by cough, pneumonitis, pleural effusion

Other: Flu-like syndrome fever, chills, diaphoresis, lethargy, myalgias, arthralgias most often limited to initial therapy; hypersensi-

P

tivity reaction (angioedema, urticaria); drug is potent teratogen; its use in MOPP therapy for Hodgkin's disease is associated with a 5%-10% risk of developing acute leukemia (especially in pts having received radiation therapy)

TOXICITY AND OVERDOSE
Clinical signs: CNS events, hypersensitivity, prolonged myelosuppression
Treatment: Supportive measures (blood transfusions, hydration, nutritional supplementation, broad-spectrum antibiotic therapy if febrile, electrolyte replacement)

PATIENT CARE MANAGEMENT
Assessment
• Assess history of hypersensitivity to drug
• Assess history of previous treatment
• Assess success of previous antiemetic regimens
• Assess baseline VS; CBC, differential, platelet count; renal function (BUN, creatinine), liver function (alk phos, LDH, AST, bilirubin)
• Assess medications being taken concurrently
• Assess dietary history
Interventions
• Administer antiemetic therapy before chemotherapy
• Instruct family to administer drug at night in order to decrease nausea, vomiting
• Provide supportive therapy to maintain hemostasis, fluid, electrolyte, nutritional balance
Evaluation
• Evaluate therapeutic response (radiologic or clinical demonstration of tumor regression)
• Evaluate CBC, differential, platelet count at least weekly
• Evaluate BUN, creatinine, alk phos, LDH, AST, bilirubin regularly
• Evaluate wt at regular intervals

PATIENT AND FAMILY EDUCATION
Teach/instruct
• To have pt well hydrated before and after chemotherapy
• About importance of follow-up to monitor blood counts, serum chemistry values, urinalysis
• To take accurate temp; rectal temp contraindicated
• To notify care provider of signs of bleeding (bluising, epistaxis, bleeding gums), infection (fever, sore throat, fatigue)
Warn/advise
• About impact of body changes that may occur (hair loss, hyperpigmentation, nail ridging), how to minimize changes (wigs, caps, scarves, long sleeves)
• To avoid OTC preparations containing aspirin
• To report any alterations in behavior, sensation, perception; help to develop a plan of care to manage side effects, stress of illness or treatment
• To call care provider immediately if fever or infection noted
• That good oral hygiene with very soft toothbrush is imperative
• That dental work be delayed until blood counts have returned to baseline, with permission of caretaker
• To avoid contact with known viral or bacterial illnesses
• That close household contacts of child not receive live polio virus; inactivated form should be used
• To report exposure to chicken pox in susceptible child immediately
• To report reactivation of herpes zoster virus (shingles) immediately
• To avoid tyramine-rich foods
• To avoid alcohol consumption including cough or cold preparations
• If appropriate, ways to preserve reproductive patterns, sexuality (sperm banking, contraceptives)
Encourage
• Provision of nutritious food intake, consider nutrition consultation

• To use top anesthetics to control discomfort of mucositis; avoid spicy foods, commercial mouthwashes

STORAGE

• Stable at room temp for about 2 yrs if protected from moisture

---

prochlorperazine, prochlorperazine edisylate, prochlorperazine maleate

Brand Name(s): Compazine, Nu-Prochlor✚, PMS-Prochlorperazine✚, Stemetil✚

Classification: Antiemetic, phenothiazine

Pregnancy Category: C

AVAILABLE PREPARATIONS

Tabs: 5 mg, 10 mg, 25 mg (prochlorperazine maleate)
Cap, ext rel: 10 mg, 15 mg, 30 mg (prochlorperazine maleate)
Syr: 5 mg/ml (prochlorperazine edisylate)
Inj: 5 mg/ml (prochlorperazine edisylate)
Rectal supp: 2.5 mg, 5 mg, 25 mg (prochlorperazine)

DOSAGES AND ROUTES

• Safety and effectiveness not established in children <9 kg or <2 yr
• Use lowest possible dosage in pediatric patients to minimize incidence of EPS
• Administer ext rel caps 1-2 times/24 hr, with same total daily dosages as tabs or syr

Antiemetic

Children >10 yr: PO/PR 0.4 mg/kg/24 hr divided tid-qid; IV not recommended; IM 0.1-0.15 mg/kg/dose

Treatment of Psychoses

Children 2-12 yr: PO/PR, initially 2.5 mg 2-3 ×/24 hr, increase dosage as needed, (maximum daily dose 20 mg for children age 2-5 yr,

25 mg for children age 6-12 yr); IM 0.13 mg/kg/dose, change to PO as soon as possible

Adults: PO initial 5-10 mg 3-4 ×/24 hr, increase dosage as needed; (maximum daily dose 150 mg/24 hr); IM 10-20 mg q4h as needed, change to PO as soon as possible

MECHANISM AND INDICATIONS

Mechanism: Blocks postsynaptic mesolimbic dopaminergic receptors in brain, depresses release of hypothalamic and hypophyseal hormones
Indications: For use in treatment of acute and chronic psychosis, management of nausea and vomiting

PHARMACOKINETICS

Onset of action: PO 30-40 min; ext rel 30-40 min; PR within 60 min; IM within 10-20 min
Duration: PO 3-4 hr; ext rel 10-12 hr; PO 3-4 hr; IM 12 hr
Metabolism: Liver
Excretion: Urine

CONTRAINDICATIONS AND PRECAUTIONS

• Contraindicated with hypersensitivity to this medication or any component, hypersensitivity to phenothiazines, bone marrow depression, severe cardiac disease, coma, severe toxic CNS depression, encephalopathy, narrow-angle glaucoma, severe liver disease, seizures
• Use cautiously with chicken pox, CNS infections, dehydration, gastroenteritis, measles, history of seizures, in pts <2 yr, pregnancy, lactation, allergy to sulfites or tartrazine dye

INTERACTIONS
Drug

• Additive effects with CNS depressants, epinephrine
• Decreased effects with antacids, barbiturates
• Increased anticholinergic action with anticholinergics, antidepressants, antiparkinson drugs

Lab
- False positive phenylketonuria, urinary amylase, uroporphyrins, urobilinogen

Nutrition
- IM sol contains sulfites which may cause allergic reactions
- Do not use in sensitive pts; some products contain tartrazine (yellow dye #5)

INCOMPATIBILITIES
- Incompatible with aminophylline, amobarbital, amphotericin B, ampicillin, Ca, cephalothin, chloramphenicol, chlorothiazide, dexamethasone, dimenhydrinate, epinephrine, erythromycin, heparin, hydrocortisone, hydromorphone, kanamycin, methicillin, methohexital, midazolam, penicillin G, pentobarbital, phenobarbital, phenytoin, prednisolone, secobarbital, tetracycline, thiopental, vancomycin
- Compatible if used within 15 min after mixing in a syringe with atropine, chlorpromazine, diphenhydramine, droperidol, fentanyl, glycopyrrolate, hydroxyzine, meperidine, metoclopramide, pentazocine, promazine, promethazine
- Do not mix with other drugs in syringe or sol

SIDE EFFECTS
CNS: Euphoria, EPS, anxiety, depression, dizziness, drowsiness, neuroleptic malignant syndrome, pseudo-parkinsonian reactions, restlessness, sedation, tardive dyskinesia, seizures, tremor
CV: Arrhythmias, hypotension, orthostatic hypotension, tachycardia, sudden death, circulatory failure
DERM: Contact dermatitis, hyperpigmentation, photosensitivity, pruritus, rash
EENT: Metallic taste, retinal pigmentation, blurred vision
GI: Anorexia, constipation, cramps, diarrhea, GI upset, cholestatic jaundice, dry mouth, nausea, vomiting, wt loss
GU: Amenorrhea, galactorrhea, gynecomastia, impotence, urinary retention

HEME: Agranulocytosis, eosinophilia, hemolytic anemia, leukopenia, thrombocytopenia
RESP: Respiratory depression
Other: Anaphylactoid reactions, abnormal glucose tolerance, wt gain

TOXICITY AND OVERDOSE
Clinical signs: Anticholinergic symptoms, cardiac arrhythmias, diaphoresis, EPS, hypertension, hypotension, rigidity, unarousable sleep, tachycardia
Treatment: If PO, induce emesis or gastric lavage; do not dialyze; for EPS, use IV benztropine mesylate 0.02-0.05 mg/kg/dose or for adults 1-2 mg/dose slowly over 3-6 min; for ventricular arrhythmias, use loading dose of phenytoin 10-15 mg/kg slow IV push; for hypotension, use IV fluids and norepinephrine or phenylephrine; for rigidity, PO dantrolene 0.5 mg/kg/dose q12h; avoid epinephrine, may cause hypotension caused by phenothiazine-induced α-adrenergic blockade and unopposed epinephrine β_2 action

PATIENT CARE MANAGEMENT
Assessment
- Assess history of hypersensitivity to drug
- Obtain baseline medical history and physical exam
- Assess nausea, vomiting, ability to function in daily activities
- Assess mental status (mood, sensorium, affect, impulsiveness, suicidal ideation, thoughts)
- Obtain baseline CBC with differential and ophthal exam if use will be long term

Interventions
- Administer IM in large muscle mass
- Avoid IV administration; if absolutely necessary, administer by direct IV at maximum rate 5 mg/min
- Rinse with water, take sips of fluid, sugarless gum, hard candy for dry mouth
- Increase fluids and fiber in diet if constipation occurs

♣ Available in Canada.

• Avoid skin contact with oral sol or injection; can cause contact dermatitis

NURSING ALERT
Do not administer SC; tissue damage may occur

Monitor for dystonic reactions (spasm of neck muscles, torticollis, extensor rigidity of back muscles, opisthotonos, trismus, mandibular tics) and tardive dyskinesia

A possible side effect is neuroleptic malignant syndrome

Evaluation
• Evaluate therapeutic response (ability to function in daily activities, nausea, vomiting, psychosis)
• Evaluate for signs of neuroleptic malignant syndrome (a possible effect); symptoms include fever, fast or irregular heartbeat, fast breathing, sweating, weakness, muscle stiffness, seizures, loss of bladder control; if these occur, obtain medical intervention immediately; monitor VS, ECG, urine output, renal function; symptom management with medications, hydration, cooling blankets
• Evaluate mental status (mood, sensorium, affect, impulsiveness, suicidal ideation, thoughts)
• Monitor respiratory status
• Monitor for dystonic reactions and neuroleptic malignant syndrome
• If used long term, monitor CBC with differential and ophthal status

PATIENT AND FAMILY EDUCATION
Teach/instruct
• To take as directed at prescribed intervals for prescribed length of time
• To make sure medication is swallowed
• That this medication is most helpful when used as part of a comprehensive, multimodal treatment program if used for psychosis

• Not to discontinue medication without prescriber approval
• To immediately report to prescriber symptoms of dystonia, tardive dyskinesia, neuroleptic malignant syndrome
Warn/advise
• That medication may cause drowsiness; be careful on bicycles, skates, skateboards, while driving, with other activities requiring alertness
• To stay out of direct sunlight (especially between 10 AM and 3 PM) if possible; if pt must be outside, to wear protective clothing, hat, sunglasses; to put on sunblock that has a skin protection factor (SPF) ≥15

STORAGE
• Store at room temp

proparacaine hydrochloride
Brand Name(s): Ak-Taine, Alcaine✣, Diocane✣, Kainair, Ocu-Caine, Opthaine, Ophthetic✣
Classification: Anesthetic, ophthalmic (local)
Pregnancy Category: C

AVAILABLE PREPARATIONS
Ophthal: 0.5% drops

ROUTES AND DOSAGES
Children and adults: Ophthal, instill 1 gtt of 0.5% sol 30 sec before diagnostic test, procedure, or suture removal; may repeat q 5-10 min for 5-7 doses (Safety and effectiveness not established in children. Dosage represents accepted standard practice recommendations. Drug has been used as a top anesthetic in children.)

MECHANISM AND INDICATIONS
Mechanism: Inhibits initiation and transmission of nerve impulses in neuronal membrane
Indications: Used to anesthetize the eye for tonometry or gonios-

✣ Available in Canada.

copy for removal of foreign bodies, sutures, or diagnostic conjunctival scraping

PHARMACOKINETICS
Onset: 13-30 sec
Duration: ≥15 min (increases with repeated doses)

CONTRAINDICATIONS AND PRECAUTIONS
• Contraindicated with known hypersensitivity to drug
• Use cautiously with ocular inflammation or infection, cardiac disease, hyperthyroidism

INTERACTIONS
Drug
• None known
Lab
• Inhibited growth of certain organisms possible, altering cultures taken for eye infections (may be prevented by using new, unopened bottle before culture)

SIDE EFFECTS
CNS: Muscle twitching, convulsions, CNS stimulation or depression, weakness (all rare)
CV: Irregular heartbeat (rare)
DERM: Rash, drying, and cracking if drug contacts skin (especially fingertips), increased sweating (rare)
EENT: Stinging, burning, conjunctival redness (may last several hr after application); immediate hypersensitivity reaction (rare): diffuse epithelial keratitis, sloughing of necrotic epithelium, corneal filaments, iritis, blurred vision (rare)
Other: Systemic toxicity (rare)

PATIENT CARE MANAGEMENT
Assessment
• Assess history of hypersensitivity to this and related drugs
Interventions
• Do not use if sol is amber in color
Evaluations
• Evaluate therapeutic response (eye is anesthetized sufficiently for procedure)

PATIENT AND FAMILY EDUCATION
Teach/instruct
• Not to rub eye because a corneal abrasion could occur
• That blink reflex is temporarily eliminated
Warn/advise
• To protect child's eye from injury after instillation because the cornea is anesthetized and blink reflex is temporarily absent
• To notify care provider of hypersensitivity, side effects

STORAGE
• Store at room temp
• Protect from light, avoid freezing
• Refrigerate open containers to prevent amber discoloration in sol

---

propoxyphene
Brand Name(s): Dextropropoxphene, Darvon, Darvon-N, Darvon Pulvules, Dolene, Dorpahen, Doxaphene, Profene, Pro Pox, Propoxycon, Propoxyhene HCI

Classification: Narcotic analgesic, opiate agonist

Controlled Substance Schedule IV

Pregnancy Category: C

AVAILABLE PREPARATIONS
Oral susp: 10 mg/ml; 50 mg/5 ml
Tabs (film coated): 100 mg
Caps: 32 mg, 65 mg

ROUTES AND DOSAGES
Children >12 yr and adults: PO (hydrochloride) 65 mg q4h prn (maximum 390 mg/24 hr); PO (napsylate) 100 mg q4h prn (maximum 600 mg/24 hr)

MECHANISM AND INDICATIONS
Mechanism: Depresses pain impulse transmission at spinal cord level by interacting with opioid receptors; alters perception of and response to painful stimuli while

---

producing generalized CNS depression

Indications: Used to treat mild-to-moderate pain

PHARMACOKINETICS
Onset: 15-60 min
Peak: 2-3 hr
Distribution: Widely distributed
Half-life: 6-12 hr
Duration: 4-6 hr
Metabolism: Liver
Excretion: Urine

CONTRAINDICATIONS AND PRECAUTIONS
• Contraindicated with hypersensitivity to drug or aspirin products (some preparations contain aspirin); respiratory depression, comatose, increased CSF pressure; in children
• Use cautiously with head trauma; hepatic, renal, or pulmonary disease; increased ICP, respiratory depression, hypothyroidism, adrenal insufficiency, undiagnosed abdominal pain, asthma, seizures, atrial flutter, tachycardia, colitis, pregnancy, lactation

INTERACTIONS
Drug
• Increased risk of coma, respiratory depression, hypotension (may even result in unpredictable fatal reaction) with use of MAOIs
• Additive CNS depression with alcohol, antihistamines, sedatives or hypnotics
• Withdrawal symptoms with partial antagonists (buprenorphine, butorphanol, nalbuphine, pentazocine)
• Increased effects of neuromuscular-blocking agents possible
• Antagonized action possible with phenothiazines
• Increased effects with dextroamphetamine
• Decreased effects of diuretics possible in CHF
Lab
• Increased serum amylase, lipase (delay drawing blood for these tests for 24 hr after administration)

• False positive urine glucose
• Decreased serum and urine 17-KS and 17-OHCS
• Increased AST, ALT, LDH, bilirubin, alk phos
• Delayed gastric emptying time
• Increased CSF pressure

SIDE EFFECTS
CNS: Sedation, confusion, headache, euphoria, dizziness, lightheadedness, weakness, drowsiness, insomnia, dysphoria, paradoxical excitement, convulsions, hyperthermia, hallucinations, agitation, seizures
CV: Hypotension, palpitation, bradycardia, arrhythmias, cardiovascular collapse
DERM: Rash, urticaria, pruritus, flushing, sweating, bruising
ENDO: Hypoglycemia
EENT: Miosis, diplopia, blurred vision, tinnitus, ototoxicity
GI: Nausea, vomiting, abdominal pain, constipation, anorexia, cramps, hepatotoxicity
GU: Urinary retention, dysuria, nephrotoxicity
HEME: Hemolytic anemia, leukopenia, neutropenia, disseminated intravascular coagulation
RESP: Respiratory depression, pulmonary edema
Other: Tolerance, physical and psychological dependence

P

TOXICITY AND OVERDOSE
Clinical signs: Respiratory depression
Treatment: Supportive care; naloxone (dose may need to be repeated); vasopressors

PATIENT CARE MANAGEMENT
Assessment
• Assess history of hypersensitivity to propoxyphene, related drugs
• Assess baseline VS, renal function (BUN, creatinine, I&O), CNS changes, respiratory function
• Assess pain (type, location, intensity)
Interventions
• May be administered with food or milk to decrease GI irritation

---

• Do not crush tabs or caps
• Determine dosing interval by pt response; administer when pain is not too severe to enhance it effectiveness; coadministration with non-narcotic analgesics may have additive analgesic effects and permit lower narcotic dosages
• Institute safety measures (supervise ambulation, raise side rails, call light within reach)

NURSING ALERT
Not to be used in children <12 yr

Provide naloxone in case of overdose.

Evaluation
• Evaluate therapeutic response (decrease in pain without significant alteration in LOC, respiratory status)
• Monitor VS, pain control 30-60 min after administration, CNS changes
• Evaluate for side effects, hypersensitivity

PATIENT AND FAMILY EDUCATION
Teach/instruct
• To take as directed at prescribed intervals for prescribed length of time
• About best time to take medication (if ordered prn)
• Not to crush tabs or cap
• That increased intake of fluids and bulk, increased activity, stool softeners, laxatives may minimize constipating effects
Warn/advise
• That drug may cause drowsiness, dizziness, orthostatic hypotension; make position changes slowly, seek assistance with ambulation
• That tolerance or dependence may develop with long term use
• To avoid OTC medications, alcohol, other CNS depressants
• To notify care provider of hypersensitivity, side effects
Encourage
• To drink adequate fluids, cough-

ing, movement, deep breathing exercises to avoid respiratory stasis
STORAGE
• Store at room temp
• Protect from light

---

propranolol, propranolol hydrochloride

Brand Name(s): Apo-Propranalol✤, Inderal✤, Inderal-LA✤, Ipran, Nu-Propranolol✤, PMS-Proprandol✤, Propranolol HCL, Propranolol Intensol

Classification: Nonselective β-adrenoceptor blocking agent, antihypertensive, antiarrhythmic agent, class II

Pregnancy Category: C

AVAILABLE PREPARATIONS
Oral sol: 4 mg/ml, 8 mg/ml
Oral sol, concentrated: 80 mg/ml
Tabs: 10 mg, 20 mg, 40 mg, 60 mg, 80 mg, 90 mg
Tabs, ext rel: 80 mg, 120 mg, 160 mg
Caps, ext rel: 60 mg, 80 mg, 120 mg, 160 mg
Inj: 1 mg/1 ml

DOSAGES AND ROUTES
Arrhythmias
Children: PO 0.5-4 mg/kg/24 hr divided q6-8h (maximum 60 mg/24 hr); IV 0.01-0.1 mg/kg/dose slow IV push, may repeat q6-8h prn (maximum for infants 1 mg/dose, for children 3 mg/dose)
Adults: PO 10-30 mg/dose q6-8h; IV 1 mg/dose q 5 min (maximum dose 5 mg)
Hypertension
Children: PO 0.5-1 mg/kg/24 hr divided q6-12h, may increase q 3-5 days (maximum dose 2 mg/kg/ 24 hr)
Adults: PO 40 mg/dose bid, increase 10-20 mg/dose q 3-7 days (maximum 480 mg/24 hr)

✤ Available in Canada.

Tetralogy Spells
Children and adults: IV treatment 0.15-0.25 mg/kg/dose slow IV push, may repeat once in 15 min (maximum dose 10 mg), PO maintenance 1-2 mg/kg/dose q6h, may increase q24h (maximum 5 mg/kg/24 hr)

Thyrotoxicosis
Neonates: PO 2 mg/kg/24 hr divided q6-12h
Adults: PO 10-40 mg qid

Migraine Headache Prophylaxis
Children: PO 0.6-1.5 mg/kg/24 hr divided tid, or children <35 kg 10-20 mg tid, or >35 kg 20-40 mg tid)
Adults: PO 80 mg/24 hr divided tid-qid, may increase by 20-40 mg/dose q 3-4 wk (maximum 160-240 mg/24 hr)

Stage Fright; Adjunctive Treatment of Anxiety
Children and adults: PO single dose 10-40 mg 20-30 min before the anxiety-provoking situation

IV administration
- Recommended concentration: 1 mg/ml
- Maximum concentration: 1 mg/ml
- IV push rate: Do not exceed 1 mg/min for adults; administer slow IV over 10 min in children

MECHANISM AND INDICATIONS
Mechanism: Reduces peripheral autonomic tone and minimizes somatic symptoms of anxiety (including palpitations, tremulousness, sweating, blushing)
Antiarrythmic mechanism: Reduces HR, prevents increases in HR secondary to exercise; decreases myocardial contractility, cardiac output, SA/AV node conduction
Antihypertensive mechanism: Thought to decrease B/P by blocking adrenergic receptors, thereby decreasing CNS sympathetic outflow and suppressing renin release
Indications: For use in treating chronic stable angina pectoris, arrhythmias, cyanotic spells of tetralogy of Fallot, neuroleptic-induced akathisia, generalized anxiety, hypertension, lithium-induced tremor, migraine, prevention of migraine, prevention of MI, panic disorder, performance anxiety, pheochromocytoma, posttraumatic stress disorder, rage outbursts, impulsive violence in pts with organic brain syndromes; used with benzodiazepines in ethanol withdrawal

PHARMACOKINETICS
Onset of action: PO 0.5-2 hr; IV 2 min
Peak: PO 1-1.5 hr; IV 15 min
Half-life: Immediate rel 3-6 hr; children 3.9-6.4 hr; sus rel 8-11 hr
Duration: PO 6 hr
Metabolism: Liver
Excretion: Urine

CONTRAINDICATIONS AND PRECAUTIONS
- Contraindicated with hypersensitivity to this medication or any component, asthma, bradycardia, cardiogenic shock, uncompensated CHF, history of cardiovascular disease, depression, history of diabetes, 2nd- or 3rd-degree heart block, Raynaud syndrome
- Use cautiously with angina pectoris, breast feeding, children, COPD, DM, hyperthyroidism, hypotension, kidney disease, liver disease, myasthenia gravis, peripheral vascular disease, pregnancy

INTERACTIONS
Drug
- Increased effects of reserpine, digitalis, neuromuscular blocking agents
- Decreased action with phenobarbital, rifampin
- Increased β-blocking effect with cimetidine, aluminum-containing antacid
- Decreased β-blocking effects with norepinephrine, isoproterenol, barbiturates, rifampin, dopamine, dobutamine, tobacco smoking
- Increased negative inotropic effects with verapamil, disopyramide

• Increased hypotension with quinidine, haloperidol, hydralazine
• Inhibited action of sympathomimetics, xanthines possible
• AV block with digitalis, Ca channel blockers
Lab
• Increased serum K⁺, uric acid, ALT, AST, alk phos, LDH, BUN
• Decreased BG

INCOMPATIBILITIES
• Inj incompatible with any drug in sol or syringe

SIDE EFFECTS
CNS: Depression, disorientation, dizziness, vivid dreams, fatigue, hallucinations, insomnia, lethargy, lightheadedness, paresthesias, sedation, weakness
CV: Bradycardia, hypotension, AV block, CHF, palpitations, peripheral vascular insufficiency, vasodilation
DERM: Itching, rash
EENT: Dry eyes, laryngospasm, sore throat, blurred vision
GI: Colitis, constipation, cramps, diarrhea, dry mouth, gastric pain, hepatomegaly, nausea, acute pancreatitis, vomiting
GU: Impotence, decreased libido, sexual dysfunction, UTIs
HEME: Agranulocytosis, thrombocytopenia
RESP: Bronchospasm, respiratory dysfunction
Other: Arthralgia, cold extremities, dyspnea, facial swelling, fever, hyperglycemia, hypoglycemia, joint pain, muscle cramps, muscle pain, Raynaud's phenomenon, wt change

TOXICITY AND OVERDOSE
Clinical signs: Bradycardia, bronchospasm, severe hypotension, heart failure
Treatment: Induce vomiting in conscious pt or gastric lavage; inactivated charcoal to reduce absorption; supportive care; treat bradycardia with atropine and/or isoproterenol; treat cardiac failure with diuretics and digoxin, hypotension with epinephrine; treat

bronchospasm with aminophylline, isoproterenol

PATIENT CARE MANAGEMENT
Assessment
• Assess history of hypersensitivity to drug
• Obtain baseline pulse, B/P, respirations, AST, ALT, bilirubin
• Obtain fasting BG if family has a history of diabetes
Interventions
• PO usually divided into 3 daily doses
• Rinse with water, take sips of fluid, sugarless gum, hard candy for dry mouth
• Administer PO with 8 oz water on an empty stomach
• Increase fluids and fiber in diet if constipation occurs
• Do not discontinue drug abruptly; taper dose gradually over 2 wk
Evaluation
• Evaluate therapeutic response (decreased arrhythmias, decreased blood pressure, ability to function in daily activities, to sleep throughout the night, resolution of target symptoms)
• Evaluate mental status (mood, sensorium, affect, impulsiveness, suicidal ideation, psychiatric symptoms)
• Evaluate for headache, lightheadedness
• Monitor pulse, B/P; in adolescents, B/P should be kept >90/60 mm Hg, pulse >60
• Monitor AST, ALT, bilirubin, ECG, wt for gain of >5 lb
• Monitor I&O; obtain CrCl if kidney damage is diagnosed
• Decrease dosage over 2 wk when discontinuing to prevent cardiac damage

PATIENT AND FAMILY EDUCATION
Teach/instruct
• To take as directed at prescribed intervals for prescribed length of time
• Not to stop taking medication without prescriber approval; do not discontinue suddenly

✤ Available in Canada.

- To increase fluids and fiber in diet if constipation occurs
- To take medicine at the same time every day
- To avoid OTC drugs unless approved by prescriber

Warn/advise
- That medication may cause dizziness; be careful on bicycles, skates, skateboards, while driving, with other activities requiring alertness
- To report signs of hypoglycemia to care provider

STORAGE
- Store at room temp in tightly sealed, light-resistant container

---

propylthiouracil (PTU)
Brand Name(s): Propylthiouracil, Propyl-Thyracil✤

Classification: Thyroid hormone antagonist

Pregnancy Category: D

AVAILABLE PREPARATIONS
Tabs: 50 mg

ROUTES AND DOSAGES
Neonates: 5-10 mg/kg/24 hr divided q8h
Children: 5-7 mg/kg/24 hr divided q8h; or 50-150 mg/24 hr divided q8h (for children 6-10 yr); or 150-300 mg/24 hr divided q8h (for children >10 yr); for maintenance, ⅓-⅔ of initial dose divided q8h-12h after 2 mo on effective initial dosage
Adults: Initially, 300-450 mg/24 hr divided q8h; for maintenance, 100-150 mg/24 hr divided q8-12h

MECHANISM AND INDICATIONS
Antithyroid mechanism: Inhibits synthesis of thyroid hormone and iodothyronine; also inhibits peripheral deiodination of thyroxine to triiodothyronine
Indications: Hyperthyroidism, preparation for thyroidectomy

PHARMACOKINETICS
Onset of action: 30-40 min
Peak: 1-1.5 hr
Half-life: 1-2 hr
Metabolism: Liver
Excretion: Urine

CONTRAINDICATIONS AND PRECAUTIONS
- Contraindicated with hypersensitivity to drug, pregnancy, lactation
- Use cautiously with other drugs that cause bone marrow suppression, infection, hepatic disease, bone marrow depression

INTERACTIONS
Drug
- Dosage may need adjustment with adrenocorticoids, ACTH
- Increased risk of agranulocytosis with bone marrow depressants
- Increased risk of hepatotoxicity with hepatotoxic agents
- Increased hypothyroid effects with iodinated glycerol, lithium, potassium iodide
- Increased anticoagulant effect with heparin, oral anticoagulants

Lab
- Altered selenomethionine, protime, AST, ALT, lactic dehydrogenase, liothyronine uptake

SIDE EFFECTS
CNS: Drowsiness, headache, vertigo, fever, paresthesias, depression
DERM: Rash, urticaria, pruritus, alopecia, hyperpigmentation, lupus-like syndrome, exfoliative dermatitis
GI: Diarrhea, nausea, vomiting, epigastric distress, sialadenopathy, jaundice, hepatitis, loss of taste
GU: Nephritis
HEME: Agranulocytosis, leukopenia, thrombocytopenia, hypoprothrombinemia, lymphadenopathy, bleeding, vasculitis, periarteritis
Other: Arthralgia, myalgia, edema, nocturnal muscle cramps

TOXICITY AND OVERDOSE
Clinical signs: Nausea, vomiting, epigastric distress, fever headache, arthralgia, pruritus, edema, pancytopenia

P

Treatment: Discontinue drug if hematologic symptoms, hepatitis, fever, exfoliative dermatitis; supportive treatment as indicated (may include antibiotics, transfusion of whole blood)

PATIENT CARE MANAGEMENT

Assessment
• Assess history of hypersensitivity
• Assess pulse, B/P, temp, I&O, T_3, T_4, TSH, CBC, ALT, AST, bilirubin, signs of hyperthyroidism or hypothyroidism

Interventions
• Tab may be crushed, mixed with food or fluid; administer with meals to reduce GI distress
• Administer at consistent times to maintain drug level
• Discontinue 4 wk before radioactive iodine uptake test
• β blocker (propanolol) may be used to decrease peripheral signs of hyperthyroidism

---

NURSING ALERT

Can cause agranulocytosis; pts complaining of fever, sore throat, or mouth sores should be evaluated immediately

---

Evaluation
• Evaluate therapeutic response (Wt gain; decreased pulse, B/P, T_4)
• Evaluate signs of overdose (peripheral edema, heat intolerance, diaphoresis, palpitations, arrhythmias, severe tachycardia, increased temp, CNS irritability)
• Monitor for signs of bone marrow suppression (sore throat, fever, fatigue)
• Evaluate signs of hypersensitivity (rash, enlarged cervical lymph nodes)
• Evaluate signs of hypoprothrombinemia (bleeding, petechiae, ecchymosis)
• Evaluate signs of bone marrow depression (sore throat, fever, fatigue)
• Monitor CBC, pulse, B/P

PATIENT AND FAMILY EDUCATION

Teach/instruct
• To take as directed at prescribed intervals for prescribed length of time

Warn/advise
• To notify care provider of hypersensitivity, side effects (especially rash, sore throat, fever, mouth sores)
• To notify care provider of symptoms of hypothyroidism or hyperthyroidism
• That response may take several mo of therapy
• To avoid use of OTC or any medications (particularly those containing iodine) unless directed by care provider
• To avoid iodized salt, soy beans, tofu, turnips, some seafood, breads
• Not to discontinue medication abruptly; thyroid crisis may occur

STORAGE
• Store at room temp
• Protect from heat, humidity, light

---

protamine sulfate
Brand Name(s): Protamine
Classification: Heparin antagonist
Pregnancy Category: C

AVAILABLE PREPARATIONS
Inj: 10 mg/ml

ROUTES AND DOSAGES
Children and adults: Dosage based on venous coagulation studies (PT/INR), route of administration of heparin, and time elapsed since heparin administered; IV 1-1.5 mg protamine per each 100 U of heparin administered in preceding 3-4 hr; maximum dose 50 mg
IV administration
• Recommended concentration: Dilute 50 mg/5 ml SW
• IV push rate: ≤20 mg over 1-3 min
• Intermittent infusion rate: May dilute with equal volume NS or

---

D_5W, using pump, run over 2-3 hr, titrate to desired PT/INR level

MECHANISM AND INDICATIONS
Mechanism: Binds with heparin to make it ineffective
Indications: For use in heparin overdose

PHARMACOKINETICS
Onset of action: 30-60 sec, neutralization of heparin in 5 min

CONTRAINDICATIONS AND PRECAUTIONS
• Contraindicated with hypersensitivity
• Use cautiously with fish allergy; in children, during lactation

INTERACTIONS
Nutrition
• Allergic reaction possible in pts with fish allergy

INCOMPATIBILITIES
• Incompatible with any drug in sol or syringe

SIDE EFFECTS
CNS: Lethary
CV: Hypotension, bradycardia, flushing
GI: Nausea, vomiting, anorexia
HEME: Bleeding, heparin rebound with bleeding within 8-9 hr and 18 hr after protamine dose
RESP: Dyspnea
Other: Hypersensitivity with urticaria, angioedema, anaphylaxis

TOXICITY AND OVERDOSE
Clinical signs: Severe hypotension and anaphylaxis may follow rapid administration
Treatment: Supportive care, administer vasopressors, fluids, antihistamines

PATIENT CARE MANAGEMENT
Assessment
• Assess history of hypersensitivity to drug and fish
• Assess baseline VS, B/P
• Assess adequacy of blood volume and fluid status
• Assess coagulation studies PT/INR
Interventions
• Treatment for shock should be available

Evaluation
• Evaluate therapeutic response (decreased bleeding)
• Monitor VS, B/P frequently during treatment
• Monitor blood coagulation studies (PT/INR)
• Monitor signs of allergic reaction
• Monitor for increased bleeding (heparin rebound), 8-9 hr and 18 hr after administration of protamine

PATIENT AND FAMILY EDUCATION
Warn/advise
• That transitory flushing may occur after administration; possibility of allergic reaction
Provide
• Support and reassurance during treatment

STORAGE
• Store in refrigerator

---

pyrantel pamoate
Brand Name(s): Antiminth, Combantrin✤, Pin-X, Reese's Pinworm
Classification: Anthelmintic
Pregnancy Category: C

AVAILABLE PREPARATIONS
Susp: 250 mg/5 ml

ROUTES AND DOSAGES
Roundworm, Pinworm
Children and adults: PO 11 mg/kg as a single dose (maximum 1 g); for pinworm, repeat in 2 wk
Hookworm
Children and adults: 11 mg/kg/24 hr qd for 3 days (maximum 1 g/24 hr)

MECHANISM AND INDICATIONS
Mechanism: Causes the release of acetylcholine and inhibits cholinesterase, paralyzing worms
Indications: Used to treat roundworm, pinworm

PHARMACOKINETICS
Peak: 1-3 hr

✤ Available in Canada.

Metabolism: Liver
Excretion: Feces, urine

CONTRAINDICATIONS AND PRECAUTIONS
• Contraindicated with known hypersensitivity to pyrantel pamoate
• Use cautiously with malnourished, dehydrated or anemic pts; hepatic disease, children < 2 yr, pregnancy

INTERACTIONS
Drug
• Mutually antagonistic effects with piperazine
Lab
• Transient elevation in liver function tests (ALT, AST)

SIDE EFFECTS
CNS: Headache, vertigo, drowsiness, fever, weakness
DERM: Rash
GI: Anorexia, nausea, vomiting, cramps, diarrhea

TOXICITY AND OVERDOSE
Clinical signs: Cardiovascular or respiratory problems
Treatment: Induce emesis or gastric lavage; follow with activated charcoal; supportive care

PATIENT CARE MANAGEMENT
Assessment
• Assess history of hypersensitivity to pyrantel pamoate
• Assess stool sample for eggs and worms; for pinworms, obtain test when child is sleeping (worms migrate to perianal area); separate buttocks and press sticky side of scotch tape to anal area
• Assess baseline hepatic function (ALT, AST, bilirubin)
Interventions
• Shake susp well
• Use appropriate hygiene techniques (especially good handwashing)
• Administer with fruit juice, milk, or food to avoid GI distress
Evaluation
• Evaluate therapeutic response (expulsion of worms)
• Evaluate stool for presence of eggs, worms, occult blood
• Monitor hepatic function (ALT, AST, bilirubin)
• Evaluate spread of infection to other household members; treat as necessary
• Evaluate for side effects, hypersensitivity (rash)
• Monitor for 3 negative stool cultures after treatment

PATIENT AND FAMILY EDUCATION
Teach/instruct
• To take as directed at prescribed intervals for prescribed length of time
• About proper hygiene procedures (especially good handwashing techniques)
• About how to prevent reinfection; to change undergarments and bed linens; to wash clothes and linens in hot water; not to shake bed linens into the air; to frequently cleanse perianal area
• To clean toilet every day with disinfectant
• To wash all fruits and vegetables before eating
• To drink fruit juice (aids in worm expulsion by eliminating accumulation in intestinal mucosa)
Warn/advise
• To notify care provider of hypersensitivity
• That all family members to be evaluated and treated
Encourage
• To comply with treatment regime

STORAGE
• Store at room temp in tight container

---

pyrazinamide
Brand Name(s): PMS-Pyrazinamide✤, Pyrazinamide, Tebrazid✤

Classification: Antitubercular (pyrazinoic acid amine/nicoturimide analog)

Pregnancy Category: C

AVAILABLE PREPARATIONS
Tabs: 500 mg

ROUTES AND DOSAGES
Children: PO 15-40 mg/kg/24 hr divided q12-24h (maximum 2 g/24 hr)
Adults: PO 15-30 mg/kg/24 hr divided tid-qid (maximum 2 g/24 hr)

MECHANISM AND INDICATIONS
Antibiotic mechanism: Interferes with lipid, nucleic acid biosynthesis
Indications: Effective against *Mycobacterium tuberculosis;* used as adjunct therapy in tuberculosis

PHARMACOKINETICS
Peak: 2 hr
Distribution: Crosses blood–brain barrier
Half-life: 9-10 hr
Metabolism: Liver
Excretion: Urine

CONTRAINDICATIONS AND PRECAUTIONS
• Contraindicated with known hypersensitivity to pyrazinamide; with severe hepatic impairment
• Use cautiously with children < 13, impaired renal function, gout, diabetes, history of peptic ulcer, pregnancy

INTERACTIONS
Drug
• Decreased serum concentrations of isoniazid
Lab
• Possible interference with urine ketone determinations
• Decreased 17-KS levels
• Increased PBI

SIDE EFFECTS
CNS: Neuromuscular blockade
DERM: Maculopapular rash, photosensitivity (skin discolors reddish-brown)
ENDO/METAB: Interference with DM control, hyperuricemia
GI: Anorexia, nausea, vomiting, hepatitis, jaundice
GU: Dysuria
HEME: Sideroblastic anemia, increased risk of bleeding
Other: Fever, malaise, arthralgia, porphyria

TOXICITY AND OVERDOSE
Clinical signs: Hepatotoxicity
Treatment: If ingested within 4 hr, induce vomiting or perform gastric lavage, followed by activated charcoal; supportive care; hemodialysis

PATIENT CARE MANAGEMENT
Assessment
• Assess history of hypersensitivity to pyrazinamide
• Obtain C&S; may begin therapy before obtaining results
• Assess hepatic function (ALT, AST, bilirubin), renal function (BUN, creatinine, I&O), hematologic function (CBC, differential, platelet count)
Interventions
• Administer PO with meals to reduce GI distress; tab may be crushed, mixed with food or fluid; administer with generous amounts of water to prevent renal damage
• Maintain age-appropriate fluid intake

> **NURSING ALERT**
> Discontinue drug if signs of hypersensitivity or hepatic impairment develop

Evaluation
• Evaluate therapeutic response (decreased TB symptoms, negative culture)
• Monitor hepatic function (ALT, AST, bilirubin), renal function (BUN, creatinine, I&O), hematologic function (CBC, differential, platelet count)
• Monitor serum uric acid; uricosuric agent may be necessary
• Monitor for hepatic impairment (anorexia, jaundice, dark urine, malaise, fatigue, liver tenderness)
• Monitor DM control

PATIENT AND FAMILY EDUCATION
Teach/instruct
• To take as directed at prescribed intervals for prescribed length of time

---

✚ Available in Canada.

Warn/advise
• To notify care provider of hypersensitivity, side effects
• To comply with follow-up care
• To avoid use of alcohol or medications containing alcohol
• That skin may discolor reddish-brown
• To avoid direct sunlight exposure

STORAGE
• Store at room temp in tightly closed container

---

pyrethrins with piperonyl butoxide
Brand Name(s): R&C Shampoo/Conditioner♣, R&C II Spray♣, RID
Classification: Pediculicide
Pregnancy Category: C

AVAILABLE PREPARATIONS
Top: Shampoo, cream, lotion, gel

ROUTES AND DOSAGES
Children and adults: Shampoo, apply to affected area thoroughly; leave on 10 min, no longer; add water to form lather, shampoo, rinse well; a 2nd treatment must be done in 7-10 days to kill newly hatched lice; avoid contact with eyes, mucous membranes; cream, lotion, gel, apply undiluted to infested area, leave on 8-12 hr; wash thoroughly with soap and water; avoid contact with eyes, mucous membranes

MECHANISM AND INDICATIONS
Mechanism: Kills head lice (*Pediculus capitis*), body lice (*Pediculus humanus*), pubic crab lice (*Pediculus pubis*), and eggs by affecting parasites' nervous system, causing paralysis and death
Indications: Used to treat head, body, pubic lice

PHARMACOKINETICS
Absorption: Poorly absorbed through skin
Metabolism: Rapid

Excretion: Urine

CONTRAINDICATIONS AND PRECAUTIONS
• Contraindicated with known hypersensitivity to pyrethrins, inflammation, abrasions of skin
• Use cautiously with ragweed-sensitive persons, infants, young children; pregnancy, lactation

SIDE EFFECTS
DERM: Irritation, pruritus, urticaria, eczema

TOXICITY AND OVERDOSE
Clinical signs: Skin irritation
Treatment: Wash off thoroughly; discontinue use; notify care provider

PATIENT CARE MANAGEMENT
Assessment
• Assess history of hypersensitivity to pyrethrins or piperonyl butoxide
• Carefully inspect all hair and skin for infestation; lice will cause intense itching
Interventions
• Take proper isolation precautions if child is hospitalized during infestation
• Administer top corticosteroids, antibiotics, antihistamines, as ordered
Evaluation
• Evaluate therapeutic response (decreased nits, crusts)
• Evaluate all family members for 2 wk for infestation; if positive, treat with product
• Evaluate for side effects (skin irritation)

PATIENT AND FAMILY EDUCATION
Teach/instruct
• To use as directed at prescribed intervals for prescribed length of time
• That all family members must understand this is a contagious condition, why it is necessary to treat
Warn/advise
• To notify care provider of hypersensitivity, side effects

♣ Available in Canada.

- That all personal clothing and bedding must be washed in hot water or dry cleaned; all personal articles such as hair care items need to be cleaned in a solution of the drug
- That a fine tooth nit comb should be used to remove dead lice or nits from hair
- That pubic lice may be transmitted sexually; all sexual partners must be treated simultaneously
- To flush with water immediately if in contact with eyes
- To notify schools and day care facilities
- To consult care provider with infestation of eyebrows or lashes
- That itching may continue for 4-6 wk
- To reapply drug if accidentally washed off

Encourage
- That children should be instructed not to borrow clothes, brushes, combs

STORAGE
- Store at room temp
- Do not reuse empty container

---

pyridostigmine bromide

Brand Name(s): Mestinon♣, Mestinon SR♣, Regonol♣

Classification: Muscle stimulant; (cholinesterase inhibitor)

Pregnancy Category: C

AVAILABLE PREPARATIONS
Tabs: 60 mg
Tabs (timed rel): 180 mg
Syr: 60 mg/5 ml
Inj: 5 mg/ml

ROUTES AND DOSAGES
Children: PO 7 mg/kg/24 hr in 5-6 divided doses; IM/IV 0.05-0.15 mg/kg/dose, maximum single dose 10 mg
Adults: PO initial 60 mg tid, maintenance 60 mg-1.5 g/24 hr; IM/IV 2 mg q2-3h or ⅓₀th of PO dose

Reversal of Nondepolarizing Neuromuscular Blocker
Children: IM/IV 0.1-0.25 mg/kg/dose preceded by atropine or glycopyrrolate
Adults: IM/IV 10-20 mg preceded by atropine or glycopyrrolate
IV administration
- Infusion rate: Administer slowly over 2-4 min direct IV

MECHANISM AND INDICATIONS
Mechanism: Inhibits destruction of acetylcholine, which increases concentration at sites where acetylcholine is released; this facilitates transmission of impulses across myoneural junction
Indications: Used as an antagonist to the non-depolarizing neuroblocking agents; in treatment of myasthenia gravis

PHARMACOKINETICS
Absorption: Poorly absorbed from GI tract
Distribution: May cross placenta in large doses
Onset of action: PO 30-45 min; IV 2-5 min; IM 15 min
Duration: PO 3-6 hr; IV 2-3 hr; depends on pt's physical and emotional status, disease severity
Metabolism: Liver; not hydralzed by cholinesterase
Excretion: Urine

CONTRAINDICATIONS AND PRECAUTIONS
- Contraindicated with known hypersensitivity to pyridostigmine or bromides; GI or GU obstruction, bradycardia
- Use with caution with asthma, seizures, peptic ulcer, pregnancy; may exacerbate vagotonia, hyperthyroidism, cardiac dysfunction

INTERACTIONS
Drug
- Decreased action of pyridostigmine with aminoglycosides, anesthetics, mecamylamine, polymyxin, magnesium, corticosteroids, antiarrhythmics, procainamide, quinidine
- Prolonged respiratory depression possible with succinylcholine

P

• Decreased B/P possible with ganglionic blockers (such as mecamylamine)

• Decreased action of gallamine, metocurine, pancuronium, tubocurarine, atropine

SIDE EFFECTS

CNS: Headache (with high dosages), dizziness, weakness, convulsions, incoordination

CV: Tachycardia, bradycardia, AV block, hypotension (rare), ECG changes, cardiac arrest, syncope

DERM: Rash, excessive sweating

GI: Abdominal cramps, nausea, vomiting, diarrhea, excessive salivation

GU: Frequency, urgency, incontinence

EENT: Miosis, blurred vision, visual changes, increased tearing

RESP: Respiratory depression, bronchospasm, constriction, laryngospasm, respiratory arrest

Other: Thrombophlebitis (with IV administration); muscle cramps

TOXICITY AND OVERDOSE

Clinical signs: Nausea, vomiting, diarrhea, blurred vision, miosis, excessive tearing, bronchospasm, increased bronchial secretions, hypotension, incoordination, excessive sweating, muscle weakness, cramps, bradycardia, tachycardia, restlessness, agitation

Treatment: Supportive, symptomatic care; support respiratory effort; atropine may be given to block muscarinic effects, but this will not counter muscle paralysis and care must be taken to avoid overdose of atropine, this could lead to bronchial plug formation

PATIENT CARE MANAGEMENT

Assessment

• Assess history of hypersensitivity to pyridostigmine or bromides

• Assess for preexisting conditions in order to avoid potential side effects

• Assess pt needs carefully; dosage must be individualized according to severity of disease and response of pt

• Be aware of all other medications to avoid potential interactions

Interventions

• Administer PO dose with food or milk to decrease GI irritation

• Sus rel tab should be swallowed whole, not crushed or chewed

• Discontinue all other cholinergic drugs during therapy to avoid risk of additive toxicity

• Monitor VS q8h

• Observe closely for cholinergic reaction (particularly with parenteral preparations)

• Atropine should be readily available to treat hypersensitivity reactions

• Prolonged use may result in decreased response; may restore response by reducing dosage or discontinuing the drug for a few days

• Administer concurrently with atropine prn to relieve or eliminate adverse reaction; however, atropine may mask some of the symptoms of pyridostigmine overdose

Evaluation

• Evaluate therapeutic response (increased muscle strength, hand grip, improved gait, decrease in labored breathing)

• Monitor regularly for drug effectiveness

• Monitor for potential side effects

• If muscle weakness is severe, try to differentiate whether it is result of drug toxicity or exacerbation of myasthenia gravis (administer a test dose of edrophonium IV; if weakness is drug-induced it will aggravate weakness, if disease-related it will be temporarily relieved)

PATIENT AND FAMILY EDUCATION

Teach/instruct

• To take with food or milk to decrease adverse GI effects

• To take sus-rel form at same time daily; swallow whole, do not crush

• About need to take drug exactly as prescribed; take a missed dose as soon as possible; but if it is almost time for next dose, eliminate missed dose and return to usual schedule; do not double dose

Warn/advise
• About potential side effects, encourage to report should any of these occur

Encourage
• To keep a record of changes in muscle strength, (particularly noting times of greatest weakness in order to individualize dosage to pt need)

STORAGE
• Store at room temp
• Avoid direct heat, protect from light

---

pyridoxine hydrochloride (vitamin B₆)

Brand Name(s): Beesix, Nestrex, Vitamin B₆✤

Classification: Water soluble vitamin

Pregnancy Category: A

AVAILABLE PREPARATIONS
Tabs: 10 mg, 25 mg, 50 mg, 100 mg, 200 mg, 250 mg, 500 mg
Inj: 100 mg/ml

ROUTES AND DOSAGES
• Safety and effectiveness not well established for children. Dosages represent accepted standard practice recommendations.

Dietary Supplement
See Appendix F, Table of Recommended Daily Dietary Allowances

Vitamin B₆ Deficiency
Children: PO 5-25 mg/24 hr × 3 wks
Adults: PO 10-20 mg × 3 wk to correct deficiency

Prevention of Vitamin B₆ Deficiency During Isoniazid Therapy
Infants: PO 0.1-0.5 mg qd
Children: PO 0.5-1.5 mg qd
Adults: PO 25-50 mg qd

Seizures Related to B₆ Deficiency
Children and adults: IV/IM 100 mg × 1

Treatment of Drug-Induced Neuritis
Children: PO 10-50 mg/24 hr
Adults: PO 100-200 mg/24 hr

Inborn Errors of Metabolism or Vitamin B₆-Responsive Anemia
Children: PO 10-100 mg qd; IV/IM initial 100 mg, maintenance 2-10 mg qd
Adults: PO/IV/IM initial up to 600 mg, maintenance 50 mg qd

IV administration
• Recommended concentration: Direct IV undiluted at rate of ≤50 mg/min in D_5W, NS
• Do not mix with $NaHCO_3$

MECHANISM AND INDICATIONS
Mechanism: Acts as a coenzyme in carbohydrate, protein, and fat metabolism; participates in amino acid decarboxylation in protein synthesis, helps to convert tryptophan to niacin or serotonin; requirements for pyridoxine increase with amount of protein in diet
Indications: Treatment and prevention of pyridoxine deficiency, vitamin B₆-dependent seizures, as adjunct to treatment of isoniazid toxicity; it is unusual for pyridoxine deficiency to occur alone and the condition may be indicative of other vitamin deficiencies

PHARMACOKINETICS
Half-life: 2-3 wk
Metabolism: Liver
Excretion: Urine

CONTRAINDICATIONS AND PRECAUTIONS
• Contraindicated with drug sensitivity or allergy; IV contraindicated with heart disease
• Use cautiously with children, pregnancy, lactation

INTERACTIONS
Drug
• Increased need with isoniazid therapy, estrogen-containing con-

P

---

traceptives, cycloserine, hydralazine
- Decreased levodopa effects
- Decreased therapeutic levels of phenobarbital and phenytoin

Lab
- False positive urobilinogen using Ehrich's reagent
- Increased liver function tests
- Decreased folic acid levels

INCOMPATIBILITES
- Alkaline sol, iron salts

SIDE EFFECTS
CNS: Headache, paresthesias, somnolence, seizures (with IV administration)
DERM: Numbing or tingling of skin, fingers, toes, around the mouth
GI: Nausea
Local: Burning at injection site
Other: Unstable gait, decreased sensation

TOXICITY AND OVERDOSE
Clinical signs: Ataxia, sensory neuropathy
Treatment: Discontinue therapy; provide supportive care

PATIENT CARE MANAGEMENT
Assessment
- Assess history of hypersensitivity to pyridoxine
- Assess need for medication; obtain pyridoxine levels
- Obtain diet history (pyridoxine deficiency rarely occurs alone)
- Assess protein consumption as excessive intake requires additional vitamin B$_6$
- Assess for concurrent use of other medications

Interventions
- PO preferred; may be administered with food
- Pts receiving levodopa should not exceed 5 mg/24 hr of pyridoxine
- Rotate IM sites; burning or stinging may occur at site; Z-track method to reduce pain

- Initial IV administration should be accompanied by EEG monitoring

> **NURSING ALERT**
> Ensure need for medication
>
> Monitor seizure activity in newborns; expect cessation after 2-3 min; monitor neurological side effects with chronic high dosage

Evaluation
- Evaluate therapeutic response (decreased symptoms of deficiency, e.g., absence of nausea, vomiting, skin lesions, glossitis, stomatitis, edema, seizures, irritability, paresthesia)

PATIENT AND FAMILY EDUCATION
Teach/instruct
- To take as directed at prescribed intervals for prescribed length of time
- To evaluate other medications or OTC drugs for interactions

Warn/advise
- To notify care provider of hypersensitivity, side effects

Encourage
- Explain the importance of a balanced diet; see Appendix F for RDAs; most people taking a varied diet do not need vitamin supplements, those who are malnourished, on various medications, or have a high protein intake may benefit from a supplement; common sources of pyridoxine are yeast, wheat germ, bananas, legumes, fish, chicken, liver, kidney, pork, beans, oats, whole wheat products, nuts

STORAGE
- Store at room temp in an airtight, light-resistant container
- Protect from freezing

pyrimethamine

Brand Name(s): Daraprim✤,
Fansidar

Classification: Antimalarial

Pregnancy Category: C

AVAILABLE PREPARATIONS
Tabs: 25 mg
Tabs (Fansidar): 25 mg pyrimethamine, 500 mg sulfadiazine

ROUTES AND DOSAGES
Malaria Chemoprophylaxis
Children <4 yr: PO 6.25 mg q wk; begin 2 wk before entering endemic area; continue through stay and for 6-10 wks after return
Children 4-10 yr: PO 12.5 mg q wk; begin 2 wk before entering endemic area; continue through stay and for 6-10 wks after return
Children >10 yr and adults: PO 25 mg q wk; begin 2 wk before entering endemic area; continue through stay and for 6-10 wks after return
Chloroquine-Resistant *P. falciparum* Malaria (in Conjunction with Quinine and Sulfadiazine)
Children <10 kg: PO 6.25 mg/24 hr qd × 3 days
Children 10-20 kg: PO 12.5 mg/24 hr qd × 3 days
Children 20-40 kg: PO 25 mg/24 hr qd × 3 days
Adults: PO 25 mg bid × 3 days
Toxoplasmosis (with Sulfadiazine or Trisulfapyrimidines)
Children: PO 2 mg/kg/24 hr divided q12h × 3 days, then 1 mg/kg/24 hr qd or divided bid × 4 wk
Adults: PO 50-75 mg/24 hr × 1-3 wk, then 25-37.5 mg/24 hr × 4-5 wk or 25-50 mg/24 hr × 3-4 wk

MECHANISM AND INDICATIONS
Mechanism: Blocks two enzymes involved in the biosynthesis of folic acid within the parasites
Indications: Used to prevent and treat malaria (*Plasmodiam falciparum*)

PHARMACOKINETICS
Peak: 1.5-8 hr
Distribution: Concentrates in kidneys, lungs, liver, spleen
Half-life: 54-231 hr
Metabolism: Liver
Excretion: Urine

CONTRAINDICATIONS AND PRECAUTIONS
• Contraindicated with known hypersensitivity to pyrimethamine, infants < 2 mo, pregnancy (at term), chloroquine-resistant malaria, megaloblastic anemia caused by folate deficiency
• Use cautiously with impaired renal or hepatic function, severe asthma, pregnancy, lactation, seizure disorders, blood dyscrasias

INTERACTIONS
Drug
• Additive adverse effects with use of sulfonamides, co-trimoxazole
• Decreased effectiveness against toxoplasmosis with para-aminobenzoic acid
Lab
• Possible decreased WBC, RBC, platelet counts

SIDE EFFECTS
CNS: Ataxia, seizures, tremors, fatigue, fever, irritability
CV: Shock
DERM: Rash, photosensitivity, Stevens-Johnson syndrome
GI: Anorexia, vomiting, cramping, diarrhea, gastritis
GU: Hematuria
HEME: Megaloblastic anemia, leukopenia, thrombocytopenia, agranulocytosis, pancytopenia, folic acid deficiency
RESP: Respiratory failure

TOXICITY AND OVERDOSE
Clinical signs: Anorexia, vomiting, seizures
Treatment: Gastric lavage, followed by cathartic, hydration, and supportive care; seizure control; monitor renal, hematologic function

P

✤ Available in Canada.

PATIENT CARE MANAGEMENT
Assessment
• Assess history of hypersensitivity to pyrimethamine
• Assess history of travel or exposure
• Obtain blood studies to identify organism
• Assess baseline hematologic function (CBC, differential, platelet count), folic acid
Interventions
• Administer with meals to avoid GI distress; may be crushed, mixed with a small amount of food or fluids
• Tab should be taken on same day each week when used for malaria prophylaxis
• Maintain age-appropriate hydration
• Administer leucovorin as ordered to prevent or treat folic acid deficiency

> **NURSING ALERT**
> Fatalities have occurred because of severe reactions; discontinue at first sign of rash, reduction in blood counts, or occurrence of active bacterial or fungal infections

Evaluation
• Evaluate therapeutic response (decreased symptoms of malaria)
• Periodic blood samples to check on disease progress
• Evaluate UA for crystalluria
• Evaluate for side effects, hypersensitivity (vomiting, anorexia, seizures, blood dyscrasias)
• Evaluate CBC, platelets twice weekly while taking drug
• Monitor for toxicity (vomiting, anorexia, seizures, blood dyscrasias, glossitis)

PATIENT AND FAMILY EDUCATION
Teach/instruct
• To take as directed at prescribed intervals for prescribed length of time
• To report visual problems, fever, fatigue, bruising, bleeding
Warn/advise
• To notify care provider of hypersensitivity
• To take precautions for mosquito control while in infested area
• Not to become pregnant or breastfeed while on drug
• To call care provider at first sign of an infection (sore throat, fever, cough, arthralgia, pallor), blood dyscrasia (visual problems, fever, fatigue, bruising, bleeding)
Encourage
• To comply with medication regime

STORAGE
• Store at room temp in tight, light-resistant containers (drug darkens with light exposure)

---

quinacrine hydrochloride
Brand Name(s): Atabrine Hydrochloride

Classification: Anthelmintic, antimalarial agent

Pregnancy Category: C

AVAILABLE PREPARATIONS
Tabs: 100 mg

ROUTES AND DOSAGES
Giardia
Children: PO 6 mg/kg/24 hr divided q8h × 5-7 days (maximum 300 mg/24 hr)

Adults: PO 100 mg tid × 5-7 days

Tapeworm
Children: Take 300 mg $NaHCO_3$ with each dose to reduce nausea and vomiting; 5-10 yr, PO 100 mg q 10 min × 4 doses; 11-14 yr, PO 200 mg q 10 min × 3 doses

Adults: Take 600 mg $NaHCO_3$ with each dose to reduce nausea and vomiting; PO 200 mg q 10 min × 4 doses

Dwarf Tapeworm
Children: Take 15 g sodium or magnesium sulfate the night be-

---

fore quinacrine administration; 4-8 yr, PO 200 mg initially, then 100 mg before breakfast × 3 days; 8-10 yr, PO 300 mg initially, then 100 mg bid × 3 days; 11-14 yr, PO 400 mg initially, then 100 mg tid × 3 days

Adults: Take 30 g sodium or magnesium sulfate the night before quinacrine administration; PO 900 mg in 3 divided doses q 20 min followed 1½ hr later by saline cathartic; then 100 mg tid × 3 days

Malaria Suppression

Children <8 yr: Begin 2 wk before entering endemic area and continue 3-4 wk after departure; PO 50 mg/24 hr for 1-3 mo

Children ≥8 yr and adult: Begin 2 wk before entering endemic area and continue 3-4 wk after departure; PO 100 mg/24 hr for 1-3 mo

MECHANISM AND INDICATIONS

Mechanism: Causes worm scolex to detach from GI tract

Indications: Used to treat giardiasis; as an alternative treatment of cestodiasis (tapeworm); and as a reserve agent for suppression and chemoprophylaxis for malaria

PHARMACOKINETICS

Peak: 8 hr

Distribution: High protein binding, crosses placenta

Half-life: 120 hr

Metabolism: Liver

Excretion: Urine

CONTRAINDICATIONS AND PRECAUTIONS

• Contraindicated with known hypersensitivity to quinacrine or any component; porphyria, psoriasis

• Use cautiously with renal, cardiac, hepatic disease; seizures, alcoholism, elderly, psychosis, G-6-PD deficiency (hemolysis may occur), children <12 yr, pregnancy

INTERACTIONS

Drug

• Increased toxicity with primaquine, hepatotoxic drugs

• Increased serum primaquine (may be toxic)

• Disulfiram-like reaction with alcohol

Lab

• False positive with adrenal function tests possible

• Increased 17-OHCS

SIDE EFFECTS

CNS: Vertigo, psychosis, restlessness, seizures, headache, behavior changes

DERM: Urticaria, yellow pigmentation of skin, exfoliation, dermatitis

EENT: Oral irritation, retinopathy, corneal deposits

GI: Nausea, vomiting, diarrhea, hepatitis, anorexia

GU: Brown coloring of urine

HEME: Aplastic anemia, agranulocytosis

TOXICITY AND OVERDOSE

Clinical signs: Restlessness, psychic stimulation, seizures, nausea, vomiting, abdominal cramps, diarrhea, hypotension, arrhythmia, yellow skin

Treatment: Gastric lavage, induced vomiting, supportive care; force fluids

PATIENT CARE MANAGEMENT

Assessment

• Assess history of hypersensitivity to quinacrine

• Assess stool culture for diagnosis

• Assess baseline hematologic function (CBC, differential, platelet count), hepatic function (ALT, AST, bilirubin), ophthal exams

Interventions

• Tabs are bitter; try mixing with sweet food or fluid

• Restrict pt to a bland, non-fat, non-residue diet 1-2 days before initiating treatment; pt should fast after the evening meal before treatment; administer saline cathartic and cleansing enemas before treatment and 1-2 hr after quinacrine use to expel worms for examination

• Administer after meals with a full glass of water or juice

Q

• Administer prn by duodenal tube (for pork tapeworm) to prevent vomiting
• Use proper hygiene techniques after BM

> **NURSING ALERT**
> Monitor for any drug-induced behavior changes and psychosis; may last up to 4 wk after treatment

Evaluation
• Evaluate therapeutic response (expulsion of worms)
• Collect all stools for the first 48 hr of treatment to examine for scolex (yellow tapeworm)
• Monitor stools during entire treatment to examine for worm segment; worms usually pass 4-10 hr after treatment
• Evaluate spread of infection to other household members; treat as needed
• Evaluate for side effects, hypersensitivity (rash, visual disturbances)
• Monitor hematologic function (CBC, differential, platelet count), hepatic function (ALT, AST, bilirubin), ophthal exams
• Evaluate stools 2 wk after last dose for giardiasis; should have 3 negative stool cultures
• Monitor for behavior changes

PATIENT AND FAMILY EDUCATION
Teach/instruct
• To take as directed at prescribed interval for prescribed length of time
• About appropriate hygiene techniques after BM (especially handwashing)
• To clean toilet qd with green disinfectant solution
Warn/advise
• To notify care provider of hypersensitivity (visual disturbances, rashes, behavior changes)
• That skin, urine may turn deep yellow
• To comply with long-term regime

• Not to drink alcohol during treatment
Encourage
• To compliance with follow-up visits

STORAGE
• Store at room temp in a tight container

---

quinidine gluconate, quinidine polygalacturonate, quinidine sulfate

Brand Name(s): Quinidine gluconate: Duraquin, Quinaglute Duratabs, Quinalin, Quinate ✤, Quinidine Gluconate Injection ✤; quinidine polygalacturonate: Cardioquin; quinidine sulfate: Apo-quinidine, Cin-quin, Novoquinidin, Quinidex Extentabs, Quinora

Classification: Antiarrhythmic

Pregnancy Category: C

AVAILABLE PREPARATIONS
Tabs: 275 mg (polygalacturonate); 100 mg, 200 mg, 300 mg (sulfate)
Tabs, sus rel: 324 mg (gluconate)
Tabs, sus action: 300 mg (sulfate)
Caps: 200 mg, 300 mg (sulfate)
Inj: 80 mg/ml (gluconate); 190 mg/ml, 200 mg/ml (sulfate)

ROUTES AND DOSAGES
Children: PO (sulfate) 2 mg/kg test dose, then 15-60 mg/kg/24 hr divided q4-6h; maximum dose 200 mg; IV not recommended
Adults: Test dose 200 mg once to check for idiosyncratic reaction; PO (sulfate) 100-600 mg/dose q4-6h, titrate to desired effect; PO (gluconate) 324-972 mg q8-12h; PO (polygalacturonate) 275 mg q8-12h; IM 400 mg/dose q4-6h; IV 200-400 mg/dose
IV administration
• Recommended concentration: 16 mg/ml

✤ Available in Canada.

- Maximum concentration: 16 mg/ml
- IV push rate: 1 ml/min

MECHANISM AND INDICATIONS

Antiarrhythmic mechanism: Prolongs action potential duration and refractory period, thereby decreasing myocardial excitability and conduction velocity; shortens AV node refractory period; may increase AV node conductivity; prolongs QRS duration and QT interval

Indications: PAT, PVCs, atrial arrhythmias, ventricular tachycardia

PHARMACOKINETICS

Onset of action: 1-3 hr
Peak: 0.5-6 hr
Half-life: 6-7 hr
Metabolism: Liver
Excretion: Urine

CONTRAINDICATIONS AND PRECAUTIONS

- Contraindicated with known hypersensitivity, complete heart block, intraventricular conduction defects, myasthenia gravis, blood dyscrasias
- Use cautiously with CHF; renal, hepatic disease; respiratory depression, incomplete heart block, hypotension, asthma, muscle weakness, fever

INTERACTIONS

Drug

- Increased effects of digoxin, coumadin, anticholinergic agents
- Increased effects of quinidine with cimetidine, propranolol, thiazides, $NaHCO_3$, carbonic anhydrase inhibitors, antacids, hydroxide suspensions
- Decreased effects of quinidine with barbiturates, phenytoin, rifampin, nifedipine
- Additive cardiac effects with phenothiazines, reserpine, amiodarone, lidocaine, procainamide

Lab

- Increased CPK

INCOMPATABILITIES

- Incompatible with any medication in sol or syringe

SIDE EFFECTS

CNS: Dizziness, headache, restlessness, confusion, psychosis, irritability, syncope, cold sweats
CV: Hypotension, PVCs, bradycardia, heart block, cardiovascular collapse or arrest, arrhythmias, ECG changes
DERM: Edema, rash, urticaria, photosensitivity, pruritus
EENT: Tinnitus, blurred vision, hearing loss, mydriasis, disturbances in color vision
GI: Anorexia, nausea, vomiting, diarrhea, hepatic dysfunction, abdominal pain
RESP: Asthma, respiratory arrest
Other: Hemolytic anemia, thrombocytopenia, agranulocytosis, fever, lupus, hypothrombinemia

TOXICITY AND OVERDOSE

Clinical signs: Severe hypotension, seizures, ventricular dysrhythmias
Treatment: Induce emesis, gastric lavage, activated charcoal for recent ingestion; supportive measures as necessary; may administer norepinephrine or metaraminol to reverse hypotension; cardiac pacing or isoproteronol may be administered; IV infusion of ⅙ molar sodium lactate sol or hemodialysis for severe cardiotoxicity

PATIENT CARE MANAGEMENT

Assessment

- Assess history of hypersensitivity to drug
- Assess baseline VS, B/P, ECG
- Assess baseline liver function tests (AST, ALT, bilirubin)

Interventions

- Use IV route only in emergencies
- Do not use if medication is discolored
- Treat with digoxin before administration when using for atrial arrhythmias

Evaluation

- Evaluate therapeutic response (decreased arrhythmias)
- Evaluate for side effects, hypersensitivity
- Monitor VS, B/P, ECG regularly

• Titrate medication based on pt response and blood levels
• Evaluate CBC, liver function (AST, ALT, bilirubin) regularly
• Monitor digoxin level in pts taking digoxin

PATIENT AND FAMILY EDUCATION
Teach/instruct
• To take as directed at prescribed intervals for prescribed length of time
Warn/advise
• To notify care provider of hypersensitivity, side effects
Encourage
• Compliance with follow-up care as indicated

STORAGE
• Store at room temp

---

quinine sulfate
Brand Name(s): Formula Q, Legatrin, M-Kya, Quinamm, Quinite, Quiphile, Q-Vel

Classification: Antimalarial

Pregnancy Category: X

AVAILABLE PREPARATIONS
Caps: 130 mg, 195 mg, 200 mg, 300 mg, 325 mg
Tabs: 260 mg, 325 mg

ROUTES AND DOSAGES
Children: PO 25 mg/kg/24 hr divided q8h × 3-7 days in conjunction with another agent (maximum 2 g/24 hr)
Adults: PO 650 mg q8h × 10 days given with pyrimethamine 25 mg q12h × 3 days, with sulfadiazine 500 mg qid × 5 days

MECHANISM AND INDICATIONS
Mechanism: Inhibits parasitic replication and transcription of DNA to RNA by forming complexes with DNA of parasite
Indications: Used to treat chloroquine-resistant/*Plasmodium falciparum* malaria

PHARMACOKINETICS
Peak: 1-3 hr
Distribution: Widely distributed to most body tissues (except brain)
Half-life: 4-5 hr
Metabolism: Liver
Excretion: Urine

CONTRAINDICATIONS AND PRECAUTIONS
• Contraindicated with known hypersensitivity to quinine or any component, G-6-PD deficiency, retinal field changes, pregnancy
• Use cautiously with cardiac arrhythmias, myasthenia gravis, blood dyscrasia, severe GI disease, neurologic disease, severe hepatic disease, psoriasis, tinnitus

INTERACTIONS
Drug
• Increased plasma levels of digoxin
• Increased half-life with use of cimetidine
• Increased effects of neuromuscular blocking agents, warfarin, other anticoagulants
• Decreased absorption with antacids containing aluminum
• Decreased renal excretion with $NaHCO_3$, acetazolamide
Lab
• Increased 17-KS
• Interference with 17-OHCS

SIDE EFFECTS
CNS: Fever
CV: Flushing, anginal symptoms
DERM: Rash, pruritus
EENT: Visual disturbances, tinnitus, impaired hearing
ENDO/METAB: Hypoglycemia
GI: Nausea, vomiting, epigastric pain, hepatitis
HEME: Hemolysis, thrombocytopenia
RESP: Dyspnea
Other: Hypersensitivity reactions

TOXICITY AND OVERDOSE
Clinical signs: Tinnitus, vertigo, headache, fever, rash, cardiovascular effects, GI distress, blindness, confusion, seizures
Treatment: Gastric lavage followed by supportive measures; severe reactions may require epineph-

---

✤ Available in Canada.

rine, corticosteroids, hemodialysis, vasodilator therapy

PATIENT CARE MANAGEMENT
Assessment
• Assess history of hypersensitivity to quinine sulfate
• Obtain history of travel and exposure
• Obtain blood studies to identify organism
• Obtain baseline hematologic function (CBC, differential, platelet count), hepatic function (ALT, AST, bilirubin)
Interventions
• Administer at same time each day to maintain drug level
• Administer after meals to minimize GI distress; swallow whole; tab should not be crushed or chewed because of its bitter taste and irritating effect on mucosa
Evaluation
• Evaluate therapeutic response (decreased symptoms of malaria)
• Monitor for any signs of tinnitus, hearing loss, rash, visual disturbance during therapy
• Evaluate side effects, hypersensitivity (nausea, visual disturbances, tinnitus, headache)
• Monitor CBC, platelets, hepatic function (ALT, AST, bilirubin), ophthal exam, BG
• Monitor serum concentration; 10 mg/ml may be considered toxic

PATIENT AND FAMILY EDUCATION
Teach/instruct
• To take as directed at prescribed intervals for prescribed length of time
• To avoid all OTC preparations, tonic water
Warn/advise
• To notify care provider of hypersensitivity, side effects
• To report visual and hearing disturbances immediately
• To take precautions for mosquito control in infested areas

Encourage
• To comply with medication regime
STORAGE
• Store at room temp
• Protect from light

---

rabies immune globulin, human (RIG)
Brand Name(s): Hyperab✤, Imogam✤
Classification: Rabies prophylaxis agent (immune serum)
Pregnancy Category: C

AVAILABLE PREPARATIONS
Inj: 150 IU/ml in 2 ml or 10 ml vials

ROUTES AND DOSAGES
Children and adults: IM 20 IU/kg administered at same time as first rabies vaccine; infiltrate wound with ½ dose, then administer remainder IM

MECHANISM AND INDICATIONS
Immunization mechanism: Provides passive immunity to rabies
Indications: Used for treatment of persons exposed to rabies

PHARMACOKINETICS
Peak: 2-13 days (appears in serum within 24 hr)
Half-life: 24 days

CONTRAINDICATIONS AND PRECAUTIONS
• Contraindicated with known hypersensitivity to equine products and thimerosal
• Use cautiously with history of systemic allergic reactions to human immune globulin, pregnancy

INTERACTIONS
Drug
• Interference with response to live vaccines possible (e.g., MMR);

do not administer live vaccines within 3 mo after RIG administration
• Interference with active immunity expected from rabies vaccine possible; do not administer repeated doses of RIG once vaccine treatment has been initiated
• Interference with immune response possible with corticosteroids, immunosuppressant agents

INCOMPATIBILITIES
• Do not administer rabies vaccine and RIG in same syringe or in same part of body

SIDE EFFECTS
CNS: Headache, malaise
Local: Pain, redness, induration at injection site
Other: Fever, anaphylaxis

PATIENT CARE MANAGEMENT
Assessment
• Obtain complete history of animal bites, rabies prophylaxis to date; do not administer repeated doses of RIG after rabies vaccine is started; pts previously immunized with a tissue culture-derived rabies vaccine and those who have confirmed adequate rabies antibody titers should receive only the vaccine
• Ascertain most recent tetanus immunization date
• Assess history of hypersensitivity to thimerosal, human immune globulin

Interventions
• Infiltrate up to ½ of dose IM in the area around wound if anatomically feasible; administer remaining dose IM in upper outer quadrant of gluteal area
• Do not administer rabies vaccine and RIG in same syringe or in same part of body
• Emergency resuscitative equipment should be made readily available for possible anaphylaxis
• Administer tetanus booster as indicated

> **NURSING ALERT**
> Do not administer RIG and rabies vaccine in same syringe or in same part of body

Evaluation
• Monitor for allergic reaction (dyspnea, skin eruptions, pruritus); reaction may occur up to 12 days after administration

PATIENT AND FAMILY EDUCATION
Warn/advise
• To notify care provider of hypersensitivity, side effects
• That RIG provides antibodies for immediate protection against rabies; immunity to rabies develops about 1 wk after vaccine is given
• That a mild analgesic (acetaminophen) may alleviate discomfort, fever
• That allergic reaction may occur up to 12 days after administration

STORAGE
• Store in refrigerator; do not freeze

---

rabies vaccine, human diploid cell
Brand Name(s): HDCV, Imovax, Rabies vaccine, Rabies Vaccine Absorbed (RVA)

Classification: Rabies prophylaxis agent

Pregnancy Category: C

AVAILABLE PREPARATIONS
Inj: 2.5 IU/ml single-dose vial

ROUTES AND DOSAGES
Postexposure Prophylaxis
Children and adults: IM 1.0 ml on first day of treatment, then on days 3, 7, 14, and 28 if previously unimmunized; administer 1.0 ml on days 1 and 3 to previously immunized pts

---

MECHANISM AND INDICATIONS

Immunization mechanism: Induces antibody formation against rabies

Indications: Used prophylactically for treatment of persons exposed to rabies

PHARMACOKINETICS

Onset of action: Antibody present within 7-10 days of first dose

Therapeutic level: 1:5 titer by rapid fluorescent focus inhibition test or 0.5 IU/ml

CONTRAINDICATIONS AND PRECAUTIONS

• No known specific contraindications

• Use cautiously with history of hypersensitivity to rabies vaccine or to neomycin, pregnancy

INTERACTIONS

Drug

• Interference possible with immune response to rabies vaccine with corticosteroids, immunosuppressant agents

INCOMPATIBILITIES

• Do not administer rabies vaccine and rabies immune globulin (RIG) in same syringe or in same part of body

SIDE EFFECTS

CNS: Headache, malaise

Local: Pain, redness, induration at injection site

Other: Fever, anaphylaxis

PATIENT CARE MANAGEMENT

Assessment

• Obtain complete history of animal bite, rabies prophylaxis to date

• Ascertain date of most recent tetanus immunization

• Assess history of hypersensitivity to rabies vaccine, neomycin

Interventions

• Administer IM in lateral thigh, deltoid muscle, or upper outer quadrant of gluteal area, depending on pt's age; discard if blood appears on aspiration; prepare injection again and administer in a different site

• Do not administer rabies vaccine and RIG in same syringe or in same part of body

• Emergency resuscitative equipment should be made readily available for possible anaphylaxis

• Administer tetanus booster as indicated

> **NURSING ALERT**
> Do not administer rabies vaccine and RIG in same syringe or in same part of body

Evaluation

• Monitor for 20 min after administration for signs of anaphylaxis (urticaria, dyspnea, wheezing, drop in B/P)

PATIENT AND FAMILY EDUCATION

Warn/advise

• To notify care provider of hypersensitivity, side effects

• That immunity to rabies develops about 1 wk after vaccine is administered; RIG provides antibodies for immediate protection

• To comply with subsequent appointments for vaccine to receive adequate treatment

• That a mild analgesic (acetaminophen) may alleviate discomfort, fever

STORAGE

• Store in refrigerator; do not freeze

R

---

ranitidine

Brand Name(s): Apo-Ranitidine, Zantac, Zantac-C

Classification: Antihistamine, H_2-receptor antagonist

Pregnancy Category: B

AVAILABLE PREPARATIONS

Elixir: 15 mg/ml

Tabs: 150 mg, 300 mg

Caps, GEL dose: 150 mg, 300 mg

Tabs: 150 mg EFFERdose

Granules: 150 mg EFFERdose

✤ Available in Canada.

Inj: 25 mg/ml, 50 mg/ml (premixed)

ROUTES AND DOSAGES
Duodenal or Gastric Ulcer
Infants and children: PO 2-4 mg/kg/dose tid up to 300 mg/24 hr or 6 mg/kg/24 hr; IV 1-2 mg/kg/24 hr divided q6-8h (Safety and effectiveness not established. Dosage represents accepted standard practice recommendations.)

Adults: PO 150 mg bid or 300 mg qhs; 150 mg qhs for prophylaxis; 150 mg bid for gastric ulcer; IM/IV 50 mg q6-8h (maximum 400 mg/24 hr)

Gastroesophageal Reflux
Infants and children: PO 2-8 mg/kg/dose tid (Safety and effectiveness not established. Dosage represents accepted standard practice recommendations.)

Adults: PO 150 mg bid

Gastric Hypersecretory Conditions
Adults: PO 150 mg bid; for severe cases, administer up to 6 g/24 hr; IM/IV 50 mg tid-qid

Prophylaxis of Aspiration Pneumonitis
Adults: IM/IV 50 mg 45-60 min before induction of general anesthesia

IV administration
• Recommended concentration: Dilute in D_5W, $D_{10}W$, LR, NS, $NaHCO_3$; 50 mg in 20 ml for IV push, 50 mg in 100 ml for intermittent infusion
• Maximum concentration: 2.5 mg/ml for IV push, 0.5 mg/ml for intermittent infusion
• IV push rate: Over ≥5 in
• Intermittent infusion rate: Over 15-20 min
• Continuous infusion: Adults 6.25 mg/hr; gastric hypersecretory conditions, begin infusion at 1 mg/kg/hr; increase by 0.5 mg/kg/hr increments (if gastric output >10 mEq/hr or if pt is symptomatic) up to 2.5 mg/kg/hr

MECHANISM AND INDICATIONS
Mechanism: Reversible competitive antagonist of the actions of histamine on the H_2 receptor resulting in a decrease of histamine-mediated basal and nocturnal gastric acid secretion by the parietal cell

Indications: Used as therapy for gastric or duodenal ulcer, GERD, pathological hypersecretory conditions, prevention of duodenal ulcer, prevention of GI bleeding in critically ill pts; investigational use for treatment of upper GI bleeding, prevention and treatment of acute upper GI-induced ulceration and bleeding in critically ill pts, prophylaxis of pulmonary aspiration of acid during anesthesia

PHARMACOKINETICS
Onset of action: Rapidly absorbed from the GI tract
Peak: PO 2-3 hr; IM 15 min
Half-life: PO 2.5 hr; IV 2-2.5 hr
Metabolism: Liver
Excretion: Urine, feces

CONTRAINDICATIONS AND PRECAUTIONS
• Contraindicated with hypersensitivity to ranitidine or other H_2-receptor antagonists; history of acute porphyria
• Use cautiously with renal or hepatic impairment, pregnancy, lactation

INTERACTIONS
Drug
• Altered bioavailability of drugs, dosage forms (enteric-coated) with pH dependent absorption possible
• Prevention of degradation of acid-labile drugs possible
• Impaired absorption of ketoconazole
• Increased blood alcohol levels possible
• Interference with hepatic metabolism of glipizide, glyburide, metoprolol, midazolam, nifedipine, phenytoin, theophylline, warfarin, procainamide possible
• Increased risk of neutropenia, other blood dyscrasias with bone marrow depressants possible
• Impaired absorption with antacids, sucralfate

♣ Available in Canada.

Lab
- Increased serum transaminase, AST, creatinine possible
- Decreased WBC, RBC, platelet count possible
- False positive urine protein with Multistix possible
- False negative allergy skin test possible
- Antagonism of pentagastrin and histamine in evaluation of gastric acid secretory function possible

Nutrition
- Vitamin B_{12} deficiency possible in pts requiring long-term therapy and who are likely to have impaired secretion of intrinsic factor (severe fundic gastritis)

INCOMPATIBILITIES
- Chlorpromazine, clindamycin, hydroxyzine, lorazepam, methotrimeprazine, opium alkaloids, phenobarbital

SIDE EFFECTS
CNS: Headache, malaise, dizziness, somnolence, insomnia, vertigo; rarely hallucination, blurred vision, reversible confusion
CV: Arrhythmias (rare)
DERM: Rash
GI: Constipation, diarrhea, nausea, vomiting, abdominal discomfort; rarely pancreatitis, hepatitis (with or without jaundice)
HEME: Rarely leukopenia, granulocytopenia, thrombocytopenia
Other: Anaphylaxis (rare)

TOXICITY AND OVERDOSE
Clinical signs: Limited experience exists with overdose; reported associated transient adverse side effects have been similar to those seen in normal clinical use
Treatment: Induce vomiting or perform gastric lavage; dialysis removes ranitidine from circulation; for seizures treat with IV diazepam; for bradycardia, treat with atropine; for ventricular arrhythmias, treat with lidocaine

PATIENT CARE MANAGEMENT
Assessment
- Assess history of hypersensitivity to ranitidine, other H_2-receptor antagonists
- Assess baseline renal function (BUN, creatinine), hepatic function (ALT, AST, bilirubin), gastric pH, abdominal symptoms

Interventions
- May be administered PO without regard to meals; tab may be crushed, mixed with food or fluid
- Do not administer within 1 hr of antacids
- Do not administer within 2 hr of ketoconazole
- Do not administer IV too rapidly (<5 min); may result in cardiac arrhythmias, hypotension, cardiac arrest
- Do not administer if sol is discolored or contains precipitate

> **NURSING ALERT**
> Do not administer rapid IV (<5 min); may result in arrhythmias, hypotension, cardiac arrest

Evaluation
- Evaluate therapeutic response (decreased abdominal pain)
- Evaluate for hypersensitivity, side effects
- Monitor for signs of GI bleeding (melena, brown-tinged or coffee-ground emesis)
- Evaluate gastric pH (>5 indicative of therapeutic response); VS with IV push administration
- Evaluate renal function (BUN, creatinine), hepatic function (ALT, AST, bilirubin)

PATIENT AND FAMILY EDUCATION
Teach/instruct
- To take as directed at prescribed intervals for prescribed length of time
- To continue taking even after symptoms subside

Warn/advise
- To notify care provider of hypersensitivity, side effects
- To avoid smoking, caffeine, alcohol (which may exacerbate symptoms)
- To avoid OTC drugs unless directed by care provider

R

STORAGE
- Store all forms at room temp
- Protect from light
- Diluted sol stable 48 hr at room temp

---

reserpine
Brand Name(s): Novoreserpine, Serpalan, Serpasil✿
Classification: Antihypertensive
Pregnancy Category: D

AVAILABLE PREPARATIONS
Tabs: 0.1 mg, 0.2 mg, 0.25 mg, 1 mg
Caps, time rel: 0.5 mg
Inj: 2.5 mg/ml

ROUTES AND DOSAGES
Hypertension
Children: PO 10-20 mcg/kg/24 hr divided q12h, maximum 0.25 mg/24 hr
Adult: PO/IV 0.25-0.5 mg qd for 1-2 wk, then 0.1-0.25 mg qd for maintainance
Psychiatric Disorders
Adult: PO/IV 0.5 mg/24 hr; maximum dose 1 mg
IV administration
- Recommended concentration: 2.5 mg/ml
- Maximum concentration: 2.5 mg/ml
- IV push rate: Over 1 min

MECHANISM AND INDICATIONS
Antihypertensive mechanism: Inhibits norepinephrine release, thereby depleting norepinephrine stores in adrenergic nerve endings
Indications: Hypertension, relief in agitated psychotic states

PHARMACOKINETICS
Onset of action: 1½-2 hr
Peak: 4 hr
Half-life: 50-100 hr
Metabolism: Liver
Excretion: Urine, feces

CONTRAINDICATIONS AND PRECAUTIONS
- Contraindicated with hypersensitivity to medication, depression or suicidal tendencies, active peptic ulcer, ulcerative colitis
- Use cautiously with seizure disorders, renal disease

INTERACTIONS
Drug
- Increased hypotension with diuretics, β-blockers, methotrimeprazine
- Arrhythmias with cardiac glycosides
- Increased cardiac depression with quinidine, procainamide
- Excitation, hypertension with MAOIs
- Increased CNS depression with barbituates, alcohol, narcotics
- Increased pressor effects of epinephrine, isoproterenol, norepinephrine
- Decreased pressor effects with ephedrine, amphetamines
Lab
- Increased VMA, 5-HIAA excretion
- Interference with 17-OHCS, 17-KS

INCOMPATIBILITIES
- None

SIDE EFFECTS
CNS: Lethargy, fatigue, drowsiness, dizziness, depression, anxiety, headaches, dreams, nightmares, convulsions, parkinsonism
CV: Bradycardia, chest pain, arrhythmias
DERM: Rash, purpura, alopecia, flushing, pruritus, ecchymosis, thrombocytopenia
EENT: Blurred vision, lacrimation, miosis, ptosis, epistaxis
GI: Nausea, vomiting, cramps, anorexia, peptic ulcer, dry mouth, increased appetite
GU: Dysuria, nocturia, impotence, edema, breast engorgement, galactorrhea, gynecomastia
RESP: Bronchospasm, dyspnea, cough, rales
Other: Prolonged bleeding time

TOXICITY AND OVERDOSE
Clinical signs: Severe hypotension, bradycardia
Treatment: Gastric lavage; IV atropine for bradycardia; supportive measures as necessary

---

✿ Available in Canada.

PATIENT CARE MANAGEMENT
Assessment
- Assess history of hypersensitivity to drug
- Assess baseline BUN, creatinine
- Assess hydration status
Interventions
- Administer with food to minimize gastric irritation
- Supervise position change and ambulation
Evaluation
- Evaluate therapeutic response (decreased B/P)
- Evaluate for side effects, hypersensitivity
- Monitor VS, B/P, wt, hydration status regularly
- Monitor for signs of CHF

PATIENT AND FAMILY EDUCATION
Teach/instruct
- To take as directed at prescribed intervals for prescribed length of time
Warn/advise
- To notify care provider of hypersensitivity, side effects
- To avoid hazardous activities if drowsiness occurs
- Not to discontinue abruptly
- To avoid cough and cold preparations unless directed by care provider
- That impotence and gynecomastia may occur, but they are reversible
- To make position changes to minimize orthostatic hypotension

STORAGE
- Store at room temp in tightly sealed, light-resistant container

---

ribavirin
Brand Name(s): Virazole✤

Classification: Antiviral, inhalation therapy (synthetic nucleoside)

Pregnancy Category: X

AVAILABLE PREPARATIONS
Powder for aerosol: 6 g/100 ml

ROUTES AND DOSAGES
Infants and young children: Inhal 1 vial per treatment day, sol 20 mg/ml delivered via Viratek Small Particle Aerosol Generator (SPAG-2) resulting in mist concentration of 190 mg/L; flow rate 12.5 L of mist per min over 12-18 hr for 3-7 days

MECHANISM AND INDICATIONS
Antiviral mechanism: Inhibits replication of RNA and DNA viruses, influenza virus RNA polymerase activity, and viral protein synthesis

Indications: Effective against RNA and DNA viruses; primarily used for treatment of severe lower respiratory tract respiratory syncytial virus infections in pts with underlying compromising condition (prematurity, bronchopulmonary dysplasia, congenital heart disease, immunodeficiency, immunosuppression)

PHARMACOKINETICS
Peak: 1-1½ hr after administration

Distribution: Highest concentration in respiratory tract, erythrocytes

Half-life: Respiratory tract secretions 2 hr; plasma 6.5-11 hr

Metabolism: Intracellular

Excretion: Urine, feces

CONTRAINDICATIONS AND PRECAUTIONS
- Contraindicated with known hypersensitivity to ribavirin, women of childbearing age, pregnancy, lactation
- Use cautiously with COPD, asthma, pts requiring ventilatory assistance (precipitate in equipment may interfere with ventilation)

INTERACTIONS
Drug
- Antagonized antiviral activity of zidovudine

✤ Available in Canada.

Lab
• Transient elevations of liver function tests, bilirubin

SIDE EFFECTS
CV: Hypotension, cardiac arrest
DERM: Rash, skin irritation
EENT: Conjunctivitis, erythema at eyelids
HEME: Anemia, reticulocytosis
RESP: Mild bronchospasm, worsening of respiratory function
Other: Irritability (crying in infants, young children), hypoactivity

PATIENT CARE MANAGEMENT
Assessment
• Obtain viral cultures per agency collection policy; confirm respiratory syncytial virus infection within 24 hr of start of treatment
• Assess nursing, health care staff, visitors for risk of pregnancy; exclude anyone who is currently or may be pregnant or lactating or who is planning a pregnancy within next 3 mos; drug may absorb to contact lenses
Interventions
• Administer via SPAG-2 only; do not use any other aerosol-generating equipment; review operation of device
• Reconstitute 6 g vial with 50-100 ml SW for injection (without preservatives); do not use bacteriostatic water or any other water containing a antimicrobial agent; do not use if sol contains precipitate or is discolored; transfer aseptically to sterile 500 ml Erlenmeyer flask and further dilute with SW without preservatives to 300 ml for final concentration of 20 mg/ml; attach face mask, hood, or O$_2$ tent
• Do not administer any other aerosol medications
• Provide appropriate respiratory and fluid therapy
• Provide appropriate emotional support to child who may be frightened by respiratory difficulty or isolation

NURSING ALERT
Use only SPAG-2 for administration

Use only SW for injection (without preservatives) for reconstitution

Discontinue with sudden respiratory deterioration

Evaluation
• Evaluate therapeutic response (decreased symptoms of infection)
• Monitor ventilated pts carefully for adequate ventilation, gas exchange, or precipitate in equipment at least q2h
• Monitor respiratory status closely
• Monitor hematologic function (CBC, differential, platelet count), hydration status

PATIENT AND FAMILY EDUCATION
Teach/instruct
• About rationale for therapy
Warn/advise
• To notify care provider of hypersensitivity, side effects

STORAGE
• Store at room temp
• Reconstituted sol stable 24 hr at room temp

---

riboflavin (vitamin B$_2$)
Brand Name(s): Riobin-50, Vitamin B$_2$ ✤
Classification: Water soluble vitamin
Pregnancy Category: A

AVAILABLE PREPARATIONS
Tabs: 5 mg, 10 mg, 25 mg, 50 mg, 100 mg
Caps: 10 mg, 25 mg, 50 mg, 100 mg
ROUTES AND DOSAGES
• See Appendix F, Table of Recommended Daily Dietary Allowance

---

✤ Available in Canada.

Deficiency

Children <12 yr: PO 3-10 mg/24 hr in divided doses

Children >12 yr and adults: PO 5-30 mg/24 hr in divided doses

MECHANISM AND INDICATIONS

Mechanism: Acts as a coenzyme to form adenine dinucleotide (FAD) and flavin mononucleotide (FMN), important in protein and energy metabolism; deficiency symptoms manifest clinically as glossitis, normochromic anemia, cheilosis, angular stomatitis, eye symptoms

Indications: Treatment and prevention of riboflavin deficiency or adjunct to thiamin treatment for polyneuritis and cheilosis; deficiency rarely occurs alone and is generally associated with other vitamin, mineral, and protein deficiencies

PHARMACOKINETICS

Half-life: 66-84 min

Metabolism: Liver, GI tract

Excretion: Urine

Absorption: Increases when administered with food, decreases with liver dysfunction or biliary obstruction

CONTRAINDICATIONS AND PRECAUTIONS

• No significant contraindications
• Use cautiously with pregnancy

INTERACTIONS

Drug

• Increased need for riboflavin with phenothiazines, tricyclic antidepressants, oral contraceptives
• Delayed absorption rate with propantheline bromide, but increased total amount absorbed
• Decreased action of tetracycline

Lab

• False elevation of urine catecholamines

SIDE EFFECTS

GU: Bright yellow urine

TOXICITY AND OVERDOSE

No information available

PATIENT CARE MANAGEMENT

Assessment

• Assess history of hypersensitivity to riboflavin
• Obtain baseline CBC, urinary riboflavin, and erythrocyte riboflavin to assess for deficiency
• Dietary assessment to evaluate possibility that other vitamin deficiencies may exist

Interventions

• Administer with food to increase absorption

NURSING ALERT

Avoid megadosing

Evaluation

• Evaluate therapeutic response (normal serum vitamin B₁₂ levels)
• Evaluate for side effects, hypersensitivity
• Newborns receiving phototherapy should be closely monitored; riboflavin is sensitive to light, may decompose during therapy

PATIENT AND FAMILY EDUCATION

Teach/instruct

• To take as directed at prescribed intervals for prescribed length of time

Warn/advise

• To notify care provider of hypersensitivity, side effects
• That drug may cause a yellow discoloration of the urine
• To avoid megadosing

Encourage

• Balanced diet to ensure adequate vitamin intake; common sources of riboflavin are meats, poultry, fish, milk products, fortified cereals, yeast, green vegetables

STORAGE

• Store at room temp in airtight, light-resistant container

rifampin
Brand Name(s): Rifadin, Rimactane♣, Rofact♣
Classification: Antibiotic, antitubercular
Pregnancy Category: C

AVAILABLE PREPARATIONS
Caps: 150 mg, 300 mg
Inj: 600 mg

ROUTES AND DOSAGES
Tuberculosis
Children: PO/IV 10-20 mg/kg/dose qd or twice weekly (maximum 600 mg/dose)
Adults: PO/IV 10 mg/kg/dose qd or twice weekly (maximum 600 mg/dose)
Haemophilus influenzae **Prophylaxis**
Neonates <1 mo: PO/IV 10 mg/kg/24 hr qd for 4 days
Infants and children: PO/IV 20 mg/kg/24 hr qd for 4 days (maximum 600 mg/dose)
Adults: PO/IV 600 mg qd for 4 days
Meningococcal Prophylaxis
Neonates <1 mo: PO/IV 10 mg/kg/24 hr divided q12h for 2 days
Infants and children: PO/IV 20 mg/kg/24 hr divided q12h for 2 days
Adults: PO/IV 600 mg q12h for 2 days
IV administration
• Recommended concentration: 1.2 mg/ml in SW
• Maximum concentration: 6 mg/ml
• Intermittent infusion rate: Over 3 hr

MECHANISM AND INDICATIONS
Antibiotic mechanism: May be bactericidal or bacteriostatic; inhibits bacterial RNA synthesis by binding to the β subunit of DNA-dependent RNA polymerase, blocking RNA transcription
Indications: Effective against *Mycobacterium tuberculosis, M. bovis, M. marinum, M. kansasii,* some strains of *M. fortuitum, M. avium, M. intracellulare,* and many gram-positive and some gram-negative bacteria; used to treat tuberculosis, to eliminate meningococci from asymptomatic carriers, and for prophylaxis of *Haemophilus influenzae* type B infection

PHARMACOKINETICS
Peak: 2-4 hr
Distribution: Widely distributed including CSF
Half-life: 3-4 hr
Metabolism: Liver
Excretion: Feces, urine

CONTRAINDICATIONS AND PRECAUTIONS
• Contraindicated with known hypersensitivity to rifampin
• Use cautiously with hepatic impairment, alcoholism, pts taking other hepatotoxic drugs, pregnancy, lactation

INTERACTIONS
Drug
• Decreased plasma concentrations of verapamil, methadone, digoxin, cyclosporine, corticosteroids, oral anticoagulants, theophylline, barbiturates, chloramphenicol, ketoconazole, oral contraceptives, quinidine, halothane
• Increased risk of hepatotoxicity with use of isoniazid, alcohol
• Decreased serum concentrations with paraaminosalicylate
Lab
• Interference with serum folate, vitamin B_{12} assays, gall bladder studies
• Elevated liver function tests (ALT, AST), serum uric acid
• Decreased vitamin D levels
Nutrition
• Cap contents unstable when mixed in fluids; pharmacist can prepare stable susp

INCOMPATIBILITIES
• Media containing sodium lactate

SIDE EFFECTS
CNS: Headache, fatigue, drowsiness, ataxia, dizziness, mental confusion, generalized numbness
DERM: Pruritus, urticaria, rash

♣ Available in Canada.

EENT: Visual disturbances, conjunctivitis
ENDO / METAB: Hyperuricemia
GI: Epigastric distress, anorexia, nausea, vomiting, abdominal pain, diarrhea, flatulence, sore mouth and tongue, pseudomembranous colitis, hepatotoxicity, transient elevations in liver function tests
HEME: Thrombocytopenia, transient leukopenia, hemolytic anemia
Local: Phlebitis, thrombophlebitis with IV injections
Other: Flu-like syndrome, red–orange discoloration of skin, sweat, tears, urine, feces

TOXICITY AND OVERDOSE
Clinical signs: Nausea, vomiting, lethargy; hepatotoxicity (hepatomegaly, jaundice, loss of consciousness, elevated liver function tests and bilirubin)
Treatment: Gastric lavage followed by activated charcoal, forced diuresis; bile drainage; supportive care

PATIENT CARE MANAGEMENT
Assessment
• Assess history of hypersensitivity to rifampin
• Obtain C&S; may begin therapy before obtaining results
• Assess hepatic function (ALT, AST, bilirubin), renal function (BUN, creatinine, I&O), hematologic function (CBC, differential, platelet count)
Interventions
• Administer PO 1 hr before or 2 hr after meals; may be administered with food to reduce GI distress; shake susp well before administering; caps may be taken apart, mixed with food or fluids
• Do not premix IV with other medications; infuse separately
• Use large vein with small bore-needle to reduce local reaction; rotate site q48-72h

• Maintain age-appropriate fluid intake

NURSING ALERT
Discontinue drug if signs of hypersensitivity, hepatotoxicity, pseudomembranous colitis develop

Evaluation
• Evaluate therapeutic response (decreased TB symptoms, negative culture)
• Monitor hepatic function (ALT, AST, bilirubin), renal function (BUN, creatinine, I&O), hematologic function (CBC, differential, platelet count), electrolyte status
• Monitor for hepatic impairment (anorexia, jaundice, dark urine, malaise, fatigue, liver tenderness)
• Evaluate IV site for vein irritation

PATIENT AND FAMILY EDUCATION
Teach/instruct
• To take as directed at prescribed intervals for prescribed length of time
Warn/advise
• To notify care provider of hypersensitivity, side effects
• To comply with follow-up care
• To avoid use of alcohol or medications containing alcohol
• That sweat, tears, urine, feces may be discolored red-orange; soft contact lenses may be permanently discolored
• That female pts should use alternative contraception (because medication may decrease effectiveness of oral contraceptives)

STORAGE
• Store at room temp in tightly closed containers
• Protect from light
• Reconstituted IV sol stable at room temp 24 hr

R

rocuronium bromide
Brand Name(s): Zemuron
Classification: Neuromuscular blocking agent (non-depolarizing)
Pregnancy Category: C

AVAILABLE PREPARATIONS
Inj: 10 mg/ml

ROUTES AND DOSAGES
Infants > 3 mo and children ≤12 yr: IV, initially 0.6 mg/kg; for maintenance of neuromuscular blockade, 0.075-0.125 mg/kg prn
Adults: IV, initially 0.6 mg/kg; for maintenance of neuromuscular blockade, 0.1-0.2 mg/kg prn to maintain neuromuscular blockade
IV administration
• Recommended concentration: May be given undiluted
• IV push rate: over 2 min

MECHANISM AND INDICATIONS
Mechanism: Interrupts transmission of nerve impulse at the skeletal neuromuscular junction; antagonizes acetylcholine by competitively binding to cholinergic sites on motor endplates, resulting in muscle paralysis; reversible with edrophonium, neostigmine, and physostigmine
Indications: Used as an adjunct in surgical anesthesia to facilitate endotracheal intubation and skeletal muscle relaxation during mechanical ventilation or surgery

PHARMACOKINETICS
Onset: Within 1 min
Peak: 1 min (range 0.5-3.3 min)
Recovery: Begins in 24-68 min when anesthesia is balanced
Half-life: 71-203 min
Metabolism: In plasma by nonspecific esterases and nonenzymatic reactions
Excretion: Urine, bile

CONTRAINDICATIONS AND PRECAUTIONS
• Contraindicated with known hypersensitivity to rocuronium

• Use cautiously with pregnancy, lactation, renal and hepatic disease, children <2 yr, fluid or electrolyte imbalances, neuromuscular disease, dehydration, respiratory diseases

INTERACTIONS
Drug
• Increased neuromuscular blockade with use of aminoglycosides, bacitracin, vancomycin, tetracyclines, polymyxins, colistin, sodium colistimethate, quinidine, local anesthetics, enflurane, isoflurane, halothane, magnesium sulfate
• Decreased neuromuscular blockade with use of carbamazepine, phenytoin
Lab
• None known

INCOMPATIBILITES
• Do not mix with alkaline solutions, barbiturates in syringe; do not administer simultaneously during IV infusion through same needle

SIDE EFFECTS
CVS: Brachycardia, tachycardia, increased or decreased BP
DERM: Rash, flushing, pruritus, urticaria
EENT: Increased secretions, salivation
MS: Weakness
RESP: Prolonged apnea, bronchospasms, cyanosis, respiratory depression
Other: Endogenous histamine release may occur (noted clinically as erythema, hypotension, and either brachycardia or tachycardia)

TOXICITY AND OVERDOSE
Clinical signs: Prolonged apnea, bronchospasm, cyanosis, respiratory depression
Treatment: Supportive care; mechanical ventilation may be required; anticholinesterases to reverse neuromuscular blockade; edrophonium or neostigmine, atropine

---

♣ Available in Canada.

PATIENT CARE MANAGEMENT
Assessment
• Assess history of hypersensitivity to rocuronium bromide
• Assess for preexisting conditions requiring caution (pregnancy, lactation, renal or hepatic disease, fluid or electrolyte imbalance, neuromuscular disease, dehydration, respiratory disease
• Assess electrolytes (Na, K⁺) before procedure (electrolyte imbalances may increase action of drug)

Interventions
• Monitor vital signs (pulse, respirations, airway, B/P) until fully recovered; characteristics of respirations (rate, depth, pattern); strength of hand grip
• Monitor therapeutic response (noting paralysis of jaw, eyelid, head, neck, rest of the body)
• Monitor I&O for urinary frequency, hesitancy, retention
• Monitor for allergic reactions (rash, fever, respiratory distress, pruritus); *drug should be discontinued*
• Instill artificial tears (q2h) and covering to eyes to protect cornea

---

NURSING ALERT

Should be administered only by experienced clinicians familiar with actions and complications of drug

Only administer in facilities where intubation, artifical respiration, O₂ therapy and antagonists are immediately available

---

Evaluation
• Monitor effectiveness of neuromuscular blockade (degree of paralysis); use nerve stimulator
• Monitor for recovery (including decreased paralysis of face, diaphragm, arm, rest of the body)

PATIENT AND FAMILY EDUCATION
Warn/advise
• Provide reassurance to patient if communication is difficult during recovery; inform pt that often postoperative stiffness occurs is normal and will subside

STORAGE
• Store in refrigerator
• Use within 30 days of removing from refrigeration to room temp

---

salicylic acid

Brand Name(s): Acnex❀, Compound W❀, Compound W Plus❀, Duofilm, Duofort❀, Duoplant for Feet, Freezone, Keralyt❀, Mediplast, Occlusal❀, Occlusal-HP❀, P&S Shampoo, Sal-Acid, Salicylic Acid Soap❀, Sebcur❀, Soluver❀, Soluver Plus❀, Trans-Plantar❀, Trans-Ver-Sal❀, X-Seb❀

Classification: Keratolytic agent

Pregnancy Category: C

AVAILABLE PREPARATIONS
Cream: 2%, 2.5%, 10%
Gel: 5%, 6%, 17%
Liq: 13.6%, 16.7%, 17%
Lotion: 2%
Oint: 25%, 40%, 60%
Plaster: 15%, 40%
Pledgets: 0.5%, 2%
Shampoo: 2%, 4%

ROUTES AND DOSAGES
Children and adults: Top lotion, cream, gel, apply thin layer to affected area qd-bid; plaster, cut to size of callus or corn, apply, leave in place 48 hr, do not exceed 5 applications in 14 days; shampoo, initially use qd-qod then 1-2 times per week to maintain control, apply to wet hair, massage into scalp, rinse thoroughly; sol, apply thin layer to wart with applicator qd for 1 wk or until wart removed

S

MECHANISM AND INDICATIONS

Mechanism: Increases hydration of stratum corneum, causing skin to swell, soften, desquamate

Indications: For use in controlling seborrheic dermatitis, psoriasis, dandruff; used to remove warts, corns, calluses

PHARMACOKINETICS

Absorption: Cutaneous

Peak: 5 hr when applied with occlusive dressing

Excretion: Urine

CONTRAINDICATIONS AND PRECAUTIONS

• Contraindicated with known sensitivity, in children <2 yr
• Use cautiously with diabetes

INTERACTIONS

• None reported

SIDE EFFECTS

CNS: Salicylism (hearing loss, tinnitus, headache, confusion, dizziness, lethargy)

DERM: Erythema, scaling, drying

Local: Irritation, burning

TOXICITY AND OVERDOSE

Clinical signs: Salicylism (see Side Effects)

Treatment: Discontinue medication, call care provider

PATIENT CARE MANAGEMENT

Assessment

• Assess history of hypersensitivity to drug
• Assess for appropriateness of treatment

Interventions

• Soak lesions in water for 5 min before applying
• Do not use on inflamed, open skin
• Wash hands after each treatment
• Use occlusive covering when possible to increase absorption

Evaluation

• Evaluate therapeutic response (decrease in size of lesions, dandruff)
• Monitor for signs of salicylism

• Monitor for hypersensitivity

PATIENT AND FAMILY EDUCATION

Teach/instruct

• To use as directed at prescribed intervals for prescribed length of time
• To avoid application to large surface areas
• To avoid contact with eyes, mucus membranes
• To cover surrounding skin with petroleum jelly when using 10% sol

STORAGE

• Store at room temp

---

salmeterol xinafoate

Brand Name(s): Serevent

Classification: Bronchodilator

Pregnancy Category: C

AVAILABLE PREPARATIONS

Inh: 13 g canister containing 120 metered doses, 6.5 g canister containing 60 metered doses; each dose delivers 21 mcg salmeterol from the actuator

ROUTES AND DOSAGES

Maintenance of Bronchodilation/Prevention of Asthma

Children >12 yr and adults: 2 inhalations (41 mcg salmeterol) q12hr

Prevention of Exercise-Induced Asthma

Children >12 yr and adults: 2 inhalations (41 mcg salmeterol) 30-60 min before exercise; *do not use again for 12 hr*

MECHANISM AND INDICATIONS

Mechanism: β-adrenergic agonist causing relaxation of bronchial smooth muscle; also inhibits release of mediators of hypersensitivity, especially in mast cells

Indications: For use in long-term, twice-daily administration in maintenance treatment of asthma

---

or in prevention of exercise-induced bronchospasm

PHARMACOKINETICS

Onset of action: Immediate upon inhalation
Peak: 45 min
Half-life: 5.5 hr
Metabolism: Lungs, liver
Excretion: Feces

CONTRAINDICATIONS AND PRECAUTIONS

• Contraindicated with hypersensitivity to drug or its components
• Use cautiously with cardiovascular disorders (especially arrhythmias, coronary insufficiencies, hypertension); convulsive disorders, thyrotoxicosis, other sympathomimetic drugs; pregnancy, lactation

INTERACTIONS

Drug

• Increased cardiovascular effects (tachycardia, palpitations, arrhythmias) with tricyclic antidepressants, MAOIs
• Increased sympathomimetic effects (increased B/P, HR) with other sympathomimetic drugs (other β agonists)

SIDE EFFECTS

CNS: Headache, nervousness, malaise, fatigue
CV: Tachycardia, palpitations
DERM: Rash, skin eruption
GI: Nausea, vomiting, diarrhea, abdominal pain
GU: dysmenorrhea
RESP: URI, tracheitis, bronchitis, pharyngitis, paradoxical bronchospasm

TOXICITY AND OVERDOSE

Clinical signs: Tachycardia, arrhythmia, tremor, headache, muscle cramps, prolonged QT interval, hypokalemia, hyperglycemia, chest pain
Treatment: Discontinue drug; consider β-adrenergic blocking agent (however, pt must be watched for bronchospasm); place pt on cardiac monitor; provide supportive care

PATIENT CARE MANAGEMENT

Assessment

• Assess history of hypersensitivity to this and related drugs
• Assess respiratory status, baseline VS

Interventions

• See Chapter 3 for discussion of inhaler instructions; shake well before using
• Maintain age-appropriate fluid intake
• Offer sips of fluid or chewing gum for dry mouth

NURSING ALERT
Discontinue use if paradoxical bronchospasm occurs

Evaluation

• Evaluate therapeutic response (decreased bronchospasm, cough, wheeze)
• Evaluate for side effects, hypersensitivity
• Evaluate VS, respiratory rate, quality of respiratory status (peak flow meter results) if indicated; dyspnea or wheezing that continues or occurs after administration

PATIENT AND FAMILY EDUCATION

Teach/instruct

• To use as directed at prescribed intervals for prescribed length of time
• About proper use and care of inhaler
• That drug is not for use in treating acute symptoms; it is a long-acting therapy
• Not to exceed recommended dosage; drug effects last for 12 hr; exceeding recommended dosage can lead to toxicity
• Not to take other prescription or OTC drugs unless directed by care provider

Warn/advise

• Notify care provider of hypersensitivity, side effects (especially palpitations, chest pain, arrhythmias)

S

- To discontinue drug and notify care provider if paradoxical bronchospasm occurs
- To notify care provider if symptoms persist or worsen
- Not to use other β-adrenergic drugs unless directed by care provider
- To avoid getting aerosol in eyes
- To rinse with or drink water to avoid dry mouth
- To avoid smoking or contact with second-hand smoke, persons with respiratory infections

STORAGE
- Store at room temp away from heat and sun
- Do not puncture canisters

---

sargramostim
Brand Name(s): GM-CSF, Leukine

Classification: Human granulocyte-macrophage colony stimulating factor

Pregnancy Category: C

AVAILABLE PREPARATIONS
Inj: 250 mcg, 500 mcg powder

ROUTES AND DOSAGES
Myeloid Reconstitution Following Autologous Bone Marrow Transplantation
Children and adults: IV 250 mcg/m^2/24 hr (60-1000 mcg/m^2/24 hr) for 21 days; 2-hr infusions begun 2-4 hr after bone marrow infusion but not <24 hr after last dose of chemotherapy or 12 hr after last dose of radiation therapy
Engraftment Delay or Failure Following Bone Marrow Transplantation
Children and adults: IV/SC 250 mcg/m^2/24 hr for 14 days as 2 hr infusion or SC injection; repeat course of treatment if engraftment has not occurred within 7 day rest; if no evidence of engraftment after another 7 day rest, repeat course with 500 mcg/m^2/24 hr for 14 days; if still no evidence of engraftment, it is unlikely that any will occur

Following Standard Chemotherapy
Children and adults: IV/SC 125 mcg/m^2/24 hr for 7-14 days
Treatment of Febrile Neutropenia Resulting from Myelosuppression
Children and adults: SC/IV 5-6 mcg/kg/24 hr for 7-14 days as SC daily dose or continuous IV infusion (rare)
Treatment of Myelodysplastic Syndrome
Children and adults: IV 120-240 mcg/m^2/24 hr for 14-21 days as 12 hr IV infusion, interval dosing repeated in cyclic fashion
IV administration
- Recommended concentration: Reconstitute with 1 ml SW; mix in NS for infusion; if less than 10 mcg/ml, 1 ml of 5% albumin must be added to each 50 ml of infusate to prevent absorption of drug to components of IV system

MECHANISM AND INDICATIONS
Mechanism: Product of recombinant DNA technology that stimulates proliferation and differentiation of hematopoietic progenitor cells; activates mature granulocytes and macrophages; increases number of stem cells circulating in peripheral blood; increases cytotoxicity of monocytes to certain neoplastic cell lines; activates polymorphonuclear neutrophils to inhibit growth of certain tumor cells
Indications: Used to accelerate engraftment in pts undergoing autologous bone marrow transplantation; to treat engraftment delay or failure following bone marrow transplantation; to increase number of circulating stem cells in peripheral blood aiding in leukophoresis harvesting; to increase WBC count in myelodysplastic syndrome and in AIDS patients receiving zidovudine; to decrease length of nadir following myelosuppressive chemotherapy; and to correct neutropenia in aplastic anemia

---

✤ Available in Canada.

PHARMACOKINETICS

Onset of action: 5 min
Peak: 2 hr
Half-life: Biphasic; initial 12-17 min, terminal 2 hr
Excretion: Clearance slowest after 2 hr IV infusion; very little drug excreted intact in urine

CONTRAINDICATIONS AND PRECAUTIONS

• Contraindicated with sensitivity to drug, yeast-derived products, or any component of protein; pts with myeloid leukemia blasts in bone marrow or peripheral blood; within 24-hr period before or after chemotherapy, or a 12 hr period before or after radiation therapy; GM-CSF theoretically could act as growth factor for underlying malignancy (particularly myeloid tumors) and drug should be discontinued if disease progression is noted
• Use cautiously with pregnancy, lactation

INTERACTIONS

• Potentiation of myeloproliferative effects by lithium, corticosteroids possible

INCOMPATIBILITIES

• No other drug should be added to infusion

SIDE EFFECTS

CV: Fluid retention (including peripheral edema, capillary leak syndrome, pericardial effusion); occasional transient supraventricular arrhythmia; potential damage to vascular epithelium (causes high concentration of growth factor at tip of catheter that may result in local accumulation of activated granulocytes)
DERM: Mild local reaction at SC injection site (including erythema, inflammation, rash)
GI: Diarrhea, transient increase in bilirubin, hepatic enzymes
GU: Increase in serum creatinine in pts with preexisting renal disease
RESP: Sequestration of granulocytes in pulmonary circulation with resultant dyspnea, pleural effusion
Other: Malaise, headache, arthralgia, myalgia, fever 60-90 min directly following IV administration, chills, bone pain commonly described as dull ache in flank, long bones of children with intensity that peaks just before 2 waves of neutrophils released from marrow (at 1-2 hr and at 12-24 hr).

TOXICITY AND OVERDOSE

• Maximum dosage has not been established

PATIENT CARE MANAGEMENT

Assessment

• Assess history of hypersensitivity to GM-CSF, yeast products
• Assess baseline CBC, differential, platelet counts
• Assess baseline renal function (BUN, creatinine), liver function (alk phos, LDH, AST, bilirubin)
• Assess history of previous treatment with growth factors, side-effects, route of administration, efficacy

Interventions

• Provide supportive measures to maintain hemostasis, fluid, electrolyte, nutritional status
• Transfuse with RBCs, platelets as appropriate

> **NURSING ALERT**
> Drug must be diluted in NS for infusion; in order to prevent adsorption of drug to IV bag or tubing in sols with <10 mcg GM-CSF/ml NS, 1 ml of 5% albumin must be added to each 50 ml NS sol before GM-CSF added

Evaluation

• Evaluate therapeutic response (WBC recovery)
• Monitor CBC, differential, platelet count at least once a week
• Monitor renal function (BUN, creatinine), liver function (alk phos, LDH, AST, bilirubin) biweekly

• Evaluate for signs, symptoms of increased fluid retention

PATIENT AND FAMILY EDUCATION
Teach/instruct
• To have pt well hydrated before and after chemotherapy
• About the importance of follow-up to monitor blood counts, serum chemistry values
• To take an accurate temp, rectal temp contraindicated
• To notify care provider of signs of bleeding (bruising, epistaxis, bleeding gums) infection (fever, sore throat, fatigue)
Warn/advise
• About impact of body changes that may occur (hair loss, hyperpigmentation, nail ridging), how to minimize changes (wigs, caps, scarves, long sleeves)
• To avoid OTC preparations containing aspirin
• To report any alterations in behavior, sensation, perception; help to develop a plan of care to manage side effects, stress of illness or treatment
• To report any signs of dyspnea or respiratory distress
• To report any pain, inflammation, swelling at injection site
• That good oral hygiene with very soft toothbrush is imperative
• That dental work be delayed until blood counts return to baseline, with permission of caretaker
• To avoid contact with known viral and bacterial illnesses
• That close household contacts of child not be immunized with live polio virus; use inactivated form
• That children on chemotherapy not receive immunizations until immune system recovers sufficiently to mount necessary antibody response
• To report exposure to chicken pox in susceptible child immediately
• To report reactivation of herpes zoster virus (shingles) immediately

• If appropriate, ways to preserve reproductive patterns, sexuality (sperm banking, contraceptives)
Encourage
• Provision of nutritious food intake; consider nutritional consultation

STORAGE
• Unopened vials should be refrigerated
• Reconstituted vial should be entered only once for single dose

---

scopolamine, scopolamine hydrobromide
Brand Name(s): Isopto, Hyoscine, Transderm Scop, Transderm-V✤

Classification: Antimuscarinic, antiemetic/antivertigo agent; antiparkinsonian agent, cycloplegic mydriatic anticholinergic

Pregnancy Category: C

AVAILABLE PREPARATIONS
Disc, transdermal: 1.5 mg/disc
Inj: 0.3 mg/ml, 0.4 mg/ml, 0.86 mg/ml, 1 mg/ml (scopolamine hydrobromide)
Ophthal sol: 0.25% (scopolamine hydrobromide)

ROUTES AND DOSAGES
Preoperative Medication
Children: IM/SC 6 mcg/kg/dose (maximum 0.3 mg/dose), or 0.2 mg/m^2; may be repeated q6-8h
Adults: IM/IV/SC 0.3-0.65 mg; may be repeated q4-6h
Motion Sickness
Children >12 yr and adults: Transdermal, apply 1 disc behind ear at least 4 hr before exposure and q 3 days prn
Refraction
Children: Ophthal, instill 1 gtt to eye(s) bid for 2 days before procedure

---

Adults: Ophthal, instill 1 gtt to eye(s) 1 hr before procedure

Iridocyclitis

Children: Ophthal, instill 1 gtt to eye(s) tid

Adults: Ophthal, instill 1-2 gtt to eye(s) tid

MECHANISM AND INDICATIONS

Mechanism: Acts to block the action of acetylcholine at parasympathetic sites in smooth and cardiac muscle, secretory glands and CNS; increases cardiac output, dries secretions, antagonizes histamine and serotonin

Indications: Used as a preoperative medication to decrease salivation and respiratory secretions, produce amnesia; in treatment of iridocyclitis; to prevent nausea and vomiting from motion

PHARMACOKINETICS

Onset of action: Ophthal sol 20-30 min; IM 1-2 hr; transdermal patch slow-release (5 mcg/hr) over a 3-day period; after application there is an initial priming dose (140 mcg) delivered from the adhesive layer of the system which saturates the skin binding sites and brings plasma concentration to a steady-state level rapidly

Duration: Ophthal sol 3-7 days; IM 8 hrs; transdermal patch 3 days (5 mcg/hr)

Metabolism: Liver

Excretion: Urine

CONTRAINDICATIONS AND PRECAUTIONS

• Contraindicated with known hypersensitivity to scopolamine or any components, with narrow-angle glaucoma, renal and hepatic dysfunction; in children (transdermal)

• Use cautiously in infants, children, and elderly (transdermal); with GI tract obstruction secondary to the relaxation of smooth muscle; with pregnancy, lactation

INTERACTIONS

Drug

• Additive adverse effects with other anticholinergic agents

• Increased CNS effects with CNS depressants (alcohol, tranquilizers, sedative-hypnotics)

• Decreased oral absorption with antacids; should be administered at least 1 hr before scopolamine

• Decreased GI absorption of many other drugs (such as levodopa, ketoconazole)

• Increased digoxin serum levels

• Interaction with oral K^+; may cause K^+-induced GI ulcerations

SIDE EFFECTS

• Adverse systemic effects may occur with top and ophthal preparations as well as parenteral

CNS: Disorientation drowsiness, hallucinations, confusion, psychosis, delirium, anaphylaxis

CV: Tachycardia, palpitations

DERM: Allergic reaction to the patch

EENT: Dry mouth, blurred vision, cycloplegia, mydriasis, photophobia, increased intraocular pressure

GI: Constipation

GU: Urinary retention

TOXICITY AND OVERDOSE

Clinical signs: Rare, but have occurred, particularly in children (more susceptible to adverse effects); dilated pupils, flushed skin, tachycardia, hypertension, ECG abnormalities, CNS manifestations that resemble acute psychosis, CNS depression, circulatory collapse, respiratory failure

Treatment: Supportive, symptomatic care; support respiration; if symptoms are severe, initiate supportive treatment; physostigmine 1-2 mg (0.5 mg or 0.02 mg/kg for child) given either SC or IV slowly to reverse the toxic effects

PATIENT CARE MANAGEMENT

Assessment

• Assess history of hypersensitivity to scopolamine or any components

• Assess for preexisting conditions in order to avoid potential side effects

• Be aware of all other medica-

---

tions to avoid potential interactions

Interventions
• Observe closely for adverse effects (especially with parenteral forms)
• Physostigmine should be made available to reduce or reverse hypersensitivity reactions
• Keep pt in bed at least 1 hr after administration of parenteral dose to prevent postural hypotension
• For ophthal installation, have pt lie down or tilt head back; after instillation, gently pinch nasal bridge for 1-2 min to reduce systemic absorbtion; wait at least 5 min before instilling other eye preparations
• Apply transdermal patch behind ear the day before traveling; do not remove for 72 hr; wash hands before and after application

Evaluation
• Evaluate therapeutic response (decreased secretions, decreased symptoms of motion sickness, decreased symptoms of iritis)
• Monitor regularly for drug effectiveness
• Monitor for potential side effects

PATIENT AND FAMILY EDUCATION
Teach/instruct
• About how to instill ophthal medications; apply transdermal patch

Warn/advise
• About potential side effects; to report to care provider should any of these occur (particularly changes in vision, severe dizziness)
• About potential drug interactions with OTC medications, to avoid using these with scopolamine
• To read all OTC medication labels; if scopolamine is found in the product avoid its use
• To avoid activities that are hazardous or require alertness (drowsiness and dizziness may occur)

STORAGE
• Store transdermal at room temp

• Store ophthal sol at room temp; protect from light

---

secobarbital, secobarbital sodium

Brand Name(s): Secobarbital Sodium, Seconal Sodium✙, Seconal Sodium Pulvules, Secretin-Ferring

Classification: Sedative, hypnotic, barbiturate

Controlled Substance Schedule II

Pregnancy Category: D

AVAILABLE PREPARATIONS
Tabs: 100 mg
Caps: 50 mg, 100 mg
Inj: 50 mg/ml
Powder, rectal supp: 200 mg

DOSAGES AND ROUTES
Preoperative Sedation
Children: PO 50-100 mg 1-2 hr before surgery; PR 4-5 mg/kg 1-2 hr before surgery
Adults: PO 200-300 mg 1-2 hr before surgery
Insomnia
Children: IM 3-5 mg/kg, maximum dose 100 mg; PR 4-5 mg/kg
Adults: PO/IM 100-200 mg hs
Acute Psychotic Agitation
Children: IM/IV 5.5 mg/kg q3-4h
Adults: IM/IV 5.5 mg/kg q3-4h
Status Epilepticus
Children and adults: IM/IV 250-350 mg or 5 mg/kg
IV administration
• Recommended concentration: Dilute with SW for injection; rotate rather than shake sol
• IV push rate: Administer ≤50 mg over 1 min, titrate IV to pt response

MECHANISM AND INDICATIONS
Mechanism: Depresses neurons in the reticular activating system in brain stem, posterior hypothalamus, and limbic structures
Indications: For use in preoperative sedation, treatment of insom-

---

nia, status epilepticus, acute tetanus convulsions

PHARMACOKINETICS
Onset of action: IM 10-15 min; PR slow
Duration: IM 4-6 hr; PR 3-6 hr
Half-life: 15-40 hr
Metabolism: Liver
Excretion: Urine

CONTRAINDICATIONS AND PRECAUTIONS
• Contraindicated with hypersensitivity to this medication or any component; hypersensitivity or addiction to barbiturates, severe liver impairment, porphyria, uncontrolled severe pain, respiratory depression
• Use cautiously with anemia, hypertension, kidney disease, liver disease, acute or chronic pain, lactation, elderly

INTERACTIONS
Drug
• Increased CNS depression with alcohol, MAOIs, sedatives, narcotics
• Decreased effects of oral anticoagulants, corticosteroids, griseofulvin, quinidine
• Decreased half-life of doxycycline
Nutrition
• Pt should not drink alcohol

INCOMPATIBILITIES
• Do not mix with other drugs in sol or syringe

SIDE EFFECTS
CNS: Drowsiness, hangover, lethargy, CNS depression, mental depression, dependence, dizziness, light-headedness, slurred speech, stimulation
CV: Bradycardia, hypotension
DERM: Rash, abscess at injection site, angioedema, hives, pain, thrombophlebitis, Stevens-Johnson syndrome
GI: Constipation, diarrhea, nausea, vomiting
HEME: Agranulocytosis, megaloblastic anemia, thrombocytopenia
RESP: Apnea, bronchospasm, laryngospasm, respiratory depression,

TOXICITY AND OVERDOSE
Clinical signs: Cold clammy skin, cyanosis of lips, hypotension, insomnia, nausea, pulmonary constriction, vomiting, hallucinations, delirium, weakness
Treatment: Monitor VS, I&O, provide warming blanket; administer lavage and activated charcoal if PO; administer hemodialysis

PATIENT CARE MANAGEMENT
Assessment
• Assess history of hypersensitivity to drug
• Assess for pain; secobarbital may cause severe stimulation if pain is present
• Obtain baseline mental status (including short- and long-term memory)
• Obtain baseline AST, ALT, bilirubin, Hct, Hgb, RBCs, serum folate
• Obtain baseline pro-time if taking anticoagulants
• Obtain baseline vitamin D with long-term therapy
Interventions
• Ensure that PO form is swallowed
• Administer PO on empty stomach for best absorption; may administer crushed or whole
• Administer ½-1 hr before hs for insomnia
• Administer after a cleansing enema if given PR preoperatively in children
• Do not use if sol is cloudy or contains precipitate
• Do not inject more than 5 ml in one site
• Administer IM deep in large muscle mass to prevent tissue sloughing and abscesses
• Administer IV only if resuscitative equipment is available
• Administer within 30 min of mixing
• Monitor VS after IM or IV q 30 min for 2 hr
• Complementary insomnia interventions (reading, exercise several hr before hs, warm bath,

S

warm milk, TV, self-hypnosis, deep breathing)
• Safety precautions (siderails up, night light, call bell within reach, remove cigarettes)
• Do not administer for more than 14 days; tolerance may develop

Evaluation
• Evaluate therapeutic response (sleep, sedation, seizures)
• Evaluate mental status (including short- and long-term memory)
• Monitor respiratory status; hold secobarbital if respirations are <10/min or if pupils are dilated
• Monitor AST, ALT, bilirubin, Hct, Hgb, RBCs, serum folate
• Secobarbital is usually discontinued if liver studies are increased
• Monitor for symptoms of blood dyscrasias (fever, sore throat, bruising, rash, jaundice, epistaxis)
• Monitor vitamin D if on long-term therapy
• Monitor PT if taking anticoagulants
• Monitor for perianal irritation if suppository is used
• Monitor for signs of physical dependency (more frequent requests for medication, shakes, anxiety)

PATIENT AND FAMILY EDUCATION
Teach/instruct
• To take as directed at prescribed intervals for prescribed length of time
• To ensure medication is swallowed
• Not to discontinue medication without prescriber approval; not to discontinue quickly after long-term use, dosage should be tapered over 1-2 wk
• To avoid ingesting alcohol, other CNS depressants
• That effects may take 2 nights to be noticed if taken for insomnia
• That hangover is common
• About insomnia interventions (reading, exercise several hr before bedtime, warm bath, warm milk, TV, self-hypnosis, deep breathing)

• To keep this and all medications out of reach of children

Warn/advise
• That medication may cause drowsiness; be careful on bicycles, skates, skateboards, while driving, with other activities requiring alertness
• That physical dependency may occur if used for 45-90 days

STORAGE
• Store in refrigerator

---

sertraline
Brand Name(s): Zoloft✤
Classification: Antidepressant
Pregnancy Category: B

AVAILABLE PREPARATIONS
Tabs: 50 mg, 100 mg

ROUTES AND DOSAGES
• Safety and effectiveness in children not established
Adults: PO 50 mg qd either in AM or PM; may increase to maximum 200 mg/24 hr; do not change dose at intervals of <1 wk; therapeutic doses 50-200 mg/24 hr

MECHANISM AND INDICATIONS
Mechanism: Blocks uptake of serotonin in neurons of the CNS
Indications: For use in treatment of depression in adolescents and adults, treatment of anorexia and obsessive compulsive disorder; major depressive disorder in adolescents and adults, particularly when there may be a greater risk of drug overdose

PHARMACOKINETICS
Peak: 6-10 hr
Half-life: 1-2 days
Excretion: Urine

CONTRAINDICATIONS AND PRECAUTIONS
• Contraindicated with hypersensitivity to this medication or any component
• Use cautiously with history of

---

attempted suicide, illness, kidney disease, liver disease, mania, history of seizures, pregnancy, lactation

INTERACTIONS
Drug
• Increased effects of alcohol, other CNS depressants, diazepam, tolbutamide, warfarin
• Hypertensive crisis, high fever, seizures if taken at the same time as or within 14 days of MAOIs
• Interacts with digitoxin, lithium
Lab
• Increased serum bilirubin, BG alk phos
• Decreased VMA, 5-HIAA
• False increase in urinary catecholamines
Nutrition
• Do not drink alcohol

SIDE EFFECTS
CNS: Anxiety, decreased concentration, confusion, dizziness, drowsiness, fatigue, headache, insomnia, mania, nervousness, paresthesia, restlessness, somnolence, stimulation, tremor, twitching
CV: Chest pain, palpitations, tachycardia
DERM: Hives, itching, rash, flushing or redness of skin with feeling of warmth or heat
EENT: Dry mouth, runny nose, taste changes, thirst, sore throat, tinnitus, blurred vision, vision changes
GI: Anorexia, increased appetite, constipation, diarrhea, dry mouth, gas, indigestion, nausea, pain, stomachache, stomach or abdominal cramps, vomiting
GU: Menstrual problems, decreased libido; male sexual dysfunction, urinary frequency, pain with urination
Other: Fever, hot flashes, back pain, muscle pain, increased muscle tension, excessive sweating, yawning

PATIENT CARE MANAGEMENT
Assessment
• Assess history of hypersensitivity to drug
• Assess ability to function in daily activities, to sleep throughout the night, depression
• Assess mental status (affect, mood, sensorium, impulsiveness, suicidal ideation, thoughts)
• Obtain a medical history and general medical examination (including orthostatic B/P)
Interventions
• Administer qd, either in AM or PM
• Pt may crush tabs if unable to swallow whole
• Increase fluids and fiber in diet if constipation occurs
• Take with food or milk if GI symptoms occur
• Rinse with water, take sips of fluid, sugarless gum, or hard candy for dry mouth
• Pt should not drink alcohol
• Withdrawal symptoms occur if discontinued abruptly (headache, nausea, vomiting, muscle pain, weakness)

> **NURSING ALERT**
> Do not take at the same time as or within 14 days of MAOIs; may cause a hypertensive crisis, high fever, seizures

Evaluation
• Evaluate therapeutic response (ability to function in daily activities, to sleep throughout the night, depression)
• Evaluate mental status (affect, mood, sensorium, impulsiveness, panic, suicidal ideation, thoughts)
• Monitor orthostatic B/P; if B/P drops 20 mm Hg, hold sertraline and notify prescriber
• Monitor for constipation
• Monitor wt

PATIENT AND FAMILY EDUCATION
Teach/instruct
• To take as directed at prescribed

intervals for prescribed length of time
- That medicine sometimes must be taken for 2-4 wks before improvement is noticed
- That this medication is most helpful when used as part of a comprehensive multimodal treatment program
- About the importance of returning for follow-up visits
- Not to discontinue medication without prescriber approval

Warn/advise
- To avoid ingesting alcohol, other CNS depressants (antihistamines, medicine for allergies or colds, sedatives, tranquilizers, sleeping medicine, prescription pain medicine, narcotics, barbiturates, medicine for seizures, muscle relaxants, or anesthetics, including some dental anesthetics)
- That medication may cause drowsiness; be careful on bicycles, skates, skateboards, while driving, with other activities requiring alertness
- To notify prescriber if pregnant, if breastfeeding or if planning pregnancy
- Not to discontinue medication quickly after long-term use; sudden discontinuation may cause headache, nausea, vomiting, muscle pain, weakness

STORAGE
- Store away from heat, direct light, moisture

---

silver nitrate

Brand Name(s): Dey Drops Silver Nitrate

Classification: Ophthalmic antiseptic

Pregnancy Category: C

AVAILABLE PREPARATIONS
Ophthal sol: 1% (wax ampuls)

ROUTES AND DOSAGES
Prevention of Gonorrheal Ophthalmia Neonatorum
Neonates: Ophthal, instill 2 gtt immediately after birth (no later than 1 hr after birth) into conjunctival sac of each eye as a single dose; do not irrigate eyes after instillation

MECHANISM AND INDICATIONS
Antiseptic mechanism: Bacteriostatic, germicidal; free silver ions precipitate bacterial proteins
Indications: Used in preventing gonorrheal ophthalmia neonatorum

PHARMACOKINETICS
Absorption: Not readily absorbed from mucous membranes

CONTRAINDICATIONS AND PRECAUTIONS
- Contraindicated with hypersensitivity to silver nitrate or any component
- Use cautiously as repeated instillation can cause cauterization of cornea and blindness; in pregnancy

SIDE EFFECTS
EENT: Cauterization of cornea, blindness, periorbital edema, chemical conjunctivitis, temporary staining of lids, surrounding tissue

TOXICITY AND OVERDOSE
Clinical signs: Dizziness, seizures, mucous membrane irritation, nausea, vomiting, diarrhea, methemoglobinemia, dermatitis, rash, hypochloremia with associated hyponatremia
Treatment: For oral overdose: dilution with 4-8 oz of water, sodium chloride by lavage, activated charcoal or cathartic, supportive care; for eye overexposure: tepid water irrigation for at least 15 min; for dermal overexposure: wash twice with soap and water

PATIENT CARE MANAGEMENT
Assessment
- Assess history of hypersensitivity to silver nitrate or any component
- Assess eye for redness, discharge, swelling

✤ Available in Canada.

Interventions
• Do not use if sol is discolored or contains a precipitate
• Wash hands before and after application, cleanse crusts or discharge from eye before application; wipe excess medication from eye; do not flush medication from eye

Evaluation
• Monitor eye for swelling, redness, drainage, itching, lacrimation

PATIENT AND FAMILY EDUCATION
Teach/instruct
• That use of ophthal antiseptic is required by law in most states

Warn/advise
• To notify care provider of hypersensitivity, side effects
• That sol may temporarily discolor neonate's eyelids, stain skin or clothing

STORAGE
• Store wax ampules at room temp
• Protect from heat, light

---

silver sulfadiazine
Brand Name(s): Flamazine♣, Silvadene, SSD♣
Classification: Topical antibiotic
Pregnancy Category: C (D if near term)

AVAILABLE PREPARATIONS
Cream: 10 mg/g

ROUTES AND DOSAGES
Children and adults: Top, apply 1/16″ qd-bid

MECHANISM AND INDICATIONS
Mechanism: Interferes with bacterial cell membrane and wall synthesis
Indications: For use in prevention and treatment of 2nd- and 3rd-degree burns; bacteriostatic against gram-positive and gram-negative organisms

PHARMACOKINETICS
Absorption: Limited with top use
Excretion: Urine

CONTRAINDICATIONS AND PRECAUTIONS
• Contraindicated with pregnancy, lactation, infants <2 mo (causes kernicterus)
• Use cautiously with known hypersensitivity, allergies to other sulfonamides, liver and renal impairment

INTERACTIONS
Lab
• Decreased neutrophil count if used extensively for long periods

SIDE EFFECTS
DERM: Rash, stinging, pain, erythema, urticaria
HEME: Reversible leukopenia

TOXICITY AND OVERDOSE
Clinical signs: Increased dermatologic side effects if over-applied
Treatment: Discontinue drug and clean skin thoroughly

PATIENT CARE MANAGEMENT
Assessment
• Assess history of hypersensitivity to drug
• Assess baseline wound appearance
• Assess baseline VS, wt, CBC

Interventions
• Apply aseptically to clean, debrided wounds using sterile gloves
• Keep burned areas covered with cream at all times
• Avoid contact with eyes, mucous membranes
• Premedicate for painful dressing changes prn

Evaluation
• Evaluate therapeutic response (wound healing, granulation tissue)
• Monitor CBC, renal function (BUN, creatinine)
• Evaluate dermatologic side effects
• Monitor for superinfection

♣ Available in Canada.

PATIENT AND FAMILY EDUCATION
Teach/instruct
• To use as directed at prescribed intervals for prescribed length of time
• That treatment may continue until pt is ready for skin grafting
• Teach appropriate burn care technique and drug application for home treatment
• About side effects; to call care provider if they occur
• About signs of superinfection; to call care provider if they occur

STORAGE
• Store at room temp in light-resistant containers
• Avoid excess heat

---

sodium bicarbonate injection (NaHCO₃)

Brand Name(s): Neut

Classification: Systemic and urinary alkalizing agent

Pregnancy Category: C

AVAILABLE PREPARATIONS
Inj: 4% (2.4 mEq/5 ml), 4.2% (5 mEq/5 ml), 5% (297.5 mEq/500 ml), 7.5% (8.92 mEq/10 ml, 44.6 mEq/50 ml), 8.4% (10 mEq/10 ml, 50 mEq/50ml

ROUTES AND DOSAGES
Cardiac Arrest
Children ≤2 yr: IV 0.5-1 mEq/kg IV bolus of 4.2% sol; may repeat q 10 min depending on ABG, not to exceed 8 mEq/kg/24 hr
Children >2 yr and adults: IV bolus 1 mEq/kg (7.5% or 8.4% sol), followed by 0.5 mEq/kg q 10 min depending on ABG
Urinary Alkalization
Children: IV 1-10 mEq/kg/24 hr divided q4h
Adults: 48 mEq PO followed by 12-24 mEq q4h
Metabolic Acidosis
Children and adults: IV 2-5 mEq/kg infused over 4-8 hr, depending on blood pH and CO_2

IV administration
• Recommended concentration: May administer undiluted injection to children; for infants dilute 1 mEq/ml sol 1:1 with SW
• IV push rate: May administer as direct IV bolus

MECHANISM AND INDICATIONS
Mechanism: Dissociates into sodium (Na^+) and bicarbonate (HCO_3^-) to neutralize hydrogen ion concentration and increase blood and urinary pH
Indications: For use as adjunct to advanced cardiac life support, metabolic acidosis, urinary alkalinization

PHARMACOKINETICS
Onset of action: 15 min
Duration: 1-2 hr
Excretion: Urine

CONTRAINDICATIONS AND PRECAUTIONS
• Contraindicated with alkalosis, hypocalcemia, unknown abdominal pain, inadequate ventilation during CPR, excess chloride losses, renal disease
• Use cautiously with CHF, cirrhosis, toxemia, ascites, children <2 yr, lactation

INTERACTIONS
Drug
• Increased effects of amphetamines, quinine, quinidine, pseudoephedrine, flecainide
• Decreased effects of lithium, chloprapramide, barbiturates, salicylates
Lab
• Increased urinary urobilinogen
• False positive urine protein, blood lactate

INCOMPATIBILITIES
• Avoid mixing in IV with atropine, Ca, carmustine, cefotaxime, chlorpromazine, cisplatin, codeine, corticotropin, dobutamine, dopamine, epinephrine, glycopyrrolate, hydromorphone, idarubicin, insulin, isoproterenol, labetalol, levarterenol, levorphanol, lincomycin, LR, Mg, meperidine, mehtadone, methicillin, metoclo-

---

pramide, morphine, penicillin, pentobarbital, pentazocine, phenobarbital, K^+ procaine, promazine, R, secobarbital, streptomycin, succinylcholine, sulfate, tetracycline, thiopental, tubocurarine, vancomycin

SIDE EFFECTS
CNS: Confusion, headache, irritability, tremors, seizures
CV: Fluid retention, edema, irregular pulse
GU: Renal calculi
METAB: Alkalosis
RESP: Decreased respiratory rate

TOXICITY AND OVERDOSE
Clinical signs: Depressed consciousness, lethargy, arrhythmias, seizures
Treatment: Correct electrolyte, fluid, and pH abnormalities

PATIENT CARE MANAGEMENT
Assessment
• Assess history of hypersensitivity to drug
• Assess VS, B/P, rhythm, depth of respiration
• Assess I&O, wt, edema
• Assess electrolytes, blood and urine pH, PO_2, HCO_3^- and ABGs
• Assess extravasation; tissue sloughing and necrosis may occur
Interventions
• May administer IV undiluted to children
• Dilute 1 mEq/ml sol 1:1 with SW for IV in infants
• Ensure adequate ventilation during administration
Evaluation
• Evaluate therapeutic response (normal ABGs, electrolytes, blood pH, HCO_3^-)
• Evaluate for signs, symptoms of alkalosis (confusion, irritability, decreased respiratory rate, hyperreflexia, irregular pulse)

PATIENT AND FAMILY EDUCATION
Teach/instruct
• About need for drug
• Provide support during critical situations

STORAGE
• In tightly closed containers at room temp; note expiration date
• Do not use if sol has precipitated

---

sodium polystyrene sulfonate

Brand Name(s): Kayexalate❦, PMS-Sodium❦, Polysterene Sulfate❦, SPS Suspension❦

Classification: Potassium removing resin

Pregnancy Category: C

AVAILABLE PREPARATIONS
Powder: 454 g (3.5 g/5ml)
Susp: 15 g/60 ml (contains 21.5 ml sorbitol per 60 ml)

ROUTES AND DOSAGES
Neonates: PO, PR 1 g/kg q 20 min prn
Children: PO 1 g/kg q6h *or* PR q2-6h
Adults: PO 15 g qd-qid or PR 30-50 g q6h prn as retention enema
• Drug delivers 1 mEq Na for each mEq K^+ removed

MECHANISM AND INDICATIONS
Mechanism: Removes K by exchanging K^+ for Na in large intestine
Indications: For use in hyperkalemia

PHARMACOKINETICS
Onset of action: Hr to days
Absorption: Minimal; Na exchanged for K^+ in large intestine
Excretion: Feces

CONTRAINDICATIONS AND PRECAUTIONS
• Contraindicated with hypokalemia
• Use cautiously with renal failure, pts whose Na intake is restricted (CHF, severe hypertension, severe edema)

INTERACTIONS
Drug
• Metabolic alkalosis in pts with renal failure with antacids

S

❦ Available in Canada.

- Alkalosis possible with laxatives containing Mg or aluminum

Lab

- Altered serum Ca and Mg levels

SIDE EFFECTS

CV: ECG abnormalities

GI: Constipation, anorexia, nausea, vomiting, diarrhea, fecal impaction, gastric irritation

METAB: Na retention, electrolyte imbalances

TOXICITY AND OVERDOSE

Clinical signs: Hypokalemia (muscle weakness, irritability, confusion, ECG changes)

Treatment: Discontinue drug; administer K⁺ supplement, diuretics

PATIENT CARE MANAGEMENT

Assessment

- Assess history of hypersensitivity to drug
- Assess VS, B/P
- Assess for signs, symptoms of hyperkalemia
- Assess serum K⁺

Interventions

- Mix PO, NG with water or sorbitol; serve chilled
- Mix PR with warm sorbitol or water; administer by high sigmoid enema, retain in rectum for several hr, cleanse colon with non-Na sol to remove drug

Evaluation

- Evaluate therapeutic response (K⁺ with normal limits)
- Evaluate serum, Na, Ca, Mg, acid–base balance
- Monitor bowel activity for constipation or diarrhea

PATIENT AND FAMILY EDUCATION

Teach/instruct

- To maintain low K⁺ diet
- About necessity of retaining enema as long as possible

STORAGE

- Store freshly prepared sol for 24 hr at room temp

---

somatrem

Brand Name(s): Protropin✤

Classification: Human growth hormone (pituitary hormone)

Pregnancy Category: C

AVAILABLE PREPARATIONS

Lyophilized powder: 5, 10 mg/vial

ROUTES AND DOSAGES

Growth Hormone Deficiency

Children and adults: IM/SC, up to 0.1 mg/kg three × per wk or divided as 0.05 mg/kg six × per wk; not to exceed 0.3 mg/kg/wk; discontinue when pt has achieved satisfactory adult height, when epiphyses are fused, or when pt no longer responds to treatment

MECHANISM AND INDICATIONS

Growth stimulation mechanism: Structurally identical to naturally occurring human growth hormone (GH) plus one additional amino acid (methionine); stimulates linear growth of bone, muscle, and organs

Indications: Replacement of endogenous GH (hypopituitarism, following cranial irradiation, trauma)

PHARMACOKINETICS

Half-life: 20-30 min

Metabolism: Liver

Excretion: Urine

CONTRAINDICATIONS AND PRECAUTIONS

- Contraindicated with hypersensitivity to GH or benzyl alcohol, active neoplasia, with closed epiphyses
- Use cautiously in pts with treated tumors or neoplasia; with family history of diabetes; with pregnancy

INTERACTIONS

Drug

- Inhibited growth possible with glucocorticoids
- Accelerated closure of epiphysis possible with anabolic steroids,

---

thyroid hormone, estrogens, androgens

Lab

- Reduced glucose tolerance
- Altered thyroid function tests possible

SIDE EFFECTS

CNS: Headache, pseudotumor cerebri (intracranial hypertension)

ENDO: Hyperglycemia, hypothyroidism

MS: Slipped capital femoral epiphysis

Local: Pain and swelling at injection site

Other: Antibodies to GH

TOXICITY AND OVERDOSE

Clinical signs: Gigantism, acromegalic features, organ enlargement, diabetes, atherosclerosis, hypertension

Treatment: Discontinue drug

PATIENT CARE MANAGEMENT

Assessment

- Assess history of hypersensitivity to GH or benzyl alcohol
- Assess for biochemical evidence of GH deficiency, baseline thyroid function tests, bone age, status of preexisting brain tumor (if applicable)

Interventions

- Do not shake after reconstituting IM/SC; do not use if sol is discolored or cloudy
- Injection is painful; rotate injection sites

Evaluation

- Evaluate therapeutic response (increased growth velocity over pre-treatment rate)
- Monitor growth q 3-4 mo using stadiometer
- Monitor for signs of glucose intolerance, increased intracranial pressure, slipped capital femoral epiphysis
- Monitor thyroid tests and bone age yearly

PATIENT AND FAMILY EDUCATION

Teach/instruct

- To take as directed at prescribed intervals for prescribed length of time

Warn/advise

- To notify care provider of hypersensitivity, side effects
- That increased appetite may be experienced along with increased growth
- To comply with follow-up care

STORAGE

- Refrigerate powder and reconstituted sol
- Reconstituted drug must be used within 14 days

---

somatropin

Brand Name(s): Humatrope❧, Nutropin❧

Classification: Human growth hormone (pituitary hormone)

Pregnancy Category: C

AVAILABLE PREPARATIONS

Lyophilized powder: 5, 10 mg/vial

ROUTES AND DOSAGES

Growth Hormone Deficiency

- Individualize dosage and administration schedule for each pt

Children and adults: Nutropin: SC, total of 0.3 mg/kg weekly

Humatrope: SC/IM up to 0.06 mg/kg 3 times per week

Chronic Renal Insufficiency (CRI)

Children and adults: Nutropin: SC, total of 0.35 mg/kg weekly; see interventions for timing of dose for dialysis pts

MECHANISM AND INDICATIONS

Growth stimulation mechanism: Structurally identical to naturally occurring human growth hormone (GH); stimulates linear growth of bone, muscle, and organs

Indications: Replacement of endogenous GH (hypopituitarism, following cranial irradiation, trauma), growth failure associated with chronic renal insufficiency up to the time of transplant

S

PHARMACOKINETICS
Peak: 7.5 hr
Half-life: 20-30 min
Metabolism: Liver
Excretion: Urine

CONTRAINDICATIONS AND PRECAUTIONS
• Contraindicated with hypersensitivity to GH or *m*-cresol, glycerin, benzyl alcohol; pts with fused epiphyses, active neoplasia
• Use cautiously in pts with treated tumors or neoplasia; with family history of diabetes; with pregnancy

INTERACTIONS
Drug
• Inhibited growth possible with glucocorticoids
• Accelerated closure of epiphyses possible with anabolic steroids, thyroid hormone, estrogens, androgens
Lab
• Reduced glucose tolerance
• Altered thyroid function tests possible
• Increased inorganic PO_4, alk phos, parathyroid hormone

SIDE EFFECTS
CNS: Headache, pseudotumor cerebri (intracranial hypertension)
ENDO: Hyperglycemia, hypothyroidism
MS: Slipped capital femoral epiphysis
Local: Pain and swelling at injection site
Other: Antibodies to GH

TOXICITY AND OVERDOSE
Clinical signs: Gigantism, acromegalic features, organ enlargement, diabetes, atherosclerosis, hypertension
Treatment: Discontinue drug

PATIENT CARE MANAGEMENT
Assessment
• Assess history of hypersensitivity to GH, *m*-cresol, glycerin, benzyl alcohol
• Biochemical evidence of GH deficiency, baseline thyroid function tests, bone age, status of preexisting brain tumor (if applicable)
Interventions
• Do not shake vial; do not use if sol is discolored or cloudy
• Injection is painful; rotate injection sites
• Administer somatropin at hs or at least 3-4 hr after hemodialysis to prevent hematoma caused by heparin
• With chronic cycling peritoneal dialysis (CCPD), administer in AM after dialysis
• With chronic ambulatory peritoneal dialysis (CAPD) administer at hs at time of overnight exchange
Evaluation
• Evaluate therapeutic response (increased growth velocity over pre-treatment rate)
• Monitor thyroid function tests, bone age yearly
• Monitor growth q 3-4 mo using stadiometer
• Monitor for symptoms of glucose intolerance, increased intracranial pressure, slipped capital femoral epiphysis

PATIENT AND FAMILY EDUCATION
Teach/instruct
• To take as directed at prescribed intervals for prescribed length of time
Warn/advise
• To notify care provider of hypersensitivity, side effects
• That increased appetite may be experienced along with increased growth
• To comply with follow-up care
STORAGE
• Refrigerate powder and reconstituted sol
• Reconstituted drug must be used within 14 days

spectinomycin hydrochloride

Brand Name(s): Trobicin ✤

Classification: Antibiotic (aminocyclitol)

Pregnancy Category: B

AVAILABLE PREPARATIONS
Inj: 2 g, 4 g

ROUTES AND DOSAGES
Uncomplicated Gonorrhea
Children: IM 40 mg/kg/dose once; usually used for children allergic to cephalosporins or penicillins; children >8 yr may be treated with oral tetracycline
Adults: IM 2-4 g once
Disseminated Gonorrhea
Adults: 2 g bid for 3-7 days

MECHANISM AND INDICATIONS
Antibiotic mechanism: Bacteriostatic; inhibits protein synthesis by binding to 30S ribosomal subunits
Indications: Effective against many gram-positive and gram-negative organism; primarily used against penicillin-resistant *Neisseria gonorrhoeae*

PHARMACOKINETICS
Peak: 1-2 hr
Half-life: 1-3 hr
Metabolism: Unknown
Excretion: Urine

CONTRAINDICATIONS AND PRECAUTIONS
• Contraindicated with known hypersensitivity to spectinomycin
• Use cautiously with infants, children, pregnancy, pts with strong history of drug allergies

INTERACTIONS
Lab
• Increased BUN, AST, serum alk phos
• Decreased Hgb, Hct, CrCl

SIDE EFFECTS
CNS: Insomnia, dizziness
DERM: Urticaria, rash, pruritus
GI: Nausea, vomiting
GU: Decreased urine output
Local: Pain at injection site
Other: Fever, chills

PATIENT CARE MANAGEMENT
Assessment
• Assess history of hypersensitivity to spectinomycin, other drugs
• Obtain C&S; may begin therapy before obtaining results
• Assess hematologic function (CBC, differential, platelet count), hepatic function (ALT, AST, bilirubin) if multiple doses will be given
Interventions
• Administer IM deeply into upper outer quadrant of buttocks; administer no more than 5 ml per injection site; rotate injection sites
• Maintain age-appropriate fluid intake
• Continue medication for full course of treatment
Evaluation
• Evaluate therapeutic response (decreased symptoms of infection)
• Evaluate hematologic function (CBC, differential, platelet count), hepatic function (ALT, AST, bilirubin) following multiple doses
• Obtain gonorrhea culture after treatment (lack of response to drug usually indicates reinfection); serologic test for syphilis 3 mo after treatment (spectinomycin may mask signs of incubating syphilis)
• Observe for signs of superinfection (perineal itching, fever, malaise, redness, pain, swelling, drainage, rash, diarrhea, sore throat, change in cough or sputum)
• Evaluate IM site for tissue damage

PATIENT AND FAMILY EDUCATION
Teach/instruct
• To take as directed at prescribed intervals for prescribed length of time
• About methods to prevent transmission of sexually transmitted diseases
Warn/advise
• To notify care provider of hyper-

sensitivity, side effects, superinfection
• That sexual partner needs to be evaluated and treated

STORAGE
• Store powder at room temp
• Reconstituted parenteral sol stable at room temp 24 hr

---

spironolactone

Brand Name(s): Aldactone✤, Novo-Spiroton✤

Classification: K^+-sparing diuretic

Pregnancy Category: D

AVAILABLE PREPARATIONS
Tabs: 25 mg, 50 mg, 100 mg

ROUTES AND DOSAGES
Edema and Hypertension
Children: PO 1.5-3.3 mg/kg/24 hr divided qd-qid or 60 mg/m^2/24 hr divided bid-qid
Adults: PO 25-200 mg/24 hr divided bid

Diagnosis of Primary Hypoaldosteronism
Children: PO 125-375 mg/m^2/24 hr divided bid × 24 hr
Adults: PO 400 mg/24 hr in 1-2 divided doses

MECHANISM AND INDICATIONS
Edema and hypertension mechanisms: Inhibits aldosterone effects in kidneys increasing Na and H_2O excretion and decreasing K^+ excretion
Mechanism for diagnosis of primary hypoaldosteronism: Inhibits effects of aldosterone; correction of hypertension and hypokalemia when taking drug is presumed to be evidence of primary hypoaldosteronism
Indications: For treatment of edematous conditions (CHF, cirrhosis, nephrotic syndrome), hypertension, hypokalemia, primary hypoaldosteronism

PHARMACOKINETICS
Onset of action: Gradual; maximum diuretic effect occurs 3 days after drug started
Half-life: 13-24 hr (qd-bid dosing), 9-16 hr (qid dosing)
Metabolism: Liver
Excretion: Urine and bile

CONTRAINDICATIONS AND PRECAUTIONS
• Contraindicated with renal failure, anuria, hyperkalemia ($K^+ > 5.5$), other K^+-sparing diuretics or K^+ supplements
• Use cautiously with hepatic or renal dysfunction, diabetes, metabolic or respiratory acidosis, lactation

INTERACTIONS
Drug
• Increased hypotensive effects with other antihypertensives
• Increased risk of hyperkalemia with captopril, K^+ supplements
• Increased diuresis with other diuretics
• Decreased hypertensive effects with NSAIDs, estrogen, aspirin
Lab
• Falsely elevated serum digoxin levels
• Increased BG in diabetics
• Altered plasma and urinary 17-OHCS levels

SIDE EFFECTS
CNS: Lethargy, headache, dizziness
CV: Arrhythmia (from hyperkalemia)
DERM: Urticaria, rash, sweating
GI: Anorexia, nausea and vomiting, dry mouth, thirst, diarrhea
METAB: Hyperkalemia, dehydration, acidosis, hyponatremia
Other: Gynecomastia in males

TOXICITY AND OVERDOSE
Clinical signs: Dehydration, electrolyte disturbance
Treatment: Discontinue drug; restrict K^+ in diet; administer glucose and insulin or $NaHCO_3$; may administer Kayexalate

---

✤ Available in Canada.

PATIENT CARE MANAGEMENT
Assessment
• Assess history of hypersensitivity to drug
• Assess baseline and ongoing VS, B/P, wt
• Assess baseline and ongoing electrolytes, BUN, ECG
Interventions
• May crush tabs and administer in flavored syrup
• Measure daily I&O
• Observe for signs of hyperkalemia (cardiac arrhythmias, confusion, weakness)
• Assure safe environment in case dizziness, hypotension occur
Evaluation
• Evaluate therapeutic response (effective diuresis)
• Evaluate for symptoms of toxicity
• Evaluate for edema
• Evaluate blood studies, especially electrolytes (K$^+$); report abnormal results to care provider

PATIENT AND FAMILY EDUCATION
Teach/instruct
• To take as directed at prescribed intervals for prescribed length of time
• To avoid foods high in K$^+$ (citrus fruits, bananas, raisins, potatoes)
• To administer drug with meals
• To notify care provider if unusual symptoms occur (weakness, fatigue, muscle cramps, nausea, vomiting, diarrhea, palpitations, mental confusion, rash)
• About importance of regular medical care while taking this drug
Warn/advise
• To call care provider if edema, excess diuresis occurs
• That dizziness may occur; use caution when rising quickly, driving; avoid hazardous activities

STORAGE
• Store at room temp in light-resistant containers

---

stavudine
Brand Name(s): Zerit
Classification: Antiretroviral
Pregnancy Category: C

AVAILABLE PREPARATIONS
Caps: 15 mg, 20 mg, 30 mg, 40 mg

ROUTES AND DOSAGES
• Safety and effectiveness in children not established
Adults: <60 kg: PO 30 mg bid q12h
Adults: >60 kg: PO 40 mg bid q12h

MECHANISM AND INDICATIONS
Mechanism: Inhibits HIV replication by causing DNA chain termination and reducing synthesis of mitochondrial DNA
Indications: For use in treatment of adults with advanced HIV infection who are intolerant of approved, standard clinical therapies or have shown clinical deterioration while on such therapies; no current data is available on long-term effects of stavudine therapy on progression of HIV disease

PHARMACOKINETICS
Onset of action: Rapid
Peak: 1 hr
Half-life: 1.44 hr
Metabolism: Unknown
Excretion: Urine

CONTRAINDICATIONS AND PRECAUTIONS
• Contraindicated with hypersensitivity to drug or its components, lactation
• Use cautiously with pregnancy, children (limited clinical data available), hepatic and renal dysfunction

INTERACTIONS
Lab
• Increased AST, ALT, alk phos, bilirubin
• Decreased absolute neutrophil count

S

SIDE EFFECTS

CNS: Peripheral neuropathy, headache, insomnia, anxiety, depression, nervousness, confusion
CV: Chest pain, vasodilation, hypertension, peripheral vascular disorder, syncope
DERM: Rash, sweating, pruritis, urticaria
ENDO/METAB: Wt loss
EENT: Conjunctivitis, blurred vision
GI: Diarrhea, nausea, vomiting, abdominal pain, anorexia, dyspepsia, constipation, pancreatitis
GU: Dysuria, genital pain, dysmenorrhea, vaginitis, urinary frequency, hematuria, impotence
HEME: Lymphadenopathy, anemia, neutropenia, leukopenia, thrombocytopenia
RESP: Dyspnea
Other: Chills, fever, back pain, malaise, myalgia, arthralgia

TOXICITY AND OVERDOSE

Clinical signs: With chronic overdose, hepatic toxicity, exaggerated peripheral neuropathy, pancreatitis
Treatment: Supportive care

PATIENT CARE MANAGEMENT
Assessment

• Assess history of hypersensitivity to drug and its components
• Assess baseline T cell studies, CBC, differential
• Assess baseline liver function (AST, ALT, bilirubin, alk phos), renal function (BUN, creatinine)
• Assess for history of peripheral neuropathy; pts with this history are at increased risk of developing neuropathy
• Assess baseline wt

Interventions

• May administer caps with or without food
• Caps should be administered q12h

NURSING ALERT

Stavudine is indicated for use in the treatment of adults with advanced HIV infection who are intolerant of approved, standard clinical therapies or who have shown clinical deterioration while on such therapies

Can cause peripheral neuropathy; notify care provider if symptoms occur

---

Evaluation

• Evaluate therapeutic response (improved T cell counts)
• Evaluate for side effects, hypersensitivity
• Monitor liver function (AST, ALT, bilirubin, alk phos), renal function (BUN, creatinine)
• Monitor baseline T cell studies, CBC, differential
• Evaluate for development of peripheral neuropathy; stop drug and notify care provider
• Monitor wt

PATIENT AND FAMILY EDUCATION
Teach/instruct

• To take as directed at prescribed intervals for prescribed length of time
• About side effects (especially peripheral neuropathy); to notify care provider
• That treatment with drug is not a first-line treatment and should be used only when standard antiretroviral therapy is not tolerated, is contraindicated, or if pt has deteriorated on standard therapies
• That opportunistic infections and HIV-related complications can still occur while taking medication

Warn/advise

• To notify care provider of numbness, burning, tingling, pain or weakness in feet or hands

Encourage

• Intake of nutritious meals; consider nutrition consultation

---

• To verbalize fears, concerns; consider social work consultation

STORAGE
• Store at room temp in tightly closed container

---

streptomycin sulfate
Classification: Antibiotic (aminoglycoside)
Pregnancy Category: D

AVAILABLE PREPARATIONS
Inj: 400 mg/ml, 500 mg/ml in 1 g or 5 g vials

ROUTES AND DOSAGES
Neonates: IM 10-20 mg/kg/24 hr qd
Infants: IM 20-30 mg/kg/24 hr divided q12h
Children: 20-40 mg/kg/24 hr divided q6-12h; maximum 2 g/24 hr
Adults: IM 15 mg/kg/24 hr divided q12h; maximum 2 g/24 hr
Tuberculosis
Infants: IM 20-30 mg/kg/24 hr divided q12h for 7-10 days; maximum 2 g/24 hr
Children: IM 20-40 mg/kg/24 hr divided q12-24h for 7-10 days; maximum 2 g/24 hr or 1 g/dose
Adults: IM 15 mg/kg/24 hr divided q12h for 7-10 days; maximum 2 g/24 hr
Enterococcal Endocarditis
Adults: IM 1 g q12h for 2 wk, then 500 mg q12h for 4 wk
Streptococcal Endocarditis
Adults: IM 1 g q12h for 1 wk, then 500 mg q12h for 1 wk

MECHANISM AND INDICATIONS
Antibiotic mechanism: Bactericidal; inhibits bacterial protein synthesis by binding directly to the 30S ribosomal subunit
Indications: Effective against *Mycobacterium tuberculosis, Yersinia pestis, Brucella, Haemophilus influenzae, Klebsiella pneumoniae, E. coli, Enterobacter aerogenes, Streptococcus viridans, Francisella tularensis, Proteus;* used to treat active tuberculosis, streptococcal or enterococcal endocarditis, mycobacterial infections, brucellosis

PHARMACOKINETICS
Peak: 1-2 hr
Distribution: Into most body tissues and extracellular fluids
Half-life: Neonates 4-10 hr, adults: 2-4.7 hr
Metabolism: Not metabolized
Excretion: Urine, bile
Therapeutic level: Peak 15-40 mcg/ml, trough <5 mcg/ml

CONTRAINDICATIONS AND PRECAUTIONS
• Contraindicated with known hypersensitivity to streptomycin or any other aminoglycoside, renal failure
• Use cautiously with neonates and infants (because of renal immaturity) impaired renal function, dehydration, 8th cranial nerve impairment, myasthenia gravis, parkinsonism, hypocalcemia, pregnancy, lactation

INTERACTIONS
Drug
• Increased risk of nephrotoxicity, ototoxicity, neurotoxicity with methoxyflurane, polymixin B, vancomycin, capreomycin, cisplatin, cephalosporins, amphotericin B, other aminoglycosides
• Increased risk of ototoxicity with ethacrynic acid, furosemide, bumetanide, urea, mannitol
• Masked symptoms of ototoxicity with dimenhydrinate, other antiemetic or antivertigo drugs
• Synergistic antimicrobial activity against certain organisms with penicillins
• Increased risk of neuromuscular blockade with general anesthetics or neuromuscular blocking agents such as succinylcholine, tubocurarine
• Increased effects of oral anticoagulants
• Inactivated when administered with parenteral penicillins (such as carbenicillin, ticarcillin)
Lab
• Increased LDH, BUN, nonprotein N, serum creatinine levels

S

- Increased urinary excretion of casts
- Decreased serum Na

INCOMPATIBILITIES

- Amphotericin B, carbenicillin, cephalothin, erythromycin, heparin, ticarcillin

SIDE EFFECTS

CNS: Headache, lethargy, neuromuscular blockade
EENT: Ototoxicity (tinnitus, vertigo, hearing loss)
GI: Diarrhea
GU: Some nephrotoxicity (less frequent than with other aminoglycosides)
HEME: Transient agranulocytosis
Local: Pain, irritation, sterile abscesses at injection site
Other: Hypersensitivity reactions (rash, fever, urticaria, angioneurotic edema, anaphylaxis), bacterial or fungal superinfection

TOXICITY AND OVERDOSE

Clinical signs: Ototoxicity, nephrotoxicity, neuromuscular toxicity
Treatment: Supportive care, hemodialysis or peritoneal dialysis; neuromuscular blockade reversed with Ca salts or anticholinesterases

PATIENT CARE MANAGEMENT

Assessment

- Assess history of hypersensitivity to streptomycin or other aminoglycosides
- Obtain C&S; may begin therapy before obtaining results
- Assess renal function (BUN, creatinine, I&O), baseline wt, hearing tests before beginning therapy

Interventions

- Protect hands when preparing medication, drug irritates skin
- Sol should be colorless or clear to very pale yellow; do not use if dark yellow, cloudy, or containing precipitates
- Administer streptomycin at least 1 hr before or after other antibiotics (penicillins, cephalosporins)
- IM concentration should not exceed 500 mg/ml

- Injection may be painful; administer deeply into large muscle mass and rotate injection site; do not inject more than 2 g of drug per injection site
- Maintain age-appropriate fluid intake
- Supervise ambulation, other safety measures with vestibular dysfunction
- Obtain drug levels after 3rd dose (sooner in neonates or pts with rapidly changing renal function); peak levels drawn 1 hr after IM injection; trough just before next dose

> **NURSING ALERT**
> Discontinue drug if signs of ototoxicity, nephrotoxicity, hypersensitivity develop

Evaluation

- Evaluate therapeutic response (decreased symptoms of infection)
- Evaluate renal function (BUN, creatinine, I&O), daily wts, hearing evaluations
- Observe for signs of superinfection (perineal itching, diaper rash, fever, malaise, redness, pain, swelling, drainage, rash, diarrhea, sore throat, change in cough or sputum)
- Evaluate IM site for tissue damage

PATIENT AND FAMILY EDUCATION

Teach/instruct

- To take as directed at prescribed intervals for prescribed length of time

Warn/advise

- To notify care provider of hypersensitivity, side effects, superinfection

STORAGE

- Store powder at room temp
- Depending on manufacturer, reconstituted sol stable 2-4 wk refrigerated

---

✤ Available in Canada.

succimer

Brand Name(s): Chemet

Classification: Antidote (lead toxicity)

Pregnancy Category: C

AVAILABLE PREPARATIONS
Caps: 100 mg

ROUTES AND DOSAGES
Children: PO 10 mg/kg/dose or 350 mg/m^2/dose q8h for 5 days, then 10 mg/kg/dose or 350 mg/m^2/dose q12h for 14 days

MECHANISM AND INDICATIONS
Antidote mechanism: Binds with ions of lead to form a water-soluble complex that is excreted in urine
Indications: Used to treat lead poisoning in children with blood lead levels >45 mcg/dl

PHARMACOKINETICS
Peak: 1-2 hr
Metabolism: Extensive to mixed succimer-cysteine disulfides
Excretion: Feces, urine

CONTRAINDICATIONS AND PRECAUTIONS
• Contraindicated with hypersensitivity to succimer
• Use cautiously with renal or hepatic impairment, children <1 yr, pregnancy, lactation

INTERACTIONS
Drug
• Do not use concomitantly with edetate calcium disodium or penicillamine
Lab
• Falsely increased serum creatinine phosphokinase
• False positive urine ketones with Ketostix
• Falsely decreased uric acid

SIDE EFFECTS
DERM: Rash, urticaria
GI: Nausea, vomiting, diarrhea, anorexia, metallic taste, increased liver function tests, cholesterol
GU: Sulfurous odor to urine, hemorrhoidal symptoms

Other: Flu-like symptoms, sulfurous odor to breath

TOXICITY AND OVERDOSE
Clinical signs: No information available
Treatment: Supportive care; induced vomiting or gastric lavage followed by activated charcoal

PATIENT CARE MANAGEMENT
Assessment
• Assess history of hypersensitivity to succimer
• Assess renal function (BUN, creatinine, I&O), hepatic function (ALT, AST, bilirubin), blood lead concentration
• Identify lead sources in child's environment
Interventions
• Caps may be taken apart, mixed with food or fluid
• Maintain age-appropriate fluid intake
Evaluation
• Evaluate therapeutic response (decreased blood lead concentration)
• Monitor renal function (BUN, creatinine, I&O), hepatic function (ALT, AST, bilirubin), hydration status
• Monitor for allergic reactions (rash, pruritus, urticaria)

PATIENT AND FAMILY EDUCATION
Teach/instruct
• To take as directed at prescribed intervals for prescribed length of time
• About sources of lead poisoning, ways to prevent further exposure or poisoning
Warn/advise
• To notify care provider of hypersensitivity, side effects
• To comply with follow-up care to monitor blood lead concentrations, neurologic or developmental status

STORAGE
• Store at room temp

S

succinylcholine chloride

Brand Name(s): Anectine✤, Anectine Flo-Pack, Brevidil M (Bromide Salt), Min-I-Mix, Quelicin, Quelicin Chloride Injection✤, Scaline, Succinycholine Chloride Min-I-Mix, Sucostrin, Sux-Cert

Classification: Neuromuscular blocking agent (depolarizing)

Pregnancy Category: C

AVAILABLE PREPARATIONS
Inj: 20 mg/ml, 50 mg/ml, 100 mg/ml
Powder for inj: 100 mg, 500 mg, 1 g

ROUTES AND DOSAGES
Older children and adolescents: IV Loading for intubation or short surgical procedures, 1-2 mg/kg; 1 mg/kg recommended; maintenance: 0.3-0.6 mg/kg q5-10 min prn; IM 2.5-4 mg/kg (maximum 150 mg)
Adults: IV 0.3-1.1 mg/kg/dose once, then maintenance 0.04-0.07 mg/kg q5-10 min prn; IM 2.5-4 mg/kg (maximum 150 mg/dose)

IV administration
• Recommended concentration: 20 mg/ml for IV push; flush needle/catheter with D_5W or NS after administration
• Maximum concentration: 20 mg/ml for IV push
• IV push rate: Over 10-30 sec
• Continuous infusion: Not routinely recommended for children; may be used for neuromuscular relaxation for infants

MECHANISM AND INDICATIONS
Mechanism: Acts to interrupt transmission of nerve impulse at neuromuscular skeletal junction; acts to depolarize membrane by opening channels in the same manner as acetylcholine, producing depolarization of the motor endplate at the myoneural junctions
Indications: Used as an adjunct to general anesthesia to facilitate tracheal intubation, to promote skeletal muscle relaxation during surgery or mechanical ventilation

PHARMACOKINETICS
Onset of action: IV 30-60 sec; IM 2-3 min
Peak: IV 2-3 min
Duration: IV 6-10 min
Metabolism: Hydrolyzed by plasma pseudocholinesterase
Excretion: Urine

CONTRAINDICATIONS AND PRECAUTIONS
• Contraindicated with known hypersensitivity; pts with malignant hyperthermia; myopathies associated with elevated serum creatinine values; narrow-angle glaucoma; penetrating eye injuries; disorders of plasma pseudocholinesterase
• Use cautiously with pregnancy, lactation, children <2 yr, fluid and electrolyte imbalances, dehydration; neuromuscular, cardiac, respiratory, collagen diseases; glaucoma, eye surgery, penetrating eye wounds; severe burns, fractures (fasciculations may increase damage); elderly or debilitated pts
• Injectable sol may contain benzyl alcohol as a preservative; administration of benzyl alcohol at 99-234 mg/kg has been associated with a fatal gasping syndrome in neonates; clinical signs include metabolic acidosis, hypotension, CNS depression, cardiovascular collapse

INTERACTIONS
Drug
• Increased neuromuscular blockade with aminoglycosides, clindamycin, lincomycin, quinidine, local anesthetics, polymyxin antibiotics, lithium, narcotic analgesics, thiazides, enflurane, isoflurane
• Arrhythmias possible with theophylline

INCOMPATIBILITIES
• Incompatible with barbiturates,

---

chlorpromazine, nafcillin, alkaline sol

SIDE EFFECTS

CV: Bradycardia, tachycardia, increased or decreased B/P, sinus arrest, arrhythmias
DERM: Rash, urticaria, flushing, pruritis
EENT: Increased secretions; increased intraocular pressure
HEME: Myoglobulinemia
MS: Weakness, fasciculations, prolonged relaxation, muscle pain
RESP: Prolonged apnea, bronchospasm, cyanosis, respiratory depression
Other: Endogenous histamine release may occur with tubocurarine chloride, noted clinically as erythema, hypotension, either bradycardia or tachycardia

TOXICITY AND OVERDOSE

Clinical signs: Prolonged apnea, bronchospasm, cyanosis, respiratory depression
Treatment: Anticholinesterase to reverse neuromuscular blockade (edrophonium or neostigmine, atropine); monitor VS; mechanical ventilation may be required

PATIENT CARE MANAGEMENT

Assessment

• Assess for history of hypersensitivity to succinylcholine
• Assess for preexisting conditions that would contraindicate use of succinylcholine
• Assess for electrolyte imbalances particularly K^+ and Mg (may increase action of drug, particularly in patients with trauma or neuromuscular disease)
• Monitor therapeutic response (paralysis of jaw, eyelid, head, neck, rest of the body)

Interventions

• Monitor for allergic reactions (rash, fever, respiratory distress, pruritus) drug should be discontinued
• Monitor VS (pulse, respirations, airway, B/P) until fully recovered; characteristics of respirations (rate, depth, pattern); strength of hand grip
• Monitor I&O for urinary frequency, hesitancy, retention
• Tachyphylaxis and phase II nerve block may occur during continuous infusion to infants/children; bradyarrhythmias may occur; prophylactic atropine (0.01-0.03 mg/kg) may be used with or during succinylcholine administration
• Administer deep IM (preferably high in deltoid)

NURSING ALERT

Injectable sol may contain benzyl alcohol as a preservative; administration of benzyl alcohol at 99-234 mg/kg has been associated with a fatal gasping syndrome in neonates; clinical signs include metabolic acidosis, hypotension, CNS depression, cardiovascular collapse

---

Evaluation

• Monitor effectiveness of neuromuscular blockade (degree of paralysis); use nerve stimulator
• Monitor for recovery (including decreased paralysis of face, diaphragm, arm, rest of the body)

PATIENT AND FAMILY EDUCATION

Teach/instruct

• Provide reassurance if communication is difficult during recovery

STORAGE

• Store sol in refrigerator; powder at room temp in a tightly closed container

S

sucralfate

Brand Name(s): Apo-Sucralfate✤, Carafate, Novo-Sucralate✤, Sulcrate✤, Sulcrate Suspension Plus✤

Classification: Antiulcer agent; gastric mucosa protectant

Pregnancy Category: B

AVAILABLE PREPARATIONS
Oral susp: 500 mg/5 ml
Tabs: 1 g

ROUTES AND DOSAGES
Duodenal/Gastric Ulcer
Infants and children: PO 40-80 mg/kg/24 hr divided q6h
Adults: PO tabs and susp, treatment, 1 g qid 1 hr ac, hs; prophylaxis, tabs 1 g bid on an empty stomach
Gastroesophageal Reflux
Infants and children: PO 40-80 mg/kg/24 hr divided q6h
Adults: PO susp 1 g qid 1 hr ac, hs

MECHANISM AND INDICATIONS
Mechanism: Thought to form an ulcer-adherent complex with proteinaceous exudate at ulcer site, protecting it against further acid attack; also creates viscous, adhesive barrier on the surface of intact mucosa of stomach and duodenum
Indications: Short-term treatment of duodenal ulcers and in prevention of recurrence; investigational uses include short-term treatment of benign gastric ulcer; prophylaxis and treatment of stress-related mucosal damage; treatment of GERD; relief of GI symptoms associated with use of NSAIDs treatment of rheumatoid arthritis

PHARMACOKINETICS
Absorption: Largely unabsorbed; acts locally in GI tract
Excretion: Feces, urine

CONTRAINDICATIONS AND PRECAUTIONS
• Use cautiously with sensitivity to sucralfate, dysphagia, GI tract obstruction disease, renal failure, pregnancy, lactation

INTERACTIONS
Drug
• Interference with binding of sucralfate to mucosa with aluminum-containing medications and antacids
• Impaired absorption of cimetidine, ranitidine, ciprofloxacin, norfloxacin, ofloxacin, digoxin, theophylline, phenytoin, oral tetracyclines possible
Lab
• Increased serum aluminum concentrations possible in pts with renal insufficiency

SIDE EFFECTS
CNS: Dizziness or lightheadedness; drowsiness
DERM: Skin rash, hives, or itching (hypersensitivity)
GI: Constipation (most common); diarrhea; dry mouth; indigestion; nausea; stomach cramps or pain
Other: Backache

PATIENT CARE MANAGEMENT
Assessment
• Assess history of hypersensitivity to sucralfate
• Assess renal function (BUN, creatinine)
• Assess baseline GI function
Interventions
• Shake susp well before administering each dose
• Tabs should be taken with water, should not be crushed or chewed; may be dissolved by placing in distilled water and allowing to stand for 15-20 min
• Administer on an empty stomach 1 hr ac and hs
• Do not administer antacids within ½ hr before or after sucralfate dose
Evaluation
• Evaluate therapeutic response (absence of pain or GI complaints)
• Evaluate for hypersensitivity, side effects
• Evaluate GI function; particularly monitor for constipation

---

✤ Available in Canada.

• Evaluate serum aluminum levels in pts with renal insufficiency

PATIENT AND FAMILY EDUCATION
Teach/instruct
• To take as directed at prescribed intervals for prescribed length of time
• That sucralfate is properly taken on an empty stomach, 1 hr ac; tab should not be chewed or crushed
• To continue taking drug even after symptoms subside
• To ensure sufficient fluid intake and encourage a generous fiber intake (a common side effect of sucralfate may be constipation)
Warn/advise
• To notify care provider if hypersensitivity or side effects occur
• To avoid smoking, caffeine, or alcohol, which may exacerbate symptoms

STORAGE
• Store at room temp in a tight container

---

sulfacetamide sodium
Brand Name(s): AK-Sulf Forte, AK-Sulf Ointment, Bleph-10, Bleph-10 Liquifilm✤, Cetamide, Dio-Sulf✤, Isopto Cetamide, Ophtho-Sulf✤, Sodium Sulamyd✤, Sulf-10, Sulfex✤

Classification: Antibiotic (sulfonamide)

Pregnancy Category: C

AVAILABLE PREPARATIONS
Ophthal sol: 10%, 15%, 30%
Ophthal oint: 10%

ROUTES AND DOSAGES
Infants, children, and adults: Ophthal sol, instill 1-2 gtt 10% sol into conjunctival sac q2-3h during day, less frequently at night; or 1-2 gtt 15% sol into conjunctival sac q1-2h initially, increasing interval as condition responds; or instill 1 gtt 30% sol q2h; ophthal oint, instill ½-1″ strip into conjunctival sac qid and hs; may use drops during day and oint at night

MECHANISM AND INDICATIONS
Antibiotic mechanism: Inhibits folic acid synthesis by preventing para-aminobenzoic acid (PABA) use, required for bacterial growth
Indications: Conjunctivitis, superficial eye infections, corneal ulcers

PHARMACOKINETICS
Half-life: 7-13 hr
Excretion: Urine

CONTRAINDICATIONS AND PRECAUTIONS
• Contraindicated with known hypersensitivity to sulfonamides or to any ingredients in preparation
• Use cautiously to avoid overgrowth of non-susceptible organisms during long-term therapy; with pregnancy

INTERACTIONS
Drug
• Decreased antibacterial activity with use of tetracaine, other local anesthetics
• Do not use with silver preparations

SIDE EFFECTS
EENT: Blurred vision, temporary burning and stinging, hyperemia, epithelial keratitis
Other: Hypersensitivity, including itching or burning, headache, overgrowth of non-susceptible organisms, Stevens-Johnson syndrome, sensitivity to light, systemic lupus erythematosus

PATIENT CARE MANAGEMENT
Assessment
• Assess history of hypersensitivity to sulfonamides or any other ingredients
• Obtain C&S; may begin therapy before obtaining results
• Assess eye for redness, drainage, swelling
Interventions
• Wash hands before and after instillation; cleanse crusts or dis-

S

✤ Available in Canada.

charge from eye before instillation; wipe excess medication from eye; do not flush medication from eye
• Wait 10 min before administering another eye preparation

NURSING ALERT
Discontinue drug if signs of sensitivity develop

Evaluation
• Evaluate therapeutic response (decreased symptoms of infection)
• Observe for allergic reaction (itching, lacrimation, redness, swelling)

PATIENT AND FAMILY EDUCATION
Teach/instruct
• To take as directed at prescribed intervals for prescribed length of time
Warn/advise
• To notify care provider of hypersensitivity, side effects, superinfection
• Not to share towels, wash cloths, linens, eye make-up, with family member being treated
• Instillation of oint may cause blurred vision

STORAGE
• Store at room temp

---

sulfadiazine
Brand Name(s): Microsulfon

Classification: Antibiotic (sulfonamide)

Pregnancy Category: B (D at term)

AVAILABLE PREPARATIONS
Tabs: 500 mg

ROUTES AND DOSAGES
Infants >2 mo and children: PO loading dose, 75 mg/kg or 2 g/m^2 once; maintenance 150 mg/kg/24 hr divided q6h (maximum 6 g/24 hr)
Adults: PO loading dose, 2-4 g once; maintenance 1 g q4-6h

Congenital Toxoplasmosis
Children and adults: PO (with pyrimethamine and folic acid) 85 mg/kg/24 hr divided q6h for 6 mo
Malaria
Children: PO (with quinine and pyrimethamine) 100-200 mg/kg/24 hr divided qid for 5 days
Adults: PO (with quinine and pyrimethamine) 500 mg qid for 5 days
Toxoplasmosis
Infants: PO (with pyrimethamine): 25 mg/kg/dose qid for 3-4 wk
Children: PO (with pyrimethamine): 25-50 mg/kg/dose qid for 3-4 wk
Adults: PO (with pyrimethamine): 2-8 g/24 hr divided qid for 3-4 wk

MECHANISM AND INDICATIONS
Antibiotic mechanism: Bacteriostatic; prevents bacterial cell synthesis of essential nucleic acids by inhibiting formation of dihydrofolic acid from paraminobenzoic acid (PABA)
Indications: Effective against gram-positive organisms including *Staphylococcus* and *Streptococcus, Chlamydia trachomatis,* many Enterobacteriaceae, and some strains of *Toxoplasma gondii* and *Plasmodium;* used to treat UTIs, adjunctive in malaria, toxoplasmosis

PHARMACOKINETICS
Peak: 2 hr
Distribution: To most tissues including CSF
Half-life: 8-10 hr
Metabolism: Liver
Excretion: Urine

CONTRAINDICATIONS AND PRECAUTIONS
• Contraindicated with infants <2 mo (may cause kernicterus); with known hypersensitivity to sulfadiazine, sulfonamides, drugs containing sulfur (thiazides, furosemide, oral hypoglycemics); with severe renal or hepatic dysfunction, porphyria, term pregnancy
• Use cautiously with mild or moderate renal or hepatic impair-

---

✤ Available in Canada.

ment, urinary obstruction, severe allergies, asthma, blood dyscrasias, G-6-PD deficiency, early pregnancy

INTERACTIONS

Drug

• Increased anticoagulant effect with oral anticoagulants
• Increased hypoglycemic response with sulfonylurea agents
• Increased serum concentrations of methotrexate
• Decreased hepatic clearance of phenytoin
• Decreased effectiveness of oral contraceptives
• Synergistic antibacterial effects with trimethoprim, pyrimethamine
• Decreased antibacterial effectiveness with PABA derivatives
• Increased risk of crystalluria with urine-acidifying agents

Nutrition

• Decreased absorption if administered with food

SIDE EFFECTS

CNS: Headache, mental depression, seizures, hallucinations
DERM: Erythema multiforme (Stevens-Johnson syndrome), generalized skin eruption, epidermal necrolysis, exfoliative dermatitis, photosensitivity, urticaria, pruritus
GI: Nausea, vomiting, diarrhea, abdominal pain, anorexia, stomatitis, jaundice
GU: Toxic nephrosis with oliguria and anuria, crystalluria, hematuria
HEME: Agranulocytosis, aplastic anemia, megaloblastic anemia, thrombocytopenia, leukopenia, hemolytic anemia
Other: Hypersensitivity, serum sickness, drug fever, anaphylaxis, bacterial or fungal superinfection

TOXICITY AND OVERDOSE

Clinical signs: Dizziness, drowsiness, headache, unconsciousness, anorexia, abdominal pain, nausea, vomiting; more severe complications are hemolytic anemia, agranulocytosis, dermatitis, acidosis, sensitivity reactions, jaundice

Treatment: If ingested within 4 hr, perform gastric lavage, followed by correction of acidosis, forced fluids, and urinary alkalinization to increase excretion; treatment of renal failure, severe hematologic toxicity; supportive care

PATIENT CARE MANAGEMENT

Assessment

• Assess history of hypersensitivity to sulfonamides or any drug containing sulfur
• Obtain C&S; may begin therapy before obtaining results
• Assess hematologic function (CBC, differential, platelet count), renal function (BUN, creatinine, I&O), particularly for long-term therapy; bowel pattern

Interventions

• Administer PO 1 hr ac or 2 hr after meals; may administer with small amount of food if nausea develops; tab may be crushed, mixed with food or fluid; administer with generous amount of water to prevent crystalluria
• Maintain age-appropriate fluid intake

> **NURSING ALERT**
> Discontinue drug if signs of toxicity or hypersensitivity, blood dyscrasias, crystalluria or renal abnormalities, pseudomembranous colitis develop

Evaluation

• Evaluate therapeutic response (decreased symptoms of infection)
• Evaluate hematologic function (CBC, differential, platelet count), renal function (BUN, creatinine, I&O); maintain alkaline urine to prevent crystalluria
• Monitor for blood dyscrasias (skin rash, fever, sore throat, bruising, bleeding, fatigue, joint pain)
• Observe for allergic reaction (rash, dermatitis, urticaria, pruritus, dyspnea, bronchospasm)
• Observe for signs of superinfection (perineal itching, diaper rash,

S

fever, malaise, redness, pain, swelling, drainage, rash, diarrhea, sore throat, change in cough or sputum)

PATIENT AND FAMILY EDUCATION
Teach/instruct
• To take as directed at prescribed intervals for prescribed length of time
Warn/advise
• To notify care provider of hypersensitivity, side effects, superinfection
• To avoid sunlight or use sunscreen during treatment
• To avoid OTC medications (particularly aspirin, vitamin C) unless prescribed by care provider
• That female pts need to use alternate forms of contraception; medication may decrease effectiveness of oral contraceptives

STORAGE
• Store at room temp
• Protect from light

---

sulfamethoxazole
Brand Name(s): Apo-Sulfamethoxazole✦, Gamazole, Gantanol, Gantanol DS, Methanoxanol

Classification: Antibiotic (sulfonamide)

Pregnancy Category: B (D at term)

AVAILABLE PREPARATIONS
Oral susp: 500 mg/5 ml
Tabs: 500 mg, 1 g

ROUTES AND DOSAGES
Infants >2 mo and children: PO loading dose, 50-60 mg/kg once; maintenance 25-30 mg/kg/dose bid (maximum 75 mg/kg/24 hr)
Adults: PO loading dose, 2 g once; maintenance 1 g bid (tid for severe infections)

MECHANISM AND INDICATIONS
Antibiotic mechanism: Bacteriostatic; prevents bacterial cell synthesis of essential nucleic acids of inhibiting formation of dihydrofolic acid from para-aminobenzoic acid (PABA)
Indications: Effective against some gram-positive organisms, *Chlamydia trachomatis,* many Enterobacteriaceae, and some strains of *Toxoplasma* and *Plasmodium;* used to treat UTIs, systemic infections, lymphogranuloma venereum

PHARMACOKINETICS
Peak: 3-4 hr
Distribution: To most tissues, including CSF
Half-life: 7-12 hr
Metabolism: Liver
Excretion: Urine

CONTRAINDICATIONS AND PRECAUTIONS
• Contraindicated in infants <2 mo (may cause kernicterus), pts with known hypersensitivity to sulfamethoxazole, sulfonamides, drugs containing sulfur (thiazides, furosemide, oral hypoglycemics),severe renal or hepatic dysfunction, porphyria, term pregnancy
• Use cautiously in pts with mild-to-moderate renal or hepatic impairment, urinary obstruction, severe allergies, asthma, blood dyscrasias, G-6-PD deficiency, early pregnancy

INTERACTIONS
Drug
• Increased anticoagulant effect with oral anticoagulants
• Increased hypoglycemic response with sulfonylurea agents
• Increased serum concentrations of methotrexate
• Decreased hepatic clearance of phenytoin
• Decreased effectiveness of oral contraceptives
• Synergistic antibacterial effects with trimethoprim, pyrimethamine
• Decreased antibacterial effectiveness with PABA derivations
• Increased risk of crystalluria with urine-acidifying agents

---

✦ Available in Canada.

Nutrition
• Decreased absorption if administered with food

SIDE EFFECTS
CNS: Headache, mental depression, seizures, hallucinations
DERM: Erythema multiforme (Stevens-Johnson syndrome), generalized skin eruption, epidermal necrolysis, exfoliative dermatitis, photosensitivity, urticaria, pruritus
GI: Nausea, vomiting, diarrhea, abdominal pain, anorexia, stomatitis, jaundice
GU: Toxic nephrosis with oliguria and anuria, crystalluria, hematuria
HEME: Agranulocytosis, aplastic anemia, megaloblastic anemia, thrombocytopenia, leukopenia, hemolytic anemia
Other: Hypersensitivity, serum sickness, drug fever, anaphylaxis, bacterial or fungal superinfection

TOXICITY AND OVERDOSE
Clinical signs: Dizziness, drowsiness, headache, unconsciousness, anorexia, abdominal pain, nausea, vomiting; more severe complications are hemolytic anemia, agranulocytosis, dermatitis, acidosis, sensitivity reactions, jaundice
Treatment: If ingested within 4 hr, perform gastric lavage, followed by correction of acidosis, forced fluids, and urinary alkalinization to increase excretion; treatment of renal failure, severe hematologic toxicity; supportive care

PATIENT CARE MANAGEMENT
Assessment
• Assess history of hypersensitivity to sulfonamides or any drug containing sulfur
• Obtain C&S; may begin therapy before obtaining results
• Assess hematologic function (CBC, differential, platelet count), renal function (BUN, creatinine, I&O), particularly for long-term therapy; bowel pattern
Interventions
• Administer PO 1 hr ac or 2 hr after meals; may administer with small amount of food if nausea develops; shake susp well before administering; tab may be crushed, mixed with food or fluid; administer with generous amount of water to prevent crystalluria
• Maintain age-appropriate fluid intake

> **NURSING ALERT**
> Discontinue drug if signs of toxicity or hypersensitivity, blood dyscrasias, crystalluria or renal abnormalities, pseudomembranous colitis develop

Evaluation
• Evaluate therapeutic response (decreased symptoms of infection)
• Evaluate hematologic function (CBC, differential, platelet count), renal function (BUN, creatinine, I&O); maintain alkaline urine to prevent crystalluria
• Monitor for blood dyscrasias (skin rash, fever, sore throat, bruising, bleeding, fatigue, joint pain)
• Observe for allergic reaction (rash, dermatitis, urticaria, pruritus, dyspnea, bronchospasm)
• Observe for signs of superinfection (perineal itching, diaper rash, fever, malaise, redness, pain, swelling, drainage, rash, diarrhea, sore throat, change in cough or sputum)

PATIENT AND FAMILY EDUCATION
Teach/instruct
• To take as directed at prescribed intervals for prescribed length of time
Warn/advise
• To notify care provider of hypersensitivity, side effects, superinfection
• To avoid sunlight or use sunscreen during treatment
• To avoid OTC medications (particularly aspirin, vitamin C) unless prescribed by care provider
• That female pts need to use alternate forms of contraceptives; medication may decrease effectiveness of oral contraceptives

S

✦ Available in Canada.

STORAGE
- Store at room temp
- Protect from light

sulfasalazine

Brand Name(s): Azaline, Azulfidine, Azulfidine En-Tabs, Salazopyrin♣, Salazopyrin En-Tabs♣, S.A.S.♣, S.A.S.-500

Classification: Antibiotic (sulfonamide)

Pregnancy Category: B (D at term)

AVAILABLE PREPARATIONS
Oral susp: 250 mg/5 ml
Tabs: 500 mg
Tabs, enteric-coated: 500 mg

ROUTES AND DOSAGES
Children >2 yr: PO initial dose 40-60 mg/kg/24 hr divided q4-6h; maintenance 30 mg/kg/24 hr divided qid; maximum 2 g/24 hr
Adults: PO initial 3-4 g/24 hr divided q4-6h; maintenance 2 g/24 hr divided q6h

MECHANISM AND INDICATIONS
Antibiotic mechanism: Exact mechanism of action against ulcerative colitis unknown; acts as a prodrug to deliver sulfapyridine and 5-aminosalicylic acid to the colon; appears to reduce *Clostridium* and *E. coli* in the feces
Indications: Used to treat ulcerative colitis

PHARMACOKINETICS
Peak: 1.5-6 hr
Half-life: 5-10 hr
Metabolism: Liver
Excretion: Urine

CONTRAINDICATIONS AND PRECAUTIONS
- Contraindicated in infants, children less than 2 yr; with known hypersensitivity to sulfasalazine, sulfonamides, or drugs containing sulfur (thiazides, furosemide, oral hypoglycemics), severe renal or hepatic dysfunction or porphyria, term pregnancy, intestinal or urinary tract obstruction
- Use cautiously with mild-to-moderate renal or hepatic impairment, severe allergies, asthma, blood dyscrasias, G-6-PD, deficiency early pregnancy

INTERACTIONS
Drug
- Increased anticoagulant effect with oral anticoagulants
- Increased hypoglycemic response with sulfonylurea agents
- Increased serum concentration of methotrexate
- Decreased hepatic clearance of phenytoin
- Decreased effectiveness of oral contraceptives
- Increased risk of crystalluria with urine-acidifying agents
- Decreased absorption of digoxin, folic acid
- Decreased absorption of iron
- Decreased effectiveness with antibiotics that alter intestinal flora
- Increased systemic absorption, risk of toxicity with antacids

Nutrition
- Decreased absorption if given with food

SIDE EFFECTS
CNS: Headache, mental depression, seizures, hallucinations, tinnitus
DERM: Erythema multiforme (Stevens-Johnson syndrome), generalized skin eruptions, epidermal necrolysis, exfoliative dermatitis, photosensitivity, urticaria, pruritus
GI: Nausea, vomiting, diarrhea, abdominal pain, anorexia, stomatitis, jaundice
GU: Toxic nephrosis with oliguria and anuria, crystalluria, hematuria, oligospermia, infertility
HEME: Agranulocytosis, aplastic anemia, megaloplastic anemia, thrombocytopenia, leukopenia, hemolytic anemia
Other: Hypersensitivity, serum sickness, drug fever, anaphylaxis, bacterial or fungal superinfection

---

♣ Available in Canada.

TOXICITY AND OVERDOSE
Clinical signs: Dizziness, drowsiness, headache, unconsciousness, anorexia, abdominal pain, nausea, vomiting; more severe complications are hemolytic anemia, agranulocytosis, dermatitis, acidosis, sensitivity reactions, jaundice
Treatment: If ingested within 4 hr, perform gastric lavage, followed by correction of acidosis, forced fluids, and urinary alkalinization to increase excretion; treatment of renal failure, severe hematologic toxicity; supportive care

PATIENT CARE MANAGEMENT
Assessment
• Assess history of hypersensitivity to sulfonamides or any drug containing sulfur
• Obtain C&S; may begin therapy before obtaining results
• Assess hematologic function (CBC, differential, platelet count), renal function (BUN, creatinine, I&O), particularly for long-term therapy; bowel pattern
Interventions
• Administer PO 1 hr ac or 2 hr after meals; may administer with small amount of food if nausea develops; shake susp well before administering; regular tab may be crushed, mixed with food or fluid, do not crush enteric-coated tablet; administer with generous amount of water to prevent crystalluria
• Do not administer antacids concurrently with enteric-coated tablets; absorption may be altered
• Maintain age-appropriate fluid intake

> **NURSING ALERT**
> Discontinue drug if signs of toxicity or hypersensitivity, blood dyscrasias, crystalluria or renal abnormalities, pseudomembranous colitis develop

Evaluation
• Evaluate therapeutic response (decreased symptoms of infection)

• Evaluate hematologic function (CBC, differential, platelet count), renal function (BUN, creatinine, I&O), folic acid for possible deficiency; maintain alkaline urine to prevent crystalluria
• Monitor for blood dyscrasias (skin rash, fever, sore throat, bruising, bleeding, fatigue, joint pain)
• Observe for allergic reaction (rash, dermatitis, urticaria, pruritus, dyspnea, bronchospasm)
• Observe for signs of superinfection (perineal itching, diaper rash, fever, malaise, redness, pain, swelling, drainage, rash, diarrhea, sore throat, change in cough or sputum)
• Monitor skin, urine for a normal change to orange-yellow color
• Monitor stools for possible passage of enteric-coated tabs without disintegrating; notify care provider

PATIENT AND FAMILY EDUCATION
Teach/instruct
• To take as directed at prescribed intervals for prescribed length of time
Warn/advise
• To notify care provider of hypersensitivity, side effects, superinfection
• To avoid sunlight or use sunscreen during treatments
• To avoid OTC medications (particularly aspirin, vitamin C) unless prescribed by care provider
• That female pt need to use alternate contraception; medication may decrease effectiveness of oral contraceptives
• That urine or skin may turn orange-yellow while taking this medication

STORAGE
• Store at room temp
• Protect from light

S

sulfisoxazole

Brand Name(s): Gantrisin, Gulfasin, Lipo Gantrisin

Classification: Antibiotic (sulfonamide)

Pregnancy Category: B (D at term)

AVAILABLE PREPARATIONS

Syr: 500 mg/5 ml
Oral susp: 500 mg/5 ml
Tabs: 500 mg
Ophthal oint, sol: 4%

ROUTES AND DOSAGES

Infants >2 mo and children: PO loading dose 75 mg/kg or 2 g/m^2 once; maintenance 150 mg/kg/24 hr divided q4-6h (maximum 6 g/24 hr); ophthal oint, instill 1 cm strip into conjunctival sac q8h; ophthal sol, instill 1-2 gtt into conjunctival sac q8h

Adults: PO loading dose 2-4 g once; maintenance 4-8 g/24 hr divided q4-6h (maximum 8 g/24 hr); ophthal oint, instill 1 cm strip into conjunctival sac q8h; ophthal sol, instill 1-2 gtt into conjunctival sac q8h

Otitis Media Prophylaxis
Children and adults: PO 50-75 mg/kg/24 hr divided bid

Rheumatic Fever Prophylaxis
Children ≤30 kg: PO 500 mg qd
Children ≥30 kg and adults: PO 1 g qd

MECHANISM AND INDICATIONS

Antibiotic mechanism: Bacteriostatic; prevents bacterial cell wall synthesis of essential nucleic acids by inhibiting formation of dihydrofolic acid from para-aminobenzoic acid (PABA)

Indications: Effective against grampositive and gram-negative organisms including *Staphylococcus, Streptococcus, E. coli, Proteus, Haemophilus influenzae, Chlamydia trachomatis,* many Enterobacteriaceae, some strains of *Toxoplasma* and *Plasmodium;* used to treat urinary tract, eye, and systemic infections, chancroid, toxo-plasmosis, acute otitis media, lymphogranuloma venereum

PHARMACOKINETICS

Peak: 2-4 hr
Distribution: Crosses blood–brain barrier; distributed in extracellular space
Half-life: 4.6-7.8 hr
Metabolism: Liver
Excretion: Urine

CONTRAINDICATIONS AND PRECAUTIONS

• Contraindicated with infants <2 mo (may cause kernicterus); with known hypersensitivity to sulfisoxazole, sulfonamides, or drugs containing sulfur (thiazides, furosemide, oral hypoglycemics); with severe renal or hepatic dysfunction, porphyria, term pregnancy
• Use cautiously with mild-to-moderate renal or hepatic impairment, urinary obstruction, severe allergies, asthma, blood dyscrasias, G-6-PD deficiency, early pregnancy

INTERACTIONS

Drug
• Increased anticoagulant effect with oral anticoagulants
• Increased hypoglycemic response with sulfonylurea agents
• Increased serum concentrations of methotrexate
• Decreased hepatic clearance of phenytoin
• Decreased effectiveness of oral contraceptives
• Synergistic antibacterial effects with trimethoprim, pyrimethamine
• Decreased antibacterial effectiveness with PABA derivations
• Increased risk of crystalluria with urine-acidifying agents

Nutrition
• Decreased absorption if administer with food

SIDE EFFECTS

CNS: Headache, mental depression, seizures, hallucinations, kernicterus
DERM: Erythema multiforme (Stevens-Johnson syndrome), generalized skin eruptions, epidermal

---

necrolysis, exfoliative dermatitis, photosensitivity, urticaria, pruritus

GI: Nausea, vomiting, diarrhea, abdominal pain, anorexia, stomatitis, jaundice

HEME: Agranulocytosis, aplastic anemia, megaloblastic anemia, thrombocytopenia, leukopenia, hemolytic anemia

Other: Hypersensitivity, serum sickness, drug fever, anaphylaxis, bacterial/fungal superinfection

TOXICITY AND OVERDOSE

Clinical signs: Dizziness, drowsiness, headache, unconsciousness, anorexia, abdominal pain, nausea, vomiting; more severe complications are hemolytic anemia, agranulocytosis, dermatitis, acidosis, sensitivity reactions, jaundice

Treatment: If ingested within 4 hr, perform gastric lavage, followed by correction of acidosis, forced fluids, and urinary alkalinization to increase excretion; treatment of renal failure, severe hematologic toxicity; supportive care

PATIENT CARE MANAGEMENT

Assessment

• Assess history of hypersensitivity to sulfonamides or any drug containing sulfur

• Obtain C&S; may begin therapy before obtaining results

• Assess hematologic function (CBC, differential, platelet count), renal function (BUN, creatinine, I&O), particularly for long-term therapy; bowel pattern

• Assess eye for redness, drainage, swelling

Interventions

• Administer PO 1 hr ac or 2 hr after meals; may administer with small amount of food if nausea develops; shake susp well before administering; tab may be crushed, mixed with food or fluid; administer with generous amount of water to prevent crystalluria

• See Chapter 2 regarding ophthal instillation; wash hands before and after instillation, cleanse crusts or discharge from eye before instillation; wipe excess medication from eye; do not flush medication from eye

• Maintain age-appropriate fluid intake

> **NURSING ALERT**
> Discontinue drug if signs of toxicity or hypersensitivity, blood dyscrasias, crystalluria or renal abnormalities, pseudomembranous colitis develop

Evaluation

• Evaluate therapeutic response (decreased symptoms of infection)

• Evaluate hematologic function (CBC, differential, platelet count), renal function (BUN, creatinine, I&O); maintain alkaline urine to prevent crystalluria

• Monitor for blood dyscrasias (skin rash, fever, sore throat, bruising, bleeding, fatigue, joint pain)

• Observe for allergic reaction (rash, dermatitis, urticaria, pruritus, dyspnea, bronchospasm)

• Observe for signs of superinfection (perineal itching, diaper rash, fever, malaise, redness, pain, swelling, drainage, rash, diarrhea, sore throat, change in cough or sputum)

PATIENT AND FAMILY EDUCATION

Teach/instruct

• To take as directed at prescribed intervals for prescribed length of time

Warn/advise

• To notify care provider of hypersensitivity, side effects, superinfection

• Not to share towels, wash cloths, linens, eye make-up with family members being treated with ophthal form

• To avoid sunlight or use sunscreen during treatment

• To avoid OTC medications (particularly aspirin, vitamin C) unless prescribed by care provider

• That female pts need to use alternate forms of contraception;

S

medication may decrease effectiveness of oral contraceptives

STORAGE
- Store all forms at room temp
- Protect from light

---

tamoxifen citrate

Brand Name(s): Alphe-Tamoxifen, Apo-Tamox✹, Nolvadex✹, Nolvadex-D✹, Nova-Tamoxifen✹, Tamofen✹, Tamone✹, Tamoplex

Classification: Antiestrogen

Pregnancy Category: C

AVAILABLE PREPARATIONS
Tabs: 10 mg, 20 mg
Tabs, enteric coated: 10 mg, 20 mg

ROUTES AND DOSAGES
- Drug may vary in response to diagnosis, extent of disease, concurrent or previous therapy, protocol guidelines, physiologic parameters; consult current literature, protocol recommendations

Adjunct Therapy in Breast Cancer after Surgery
PO 10 mg bid or 20 mg qd (no more than 2 yr duration); in advanced breast cancer, 20-40 mg/24 hr divided bid

MECHANISM AND INDICATIONS
Mechanism: A non-steroidal antiestrogen which binds to estrogen receptors, forming an abnormal complex that migrates to the cell nucleus and inhibits DNA synthesis
Indications: Relatively nontoxic; used to treat estrogen-dependent tumors (such as breast cancer)

PHARMACOKINETICS
Onset of action: 4-10 wk; but may take mo
Peak: 3-6 hr
Half-life: 7 days
Metabolism: Liver
Absorption: Slowly following PO administration

Excretion: Feces; small amounts in urine

CONTRAINDICATIONS AND PRECAUTIONS
- Contraindicated with known hypersensitivity to drug, pregnancy, lactation

INTERACTIONS
Drug
- Avoid taking antacids when taking enteric coated tabs
Lab
- Prolonged PTT possible with concurrent warfarin tamoxifen therapy

SIDE EFFECTS
EENT: Retinopathy, decreased visual acuity, corneal opacities
DERM: Rash
ENDO/METAB: Hypercalcemia
GI: Nausea, vomiting, anorexia, fatty liver, cholestasis
GU: Vaginal discharge and bleeding, pruritus vulvae, leaking breast, drug-induced menstrual irregularities, loss of libido, impotence
HEME: Transient fall in WBC or platelet count
Other: Temporary bone or tumor pain, hot flashes, exacerbation of pain from osseous metastasis, headache, dizziness, leg cramps, edema, cough

TOXICITY AND OVERDOSE
Clinical signs: Acute neurotoxicity manifested by tremor, hyperreflexia, unsteady gait, dizziness with high dosages
Treatment: In discontinuing drug, adverse effects disappear in 2-5 days

PATIENT CARE MANAGEMENT
Assessment
- Assess history of hypersensitivity to tamoxifen
- Assess baseline VS, CBC, differential, platelet count, lipid and Ca levels, liver function (ALT, AST, LDH, bilirubin)
- Assess for signs or symptoms of hair loss, edema, skin rash
- Assess for signs or symptoms of infection (fever, fatigue, sore

---

✹ Available in Canada.

throat), bleeding (easy bruising, nose bleeds, bleeding gums)

• Assess success of previous antiemetic therapy

• Assess history of previous treatment with special attention to other therapies that may predispose pt to hepatic and hematologic dysfunction

Interventions

• Premedicate with antiemetics and continue periodically throughout chemotherapy

• Enteric coated tabs should be swallowed whole; do not crush or chew; do not administer antacids within 2 hr of enteric coated tabs

• Encourage small, frequent feedings of foods pt likes

• Provide supportive measures to maintain hemostasis, fluid and electrolyte balance, nutritional support

---

NURSING ALERT

Instruct pt to swallow enteric-coated tabs whole without crushing or chewing; not to take antacids within 2 hr after tamoxifen

Pt may experience bone pain during therapy; encourage use of analgesics

---

Evaluation

• Evaluate therapeutic response (decreased tumor size, spread of malignancy)

• Evaluate CBC, differential, platelet count, liver function (ALT, AST, LDH, bilirubin), lipids, Ca at given intervals after chemotherapy

• Evaluate for signs or symptoms of infection (fever, fatigue, sore throat), bleeding (easy bruising, nose bleeds, bleeding gums)

• Evaluate for side effects and response to antiemetic regimen

PATIENT AND FAMILY EDUCATION

Teach/instruct

• To have pt well-hydrated before and after chemotherapy

• About importance of follow-up to monitor blood counts, serum chemistry values, drug blood levels

• To take accurate temp, rectal temp contraindicated

• To notify care provider of signs of bleeding (bruising, epistaxis, bleeding gums), infection (fever, sore throat, fatigue)

Warn/advise

• About impact of body changes that may occur (hair loss, hyperpigmentation, nail ridging), how to minimize changes (wigs, caps, scarves, long sleeves)

• To avoid OTC products containing aspirin

• To report any alterations in behavior, sensation, perception; help to develop a plan of care to manage side effects, stress of illness or treatment

• To monitor bowel function and call if abdominal pain or constipation noted

• That good oral hygiene with very soft toothbrush is imperative

• That dental work be delayed until blood counts return to baseline, with permission of care provider

• To avoid contact with known viral or bacterial illnesses

• That household contacts of child not be immunized with live polio virus; inactivated form should be used

• That child not receive immunizations until immune system recovers sufficiently to mount needed antibody response

• To report exposure to chicken pox in susceptible child immediately

• To report reactivation of herpes zoster virus (shingles) immediately

• If appropriate, ways to preserve reproductive patterns, sexuality (sperm banking, contraceptives)

• About signs or symptoms of possible "flare" reactions (bone or tumor pain), to report them immediately

• About possibility of nausea, vomiting, anorexia

• To report headache, dizziness, light-headedness, any visual changes
• About signs or symptoms of hypercalcemia (nausea, vomiting, weakness, constipation, loss of muscle tone, malaise, decreased urine output), to report them immediately
• That acute exacerbation of bone pain during tamoxifen usually indicates drug will produce a good response; use of analgesics will help relieve pain

Encourage
• Provision of nutritious food intake; consider nutritional consultation
• To comply with bowel management program
• To use top anesthetics to control discomfort of mucositis; avoid spicy foods, commercial mouthwashes
• That women need to have regular gynecologic exams because of increased risk of uterine cancer associated with tamoxifen

STORAGE
• Store at room temp in tight-fitting containers
• Protect from light

---

teniposide

Brand Name(s): VM-26, Vumon, Vumon Parenteral✢

Classification: Plant alkaloid (derivative of mandrake plant); investigational agent

Pregnancy Category: D

AVAILABLE PREPARATIONS
Inj: 50 mg/5ml (10 mg/ml in 5 ml ampules)

ROUTES AND DOSAGE
• Drug may vary in response to diagnosis, extent of disease, concurrent or previous therapy, protocol guidelines, physiologic parameters; consult current literature, protocol recommendations

Non–Hodgkin's Lymphyoma
Children and adolescents: IV 30 mg/m^2/24 hr for 10 days or q 5 days; 50-100 mg/m^2 q wk as a single agent; 60-70 mg/m^2 q wk in combo with other agents

Recurrent ALL
Children and adolescents: IV 165 mg/m^2 2 × per wk for 8-9 doses (4 wk) (in combination with cytosine arabinoside); 250 mg/m^2 q wk for 4-8 wk (in combination with vincristine and prednisone)

Neuroblastoma (Investigational)
Children and adolescents: IV 130-180 mg/m^2 q wk as single agent; 100 mg/m^2 once q 21 days in combo with other agents

IV administration
• Recommended concentration: Dilute with D$_5$W or NS to concentration of 0.1, 0.2, 0.4, or 1 mg/ml
• Infusion rate: Slow, over 45-60 min if hypotensive reaction occurs, stop infusion, then restart at a slower rate after appropriate treatment, monitoring carefully; chemical phlebitis may also occur if infused too rapidly or not diluted properly
• Do not give IV push

MECHANISM AND INDICATIONS
Mechanism: A semisynthetic derivative of podophyllotoxin which is cell-cycle specific in late S phase, early G-2 phase causing arrest of cell division in mitosis and causing breaks in DNA; inhibits uptake of thymidine into DNA so DNA synthesis is impaired
Indications: Used to treat refractory ALL and AML; investigational agent used in neuroblastoma and non-Hodgkin's protocols

PHARMACOKINETICS
Absorption: Instantaneous peak plasma concentration
Distribution: Highly protein bound; limits distribution within the body
Half-life: Terminal elimination half-life 6-10 hr in bi-exponential decay; 20-48 hr in those with

---

✢ Available in Canada.

triphasic characteristics; distribution half-life about 1 hr
Metabolism: Liver
Excretion: Bile, urine

CONTRAINDICATIONS AND PRECAUTIONS

• Contraindicated with known hypersensitivity to the drug or to polyoxyethylated castor oil or injection vehicle; with pts in whom previous use has proven ineffective; with severely depressed bone marrow function, active infections (especially chicken pox or herpes zoster), pregnancy, lactation
• Use cautiously with history of mild-to-moderate sensitivity to the drug, Down Syndrome (may be particularly sensitive to myelosuppressive chemotherapy)

INTERACTIONS
Drug
• Increased toxicity possible with tolbutamide, sodium salicylate, sulfamethizole
• Increased clearance of plasma methotrexate, increased intracellular methotrexate levels when given together
Lab
• Increased plasma clearance and increased intracellular levels of methotrexate possible

INCOMPATIBILITIES
• Physically incompatible with heparin
• Should not be mixed with other drugs during administration

SIDE EFFECTS
CNS: Somnolence, lethargy
CV: Hypotension from rapid infusion, tachycardia
GI: Nausea, vomiting, mucositis, diarrhea
HEME: Myelosuppression (dose limiting), leukopenia, neutropenia, thrombocytopenia, anemia; secondary ANLL has been reported in pts who receive VM-26
Other: Alopecia (rare), phlebitis at injection site with extravasation, hypersensitivity reactions (chills, fever, urticaria, tachycardia, bronchospasm, dyspnea, hypotension, flushing)

TOXICITY AND OVERDOSE
Clinical signs: Anticipated complications of overdose are secondary to bone marrow suppression
Treatment: Supportive care with blood products and antibiotics as needed

PATIENT CARE MANAGEMENT
Assessment
• Assess history of hypersensitivity to teniposide and related drugs
• Assess baseline CBC, differential, platelet count, renal function (BUN, creatinine, I&O), hepatic function (ALT, AST, LDH, bilirubin, alk phos)
• Assess baseline VS
• Assess baseline pulmonary, cardiac, urinary function
• Assess motor and sensory function before administration
• Assess success of previous antiemetic regimen
• Assess history of previous treatment with special attention to other therapies that might predispose pt to renal, hepatic, pulmonary, cardiac dysfunction
Interventions
• Monitor VS (especially B/P) q 15 min during infusion; if systolic B/P falls below 90 mm Hg, stop infusion and notify care provider
• Premedicate with antiemetics and continue prophylactically for 24 hr after chemotherapy to decrease nausea and vomiting
• Take precautions to avoid extravasation; administer through central line or carefully use peripheral IV and monitor closely during infusion
• Offer small, frequent feedings of foods pt likes
• Administer IV fluids until pt is able to resume normal PO intake
• Provide supportive measures to maintain hemostasis, fluid and electrolyte balance, nutritional support

T

✤ Available in Canada.

NURSING ALERT
Must be administered by slow IV infusion to prevent hypotension (over at least 30-60 min); do not administer IV push

If hypotension occurs, stop infusion until B/P normalizes, then restart at slower rate

Avoid extravasation; administer through central line or carefully use peripheral IV, monitor closely during infusion

Evaluation
• Evaluate therapeutic response (remission of ALL, AML)
• Monitor CBC, differential, platelet count, renal function (BUN, creatinine, I&O), hepatic function (ALT, AST, LDH, bilirubin, alk phos), cardiac, pulmonary function at given intervals after chemotherapy
• Evaluate for signs or symptoms of infection (fever, fatigue, sore throat), bleeding (easy bruising, nosebleeds, bleeding gums)
• Evaluate side effects and response to antiemetic regimen

PATIENT AND FAMILY EDUCATION
Teach/instruct
• To have pt well-hydrated before and after chemotherapy
• About importance of follow-up to monitor blood counts, serum chemistry values, drug blood values
• To take accurate temp; rectal temp contraindicated
• To notify care provider of signs of bleeding (bruising, epistaxis, bleeding gums), infection (fever, sore throat, fatigue)
Warn/advise
• About impact of body changes that may occur (hair loss, hyperpigmentation, nail ridging), how to minimize changes (wigs, caps, scarves, long sleeves)
• To avoid OTC products containing aspirin

• To report any alterations in behavior, sensation, perception; help to develop a plan of care to manage side effects, stress of illness or treatment
• To monitor bowel function and call if abdominal pain, constipation noted
• To immediately report any pain, discoloration at injection site (parenteral forms)
• That good oral hygiene with very soft toothbrush is imperative
• That dental work be delayed until blood counts return to baseline, with permission of care provider
• To avoid contact with known viral or bacterial illnesses
• That household contacts of child not be immunized with live polio virus; inactivated form should be used
• That child not receive immunizations until immune system recovers sufficiently to mount needed antibody response
• To report exposure to chicken pox in susceptible child immediately
• To report reactivation of herpes zoster virus (shingles) immediately
• If appropriate, ways to preserve reproductive patterns, sexuality (sperm banking, contraceptives)
Encourage
• Provision of nutritious food intake; consider nutritional consultation
• To comply with bowel management program
• To use top anesthetics to control discomfort of mucositis; avoid spicy foods, commercial mouthwashes

STORAGE
• Intact vials stable several yr at room temp, protected from light
• Do not refrigerate diluted sol; 1 mg/ml dilution stable at room temp 4 hr; all other dilutions stable at room temp 24 hr

terbutaline sulfate

Brand Name(s): Brethine, Brethaire, Bricanyl, Bricanyl Tablets♣, Bricanyl Turbuhaler♣

Classification: Bronchodilator (adrenergic, β_2-agonist)

Pregnancy Category: B

AVAILABLE PREPARATIONS
Tabs: 2.5 mg, 5 mg
Aerosol inhaler: 200 mcg/metered spray
Inhal sol: Injectable product may be used for nebulization
Inj: 1 mg/ml

ROUTES AND DOSAGES
• Safety and effectiveness in children not established; dosage represents accepted standard practice recommendations
Children <12 yr: PO, initially 0.05 mg/kg/dose tid, then increase prn (maximum 0.15 mg/kg/dose tid or 5 mg/24 hr); SC 0.005-0.01 mg/kg/dose q 15-20 min × 2 (maximum 0.4 mg/dose)
Children >12 yr and adult: PO 2.5 mg/dose tid or 0.05 mg/kg/dose tid (maximum 7.5 mg/24 hr); maintenance usually 5 mg or 0.075 mg/kg/dose tid-qid (maximum 15 mg/24 hr); SC 0.25 mg/dose q15-30 min prn × 1 (maximum 0.5 mg/4 hr period)
Children <2 yr: Aerosol inhal, 2 inhalations (400 mcg) q4-6h with 1 min elapsing between inhalations; nebulization, 0.5 mg in 2.5 ml NS
Children 2-9 yr: Aerosol inhal, 2 inhalations (400 mcg) q4-6h with 1 min elapsing between inhalations; nebulization, 1 mg in 2.5 ml NS
Children >9 yr and adult: Aerosol inhal, 2 inhalations (400 mcg) q4-6h with 1 min elapsing between inhalations; nebulization, 1.5 mg in 2.5 ml NS

MECHANISM AND INDICATIONS
Bronchodilator mechanism: Acts directly on β_2-adrenergic receptors of the lungs, uterus, vascular muscles; relaxation of bronchial muscles relieves bronchospasm and reduces airway resistance
Indications: To prevent and treat reversible obstructive bronchospasm of asthma, bronchitis, emphysema

PHARMACOKINETICS
Onset of action: PO 0.5-2 hr; aerosol inhal 5-30 min; SC 30-60 min
Half-life: PO 4-8 hr; aerosol inhal 3-4 hr; SC 1.5-4 hr
Metabolism: Liver
Excretion: Urine, feces

CONTRAINDICATIONS AND PRECAUTIONS
• Contraindicated with known hypersensitivity to the drug, any components, or other sympathomimetic amines
• Use cautiously with asthma, DM, hyperthyroidism, hypertension, history of seizures or cardiac disease (especially if associated with arrhythmias); pregnancy, lactation

INTERACTIONS
Drug
• Decreased bronchodilation effect with propranolol or other β-adrenergic blockers
• Increased cardiovascular effects within 14 days of MAOIs
• Increased cardiovascular effects with other sympathomimetic agents (epinephrine)
Lab
• Elevated liver enzymes (rare)
• Changes in ECG readings

SIDE EFFECTS
CNS: Nervousness, tremor, headache, drowsiness, vertigo, insomnia, anxiety, restlessness, lethargy, irritability
CV: Increased heart rate, palpitations, hypertension, hypotension, chest pain, angina, arrhythmias, peripheral vasodilation; hypersensitivity vasculitis (CV effects most pronounced with SC route, least pronounced with aerosol route)
DERM: Sweating, flushed feeling
EENT: Tinnitus, unusual taste,

T

drying or irritation of nose and oropharynx

GI: Nausea, vomiting

Local: Pain at injection site

RESP: Wheezing, chest discomfort

Other: Muscle cramps, wheezing, chest discomfort, hypersensitivity reactions

TOXICITY AND OVERDOSE

Clinical signs: Exaggeration of common side effects (particularly arrhythmias, seizures, nausea and vomiting); hyperglycemia and increased insulin levels followed by hypoglycemia; hypokalemia in early stages

Treatment: No specific antidote; discontinue therapy; requires supportive measures; empty the stomach by induced emesis in alert pt who has taken excess oral medication, follow with gastric lavage; in unconscious pt secure airway with cuffed endotracheal tube before beginning lavage, do not induce emesis; instillation of activated charcoal may help reduce absorption of the drug; maintain adequate airway and respiratory exchange; provide cardiac and respiratory support prn; observe until symptom-free; monitor VS and electrolyte levels

PATIENT CARE MANAGEMENT

Assessment

• Assess history of hypersensitivity to terbutaline, related drugs

• Assess respiratory status, VS

Interventions

• Tabs can be crushed, mixed with small amounts of food or fluid; do not crush ext rel tabs; administer with meals if gastric irritation results

• Do not use SC sol if containing precipitates or discolored

• Administer SC injection in lateral deltoid area; may repeat if no clinical improvement within 15-30 min of first dose; do not administer a third dose

• See Chapter 3 for discussion of inhaler, or nebulizer use

• Shake inhaler well before use

• Manufacturer recommends 1 min between first and second inhalations

• Offer sips of fluids for dry mouth

• Maintain age-appropriate fluid intake

• Report any difficulty breathing that persists 1 hr after treatment, if symptoms return within 4 hr, if status worsens, or if chest pain or dizziness occurs

---

NURSING ALERT

Double-check SC dosage carefully to avoid decimal point error

Discontinue if hypersensitivity reactions or paradoxical bronchospasm occur

---

Evaluation

• Evaluate therapeutic response (improved respiratory effort)

• Evaluate for hypersensitivity, adverse effects

• Evaluate respiratory status, VS, fluid status

• Evaluate HR, B/P (particularly after SC route)

• Evaluate HR, B/P before each dose if pt has arrhythmias

• Evaluate for signs of toxicity

PATIENT AND FAMILY EDUCATION

Teach/instruct

• To use as directed at prescribed intervals for prescribed length of time

• To begin treatment promptly with first symptoms

• About correct use and care of inhaler or nebulizer

• To wait 1 full min after inhalation to be sure of necessity of second dose

• That increased fluid intake facilitates clearing of secretions

• To rinse mouth or drink water to avoid dryness and throat irritation

Warn/advise

• Not to use more than prescribed amount or more frequently than prescribed

• Not to administer simultaneously with steroids or other adrenergics because of risk of excess cardiac stimulation

---

- To alternate with administration of steroids or adrenergics; wait 15 min between use of steroid inhaler and inhaled terbutaline
- To notify provider if side effects occur (especially chest pain or dizziness), if no relief obtained from dose, or if symptoms worsen
- That paradoxical bronchospasm may occur with repeated use or overuse of inhaler or nebulizer
- To discontinue medication and contact provider if paradoxical bronchospasm occurs
- That overuse can lead to tachycardia, palpitations, headache, nausea, dizziness, loss of effectiveness, possible paradoxical bronchospasm and cardiac arrest
- That long term use may lead to decreased effectiveness
- That saliva and sputum may appear pink
- To avoid smoking and contact with second-hand smoke
- To avoid contact with persons with respiratory infections

STORAGE

- Store tabs in light-resistant containers, ampules for injection/inhalation in original carton until dispensed
- Store at room temp
- Do not puncture aerosol canister, do not place near heat or open flame
- Keep out of reach of children

---

terfenadine

Brand Name(s): Apo-Terfenedine✤, Novo-Terfenedine✤, Seldane✤

Classification: Antihistamine

Pregnancy Category: C

AVAILABLE PREPARATIONS
Tabs: 60 mg

ROUTES AND DOSAGES
Children 3-6 yr: 15 mg bid (Safety and effectiveness not established. Dosage represents accepted standard practice recommendations.)
Children 6-12 yr: 30 mg bid (Safety and effectiveness not established. Dosage represents accepted standard practice recommendations.)
Children >12 yr and adults: 60 mg bid

MECHANISM AND INDICATIONS
Antihistamine mechanism: Competes with histamine for H_1-receptor site; blocks histamine, thus decreasing allergic response
Indications: Used to treat seasonal and perennial allergic rhinitis, other allergic symptoms

PHARMACOKINETICS
Peak: 3-6 hr
Half-life: Biphasic; distribution 3.5 hr, elimination 16-23 hr
Metabolism: Liver
Excretion: Feces, urine

CONTRAINDICATIONS AND PRECAUTIONS
- Contraindicated with known hypersensitivity to terfenadine or any component, severe hepatic dysfunction; with concomitant use of ketoconazole, itraconazole, clarithromycin, erythromycin, troleandomycin
- Use cautiously with asthma, lower respiratory diseases, pregnancy

INTERACTIONS
Drug
- Reduced hepatic metabolism, resulting in life-threatening cardiac arrhythmias with ketoconazole, itraconazole, clarithromycin, erythromycin, troleandomycin; reduced hepatic metabolism possible with azithromycin
Lab
- False negative skin allergy tests
Nutrition
- Taking terfenadine with grapefruit juice impairs hepatic metabolism.

SIDE EFFECTS
CNS: Fatigue, dizziness, headache, nervousness, insomnia
CV: Life-threatening arrhythmias; prolongs QT interval
DERM: Rash

✤ Available in Canada.

GI: Nausea, vomiting, dry mouth, elevated liver function tests, jaundice
RESP: Cough, sore throat
Other: Hypersensitivity, wt gain

TOXICITY AND OVERDOSE
Clinical signs: Headache, nausea, confusion, syncope, seizures, cardiac arrhythmias
Treatment: Induce vomiting or perform gastric lavage; supportive care

PATIENT CARE MANAGEMENT
Assessment
• Assess history of hypersensitivity to terfenadine, any component
• Assess renal function (BUN, creatinine, I&O), hepatic function (ALT, AST, bilirubin), hematologic function (CBC, differential, platelet count) for long-term therapy
Interventions
• Administer PO with meals to reduce GI distress; tab may be crushed, mixed with food or fluid
• Provide sugarless hard candy, gum, frequent oral care for dry mouth

---

NURSING ALERT
Do not exceed recommended dosage; life-threatening arrhythmias may develop

---

Evaluation
• Evaluate therapeutic response (decreased allergy symptoms)
• Monitor respiratory status (change in secretions, wheezing, chest tightness)

PATIENT AND FAMILY EDUCATION
Teach/instruct
• To take as directed at prescribed intervals for prescribed length of time
Warn/advise
• To notify care provider of hypersensitivity, side effects
• Not to exceed recommended dosage
• To avoid hazardous activities if drowsiness occurs (bicycles, skateboards, skates)

• To avoid use of alcohol, medications containing alcohol, CNS depressants

STORAGE
• Store at room temp in light-resistant, tight container

---

testosterone, testosterone cypionate, testosterone enanthate, testosterone proprionate

Brand Name(s): Testosterone Andro 100, Andronaq-50, Histerone, Testaqua, Testoject-50; testosterone cypionate: Andro-Cyp 100, Andro-Cyp 200, Andronate, dep Andro 100, dep Andro 200, Depo-Testosterone, Depo-Testosterone Cypionate✢, Duratest, Testa-C, Testoject LA; testosterone enanthate: Andro LA 200, Andryl, Delatestryl✢, Everone, Testone LA, Testrin-PA; testosterone propionate: Testex

Classification: Androgen replacement, antineoplastic (androgen)

Controlled Substance Schedule III

Pregnancy Category: X

AVAILABLE PREPARATIONS
Inj: 25 mg/ml, 50 mg/ml, 100 mg/ml (testosterone, aqueous susp); 50 mg/ml, 100 mg/ml, 200 mg/ml; (testosterone cypionate, in oil; 100 mg/ml, 200 mg/ml (testosterone enanthate, in oil); 25 mg/ml, 50 mg/ml, 100 mg/ml (testosterone propionate, in oil)

ROUTES AND DOSAGES
Male Hypogonadism
Children: Initiation of pubertal growth, IM 40-50 mg/m^2/dose (testosterone cyprionate or enanthate ester) monthly until growth rate falls to prepubertal levels; during terminal growth phase, 100 mg/

✢ Available in Canada.

m²/dose (testosterone cyprionate or enanthate ester) monthly until growth ceases; maintenance virilizing dose, 100 mg/m²/dose (testosterone cyprionate or enanthate ester) twice monthly

Adults: IM 10-25 mg 2-3 ×/wk (testosterone or testosterone propionate) or 50-400 mg q 2-4 wk (testosterone cypionate or enanthate)

Delayed Puberty
Children: IM 40-50 mg/m²/dose monthly (testosterone cypionate or enanthate) for 6 months

Postpubertal Cryptorchism
Children and adults: IM 10-25 mg 2-3 ×/wk (testosterone or testosterone propionate)

MECHANISM AND INDICATIONS
Androgen mechanism: Binds with androgen receptors to promote growth and development of male sexual organs and secondary sexual characteristics
Indications: Hypogonadism, constitutional delay of growth and puberty in males

PHARMACOKINETICS
Half-life: 10-100 min
Metabolism: Liver
Excretion: Urine

CONTRAINDICATIONS AND PRECAUTIONS
• Contraindicated with severe renal or cardiac disease, hepatic disease, hypersensitivity, pregnancy, lactation, undiagnosed genital bleeding, male breast cancer or prostatic cancer
• Use cautiously with DM, anticoagulant therapy

INTERACTIONS
Drug
• Potentiates warfarin-type anticoagulants
• Increased oxyphenbutazone concentrations possible

Lab
• Increased LFTs, PT, serum creatinine, Na, K⁺, Ca, PO₄, cholesterol
• Altered thyroid function tests, serum 17-KS

SIDE EFFECTS
CNS: Headache, anxiety, dizziness, fatigue, paresthesias, depression
CV: Edema, hypertension
DERM: Acne, oiliness, hirsutism, flushing, sweating, male pattern baldness
GI: Nausea, vomiting, diarrhea, gastroenteritis, constipation, wt gain, cholestatic jaundice, change in appetite
GU: Bladder irritability, testicular atrophy, hematuria, priapism, phallic enlargement, gynecomastia, impotence, epididymitis
MS: Premature epiphyseal closure
Local: Pain at injection site, induration, postinjection furunculosis

TOXICITY AND OVERDOSE
No information available

PATIENT CARE MANAGEMENT
Assessment
• Assess history of hypersensitivity to testosterone, related drugs
• Assess growth rate, bone age, pubertal status (Tanner Stage), wt, Na, Cl, Ca, ALT, AST, bilirubin

Interventions
• Warming sol to room temp, shaking will help dissolve crystals
• Administer IM deep in upper outer quadrant of gluteal muscle

> **NURSING ALERT**
> Potential for abuse by athletes and body builders; warn pts that testosterone does not improve athletic performance
>
> Store in a secure place

Evaluation
• Evaluate therapeutic response (monitor pubertal status and bone age for appropriate progression; increased growth velocity may occur as puberty progresses)
• Evaluate signs of virilization in females (increased libido, deepening of voice, breast tissue, enlarged clitoris, menstrual irregularities), gynecomastia, impotence, testicular atrophy in males
• Monitor for signs of hypoglycemia in diabetics

T

- Monitor for edema, hypertension, cardiac symptoms, jaundice
- Monitor bone age q 6 mo (bone age advancement should not exceed increase in linear growth)
- Monitor priapism (may need to decrease dosage)
- Monitor K^+, Na, Cl, Ca, ALT, AST, bilirubin
- Monitor for signs of hypercalcemia (lethargy, polyuria, polydipsia, nausea, vomiting, constipation)

PATIENT AND FAMILY EDUCATION
Teach/instruct
- To take as directed at prescribed intervals for prescribed length of time
- About anticipated changes in body image with adolescents

Warn/advise
- To notify care provider of hypersensitivity, side effects (GI distress, diarrhea, jaundice, priapism, menstrual irregularities)
- Not to discontinue medication suddenly
- That side effects are reversible with discontinuation of medication
- That sexually active pts need to practice contraception when taking this medication
- About dangers of using steroids to improve athletic performance

STORAGE
- Store at room temp

---

tetracaine hydrochloride

Brand Name(s): Pontocaine✤

Classification: Ophthalmic anesthetic

Pregnancy Category: C

AVAILABLE PREPARATIONS
Ophthal sol: 0.5%
Ophthal oint: 0.5%

ROUTES AND DOSAGES
Children: Ophth, safety and effectiveness not established

Adults: Sol, instill 1-2 gtt just before procedure; oint, apply ½-1 inch to lower conjunctival fornix

MECHANISM AND INDICATIONS
Anesthetic mechanism: Decreases permeability of neuronal membrane to Na ions, thus blocking generation and conduction of sensory, motor, and autonomic nerve fibers
Indications: Used as a local anesthetic in eye for various diagnostic and examination purposes

PHARMACOKINETICS
Onset of action: Within 60 sec
Duration: 15-20 min
Metabolism: Liver
Excretion: Urine

CONTRAINDICATIONS AND PRECAUTIONS
- Contraindicated with known hypersensitivity to tetracaine, any component, or ester-type local anesthetics (benzocaine, procaine)
- Use cautiously with plasma cholinesterase deficiency, ocular secondary bacterial infection, pregnancy

INTERACTIONS
Drug
- Decreased antibacterial action of sulfonamides
- Increased risk of toxicity, anesthetic effect with cholinesterase inhibitors

Lab
- Inhibition of bacterial growth on cultures possible

SIDE EFFECTS
DERM: Rash, drying, cracking with skin contact
EENT: Stinging, burning, blurred vision, lacrimation, photophobia, conjunctival redness

PATIENT CARE MANAGEMENT
Assessment
- Assess history of hypersensitivity to tetracaine, any component, ester-type local anesthetics

Interventions
- Sol should be clear, without crystals

✤ Available in Canada.

- See Chapter 2 regarding instillation; wash hands before, after application, cleanse crusts or discharge from eye before application; wipe excess medication from around eye; do not rub eye or flush medication from eye
- Provide protective covering for eye while cornea is anesthetized and blink reflex is absent

Evaluation
- Monitor for signs of hypersensitivity (diffuse epithelial keratites, sloughing of necrotic epithelium, corneal filaments, iritis)
- Monitor delayed corneal epithelial healing with prolonged use

PATIENT AND FAMILY EDUCATION
Warn/advise
- To notify care provider of hypersensitivity, side effects
- Not to touch or rub eye after instillation until after anesthesia has worn off
- To notify care provider if any change in vision occur

STORAGE
- Store at room temp in tightly closed container
- Protect from light
- Do not freeze

---

tetracycline hydrochloride

Brand Name(s): Achromycin, Achromycin V✤, Apo-Tetra✤, Novo-Tetra✤, Nu-Tetra✤, Panmycin, Sumycin, Tetracyn, Topicycline (topical)

Classification: Antibiotic (tetracycline)

Pregnancy Category: D

AVAILABLE PREPARATIONS
Oral susp: 125 mg/5 ml
Tabs, film-coated: 250 mg, 500 mg
Caps: 100 mg, 250 mg, 500 mg
Ophthal: 1% susp, oint
Top: 0.22% sol, 3% oint

ROUTES AND DOSAGES
- Not recommended for children <8 yr
Children >8 yr: PO 25-50 mg/kg/24 hr divided q6h (maximum 2 g/24 hr)
Adults: PO 250-500 mg q6h

Prophylaxis of Ophthalmia Neonatorum
Ophthal, 1-2 gtt of suspension or 0.5-2 cm strip of ointment into conjunctival sac within 1 hr of delivery

Ocular Infections
Ophthal, 1-2 gtt of suspension or 0.5-2 cm strip of ointment into conjunctival sac bid-qid

Acne Vulgaris
Top sol, after cleansing skin, apply quantity sufficient to thoroughly wet area affected by acne bid; top oint, after cleansing skin, apply sparingly to infected areas 2-5 ×/24 hr

MECHANISM AND INDICATIONS
Antibiotic mechanism: Bacteriostatic; inhibits bacterial protein synthesis by binding reversibly to ribosomal subunits
Indications: Effective against gram-positive and gram-negative organisms including *Mycoplasma, Rickettsia, Chlamydia,* and spirochetes; used to treat syphilis, *Chlamydia trachomatis,* lymphogranuloma venereum, mycoplasma pneumonia, early stages of Lyme disease, rickettsial infections; consider alternative agent to treat *Neisseria gonorrhoeae* because of its high level of resistance

PHARMACOKINETICS
Peak: 2-4 hr
Distribution: Widely distributed
Half-life: 6-12 hr
Metabolism: Liver
Excretion: Urine, feces

CONTRAINDICATIONS AND PRECAUTIONS
- Contraindicated with pregnancy, lactation, children <8 yr (because of risk of permanent discoloration of teeth, enamel defects, retardation of bone growth), with known

hypersensitivity to any tetracycline
• Use cautiously with impaired renal or hepatic function, diabetes insipidus

INTERACTIONS
Drug
• Decreased bactericidal effects of penicillins
• Increased effects of oral anticoagulants
• Decreased absorption with antacids containing aluminum, Ca, or Mg, laxatives containing Mg, oral iron, zinc, $NaHCO_3$
• Increased effects of digoxin
• Increased risk of nephrotoxicity from methoxyflurane
Lab
• False positive urine catecholamines
Nutrition
• Decreased oral absorption if given with food or dairy products

SIDE EFFECTS
CNS: Dizziness, headache, increased intracranial pressure
CV: Pericarditis
DERM: Maculopapular and erythematous rashes, urticaria, photosensitivity, increased pigmentation, discolored nails; with top use, temporary stinging or burning on application, slight yellowing of treated skin, severe dermatitis, fluorescence of treated skin under black light
EENT: Sore throat; with ophthal, eye itching
GI: Anorexia, epigastric distress, nausea, vomiting, diarrhea, glossitis, dysphagia, stomatitis, pseudomembranous colitis, inflammatory anogenital lesions, hepatotoxicity (with large IV doses)
GU: Reversible nephrotoxicity with outdated tetracycline
HEME: Neutropenia, eosinophilia
METAB: Elevated BUN
Other: Hypersensitivity, bacterial/fungal superinfection

TOXICITY AND OVERDOSE
Clinical signs: GI disturbance
Treatment: Antacids; if ingested within 4 hr, empty stomach by gastric lavage; supportive care

PATIENT CARE MANAGEMENT
Assessment
• Assess history of hypersensitivity to tetracyclines
• Obtain C&S; may begin therapy before obtaining results
• Assess renal function (BUN, creatinine, I&O), hepatic function (ALT, AST, bilirubin), hematologic function (CBC, differential, platelet count) (particularly for long term therapy), bowel pattern
• Assess eye, skin (for redness, discharge, swelling)
Interventions
• Check expiration dates; nephrotoxicity may result from outdated tetracycline
• If pt is receiving concurrent penicillins, administer penicillins at least 1 hr before tetracycline
• Administer PO 1 hr before or 2 hr after meals; administer with water to prevent esophageal irritation; do not administer within 1 hr of hs to prevent esophageal reflux; do not administer with milk or dairy products, $NaHCO_3$, oral iron, zinc, antacids
• Shake susp well before administering; film-coated tabs must be swallowed whole; caps may be taken apart, mixed with food or fluid
• See Chapter 2 regarding ophthal instillation; wash hands before and after application, cleanse crusts or discharge from eye before application; wipe excess medication from eye; do not flush medication from eye; for prophylaxis of ophthalmia neonatorum, use new single unit tube for each neonate
• Wash hands before and after top application; before application, cleanse area with soap and water then dry well; apply sol quantity sufficient to thoroughly wet affected area; apply ointment sparingly to infected area
• Maintain age-appropriate fluid intake

✤ Available in Canada.

NURSING ALERT
Discontinue drug if signs of toxicity, hypersensitivity, renal dysfunction, superinfection, erythema to sun or ultraviolet exposure, pseudomembranous colitis develop

Evaluation
• Evaluate therapeutic response (decreased symptoms of infection)
• Monitor for signs of superinfection (perineal itching, diaper rash, fever, malaise, redness, pain, swelling, drainage, rash, diarrhea, sore throat, change in cough or sputum)
• Observe for signs of allergic reaction (rash, pruritus, angioedema)
• Monitor bowel pattern; diarrhea may be symptomatic of pseudomembranous colitis
• Monitor renal function (BUN, creatinine, I&O), hepatic function (ALT, AST, bilirubin), hematologic function (CBC, differential, platelet count)

PATIENT AND FAMILY EDUCATION
Teach/instruct
• To take as directed at prescribed intervals for prescribed length of time
Warn/advise
• To notify care provider of hypersensitivity, side effects, superinfection
• Not to use outdated medications
• To avoid sun or ultraviolet light exposure
• Not to share towels, wash cloths, linens, eye make-up with family member being treated with ophthal forms
• Avoid use of OTC creams, ointments, lotions while using top forms (unless directed by care provider)

STORAGE
• Store tabs, caps, ophthalmic, top at room temp in airtight, light-resistant containers

• Reconstituted oral susp stable refrigerated 14 days

---

theophylline, theophylline sodium glycinate (49% anhydrous theophylline)

Brand Name(s): Theophylline: Aerolate, Apo-Theo LA✤, Aquaphyllin, Asmalix, Bronkodyl, Constant-T, Elixicon, Elixophyllin, Pulmophylline✤, Quibron-T✤, Quibron-SR✤, Respbid, Slo-Bid✤, Slo-Phyllin, Sustaire, Theo-24, Theobid, Theochron, Theochron-SR✤, Theoclear, Theodur✤, Theolair✤, Theospan-SR, Theo-SR✤, Theovent, Theox, Uniphyl✤ (and more); theophylline sodium glycinate (49% anhydrous theophylline); Synophylate

Classification: Bronchodilator (xanthine derivative)

Pregnancy Category: C

AVAILABLE PREPARATIONS
Many preparations and dosage forms exist, including elixir, sol, syr, tabs (immediate and controlled release), and caps (immediate and timed release); combination forms are also available

ROUTES AND DOSAGES
IV: See aminophylline (theophylline ethylenediamine)
Neonatal Apnea
PO (immediate release) loading dose 5 mg/kg/dose (use immediate-release oral products for loading dose); then 1-2 mg/kg/24 hr divided q8-12h in preterm neonates (<36 wk) or 2-4 mg/kg/24 hr divided q8-12h in neonates ≥36 wk gestation
Bronchospasm
PO (immediate release) loading dose 0.8 mg/kg/dose for each 2 mcg/ml desired increase in serum

theophylline level; in emergency situations when no serum level available, can give 2.5 mg/kg/dose (use immediate-release oral products for loading dose); for maintenance, dose by age; maximum dose 900 mg/24 hr; may use sus rel preparations, using same dose, but divided bid-tid; further dose adjustments should be based on serum levels; for maintenance, 3-6 mg/kg/24 hr divided q8h (infants 0-2 mo), 6-15 mg/kg/24 hr divided q6h (infants 2-6 mo), 15-22 mg/kg/24 hr divided q4-6h (infants 6-12 mo), 22 mg/kg/24 hr divided q6h (children 1-9 yr), 20 mg/kg/24 hr divided q6h (children 9-11 yr), 18 mg/kg/24 hr divided q6h (children 12-16 yr), 13 mg/kg/24 hr divided q6h (adults)

MECHANISM AND INDICATIONS

Bronchodilator mechanism: Relaxes smooth muscle particularly bronchial airways and pulmonary blood vessels, producing reversal of bronchospasm, increasing respiratory flow rates and vital capacity; increases sensitivity of the medullary respiratory center to CO_2, decreasing apneic episodes in neonates; prevents diaphragmatic fatigue, thereby improving contractility in COPD

Indications: Used to treat bronchospasm of bronchial asthma, bronchitis, pulmonary emphysema, other COPDs, and neonatal apnea

PHARMACOKINETICS

Peak: PO sol 1 hr; tabs immediate release, 2 hr; chewable tabs 1-1.5 hr; enteric coated 5 hr; ext rel or caps 4-7 hr; IV within 30 min
Half-life: Premature 30 hr; newborn-6 mo >25-30 hr; infants >1 yr 6.9 hr; children 3.4-3.7 hr; adult non-smoker, uncomplicated asthma, 6.5-10.9 hr; smoker 1-2 packs per day 4-5 hr; COPD, cardiac failure, liver disease >24 hr
Metabolism: Liver
Excretion: Urine
Therapeutic level: Bronchodilation, 10-20 mcg/ml; respiratory stimulation, 6-13 mcg/ml; toxic concentrations, ≥20 mcg/ml (for bronchodilation and respiratory stimulation, therapeutic response may be seen at 5-10 mcg serum level and some toxicity noted at 15-20 mcg/ml, therefore close monitoring and individualized dosage adjustment is indicated)
• Guidelines for drawing therapeutic level: IV bolus (see aminophylline); IV continuous infusion (see aminophylline); PO (liquid, fast-release tablet), peak 1 hr after administration after at least 1 day of therapy, trough just before administration after at least 1 day of therapy; PO (slow-release product), peak 4 hr after administration after at least 1 day of therapy, trough just before administration after at least 1 day of therapy; in pts with a prolonged half-life, draw levels after 48-72 hr of therapy

CONTRAINDICATIONS AND PRECAUTIONS

• Contraindicated with uncontrolled arrhythmia, xanthine (caffeine) hypersensitivity, active peptic ulcer disease, seizure disorder (unless on appropriate anticonvulsants)
• Use cautiously with compromised circulatory or cardiac function, diabetes, glaucoma, hyperthyroidism, peptic ulcer, GERD, renal or hepatic disease, cor pulmonale, hypoxemia, smokers and those who have quit within previous 2 yr, sulfite sensitivity, sustained high fever, infants, children, adolescents, lactation (drug is excreted in breast milk and may cause insomnia, fretfulness, irritability; known potential for toxicity in the breastfed infant exists)

INTERACTIONS

Drug
• Increased serum concentration of theophylline with allopurinol, cimetidine, ciprofloxacillin, ephedrine, other sympathomimetics, erythromycin, oral contraceptives, propranolol, ranitidine, thiabendazole, troleandomycin (because of

decreased hepatic clearance of theophylline)

• Decreased serum concentration of theophylline with corticosteroids, lithium, barbiturates, phenytoin, carbamazepine, phenobarbital, primidone, rifampin, IV isoproterenol; tobacco, marijuana

• Antagonistic effect seen with β-adrenergic blockers (propranolol) and bronchospasm may result if combination used

• Decreased sedative effect of propofol

• Increased potential for toxicity with cardiac glycosides

• Decreased effect of lithium, furosemide

• Increased potential for seizures with ketamine

Lab

• Increased serum uric acids possible

• Falsely elevated theophylline levels possible with furosemide, phenbutazone, probenecid, theobromine, caffeine, tea, chocolate, cola drinks, acetaminophen, depending on analytical methods used

Nutrition

• Increased serum concentration of theophylline with high carbohydrate diet

• Decreased serum concentration of theophylline with high protein, low carbohydrate diets and charcoal-broiled foods

INCOMPATIBILITIES

• See aminophylline

SIDE EFFECTS

CNS: Anxiety, restlessness, headache, dizziness, nervousness, depression, irritability, insomnia, muscle twitching, seizure

CV: Palpitations, arrhythmias, sinus tachycardia, extrasystoles, chest pain, flushing, decreased B/P, circulatory failure, cardiac arrest

DERM: Urticaria, exfoliative dermatitis, rash

GI: Nausea, GI upset, vomiting, anorexia, bitter aftertaste, epigastric pain, diarrhea, GERD

GU: Urinary retention

RESP: Tachypnea, respiratory arrest

Local: Redness, pain at IV site

Other: Hyperglycemia, inappropriate ADH

TOXICITY AND OVERDOSE

Clinical signs: Behavior changes, insomnia, headaches, flushing, dizziness, increasing irritability, anorexia, severe nausea or vomiting, seizure, abdominal pain, increased respiratory or HR, irregular heart beat, weakness, black or bloody stools, vomiting of dark (dry blood) emesis or blood, urinary urgency, falling blood pressure; *onset of toxicity may be sudden and severe, with seizure, arrhythmia, even death as a first sign*

Treatment: Charcoal hemoperfusion may be indicated in severe overdose (level >40 mcg/ml); otherwise induce emesis (except in pts with impaired LOC), then administer activated charcoal q4h (taking precautions to prevent aspiration) and cathartics; treat seizure with IV diazepam; treat arrhythmias with lidocaine; support cardiac and respiratory systems, provide adequate hydration

PATIENT CARE MANAGEMENT

Assessment

• Assess history of hypersensitivity to theophylline, related drugs

• Assess respiratory status

• Assess baseline VS

• Assess for risks of toxicity (age, smoking, drug use, medical history; medication history, especially any theophylline; time of last dose)

• Obtain height, wt

Interventions

• Administer PO at equally-spaced intervals

• Can administer with food if GI distress occurs; do not crush timed rel preparations or allow pt to chew; plain tabs may be crushed, administered with food or fluids; chewable form should be chewed, not swallowed whole

• Maintain age-appropriate fluid intake

✦ Available in Canada.

- PO dose can be administered via NG tube
- See aminophylline for IV interventions
- Calculate drug dosage based on lean body wt (drug does not distribute to fatty tissue)
- Notify care provider for levels ≥20 mcg/ml
- Monitor closely when changing from one route of administration to another; wait 4-6 hr after discontinuing IV therapy to start oral therapy

---

NURSING ALERT

Rapid IV administration can lead to severe or fatal acute circulatory failure

Serious toxicity is not reliably preceded by less-severe side effects

Do not attempt to maintain any dosage that is not well tolerated

Individualization of dosage necessary

Some commercial products contain sulfites, which may produce hypersensitivity reactions in sensitive pts

---

Evaluation
- Evaluate therapeutic response (improved respiratory effort)
- Evaluate peak serum levels frequently in infants and young children
- Evaluate peak serum levels at least q 6 mo for maintenance therapy and more frequently for acute indications
- Evaluate respiratory status, VS, I&O
- Evaluate for signs or symptoms of toxicity
- Evaluate arterial or capillary blood gases (if appropriate)
- Evaluate number and severity of apnea spells (if used to treat neonatal apnea)
- Evaluate children closely for CNS effects (nervousness, restlessness, insomnia, hyperreflexia, twitching, convulsions)

PATIENT AND FAMILY EDUCATION
Teach/instruct
- To use only prescribed amount of drug; carefully review dosage schedule and preparation
- To avoid other medications (especially those for pulmonary disorders) unless prescribed
- To take any missed dose as soon as possible, but *not* to double the dose
- That drug should be taken at regular intervals to maintain blood levels
- That oral preparations should be taken with a full glass of water
- Not to crush or chew sus/ext rel tabs; plain tabs may be crushed, taken with food or fluid
- That some timed rel caps can be opened and sprinkled on a spoonful of applesauce or pudding, then swallowed without chewing and follow with juice or water
- That medication may be given with food if GI upset occurs with liquid or non–sus rel forms
- About follow-up appointments, lab appointments for monitoring blood levels; emphasize importance of compliance
- That some elixir preparations contain alcohol

Warn/advise
- About adverse effects and signs of toxicity (nausea or vomiting, restlessness, tachycardia, irregular heartbeat, seizure) and advise to contact provider immediately if any of these occur
- To avoid drinking large amounts of coffee, tea, cola, cocoa, or eating large amounts of chocolate with this medication to avoid increased potential for adverse effects
- That smoking decreases effectiveness of drug
- That dizziness may occur, to take precautions to avoid falls
- Not to change brands because all forms are not equivalent
- To notify care provider if flu

✤ Available in Canada.

symptoms occur; a dosage change may be indicated

STORAGE
- Store at room temp in tightly closed container
- Keep out of reach of children

---

thiabendazole
Brand Name(s): Mintezol✤
Classification: Anthelmintic
Pregnancy Category: C

AVAILABLE PREPARATIONS
Susp: 500 mg/ml
Tabs, chewable: 500 mg

ROUTES AND DOSAGES
Children and adults: PO 50 mg/kg/24 hr divided q12h × 2-5 days (maximum 3 g/24 hr)

MECHANISM AND INDICATIONS
Mechanism: Interferes with enzyme activity of parasite
Indications: Used to treat cutaneous larva migrans, roundworm, pinworm, whipworm, threadworm and trichinosis, hookworm

PHARMACOKINETICS
Peak: 1-2 hr
Metabolism: Liver
Excretion: Urine, feces

CONTRAINDICATIONS AND PRECAUTIONS
- Contraindicated with known hypersensitivity to thiabendazole
- Use cautiously with renal or hepatic impairment, malnutrition, anemia, dehydration, pregnancy, lactation, children <14 kg

SIDE EFFECTS
CNS: Drowsiness, vertigo, seizures, fever, headache, chills, hallucination, flushing
CV: Hypotension, bradycardia
DERM: Rash, Stevens-Johnson syndrome, erythema, pruritus
EENT: Tinnitus, blurred vision
GI: Nausea, vomiting, diarrhea, hepatotoxicity, anorexia, jaundice
GU: Urine malodor, nephrotoxicity, hematuria, enuresis

HEME: Leukopenia

TOXICITY AND OVERDOSE
Clinical signs: Visual disturbances, altered mental status
Treatment: If ingested within 4 hr, induce emesis or gastric lavage followed by activated charcoal; supportive care

PATIENT CARE MANAGEMENT
Assessment
- Assess history of hypersensitivity to thiabendazole
- Obtain pinworm test at night when child is sleeping (worms migrate to perianal area); carefully separate buttocks and press sticky side of scotch tape to anal area
- Obtain stool samples for other parasites
- Assess for dehydration, malnutrition before therapy
- Assess baseline renal function (BUN, creatinine, I&O), hepatic function (ALT, AST, bilirubin), hematologic function (CBC, differential, platelet count)
- Assess concurrent use of other drugs metabolized by liver

Interventions
- Administer after meals; tab must be chewed, not swallowed whole
- Use appropriate hygiene techniques (especially handwashing)

Evaluation
- Evaluate therapeutic response (expulsion of worms)
- Evaluate spread of infection to other household members and treat as necessary
- Evaluate for side effects, hypersensitivity (rash, headache, nausea)
- Monitor renal function (BUN, creatinine, I&O), hepatic function (ALT, AST, bilirubin)

PATIENT AND FAMILY EDUCATION
Teach/instruct
- To take as directed at prescribed intervals for prescribed length of time
- About proper hygiene procedures (especially good handwashing techniques)

T

✤ Available in Canada.

• How to prevent reinfection (change undergarments and bed linens, wash clothes and linens in hot water; not to shake bed linens into the air; to frequently cleanse perianal area)
• To clean toilet every day with disinfectant
• To wash all fruits and vegetables before eating
• To drink fruit juice (aids in worm expulsion by eliminating accumulation in intestinal mucosa)
Warn/advise
• To notify care provider of hypersensitivity
• That all family members need to be evaluated and treated
• To avoid hazardous activities; drowsiness may occur
Encourage
• To comply with treatment regime

STORAGE
• Store at room temp in tight container

---

thiamine hydrochloride (vitamin B₁)
Brand Name(s): Betakin✤, Betalin S, Bewan✤, Biamine, Thiamin Hydrochloride Injection✤, Vitamin B₁✤
Classification: Water soluble vitamin
Pregnancy Category: A (C if dosage exceeds RDA)

AVAILABLE PREPARATIONS
Tabs: 5 mg, 10 mg, 25 mg, 50 mg, 100 mg, 250 mg, 500 mg
Elixir: 2.25 mg/ml
Inj: 100 mg/ml, 200 mg/ml

ROUTES AND DOSAGES
• See Appendix F, Table of Recommended Daily Dietary Allowances
Supplementation
Infants: 0.3-0.5 mg/24 hr
Children: 0.5-1 mg/24 hr
Adults: 1-2 mg/24 hr

Bereberi
Children: PO 10-50 mg/24 hr qd × 2 wk, then 5-10 mg/24 hr qd for 1 mo; IV/IM 10-25 mg/24 hr qd
Adults: IM 5-30 mg tid × 2 wk, then PO 5-30 mg/24 hr qd or divided tid for 1 mo
IV administration
• Recommended concentration: 100 mg/ml
• IV infusion: Dilute or undiluted at rate of <100 mg/5 min or more
• Continuous infusion rate: May be added to maintenance infusions

MECHANISM AND INDICATIONS
Mechanism: Coenzyme important in carbohydrate and energy metabolism; vitamin requirements will increase with carbohydrate intake; vitamin B₁ deficiency can occur within 3 wk of total absence of dietary thiamine; deficiency is characterized by depression, decreased concentration, neuritis, nausea and vomiting, changes in vision, fever and SOB
Indications: Treatment and prevention of vitamin B₁ deficiency, also known as beriberi

PHARMACOKINETICS
Metabolism: Liver
Excretion: Urine

CONTRAINDICATIONS AND PRECAUTIONS
• Contraindicated with hypersensitivity to thiamin
• Use cautiously with Wernicke's encephalopathy, pregnancy

INTERACTIONS
Drug
• Increased effects of neuromuscular blocking agents possible
Lab
• False uric acid, urobilinogen possible

INCOMPATIBILITIES
• Carbonates, citrates, barbiturates, sulfites, erythromycin lactobionate

SIDE EFFECTS
CNS: Weakness, restlessness
CV: Fluid retention, edema

✤ Available in Canada.

DERM: Itching, hives, sweating, warmth, pruritis
GI: Nausea, diarrhea
Other: SOB, pulmonary edema, anaphylaxis with IV administration, sweating, tightness of throat

TOXICITY AND OVERDOSE
Clinical signs: Large doses of IV vitamin may produce neuromuscular blockade and cause neurologic symptoms
Treatment: Supportive care

PATIENT CARE MANAGEMENT
Assessment
• Assess history of hypersensitivity to thiamine; consider ID test before IV administration
• Review medical history; for pts with Wernicke's encephalopathy, thiamine should be administered before IV administration of glucose to avoid worsening of this condition
• Obtain dietary history; evaluate fad or unusual dietary habits; single-vitamin deficiency is rare, other vitamin deficiencies should be suspected
• Assess for use of alcohol
Interventions
• Administer IV slowly
• For pts with Wernicke's encephalopathy with suspected thiamine deficiency, administer thiamine before a glucose load
• Rotate IM injection site; may become sore
• Provide diet to assure adequate thiamine intake

NURSING ALERT
Thiamine is unstable in neutral or alkaline sols; do not use in combination with carbonates, citrates, barbiturates, or erythromycin lactobionate IV; also incompatible with sols containing sulfites

Sensitivity reactions can occur; consider ID test before IV administration

Evaluation
• Evaluate therapeutic response

(normal serum thiamine levels, decreased symptoms of deficiency)
• Monitor for signs of hypersensitivity (neuritis, heart failure within hrs of IV administration)
• Monitor dietary intake with specific attention to whole wheat products, brewer's yeast, enriched or fortified breads and cereals, seed, and legumes

PATIENT AND FAMILY EDUCATION
Teach/instruct
• To take as directed at prescribed intervals for prescribed length of time
• To evaluate other medication/OTC drugs for interactions
Warn/advise
• To notify care provider if hypersensitivity, side effects are noted
• To supplement the RDAs (see Appendix F) if needed; megadosing is not recommended
• That thiamine requirements are increased with increased intake of carbohydrates
Encourage
• To eat a balanced diet; most people who eat a varied diet generally do not require supplemental vitamins; common sources of thiamine are pork, organ meats, whole wheat flour, brewer's yeast, enriched and fortified breads and cereals, seeds, legumes

STORAGE
• Store in a tightly sealed, light-resistant, non-metallic container
• Protect IV form from freezing

T

6-thioguanine
Brand Name(s): Lanvis✦, Tabloid
Classification: Antineoplastic, antimetabolite; cell cycle phase specific (S phase)
Pregnancy Category: D

AVAILABLE PREPARATIONS
Tabs: 40 mg

ROUTES AND DOSAGES
• Dosage may vary in response to diagnosis, extent of disease, concurrent or previous therapy, protocol guidelines, physiological parameters; consult current literature, protocol recommendations

Infants <3 yr: PO 3.3 mg/kg/24 hr divided bid × 4 days

Children >3 yr and adults: PO, initial dose 2 mg/kg/24 hr or 75-100 mg/m^2/24 hr (calculated to nearest 20 mg); maintenance, 2-3 mg/kg/24 hr or 100 mg/m^2/24 hr

MECHANISM AND INDICATIONS
Mechanism: Exact mechanism unknown; structurally similar to purine bases and is substituted in nucleotide synthesis; substitution results in blockage of synthesis and use of purine nucleotides, which in turn results in inhibition of DNA and RNA synthesis

Indications: Used in combination with other agents for remission induction, consolidation, and maintenance therapy for ANLL; may also be used in ALL

PHARMACOKINETICS
Peak: Uncertain; 2-12 hr after ingestion

Distribution: Incomplete, erratic with PO administration 30%-50% of dose enters systemic circulation

Half-life: Initial phase 15 min; terminal: 11 hr

Metabolism: Primarily in liver

Excretion: Urine, as metabolite

CONTRAINDICATIONS AND PRECAUTIONS
• Contraindicated with hypersensitivity history to drug, pregnancy, lactation, active infections, especially chicken pox, herpes zoster; previously demonstrated resistance to 6-mercaptopurine or 6-thioguanine therapy (complete cross-resistance generally)
• Use cautiously with impaired hepatic function, stomatitis, diarrhea (if severe, may require dosage reduction)

INTERACTIONS
Drug
• Unlike 6-mercaptopurine, does not require dosage adjustment if allopurinol is being administered concurrently
• Increased toxicity possible with busulfan
• Increased therapeutic effect of nitrosoureas possible by enhancing alkylating potential

Lab
• Increased blood, urine concentration of uric acid possible

SIDE EFFECTS
EENT: Nasal congestion, rhinorrhea with higher dosage regimens

GI: Nausea, vomiting, diarrhea, stomatitis, anorexia; reversible cholestatic jaundice, hepatovenoocclusive disease; esophageal varices described in individual also receiving busulfan

GU: Crystalluria, increased serum creatinine; can cause transient renal dysfunction with increased BUN, creatinine

HEME: Neutropenia, thrombocytopenia

TOXICITY AND OVERDOSE
Clinical signs: Prolonged myelosuppression, jaundice, severe stomatitis, severe diarrhea

Treatment: Supportive measures (including blood transfusions, hydration, nutritional supplementation, broad-spectrum antibiotic coverage [if febrile], electrolyte replacement)

PATIENT CARE MANAGEMENT
Assessment
• Assess history of hypersensitivity to drug
• Assess history of previous chemotherapy, radiation therapy with attention to those that might predispose pt to hepatic dysfunction

---

♣ Available in Canada.

- Assess baseline VS, hematologic function (CBC, differential, platelet count), renal function (BUN, creatinine, I&O) hepatic function (uric acid, bilirubin, alk phos, LDH, AST, ALT)
- Assess success of previous antiemetic therapy

Interventions

- Administer antiemetic therapy 30 min before chemotherapy if initiated
- Administer between meals to facilitate absorption
- Monitor I&O; provide IV hydration until child is able to resume normal PO intake
- Provide supportive measures to maintain hemostasis, fluid, electrolyte, nutritional status

Evaluation

- Evaluate therapeutic response (tumor regression)
- Evaluate hematologic function (CBC, differential, platelet count) at least q wk
- Evaluate renal function (BUN, creatinine, I&O), hepatic function (bilirubin, uric acid, alk phos, LDH, AST, ALT) at regular intervals

PATIENT AND FAMILY EDUCATION

Teach/instruct

- To take as directed at prescribed intervals for prescribed length of time
- To have patient well hydrated before and after chemotherapy
- About the importance of follow-up to monitor blood counts, serum chemistry values
- To take accurate temp; rectal temp contraindicated
- To notify care provider of signs of bleeding (bruising, epistaxis, bleeding gums), infection (fever, sore throat, fatigue)

Warn/advise

- About impact of body changes that may occur (hair loss, hyperpigmentation, nail ridging), how to minimize changes (wigs, caps, scarves, long sleeves)

- To avoid OTC preparations containing aspirin
- To report any alterations in behavior, sensation, perception; help to develop a plan of care to manage side effects, stress of illness and treatment
- To monitor bowel function and call if abdominal pain, constipation noted
- That good oral hygiene with very soft toothbrush is imperative
- That dental work be delayed until blood work returns to normal, with permission of caretaker
- To avoid contact with known viral and bacterial illnesses
- That close household contacts of child not be immunized with live polio virus; use inactivated form
- That children receiving chemotherapy should not receive immunizations until immune system recovers sufficiently to mount necessary antibody response
- To report exposure to chicken pox in susceptible child immediately
- To report reactivation of herpes zoster virus (shingles) immediately
- If appropriate, ways to preserve reproductive patterns, sexuality (sperm banking, contraceptives)

Encourage

- Provision of nutritious food intake; consider nutrition consultation
- To use top anesthetics or systemic analgesics to control discomfort of mucositis; avoid spicy foods, commercial mouthwashes

STORAGE

- Tabs should be stored at room temp
- Protect from moisture

T

thiopental sodium

Brand Name(s): Pentothal Sodium✤, Thiopental Sodium

Classification: Anticonvulsant, barbiturate, general anesthetic, sedative

Controlled Substance Schedule III

Pregnancy Category: C

AVAILABLE PREPARATIONS
Susp, rectal: 400 mg/g
Inj: 250 mg, 400 mg, 500 mg, 1 g, 2.5 g, 5 g

DOSAGES AND ROUTES
Induction Anesthesia
• IV, to be administered by anesthesiologist
Sedation
Children: PR 5-10 mg/kg/dose
Adults: PR 3-4 g/dose
Increased Intracranial Pressure
Children: IV 1.5-5 mg/kg/dose; may increase to control intracranial pressure

MECHANISM AND INDICATIONS
Mechanism: Interferes with transmission of impulses in reticular-activating system of the brain to produce anesthesia
Indications: For use as induction anesthesia, short general anesthesia, adjunct for intubation in head injury; control of convulsive states, treatment of elevated intracranial pressure

PHARMACOKINETICS
Onset of action: IV 30-60 sec
Duration: 5-30 min
Half-life: IV, adults 3-11.5 hr; shorter in children
Metabolism: Liver

CONTRAINDICATIONS AND PRECAUTIONS
• Contraindicated with hypersensitivity to this medication or any component, status asthmaticus, hepatic or intermittent porphyrias
• Use cautiously with asthma, severe cardiovascular disease, CNS depressants, hypotension, increased intracranial pressure, kidney disease, liver disease, myasthenia gravis, pharyngeal infections

INTERACTIONS
Drug
• Increased action of CNS depressants

INCOMPATIBILITIES
• Incompatible with amikacin, aminophylline, atracurium, atropine sulfate, benzquinamide, cephalothin, cephapirin, cimetidine, clindamycin, chlorpromazine, codeine, dimenhydrinate, diphenhydramine, doxapram, droperidol, ephedrine, glycopyrrolate, hydromorphone, insulin, levarterenol, levorphanol, magnesium sulfate, meperidine, methadone, methylprednisolone, morphine, penicillins, procaine, prochlorperazine, promazine, promethazine, $NaHCO_3$ succinylcholine, tetracycline, tubocurarine, Ca, R

SIDE EFFECTS
CNS: Retrograde amnesia, prolonged somnolence
CV: Decreased cardiac output, arrhythmias, hypotension, tachycardia
DERM: Chills, necrosis, pain at injection site, shivering
EENT: Coughing, sneezing
GU: Decreased urine output
RESP: Apnea, bronchospasm, laryngospasm, respiratory depression
Other: Anaphylaxis, muscle irritability

TOXICITY AND OVERDOSE
• Thiopental is usually not used for procedures lasting more than 15-20 min because it is lipid soluble and redistributes into fat stores, prolonging recovery

PATIENT CARE MANAGEMENT
Assessment
• Assess history of hypersensitivity to drug
• Monitor respiratory rate, HR, B/P q 3-5 min during IV administration and q4h postoperatively

---

✤ Available in Canada.

Interventions

- IV to be administered by anesthesiologist for induction of anesthesia
- Administer only if crash cart and resuscitative equipment are nearby
- Use nitroprusside or chloroprocaine to decrease pain and increase circulation if extravasation occurs

---

NURSING ALERT

Ensure patent IV access; extravasation or intraarterial injection causes necrosis because the pH is 10.6

Rapid IV injection may cause hypotension or decreased cardiac output

---

Evaluation

- Evaluate therapeutic response (maintenance of anesthesia)
- Monitor for arrhythmias or myocardial depression

PATIENT AND FAMILY EDUCATION

Encourage

- Provide support as needed

STORAGE

- Store at room temp
- Protect from heat and light

---

thioridazine hydrochloride

Brand Name(s): Apo-Thioridazine✿, Mellaril✿, Mellaril-S, Thioridazine HCL

Classification: Antipsychotic agent, phenothiazine

Pregnancy Category: C

AVAILABLE PREPARATIONS

Oral susp: 25 mg/5 ml, 100 mg/5 ml; not available as generic
Tabs: 10 mg, 15 mg, 25 mg, 50 mg, 100 mg, 150 mg, 200 mg; available as generic

Concentrate: 30 mg/ml, 100 mg/ml; available as generic

DOSAGES AND ROUTES

- Do not use in children <2 yr

Children >2 yr: PO, range 0.5-3 mg/kg/24 hr divided bid-tid; usual 1 mg/kg/24 hr

Behavior Problems

Children >2 yr: PO initial 10 mg bid-tid, increase gradually

Severe Psychoses

Children >2 yr: PO initial 25 mg bid-tid, increase gradually if child is hospitalized; maximum 3 mg/kg/24 hr

Psychoses

Children >12 yr and adults: PO initial 25-100 mg tid with gradual increments prn; maintenance dose 10-200 mg bid-qid; maximum 800 mg/24 hr divided bid-qid

Depressive Disorders, Dementia

Children >12 yr and adults: PO initial 25 mg tid; maintenance 20-200 mg/24 hr

MECHANISM AND INDICATIONS

Mechanism: Blocks dopamine receptors in the CNS; depresses cerebral cortex, hypothalamus, and limbic system, which control activity; has strong anticholinergic and sedative effects; has weak extrapyramidal and antiemetic effects

Indications: For use in the management of psychotic disorders (including schizophrenia); severely aggressive disorders; combative, aggressive children with attention deficit disorder; depression; organic brain disease; adjunct in alcohol withdrawal

PHARMACOKINETICS

Onset of action: Full therapeutic effect takes about 5 days of continual, regular doses to achieve; PO erratic
Peak: PO 2-4 hr
Distribution: Crosses blood–brain barrier
Half-life: 26-36 hr
Metabolism: Liver
Excretion: Urine

✿ Available in Canada.

CONTRAINDICATIONS AND PRECAUTIONS

• Contraindicated with hypersensitivity to thioridazine or any component, to other phenothiazines; agranulocytosis, blood dyscrasias, bone marrow depression, brain damage, cardiac arrhythmias, severe cardiac disease, coma, severe CNS depression, narrow-angle glaucoma, severe liver disease, history of tardive dyskinesia, history of neuroleptic malignant syndrome

• Use cautiously with acute illness, taking antineoplastics, cardiac disease, cardiovascular disease, dehydration, hypertension, hypocalcemia, previous reaction to insulin, kidney disease, liver disease, seizures, pregnancy, lactation

INTERACTIONS

Drug

• Increased sedation with alcohol, barbiturate anesthetics, CNS depressants

• Acute encephalopathy-like syndrome with lithium (rare)

• Decreased effects of lithium, levodopa

• Increased cardiac arrhythmias with tricyclic antidepressants

• Hypotension with epinephrine; do not administer together

• Decreased absorption of thioridazine with aluminum hydroxide or magnesium hydroxide antacids

• Increased effects of alcohol, β-adrenergic blockers

• Increased anticholinergic effects with anticholinergics

• Masking of toxic effects of antineoplastic drugs (nausea and vomiting)

• Decreased metabolism of phenytoin

• Additive hypotensive effects with β-adrenergic blockers

• Increased excretion of thioridazine with phenobarbital

Lab

• Increased alk phos, bilirubin, BG, cardiac enzymes, cholesterol, cholinesterase, ^{131}I, liver function tests, PBI, prolactin, transaminases

• Decreased blood and urine hormones

• False negative pregnancy tests, urinary steroids

• False positive pregnancy tests, amylase, 5-hydroxyindoleacetic acid, phenylketonuria, porphobilinogens, urinary amylase, uroporphyrins, urobilinogen

• Urine may turn red

Nutrition

• Possible sensitivity to tabs containing yellow dye #5 (tartrazine); some individuals are sensitive to this component

SIDE EFFECTS

CNS: Dystonic reactions, headache, seizures, anxiety, confusion, depression, drowsiness, insomnia, restlessness, sedation, altered central temperature regulation, weakness

CV: Arrhythmias, cardiac arrest, ECG changes, hypotension, orthostatic hypotension, syncope, tachycardia

DERM: Rash, contact dermatitis, hives, hyperpigmentation, itching, photosensitivity

EENT: Dry eyes, glaucoma, blurred vision, possibly reversible decreased visual acuity; in dosages >800 mg/24 hr, retinitis pigmentosa

GI: Anorexia, constipation, dry mouth, nausea, vomiting, diarrhea, GI upset, cholestatic jaundice after 2-4 wk of therapy, paralytic ileus, wt gain

GU: Urinary retention

HEME: Agranulocytosis, anemia, aplastic anemia, eosinophilia, leukocytosis, leukopenia, thrombocytopenia

RESP: Bronchospasm, dyspnea, laryngospasm, respiratory depression

Other: Amenorrhea, anaphylactoid reactions, galactorrhea, glycosuria, gynecomastia, wt gain

TOXICITY AND OVERDOSE

Clinical signs: CNS depression (deep, unarousable sleep, possible coma), hypotension or hyperten-

---

✦ Available in Canada.

sion, EPS, abnormal involuntary muscle movements, agitation, seizures, arrhythmias, ECG changes, hypothermia or hyperthermia, autonomic nervous system dysfunction

Treatment: Provide an airway; if taken PO, emesis or gastric lavage, do not induce vomiting or dialyze; use IV benztropine mesylate 0.02-0.05 mg/kg/dose or for adults 1-2 mg/dose slowly over 3-6 min for EPS; use loading dose of phenytoin 10-15 mg/kg slow IV push for ventricular arrhythmias; IV fluids and norepinephrine or phenylephrine for hypotension, avoid epinephrine which may cause hypotension because of phenothiazine-induced α-adrenergic blockade and unopposed epinephrine β-adrenergic action; rigidity may be helped by dantrolene PO 0.5 mg/kg/dose q12h

PATIENT CARE MANAGEMENT
Assessment
• Assess hypersensitivity history to drug
• Assess behavior, depression, ability to function in daily activities, to sleep throughout the night
• Assess mental status (mood, sensorium, affect, impulsiveness, suicidal ideation, thoughts)
• Obtain baseline eye exam, CBC, liver function (ALT, AST, bilirubin), UA
• Obtain baseline physical exam (including B/P, ECG); rule out acute illness or dehydration

Interventions
• Avoid skin contact with oral susp or concentrate; may cause contact dermatitis
• Dilute oral concentrate with citrus juice, milk, carbonated beverage, or water before administration
• Administer with food or milk if GI symptoms occur
• Increase fluids and fiber in diet if constipation occurs
• Rinse with water, take sips of fluid, sugarless gum, hard candy for dry mouth

• Decrease stimulation by dimming lights, avoiding loud noises
• Obtain order for an antiparkinsonian agent if EPS occurs

NURSING ALERT
A possible side effect is neuroleptic malignant syndrome; if this occurs, obtain medical intervention immediately

Evaluation
• Evaluate therapeutic response (behavior, depression, ability to function in daily activities, to sleep throughout the night)
• Monitor for signs of neuroleptic malignant syndrome; symptoms include fever, fast or irregular heartbeat, fast breathing, sweating, weakness, muscle stiffness, seizures, loss of bladder control; obtain medical intervention immediately; monitor vital signs, ECG, urine output, renal function; manage symptoms with medications, hydration, and cooling blankets
• Evaluate mental status (mood, sensorium, affect, impulsiveness, suicidal ideation, delusions, hallucinations, paranoia, thought patterns, speech)
• Monitor urine bilirubin q wk for the first month
• Monitor orthostatic B/P and report B/P drops of 30 mm Hg to prescriber
• Monitor monthly bilirubin, CBC, UA, alk phos, transaminase, urine glucose, skin turgor, constipation
• Monitor for neuroleptic malignant syndrome (altered mental status, muscle rigidity, increased CPK, hyperthermia)
• Monitor hydration, orientation, LOC, reflexes, gait, coordination, VS, ECG
• Monitor q 3 mo for tardive dyskinesia, akathisia, pseudoparkinsonism
• Obtain periodic eye exams for retinitis pigmentosa with long-term therapy or on dosages above 800 mg/24 hr

T

PATIENT AND FAMILY EDUCATION
Teach/instruct
• To take as directed at prescribed intervals for prescribed length of time
• That medication is most helpful when used as part of a comprehensive multimodal treatment program
• That to achieve full therapeutic effect takes about 5 days of continuous, regular doses
• To ensure medication is swallowed
• That urine may turn red
• Not to discontinue medication without prescriber approval
• To keep this and all medications out of reach of children
Warn/advise
• To avoid OTC preparations (e.g., cough, hay fever, cold, antacids) unless approved by prescriber
• That this medication may cause drowsiness; be careful on bicycles, skates, skateboards, while driving, with other activities requiring alertness
• To report continued insomnia, fainting, altered mental status, muscle rigidity, sore throat, malaise, fever, bleeding, mouth sores
• To stay out of direct sunlight, especially between 10 AM and 3 PM (if possible); if pt must be outside, to wear protective clothing, a hat, sunglasses; to put on sun block that has a skin protection factor (SPF) of ≥15
• To use caution when exposed to heat; may impair body's adaptation to hot environments, increasing risk of heat stroke; avoid saunas, hot tubs, hot baths

STORAGE
• Store at room temp in a tightly closed, light-resistant container
• Avoid freezing
• Avoid contact with skin

---

thyroglobulin
Brand Name(s): Proloid
Classification: Thyroid hormone
Pregnancy Category: A

AVAILABLE PREPARATIONS
Tabs: 32 mg, 65 mg, 100 mg, 130 mg, 200 mg

ROUTES AND DOSAGES
Infants 1-4 mo: PO 15-30 mg qd, increased at 2 wk intervals; usual maintenance dose 30-45 mg qd
Infants 4-12 mo: PO 60-80 mg qd
Children >1 yr: PO 60-180 mg based on response
Adults: PO 32-200 mg/24 hr

MECHANISM AND INDICATIONS
Thyrotropic mechanism: Increases metabolic rates of tissues and regulates growth; essential for normal neurologic development in the first 2-3 yr of life
Indications: Replacement of endogenous thyroid hormone

PHARMACOKINETICS
Peak: 12-48 hr
Half-life: 6-7 days
Metabolism: Liver, kidneys, intestines, peripheral tissues
Excretion: Feces

CONTRAINDICATIONS AND PRECAUTIONS
• Contraindicated with adrenal insufficiency, acute MI, thyrotoxicosis, hypersensitivity to beef or pork
• Use cautiously with angina, cardiovascular disease, diabetes, corrected adrenal insufficiency, pregnancy, lactation

INTERACTIONS
Drug
• Decreased absorption with cholestyramine, colestipol
• Increased effects of anticoagulants, sympathomimetics, tricyclic antidepressants, catecholamines
• Altered dosage requirements with adrenocorticoids, insulin, estrogens, hepatic enzyme inducers (phenytoin)

Lab
• Altered thyroid function tests

SIDE EFFECTS
CNS: Insomnia, tremors, nervousness, headache
CV: Tachycardia, palpitations, arrhythmias, angina, hypertension, widened pulse pressure, cardiac arrest
DERM: Allergic skin rashes, hair loss in initial treatment phase
GI: Nausea, diarrhea, change in appetite
GU: Menstrual irregularities
Other: Sweating, wt loss, heat intolerance

TOXICITY AND OVERDOSE
Clinical signs: Signs of hyperthyroidism are wt loss, anxiety, tachycardia, arrhythmias, insomnia, diarrhea, heat intolerance
Treatment: Discontinue treatment until symptoms resolve; reinstitute therapy at a lower dosage; for acute massive overdose, decrease GI absorption and counteract central and peripheral effects; use gastric lavage, induce emesis, activated charcoal; symptomatic and supportive treatment for cardiac and respiratory symptoms; β-blockers can be used to counter increased sympathetic activity

PATIENT CARE MANAGEMENT
Assessment
• Assess history of hypersensitivity to thyroglobulin, pulse, B/P, I&O, height, wt, dry skin, constipation, cold intolerance, baseline T_3, T_4, TSH
Interventions
• Tabs may be crushed, mixed with food or fluid; do not administer with soy formulas
• Administer qd at consistent time; administer in AM to reduce sleeplessness
• Stop medication 4 wk before radioactive iodine uptake test
Evaluation
• Evaluate therapeutic response (absence of depression, increased wt loss, diuresis, absence of constipation, peripheral edema, cold intolerance, pale, cool dry skin,

brittle nails, alopecia, coarse hair, menorrhagia, night blindness, paresthesias, syncope, stupor, coma, rosy cheeks)
• Monitor pulse, BP, growth (including head circumference in infants), bone age, development, thyroid function tests
• Monitor for signs of overdose (nervousness, excitability, irritability, tachycardia, palpitations, angina pectoris, hypertension, nausea, diarrhea, wt loss, heat intolerance)

PATIENT AND FAMILY EDUCATION
Teach/instruct
• To take as directed at prescribed intervals for prescribed length of time
Warn/advise
• To notify care provider of hypersensitivity, side effects (hyperthyroidism or hypothyroidism)
• That temporary hair loss will occur in children
• Not to switch brands unless directed by care provider
• To avoid use of OTC or any medications (particularly those containing iodine) unless directed by care provider
• To avoid iodine food, iodized salt, soy beans, tofu, turnips, some seafood and breads
• To comply with follow-up care

STORAGE
• Store at room temp, protected from heat, humidity, light

T

thyroid USP

Brand Name(s): Armour Thyroid, Dathroid, Delcoid, SPT, Thermoloid, Thyrar, Thyrocine, Thyroid Strong, Thyroteric

Classification: Thyroid hormone

Pregnancy Category: A

AVAILABLE PREPARATIONS
Tabs: 16 mg, 32 mg, 65 mg, 98 mg, 130 mg, 195 mg, 260 mg, 325 mg

Tabs enteric coated: 32 mg, 65 mg, 130 mg
Tabs (bovine origin): 32 mg, 65 mg, 130 mg
Caps (porcine origin): 65 mg, 130 mg, 195 mg, 325 mg

ROUTES AND DOSAGES
Infants 1-4 mo: PO 15-30 mg qd, increased at 2 wk intervals; usual maintenance dose 30-45 mg qd
Infants 4-12 mo: PO 30-60 mg qd
Children >1 yr and adults: PO 60-180 mg based on response

MECHANISM AND INDICATIONS
Thyrotropic mechanism: Increases metabolic rates of tissues and regulates growth; essential for normal neurologic development in the first 2-3 yr of life
Indications: Replacement of endogenous thyroid hormone

PHARMACOKINETICS
Peak: 12-48 hr
Half-life: 6-7 days
Metabolism: Liver, kidneys, intestines, peripheral tissues
Excretion: Feces

CONTRAINDICATIONS AND PRECAUTIONS
• Contraindicated with adrenal insufficiency, acute MI, thyrotoxicosis, hypersensitivity to beef or pork
• Use cautiously with angina, cardiovascular disease, diabetes, corrected adrenal insufficiency, pregnancy, lactation

INTERACTIONS
Drug
• Decreased absorption with cholestyramine, colestipol
• Increased effects of anticoagulants, sympathomimetics, tricyclic antidepressants, catecholamines
• Altered dosage requirements with adrenocorticoids, insulin, estrogens, hepatic enzyme inducers (phenytoin)
Lab
• Altered thyroid function tests

SIDE EFFECTS
CNS: Insomnia, tremors, nervousness, headache
CV: Tachycardia, palpitations, arrhythmias, angina, hypertension, widened pulse pressure, cardiac arrest
DERM: Allergic skin rashes, hair loss in initial treatment phase
GI: Nausea, diarrhea, change in appetite
GU: Menstrual irregularities
Other: Sweating, wt loss, heat intolerance

TOXICITY AND OVERDOSE
Clinical signs: Signs of hyperthyroidism are wt loss, anxiety, tachycardia, arrhythmias, insomnia, diarrhea, heat intolerance
Treatment: Discontinue treatment until symptoms resolve, reinstitute therapy at a lower dosage; for acute massive overdose, decrease GI absorption and counteract central and peripheral effects; use gastric lavage, induce emesis, activated charcoal; symptomatic and supportive treatment for cardiac and respiratory symptoms; β-blockers can be used to counter increased sympathetic activity

PATIENT CARE MANAGEMENT
Assessment
• Assess history of hypersensitivity to thyroid, beef, pork products
• Assess pulse, B/P, I&O, height, wt, dry skin, constipation, cold intolerance, baseline T_3, T_4, TSH
Interventions
• Tabs may be crushed, mixed with food or fluid; do not administer with soy formulas
• Administer qd at consistent time; administer in AM to reduce sleeplessness
• Stop medication 4 wk before radioactive iodine uptake test
Evaluation
• Evaluate therapeutic response: absence of depression; increased wt loss; diuresis; absence of constipation; peripheral edema; cold intolerance; pale, cool dry skin; brittle nails; alopecia; coarse hair; menorrhagia; night blindness; par-

esthesias; syncope; stupor; coma; rosy cheeks
- Monitor pulse, B/P
- Monitor growth (including head circumference in infants), bone age, development, thyroid function tests
- Monitor for signs of overdose (nervousness, excitability, irritability, tachycardia, palpitations, angina pectoris, hypertension, nausea, diarrhea, wt loss, heat intolerance)

PATIENT AND FAMILY EDUCATION
Teach/instruct
- To take as directed at prescribed intervals for prescribed length of time

Warn/advise
- To notify care provider of hypersensitivity, side effects
- To notify care provider of symptoms of hypothyroidism or hyperthyroidism
- That temporary hair loss will occur in children
- Not to switch brands unless directed by care provider
- To avoid use of OTC or any medications (particularly those containing iodine) unless directed by care provider
- To avoid iodine food, iodized salt, soy beans, tofu, turnips, some seafood and breads
- To comply with follow-up care

STORAGE
- Store at room temp
- Protect from heat, humidity, light

---

ticarcillin disodium
Brand Name(s): Ticar✦

Classification: Antibiotic (extended-spectrum penicillin)

Pregnancy Category: B

AVAILABLE PREPARATIONS
Inj: 1 g, 3 g, 6 g, 20 g, 30 g

ROUTES AND DOSAGES
Neonates ≤4 wk, <1200 g: IV 150 mg/kg/24 hr divided q12h
Neonates ≤7 days, <2000 g: IV 150 mg/kg/24 hr divided q12h
Neonates >7 days, <2000 g: IV 225 mg/kg/24 hr divided q8h
Neonates ≤7 days, >2000 g: IV 225 mg/kg/24 hr divided q8h
Neonates >7 days, >2000 g: IV 300 mg/kg/24 hr divided q6-8h
Infants and children <40 kg: IM/IV 200-300 mg/kg/24 hr divided q4-6h; maximum 24-30 g/24 hr
Adults: IM/IV 200-300 mg/kg/24 hr divided q4-6h; maximum 24-30 g/24 hr

Uncomplicated Urinary Tract Infection
Children <40 kg: IM/IV 50-100 mg/kg/24 hr divided q6-8h
Adults: IM/IV 1 g q6h (maximum IM dose 2 g/injection)

Cystic Fibrosis
IM/IV 300-600 mg/kg/24 hr divided q4-6h

IV administration
- Recommended concentration: 10-100 mg/ml in D_5W, LR, NS
- Maximum concentration: 100 mg/ml; ≤50 mg/ml preferred for peripheral infusion to avoid vein irritation
- IV push rate: Over 30-120 min (10-20 min in neonates)
- Intermittent infusion rate: Over 30 min; may be infused ≤120 min

MECHANISM AND INDICATIONS
Antibiotic mechanism: Bactericidal; inhibits bacterial cell wall synthesis by adhering to bacterial penicillin-binding proteins
Indications: Effective against many gram-positive and gram-negative organisms including *Staphylococcus aureus, Streptococcus pneumoniae, Str. faecalis, Neisseria gonorrhoeae, Clostridium perfringens, C. tetani, Bacteroides, E. coli, Proteus mirabilis, P. vulgaris, Salmonella, Morganella morganii, Enterobacter, Pseudomonas aeruginosa,* and *Serratia;* used to treat

T

septicemia, meningitis, and respiratory tract, urinary tract, intra-abdominal, skin, and soft tissue infections

PHARMACOKINETICS
Peak: IM, neonates 1 hr; older children 0.5-1.5 hr; IV, from end of infusion to 30 min
Distribution: Good CNS concentrations only with inflamed meninges
Half-life: Neonates 1.3-5.6 hr; older children 0.9 hr
Metabolism: Liver
Excretion: Urine, bile

CONTRAINDICATIONS AND PRECAUTIONS
• Contraindicated with known hypersensitivity to ticarcillin, penicillins, cephalosporins
• Use cautiously with impaired renal function, history of bleeding problems, hypokalemia, Na restriction, pregnancy

INTERACTIONS
Drug
• Synergistic antimicrobial activity against certain organisms with aminoglycosides, clavulanic acid
• Increased serum concentrations with probenecid
• Increased serum concentrations of methotrexate
• Decreased effectiveness with tetracyclines, erythromycins, chloramphenicol
• Increased risk of bleeding with anticoagulants
Lab
• False positive urine protein except with those tests using bromophenol blue—Albustix, Albutest, Multistix
• Increased liver function tests
• False positive Coombs' test

INCOMPATIBILITIES
• Aminoglycosides, amphotericin B, tetracyclines

SIDE EFFECTS
CNS: Neuromuscular irritability, seizures
ENDO / METAB: Hypokalemia
GI: Nausea, diarrhea, vomiting, pseudomembranous colitis
GU: Acute interstitial nephritis
HEME: Leukopenia, neutropenia, eosinophilia, thrombocytopenia, hemolytic anemia, bleeding at high dosages
Local: Pain at injection site; phlebitis, vein irritation with IV injection
Other: Hypersensitivity reactions (rash, pruritus, urticaria, chills, fever, edema, anaphylaxis), bacterial or fungal superinfection

TOXICITY AND OVERDOSE
Clinical signs: Neuromuscular hypersensitivity; seizures may result from high CNS concentrations
Treatment: Supportive care; hemodialysis

PATIENT CARE MANAGEMENT
Assessment
• Assess history of hypersensitivity to ticarcillin, penicillins, cephalosporins
• Obtain C&S; may begin therapy before obtaining results
• Assess renal function (BUN, creatinine, I&O), hepatic function (ALT, AST, bilirubin), hematologic function (CBC, differential, platelet count), K^+ levels (with long-term therapy)
Interventions
• Administer penicillins at least 1 hr before bacteriostatic antibiotics (tetracyclines, erythromycins, chloramphenicol)
• Do not reconstitute IM with bacteriostatic preparations containing benzyl alcohol for neonates
• Injection is painful; administer slowly and deeply into large muscle mass, rotate injection site
• Do not premix IV with other medications (particularly aminoglycosides); infuse separately
• Use large vein with small-bore needle to reduce local reaction; rotate site q48-72h
• Maintain age-appropriate fluid intake

✤ Available in Canada.

NURSING ALERT
Discontinue drug if signs of hypersensitivity, bleeding complications, pseudomembranous colitis develop

Do not infuse rapidly; seizures may result

ticarcillin disodium/ clavulanate potassium

Brand Name(s): Timentin

Classification: Antibiotic (extended-spectrum penicillin)

Pregnancy Category: B

Evaluation
- Evaluate therapeutic response (decreased symptoms of infection)
- Monitor for signs of superinfection (perineal itching, diaper rash, fever, malaise, redness, pain swelling, drainage, rash, diarrhea, sore throat, change in cough or sputum)
- Observe for signs of allergic reaction (wheezing, tightness in chest, urticaria), especially within 20-30 min of first dose
- Monitor bowel pattern; diarrhea may be symptomatic of pseudomembranous colitis
- Monitor renal function (BUN, creatinine, I&O), hepatic function (ALT, AST, bilirubin), electrolyte levels (particularly K^+, Na)
- Monitor for signs of bleeding (ecchymosis, bleeding gums, hematuria, daily stool guaiac); monitor PT and platelet counts
- Evaluate IM site for tissue damage, IV site for vein irritation

PATIENT AND FAMILY EDUCATION
Teach/instruct
- To take as directed at prescribed intervals for prescribed length of time
Warn/advise
- To notify care provider of hypersensitivity, side effects, superinfection

STORAGE
- Store powder at room temp
- Reconstituted sol stable at room temp 72 hr, refrigerated 14 days

AVAILABLE PREPARATIONS
Inj: 3 g ticarcillin, 100 mg clavulanic acid

ROUTES AND DOSAGES
Children >15 mo: IV 200-300 mg/kg/24 hr divided q4-6h (dosages based on ticarcillin component)
Adults: IV 3.1 g q4-6h, infused over 30 min (dosages based on ticarcillin component)
IV administration
- Recommended concentration: 10-50 mg/ml in D_5W, LR, NS
- Maximum concentration: 100 mg/ml of ticarcillin
- Intermittent infusion rate: Over 30 min

MECHANISM AND INDICATIONS
Antibiotic mechanism: Bactericidal; inhibits bacterial cell wall synthesis by adhering to bacterial penicillin-binding proteins; clavulanic acid has weak bactericidal activity but prevents inactivation of ticarcillin and broadens its bactericidal spectrum by binding irreversibly with certain β-lactamase
Indications: Effective against many gram-positive and gram-negative organisms including *Staphylococcus aureus, Streptococcus pneumoniae, Str. faecalis, Neisseria gonorrhoeae, Clostridium perfringens, C. tetani, Bacteroides, E. coli, Proteus mirabilis, Salmonella, Morganella morganii, Enterobacter, Pseudomonas aeruginosa, Serratia;* used to treat septicemia, lower respiratory tract, urinary tract, skin, soft tissue, bone, and joint infections

PHARMACOKINETICS
Peak: End of infusion
Distribution: Widely distributed;

T

highest concentrations in urine, bile

Half-life: 1 hr

Metabolism: Liver

Excretion: Urine, bile

CONTRAINDICATIONS AND PRECAUTIONS

• Contraindicated with known hypersensitivity to ticarcillin, clavulanic acid, penicillins, cephalosporins, in neonates

• Use cautiously with impaired renal function, history of bleeding problems, hypokalemia, Na restriction, pregnancy

INTERACTIONS

Drug

• Synergistic antimicrobial activity against certain organisms with aminoglycosides

• Increased serum concentrations with probenecid

• Increased serum concentrations of methotrexate

• Decreased effectiveness with tetracyclines, erythromycins, chloramphenicol

Lab

• False positive urine protein except with those tests using bromophenol blue—Albustix, Albutest, Multi Stix

• Increased liver function tests

• False positive Coombs' test

INCOMPATIBILITIES

• Aminoglycosides, amikacin, $NaHCO_3$

SIDE EFFECTS

CNS: Neuromuscular irritability, seizures

ENDO/METAB: Hypokalemia

GI: Nausea, diarrhea, vomiting, pseudomembranous colitis

HEME: Leukopenia, neutropenia, eosinophilia, thrombocytopenia, hemolytic anemia, bleeding at high dosages

Local: Vein irritation, phlebitis

Other: Hypersensitivity reactions (rash, pruritus, urticaria, chills, fever, edema, anaphylaxis), bacterial or fungal superinfection

TOXICITY AND OVERDOSE

Clinical signs: Neuromuscular hypersensitivity; seizures may result from high CNS concentrations

Treatment: Supportive care; hemodialysis

PATIENT CARE MANAGEMENT

Assessment

• Assess history of hypersensitivity to ticarcillin, penicillins, cephalosporins

• Obtain C&S; may begin therapy before obtaining results

• Assess renal function (BUN, creatinine, I&O), hepatic function (ALT, AST, bilirubin), hematologic function (CBC, differential, platelet count), K^+ levels (with long-term therapy)

Interventions

• Administer penicillins at least 1 hr before bacteriostatic antibiotics (tetracyclines, erythromycins, chloramphenicol)

• Do not premix IV with other medications (particularly aminoglycosides); infuse separately

• Use large vein with small-bore needle to reduce local reaction; rotate site q48-72h

• Maintain age-appropriate fluid intake

> **NURSING ALERT**
> Discontinue drug if signs of hypersensitivity, bleeding complications, pseudomembranous colitis develop
>
> Do not infuse rapidly; seizures may result

Evaluation

• Evaluate therapeutic response (decreased symptoms of infection)

• Monitor signs of superinfection (perineal itching, diaper rash, fever, malaise, redness, pain, swelling, drainage, rash, diarrhea, sore throat, change in cough or sputum)

• Observe for signs of allergic reaction (wheezing, tightness in chest, urticaria), especially within 20-30 min of first dose

• Monitor bowel pattern; diarrhea may be symptomatic of pseudomembranous colitis

---

✤ Available in Canada.

- Monitor renal function (BUN, creatinine, I&O), hepatic function (ALT, AST, bilirubin), electrolyte levels (particularly K+, Na)
- Monitor for signs of bleeding (ecchymosis, bleeding gums, hematuria, daily stool guaiac); monitor PT and platelet counts
- Evaluate IV site for vein irritation

PATIENT AND FAMILY EDUCATION
Teach/instruct
- To take as directed at prescribed intervals for prescribed length of time
Warn/advise
- To notify care provider of hypersensitivity, side effects, superinfection

STORAGE
- Store powder at room temp
- Reconstituted sol stable at room temp 6 hr, refrigerated 72 hr
- Further dilution extends stability; see package insert

---

tobramycin sulfate
Brand Name(s): Nebcin✤, Tobrex

Classification: Antibiotic (aminoglycoside)

Pregnancy Category: D

AVAILABLE PREPARATIONS
Inj: 10, 40 mg/ml
Ophthal: 0.3% oint, sol

ROUTES AND DOSAGES
Neonates 0-4 wk, <1200 g: IM/IV 2.5 mg/kg/dose q24h
Neonates ≤7 days, 1200-2000 g: IM/IV 2.5 mg/kg/dose q12-18h
Neonates ≤7 days, >2000 g: IM/IV 2.5 mg/kg/dose q12h
Neonates >7 days, 1200-2000 g: IM/IV 2.5 mg/kg/dose q12-18h
Neonates >7 days, >2000 g: IM/IV 2.5 mg/kg/dose q8h
Infants and children <5 yr: IM/IV 2.5 mg/kg/dose q8h
Children >5 yr: IM/IV 1.5-2.5 mg/kg/dose q8h

Adults: 3-6 mg/kg/24 hr divided q8h
Eye Infections
Opthal oint, instill 1 cm strip into conjunctival sac q8-12h (for severe infections, instill q3-4h); ophthal drops, instill 1-2 gtt into conjunctival sac q4h (for severe infections, instill 2 gtt q 30-60 min initially, then reduce to less-frequent intervals)

IV administration
- Recommended concentration: 10 or 40 mg/ml or dilute in appropriate volume of D5W or NS
- Maximum concentration: 40 mg/ml
- IV push rate: Not recommended
- Intermittent infusion: Over 20-30 min using a constant-rate infusion device
- Continuous infusion: Not recommended

MECHANISM AND INDICATIONS
Antibiotic mechanism: Bactericidal; inhibits bacterial protein synthesis by binding directly to the 30S ribosomal subunit
Indications: Effective against many aerobic gram-negative organisms and some aerobic gram-positive organisms including *Pseudomonas aeruginosa, E. coli, Enterobacter, Providencia, Citrobacter, Staphylococcus, Proteus, Klebsiella, Serratia;* used to treat severe systemic infections of CNS, respiratory, GI, urinary tracts, bone, skin, and soft tissue; ophthal used to treat eye infections

PHARMACOKINETICS
Peak: IM 30-60 min; IV 30-45 min after infusion
Distribution: Primarily in extracellular fluid; poor penetration into CSF
Half-life: Neonates <1200 g, 11 hr; neonates >1200 g, 2-9 hr; older infants/children, 2 hr
Metabolism: Not metabolized
Excretion: Urine, bile
Therapeutic level: Peak 4-10 mcg/ml; trough 0.5-2 mcg/ml

CONTRAINDICATIONS AND PRECAUTIONS

- Contraindicated with known hypersensitivity to tobramycin or any other aminoglycoside, renal failure
- Use cautiously with neonates and infant (because of renal immaturity), with impaired renal function, dehydration, 8th cranial nerve impairment, myasthenia gravis, parkinsonism, hypocalcemia, pregnancy, lactation

INTERACTIONS
Drug

- Increased risk of nephrotoxicity, ototoxicity, neurotoxicity with methoxyflurane, polymyxin B, vancomycin, capreomycin, cisplatin, cephalosporins, amphotericin B, other aminoglycosides
- Increased risk of ototoxicity with ethacrynic acid, furosemide, bumetanide, urea, mannitol
- Masked symptoms of ototoxicity with dimenhydrinate and other antiemetic or antivertigo drugs
- Synergistic antimicrobial activity against certain organisms with penicillins
- Increased risk of neuromuscular blockade with general anesthetics or neuromuscular blocking agents (succinylcholine, tubocurarine)
- Inactivated when given with parenteral penicillins (carbenicillin, ticarcillin)

Lab

- Increased LDH, BUN, nonprotein nitrogen, serum creatinine levels
- Increased urinary excretion of casts
- Decreased serum Na

INCOMPATIBILITIES

- Cefamandole, clindamycin, heparin; do not mix in syringe or sol with other drugs

SIDE EFFECTS

CNS: Headache, lethargy, neuromuscular blockage with respiratory depression
EENT: Ototoxicity (tinnitus, vertigo, hearing loss); with ophthal use, burning or stinging on instillation, lid itching or swelling
GI: Diarrhea, nausea, vomiting, increased AST, ALT
GU: Nephrotoxicity (cells or casts in urine, oliguria, proteinuria, decreased CrCl, increased BUN, serum creatinine, and non-protein N levels)
HEME: Anemia, agranulocytopenia
Other: Hypersensitivity reactions (eosinophilia, fever, rash, urticaria, pruritus), bacterial or fungal superinfection

TOXICITY AND OVERDOSE

Clinical signs: Ototoxicity, nephrotoxicity, neuromuscular toxicity
Treatment: Supportive care, hemodialysis or peritoneal dialysis, neuromuscular blockade reversed with Ca salts or anticholinesterases

PATIENT CARE MANAGEMENT
Assessment

- Assess history of hypersensitivity to tobramycin or other aminoglycosides
- Obtain C&S; may begin therapy before obtaining results
- Assess renal function (BUN, creatinine, I&O), baseline wt and hearing tests before beginning therapy

Interventions

- Sol should be colorless or clear to very pale yellow; do not use if it is dark yellow, cloudy, or contains precipitates
- Administer tobramycin at least 1 hr before or after other antibiotics (penicillins, cephalosporins)
- IM injection may be painful; administer deeply into large muscle mass and rotate injection site; do not inject more than 2 g per injection site
- Do not premix IV with other medications; infuse separately, flush line with D_5W or NS
- Use large vein with small-bore needle to reduce local reaction; rotate site q48-72h
- See Chapter 2 regarding ophthal instillation; wash hands before and after application, cleanse crusts or discharge from eye before

application; after instillation, apply gentle pressure to lacrimal sac for 1 minute to minimize systemic absorption; wipe excess medication from eye; do not flush medication from eye
• Maintain age-appropriate fluid intake; keep pt well hydrated to reduce risk of renal toxicity
• Supervise ambulation, other safety measures with vestibular dysfunction
• Obtain drug levels after the third dose (sooner in neonates, pts with rapidly changing renal function); peak levels drawn 30 min after end of 30-min infusion, 1 hr after IM injection; trough levels drawn just before next dose

> **NURSING ALERT**
> Discontinue drug if signs of ototoxicity, nephrotoxicity, hypersensitivity develop
> Do not administer IV push

Evaluation
• Evaluate therapeutic response (decreased symptoms of infection)
• Evaluate renal function (BUN, creatinine, I&O), daily wts, hearing evaluations
• Monitor signs of respiratory distress with IV infusion
• Observe for signs of superinfection (perineal itching, diaper rash, fever, malaise, redness, pain, swelling, drainage, rash, diarrhea, sore throat, change in cough or sputum)
• Evaluate IM site for tissue damage, IV site for vein irritation

PATIENT AND FAMILY TEACHING
Teach/instruct
• To take as directed at prescribed intervals for prescribed length of time
Warn/advise
• To notify care provider of hypersensitivity, side effects, superinfection
• Not to share towels, wash cloths, linens, eye make-up with family

members being treated with ophthal forms

STORAGE
• Store powder, ophthal at room temp
• Reconstituted sol stable refrigerated 96 hr, room temp 24 hr

---

tolazoline
Brand Name(s): Priscoline
Classification: Pulmonary antihypertensive, vasodilator
Pregnancy Category: C

AVAILABLE PREPARATIONS
Inj: 25 mg/ml in 10 ml vials
ROUTES AND DOSAGES
Neonates: IV, initially 1-2 mg/kg over 10 min (via upper body or scalp vein) followed by maintenance infusion of 1-2 mg/kg/hr
IV administration
• Recommended concentration: May dilute as desired in NS, D_5W, $D_{10}W$
• Maximum concentration: May administer undiluted
• IV push rate: 1-2 mg/kg over 10 min
• Continuous infusion rate: 1-2 mg/kg/hr
MECHANISM AND INDICATIONS
Mechanism: Relaxes vascular smooth muscle, causing decreased pulmonary vascular resistance and increased peripheral vasodilatation
Indications: Indicated in treatment of persistent vasoconstriction and hypertension of newborn
PHARMACOKINETICS
Onset of action: Within 30 min
Peak: 30-60 min
Half-life: 3-10 hr
Metabolism: Liver
Excretion: Urine
CONTRAINDICATIONS AND PRECAUTIONS
• Contraindicated with known hy-

persensitivity, with CAD or after CVA
• Use cautiously with peptic ulcer, mitral stenosis

INTERACTIONS
Drug
• Increased effects with alcohol, β-blockers, antihypertensives
Lab
• Increased liver enzymes

INCOMPATIBILITIES
• Ethacrynic acid, hydrocortisone, methyl prednisolone

SIDE EFFECTS
CNS: Headache, dizziness, paresthesias
CV: Orthostatic hypotension
DERM: Flushing, chills, sweating, increased pilomotor activity
GI: Nausea, vomiting, diarrhea, abdominal distention, increased gastric secretions, GI bleeding, gastric perforation
GU: Oliguria, hematuria
HEME: Thrombocytopenia, agranulocytosis, bone marrow suppression

TOXICITY AND OVERDOSE
Clinical signs: Flushing, hypotension, shock
Treatment: Supportive care; administer IV fluids, vasopressors (not epinephrine)

PATIENT CARE MANAGEMENT
Assessment
• Assess history of hypersensitivity to drug
• Assess VS, B/P
• Assess ABGs, electrolytes, AST, ALT, bilirubin, CBC with differential
• Assess ECG
Interventions
• Filter drug when drawing IV, may administer undiluted or dilute with NS, D_5W, $D_{10}W$; use scalp or upper limb veins
• May administer antacid to decrease gastric secretions
Evaluation
• Evaluate therapeutic response (decreased pulmonary hypertension)
• Monitor B/P continuously

• Monitor ABGs, blood pH
• Monitor for GI bleed; test stool and NG aspirate for occult blood

PATIENT AND FAMILY EDUCATION
Teach/instruct
• To report side effects
• Rationale for treatment

STORAGE
• Store at room temp in light-resistant containers

---

tolmetin
Brand Name(s): Tolectin, Tolectin DS, Tolectin 200, Tolectin 600, Tolmentin Sodium

Classification: NSAID, antipyretic

Pregnancy Category: B(D at term)

AVAILABLE PREPARATIONS
Caps: 400 mg
Tabs: 200 mg

ROUTES AND DOSAGES
Antiinflammatory
Children >2 yr: PO 20 mg/kg/24 hr divided tid-qid, then 15-30 mg/kg/24 hr divided tid-qid; maximum 30 mg/kg/24 hr
Adults: PO 400 mg tid; maximum 2 g/24 hr
Analgesic
Children >2 yr: PO 5-7 mg/kg/dose q6-8h
Adults: PO 400 mg tid; maximum 2 g/24 hr

MECHANISM AND INDICATIONS
Mechanism: Inhibits prostaglandin synthesis by decreasing an enzyme needed for biotransfer
Indications: Used in the management of inflammatory disorders, including rheumatoid arthritis, treatment of mild or moderate pain or dysmenorrhea, treatment of fever

PHARMACOKINETICS
Onset of action: Antiinflammatory, within 7 days

Peak: Analgesia 2 hr; antiinflammatory 1-2 wk
Distribution: Unknown
Half-life: 1-3.5 hr
Metabolism: Liver
Excretion: Urine

CONTRAINDICATIONS AND PRECAUTIONS
• Contraindicated with known hypersensitivity (cross sensitivity may exist with other NSAIDs, including aspirin), active GI bleeding or ulcer disease, severe renal or hepatic disease, asthma
• Use cautiously with pregnancy, lactation; bleeding, GI, cardiac disorders; peptic ulcer disease

INTERACTIONS
Drug
• Increased risk of bleeding with oral anticoagulant, cefamandole, cefoperazone, cefofetan, moxalactam, plicamycin
• Increased serum lithium level, increased risk of toxicity
• Increased risk of toxicity from methotrexate
• Increased probenecid blood levels, increased risk of toxicity
• Increased risk of GI side effects with other drugs of similar effects (corticosteroids, aspirin, other NSAIDs)
• Increased risk of adverse renal effects with gold compounds or chronic use of acetaminophen
• Increased action of coumarin, phenytoin, sulfonamides
Lab
• Prolongs bleeding time for up to 2 days after discontinuation
• Increased AST, ALT, alk phos, BUN, K^+
• Decreased Hgb, Hct possible
• False positive urinary protein tests possible
Nutrition
• Food slows in GI tract, but drug does not reduce the extent of absorption

SIDE EFFECTS
CNS: Headache, drowsiness, dizziness, insomnia, confusion, fatigue, tremors, anxiety, mood changes, depression, sleep disturbances
CV: Palpitations, tachycardia, peripheral edema, arrhythmias, hypertension
DERM: Urticaria, pruritus, sweating, rashes, purpura
EENT: Blurred vision, tinnitus, hearing loss
GI: Nausea, dyspepsia, vomiting, constipation, GI bleeding, discomfort, anorexia, diarrhea, jaundice, cholestatic hepatitis, flatulence, cramps, peptic ulcer, GI ulceration and perforation, dry mouth
GU: Renal failure, hematuria, cystitis, nephrotoxicity, oliguria, azotemia, pseudoproteinuria
HEME: Blood dyscrasias, prolonged bleeding time
Other: Muscle weakness

TOXICITY AND OVERDOSE
Clinical signs: Blurred vision, tinnitus, roaring in ears
Treatment: Empty stomach, induce vomiting or gastric lavage; activated charcoal

PATIENT CARE MANAGEMENT
Assessment
• Assess history of hypersensitivity to tolmetin, aspirin, other NSAIDs
• Assess renal function (BUN, creatinine, I&O), liver function (ALT, AST, bilirubin)
• Perform audiometric, ophthal examination
• Assess cardiac status, baseline VS
• Assess history of peptic ulcer, any GI irritation
Interventions
• Take with full glass of water; may mix with food, milk, or antacids to decrease GI irritation; tabs may be crushed, caps opened and mixed with fluids or food
• For rapid initial effect, administer 30 min before or 2 hr after meals
Evaluation
• Evaluate therapeutic response (decreased pain, stiffness in joints, swelling in joints; ability to move more easily)
• Evaluate renal function (BUN, creatinine, I&O), liver function

T

♣ Available in Canada.

(ALT, AST, bilirubin), VS, and cardiac status periodically during therapy
• Evaluate for side effects, hypersensitivity

PATIENT AND FAMILY EDUCATION
Teach/instruct
• To take as directed at prescribed intervals for prescribed length of time
• To take with full glass of water; may mix with food, milk or antacids
• That partial arthritic relief usually occurs within 7 days, but maximum effectiveness may require 1-2 wk of continuous therapy
• That antiinflammatory response may not be seen for up to 1 mo
• To drink 8 glasses of water per day
Warn/advise
• To notify care provider of hypersensitivity, side effects
• To avoid activities that require alertness until response of medication is known
• To avoid concurrent use of alcohol, aspirin, acetaminophen, steroids, other OTC medications without consultation with care provider
Encourage
• Discuss effectiveness of therapy with care provider (pts who do not respond to one NSAID may respond to another)

STORAGE
• Store at room temp

---

trazodone
Brand Name(s): Desyrel, Desyrel Dividose, Trazodone HCL

Classification: Antidepressant

Pregnancy Category: C

AVAILABLE PREPARATIONS
Tabs: 50 mg, 100 mg, 150 mg, 300 mg (generic is available)

DOSAGES AND ROUTES
• Safety and effectiveness in children <18 yr have not been established; dosage represents accepted standard practice recommendations
Children 6-18 yr: PO initial, 1.5-2 mg/kg/24 hr divided bid-tid; increase gradually 3-4 days prn; maximum 6 mg/kg/24 hr divided tid
Adolescents: PO initial, 25-50 mg/24 hr; increase to 100-150 mg/24 hr divided bid-tid
Adults: PO initial, 150 mg/24 hr divided qd-tid; may increase by 50 mg/24 hr q3-7 days; maximum 600 mg/24 hr

MECHANISM AND INDICATIONS
Mechanism: Inhibits reuptake of serotonin; minimal or no effect on reuptake of norepinephrine or dopamine
Indications: For use in treating depression; sometimes used for cocaine withdrawal, panic attacks, agoraphobia, and with other medications to manage aggressive behavior

PHARMACOKINETICS
Onset of action: 2-6 wk
Half-life: 4.4-7.5 hr
Metabolism: Liver
Excretion: Urine, feces

CONTRAINDICATIONS AND PRECAUTIONS
• Contraindicated with hypersensitivity to this medication or any component, to tricyclic antidepressants; recovery phase of MI, prostatic hypertrophy, seizures
• Use cautiously with severe depression, recent heart attack, abnormal heart rhythms, electroshock therapy, narrow-angle glaucoma, hyperthyroidism, increased intraocular pressure, history of suicide attempts, elective surgery, urinary retention

INTERACTIONS
Drug
• Increased effects with alcohol, barbiturates, benzodiazepines, CNS depressants

---

❤ Available in Canada.

• Increased trazodone serum concentration with fluoxetine
• Increased effects of epinephrine
• Decreased effects of clonidine, ephedrine, guanethidine, methyldopa
• Increased serum concentrations of digoxin, phenytoin
• Hyperpyretic crisis with seizures and hypertensive episode within 14 days of MAOI
• Interacts with anesthetics, tricyclic antidepressants, isocarboxazid, narcotics, pargyline, phenelzine, selegiline, tranylcypromine, warfarin

Lab

• Increased serum bilirubin, BG, alk phos
• Falsely elevated urinary catecholamines
• Decreased VMA, 5-HIAA

Nutrition

• Do not drink alcohol

SIDE EFFECTS

CNS: Dizziness, drowsiness, agitation, anger, anxiety, confusion, decreased concentration, disorientation, vivid dreams, excitement, EPS, fatigue, headache, hostility, incoordination, insomnia, lightheadedness, impaired memory, nervousness, nightmares, sedation, seizures, stimulation, tremors, weakness
CV: Orthostatic hypotension, arrhythmias, chest pain, ECG changes, hypertension, palpitations, tachycardia
DERM: Clamminess, hives, itching, photosensitivity, rash, sweating
EENT: Dry mouth, blurred vision, itching eyes, red eyes, bad taste in mouth, mydriasis, nasal or sinus congestion, stomatitis, tinnitus, double vision
GI: Diarrhea, appetite changes, constipation, cramps, hepatitis, jaundice, nausea, paralytic ileus, upset stomach, vomiting
GU: Urinary retention, premature ejaculation, gynecomastia, incontinence of urine, impotence, missed menstrual periods, priapism, acute renal failure, changes in sex drive, blood in urine, delayed urine flow, increased urinary frequency
HEME: Agranulocytosis, abnormal blood counts, eosinophilia, thrombocytopenia, leukopenia
RESP: Dyspnea
Other: Aches and pains, edema, fainting, weight changes

TOXICITY AND OVERDOSE

Clinical signs: Drowsiness, vomiting, priaprism, respiratory arrest, seizures, ECG changes, increased incidence or severity of any side effects
Therapeutic range: 0.5-2.5 mcg/ml (SI 1-6 mcmol/L); potentially toxic at >2.5 mcg/ml (SI >6 mcmol/L); toxic at >4 mcg/ml (SI 10 mcmol/L)
Treatment: Monitor ECG, induce emesis, lavage, administer activated charcoal, anticonvulsant

PATIENT CARE MANAGEMENT

Assessment

• Assess history of hypersensitivity to drug
• Obtain physical exam, medical history (including use of MAOIs within last 14 days)
• Assess ability to function in daily activities, to sleep throughout the night, symptoms of depression
• Assess mental status (mood, sensorium, affect, impulsiveness, suicidal ideation, thoughts)
• Obtain baseline hematologic function (CBC, leukocytes, differential, cardiac enzymes), liver function (AST, ALT, bilirubin), wt
• Obtain baseline ECG

Interventions

• Administering trazodone after meals may decrease lightheadedness and postural hypotension
• Give with food or milk if GI symptoms occur
• Rinse with water, take sips of fluid, sugarless gum, hard candy for dry mouth
• Increase fluids and fiber in diet if constipation occurs
• Give entire dose at hs if oversedation occurs during the day

T

> **NURSING ALERT**
> Do not take within 14 days of administration of MAOIs; may cause a hypertensive crisis, high fever, and seizures

Evaluation
• Evaluate therapeutic response (ability to function in daily activities, to sleep throughout the night, symptoms of depression)
• Evaluate mental status (mood, sensorium, affect, impulsiveness, suicidal ideation, thoughts)
• Monitor hematologic function (CBC, leukocytes, differential, cardiac enzymes) liver function (AST, ALT, bilirubin), wt
• Monitor ECG for flattening of T-wave, bundle branch block, AV block, arrhythmias
• Monitor for orthostatic hypotension; if systolic B/P drops 20 mm Hg hold trazodone and notify prescriber
• Monitor for rigidity, dystonia, akathisia, urinary retention, constipation

PATIENT AND FAMILY EDUCATION
Teach/instruct
• To take as directed at prescribed intervals for prescribed length of time
• To ensure that medication is swallowed
• That medicine sometimes must be taken for 2-3 wk before improvement is noticed
• That medication is most helpful when used as part of a comprehensive multimodal treatment program
• Not to discontinue medication without prescriber approval; if stopped suddenly, withdrawal symptoms include headache, nausea, vomiting, muscle pain, weakness
• To consult with prescriber or pharmacist before taking other OTC and prescription medications
Warn/advise
• To avoid ingesting alcohol, other CNS depressants

• That this medication may cause drowsiness; be careful on bicycles, skates, skateboards, while driving, with other activities requiring alertness
• To stay out of direct sunlight (especially between 10 AM and 3 PM) if possible; if pt must be outside, to wear protective clothing, hat, sunglasses; to put on sun block that has a skin protection factor (SPF) of ≥15
• To report to prescriber episodes of dizziness, lightheadedness, fainting, dry mouth, irregular heartbeat, SOB, nausea, vomiting, blood in urine
• To immediately discontinue trazodone and consult prescriber if prolonged and painful erections occur

STORAGE
• Store at room temp in a tight, light-resistant container

---

tretinoin
Brand Name(s): Retisol-A✦, Retin-A✦, Stieva-A✦, Stieva-A Forte✦, Vitamin A Acid✦, Vitinoin✦
Classification: Antiacne agent
Pregnancy Category: C

AVAILABLE PREPARATIONS
Cream: 0.025%, 0.05%, 0.1%
Gel: 0.01%, 0.025%
Sol: 0.05%

ROUTES AND DOSAGES
Adolescents and adults: Top, apply cream, gel, or sol qd, usually at hs, at least 20 min after washing and drying face; do not apply near eyes, mouth, or mucous membranes

MECHANISM AND INDICATIONS
Anti-acne mechanism: Exact mechanism unknown; it appears to act as a follicular epithelium irritant causing extrusion of come-

---

✦ Available in Canada.

dones and decreased microcomedone formation

Indications: Used for top treatment of acne vulgaris

PHARMACOKINETICS

Absorption: Limited with top application

Excretion: Minimal amount in urine

CONTRAINDICATIONS AND PRECAUTIONS

• Contraindicated with known hypersensitivity to tretinoin or vitamin A

• Use cautiously with eczema; in pts with frequent exposure to sunlight

INTERACTIONS
Drug

• Interaction possible with top medicated preparations, cleansers, soaps, products with high alcohol concentrations; preparations containing sulfur, resorcinol, or salicylic acid

SIDE EFFECTS

DERM: Localized erythema, peeling, blisters, hypopigmentation, hyperpigmentation, contact dermatitis; discontinue use if these occur

TOXICITY AND OVERDOSE

Clinical signs: Localized marked erythema, peeling, discomfort

Treatment: Discontinue drug

PATIENT CARE MANAGEMENT
Assessment

• Assess history of hypersensitivity to drug

• Assess skin for appropriateness of treatment; if skin dry, irritated, do not use this drug for acne treatment; once treatment begun, assess skin for side effects

Interventions

• Apply small amount qd at least 20 min after washing and drying face; do not apply near eyes, mouth, or mucous membranes; if skin irritation warrants, decrease frequency of drug use

• Alterations of drug vehicle (gel is most potent, sol least potent), drug concentration, dose frequency should be made by close monitoring of clinical response

Evaluation

• Evaluate clinical response (decreased acne)

• Monitor skin for side effects; modify vehicle, frequency, concentration of dose per clinical response

PATIENT AND FAMILY EDUCATION
Teach/instruct

• To use as directed at prescribed intervals for prescribed length of time

• To avoid exposure to sun (increases irritation), wear sunscreen (SPF ≥15) when exposure to sun unavoidable

• To apply to clean, dry skin at least 20 min after washing

• That therapeutic effect takes 2-3 wk and that a mild exacerbation of acne may precede therapeutic effect

• To discontinue tretinoin temporarily if severe irritation occurs, readjust dose when irritation subsides

STORAGE

• Store at room temp

T

triamcinolone, triamcinolone diacetate, triamcinolone hexacetonide

Brand Name(s): Aristocort♣, Azmocort♣, Kenacort, Kenalog♣, Kenalog-10 Injection♣, Kenalog-40 Injection♣, Kenalog in Orabase, Kenalone, Ledercort, Nasacort♣, Oracort♣, Triaderm♣, Triam-A Triamcinolone diacetate: Amcort♣, Aristocort♣, Aristocort Forte♣, Artistocort Intralesional♣, Aristocort Parenteral♣, Kenacort, Triamolone, Tristoject Triamcinolone hexacetonide: Aristospan Intraarticular, Aristospan Intralesional

Classification: Antiinflammatory, immunosuppressant

Pregnancy Category: C

AVAILABLE PREPARATIONS
Tabs: 1 mg, 2 mg, 4 mg, 8 mg (triamcinalone)
Syr: 2 mg/ml, 4 mg/ml (triamcinolone)
Triamcinolone Acetonide
Inj: 10 mg/ml (acetonide); 25 mg/ml (diacetate); 5 mg/ml (hexacetonide)
Cream, oint: 0.025%, 0.1%, 0.5%
Lotion: 0.025%, 0.1%
Aerosol (top): 0.015, 0.2 mg/2 second spray
Oral inhal: 100 mcg/metered spray

ROUTES AND DOSAGES
Adrenal Insufficiency
Children: PO 117 mcg/kg/24 hr single or divided dose
Adult: PO 4-12 mg qd single or divided dose

Severe Inflammation or Immunosuppression
Triamcinolone
Children: PO 416 mcg-1.7 mg/kg/24 hr in single or divided doses
Adults: PO 4-60 mg/24 hr in single or divided doses
Triamcinolone acetonide
Children >6 yr: IM 40 mg q 4 wk or 2.5-15 mg intraarticularly prn
Adults: IM 40-80 mg q 4 wk, or 2.5-15 mg intraarticularly prn, or up to 1 mg intralesionally prn
Triamcinolone diacetate
Children >6 yr: IM 40 mg q wk
Adults: IM 40 mg q wk or 3-40 mg intraarticularly, intrasynovially, or intralesionally q 1-8 wk
Triamcinolone hexacetonide
Adults: IM 2-20 mg intraarticularly q 3-4 wk prn
Asthma
Children: Inhal, acetonide, 1-2 inhalations tid-qid, maximum 12 inhalations/24 hr
Adults: Inhal, acetonide, 2 inhalations tid-qid, maximum 16 inhalations/24 hr
Topical Antiinflammatory
Triamcinolone
Children: Top, acetonide, 0.025% cream, lotion, oint, or 0.015% aerosol spray qd-bid; 0.1%-0.5% oint, cream, lotion qd
Adults: Top, acetonide, apply cream, lotion, oint bid-qid

MECHANISM AND INDICATIONS
Mechanism: Decreases inflammation by reducing migration of PMN leukocytes and reversal of increased capillary permeability; suppresses immune system by decreasing activity of lymphatic system
Indications: For use in severe inflammation, immunosuppression, neoplasm, asthma; collagen, respiratory, and dermatologic disorders

PHARMACOKINETICS
Peak: 1-2 hr
Half-life: 18-36 hr
Absorption: Readily absorbed PO, IM, inhal
Metabolism: Liver
Excretion: Urine

♣ Available in Canada.

CONTRAINDICATIONS AND PRECAUTIONS
• Contraindicated with known hypersensitivity to adrenocorticoid preparations, fungal infections AIDS, TB, psychosis, ITP; with live virus vaccines
• Use cautiously with DM, glaucoma, osteoporosis, CHF, ulcerative colitis, esophagitis, peptic ulcer, renal disease, pregnancy, lactation

INTERACTIONS
Drug
• Decreased action with colestipol, cholestyramine, barbiturates, rifampin, phenytoin, theophylline
• Decreased effects of anticoagulants, anticonvulsants, antidiabetic agents, vaccines, salicylates, isoniazid
• Increased side effects with alcohol, salicylates, indomethacin, amphotericin B, digitalis, cyclosporin, diuretics
• Increased action with salicylates, estrogens, indomethacin, oral contraceptive pills, ketoconazole, macrolide antibiotics
Lab
• Suppressed skin test response
• Decreased iodine uptake and protein-bound iodine in thyroid function tests
• Increased glucose and cholesterol possible
• Decreased serum K^+, Ca, thyroxine possible

SIDE EFFECTS
CNS: Fatigue, depression, flushing, sweating, headache, mood changes
CV: Facial edema, hypertension, thrombophlebitis, embolism, tachycardia
DERM: Pruritus, hypertrichosis, skin atrophy, hyper- and hypopigmentation, acne
EENT: Increased intraocular pressure, blurred vision, cataracts, fungal infections
GI: Oral candidiasis, diarrhea, nausea, increased appetite, peptic ulcer, pancreatitis
HEME: Thrombocytopenia
MS: Osteoporosis, fractures

RESP: Wheezing, cough

TOXICITY AND OVERDOSE
Clinical signs: Acute ingestion is rarely a clinical problem; chronic use causes suppression of the hypothalmic-pituitary-adrenal axis, cushingoid appearance, muscle weakness, osteoporosis
Treatment: Decrease drug (gradually if possible); sudden withdrawal may exacerbate underlying disease or may be fatal; chronic use in children may delay growth, maturation

PATIENT CARE MANAGEMENT
Assessment
• Assess for hyperglycemia, hypokalemia
• Assess wt qd; B/P, HR q4h
• Assess I&O, looking for decreased urinary output, increased fluid retention (edema)
• Assess baseline behavior
• Assess during time of physiologic stress; additional dose may be required
Interventions
• Administer PO with food or milk
• Rinse mouth and throat after inhalation
• Administer IM deep in muscle mass; rotate sites; avoid SC administration
• Avoid top administration on face

> **NURSING ALERT**
> In children, limit top application to smallest effective amount
>
> Do not abruptly decrease or withdraw drug

Evaluation
• Evaluate therapeutic response (decreased inflammatory response)
• Evaluate for signs and symptoms of infection
• Evaluate for K^+ depletion, Ca depletion
• Evaluate for edema, hypertension
• Evaluate mental status changes

• Evaluate need for continued therapy; withdraw drug very gradually

PATIENT/FAMILY EDUCATION
Teach/instruct
• To take as directed at prescribed intervals for prescribed length of time
• Not to decrease or discontinue abruptly
• About top and inhal administration
• About side effects; to call care provider if noted
• To wear medical alert identification
• To avoid OTC products unless directed by care provider
• To report sudden wt gain to care provider
• To have regular ophthal exams with long term therapy

STORAGE
• Store at room temp

---

triethanolamine polypeptide oleate

Brand Name(s): Cerumenex

Classification: Surfactant, earwax emulsifier

Pregnancy Category: C

AVAILABLE PREPARATIONS
Otic sol: 100 mg/ml

ROUTES AND DOSAGES
Children and adults: Top, tilt pt's head 45°; fill external ear canal with sol; plug with cotton; allow to remain 15-30 min; flush with warm water using bulb syringe; may repeat

MECHANISM AND INDICATIONS
Mechanism: Emulsifies and disperses impacted cerumen
Indication: Removal of impacted cerumen

PHARMACOKINETICS
Onset of action: 15-30 min
Absorption: Negligible

Excretion: Flushed out of canal with warm water

CONTRAINDICATIONS AND PRECAUTIONS
• Contraindicated with perforated tympanic membrane, known hypersensitivity to drug
• Use cautiously with otitis externa, top allergy history; avoid contact with skin, limit exposure of ear canal to 30 min maximum

INTERACTIONS
Drug
• None identified
Lab
• None identified

SIDE EFFECTS
Local: Erythema, pruritus, eczematoid reaction, contact dermatitis, skin ulcers, rash

TOXICITY AND OVERDOSE
Clinical signs: Not significant
Treatment: Discontinue drug; flush ear canal with warm water

PATIENT CARE MANAGEMENT
Assessment
• Assess for presence of cerumen in ear canal (otoscopy)
Interventions
• Tilt head 45°, fill ear canal with drug, plug with cotton for 15-30 min, gently flush with warm water with bulb syringe; may repeat if necessary
Evaluation
• Repeat otoscopy, evaluate for presence of cerumen

PATIENT AND FAMILY EDUCATION
Teach/instruct
• To use as directed at prescribed intervals for prescribed length of time
• About how to administer
• About local side effects; discontinue drug, flush with water, call care provider

STORAGE
• Store at room temp

---

triethylenethiophosphoramide

Brand Name(s): Thiotepa, Tespa
Classification: Alkylating Agent
Pregnancy Category: D

AVAILABLE PREPARATIONS
Inj: 15 mg vials

ROUTES AND DOSAGES
• Drug may vary in response to diagnosis, extent of disease, concurrent or previous therapy, protocol guidelines, physiologic parameters; consult current literature, protocol recommendations

Breast, Lung, Ovarian Cancer; Hodgkins Disease, Non-Hodgkins Lymphoma
Children and adults: IV 6 mg/m^2 (0.2-0.4 mg/kg) qd × 5 days, repeat q1-4 wk; 30-60 mg q wk depending on WBC (IV, IM, SC)

Bladder Cancer
Intrabladder 60 mg in 60 ml SW q wk for 3-4 wk, instill over 2 hr

Neoplastic Effusions
Intracavity or intratumor 0.6-0.8 mg/kg q wk

IV administration
• Recommended concentration: Reconstitute 15 mg vial with 1.5 ml SW, resulting concentration 10 mg/ml; may be further diluted with D$_5$NS, D$_5$W, LR if needed; drug is non-vesicant
• IV push rate: May be administered rapidly
• Sol may be clear to slightly opaque

MECHANISM AND INDICATIONS
Mechanism: Cell-cycle phase nonspecific; mimics a radiation-induced injury; works by selectively reacting with DNA phosphate groups to produce chromosome cross-linkage by blocking of nucleoprotein synthesis; acts as a polyfunctional alkylating agent
Indications: Used to treat Hodgkin's disease, leukemia, non-Hodgkin's lymphoma, retinoblastoma, breast cancer, ovarian cancer, bladder cancer, lung cancer

PHARMACOKINETICS
Absorption: Incompletely absorbed from GI tract; variable absorption through serous membrane; absorption through bladder mucosa 10%-100% depending upon amount instilled, extent of tumor infiltration, or mucosal inflammation (related to endoscopic surgery or radiation therapy)
Excretion: 60% in urine within 24-72 hr

CONTRAINDICATIONS AND PRECAUTIONS
• Contraindicated with known hypersensitivity, severe bone marrow, hepatic, or renal dysfunction, pregnancy, lactation
• Use cautiously with mild bone marrow suppression, renal or hepatic dysfunction

INTERACTIONS
Drug
• Increased risk of bleeding with aspirin, anticoagulants
• Increased risk of leukopenia, thrombocytopenia, anemia (bone marrow suppression) with other chemotherapeutic drugs of same mechanism (nitrogen mustard, cytoxan)
• Increased risk of toxicity if combined with radiation therapy
• Avoid drugs known to produce bone marrow depression (co-trimoxazole)
Lab
• Irreversible bone marrow suppression possible (leukopenia, thrombocytopenia, anemia)

INCOMPATIBILITIES
• Unstable in acid medium

SIDE EFFECTS
CNS: Headache, dizziness
DERM: Alopecia, hives, rash
GI: Nausea, vomiting, anorexia
GU: Amenorrhea, decreased spermatogenesis
HEME: Thrombocytopenia, neutropenia, anemia, leukopenia (begins within 5-30 days)
Other: Fever, tightness in throat,

hyperuricemia, intense pain at administration site

TOXICITY AND OVERDOSE

Clinical signs: WBC <3000 or platelets <150,000; intrathecal doses have been associated with lower extremity weakness, pain, demyelination of spinal cord in some pts

Treatment: Stop drug until WBC and platelets recover; transfuse prn

PATIENT CARE MANAGEMENT
Assessment

• Assess history of hypersensitivity to thiotepa
• Assess baseline VS, pulmonary function tests, CBC, serum electrolytes, liver function (ALT, AST, bilirubin, alk phos) before each course
• Assess sexual patterns and function before chemotherapy
• Assess baseline neurologic and mental status before administration
• Assess success of previous antiemetic therapy
• Assess history of previous treatment with special attention to other therapies that may predispose pt to neurologic, pulmonary, renal, hepatic, impairment, bone marrow depression

Interventions

• Premedicate with antiemetics; continue periodically if needed
• Do not use if sol is cloudy
• Encourage small, frequent feedings of cool, bland foods pt likes

---

NURSING ALERT

Hematologic status must be monitored closely because of effects on bone marrow (myelosuppression)

Pt should not receive any aspirin or medications containing aspirin because of increased risk of bleeding

Sol must be clear; do not use ~~t~~ is cloudy or contains a ~~....~~bitate

---

Evaluation

• Evaluate therapeutic response (decreased tumor size, spread of malignancy)
• Evaluate CBC, serum electrolytes, renal function (BUN, creatinine), liver function (ALT, AST, bilirubin, alk phos), neurologic or mental status at given intervals after chemotherapy
• Evaluate signs or symptoms of allergic reaction during administration
• Evaluate for side effects, response to antiemetic regimen
• Evaluate for signs or symptoms of infection (fever, sore throat, fatigue), bleeding (easy bruising, nosebleeds, bleeding gums)

PATIENT AND FAMILY EDUCATION
Teach/instruct

• To have pt well-hydrated before and after chemotherapy
• About importance of follow-up to monitor blood counts, serum chemistry values, drug blood values
• To take accurate temp; rectal temp contraindicated
• To notify care provider of signs of bleeding (bruising, epistaxis, bleeding gums), infection (fever, sore throat, fatigue)

Warn/advise

• About impact of body changes that may occur (hair loss, hyperpigmentation, nail ridging), how to minimize changes (wigs, caps, scarves, long sleeves)
• To avoid OTC products containing aspirin
• To report any alterations in behavior, sensation, perception; help to develop a plan of care to manage side effects, stress of illness and treatment
• To monitor bowel function and call if abdominal pain or constipation are noted
• To immediately report any pain or discoloration at injection site (parenteral forms)
• That good oral hygiene with very soft toothbrush is imperative
• That dental work be delayed

Canada.

until blood counts return to baseline, with permission of the care provider
- To avoid contact with known viral or bacterial illnesses
- That household contacts of child not be immunized with live polio virus; inactivated form should be used
- That child not receive immunizations until immune system recovers sufficiently to mount needed antibody response
- To report exposure to chicken pox in susceptible child immediately
- To report reactivation of herpes zoster virus (shingles) immediately
- If appropriate, ways to preserve reproductive patterns, sexuality (sperm banking, contraceptives)

Encourage
- Provision of nutritional food intake; consider nutrition consultation
- To comply with bowel management program
- To use top anesthetics to control discomfort of mucositis; avoid spicy foods, commercial mouthwashes

Storage
- Refrigerate vial until use
- Protect from light
- Reconstituted sol stable refrigerated 5 days

---

trifluoperazine, trifluoperazine hydrochloride

Brand Name(s): Apo-Trifluoperazine♣, Stelazine♣, Terfluzine, Trifluoperazine HCL, Triflurin

Classification: Phenothiazine, antipsychotic, neuroleptic

Pregnancy Category: C

AVAILABLE PREPARATIONS
Tabs: 1 mg, 2 mg, 5 mg, 10 mg, 20 mg
Tabs ext-rel: 1 mg, 2 mg, 5 mg, 10 mg
Concentrate: 10 mg/ml
Inj: 2 mg/ml

DOSAGES AND ROUTES
- Do not use in children under six years old
- IM not recommended for children, but 1 mg may be given qd or bid
Adults: IM 1-2 mg q4-6h
Children >6 yr: PO 1 mg qd or bid
For Psychosis
Adult: PO, initially 2-5 mg bid; usual range 15-20 mg; may require 40 mg/24 hr or more
For Nonpsychotic Anxiety
Adult: PO, initially 1-2 mg bid; maximum 5 mg/24 hr; do not administer for >12 wks

MECHANISM AND INDICATIONS
Mechanism: Blocks neurotransmission produced by dopamine at synapse, depresses the cerebral cortex, hypothalamus, and limbic system
Indications: For use in treating psychotic disorders, schizophrenia, non-psychotic anxiety

PHARMACOKINETICS
Onset of action: PO rapid; IM immediate
Peak: PO 2-3 hr; IM 1 hr
Duration: PO 12 hr; IM 12 hr
Metabolism: Liver
Excretion: Urine

CONTRAINDICATIONS AND PRECAUTIONS
- Contraindicated with hypersensitivity to this medication or any component, blood dyscrasias, cardiovascular disease, coma, glaucoma, severe liver disease
- Use cautiously with breast cancer, DM, respiratory insufficiency, prostatic hypertrophy, seizures, pregnancy, lactation

INTERACTIONS
Drug
- Increased sedation with alcohol, barbiturate anesthetics, CNS depressants
- Toxicity with epinephrine
- Decreased absorption with alu-

T

♣ Available in Canada.

minum hydroxide or magnesium hydroxide antacids
• Decreased effects of lithium, levodopa
• Increased effects of alcohol, β-adrenergic blockers
• Increased anticholinergic effects with anticholinergics

Lab
• Increased liver function tests, cardiac enzymes, cholesterol, BG, prolactin, bilirubin, PBI, cholinesterase, ^{131}I
• Decreased blood and urine hormones
• False positive PKU, pregnancy test
• False negative urinary steroids, 17-OHCS, pregnancy test

Nutrition
• Stelazine concentrate contains sulfites; individuals sensitive to sulfites should not take concentrate
• Do not drink alcohol

SIDE EFFECTS
CNS: Akathisia, dystonia, headache, pseudoparkinsonism, seizures, tardive dyskinesia
CV: Cardiac arrest, ECG changes, hypertension, orthostatic hypotension, tachycardia
DERM: Dermatitis, photosensitivity, rash
EENT: Dry eyes, dry mouth, glaucoma, blurred vision
GI: Anorexia, constipation, diarrhea, jaundice, nausea, vomiting, wt gain
GU: Amenorrhea, enuresis, gynecomastia, impotence, urinary frequency, urinary retention
HEME: Agranulocytosis, anemia, leukocytosis, leukopenia
RESP: Dyspnea, respiratory depression, laryngospasm

TOXICITY AND OVERDOSE
Clinical signs: CNS depression (deep, unarousable sleep, possible coma), hypotension or hypertension, EPS, abnormal involuntary movements, agitation, seizures, arrhythmias, ECG changes, hypothermia or hyperthermia, autonomic nervous system dysfunction
Treatment: Provide an airway; if orally ingested, lavage; do not induce vomiting

PATIENT CARE MANAGEMENT
Assessment
• Assess history of hypersensitivity to drug
• Assess ability to function in daily activities, to sleep throughout the night
• Assess mental status (mood, sensorium, affect, impulsiveness, suicidal ideation, thoughts)
• Obtain medical history, baseline physical examination
• Obtain baseline CBC, liver function studies (AST, ALT, bilirubin), UA

Interventions
• Make sure oral medication is swallowed
• Concentrate is for institutional use only; use when oral medication is preferred and other oral forms are impractical; add dose to ≥2 oz of tomato or fruit juice, milk, simple syrup, orange syrup, carbonated beverages, coffee, tea, water, semisolid foods (like soup or puddings) before use
• Pt should remain lying down for at least 30 min after IM administration
• Minimize environmental stimulation by dimming lights, avoiding loud noises
• Obtain order for antiparkinsonian agent if EPS occur
• Rinse with H_2O, take sips of fluid, sugarless gum, hard candy for dry mouth
• Increase fluids and fiber in diet if constipation occurs

NURSING ALERT
A possible side effect is neuroleptic malignant syndrome; obtain medical intervention immediately; monitor VS, ECG, urine output, renal function; symptom management with medications, hydration, cooling blankets

Monitor for dystonic reactions and tardive dyskinesia

✚ Available in Canada.

Evalution
- Evaluate therapeutic response (psychosis, ability to function in daily activities, to sleep throughout the night)
- Monitor for signs of neuroleptic malignant syndrome; symptoms include fever, fast or irregular heartbeat, fast breathing, sweating, weakness, muscle stiffness, seizures, loss of bladder control; if these occur, obtain medical intervention immediately; monitor VS, ECG, urine output, renal function; symptom management with medications, hydration, cooling blankets
- Evaluate mental status (mood, sensorium, affect, impulsiveness, suicidal ideation, hallucinations, delusions, paranoia, thoughts)
- Monitor for akathisia, tardive dyskinesia, pseudoparkinsonism, constipation, urinary retention
- Monitor skin turgor, reflexes, gait, coordination
- Monitor orthostatic hypotension; report drops of 30 mm Hg to prescriber
- Monitor CBC, liver function studies (AST, ALT, bilirubin), UA monthly
- Monitor for sore throat, malaise, fever, bleeding, mouth sores; if these occur, draw CBC and discontinue trifluoperazine

PATIENT AND FAMILY EDUCATION
Teach/instruct
- To take as directed at prescribed intervals for prescribed length of time
- To ensure that medication is swallowed
- That medicine sometimes must be taken for 3-4 wk before improvement is noticed
- That medication is most helpful when used as part of a comprehensive multimodal treatment program
- Not to discontinue medication without prescriber approval
- Not to discontinue medication quickly after long-term use
- To consult with prescriber or pharmacist before taking other OTC and prescription medications
- To report sore throat, bleeding, fever, mouth sores to prescriber
- Not to take aluminum hydroxide or magnesium hydroxide antacids
Warn/advise
- To avoid ingesting alcohol, other CNS depressants
- That medication may cause drowsiness; be careful on bicycles, skates, skateboards, while driving, with other activities requiring alertness
- To stay out of direct sunlight (especially between 10 AM and 3 PM) if possible; if pt must be outside, to wear protective clothing, hat, sunglasses; put on sun block that has a skin protection factor (SPF) ≥15
- To use caution when exposed to heat; drug may impair body's adaptation to hot environments, increasing the risk of heat stroke; avoid saunas, hot tubs, hot baths
Storage
- Store in tight, light-resistant container
- Oral sol should be stored in amber bottle
- Slight yellowing of inj or concentrate is common, does not affect potency

---

triflupromazine, triflupromazine hydrochloride

Brand Name(s): Vesprin

Classification: Phenothiazine, antipsychotic, neuroleptic

Pregnancy Category: C

AVAILABLE PREPARATIONS
Tabs: 10 mg, 25 mg
Inj: 10 mg/ml, 20 mg/ml

DOSAGES AND ROUTES
- Do not use with children <2½ years old
Psychosis
Children >2½ yr: PO 0.5-2 mg/kg/24 hr divided tid, may increase

T

to 10 mg if needed; IM 0.2-0.25 mg/kg, maximum 10 mg/24 hr
Adults: PO 10-50 mg bid-tid (depending on severity of condition), increase gradually; IM 60 mg, maximum 150 mg/24 hr

Nausea and Vomiting
Children >2½ yr: IM 0.2-0.25 mg/kg/dose, maximum 10 mg/24 hr
Adults: IM 5-15 mg, maximum 60 mg/24 hr; IV 1 mg, maximum 3 mg/24 hr

Acute Agitation
Children >2½ yr: IM 0.2-0.25 mg/kg/24 hr in divided doses, maximum 10 mg/24 hr
Adults: IM 60-150 mg/24 hr divided tid

IV administration
• Recommended concentration: Dilute IV 10 mg/9 ml of NS
• IV push rate: Administer IV ≤1 mg over 2 min

MECHANISM AND INDICATIONS
Mechanism: Blocks neurotransmission produced by dopamine at synapse, depresses cerebral cortex, hypothalamus, limbic system
Indications: For use in treating psychosis, schizophrenia, acute agitation, nausea, vomiting

PHARMACOKINETICS
Onset of action: PO erratic; IM 15-30 min
Peak: PO 2-4 hr; IM 15-20 min
Duration: PO 4-6 hr; IM 4-6 hr
Metabolism: Liver
Excretion: Urine, feces

CONTRAINDICATIONS AND PRECAUTIONS
• Contraindicated with hypersensitivity to this medication or any component, blood dyscrasias, bone marrow, depression, brain damage, coma
• Use cautiously with cardiac disease, liver disease, seizures, pregnancy, lactation

INTERACTIONS
Drug
• Increased sedation with alcohol, barbiturate anesthetics, other CNS depressants

• Toxicity with epinephrine
• Decreased absorption with aluminum hydroxide or magnesium hydroxide antacids
• Decreased effects of lithium, levodopa
• Increased effects of alcohol, β-adrenergic blockers
• Increased anticholinergic effects with anticholinergics
Lab
• Increased bilirubin, cardiac enzymes, cholesterol, cholinesterase, BG, ^{131}I, liver function tests, prolactin, PBI
• False positive pregnancy tests, PKU
• False negative urinary steroids, pregnancy tests
Nutrition
• Do not drink alcohol.

SIDE EFFECTS
CNS: Akathisia, drowsiness, dystonia, headache, pseudoparkinsonism, seizures, tardive dyskinesia
CV: Cardiac arrest, ECG changes, hypertension, orthostatic hypotension, tachycardia
DERM: Dermatitis, photosensitivity, rash
EENT: Glaucoma, blurred vision
GI: Anorexia, constipation, diarrhea, jaundice, dry mouth, nausea, vomiting, wt gain
GU: Amenorrhea, enuresis, gynecomastia, impotence, urinary frequency, urinary retention
HEME: Agranulocytosis, anemia, leukocytosis, leukopenia
RESP: Dyspnea, laryngospasm, respiratory depression

TOXICITY AND OVERDOSE
Clinical signs: CNS depression (deep, unarousable sleep, possible coma), hypotension or hypertension, EPS, abnormal involuntary muscle movements, agitation, seizures, arrhythmias, ECG changes, hypothermia or hyperthermia, autonomic nervous system dysfunction
Treatment: Provide an airway; if orally ingested, lavage; do not induce vomiting

---

✚ Available in Canada.

PATIENT CARE MANAGEMENT
Assessment
- Assess history of hypersensitivity to drug
- Obtain medical history and baseline physical assessment (including orthostatic B/P)
- Assess symptoms of psychosis, ability to function in daily activities, to sleep throughout night
- Assess mental status (mood, sensorium, affect, impulsiveness, suicidal ideation, thoughts)
- Obtain baseline CBC, liver function (ALT, AST, bilirubin), UA

Interventions
- Ensure that PO medication is swallowed
- Avoid skin contact with IM medication
- Administer IM injection into large muscle mass
- Pt should lie down for 30 min after IM injection
- Decrease environmental stimulation by dimming lights and avoiding loud noises
- Rinse with water, take sips of fluid, sugarless gum, hard candy for dry mouth
- Increase fluids and fiber in diet if constipation occurs
- Obtain order for antiparkinsonian agent if EPS occurs

> **NURSING ALERT**
> A possible side effect is neuroleptic malignant syndrome; if this occurs, obtain medical intervention immediately
>
> Monitor for dystonic reactions and tardive dyskinesia

Evaluation
- Evaluate therapeutic response (psychosis, ability to function in daily activities, to sleep throughout the night)
- Evaluate mental status (mood, sensorium, affect, impulsiveness, suicidal ideation, thoughts, hallucinations, delusions, paranoia)
- Monitor orthostatic B/P; report drops of 30 mm Hg to prescriber

- Monitor CBC, liver function (ALT, AST, bilirubin), UA monthly
- Monitor for symptoms of tardive dyskinesia
- Monitor for signs of neuroleptic malignant syndrome; symptoms include fever, fast or irregular heartbeat, fast breathing, sweating, weakness, muscle stiffness, seizures, loss of bladder control; if these occur, obtain medical intervention immediately; monitor VS, ECG, urine output, renal function; symptom management with medications, hydration, cooling blankets
- Monitor for urinary retention and constipation
- Monitor for sore throat, malaise, fever, bleeding, mouth sores; if present, draw CBC and discontinue triflupromazine

PATIENT AND FAMILY EDUCATION
Teach/instruct
- To take as directed at prescribed intervals for prescribed length of time
- To make sure medication is swallowed
- That this medication is most helpful when used as part of a comprehensive multimodal treatment program
- Not to discontinue medication without prescriber approval

Warn/advise
- That medication may cause drowsiness; be careful on bicycles, skates, skateboards, while driving, with other activities requiring alertness
- To stay out of direct sunlight (especially between 10 AM and 3 PM) if possible; if pt must be outside, to wear protective clothing, hat, sunglasses; to put on sun block that has a skin protection factor (SPF) ≥15
- To avoid ingesting alcohol, other CNS depressants
- To immediately report signs of neuroleptic malignant syndrome to prescriber (altered mental status, muscle rigidity, hyperthermia)

T

• To report sore throat, malaise, fever, bleeding, mouth sores to prescriber

Storage

• Store in a tight, light-resistant container

---

trifluridine

Brand Name(s): Viroptic✤

Classification: Antiviral (pyrimidine nucleoside)

Pregnancy Category: C

AVAILABLE PREPARATIONS

Ophthal sol: 1%

ROUTES AND DOSAGES

Children and adults: Instill 1 gtt into affected eye q2h while awake (maximum 9 gtt/24 hr) until reephithelialization of cornea occurs; then 1 gtt q4h for 7 days; do not use longer than 21 days

MECHANISM AND INDICATIONS

Antiviral mechanism: Inhibits viral DNA synthesis and replication

Indications: Used to treat primary keratoconjunctivitis and recurrent epithelial keratitis caused by herpes simplex virus types I and II

PHARMACOKINETICS

Onset of action: Response to treatment within 2-7 days; complete epithelial healing in 1-2 wk

CONTRAINDICATIONS AND PRECAUTIONS

• Contraindicated with known hypersensitivity to trifluridine

• Use cautiously with known antibiotic hypersensitivity, pregnancy

SIDE EFFECTS

EENT: Burning, stinging, mild edema of eyelid or cornea, photophobia, increased intraocular pressure

TOXICITY AND OVERDOSE

Clinical signs: No effects likely from oral ingestion

PATIENT CARE MANAGEMENT

Assessment

• Assess history of hypersensitivity to trifluridine

• Obtain C&S; may begin therapy before obtaining results

• Assess eye for redness, swelling, discharge

Interventions

• See Chapter 2 regarding ophthal instillation; wash hands before and after application, cleanse crusts or discharge from eye before application; after instillation, apply gentle pressure to lacrimal sac for 1 min to minimize systemic absorption; wipe excess medication from eye, do not flush medication from eye

> **NURSING ALERT**
> Store in refrigerator; storage at room temp may result in ocular discomfort with instillation or decreased potency

Evaluation

• Evaluate therapeutic response (decreased redness, inflammation, tearing, photophobia)

• Monitor for signs of allergic reaction (itching, excessive tearing, redness, swelling)

PATIENT AND FAMILY EDUCATION

Teach/instruct

• To take as directed at prescribed intervals for prescribed length of time

Warn/advise

• To notify care provider of hypersensitivity, side effects

• Not to share towels, washcloths, bed linens, eye makeup with family members being treated

Storage

• Store in refrigerator

✤ Available in Canada.

trimethadione

Brand Name(s): Tridione

Classification: Anticonvulsant; oxazolidinedione derivative

Pregnancy Category: D

AVAILABLE PREPARATIONS
Caps: 150 mg (chewable); 300 mg
Sol: 40 mg/ml

ROUTES AND DOSAGES
Children: PO 20-50 mg/kg/24 hr, divided q6-8h; usual maintenance dose 40 mg/kg/24 hr or 1 g/m²/24 hr divided tid or qid; do not exceed 900 mg/24 hr
Adults: PO, initial 300 mg tid; may increase by 300 mg/24 hr at weekly intervals, up to 600 mg qid

MECHANISM AND INDICATIONS
Mechanism: The exact mechanism of action is not known; however trimethadione elevates the cortical and basal seizure thresholds and reduces the synaptic response to low-frequency impulses
Indications: Considered the prototype for agents useful in the treatment of absence seizures; effective in reducing the spike and wave pattern characteristic of absence seizures; not effective in suppressing tonic–clonic seizures characterized by maximum electroshock seizure patterns

PHARMACOKINETICS
Peak: 30-120 min
Half-life: Parent drug 12-24 hr; dimethadione 6-13 days; with chronic administration the metabolite accumulates and is largely responsible for the anticonvulsant effects
Metabolism: Liver
Excretion: Urine (3% as unchanged drug)

CONTRAINDICATIONS AND PRECAUTIONS
• Contraindicated with known hypersensitivity to oxazolidinedione derivatives, hepatic and renal dysfunction, pregnancy

• Used cautiously with severe blood dyscrasias, acute intermittent diseases of the retina or optic nerves

INTERACTIONS
Drug
• Toxicity possible with mephytoin, phenacemide

SIDE EFFECTS
CNS: Drowsiness, fatigue, malaise, irritability, insomnia, dizziness, headache, paresthesias
CV: Hypertension, hypotension
DERM: Acneiform and morbilliform rash, exfoliative dermatitis, erythema multiforme, petechiae, alopecia
EENT: Diplopia, photophobia, hemeralopia, retinal hemorrhage, epistaxis
GI: Nausea, vomiting, anorexia, abdominal pain, bleeding gums
GU: Nephrosis, albuminuria, vaginal bleeding
Other: Lymphadenopathy

TOXICITY AND OVERDOSE
Clinical signs: Nausea, drowsiness, ataxia, visual disturbances; coma may follow a massive overdose
Treatment: Supportive, symptomatic care; monitor vs, I&O, intake and output electrolytes (Na, K⁺); support ventilation and pulmonary function prn; use vasopressors and IV fluids to support cardiac function and circulation; if ingestion was recent, induce emesis with ipecac in conscious pt who has intact gag reflex; if emesis contraindicated, gastric lavage with a cuffed endotracheal tube to prevent aspiration; follow with charcoal or saline cathartic; alkalinization of urine may hasten renal excretion

PATIENT CARE MANAGEMENT
Assessment
• Assess history of hypersensitivity to oxazolidinedione derivatives
• Assess for preexisting conditions that would contraindicate using trimethadione (hepatic and renal dysfunction, pregnancy)

T

✤ Available in Canada.

- Assess baseline laboratory studies, including CBC, differential and liver function (ALT, AST, bilirubin, alk phos)
- Assess seizure type and determine appropriate anticonvulsant for this type of seizure; trimethadione has only been shown to be effective in absence seizures

Interventions
- May administer with food or milk if GI upset occurs
- Initiate drug at modest dosage
- Increase the dosage and level prn to control seizures, to the point of intolerable side effects

Evaluation
- Evaluate therapeutic response (control of absence seizures)
- Evaluate neurologic status to monitor for alterations or deterioration
- Evaluate for signs and symptoms of toxicity

PATIENT AND FAMILY EDUCATION
Teach/instruct
- To take as prescribed; not to change dosage independently or withdraw the drug suddenly
- Explain process for initiating anticonvulsant drugs and need for frequent visits (especially initially)
- Encourage to take drug with food or milk if GI upset occurs

Warn/advise
- About potential side effects; encourage to report serious side effects immediately (rash, skin lesions, scotomata, joint pain, fever, sore throat, unusual bleeding or bruising)
- About additive effects when combining with CNS depressants (alcohol, antihistamines)
- That drug may cause sensitivity to bright light; sunscreens, protective clothing, sunglasses may be helpful
- That unpleasant side effects may decrease as pt becomes more used to the drug, particularly GI effects
- That drug initially may be more sedating until the pt becomes used to it; avoid hazardous tasks (bike, skates, skateboard) that require mental alertness until stabilized on the drug
- To make other health care providers aware of medications in order to avoid drug interactions
- That pregnancy should be avoided while taking this drug (has been found to be teratogenic); inform care provider immediately if pregnancy should occur while taking the drug

Encourage
- To keep a record of any seizures (seizure calendar); this will help with determining effectiveness of the drug

STORAGE
- Store at room temp

---

trimethobenzamide hydrochloride

Brand Name(s): Arrestin, Benzacot, Tegamide, T-Gen, Ticon, Tigan, Tiject-20, Triban, Tribenzagan

Classification: Antiemetic

Pregnancy Category: C

AVAILABLE PREPARATIONS
Caps: 100 mg, 250 mg
Rectal supp: 100 mg, 200 mg
Inj: 100 mg/ml

ROUTES AND DOSAGES
- PR route contraindicated in neonates and premature infants
- IM route not recommended for use in infants and children

Infants and children <15 kg: PO 15 mg/kg/24 hr divided tid-qid prn; PR 100 mg tid-qid prn
Children 15-45 kg: PO/PR 100-200 mg tid-qid prn
Adults: PO 250 mg tid-qid prn; PR/IM 200 mg tid-qid prn

MECHANISM AND INDICATIONS
Mechanism: Thought to inhibit the medullary chemoreceptor trigger zone; structurally related to etha-

nolamine antihistamines, has only a weak antihistaminic activity
Indications: Prophylaxis and treatment of nausea and vomiting; not recommended for treatment of uncomplicated vomiting in children

PHARMACOKINETICS
Onset of action: PO 10-40 min; IM 15-35 min
Duration: 3-4 hr
Metabolism: Liver
Excretion: Urine, bile

CONTRAINDICATIONS AND PRECAUTIONS
• Contraindicated with sensitivity to trimethobenzamide; pts with sensitivity to benzocaine or similar anesthetics PR form contraindicated; not recommended for treatment of uncomplicated vomiting in children; contraindicated parenterally in children, rectally in neonates, premature infants
• Use cautiously with pregnancy, lactation, in the presence of a viral illness (may contribute to the development of Reye's syndrome); with high fever, dehydration, electrolyte imbalance, encephalopathy, gastroenteritis

INTERACTIONS
Drug
• Decreased emetic response to apomorphine possible
• Additive CNS effects with apomorphine, CNS depressants (may cause opisthotonos, convulsions, coma, EPS)
• Masked signs of ototoxicity (tinnitus, dizziness, and vertigo) of other agents possible

SIDE EFFECTS
CNS: Drowsiness, convulsions, mental depression, opisthotonos, Parkinson-like syndrome, Reye syndrome, blurred vision, dizziness, headache
CV: Hypotension
DERM: Skin rash (allergic reaction)
GI: Diarrhea, jaundice, hepatotoxicity, acute hepatitis
HEME: Blood dyscrasias
Other: Sore throat, fever, fatigue, muscle cramps

TOXICITY AND OVERDOSE
Clinical signs: Severe neurologic reaction (seizures, opisthotonos, EPS)

PATIENT CARE MANAGEMENT
Assessment
• Assess hypersensitivity to trimethobenzamide, benzocaine, other related anesthetics
• Assess baseline GI symptoms
Interventions
• Caps may be broken apart, contents mixed with food or liquid for administration
• Do not administer PR to neonates or premature infants
• IV not recommended
• Do not administer IM to children
• Administer IM deeply into upper outer quadrant of gluteal area
• Institute safety measures (supervise ambulation, raise side rails)

> **NURSING ALERT**
> Antiemetic effect may mask symptoms of other conditions (e.g., increased intracranial pressure, GI infection, toxic reaction, or overdosage of other drugs)

Evaluation
• Evaluate therapeutic response (decreased nausea or vomiting)
• Evaluate for hypersensitivity, side effects
• Monitor I&O, hydration status, electrolyte balance, hepatic function (ALT, AST, bilirubin)

PATIENT AND FAMILY EDUCATION
Teach/instruct
• To take as directed at prescribed intervals for prescribed length of time
• Do not use for subsequent illnesses without specific instructions from care provider
Warn/advise
• To notify care provider of hypersensitivity, side effects

T

✤ Available in Canada.

• To avoid use of alcohol, CNS depressants
• About possible dizziness, drowsiness, light-headedness; use caution with activities requiring alertness (bike, skate, skateboard)

STORAGE
• Store caps, supps at room temp
• Do not expose unwrapped supps to direct sunlight

---

tripelennamine hydrochloride

Brand Name(s): PBZ, PBZ-SR

Classification: Antihistamine

Pregnancy Category: C

AVAILABLE PREPARATIONS
Elixir: 37.5 mg/5 ml (as citrate salt; equivalent to 25 mg/5 ml hydrochloride salt)
Tabs: 25 mg, 50 mg
Tabs, sus rel: 100 mg

ROUTES AND DOSAGES
Infants and children: PO 5 mg/kg/24 hr divided q4-6h; maximum 300 mg/24 hr; do not use sust rel tabs in infants or children
Adults: PO 25-50 mg q4-6hr (tabs) or 100 mg q8-12h (sus rel tabs); maximum 600 mg/24 hr

MECHANISM AND INDICATIONS
Antihistamine mechanism: Competes with histamine for H_1-receptor sites; blocks histamine, thus decreasing allergic response
Indications: Used to treat seasonal and perennial allergic rhinitis, other allergic symptoms

PHARMACOKINETICS
Peak: Tabs 2-3 hr
Metabolism: Liver
Excretion: Urine

CONTRAINDICATIONS AND PRECAUTIONS
• Contraindicated with hypersensitivity to tripelennamine, other H_1-receptor antagonists, or antihistamines; in neonates, premature infants, pts with asthma attacks or lower respiratory tract disease, pts who have taken MAOIs within 14 days
• Use cautiously with narrow-angle glaucoma, pyloroduodenal obstruction, bladder neck obstruction, cardiovascular disease or hypertension, in infants and children (paradoxical hyperexcitability), pregnancy

INTERACTIONS
Drug
• Intensified central depressant, anticholinergic effects with MAOIs
• Additive sedative effects with alcohol, barbiturates, tranquilizers, sleeping aids, antianxiety agents
Lab
• False negative skin allergy tests

SIDE EFFECTS
CNS: Sedation, CNS stimulation, dizziness, confusion, impaired coordination
CV: Tachycardia, hypotension
DERM: Urticaria, photosensitivity
EENT: Blurred vision, tinnitus, dry nose and throat
GI: Dry mouth, constipation, anorexia, nausea, vomiting, diarrhea
GU: Dysuria, retention
HEME: Hemolytic anemia, leukopenia, agranulocytosis
RESP: Thickened bronchial secretions
Other: Fatigue

TOXICITY AND OVERDOSE
Clinical signs: CNS depression, CNS stimulation, GI symptoms, anticholinergic symptoms
Treatment: Induce vomiting, followed by activated charcoal; gastric lavage; supportive treatment; do not give stimulants

PATIENT CARE MANAGEMENT
Assessment
• Assess hypersensitivity to tripelennamine, other H_1-receptor antagonist antihistamines
• Assess urinary output, hematologic function (CBC, differential,

---

♣ Available in Canada.

platelet count) during long-term therapy

Interventions
• Administer PO with meals to reduce GI distress; sus rel tabs should not be crushed or chewed
• Provide sugarless hard candy, gum, frequent oral care for dry mouth
• Institute safety measures (supervise ambulation, raise bed rails) because of CNS side effects

Evaluation
• Evaluate therapeutic response (decreased allergy symptoms)
• Monitor respiratory status (change in secretions, wheezing, chest tightness)
• Monitor cardiac status (palpitations, tachycardia, hypotension)

PATIENT AND FAMILY EDUCATION
Teach/instruct
• To take as directed at prescribed intervals for prescribed length of time

Warn/advise
• To notify care provider of hypersensitivity, side effects
• Not to exceed recommended dosage
• To avoid hazardous activities if drowsiness occurs (bicycles, skateboards, skates)
• To avoid use of alcohol, medications containing alcohol, CNS depressants

STORAGE
• Store at room temp in tight container

---

troleandomycin
Brand Name(s): Tao
Classification: Antibiotic (macrolide; synthetic derivative of oleandomycin)
Pregnancy Category: C

AVAILABLE PREPARATIONS
Caps: 250 mg

ROUTES AND DOSAGES
Children: PO 25-40 mg/kg/24 hr divided q6h
Adults: PO 250-500 mg qid

MECHANISM AND INDICATIONS
Antibiotic mechanism: Inhibits bacterial protein synthesis; chemically related to erythromycin
Indications: Effective against *Streptococcus pyogenes* and *Diplococcus pneumoniae;* used to treat severe upper and lower respiratory infections

PHARMACOKINETICS
Peak: 2 hr
Distribution: Distributed throughout body fluids; penetrates CSF only with inflamed meninges
Metabolism: Liver
Excretion: Bile, urine

CONTRAINDICATIONS AND PRECAUTIONS
• Contraindicated with known hypersensitivity to troleandomycin
• Use cautiously with impaired liver function, pregnancy, estrogen-containing oral contraceptives

INTERACTIONS
Drug
• Ischemic reactions possible with ergotamine-containing drugs
• Increased toxicity possible from theophylline
Lab
• Elevated liver function tests possible
• Elevated serum theophylline levels possible

SIDE EFFECTS
DERM: Urticaria, rash
GI: Abdominal cramping, allergic type of cholestatic hepatitis (prolonged or repeated treatment), jaundice, nausea, vomiting, diarrhea
Other: Anaphylaxis; bacterial or fungal superinfection

PATIENT CARE MANAGEMENT
Assessment
• Assess history of hypersensitivity to troleandomycin
• Obtain C&S

T

• Assess liver function (ALT, AST, bilirubin)

Interventions

• Administer PO 1 hr ac or 2 hr after meals; caps may be taken apart, mixed with food or fluid

• Maintain age-appropriate fluid intake

• For group A β-hemolytic streptococcal infections, provide 10-day course of treatment to prevent risk of acute rheumatic fever or glomerulonephritis

Evaluation

• Evaluate therapeutic effect (decreased symptoms of infection)

• Monitor for signs of superinfection (perineal itching, diaper rash, diarrhea, sore throat, change in cough or sputum)

• Observe for signs of allergic reaction (rash, urticaria, pruritus respiratory difficulty)

• Monitor liver function (ALT, AST, bilirubin)

• Monitor serum theophylline levels with concurrent theophylline therapy

PATIENT/FAMILY EDUCATION

Teach/instruct

• To take as directed at prescribed intervals for prescribed length of time

Warn/advise

• To notify care provider of hypersensitivity, side effects, superinfection

Encourage

• To add live-culture yogurt or buttermilk to diet to prevent intestinal superinfection

STORAGE

• Store at room temp

---

tropicamide

Brand Name(s): Diotrope✿, I-Picamide, Mydriacyl✿, Tropicacyl

Classification: Cycloplegic, mydriatic

Pregnancy Category: C

AVAILABLE PREPARATIONS
Ophthal sol: 0.5%, 1%

ROUTES AND DOSAGES

Cycloplegia

Children and adults: Ophthal instill 1-2 gtt 1% sol in OU; repeat in 5 min; exam must be performed within 30 min of repeat dose; if exam not performed in 20-30 min, instill an additional gtt

Mydriasis

Children and adults: Ophthal instill 1-2 gtt of 0.5% sol in OU 15-20 min before exam; repeat q30 min as needed

MECHANISM AND INDICATIONS

Mydriatic mechanism: Prevents sphincter muscle of iris and muscle of ciliary body from responding to cholinergic stimulation, resulting in dilation and loss of accommodation

Indications: Used in refraction, diagnostic ophthal procedures, and treatment of some cases of acute iritis, iridocyclitis, keratitis

PHARMACOKINETICS

Peak: Cycloplegia within 30 min; mydriasis 20-40 min

Duration: Cycloplegia 50 min-6 hr; mydriasis 6-7 hr

CONTRAINDICATIONS AND PRECAUTIONS

• Contraindicated with hypersensitivity to tropicamide or any components; narrow-angle glaucoma

• Use cautiously with infants and children (increased risk of cardiovascular and CNS effects); pts in whom increased intraocular pressure may occur, pregnancy

SIDE EFFECTS

CNS: Parasympathetic stimulation, drowsiness, headache, behavioral disturbances, psychotic reactions

CV: Tachycardia

EENT: Blurred vision, transient stinging, photophobia, increased intraocular pressure, follicular conjunctivitis, nose or throat dryness

GI: Mouth dryness

Other: Fever, allergic reactions

✿ Available in Canada.

TOXICITY AND OVERDOSE
Clinical signs: Dry flushed skin, dry mouth, dilated pupils, hallucinations, delirium, tachycardia, decreased bowel sounds
Treatment: Induced emesis, activated charcoal; supportive care; for severe toxicity, physostigmine, propanolol

PATIENT CARE MANAGEMENT
Assessment
• Assess history of hypersensitivity to tropicamide, any components

Interventions
• See Chapter 2 regarding instillation; wash hands before and after application, cleanse crusts or discharge from eye before application; after instillation, apply gentle pressure to lacrimal sac for 1 min to minimize systemic absorption, wipe excess medication from eye; do not flush medication from eye

NURSING ALERT
Discontinue drug if signs of behavioral changes develop

Evaluation
• Monitor for signs of CNS disturbances (psychotic reactions, behavioral changes)
• Monitor for blurred vision, photosensitivity lasting >72 hr; notify care provider

PATIENT AND FAMILY EDUCATION
Warn/advise
• To notify care provider of hypersensitivity, side effects
• Not to let child rub, blink eyes
• To wait 5 min before using other ophthal preparations
• To wear dark glasses to reduce photophobia
• Not to engage in hazardous activities until effects have subsided
• To notify care provider of any change in vision, difficulty breathing, flushing

STORAGE
• Store at room temp, tightly sealed
• Do not freeze

---

tubocurarine chloride
Brand Name(s): Tubarine, Tubocuraine
Classification: Neuromuscular blocker; curare alkaloid
Pregnancy Category: C

AVAILABLE PREPARATIONS
Inj: 3 mg/ml

ROUTES AND DOSAGES
Neonates: IV 0.1-0.4 mg/kg/dose or 4 mg/m^2/dose repeated prn to maintain desired level of muscle paralysis
Infants and children: IV 0.1-0.8 mg/kg/dose, repeat prn to maintain desired level of muscle paralysis
Adults: IV bolus 0.4-0.5 mg/kg, then 0.08-0.10 mg/kg 20-45 min after initial dose if needed for prolonged procedures

IV administration
• Recommended concentration: 3 mg/ml (commercially available) or dilute to desired concentration in D-LR, D-R, D-S, D$_5$W, D$_{10}$W, LR, NS, ½ NS, R
• Maximum concentration: 3 mg/ml
• IV push rate: Undiluted over 60-90 sec

MECHANISM AND INDICATIONS
Mechanism: Interrupts the transmission of nerve impulses at the skeletal neuromuscular junction; antagonizes acetylcholine by competitively binding to cholinergic sites on motor endplates, resulting in muscle paralysis; reversible with edrophonium, neostigmine, physostigmine
Indications: Used as an adjunct in surgical anesthesia, to facilitate endotracheal intubation and skel-

---

etal muscle relaxation during mechanical ventilation or surgery

PHARMACOKINETICS
Onset of action: 15 sec
Peak: 2-3 min
Duration: ½-1½ hr
Half-life: 1-3 hr
Metabolism: Liver; minimally in kidney
Excretion: Urine

CONTRAINDICATIONS AND PRECAUTIONS
• Contraindicated with known hypersensitivity
• Use cautiously with pregnancy, lactation, children <2 yr, fluid and electrolyte imbalances, dehydration, neuromuscular disease, respiratory disease
• Injectable solution may contain 0.9% benzyl alcohol as a preservative; administration of benzyl alcohol at 99-234 mg/kg has been associated with fatal gasping syndrome in neonates; clinical signs include metabolic acidosis, hypotension, CNS depression, cardiovascular collapse

INTERACTIONS
Drug
• Increased neuromuscular blockade with aminoglycosides, clindamycin, lincomycin, quinidine, local anesthetics, polymyxin antibiotics, lithium, narcotic analgesics, thiazides, enflurane, isoflurane
• Arrhythmias possible with theophylline
• Should not be mixed with barbiturates in sol or syringe

SIDE EFFECTS
CV: Bradycardia, tachycardia, increased or decreased B/P
DERM: Rash, urticaria, flushing, pruritis
EENT: Increased secretions
RESP: Prolonged apnea, bronchospasm, cyanosis, respiratory depression
Other: Endogenous histamine release may occur, noted clinically as erythema, hypotension, either bradycardia or tachycardia

TOXICITY AND OVERDOSE
Clinical signs: Prolonged apnea, bronchospasm, cyanosis, respiratory depression
Treatment: Supportive, symptomatic care; monitor VS; mechanical ventilation may be required; anticholinesterase to reverse neuromuscular blockade (edrophonium, neostigmine, atropine)

PATIENT CARE MANAGEMENT
Assessment
• Assess history of hypersensitivity
• Assess for preexisting conditions requiring caution
• Assess electrolytes (Na, K+); K+ and Mg imbalances may increase action of drug
Interventions
• Monitor VS (pulse, respirations, airway, B/P) q 15 min until fully recovered; characteristics of respiration (rate, depth, pattern), strength of hand grip
• Monitor therapeutic response (paralysis of jaw, eyelid, head, neck, rest of the body)
• Monitor I&O for urinary frequency, hesitancy, retention
• Monitor for allergic reactions (rash, fever, respiratory distress, pruritus); drug should be discontinued
• Instill artificial tears (q2h) and covering to eyes to protect the cornea
• Administer with diazepam or morphine when used for therapeutic paralysis because drug does not provide sedation independently
Evaluation
• Monitor for recovery (including decreased paralysis of face, diaphragm, arm, rest of the body)

PATIENT AND FAMILY EDUCATION
Encourage
• Provide reassurance to pt if communication is difficult during recovery

STORAGE
• Store in a light-resistant container
• Use only fresh sol

---

urokinase

Brand Name(s): Abbokinase
Open Cath❦

Classification: Thrombolytic
enzyme

Pregnancy Category: B

AVAILABLE PREPARATIONS
Inj: 5000 U/ml in 1 ml, 1.8-ml vials

ROUTES AND DOSAGES
Adults and children: IV for catheter clearance: Remove protective cap of univial, turn stopper gently to force diluent into lower chamber; roll or tilt gently to mix; use only clear, colorless sol, immediately after reconstitution; clean stopper with germicidal solution and withdraw contents of vial

IV administration
• Infusion rate: Instill 5000 U in each lumen over 1-2 min; leave in place for 1-4 hr, then aspirate; may repeat with 10,000 U in each lumen if 5000 U fails to clear catheter; do not infuse into pt

MECHANISM AND INDICATIONS
Mechanism: Enzyme obtained from human kidney cells; acts by converting plasminogen to plasmin; plasmin degrades fibrin clots, fibrinogen, plasma proteins
Indications: Restoration of patency of IV catheters and central venous catheters obstructed by clotted blood or fibrin strands

PHARMACOKINETICS
Distribution: Information incomplete; minute amount reaches circulation
Metabolism: Liver

CONTRAINDICATIONS AND PRECAUTIONS
• Use cautiously, avoid excessive force or suction; may rupture or collapse catheter, damage vascular epithelium

SIDE EFFECTS
RESP: Coughing, dyspnea

PATIENT CARE MANAGEMENT
Assessment
• Assess history of hypersensitivity to urokinase
• Assess that catheter is indeed blocked
• Assess position of central venous catheter tip; possibility of mass clot on catheter tip in right atrium might best be left undisturbed
Interventions
• Inject drug according to instructions
• Observe for signs or symptoms of respiratory distress
Evaluation
• Evaluate therapeutic response (clear IV line)

PATIENT AND FAMILY EDUCATION
Teach/instruct
• That catheter is flushed qd; may consider increasing to bid if occlusion is frequent problem
• To report any signs or symptoms of pain, erythema, tenderness along catheter
• To report any febrile episodes, SOB

STORAGE
• Store powder at room temp
• Use sol immediately after reconstitution

valproic acid, valproate sodium

Brand Name(s): Depakene
(valproic acid)❦, Depokote
(divalproex sodium),
Kenral-Valproic❦

Classification: Anticonvulsant; carboxylic acid derivative

Pregnancy Category: D

AVAILABLE PREPARATIONS
Caps: 250 mg (valproic acid)
Syr: 250 mg/ml (valproic acid)
Tabs, enteric coated: 125 mg, 250 mg, 500 mg (divalproex sodium)

ROUTES AND DOSAGES

Children and adults: PO, initially 15 mg/kg/24 hr divided bid or tid, may increase by 5-10 mg/kg/24 hr at weekly intervals to maximum 60 mg/kg/24 hr divided bid or tid, bid dosing recommended for enteric coated tablets; PR, dilute syrup 1:1 with water for use as a retention enema, loading dose 17-20 mg/kg, maintenance dose 10-15 mg/kg/dose q8h

MECHANISM AND INDICATIONS

Mechanism: Increases availability of γ-aminobutyric acid (GABA), an inhibitory transmitter in the brain, either by increasing the GABA brain levels or decreasing GABA catabolism; acts at postsynaptic receptor sites

Indications: Used in the management of simple and complex absence seizures; mixed seizure types, myoclonic, and generalized tonic-clonic seizures; some effectiveness in treatment of partial seizures and infantile spasms

PHARMACOKINETICS

Onset: 15-30 min
Peak: 1-4 hr; enteric-coated 3-5 hr
Half-life: Children 4-14 hr; adults 8-17 hr (increased in neonates, pts with liver disease; if given with other anticonvulsants)
Metabolism: Liver
Excretion: Urine, feces (2%-3% unchanged drug)
Therapeutic level: 50-100 mcg/ml

CONTRAINDICATIONS AND PRECAUTIONS

• Contraindicated with known hypersensitivity, history of hepatic disease; pts with congenital metabolic or seizure disorders, mental retardation (especially children <2 yr; may be at increased risk to adverse side effects

• Use cautiously with anticoagulants, multiple anticonvulsants, pregnancy, lactation

INTERACTIONS

Drug
• Additive effects of MAOIs, other CNS antidepressants, oral anticoagulants with primidone, phenobarbital possible;
• Excessive somnolence requires careful monitoring
• Exacerbated absence seizures with clonazepam

Lab
• False positive urinary ketones
• Abnormal liver function tests

SIDE EFFECTS

CNS: Sedation, emotional lability; depression, aggression, hyperactivity, psychosis, behavioral deterioration, muscle weakness, tremors, ataxia, headache, hallucinations
DERM: Alopecia
EENT: Stomatitis, hypersalivation, nystagmus, diplopia, scotomata
GI: Nausea, vomiting, indigestion, diarrhea, abdominal cramps, constipation, increased appetite, weight gain, anorexia, pancreatitis, hepatic failure
GU: Enuresis, irregular menses
HEME: Thrombocytopenia, inhibited platelet aggregation, increased bleeding time (PT), leukopenia, lymphocytosis
Other: Acute pancreatitis, elevated serum ammonia levels; rarely, fulminant hepatitis that is frequently fatal; 85% of cases were taking multiple drugs; not necessarily preceded by abnormal liver function tests

TOXICITY AND OVERDOSE

Clinical signs: Somnolence, coma
Treatment: Supportive, symptomatic care; monitor VS, fluid and electrolyte balance, urine output; naloxone may be used to reverse CNS and respiratory depression, but it may also decrease anticonvulsant effect; valproate is not dialyzable

PATIENT CARE MANAGEMENT

Assessment
• Assess for hypersensitivity
• Assess for preexisting physical condition and current medications to avoid potential interactions

---

✦ Available in Canada.

- Assess baseline laboratory studies including CBC, differential, liver function testing (ALT, AST, bilirubin, alk phos)
- Assess seizure type and determine appropriate anticonvulsant for this type of seizure
- Drug interactions are a frequent problem, particularly with drugs metabolized via the liver; care must be taken should other drugs need to be prescribed; it may be necessary to check serum levels to avoid increased decreased levels

Interventions

- Tabs should be swallowed whole to avoid mucosal irritation; may take with food, milk to decrease GI symptoms; do not give with carbonated beverage (tablet may dissolve in mouth or throat prematurely, causing mucosal irritation)
- Initiate drug at modest dosage
- Increase the dosage and level prn to control seizures, to the point of intolerable side effects
- If first drug is only partially effective, another may be initiated in the same way; if first drug is not effective, discontinue and initiate a second medication
- If break-through seizures are occurring at times of trough serum levels or toxicity at times of peak levels, increase the frequency of administration
- Measure serum levels when pt is regulated on appropriate dosage, (when the seizures are controlled with minimal side effects), to get a baseline level; also measure serum levels if there is a break-through seizure or evidence of toxicity, to determine appropriate increments in dosage, to determine peak and trough levels, if other drugs are added or removed from treatment plan, to determine compliance or monitor for changes with growth, and at occasional intervals in pts on polytherapy or high dosage monotherapy
- Do not give syr to pts on Na restriction

Evaluation

- Evaluate therapeutic response (seizure control); initially dose more frequently until seizures are controlled, then q3-6 mo, with seizure break throughs or side effects
- Evaluate neurological status to monitor for alterations or deterioration
- Evaluate for signs and symptoms of toxicity
- Evaluate anticonvulsant levels periodically
- Monitor PT/INR in pts taking anticoagulants

PATIENT AND FAMILY EDUCATION

Teach/instruct

- To take as prescribed not to change dosage independently or withdraw the drug suddenly
- About potential side effects; to report serious side effects immediately (somnolence, fever, sore throat, unusual bleeding or bruising)
- About the process for initiating anticonvulsant drugs, need for frequent visits (especially initially)
- Explain the rationale for measuring serum levels, how these should be obtained (peak/trough)
- To swallow tabs whole to avoid local mucosal irritation; may take with food to decrease GI symptoms; avoid taking with carbonated beverages (tab may dissolve prematurely, causing local irritation and unpleasant taste)

Warn/advise

- That unpleasant side effects may decrease as pt becomes more used to the drug
- That initially the drug may be more sedating until pt becomes used to it; avoid hazardous tasks (bike, skates, skateboard) that require mental alertness until stabilized on drug
- To make other health care providers aware of medications in order to avoid drug interactions
- To inform care provider if pregnancy should occur while taking drug

Encourage

- To keep a record of any seizures (seizure calendar)

✤ Available in Canada.

STORAGE
• Store at room temp

---

vancomycin hydrochloride

Brand Name(s): Lyphocin, Vancoled, Vanocin

Classification: Antibiotic (glycopeptide)

Pregnancy Category: C

AVAILABLE PREPARATIONS
Oral sol: 1g, 10 g
Caps: 125 mg, 250 mg
Inj: 500 mg, 1 g, 2 g, 5 g, 10 g

ROUTES AND DOSAGES
Neonates ≤7 days, <1000 g: IV 10 mg/kg/dose q24h
Neonates ≤7 days, 1000-2000 g: IV 10 mg/kg/dose q18h
Neonates ≤7 days, >2000 g: IV 10 mg/kg/dose q12h
Neonates >7 days, <1000 g: IV 10 mg/kg/dose q18h
Neonates >7 days, 1000-2000 g: IV 10 mg/kg/dose q12h
Neonates >7 days, >2000 g: IV 10 mg/kg/dose q8h
Infants and children: IV 10-15 mg/kg/dose q8h
Adults: PO 0.5-2 g/24 h divided q6-8h; IV 500 mg q6h or 1 g q12h (maximum 2 g/24 hr)
Antibiotic-Associated Pseudomembranous and Staphylococcal Entercolitis
Children: PO 10 mg/kg/dose q6h (maximum 500 mg/24 hr)
Adults: PO 125 mg q6h
IV administration
• Recommended concentration: 2.5-5 mg/ml in D_5LR, D_5NS, D_5W, LR, NS
• Maximum concentration: 5 mg/ml
• IV push rate: Not recommended
• Intermittent infusion rate: Over 60 min; red man or red neck syndrome usually develops during a rapid infusion or with dosages ≥15-20 mg/kg/hr; reaction dissipates in 30-60 min

MECHANISM AND INDICATIONS
Antibiotic mechanism: Hinders cell-wall synthesis by blocking glycopeptide polymerization
Indications: Effective against many gram positive organisms including *Staphylococcus* and *Enterococcus;* used to treat *S. epidermidis,* methicillin-resistant *S. aureus,* penicillin-resistant *S. pneumococcus* and other resistant strains and serious infections

PHARMACOKINETICS
Peak: IV, at end of infusion
Distribution: Widely distributed in body tissues and fluids; small amount penetrates CSF if meninges are inflamed
Half-life: Neonates, 6-10 hr; 3 mo-3 yr, 4 hr; >3 yr, 2.2-3 hr; adults, 4-8 hr
Excretion: Urine, feces
Therapeutic levels: Peak 25-40 mcg/ml; trough 5-10 mcg/ml

CONTRAINDICATIONS AND PRECAUTIONS
• Contraindicated with known hypersensitivity to vancomycin, with hearing loss
• Use cautiously with premature infants and neonates (because of renal immaturity) impaired renal function, pts receiving other nephrotoxic or ototoxic drugs, pregnancy, lactation

INTERACTIONS
Drug
• Increased risk of ototoxicity, nephrotoxicity with aminoglycosides, polymyxin B, colistin, amphotericin B, capreomycin, methoxyflurane, cisplatin, cephalosporins
Lab
• Increased BUN, serum creatinine

INCOMPATIBILITIES
• Aminophylline, amobarbital, chloramphenicol, chlorthiazide, dexamethasone, heparin, hydrocortisone, methicillin, penicillins, pentobarbital, phenobarbital, phe-

---

nytoin, prochlorperazine, secobarbital, warfarin

SIDE EFFECTS

CNS: Neurotoxicity
CV: Hypotension, tachycardia with rapid infusion
DERM: Rash
EENT: Tinnitus, deafness, ototoxicity
GI: Nausea, vomiting
GU: Nephrotoxicity
HEME: Neutropenia, eosinophilia
Local: Pain, phlebitis at IV site; tissue necrosis with extravasation
Other: Anaphylaxis, fever, chills, hypotension, flushing, rash on face, neck, trunk, and upper extremities (red neck syndrome associated with rapid infusion)

TOXICITY AND OVERDOSE

Clinical signs: Ototoxicity
Treatment: Supportive care

PATIENT CARE MANAGEMENT

Assessment

• Assess history of hypersensitivity to vancomycin
• Obtain C&S; may begin therapy before obtaining results
• Assess renal function (BUN, creatinine, I&O), hematologic function (CBC, differential, platelet count), baseline hearing test, B/P

Interventions

• May administer PO without regard to meals; shake susp well before administering; caps may be taken apart, mixed with food or fluid
• Do not mix IV with other medications; infuse separately
• Use large vein with small-bore needle to reduce local reaction; rotate site q48-72h
• Maintain age-appropriate fluid intake
• Continue medication for full course of treatment (usually 10-14 days)

> **NURSING ALERT**
>
> Discontinue drug if signs of hypersensitivity, ototoxicity develop
>
> If red neck syndrome develops, stop infusion and notify care provider
>
> Do not administer IM, IV push

Evaluation

• Evaluate therapeutic response (decreased symptoms of infection)
• Evaluate renal function (BUN, creatinine, I&O), hematologic function (CBC, differential, platelet count), daily hearing evaluations
• Monitor B/P frequently during IV infusion
• Observe for signs of superinfection (perineal itching, diaper rash, fever, malaise, redness, pain, swelling, drainage, rash, diarrhea, sore throat, change in cough or sputum)
• Evaluate IV site for thrombophlebitis, extravasation

PATIENT AND FAMILY EDUCATION

Teach/instruct

• To take as directed at prescribed intervals for prescribed length of time

Warn/advise

• To notify care provider of hypersensitivity, side effects, superinfection
• To avoid use of OTC antidiarrheals if diarrhea develops

STORAGE

• Store powder, caps at room temp in airtight containers
• Reconstituted oral sol stable 14 days refrigerated; label date and time of reconstitution
• Reconstituted parenteral sol stable 96 hr refrigerated

V

varicella zoster immune globulin (human)

Brand Name(s): VZIG

Classification: IgG class varicella antibody

Pregnancy Category: C

AVAILABLE PREPARATIONS
Inj: 125 U/2.5 ml

ROUTES AND DOSAGES
Infants and children ≤10 kg: IM 125 U

Infants and children 10.1-20 kg: IM 250 U

Infants and children 20.1-30 kg: IM 375 U

Infants and children 30.1-40 kg: IM 500 U

Infants and children >40 kg: IM 625 U

• Do not administer >2.5 ml/injection site

• Maximum benefit is achieved if administered within 96 hr of exposure

MECHANISM AND INDICATIONS
Mechanism: Provides immediate passive immunity to varicella zoster virus

Indications: Used to prevent varicella infection in exposed, susceptible individuals at greater risk of developing complications from disease; high risk groups include immunocompromised children, newborns born to mothers who develop varicella shortly before or after delivery, infants <1 yr; susceptible and immunocompromised adults

PHARMACOKINETICS
Onset of action: Immediate

Duration of protection: At least 3 wk

CONTRAINDICATIONS AND PRECAUTIONS
• Contraindicated with known hypersensitivity to thimerosal (preservative)

• Use cautiously with immunoglobulin A deficiency; pt may develop antibodies to immunoglobulin A component, creating potential for anaphylactic reactions with subsequent exposures of products containing immunoglobulin A

INTERACTIONS
Drug

• Interference with immune response to live virus vaccines possible

SIDE EFFECTS
CNS: Headache

DERM: Discomfort at injection site including pain, erythema, swelling (1 in 100 pt), rash

GI: Nausea, vomiting, diarrhea

RESP: Respiratory distress, anaphylaxis

Other: Malaise

TOXICITY AND OVERDOSE
• Not reported

PATIENT CARE MANAGEMENT
Assessment

• Assess history of susceptibility to chicken pox

• Assess varicella antibody titer to determine status before immunosuppressive chemotherapy

• Assess history of allergic reactions to previous immunizations or preparations containing thimerosal

Interventions

• Administer as deep IM injection; gluteal muscle preferred; do not administer IV

• Epinephrine should be available for possible allergic reactions

---

NURSING ALERT

VZIG distributed by the American National Red Cross in areas outside of Massachusetts; within the state of Massachusetts, distributed by Massachusetts Public Health Biologic Laboratories

Drug should never be administered IV

✦ Available in Canada.

PATIENT AND FAMILY EDUCATION
Teach/instruct
- That VZIG is *likely* to prevent occurrence of chicken pox, but pt/family must be vigilant about watching for disease
- To recognize chicken pox lesion
- That chicken pox rash may be atypical after administration of VZIG

Warn/advise
- That administration of VZIG may delay onset of disease up to 4-6 wk after exposure
- To report any suspicious rash
- That local inflammation at injection site may be treated with acetaminophen
- Not to administer live virus vaccines within 3 mo of VZIG injection

STORAGE
- Store unopened vials in refrigerator; do not freeze

---

vasopressin
Brand Name(s): Pitressin✤, Pressyn✤

Classification: Antidiuretic hormone, peristaltic stimulant, hemostatic agent, posterior pituitary hormone

Pregnancy Category: C

AVAILABLE PREPARATIONS
Inj: 20 U/ml

ROUTES AND DOSAGES
Central Diabetes Insipidus
Children: IM/SC 2.5-10 U bid-qid prn, or intranasally by spray or cotton pledgets in individualized doses
Adults: IM/SC 5-10 U bid-qid prn

MECHANISM AND INDICATIONS
Antidiuretic mechanism: Increases reabsorption of water at the renal tubules, increasing urine osmolality
Indications: Used to diagnose and treat central diabetes insipidus, post-operative abdominal distention, abdominal roentgenography

PHARMACOKINETICS
Half-life: 10-20 min
Metabolism: Liver, kidneys
Excretion: Urine

CONTRAINDICATIONS AND PRECAUTIONS
- Contraindicated with hypersensitivity, chronic nephritis with N retention
- Use cautiously with CAD, epilepsy, migraine, asthma, heart failure, pregnancy, any condition in which rapid addition of extracellular water may pose a hazard

INTERACTIONS
Drug
- Additive effects of vasopressin possible with carbamazepine, chlorpropamide, clofibrate, urea, fludrocortisone, tricyclic antidepressants
- Decreased effects with demecycline, norepinephrine, lithium, heparin, alcohol

SIDE EFFECTS
CNS: Tremor, vertigo, "pounding" in head
CV: Angina, vasoconstriction, cardiac arrest, hypertension (large doses); bradycardia, pulmonary edema, arrhythmias (intraarterial infusion)
DERM: Circumoral pallor, sweating, urticaria, cutaneous gangrene
GI: Abdominal cramps, nausea, vomiting, diarrhea, intestinal hyperactivity
GU: Uterine cramps, vulval pain, anuria
Other: Anaphylaxis, hypersensitivity, water intoxication (drowsiness, listlessness, headache, confusion)

TOXICITY AND OVERDOSE
Clinical signs: Signs of water intoxication including drowsiness, listlessness, confusion, headache, wt gain, anuria
Treatment: Water restriction and temporary withdrawal of vasopressin until polyuria occurs; severe cases may require osmotic diuresis with mannitol, hypertonic

V

✤ Available in Canada.

dextrose, or urea with or without furosemide

PATIENT CARE MANAGEMENT
Assessment
• Assess history of hypersensitivity to vasopressin, related drugs
• Assess I&O, daily wt, B/P, signs of water intoxication, signs of abdominal distention (in post-op patients)
Interventions
• Provide appropriate amounts of fluids to avoid water intoxication
Evaluation
• Evaluate therapeutic response (absence of severe thirst, decreased urine output, improvement in abdominal symptoms, LOC)
• Monitor pulse, B/P
• Monitor wt (appropriate for age; same scale at same time of day); urine osmolality (appropriate for age); serum and urine electrolytes
• Monitor signs of water intoxication (behavioral changes, lethargy, disorientation, neuromuscular irritability)

PATIENT AND FAMILY EDUCATION
Teach/instruct
• To take as directed at prescribed intervals for prescribed length of time
Warn/advise
• To notify care provider of hypersensitivity, side effects (water intoxication)
• To drink fluids with each dose to reduce possible nausea, pallor, abdominal cramps, vomiting

STORAGE
• Store at room temp

---

vecuronium bromide
Brand Name(s): Norcuron❦
Classification: Neuromuscular blocker
Pregnancy Category: C

AVAILABLE PREPARATIONS
Inj: 10 mg

ROUTES AND DOSAGES
Infants >7 wk-1 yr: Initially 0.08-0.1 mg/kg/dose; maintenance 0.05-0.1 mg/kg/dose q1h prn
Children >1 yr and adults: IV, initially 0.08-0.1 mg/kg/dose; maintenance 0.05-0.1 mg/kg/dose q1h prn; may be administered as continuous infusion at 0.1 mg/kg/hr
IV administration
• Maximum concentration: 2 mg/ml for IV push, 1 mg/ml for continuous infusion
• IV push rate: Over 30-60 sec

MECHANISM AND INDICATIONS
Mechanism: Acts to interrupt transmission of nerve impulse at the skeletal neuromuscular junction; blocks acetylcholine from binding to receptors on motor endplates, inhibiting depolarization and resulting in muscle paralysis; reversible with edrophonium, neostigmine, and physostigmine
Indications: Used as an adjunct in surgical anesthesia, to facilitate endotracheal intubation and skeletal muscle relaxation during mechanical ventilation or surgery

PHARMACOKINETICS
Onset of action: IV 15 sec
Peak: 3-5 min
Duration: 45-60 min
Half-life: 65-75 min
Metabolism: Not metabolized
Excretion: Bile, urine

CONTRAINDICATIONS AND PRECAUTIONS
• Contraindicated in known hypersensitivity
• Use cautiously with pregnancy, lactation, children <2 yr, fluid and electrolyte imbalances, dehydration, neuromuscular disease, respiratory disease, hepatic dysfunction, elderly
• Injectable sol may contain benzyl alcohol as a preservative; administration of benzyl alcohol at 99 - 234 mg/kg has been associated with a fatal gasping syndrome in neonates; clinical signs include metabolic acidosis, hypotension,

---

❦ Available in Canada.

CNS depression, cardiovascular collapse

INTERACTIONS
Drug
• Increased neuromuscular blockade with aminoglycosides, clindamycin, lincomycin, quinidine, local anesthetics, polymyxin antibiotics, lithium, narcotic analgesics, thiazides, enflurane, isoflurane
• Arrhythmias possible with theophylline

INCOMPATIBILITIES
• Do not mix with alkaline drugs

SIDE EFFECTS
CV: Bradycardia, tachycardia, increased or decreased B/P
DERM: Rash, urticaria, flushing, pruritus
EENT: Increased secretions
RESP: Prolonged apnea, bronchospasm, cyanosis, respiratory depression
Other: Endogenous histamine release may occur with tubocurarine chloride noted clinically as erythema, hypotension, either bradycardia or tachycardia

TOXICITY AND OVERDOSAGE
Clinical signs: Prolonged apnea, bronchospasm, cyanosis, respiratory depression
Treatment: Supportive, symptomatic care; monitor VS; mechanical ventilation may be required; anticholinesterase to reverse neuromuscular blockade (edrophonium or neostigmine, atropine)

PATIENT CARE MANAGEMENT
Assessment
• Assess history of hypersensitivity to vecuronium
• Assess for preexisting conditions
• Assess electrolytes (Na, K^+) before procedure (K^+, Mg imbalances may increase action of drug)
Interventions
• Administer with diazepam or morphine when used for therapeutic paralysis, drug does not provide sedation independently

• Monitor VS (pulse, respirations, airway, B/P) q15 min until fully recovered; characteristics of respirations (rate, depth, pattern); strength of hand grip
• Monitor for allergic reactions (rash, fever, respiratory distress, pruritus); *drug should be discontinued*
• Monitor I&O for urinary frequency, hesitancy, retention
• Instill artificial tears (q2h) and covering to eyes to protect cornea

> **NURSING ALERT**
> Injectable sol may contain benzyl alcohol as a preservative; administration of benzyl alcohol 99-234 mg/kg has been associated with a fatal gasping syndrome in neonates; clinical signs include metabolic acidosis, hypotension, CNS depression, cardiovascular collapse

Evaluation
• Monitor therapeutic response (paralysis of jaw, eyelid, head, neck, rest of the body)
• Monitor effectiveness of neuromuscular blockade (degree of paralysis) using nerve stimulator
• Monitor for recovery (including decreased paralysis of face, diaphragm, arm, rest of the body)

PATIENT AND FAMILY EDUCATION
Teach/instruct
• Provide reassurance if communication is difficult during recovery
• That postoperative stiffness often occurs, is normal, and will subside

STORAGE
• Refrigerate, discard in 24 hr
• Stable 5 days at room temp when reconstituted with bacteriostatic water; stable 24 hr at room temp when reconstituted with preservative free SW (avoid preservatives with neonates)

verapamil hydrochloride

Brand Name(s): Apo-Verap✤, Calan, Calan SR, Isoptin✤, Isoptin IV✤, Isoptin SR✤, Novo-Veramil✤, Nu-Verap✤, Verapamil HCL, Verapamil Injection✤, Verelan✤

Classification: Calcium channel blocker, antianginal, antihypertensive

Pregnancy Category: C

AVAILABLE PREPARATIONS
Tabs: 40 mg, 80 mg, 120 mg
Tabs, sus: 240 mg
Inj: 2.5 mg/ml

ROUTES AND DOSAGES
Children 1-16 yr: PO 4-8 mg/kg/24 hr divided tid; IV, children ≤1 yr: 0.1-0.2 mg/kg over 2-3 min; may repeat once in 30 min; maximum dose 2 mg; children 1-16 yr 0.1-0.3 mg/kg; maximum dose 5 mg
Adults: PO 240-480 mg/24 hr divided tid-qid; IV 0.075-0.15 mg/kg; may administer 0.15 mg/kg 15-30 min after initial dose

IV administration
• Recommended concentration: 0.4 mg/ml IV infusion, 0.5-2.5 mg/ml for IV push
• Maximum concentration: 2.5 mg/ml for IV push
• IV push rate: 30-60 sec
• Continuous infusion rate: 2.5-5 mcg/kg/min

MECHANISM AND INDICATIONS
Calcium channel blocker mechanism: Inhibits Ca ion influx across cell membrane during depolarization; decreases SA/AV node conduction
Antianginal mechanism: Produces relaxation of coronary vascular smooth muscle and dilates coronary and peripheral arteries; reduces afterload at rest and with exercise, thereby decreasing O_2 consumption
Antihypertensive mechanism: Dilates peripheral blood vessels, thereby decreasing B/P
Indications: Arrhythmias (esp. SVT not responsive to adenosine), chronic stable angina, vasospastic angina, hypertension

PHARMACOKINETICS
Onset of action: IV 3 min; PO variable
Peak: IV 3-5 min; PO 3-4 hr, sus rel tab 4-8 hr
Half-life: Infants 5-7 hr; adults 6-12 hr
Metabolism: Liver
Excretion: Urine (drug and metabolites)

CONTRAINDICATIONS AND PRECAUTIONS
• Contraindicated with severe hypotension, sick sinus syndrome, 2nd- or 3rd-degree heart block, severe left ventricular dysfunction, cardiogenic shock, severe CHF
• Use cautiously with hypotension, CHF, hypertrophic cardiomyopathy, hepatic or renal impairment, Wolff-Parkinson-White syndrome, renal disease, other β-blocker therapy

INTERACTIONS
Drug
• Increased effects with β-blockers, antihypertensives, cimetidine
• Increased hypotension with prazosin, quinidine
• Increased level of digoxin, theophylline, cyclosporine, carbamazepine, non-depolarizing muscle relaxants
• Decreased effects of lithium
Lab
• Increase liver function tests

INCOMPATIBILITIES
Albumin, amphotericin B, ampicillin, dobutamine, hydralazine, mezlocillin, nafcillin, oxacillin, $NaHCO_3$

SIDE EFFECTS
CNS: Dizziness, headache, drowsiness, fatigue, anxiety, insomnia, confusion, depression, weakness, light-headedness

---

✤ Available in Canada.

CV: CHF, hypotension, bradycardia, AV block, palpitations, ventricular asystole
GI: Nausea, diarrhea, constipation, gastric distress
GU: Nocturia, polyuria
RESP: Apnea

TOXICITY AND OVERDOSE
Clinical signs: Heart block, asystole, hypotension
Treatment: Supportive therapy including IV isoproterenol, norepinephrine, epinephrine, atropine, calcium gluconate; methoxamine, phenylephrine, metaraminol, dopamine, dobutamine to maintain B/P; cardioversion with lidocaine or procainamide in pts with Wolff-Parkinson-White syndrome

PATIENT CARE MANAGEMENT
Assessment
• Assess history of hypersensitivity to drug
• Assess baseline VS, B/P, ECG
• Assess baseline liver function tests (ALT, AST, bilirubin), CBC, differential
Interventions
• Monitor ECG continuously with IV administration
Evaluation
• Evaluate therapeutic response (decreased arrhythmias, decreased B/P, decreased anginal pain)
• Evaluate for side effects, hypersensitivity
• Evaluate VS, B/P, ECG regularly
• Evaluate CBC, differential, liver function (ALT, AST, bilirubin) regularly

PATIENT AND FAMILY EDUCATION
Teach/instruct
• To take as directed at prescribed intervals for prescribed length of time
Warn/advise
• To notify care provider of hypersensitivity, side effects
• To identify signs of CHF (swelling of hands and feet, SOB), to

notify care provider immediately
• Not to discontinue medication abruptly
• To avoid hazardous activities until therapy is well-established
• To limit caffeine consumption
• To avoid alcohol, OTC medication (unless directed by care provider)

STORAGE
• Store at room temp in tightly sealed, light-resistant container

---

vidarabine
Brand Name(s): ARA-A, Vira-A, Vira-A Ophthalmic✤
Classification: Antiviral (purine nucleoside)
Pregnancy Category: C

AVAILABLE PREPARATION
Inj: 200 mg/ml
Ophthal oint: 3%

ROUTES AND DOSAGES
Herpes Simplex Infection
Neonates: IV 15-30 mg/kg/24 hr qd as an 18-24 hr infusion
Herpes Simplex Encephalitis
Children and adults: IV 15 mg/kg/24 hr qd as a 12-24 hr infusion for 10 days
Herpes Zoster, Varicella Infection
Children and adults: IV 10 mg/kg/24 hr qd as a 12-24 hr infusion for 5-7 days.
Keratoconjunctivitis
Children and adults: Ophthal 1 cm strip of oint in conjunctival sac 5 times/24 hr q3h while awake until complete reepithelialization, then bid for an additional 7 days
IV administration
• Recommended concentration: 0.45 mg/ml to avoid precipitation
• Maximum concentration: 0.7 mg/ml
• Continuous infusion rate: Over 12-24 hr

V

✤ Available in Canada.

MECHANISM AND INDICATIONS

Antiviral mechanism: Inhibits viral DNA synthesis by blocking DNA polymerase

Indications: Used to treat herpes simplex encephalitis, neonatal herpes simplex virus infections, and disseminated varizella zoster in immunosuppressed patients; ophthal oint used to treat keratoconjunctivitis and epithelial keratitis caused by herpes simplex virus I and II

PHARMACOKINETICS

Distribution: Crosses into CNS
Half-life: Infants 2.4-3.1 hr; children 2.8 hr; adults 1.5 hr
Excretion: Urine

CONTRAINDICATIONS AND PRECAUTIONS

• Contraindicated with known hypersensitivity to vidarabine
• Use cautiously with renal or hepatic impairment; in pts at risk of fluid overload (cerebral edema); with pregnancy, lactation

INTERACTIONS

Drug
• Increased risk of toxicity from theophylline
• Increased neurologic side effects with allopurinol

Lab
• Elevated liver function tests, bilirubin
• Decreased Hct, Hgb, leukocyte, platelet, reticulocyte values

INCOMPATIBILITIES

• Blood, protein products

SIDE EFFECTS

CNS: Weakness, ataxia, disorientation, depression, agitation, tremors
DERM: Rash, pruritus
EENT: With ophthal oint, lacrimation, foreign body sensation, burning, photophobia, pain, sensitivity, temporary visual haze
GI: Anorexia, nausea, vomiting, diarrhea, wt loss, elevated liver function tests, bilirubin
HEME: Anemia, neutropenia, thrombocytopenia

Local: Pain, thrombophlebitis with IV injection

TOXICITY AND OVERDOSE

Clinical signs: Signs of fluid overload, risk of heart failure caused by volume of fluid needed to administer drug
Treatment: Supportive care; monitor renal, hepatic, hematologic status

PATIENT CARE MANAGEMENT

Assessment
• Assess history of hypersensitivity to vidarabine
• Obtain cultures to confirm diagnosis; EEG, CT scan
• Assess hepatic function (ALT, AST, bilirubin), renal function (BUN, creatinine, I&O), hematologic function (CBC, differential, platelet count), bowel pattern

Interventions
• Shake well before withdrawing IV dose; warming the diluting sol to 35-40° C facilitates dissolving; must be filtered with a 0.45 micron or smaller inline filter
• Rapid infusion may cause nausea and vomiting; do not administer IV push, IM, SC
• Use large vein with small-bore needle to reduce local reaction; rotate site q48-72h
• See Chapter 2 regarding ophthal instillation; wash hands before and after application, cleanse crusts or discharge from eye before application; wipe excess medication from eye; do not flush medication from eye
• Maintain age-appropriate fluid intake

NURSING ALERT

Large fluid volume required for dilution; monitor closely for signs of fluid overload

Do not administer IV push, IM, or SC

Evaluation
• Evaluate therapeutic response (decreased symptoms of infection)

- Monitor renal function (BUN, creatinine, I&O), hepatic function (ALT, AST, bilirubin), hematologic function (CBC, differential, platelet count), bowel patterns
- Monitor for signs of fluid overload, cerebral edema
- Monitor for CNS effects (tremor, disorientation, ataxia)
- Monitor theophylline levels, signs of toxicity if pt receiving concomitant theophylline
- Evaluate IV site for vein irritation

PATIENT AND FAMILY EDUCATION
Teach/instruct
- To take as directed at prescribed intervals for prescribed length of time

Warn/advise
- To notify care provider of hypersensitivity, side effects
- That vision will blur for a few minutes after instillation; then it should clear
- To wear sunglasses if photosensitivity develops
- Not to share towels, washcloths, bed linens, eye makeup with family member being treated

STORAGE
- Store at room temp
- Store ophthal oint in light-resistant, airtight container
- Diluted sol stable at room temperature 48 hr; do not refrigerate

---

vinblastine
Brand Name(s): Velban, Velbe✤

Classification: Antineoplastic, vinca alkaloid; cell cycle phase specific (effect in S-phase, expressed in M-phase)

Pregnancy Category: D

AVAILABLE PREPARATIONS
Inj: 10 mg vials of powder

ROUTES AND DOSAGES
- Dosages may vary in response to diagnosis, extent of disease, concurrent or previous therapy, protocol guidelines, physiologic parameters; consult current literature, protocol recommendations

Hodgkin's Disease
Children and adolescents: IV 3.5-6 mg/m^2/24 hr q wk for 3-6 wk

Other Malignancies
Children: IV 2.5-12.5 mg/m^2/24 hr q 7-10 days
Adults: IV 3.7-18.5 mg/m^2/24 hr q 7-10 days or 1.4-1.8 mg/m^2/24 hr for 5 days as continuous infusion

IV administration
- Recommended concentration: 1 mg/ml
- IV push rate: Over 1-2 min

MECHANISM AND INDICATIONS
Mechanism: Produces metaphase arrest by disrupting microtubules; action causes inability of chromosomal material to align correctly, blocking mitosis, producing cell death; also interferes with metabolic pathways of amino acids, inhibiting purine synthesis; interferes with DNA and DNA-dependent RNA synthesis
Indications: Hodgkin's disease, non-Hodgkin's lymphoma, neuroblastoma, Letterer-Siwe disease (histocytosis X), blast crises of CML, Kaposi's sarcoma

PHARMACOKINETICS
Distribution: Rapid, extensive binding to serum protein
Half-life: Triphasic; initial <5 min, middle 53-99 min, terminal 20-24 hr
Metabolism: Partially metabolized in liver to biologically active metabolite desacetylvinblastine
Excretion: 15%-33% intact in urine, 10%-21% intact in feces

CONTRAINDICATIONS AND PRECAUTIONS
- Contraindicated with hypersensitivity to drug, active infections (especially chicken pox or herpes zoster [shingles]), intrathecal administration, pregnancy, lactation

V

✤ Available in Canada.

INTERACTIONS
Drug
- Increased cellular uptake of methotrexate
- Decreased serum phenytoin

Lab
- Increase blood, urine concentrations of uric acid possible

SIDE EFFECTS
CNS: Symptoms less common than with vincristine; peripheral neuropathy characterized by numbness, tingling, weakness, loss of deep tendon reflexes, foot drop, ataxia, muscular cramps, neuritic pain, depression; may cause cranial nerve palsies, headache, malaise, jaw pain, seizures, vocal cord paralysis, muscular weakness involving extrinsic muscles of eyes, SIADH
CV: Hypertension, ischemic cardiac toxicity, Raynaud's phenomenon, orthostatic hypotension
GI: Nausea, vomiting occurring from 4-24 hrs after dose, diarrhea, anorexia, constipation, abdominal pain, paralytic ileus, stomatitis, ulcer, bleeding, paralytic ileus
GU: Oligospermia, aspermia, urinary retention, amenorrhea during treatment
HEME: Leukopenia with nadir occurring at 7-10 days, recovery in 7-14 days; rare effect on RBCs platelets
RESP: Dyspnea, acute bronchospasm (most often reported in pt receiving concurrent treatment with mitomycin)
Other: May cause intense pain, stinging, burning sensation at tumor site; abrupt in onset, lasting 20 min-3 hr

TOXICITY AND OVERDOSE
Clinical signs: Myelosuppression, severe mucositis, paralytic ileus, paresthesias
Treatment: Supportive measures including laxatives, blood transfusions, hydration, nutritional supplementation, broad spectrum antibiotic coverage (if febrile), electrolyte replacement

PATIENT CARE MANAGEMENT
Assessment
- Assess history of hypersensitivity to drug
- Assess history of previous treatment (especially that which may predispose to hepatic dysfunction)
- Assess baseline hematologic function (CBC, differential, platelet count)
- Assess baseline renal function (BUN, creatinine), liver function (bilirubin, alk phos, LDH, AST, ALT)
- Assess history of antiemetic success
- Assess bowel function
- Assess neurologic status

Interventions
- Administer antiemetic before chemotherapy
- Ongoing assessment of bowel function with addition of stool softener, laxatives at earliest sign of constipation; individual bowel management program should be developed early and strictly adhered to while taking drug
- Provide supportive measures to maintain hemostasis, fluid, electrolyte, nutritional status
- In event of extravasation, hyaluronidase (150 U in 1 ml NS) should be injected SC with moderate heat applied to site

Evaluation
- Evaluate therapeutic response (radiologic or clinical evidence of tumor regression)
- Evaluate hematologic function (CBC, differential, platelet count) at least weekly; evaluate renal function (BUN, creatinine), liver function (bilirubin, alk phos, LDH, AST, ALT) regularly

PATIENT AND FAMILY EDUCATION
Teach/instruct
- To have patient well hydrated before and after chemotherapy
- About importance of follow-up to monitor blood counts, serum chemistry values

---

♣ Available in Canada.

- To take accurate temp; rectal temp contraindicated
- To notify care provider of signs of bleeding (bruising, epistaxis, bleeding gums), infection (fever, sore throat, fatigue)

Warn/advise
- About impact of body changes that may occur (hair loss, hyper-pigmentation, nail ridging), how to minimize changes (wigs, caps, scarves, long sleeves)
- To avoid OTC preparations containing aspirin
- To report any alterations in behavior, sensation, perception; help to develop a plan of care to manage side effects, stress of illness or treatment
- To monitor bowel function and call care provider if abdominal pain or constipation are noted
- That good oral hygiene with very soft toothbrush is imperative
- That dental work be delayed until blood counts return to baseline, with permission of caretaker
- To avoid contact with known viral and bacterial illnesses
- That close household contacts of child not be immunized with live polio virus; use inactivated form
- That children on chemotherapy not receive immunizations until immune system recovers sufficiently to mount necessary antibody response
- To report exposure to chicken pox in susceptible child immediately
- To report reactivation of herpes zoster virus (shingles) immediately
- To immediately report any signs of pain, inflammation at injection site
- If appropriate, ways to preserve reproductive patterns, sexuality (sperm banking, contraceptives)

Encourage
- Provision of nutritious food intake; consider nutrition consultation

- To use top anesthetics to control discomfort of mucositis; avoid spicy foods, commercial mouth-washes
- To strictly adhere to bowel management program

STORAGE
- Store unopened vials in refrigerator
- Protect from light
- Drug reconstituted with bacteriostatic diluent stable for 30 days under refrigeration

---

vincristine
Brand Name(s): Oncovin✤
Classification: Antineoplastic, vinca alkaloid; cell cycle phase specific (M phase)
Pregnancy Category: D

AVAILABLE PREPARATIONS
Inj: 1 mg/ml

ROUTES AND DOSAGES
- Dosage may vary in response to diagnosis, extent of disease, concurrent or previous therapy, protocol guidelines, physiologic parameters; consult current literature and protocol recommendations
Children <10 kg or BSA <1 m^2: 0.05 mg/kg/dose q wk, then titrate dose; maximum dose 2 mg/wk
Children >10 kg or BSA ≥1 m^2: 1.0-2.0 mg/m^2/dose q wk for 3-6 wk; maximum dose 2 mg/wk
Adults: IV 0.4-1.4 mg/m^2/dose q wk; maximum dose 2 mg/wk; may repeat q wk
IV administration
- Recommended concentration: 1 mg/ml
- IV push rate: Over 1 min

MECHANISM AND INDICATIONS
Mechanism: Derived from periwinkle plant; blocks mitosis, pro-

V

---

duces metaphase arrest by disruption of microtubules (key component in formation of mitotic spindles); chromosomal material cannot align along microtubules, causing cell death; also inhibits DNA-dependent RNA synthesis
Indications: ALL, Hodgkin's disease, non-Hodgkin's lymphoma, Wilm's tumor, neuroblastoma, rhabdomyosarcoma, brain tumors, osteogenic sarcoma, Ewing's sarcoma; may also be considered for idiopathic thrombocytopenic purpura

PHARMACOKINETICS
Peak: 6-12 hr demonstrated by marked increase in number cells in mitosis
Distribution: Rapid, to all body tissues where it is bound to formed blood elements (especially RBCs, platelets); does cross blood–brain barrier, but does not achieve high concentration in CSF
Half-life: Triphasic; initial 5 min, middle 2-3 hr, terminal 85 hr
Metabolism: Primarily in liver
Excretion: Bile, feces; small amount in urine

CONTRAINDICATIONS AND PRECAUTIONS
• Contraindicated with hypersensitivity; intrathecal administration, pregnancy, lactation, pts with demyelinating form of Charcot-Marie-Tooth syndrome
• Use cautiously with underlying neurologic disorders, hepatic dysfunction

INTERACTIONS
Drug
• Stathmokinetic effect (cell cycle arrest) of drug could theoretically be used to maximize effect of other drugs in combination chemotherapy
• Additive neurotoxicity possible with other neurotoxic agents
• Increased cellular uptake of methotrexate (clinical significance not clear)
• Decreased neurotoxicity of vincristine with glutamic acid; may also interfere with therapeutic effect

• Inhibition of vincristine-induced paralytic ileus with low-dose dopamine receptor inhibitors (metoclopramide)
• Decreased hepatic clearance of vincristine possible with asparaginase, increasing neurotoxicity effect
• Occasionally SOB, bronchospasm during concurrent treatment with mitomycin
• Increased action of anticoagulants
• Decreased serum levels of digoxin, phenytoin
Lab
• Increased serum, urine concentrations of uric acid possible
• Hyperkalemia possible

SIDE EFFECTS
CNS: Jaw pain caused by trigeminal neuralgia, cranial nerve palsies, headache, hoarseness, vocal cord paralysis, depression, SIADH; peripheral neuropathy (often dose-limiting factor) including numbness, tingling of extremities, weakness, loss of deep tendon reflexes, foot-drop, wrist drop, ataxia
CV: Potent vesicant, orthostatic hypotension
EENT: Ptosis, jaw pain, diplopia, optic and extraocular neuropathy, transient cortical blindness
GI: Constipation, obstipation, paralytic ileus, abdominal pain, anorexia, stomatitis, wt loss, dysphagia, occasional nausea, vomiting
GU: Polyuria, dysuria, bladder atony, azoospermia and amenorrhea in postpubertal pts
HEME: Generally not myelosuppressive
RESP: Dyspnea, acute bronchospasm (generally when given with mitomycin-C)
Other: Fever within 6-24 hrs after injection; can be associated with anorexia, fatigue

TOXICITY AND OVERDOSE
Clinical signs: Generally neuromuscular including obstipation, severe central and peripheral neurologic effects

---

✦ Available in Canada.

Treatment: Supportive measures (including stool softeners, laxatives, hydration, nutritional supplementation)

PATIENT CARE MANAGEMENT
Assessment
- Assess history of hypersensitivity to drug
- Assess history of previous therapy that might predispose pt to hepatic dysfunction
- Assess success of previous antiemetic regimens
- Assess baseline hematologic function (CBC, differential, platelet count); baseline renal function (BUN, creatinine), liver function (bilirubin, alk phos, LDH, AST, ALT)
- Assess bowel function
- Assess neurologic status
Interventions
- Administer antiemetic therapy before chemotherapy if necessary
- Ongoing assessment of bowel function with addition of stool softeners, laxatives at earliest sign of constipation; individual bowel management program should be developed early and strictly adhered to while taking drug
- If extravasation occurs, the area may be infiltrated with hyaluronidase SC (150 U in 1 ml NS); moist heat may also be helpful

> **NURSING ALERT**
> Drug is potent vesicant and should only be administered into an unquestionably patent IV which is not positioned over a joint; if extravasation occurs, area may be infiltrated with hyaluronidase with some effect
>
> Maximum dose is 2 mg/wk, regardless of body size
>
> Inadvertent intrathecal administration of drug has been universally fatal

Evaluation
- Evaluate therapeutic response (radiologic or clinical demonstration of tumor regression)

- Evaluate hematologic function (CBC, differential, platelet count) weekly; assess renal function (BUN, creatinine), liver function (alk phos, LDH, AST, ALT) regularly

PATIENT AND FAMILY EDUCATION
Teach/instruct
- To have patient well hydrated before and after chemotherapy
- Regarding importance of follow-up to monitor blood counts, serum chemistry values, serum drug levels
- To take accurate temp; rectal temp contraindicated
- To notify care provider of signs of bleeding (bruising, epistaxis, bleeding gums), infection (fever, sore throat, fatigue)
Warn/advise
- About impact of body changes that may occur (hair loss, hyperpigmentation, nail ridging), how to minimize changes (wigs, caps, scarves, long sleeves)
- To avoid OTC preparations containing aspirin
- To report any alterations in behavior, sensation, perception; help to develop a plan of care to manage side effects, stress of illness and treatment
- To monitor bowel function, call care provider if abdominal pain, constipation noted
- To immediately report to care provider any pain, discoloration at injection site
- That good oral hygiene with very soft toothbrush is imperative
- That dental work be delayed until blood counts returns to baseline, with permission of caretaker
- To avoid contact with known viral and bacterial illnesses
- That close household contacts of child not be immunized with live polio virus; use inactivated form
- That children on chemotherapy not receive immunizations until immune system recovers sufficiently to mount necessary antibody response
- To report exposure to chicken

pox in susceptible child immediately
• To report reactivation of herpes zoster virus (shingles) immediately
• To immediately report any signs of pain, inflammation at injection site
• If appropriate, ways to preserve reproductive patterns, sexuality (sperm banking, contraceptives)
Encourage
• Provision of nutritious food intake; consider nutrition consultation
• To use top anesthetics to control discomfort of mucositis; avoid spicy foods, commercial mouthwashes
• To strictly adhere to bowel management program

STORAGE
• Undiluted drug may be stored at room temp for at least 6 mo, may also be stored in refrigerator but should be protected from light

---

vitamin A

Brand Name(s): Aquasol A✤, Del-Vi-A

Classification: Fat-soluble vitamin

Pregnancy Category: A (X if dose exceeds RDA)

AVAILABLE PREPARATIONS
Tabs: 10,000 IU
Caps: 25,000 IU, 50,000 IU
Inj: 2 ml (50,000 IU/ml);
• 1 IU Vitamin A = 0.3 mcg retinol or 0.6 mcg β-carotene; 1 RE (retinol equivalent) = 1 mcg all-trans-retinol (3.33 IU), 6 mcg (10 IU) β-carotene or 12 carotenoid provitamins

ROUTES AND DOSAGES
See Appendix F, Table of Recommended Daily Dietary Allowances
Severe Vitamin A Deficiency with Xerophthalmia
Children 1-8 yr: PO 5000 IU/kg/24 hr × 5 days
Children <8 yr: PO 500,000 IU/24 hr × 3 days, then 50,000 IU/24 hr × 14 days; maintenance 10,000-20,000 IU/24 hr × 60 days
Severe Vitamin A Deficiency
Infants <1 yr: IM 7500-15,000 IU/24 hr × 10 days
Children 1-8 yr: IM 17,500-35,000 IU/24 hr × 10 days
Children >8 yr and adults: IM/PO 100,000 IU q24h × 3 days, then 50,000 IU/24 hr × 14 days; maintenance 10,000-20,000 IU/24 hr × 60 days

MECHANISM AND INDICATIONS
Mechanism: Fat-soluble vitamin which plays a vital role in vision and maintaining the integrity of mucosal and epithelial cells; also important in bone growth and other body functions; forms include preformed vitamin A as retinol or carotene; β-carotene is converted to retinol in the intestinal mucosa
Indications: Prevention and treatment of vitamin A deficiency; deficiencies rarely occur without a concurrent medical basis, may occur with biliary tract or pancreatic disease, sprue, colitis, hepatic cirrhosis, celiac disease, regional enteritis, partial gastrectomy, cystic fibrosis

PHARMACOKINETICS
Metabolism: Liver
Excretion: Feces, urine

CONTRAINDICATIONS AND PRECAUTIONS
• Contraindicated with hypervitaminosis A, hypersensitivity to vitamin A; do not administer IV
• Use cautiously with PO use in malabsorption disorders; with kidney disease pregnancy, lactation

INTERACTIONS
Drug
• Decreased absorption with cholestyramine
• Increased plasma levels with oral contraceptives
• Decreased absorption with neomycin
• Interference with warfarin effect possible with large doses

---

✤ Available in Canada.

Lab
- Falsely elevated cholesterol, triglycerides, BUN, bilirubin
- Increased liver function tests, PT

SIDE EFFECTS
CNS: Tiredness, dizziness, irritability, headache, bulging fontanel or bulging eyes
CV: Gum bleeding
DERM: Cracking of skin, hair loss, scaling, itching, erythema; tongue, lips, gum inflammation; yellowing of skin and eyes
EENT: Miosis, papilledema
GI: Nausea, diarrhea, vomiting
GU: Hypermenorrhea
Other: Delayed growth, night sweats, joint and bone pain, swelling of legs and ankles, decreased menstrual periods, hypercalcemia, fatal anaphylaxis has occurred after IV administration

TOXICITY AND OVERDOSE
Clinical signs: Acute signs of hypervitaminosis A can be noted 8-12 hr after dose (headache, nausea, vomiting, blurred or double vision); toxicity can occur after a single dose of 25,000 IU/kg or chronic use of 4,000 IU/kg for 6-15 mo
Treatment: Discontinue drug; administer IV saline, prednisolone, calcitonin if hypercalcemia persists; monitor liver function tests; provide supportive care

PATIENT CARE MANAGEMENT
Assessment
- Assess history of hypersensitivity to vitamin A
- Determine serum levels to establish deficiency (serum levels <30 mcg/ml of retinol)
- Evaluate for presence of malabsorption; vitamin A is fat-soluble and requires bile, pancreatic lipase, and dietary fat for absorption
- Evaluate appropriateness of dosage; prolonged use of doses >25,000 IU/24 hr requires close supervision
- Assess other medications, OTC drugs that may contain vitamin A
- Obtain dietary assessment to evaluate possibility that other vitamin deficiencies may exist

Interventions
- Administer water-soluble PO form or bile salts concurrently to pts with malabsorption because of inadequate bile secretion
- Take with food; liquid preparations may be mixed with juice

---

NURSING ALERT

Assess dosage to avoid toxicity; toxicity can occur after a single dose of 25,000 IU/kg or chronic use of 4,000 IU/kg for 6-15 mo

Do not administer IV; may cause anaphylaxis

Evaluation
- Evaluate therapeutic response (decreased vitamin A deficiency symptoms)
- Monitor for side effects suggesting overdose (nausea, vomiting, headache, blurred vision)
- Monitor growth in children

PATIENT AND FAMILY EDUCATION
Teach/instruct
- To take as directed at prescribed intervals for prescribed length of time
- To evaluate other medications, OTC drugs for interactions

Warn/advise
- To notify care provider of hypersensitivity, side effects
- Do not take more than recommended dose; doses >25,000 IU should be taken only under a provider's directions
- Modify time schedule to avoid taking vitamin A with cholestyramine or other medications
- Watch for signs of toxicity or overdose; consult care provider

Encourage
- Encourage and explain importance of a balanced diet and foods high in vitamin A; common sources are cod liver, halibut, tuna, shark, sweet potatoes, carrots, green leafy vegetables, egg, whole milk products

---

✦ Available in Canada.

STORAGE
- Store in an airtight, moisture-free container
- Protect from freezing and light

---

vitamin D (chole-calciferol, vitamin D$_3$; ergocalciferol, vitamin D$_2$)

Brand Name(s): Calciferol, Drisdol, D-Vi-Sol

Classification: Fat-soluble vitamin, antihypocalcemic agent

Pregnancy Category: C

AVAILABLE PREPARATIONS
Liquid: 8,000 U/ml (as ergocalciferol)
Caps: 0.625 mg (25,000 U), 1.25 mg (50,000 U)
Tabs: 1.25 mg (50,000 U)
- 1 IU vitamin D = 0.025 mcg vitamin D$_3$

ROUTES AND DOSAGES
See Appendix F, Recommended Daily Dietary Allowances
Nutritional Rickets and Osteomalacia
Children and adults, normal GI function: PO 25-125 mcg/24 hr
Malabsorption: Children PO 250-625 mcg/24 hr; adults, PO 250-7500 mcg/24 hr
Familial Hypophosphatemia/ Vitamin D Resistant Rickets
- Take with phosphate supplements
Children: PO 1000-2000 mcg/24 hr, increase in 250-500 mcg increments at 3-4 mo intervals prn
Adults: PO 250 mcg-1500 mcg/ 24 hr
Vitamin D-Dependent Rickets
Children: PO 75-125 mcg/24 hr
Adults: PO 250 mcg-1.5 mg/24 hr
Hypoparathyroidism
- Take with calcium supplements
Children: PO 1.25-5 mg/24 hr
Adults: PO 625 mcg-5 mg/24 hr

Renal Failure
Children: PO 0.1-1 mg/24 hr
Adults: PO 0.5 mg/24 hr

MECHANISM AND INDICATIONS
Mechanism: Regulates serum Ca and phosphate concentrations by promoting absorption from the GI tract and bone resorption; important in bone development and maintenance; involved in Mg metabolism; 1.25-dihydroxyvitamin D is the most active form of Vitamin D$_3$ in stimulating intestinal Ca transport
Indications: Treatment and prevention of rickets, hypoparathyroidism, hypophosphatemia

PHARMACOKINETICS
Peak: 1 mo following daily doses
Half-life: 24 hr
Metabolism: Liver, kidneys
Excretion: Bile (feces), urine

CONTRAINDICATIONS AND PRECAUTIONS
- Contraindicated with drug hypersensitivity, hypercalcemia, malabsorption syndrome, vitamin D toxicity
- Use cautiously with impaired renal function, heart disease, renal stones, arteriosclerosis, pregnancy

INTERACTIONS
Drug
- Increased risk of cardiac arrhythmias with cardiac glycosides
- Risk of hypercalcemia in pts with hypoparathyroidism with thiazide diuretics
- Increased risk of hypermagnesemia with Mg-containing antacids
- Decreased drug effects with corticosteroids
- Increased requirements possible with chronic use of cholestyramine or mineral oil
Lab
- False increase in serum cholesterol levels
- Increased AST, ALT, bilirubin

SIDE EFFECTS

CNS: Headache, dizziness, ataxia, irritability, weakness, somnolence, seizures
CV: Hypertension, arrhythmias
DERM: Pruritus
GI: Anorexia, nausea, vomiting, diarrhea, constipation, thirst, metallic taste
GU: Polyuria, albuminuria, hypercalciuria, nocturia, renal calculi
Other: Hypercalcemia, sensitivity to light, hyperphosphatemia, calcifications of soft tissues, bone and muscle pain, wt loss, weakness, fever, psychosis

TOXICITY AND OVERDOSE

Clinical signs: Weakness, anorexia, nausea, wt loss, stiffness, hypertension, convulsion
Treatment: Check labs for hypercalcemia, hyperphosphatemia; discontinue vitamin D supplement, increase fluids, low Ca diet; supportive care; a loop diuretic may be needed to increase Ca excretion

PATIENT CARE MANAGEMENT

Assessment

• Assess history of hypersensitivity to vitamin D (especially in infants)
• Obtain baseline serum Ca, PO_4, Mg., alk phos, BUN, urine Ca, creatinine
• Assess dietary history for adequate intake of vitamin D, Ca and PO_4, adequate dietary Ca is needed for clinical response; see Appendix F for Ca requirement

Interventions

• Oral dosing preferred; tabs should be swallowed whole, not crushed or chewed
• Check dosage; intake of >60,000 U/24 hr can cause hypercalcemia
• IM preferable for those with malabsorption as bile salts are required for absorption
• Inject deeply into large muscle mass, administer slowly, rotate injection sites; avoid IV injection
• For pts with hyperphosphatemia or phosphate restrictions a binding agent may be necessary to reduce risk of metastatic calcifications and renal calculi
• Maintain age-appropriate fluid intake

NURSING ALERT

Serum Ca × PO_4 should not exceed 70 mg/dl to avoid ectopic calcification

Monitor for symptoms of toxicity (dry mouth, metallic taste, nausea may be early indicators)

Evaluation

• Evaluate therapeutic response (absence of rickets or osteomalacia, decreased bone pain, normal Ca, PO_4 levels)
• Monitor serum Ca, PO_4, Mg, BUN, alk phos, urine Ca, creatinine; serum Ca × PO_4 should not be >70 mg/dl to avoid ectopic calcification
• Evaluate for symptoms of toxicity (dry mouth, metallic taste, and nausea may be early indicators of toxicity)
• Dosage adjustment is required once clinical response goal is achieved

PATIENT AND FAMILY TEACHING

Teach/instruct

• To take as directed at prescribed intervals for prescribed length of time

Warn/advise

• To notify care provider of hypersensitivity, side effects, symptoms of toxicity (headache, weakness, vomiting, diarrhea, loss of appetite, wt loss, abdominal cramps, dry mouth, bone and muscle pain)
• To restrict Mg-containing antacids to avoid Mg overload

Encourage

• Explain the importance of a balanced diet to meet nutrient requirements; see Appendix F, Table of Recommended Daily Dietary Allowances
• That common sources of vitamin D include fortified milk and milk products, eggs, sardines, fresh water fish, chicken livers, cod liver oil

STORAGE
• Store at room temp in an air-tight container
• Protect from light, heat, moisture

---

vitamin E
(α tocopherol)

Brand Name(s): Aquasol E✤, Vita-Plus E, Vitec, Webber Water-Soluble Vitamin E✤

Classification: Fat-soluble vitamin

Pregnancy Category: C

AVAILABLE PREPARATIONS
Oral drops: 50 mg/ml
Tabs: 200 IU, 400 IU
Caps: 50 IU, 100 IU, 200 IU, 400 IU, 500 IU, 600 IU, 1000 IU
Caps, water miscible: 73.5 mg, 147 mg, 165 mg, 330 mg
• 1 IU = 1 mg dl-α tocopherol acetate; 1.1 IU = 1 mg dl-α tocopherol; 1.36 IU = 1 mg d-α tocopherol acetate; 1.49 IU = 1 mg d-α tocopherol; 1.21 IU = 1 mg d-α tocopherol acid succinate; 0.89 IU = 1 mg dl-α tocopherol acid succinate

ROUTES AND DOSAGES
See Appendix F, Table of Recommended Daily Dietary Allowances: requirement is related to average daily intake of polyunsaturated fatty acids

Vitamin E Deficiency
Neonates, premature or low birth weight infants: PO 25-50 IU/24 hr until 6-19 wk of age or 7 IU/L of formula
Children: PO 1 IU/kg/24 hr
Adults: PO 60-75 IU/24 hr, maximum 300 IU/24 hr

Cholestasis, Biliary Atresia, Fat Malabsorption
Children and adults: PO use water-soluble form 15-25 IU/kg/24 hr and decrease as levels approach normal

Cystic Fibrosis
Children and adults: PO 100-400 IU/24 hr

β-thalassemia
Children and adults: PO 750 IU/24 hr

Sickle Cell Anemia
Children and adults: PO 450 IU/24 hr

MECHANISM AND INDICATIONS
Mechanism: Prevents certain oxidative reactions in the body, protects cell membranes from damage from free radicals; protects polyunsaturated fatty acids in membranes against peroxidation and preserves RBC wall integrity; may act as cofactor in enzyme systems; requires bile for absorption
Indications: Treatment and prevention of vitamin E deficiency in premature infant and pts with impaired fat absorption

PHARMACOKINETICS
Metabolism: Liver
Excretion: Feces

CONTRAINDICATIONS AND PRECAUTIONS
• Use cautiously with pregnancy

INTERACTIONS
Drug
• Increased bleeding tendency with oral anticoagulants

SIDE EFFECTS
CNS: Fatigue, weakness, headache
DERM: Rash
EENT: Blurred vision
GI: Nausea, diarrhea, flatulence

TOXICITY AND OVERDOSE
Clinical signs: Symptoms of increased B/P
Treatment: Supportive care

PATIENT CARE MANAGEMENT
Assessment
• Assess history of hypersensitivity to vitamin E
• Assess vitamin E levels, BUN, creatinine, CBC
• Assess absorptive abilities; pt may need concurrent administration of bile salts for absorption

---

✤ Available in Canada.

- Assess dietary intake; vitamin E deficiency rarely occurs alone
- Assess for other medication usage to assure optimal utilization

Interventions
- Administer PO with or after meals if GI upset occurs; liquid forms may be given orally or mixed with food
- Water-miscible preparation is useful for prevention of vitamin E deficiency for persons with fat malabsorption
- Maintain age-appropriate fluid intake

Evaluation
- Evaluate therapeutic response (normal vitamin E levels, absence of hemolytic anemia, decreased edema)
- Evaluate for side effects (nausea, diarrhea, weakness or blurred vision), hypersensitivity

PATIENT AND FAMILY EDUCATION

Teach/instruct
- To take as directed at prescribed intervals for prescribed length of time
- That liquid vitamin may be mixed with juice or food
- To assess for other medications, OTC drugs which might affect vitamin E effects

Warn/advise
- To notify care provider of hypersensitivity, side effects

Encourage
- To discuss the importance of a balanced diet to provide essential micronutrients; common dietary sources of vitamin E include vegetable oil, green leafy vegetables, nuts, wheat germ, eggs, meat, liver, dairy products, cereal

STORAGE
- Store at room temp in airtight light-resistant container
- Protect from heat or moisture

---

warfarin
Brand Name(s): Coumadin✤, Panwarfin, Sofarin, Warfilone✤
Classification: Anticoagulant
Pregnancy Category: D

AVAILABLE PREPARATIONS
Tabs: 1 mg, 2 mg, 2.5 mg, 5 mg, 7.5 mg, 10 mg
Inj: 50 ml vial

ROUTES AND DOSAGES
Children: PO/IV 0.2 mg/kg (maximum 10 mg) × 2 days, then adjust dosage to desired INR
Adults: PO/IV 5-15 mg for 2-5 days until desired INR is reached; then 2-10 mg qd titrated to INR level

IV administration
- Recommended concentration: Dilute with diluent
- Intermittent infusion rate: Administer through Y tube or stopcock at ≤25 mg/min

MECHANISM AND INDICATIONS
Mechanism: Inhibits action of vitamin K, blocking formation of type II, VII, IX, and X clotting factors
Indications: For use in pulmonary emboli, deep vein thrombosis, MI, atrial arrhythmias, postcardiac valve replacement

PHARMACOKINETICS
Onset of action: 12-24 hr
Peak: 1½-3 days
Half-life: 1½-2½ days
Metabolism: Liver
Excretion: Urine, feces

CONTRAINDICATIONS AND PRECAUTIONS
- Contraindicated with bleeding or hemorrhagic tendencies, hemophilia, leukemia, GI ulcers, subacute bacterial endocarditis, vitamin K deficiency, recent surgery, stroke, aneurysm
- Use cautiously with liver, kidney disease, diabetes, colitis, lactation, menstruation, in pts with drainage tubes, or regional or lumbar block anesthesia

---

✤ Available in Canada.

INTERACTIONS
Drug
• Increased drug effect with amiodarone, anabolic steroids, chloramphenicol, metronidazole, clofibrate, thyroid preparations, salicylates, streptokinase, urokinase, sulfonamides, ethacrynic acid, indomethacin, allopurinol, moxalactam, cefamandole, cefotetan, miconazole, quinidine, vitamin E, alcohol intoxication
• Decreased drug effect with rifampin, barbiturates, carbamazepine, oral contraceptives, corticosteroids, griseofulvin, vitamin K, cholestyramine, chronic alcohol abuse
• Increased or decreased drug effect with chloral hydrate
Lab
• Increased PT, PTT, LDH, INR
• False negative serum theophylline level

INCOMPATIBILITIES
• Amikacin, dextrose, epinephrine, metaraminol, oxytocin, promazine, tetracycline, vancomycin

SIDE EFFECTS
DERM: Petechiae, dermatitis, rash, urticaria, necrosis, alopecia, ecchymosis
GI: Diarrhea, vomiting, abdominal cramps nausea, melena, hematemesis, paralytic ileus, intestinal obstruction, hepatitis
GU: Excessive uterine bleeding, hematuria
HEME: Leukopenia, hemorrhage, eosinophilia, agranulocytosis

TOXICITY AND OVERDOSE
Clinical signs: Hematuria, internal or external bleeding, skin necrosis
Treatment: Withhold drug; administer vitamin K, fresh frozen plasma, whole blood

PATIENT CARE MANAGEMENT
Assessment
• Assess history of hypersensitivity to drug
• Assess blood studies (Hct, platelets, occult blood in stool)
• Assess baseline PT and INR

Interventions
• Administer at same time each day
• Avoid IM injections
Evaluation
• Evaluate regularly for bleeding (epistaxis, bruises, petechiae, hematuria, melena, hematemesis)
• Evaluate PT/INR regularly, qd initially, q 2-8 wk maintenance
• Evaluate need for dosage change based on PT/INR

PATIENT AND FAMILY EDUCATION
Teach/instruct
• To take as directed at prescribed intervals for prescribed length of time
• To carry medical alert identification
• About rationale for treatment, stressing importance of complying with drug regimen and follow up
• To watch for signs of bleeding and report immediately
• About rationale for avoiding hazardous activities, contact sports; use soft bristle toothbrush
• To report all medications to care provider
• That smoking may increase dosage requirement
Warn/advise
• Not to significantly alter intake of foods containing vitamin K (broccoli, cabbage, lettuce, spinach, turnip greens, pork or beef liver, tomatoes); wide variation in intake of these may alter anticoagulant effect of warfarin

STORAGE
• Store at room temp

---

zalcitabine
Brand Name(s): Hivid✽
Classification: Antiviral (synthetic pyrimidine nucleoside analog)
Pregnancy Category: C

AVAILABLE PREPARATIONS
Tabs: 0.375 mg, 0.75 mg

✽ Available in Canada.

ROUTES AND DOSAGES
Children >13 yr and adults: PO 0.75 mg administered concomitantly with zidovudine 200 mg q8h; no need to reduce dosage for wt to 30 kg; if peripheral neuropathy exists, initiate dosage at 0.375 mg zalcitabine q8h

MECHANISM AND INDICATIONS
Antiviral mechanism: Inhibits HIV replication by the conversion of zalcitabine by cellular enzymes to an active antiviral metabolite
Indications: Used to treat pts with advanced HIV infection who are resistant to zidovudine therapy or intolerant of zidovudine

PHARMACOKINETICS
Half-life: 1.62 hr
Excretion: Urine

CONTRAINDICATIONS AND PRECAUTIONS
• Contraindicated in children <13 yr; with known hypersensitivity to zalcitabine
• Use cautiously with renal or hepatic impairment, peripheral neuropathy, pregnancy, lactation

INTERACTIONS
Drug
• Increased risk of peripheral neuropathy with other drugs that can cause peripheral neuropathy (chloramphenicol, cisplatin, dapsone, disulfiram, ethionamide, glutethimide, gold, hydralazine, iodoquinol, isoniazid, metronidazole, nitrofurantoin, phenytoin, ribavirin, vincristine
• Increased risk of peripheral neuropathy with amphotericin, foscarnet, aminoglycosides
• Increased risk of pancreatitis with drugs having potential to cause pancreatitis
Nutrition
• Decreased absorption if given with food

INCOMPATIBILITIES
• Use with didenosine not recommended

SIDE EFFECTS
CNS: Peripheral neuropathy, headache, seizures, asthma, insomnia, CNS depression, fever
CV: Hypertension, vasodilation, dysrhythmia, syncope, palpitations, tachycardia
DERM: Rash, pruritus, alopecia
EENT: Ear pain, photophobia, visual impairment
GI: Pancreatitis, diarrhea, nausea, vomiting, abdominal pain, constipation, stomatitis, elevated liver function tests
GU: Toxic nephropathy, polyuria
HEME: Leukopenia, granulocytopenia, thrombocytopenia, anemia
RESP: Cough, dyspnea

TOXICITY AND OVERDOSE
Clinical signs: Peripheral neuropathy
Treatment: Supportive care

PATIENT CARE MANAGEMENT
Assessment
• Assess history of hypersensitivity to zalcitabine
• Assess hematologic function (CBC, differential, platelet count), renal function (BUN, creatinine, I&O), hepatic function (ALT, AST, bilirubin)
Interventions
• Administer PO 1 hr before or 2 hr after meals; tab can be crushed, mixed with food or fluid
• Maintain age-appropriate fluid intake
• Administer antibiotics, antivirals as ordered to prevent opportunistic infections

> **NURSING ALERT**
> Discontinue drug if signs of pancreatitis develop
>
> Withhold drug if WBC <4000 or platelet count <75,000

Evaluation
• Evaluate therapeutic response (control of symptoms, decreased incidence of opportunistic infections)
• Monitor hematologic function (CBC, differential, platelet count);

treatment may need to be discontinued, restarted after hematologic recovery

• Monitor renal function (BUN, creatinine, I&O), hepatic function (ALT, AST, bilirubin)

• Monitor for signs of neuropathy (tingling or pain in hands and feet, distal numbness)

• Monitor for signs of pancreatitis (abdominal pain, nausea, vomiting, elevated liver function tests); treatment may need to be discontinued because condition can be fatal

• Monitor for signs of opportunistic infection (such as pneumonia, meningitis, sepsis)

PATIENT AND FAMILY EDUCATION
Teach/instruct
• To take as directed at prescribed intervals for prescribed length of time

• About HIV disease, measures to prevent transmission, reasons for medication therapy (including concomitant use of antibiotic and antiviral medications), include information that pt is still infectious during zalcitabine therapy, and that zalcitabine will not cure the illness but will control symptoms

Warn/advise
• To notify care provider of hypersensitivity, side effects, opportunistic infection

• To notify care provider if signs of infection (fever, sore throat, flu-like symptoms), signs of anemia (fatigue, headache, faintness, shortness of breath, irritability), bruising, bleeding develop

• That hair loss may occur during therapy; pt may choose to wear a wig or hairpiece

STORAGE
• Store at room temp in tightly closed container

---

zidovudine (AZT)
Brand Name(s): Apo-Zidovudine✤, Novo-AZT✤, Retrovir✤

Classification: Antiviral (thymidine analog)

Pregnancy Category: C

AVAILABLE PREPARATIONS
Syr: 50 mg/5 ml
Caps: 100 mg
Inj: 10 mg/ml

ROUTES AND DOSAGES
• Dosages may differ depending on protocol used.

Infants >3 mo/children: PO 90-180 mg/m^2/dose q6h (maximum 200 mg q6h); IV continuous infusion 0.5-1.8 mg/kg/hr, intermittent infusion 100 mg/m^2/dose q6h

Adults: PO, for asymptomatic infection, 100 mg q4h while awake (maximum 500 mg/24 hr); for symptomatic HIV infection, 200 mg q4h for 1 mo, then 100 mg q4h (maximum 600 mg/24 hr); IV 1-2 mg/kg/dose q4h

IV administration
• Recommended concentration: 1-4 mg/ml in D_5W

• Maximum concentration: 4 mg/ml

• Intermittent infusion rate: Over 60 min

MECHANISM AND INDICATIONS
Antiviral mechanism: Inhibits viral replication by interfering with the HIV viral RNA-dependent DNA polymerase

Indications: Used to treat pts with HIV infections who have had at least one confirmed episode of *Pneumocystis carinii* pneumonia, CD_4 cell counts of ≤500/mm^3, HIV-related symptoms, or are asymptomatic with evidence of HIV-related immunosuppression

PHARMACOKINETICS
Peak: 0.5-1.5 hr
Distribution: Significant penetration into CSF

Half-life: 1 hr
Metabolism: Liver
Excretion: Urine

CONTRAINDICATIONS AND PRECAUTIONS
• Contraindicated with life-threatening hypersensitivity to zidovudine
• Use cautiously with bone marrow compromise, renal or hepatic impairment, anemia or granulocytopenia, myopathy, pregnancy, lactation

INTERACTIONS
Drug
• Increased risk of granulocytopenia with acetaminophen, cimetidine, indomethacin, lorazepam, probenecid, aspirin
• Increased risk of toxicity from dapsone, pentamidine, amphotericin B, flucytosine, vincristine, vinblastine, doxorubicin, interferon
Lab
• Depression of erythrocytes, leukocytes, platelets in peripheral blood possible

INCOMPATIBILITIES
• Blood, protein products

SIDE EFFECTS
CNS: Malaise, dizziness, asthenia, manic syndrome, seizures, confusion, tremor, fever, severe headache, insomnia
DERM: Rash, blue pigmentation of nails
GI: Nausea, diarrhea, vomiting, anorexia, cholestatic hepatitis
HEME: Granulocytopenia, thrombocytopenia, leukopenia, anemia
Other: Myalgia

TOXICITY AND OVERDOSE
Clinical signs: Nausea, vomiting
Treatment: Supportive treatment

PATIENT CARE MANAGEMENT
Assessment
• Assess history of hypersensitivity to zidovudine
• Assess hematologic function (CBC, differential, platelet count), renal function (BUN, creatinine, I&O), hepatic function (ALT, AST, bilirubin), CD_4 cell count

Interventions
• Administer PO 30 min before or 1 hr after meals with a full glass of water; cap should be swallowed whole
• Do not administer IM, IV push, or by rapid infusion
• Maintain age-appropriate fluid intake
• Administer antibiotics, antivirals as ordered to prevent opportunistic infections; blood transfusions as ordered to treat anemia

---

NURSING ALERT

Temporarily discontinue drug if marked anemia or granulocytopenia develop

Do not administer IM, IV push, or by rapid infusion

Evaluation
• Evaluate therapeutic response (control of symptoms, decreased incidence of opportunistic infections)
• Monitor hematologic function (CBC, differential, platelet count) for anemia, granulocytopenia at least every 2 wk; treatment may need to be discontinued and restarted after hematologic recovery
• Monitor renal function (BUN, creatinine, I&O), hepatic function (ALT, AST, bilirubin)
• Monitor for signs or symptoms of opportunistic infection (such as pneumonia, meningitis, sepsis)
• Monitor for signs or symptoms of neurotoxicity if concomitant therapy with acyclovir

PATIENT AND FAMILY EDUCATION
Teach/instruct
• To take as directed at prescribed intervals for prescribed length of time; when drug must be taken q4h around the clock, suggest ways to avoid missing doses (set an alarm clock)
• About HIV disease, measures to prevent transmission, reasons for medication therapy (including concomitant use of antibiotic or antiviral medications); include in-

Z

---

formation that pt is still infectious during AZT therapy, that AZT will not cure illness but will control symptoms

Warn/advise

• To notify care provider of hypersensitivity, side effects, opportunistic infection (especially bruising, bleeding, poor healing, fatigue, malaise, sore throat, swollen lymph nodes, fever)

• To consult care provider before taking OTC medications (including aspirin, acetaminophen, indomethacin)

STORAGE

• Store syr, caps, undiluted vials at room temp protected from light, moisture

• Stable after dilution at room temp 8 hr, refrigerated 24 hr

APPENDIX A ═══════════

Table for Determining Body Surface Area (m²)

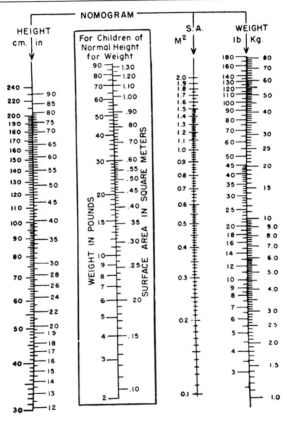

NOMOGRAM

BSA is indicated where straight line that connects height *(on the left)* and weight *(on the right)* levels intersects BSA column. Modified from data of Boyd E, by West CD. In Behrman RE, Vaughn VC, eds: *Nelson textbook of pediatrics,* ed 13, Philadelphia, 1987, WB Saunders. Reprinted with permission.

APPENDIX B ═══════════

U.S. Food and Drug Administration Pregnancy Risk Categories

CATEGORY A

Well-controlled studies in women do not demonstrate fetal risk. The risk of harm to fetus is minimal.

CATEGORY B

Animal studies do not show risk; data from studies in pregnant women or animals are insufficient to show clear evidence of risk to fetus; or studies in women have failed to demonstrate fetal harm.

CATEGORY C

Animal studies show adverse effects; however, there are no studies in women or no data available from animal or human studies. In some situations the benefits of use may outweigh the possible risks to the fetus.

CATEGORY D

Human fetal harm has been clearly demonstrated. In life-threatening illness the benefits of use may outweigh the risks to the fetus.

CATEGORY X

Human fetal harm has been clearly demonstrated. Possible risks to the fetus outweigh any possible benefit to the pregnant woman. Do not use during pregnancy.

From Keen JH, Baird MS, Allen JH: *Mosby's Critical care and emergency drug reference,* St. Louis, 1994, Mosby.

Appendix C ═══════════

Controlled Substances Classification

Controlled substances are classified by the U.S. Drug Enforcement Administration (DEA). State laws often are more stringent than federal laws.

Description of Categories

Drug Examples

Schedule I
No accepted medical use; high potential for abuse; drug may be used for research with application approved by DEA

Cannabinol: marijuana, hashish, tetrahydrocannabinol
Hallucinogens: LSD, MDA, DMT, peyote, mescaline, psilocybin

Schedule II
High abuse potential exists, with possibility for severe psychological or physical dependence

Narcotics: morphine, opium, codeine, hydromorphone, methadone, meperidine, oxycodone
Stimulants: cocaine, amphetamine, dextroamphetamine, methamphetamine, methylphenidate
Depressants: amobarbital, methaqualone, pentobarbital, phencyclidine, secobarbital
Other: Anabolic steroids

Schedule III
Abuse potential is less than that of schedule I or II drugs; misuse leads to psychologic or physical dependence

Narcotics: opiates in limited amounts and combined with other non-narcotic drugs (e.g., acetaminophen with codeine), paregoric
Depressants: barbiturates (except those listed under other schedules)

Adapted from Keen JH, Baird MS, Allen JH: *Mosby's Critical care and emergency drug reference,* St. Louis, 1994, Mosby.

Schedule IV

Abuse potential is less than that of schedule III drugs; misuse leads to psychologic or possibly physical dependence

Narcotics: pentazine, propoxyphene

Depressants: benzodiazepines, chloral hydrate, paraldehyde, phenobarbital

Schedule V

Abuse potential is less than that of schedule IV drugs; schedule V drugs contain limited amount of narcotics; category includes preparations used for coughs, diarrhea

Buprenorphine, diphenoxylate/ atropine, loperamide, antitussives containing codeine/ dihydrocodeine

Appendix D

Childhood Immunizations: Schedule and Dosages

Hepatitis B (HBV)	Birth, 2 mo, 6-18 mo Alternate schedule: 0-2 mo, 4 mo, 6-18 mo	IM 0.5 ml (check manufacturer's recommendations) SC with bleeding disorders
Diphtheria, tetanus, pertussis (DTP)	2 mo, 4 mo, 6 mo, 15-18 mo (DTP or DTaP), 4-6 yr (DTaP or DTP), 14-16 yr (Td)	IM 0.5 ml
Haemophilus influenzae type B (Hib)	2 mo, 4 mo, 6 mo, 12-15 mo (not required for Pedvax Hib [PRP-OMP])	IM 0.5 ml
Polio (OPV)	2 mo, 4 mo, 6-18 mo, 4-6 yr	PO 0.5 ml or 2 drops or entire contents of single-dose dispenser
	or	
Polio (IPV)	2 mo, 4 mo, 10-16 mo (6-12 mo after second dose), 4-6 yr	SC/IM 0.5 ml
Measles, mumps, rubella (MMR)	12-15 mo, 4-6 yr *or* 11-13 yr	SC 0.5 ml
Varicella zoster virus vaccine	12-18 mo or 11-12 yr	SC 0.5 ml (>13 yr: additional 0.5 ml 4-8 wk after initial dose)

Adapted from Committee on Infectious Diseases American Academy of Pediatrics: *1994 redbook: report of the committee on infectious diseases,* ed 23, Elk Grove Village, Ill, 1994, American Academy of Pediatrics.

APPENDIX E

Selected Oral Contraceptives for Use by Adolescents (low estrogen [30-35 mcg]/low progestin)

	Estrogen	mcg	Progestin	mg
Monophasic				
Demulen 1/35	Ethinyl estradiol	35	Ethydiacetate	1.0
Desogen	Ethinyl estradiol	30	Desogestrel	0.15
Lo-Ovral	Ethinyl estradiol	30	Norgestrel	0.3
Nordette	Ethinyl estradiol	30	Levonorgestrel	0.15
Norethin 1/35	Ethinyl estradiol	35	Norethindrone	1.0
Norinyl 1/35	Ethinyl estradiol	35	Norethindrone	1.0
Ortho-Cept	Ethinyl estradiol	30	Desogestrel	0.15
Ortho-Cyclen	Ethinyl estradiol	35	Norgestimate	0.25
Ortho-Novum 1/35	Ethinyl estradiol	35	Norethindrone	1.0
Ovcon	Ethinyl estradiol	35	Norethindrone	0.4
Multiphasic				
Ortho-Novum 7/7/7	Ethinyl estradiol	35 (7)	Norethindrone	0.5 (7)
	Ethinyl estradiol	35 (7)	Norethindrone	0.75 (7)
	Ethinyl estradiol	35 (7)	Norethindrone	1.0 (7)
Tri-Norinyl	Ethinyl estradiol	35 (7)	Norethindrone	0.5 (7)
	Ethinyl estradiol	35 (7)	Norethindrone	1.0 (9)
	Ethinyl estradiol	35 (7)	Norethindrone	0.5 (5)
Triphasil	Ethinyl estradiol	30 (6)	Levonorgestrel	0.05 (6)
	Ethinyl estradiol	40 (5)	Levonorgestrel	0.075 (5)
	Ethinyl estradiol	30 (10)		
	Levonorgestrel	0.125 (10)		

Adapted from Dickey RP: *Managing contraceptive pill patients,* ed 8, Durant, Okla, 1994, Essential Medical Information Systems, Inc.

APPENDIX F

Table of Recommended Daily Dietary Allowances

| | | WEIGHT | | HEIGHT | | PROTEIN | FAT-SOLUBLE VITAMINS | | |
	AGE (YEARS)	kg	lb	cm	in	(g)	VIT. A (µg RE)†	VIT. D (µg)‡	VIT. E (mg α TE)§
Infants	0-0.5	6	13	60	24	13	375	7.5	3
	0.5-1.0	9	20	71	28	14	375	10	4
Children	1-3	13	29	90	35	16	400	10	6
	4-6	20	44	112	44	24	500	10	7
	7-10	28	62	132	52	28	700	10	7
Males	11-14	45	99	157	62	45	1000	10	10
	15-18	66	145	176	69	59	1000	10	10
	19-24	70	154	177	70	58	1000	10	10
	25-50	70	154	178	70	63	1000	5	10
	51+	70	154	178	70	63	1000	5	10
Females	11-14	46	101	157	62	46	800	10	8
	15-18	55	120	163	64	44	800	10	8
	19-22	55	120	163	64	46	800	10	8
	23-50	55	120	163	64	50	800	5	8
	51+	55	120	163	64	50	800	5	8
Pregnant						60	1300	10	10
Lactating						65	1200	10	12

From Food and Nutrition Board, National Academy of Sciences–National Research Council, Washington, DC, 1989. From McKenry LM, Salerno E: *Pharmacology in nursing,* ed 19, St. Louis, 1992, Mosby, pp. 1270-1271.

*The allowances are intended to provide for individual variations among most normal persons as they live in the United States under usual environmental stresses. Diets should be based on a variety of common foods in order to provide other nutrients for which human requirements have been less well defined.

†Retinol equivalents, 1 Retinol equivalent = 1 µg retinol or 6 µg β carotene.

‡As cholecalciferol, 10 µg cholecalciferol = 400 IU vitamin D.

§α-Tocopherol equivalents, 1 mg d-α-tocopherol = 1 α TE.

	WATER-SOLUBLE VITAMINS							MINERALS					
	VIT. C (mg)	THIAMIN (mg)	RIBOFLAVIN (mg)	NIACIN (mg NE)‖	VIT. B$_6$ (mg)	FOLACIN¶ (µg)	VIT. B$_{12}$ (µg)	Ca (mg)	PO$_4$ (mg)	Mg (mg)	Fe (mg)	Zn (mg)	I (µg)
Infants	35	0.3	0.4	6	0.3	30	0.5	360	240	50	10	3	40
	35	0.5	0.6	8	0.6	45	1.5	540	360	70	15	5	50
Children	45	0.7	0.8	9	0.9	100	2.0	800	800	150	15	10	70
	45	0.9	1.0	11	1.3	200	2.5	800	800	200	10	10	90
	45	1.2	1.4	16	1.6	300	3.0	800	800	250	10	10	120
Males	50	1.4	1.6	18	1.8	400	3.0	1200	1200	350	18	15	150
	60	1.4	1.7	18	2	400	3.0	1200	1200	400	18	15	150
	60	1.5	1.7	19	2.2	400	3.0	800	800	350	10	15	150
	60	1.4	1.6	18	2.2	400	3.0	800	800	350	10	15	150
	60	1.2	1.4	16	2.2	400	3.0	800	800	350	10	15	150
Females	50	1.1	1.3	15	1.8	400	3.0	1200	1200	300	18	15	150
	60	1.1	1.3	14	2	400	3.0	1200	1200	300	18	15	150
	60	1.1	1.3	14	2	400	3.0	800	800	300	18	15	150
	60	1.0	1.2	13	2	400	3.0	800	800	300	18	15	150
	60	1.0	1.2	13	2	400	3.0	800††	800	300	10	15	150
Pregnant	+20	+0.4	+0.3	+2	+0.6	+400	+1.0	+400	+400	+150	**	+5	+025
Lactating	+40	+0.5	+0.5	+5	+0.5	+100	+1.0	+400	+400	+150	**	+10	+050

‖NE (niacin equivalent) is equal to 1 mg of niacin or 60 mg of dietary tryptophan.

¶The folacin allowances refer to dietary sources as determined by *Lactobacillus casei* assay after treatment with enzymes ("conjugates") to make polyglutamyl forms of the vitamin available for the test organism.

#The RDA for vitamin B$_{12}$ in infants is based on average concentration of the vitamin in human milk. The allowances after weaning are based on energy intake (as recommended).

**The increased requirement during pregnancy cannot be met by the iron content of habitual American diets nor by the existing iron stores of many women; therefore the use of 30–60 mg of supplemental iron is recommended. Iron needs during lactation are not substantially different from those of nonpregnant women, but continued supple-

APPENDIX G

Nonprescription Medications

Drug	Indications, Dosage, and Route	Remarks
Cough and cold		
brompheniramine (Dimetane)	*Antihistamine* 2 mg/5 ml, 4 mg tabs 2-6 yr: PO ½ tsp q4-6h 6-12 yr: PO 1 tsp or ½ tab q4-6h ≥12 yr: PO 2 tsp or 1 tab q4-6h	May cause drowsiness; use cautiously May cause excitability in children Use cautiously with asthma, pulmonary disease, heart disease, diabetes
chlorpheniramine (Chlor-trimeton)	*Antihistamine* 2 mg/5 ml, 4 mg tabs 2-5 yr: PO ½ tsp q4-6h 6-11 yr: PO 1 tsp or ½ tab q4-6h ≥12 yr: PO 2 tsp or 1 tab q4-6h	May cause drowsiness; use cautiously May cause excitability in children Use cautiously with asthma, pulmonary disease, heart disease, diabetes
dextromethorphan	*Cough suppressant* 10 mg/5 ml 2-6 yr: PO ½ tsp q4h 6-12 yr: PO 1 tsp q4h ≥12 yr: PO 2 tsp q4h	Use cautiously with asthma, chronic cough, or if cough is accompanied by excess mucus Do not use for >5 days; see care provider
diphenhydramine (Benadryl)	*Antihistamine* 6.25 mg/5 ml, 12.5 mg/5 ml, 25 mg caps 2-6 yr: PO ½ tsp q4-6h 6-12 yr: PO 1-2 tsp q4-6h 12 yr: PO 2-4 tsp or 1-2 caps q4-6h	May cause drowsiness; use cautiously May cause excitability in children Use cautiously with asthma, pulmonary disease, heart disease, diabetes

Drug	Indications, Dosage, and Route	Remarks
guaifenesin (Robitussin)	*Expectorant* 100 mg/5 ml 2-6 yr: PO ½-1 tsp q4h 6-12 yr: PO 1-2 tsp q4h ≥12 yr: PO 2-4 tsp q4h	Use cautiously with asthma, chronic cough, or if accompanied by excess mucus Do not use for >5 days; see care provider
oxymetazoline (Afrin, Neo-Synephrine, Maximum Strength Duration)	*Topical nasal decongestant / vasoconstrictor* 0.25% sol ≥6 yr: 2 sprays into each nostril bid 0.025% (children's strength) 2-5 yr: 2 drops into each nostril bid	Do not exceed recommended dosage Do not use for >3 days Use of dispenser by more than one person may spread infection Do not use with heart disease, hypertension, thyroid disease
phenylephrine hydrochloride (Neo-Synephrine, Dristan, Nostril, Vicks Sinus Nasal Decongestant)	*Topical nasal decongestant / vasoconstrictor* 0.25% sol ≥6 yr: 2 drops into each nostril q6h 0.125% sol 2-6 yr: 2 drops into each nostril q6h	Do not exceed recommended dosage Do not use for >3 days Use of dispenser by more than one person may spread infection Do not use with heart disease, hypertension, thyroid disease
phenylpropanolamine hydrochloride (in combination with Triaminic, Coricidin, Dimetapp, Contac, Allerest)	*Decongestant* 12.5 mg/5 ml, 12.5 mg tab 2-6 yr: PO ½ tsp q4-6h 6-12 yr: PO 1 tsp or 1 tab q4-6h ≥12 yr: PO 2 tsp or 2 tab q4-6h	Do not use with heart disease, antihistamine in hypertension, thyroid disease, diabetes, asthma May cause excitability, sleeplessness, nervousness Do not exceed recommended dosage Do not administer to pt taking medication for hypertension or depression
pseudoephedrine hydrochloride (Sudafed)	*Decongestant* 30 mg/5 ml, 30 mg tabs 2-6 yr: PO ½ tsp q4h 6-12 yr: PO 1 tsp or 1 tab q4h ≥12 yr: PO 2 tsp or 2 tabs q4h	Do not use with heart disease, hypertension, thyroid disease, diabetes, asthma May cause excitability, sleeplessness, nervousness Do not exceed recommended dosage

Drug	Indications, Dosage, and Route	Remarks
pseudoephedrine hydrochloride (Sudafed)—cont'd		Do not administer to pt taking medication for hypertension or depression
triprolidine (Actifed)	*Antihistamine* 1.25 mg/5 ml 1.25 mg tabs/caps 2-6 yr: PO ½ tsp q4-6h 6-12 yr: PO 1 tsp or 1 tab/cap q4-6h ≥12 yr: PO 2 tsp or 2 cap q4-6h	May cause drowsiness; use cautiously Do not exceed recommended dosage Use cautiously with asthma, heart disease, diabetes, thyroid disease
Gastrointestinal		
aluminum hydroxide (Gaviscon, Gelusil, Maalox Plus, WinGel)	*Antacid* Children: PO 5-15 ml qid Adults: PO 15-30 ml qid	May have laxative effect Do not use with kidney disease Do not use with Na-restricted diet
bisacodyl (Dulcolax)	*Constipation* 5 mg tabs 10 mg suppository Child: PO 0.3 mg/kg/24 hr or 5-10 mg 6 hr before desired effect <2 yr: PR 5 mg 2-11 yr: PR 5-10 mg >11 yr: PR 10 mg	Do not use in newborn period May cause nausea, abdominal cramps, vomiting Oral dose effective in 6-10 hr Rectal dose effective in 15-60 min
calcium carbonate (Tums)	*Antacid* Children: PO 5-15 ml q3-6h or 1-3 hr pc and hs >12 yr: PO chew 1-2 tabs prn, not to exceed 16 tabs/24 hr	Monitor bowel function; may cause constipation Do not take for prolonged periods
docusate (Colace)	*Constipation* Syrup: 20 mg/5 ml Sol: 10 mg/ml, 50 mg/ml 50 mg, 100 mg, 240 mg, 300 mg caps <3 yr: PO 10-40 mg qd 3-6 yr: PO 20-60 mg qd 6-12 yr: PO 40-120 mg qd >12 yr: PO 50-200 mg qd	May cause abdominal cramps Liquid may be diluted with juice to improve taste Effectiveness may decrease with long term use

Drug	Indications, Dosage, and Route	Remarks
glycerin	*Constipation* <6 yr: PR 1-1.5 g suppository >6 yr: PR 3 g suppository	May cause rectal discomfort Keep in tightly closed container
kaolin and pectin (Kaopectate)	*Mild diarrhea* 3-5 yr: PO 15 ml concentrate or 15-30 ml regular susp after each bowel movement 6-11 yr: PO 30 ml concentrate or 30-50 ml regular susp after each bowel movement >12 yr: PO 45 ml concentrate or 60 ml regular susp after each bowel movement	May cause constipation Discontinue use if diarrhea persists >48 hr Discontinue use if fever develops Do not use if there is blood in stools
loperamide (Immodium A-D)	*Diarrhea* 1 mg/5 ml liquid 2 mg caps 2-5 yr: PO one tsp after loose bowel movement; do not exceed 3 tsp/24 hr 6-8 yr: PO 2 tsp or ½ cap after loose bowel movement; do not exceed 4 tsp or 2 cap/24 hr 9-11 yr: PO 2 tsp or 1 cap after loose bowel movement; do not exceed 6 tsp or 3 cap/24 hr >11 yr: PO 4 tsp or 2 cap after loose bowel movement; do not exceed 8 tsp or 4 cap/24 hr	Do not use if diarrhea is accompanied by high fever or if there is blood in stools Do not use for >2 days May cause constipation
magaldrate (Riopan)	*Antacid* ≥6 yr: PO 1 or 2 tsp/tab between meals and at hs; do not exceed 18 tsp/tab/24 hr	Shake well May cause mild diarrhea or constipation

Drug	Indications, Dosage, and Route	Remarks
magnesium hydroxide (Di-Gel, Gelusil, Haleys M-O, Maalox Plus, Mylanta, Phillips Milk of Magnesia)	*Antacid* Children: PO 2.5-5 ml prn Adults: PO 5-15 ml prn *Constipation* 2-6 yr: PO 5-15 ml 6-12 yr: PO 15-30 ml Adults: 30-60 ml	May cause diarrhea, abdominal cramps or fluid and electrolyte changes Do not administer if abdominal pain is present
methylcellulose (Citrucel)	*Chronic constipation* Children: PO 5-10 ml in 4 oz cold liquid qd-tid Adults: PO 20 ml in 8 oz cold liquid qd-tid *Chronic diarrhea* ≥12 yr: PO 15 ml in 3 oz cold liquid qd-tid	Do not use if abdominal pain is present May cause abdominal cramps, diarrhea, nausea, vomiting Drug effect may take 2-3 days Encourage fluid intake when used as laxative
mineral oil	*Constipation* ≥4 yr: PO 5-15 ml hs	Do not administer to any child with potential for aspiration May cause nausea, vomiting, diarrhea, abdominal cramps Administer with fruit juice, applesauce, ice cream for palatability May impair absorption of fat soluble vitamins (A, D, E, K)
psyllium (Fiberall, Metamucil, Perdiem)	*Constipation, irritable bowel syndrome* Children >6 yr: PO 1 tsp (1 packet) in ½ glass liquid qd-tid Adults: PO 1-2 tsp in 8 oz liquid qd-tid	May administer in fruit juice to improve palatability May decrease appetite if administered ac Encourage fluid intake when used as laxative
senna (Gentle Nature, Senokot)	*Acute constipation* 1 mo-1 yr: PO 1.25-2.5 ml hs 1-5 yr: PO 2.5-5 ml hs 5-15 yr: PO 5-10 ml hs Adult: PO 10-15 ml hs or 2 tabs hs	May cause nausea, vomiting, abdominal cramps, diarrhea May discolor urine, feces
simethicone	*Excess gas in digestive tract* Infants: PO 0.3 ml qid after meals and hs >2 yr: PO 0.6 ml qid after meals and hs	Keep head elevated >45° to facilitate elimination of freed gas by belching Shake well

Appendix H

American Heart Association Guidelines for Bacterial Endocarditis Prophylaxis

---

Name: _____

needs protection from
BACTERIAL ENDOCARDITIS
because of an existing
HEART CONDITION

Diagnosis: _____

Prescribed by: _____

Date: _____

For Dental/Oral/Upper Respiratory Tract Procedures

I. Standard Regimen in Pts at Risk (includes those with prosthetic heart valves and other high risk pts):

Amoxicillin 3.0 g PO 1 hour before procedure, then 1.5 g 6 hr after initial dose*

For amoxicillin/penicillin-allergic pts:

Erythromycin ethylsuccinate 800 mg or erythromycin stearate 1.0 g PO 2 hr before procedure, then ½ that dose 6 hr after initial administration*

or

Clindamycin 300 mg PO 1 hr before procedure and 150 mg 6 hr after initial dose*

II. Alternative Prophylactic Regimens for Dental/Oral/Upper Respiratory Tract Procedures in Pts at Risk:

A. For pts unable to take PO medications:

Ampicillin 2.0 g IV (or IM) 30 min before procedure, then ampicillin 1.0 g IV (or IM) or amoxicillin 1.5 g PO 6 hr after initial dose*

or

For ampicillin/amoxicillin/penicillin-allergic pts unable to take PO medications:

Clindamycin 300 mg IV 30 min before procedure and 150 mg IV (or PO) 6 hr after initial dose*

B. For pts considered to be at high risk who are not candidates for the standard regimen:

Ampicillin 2.0 g IV (or IM) plus gentamicin 1.5 mg/kg IV (or IM) (not to exceed 80 mg) 30 min before procedure, followed by amoxicillin 1.5 g PO 6 hours after initial dose; alternatively, parenteral regimen may be repeated 8 hr after initial dose*

For ampicillin/amoxicillin/penicillin-allergic pts considered to be at high risk:

Vancomycin 1.0 g IV administered over one hour, starting one hour before the procedure. No repeat dose is necessary.*

*Note: Initial pediatric dosages are listed below. Follow-up PO dose should be ½ initial dose. Total pediatric dose should not exceed total adult dose:

Amoxicillin†: 50 mg/kg	Vancomycin: 20 mg/kg
Clindamycin: 10 mg/kg	Ampicillin: 50 mg/kg
Erythromycin ethylsuccinate	Gentamicin: 2.0 mg/kg
or stearate: 20 mg/kg	

For Genitourinary/Gastrointestinal Procedures

I. Standard regimen:

Ampicillin 2.0 g IV (or IM) plus gentamicin 1.5 mg/kg IV (or IM) (not to exceed 80 mg) 30 minutes before procedure, followed by amoxicillin 1.5 g PO 6 hr after initial dose; alternatively, parenteral regimen may be repeated once 8 hr after initial dose*

For amoxicillin/ampicillin/penicillin-allergic pts:

Vancomycin 1.0 g IV administered over 1 hr plus gentamicin 1.5 mg/kg IV (or IM) (not to exceed 80 mg) one hr before procedure; may be repeated once 8 hr after initial dose**

II. Alternate PO regimen for low-risk pts:

Amoxicillin 3.0 g PO one hr before procedure, then 1.5 g 6 hr after initial dose**

† The following weight ranges may also be used for the initial pediatric dose of amoxicillin:

<15 kg (33 lbs), 750 mg
15–30 kg (33–66 lbs), 1500 mg
>30 kg (66 lbs), 3000 mg (full adult dose)

Kilogram to pound conversion chart: (1 kg = 2.2 lb)

kg	lb
—	—
5	11.0
10	22.0
20	44.0
30	66.0
40	88.0
50	110.0

**Note: Initial pediatric dosages are listed below. Follow-up PO dose should be ½ initial dose. Total pediatric dose should not exceed total adult dose.

Ampicillin: 50 mg/kg	Gentamicin: 2.0 mg/kg
Amoxicillin: 50 mg/kg	Vancomycin: 20 mg/kg

Note: Antibiotic regimens used to prevent recurrences of acute rheumatic fever are inadequate for the prevention of bacterial endocarditis. In pts with markedly compromised renal function, it may be necessary to modify or omit second dose of gentamicin or vancomycin. Intramuscular injections may be contraindicated in pts receiving antioagulants.

Used with permission of the American Medical Association. Adapted from Committee on Rheumatic Fever, Endocarditis, and Kawasaki Disease: *Prevention of bacterial endocarditis: recommendations by the American Heart Association, JAMA* 264:2919, 1990. © 1990 American Medical Association (also excerpted in *J Am Dent Assoc* 122:87, 1991. Please refer to these joint American Heart Association–American Dental Association recommendations for more complete information as to which pts and which procedures require prophylaxis.

APPENDIX I

Bibliography

Alfano-Lefevre R, Blicharz ME, Fynn NM, Boyer MJ: *Drug handbook: a nursing process approach,* Redwood City, Calif, 1992, Addison-Wesley.

Chameides L: *American heart association: pediatric advanced life support,* Dallas, 1994, American Heart Association.

Benitz WE, Tatro DS: *The pediatric drug handbook,* ed 3, St. Louis, 1995, Mosby.

Bindler RM, Howry LB: *Pediatric drugs and nursing applications,* Norwalk, Conn, 1991, Appleton & Lange.

Briggs GG, Freeman RK, Yaffe SJ: *Drugs in pregnancy and lactation,* ed 4, Philadelphia, 1994, Williams and Wilkins.

Committee on Infectious Diseases, American Academy of Pediatrics: *1994 Redbook: report of the committee on infectious diseases,* ed 23, Elk Grove Village, Ill, 1994, American Academy of Pediatrics.

Dickey RP: *Managing contraceptive pill patients,* ed 8, Durant, Okla, 1994, Essential Medical Information Systems, Inc.

Dorr RT, VonHuff DD: *Cancer chemotherapy handbook,* ed 2, Norwalk, 1994, Appleton & Lange.

Drug facts and comparisons, St. Louis, 1993, A. Wolters Kluwer.

Drug information for the health care professional, ed 15, Tauton, 1995, Rand-McNally.

Fisher DS, Knobf MT: *The cancer chemotherapy handbook,* ed 3, Littleton, 1989, Year Book Medical Publishers, Inc.

Gahart BL: *Intravenous medications,* ed 11, St. Louis, 1995, Mosby.

Gilman AG, Rau TW, Nies AS, Taylor P: *Goodman and Gilman: the pharmacological basis of therapeutics,* ed 8, New York, 1990, Pergamon Press.

Handbook of pediatric drug therapy, Springhouse, 1990, Springhouse Corporation.

Johnson K: *The Harriett Lane handbook,* ed 13, St. Louis, 1993, Mosby.

Keen JH, Baird MS, Allen JH: *Mosby's critical care and emergency drug reference,* St. Louis, 1994, Mosby.

Lacy C, Armstrong LL, Lipsy RJ, Lance LL: *Drug information handbook,* Hudson, 1993, Lexi-Comp Inc.

McKenry LM, Salerno E: *Mosby's pharmacology in nursing,* ed 18, St. Louis, 1992, Mosby.

819

Nelson JD: *Pocket book of pediatric antimicrobial therapy,* ed 11, Philadelphia, 1995, Williams and Wilkins.

Nursing '95 drug handbook, Springhouse, 1995, Springhouse Corporation.

Perry MC: *The chemotherapy source book,* Philadelphia, 1992, Williams and Wilkins.

Phelps SJ, Cochran EB: *Guidelines for administration of intravenous medications to pediatric patients,* ed 4, Bethesda, Md, 1993, American Society of Hospital Pharmacists, Inc.

Physician's desk reference, ed 49, Montvale, 1995, Medical Economic Data Production Co.

Shannon MT, Wilson BA, Stang CL: *Drugs and nursing implications,* ed 8, Norwalk, Conn, 1995, Appleton & Lange.

Skidmore-Roth L: *Mosby's nursing drug reference,* St. Louis, 1995, Mosby.

Taketomo CK, Hodding JH, Kraus DM: *Pediatric dosage handbook,* ed 2, Hudson, 1992, Lexi-Comp Inc.

Trissel LA: *Handbook on injectable drugs,* ed 7, Houston, 1992, M.D. Anderson Cancer Center.

Whaley LF, Wong DL: *Nursing care of infants and children,* ed 4, St. Louis, 1991, Mosby.

APPENDIX J ═══════════

Patient and Family Education

Each drug monograph contains a Patient and Family Education section, which offers key points that should be discussed with the patients and family about a medication. Also included are several more general topics that should be included when teaching patients and families about any medication use. Each topic is not listed in every monograph because the information would be repetitive and the length of the book would be prohibitive. The following teaching topics, nonetheless, should be included in Patient Care Management.

- Explain the rationale for using the medication and the anticipated patient response to the medication.
- Teach the proper administration technique for the medication being prescribed. Information should include whether or not the oral tablet can be crushed, how to accurately measure liquid medications, how to use inhalers and nebulizers, and how to administer medications such as ear and eye drops and rectal and vaginal suppositories.
- Discuss how to prepare the patient for medication administration. Strategies include using concrete terms appropriate to the child's level of understanding, being honest with the child about unpleasant aspects of the medication, using distractions (such as tape recordings), and using relaxing techniques.
- Provide information about how often the medication should be taken and for what length of time it should be used. Discourage overusage and underusage of medications. Explain which signs and symptoms the patient or parent should use to determine when prn medications should be used.
- Instruct family member to keep all medications out of the reach of children. This is particularly important with medications requiring refrigeration; children may assume that they are food.
- Discourage parents from referring to medications as candy, particularly medications such as pleasant-tasting chewable

821

tablets or oral liquids. Children may believe that these medications are to be eaten as snacks or treats.

- Teach patients or parents to discard any unused medications; advise patients or parents never to use expired or outdated medications.
- Discuss the possible side effects and symptoms of hypersensitivity for each medication. Tell the parents which side effects are of particular concern and warrant notifying the care provider.
- Discuss specific activities to be monitored or restricted as related to specific medications. (For example, activities such as biking, skating, or skateboarding might need to be restricted if the child is experiencing drowsiness as a side effect from antihistamines, anticonvulsants, or psychotropic drugs.) Insulin doses may need to be modified as activity levels change. Certain drugs may cause drowsiness upon arising.
- Determine whether the family can afford to purchase the medication, both on an immediate basis and a long-term basis. A referral to the social work department of the health care agency when needed may be helpful.
- Provide information to the patient or parent about whom they can contact with questions about medications. This may be the primary care provider, a specialist, or a hospital clinic.
- Stress the importance of compliance with any follow-up or ongoing care. Be sure the patient or parent knows when and with whom to seek follow-up care.

Index

Page numbers followed by f
indicate figures. Page numbers
followed by t indicate tables.

Abbreviations

ā	before
abd	abdomen
ABGs	arterial blood gases
ac	before meals
ACE	angiotensin-converting enzyme
ADH	antidiuretic hormone
ADHD	attention deficit hyperactivity disorder
alk phos	alkaline phosphatase
α	alpha
ALT	alanine aminotransferase, serum
ANA	antinuclear antibodies
ARDS	adult respiratory distress syndrome
ASA	acetylsalicylic acid, aspirin
AST	aspartate aminotransferase, serum
ASHD	arteriosclerotic heart disease
AV	atrioventricular
β	beta
BG	blood glucose
bid	twice a day
BM	bowel movement
B/P	blood pressure
BUN	blood urea nitrogen
c̄	with
C	celsius (centigrade)
Ca	calcium
cap	capsules
cath	catheterization or catheterize
CBC	complete blood count
cc	cubic centimeter
CHF	congestive heart failure
Cl	chlorine
cm	centimeter
CNS	central nervous system
CO₂	carbon dioxide
CONT IV	continuous IV
COPD	chronic obstructive pulmonary disease
CPAP	continuous positive airway pressure
CPK	creatinine phosphokinase
CPR	cardiopulmonary resuscitation
CrCl	creatinine clearance
C&S	culture and sensitivity
CSF	cerebrospinal fluid
CV	cardiovascular
CVP	central venous pressure
D₅LR	dextrose 5% in Ringer's injection, lactated
D₅NS	dextrose 5% in sodium chloride 0.9%

D₅¼NS	dextrose 5% in sodium chloride 0.225%
D₅½NS	dextrose 5% in sodium chloride 0.45%
D₅R	dextrose 5% in Ringer's injection
D₅S	dextrose 5% in sodium chloride 0.9%, 0.45%, 0.225%
D₅W	dextrose 5% in water
D₁₀NS	dextrose 10% in sodium chloride 0.9%
D₁₀W	dextrose 10% in water
D₁₅W	dextrose 15% in water
D₂₀W	dextrose 20% in water
D-LR	dextrose-Ringer's injection, lactated, combination
D-R	dextrose-Ringer's injection, combination
D-S	dextrose-saline
DIR INF	direct infusion
DM	diabetes mellitus
ECG	electrocardiogram (EKG)
EDTA	ethylenediaminetetraacetic acid
EEG	electroencephalogram
EENT	ear, eye, nose, and throat
EPS	extrapyramidal symptoms
ESR	erythrocyte sedimentation rate
EXT REL	extended release
FSH	follicle-stimulating hormone
γ	gamma
g	gram
GERD	gastroesophageal reflux disorder
GI	gastrointestinal
G-6-PD	glucose-6-phosphate dehydrogenase
GTT	glucose tolerance test
gtt	drop
GU	genitourinary
H₂	histamine₂
Hct	hematocrit
HCG	human chorionic gonadotropin
HDCV	human diploid cell rabies vaccine
Hgb	hemoglobin
5-HIAA	5-hydroxyindoleacetic acid
HIV	human immunodeficiency virus (AIDS)
H₂O	water
HR	heart rate
hr	hour
hs	at bedtime
ICP	intracranial pressure